Management
of PEDIATRIC
TRAUMA

Management *of* PEDIATRIC TRAUMA

WILLIAM L. BUNTAIN, M.D.
Professor of Surgery
Chief of Pediatric Surgery
University of Kansas Medical Center
Kansas City, Kansas

W.B. SAUNDERS COMPANY
A Division of Harcourt Brace & Company   *Philadelphia   London   Toronto   Montreal   Sydney   Tokyo*

W.B. SAUNDERS COMPANY
A Division of
Harcourt Brace & Company

The Curtis Center
Independence Square West
Philadelphia, Pennsylvania 19106

Library of Congress Cataloging-in-Publication Data

Buntain, William L.

Management of pediatric trauma / William L. Buntain.—1st ed.

    p.   cm.

ISBN 0–7216–6280–3

1. Children—Wounds and injuries.   2. Children—Wounds and
injuries—Treatment.   3. Pediatric intensive care.
I. Title.   [DNLM: 1. Wounds and Injuries—in infancy &
childhood.   2. Wounds and Injuries—therapy.
WO 700 B942m 1994]

RD93.5.C4B86   1994

617.1′0083—dc20

DNLM/DLC   93–47168

Management of Pediatric Trauma   ISBN 0–7216–6280–3

Last digit is the print number: 9   8   7   6   5   4   3   2   1

Dedication

This text was developed and produced to affect and improve, where possible, the welfare and outcome of the injured child. It is hoped that all of the contributors have succeeeded in this objective, providing expertise and experience to further the knowledge and improve the management of injured children. Our efforts are commendable and usually very rewarding, but this text is dedicated to those individuals who spend their time caring for these children, making us look good, and making us proud of what they accomplish and the results we all achieve.

These unselfish and enormously dedicated persons provide the glue that holds everything together, the expertise that allows our orders to be accomplished successfully, and the sensitivity to listen to the children and their families and to report the emotional as well as the physical findings as they occur. Without their dedication, concern, empathy, sympathy, and extraordinary skills our results would be ordinary. They make the difference in the outcome. This text is dedicated with sincerest respect and admiration to

Our Critical Care Unit Nurses

For you,
Dear Mother,
Whose child will remain forever young:
For you,
Dear Mother,
My nursing philosophy is meant.

Ours is not to question why.
Ours is not to let'em die.

I'm in this institution right now because I need to feed my children. I can put up with anything for 8 hours . . . just give me a paycheck.

I'm here because any comparable income I could possibly make otherwise would be either illegal or immoral.

I'm here, dear Mother, because your little child suddenly became ill just the day before yesterday and you turned to me and my colleagues for help. Now it's 3 days before Christmas, and I stand here with your child, brain-dead in my arms. She is attached to the ventilator and the many drips: dopamine, dobutamine, TPN, arterial line, electrodes for the heart monitor, to name a few. I am an expert, I am told, at the "science" and "technology" needed to make all these life-support mechanisms work right. I have seen Death lurk over children many times and can give Him a good fight, as I have never been a complacent companion of this enemy that steals your little one away so soon. As I look into your loving, motherly eyes, I feel your pain and my heart bleeds for you. I, too, am a "Mama," yet my children are at home and full of life and vigor. I wonder why God has for another day spared me the agony you are now feeling. Your little girl feels so limp in my arms.

I invite you to sit down in the rocker I have placed close to your little one's bedside. I ask you to spread the nice soft quilt on your lap so your little daughter will be kept warm.

I gently hand you your dear little child, being careful not to disturb any of the "lifelines."

You cry.

I hold back the tears. (I must be strong for you.) I encourage you to spend a few moments rocking your baby now. I leave the room. I cry. I come back and ask if you're doing okay. You are.

A few moments pass. Daddy gets the courage to come into the room. He watches you, my dear baby's mother, as you hold your little girl in your arms. Finally he breaks into tears. He says that this is "his" little girl. He would always take her fishing on the boat because she liked fishing with Daddy so much. She'd always catch the biggest one. She'd get a little dirty, oh yes, but she was Daddy's little Tom-girl. He confides that he does not want to hold her now. He just doesn't think he can handle that. I put my arm around Dad and say, "That's okay." He knows that I know what he feels. There is a bond between us—a spiritual bond we instantly feel but do not speak, lest we break the magnitude of that brief, intimate moment.

An hour has passed now, dear Mother, and your arm grows weary, but you will rock just a few more minutes while I call for some help to transfer your little daughter back to bed. You savor those moments.

I battle a few tubes and wires, but finally get your daughter back into her comfy little bed.

You kiss her forehead and say goodbye for the night. More tears (yours and mine). You know that in the morning they will do another brain flow study to see if there is even a flicker of life in your child's brain. My gut feeling tells me that you already know there isn't. I say goodnight to you and Daddy and tell you I will take good care of your baby and to call anytime.

You are gone.

I stare at your daughter and wonder if I could have done anything else to save her life. No. I recall, everything was done right: drugs, blood, FFP, cryoprecipitate, platelets, mannitol, antibiotics, steroids, ventilatory and circulatory support. How else does one fight fulminating meningococcemia and DIC in a 2 year old? I sat by her crib and watched for all the "ominous" signs. Still, she is gone.

Who am I? I am her nurse.

I exist as a nurse for those moments when I can make a difference for the better in someone's life. This is my nursing philosophy in a nutshell. Rather simple, perhaps archaic. But true. I reflect.

I cannot make you live again, dear child, but I can help ease your passing a little for your mother and daddy. Nurses and doctors can't always fix problems. But I will do all I can to make it bearable; that is my goal as a nurse, whether it be easing postoperative pain or easing dead-baby pain. I try not to feel this doom. It's Christmastime, you know. But I can't escape feeling it. It's an enigma; it's everywhere; it's in the air.

I recall a phrase, "There but for the grace of God go I." I, as a nurse, am given the rare privilege of truly understanding this phrase and appreciating how much I truly have in my own life, outside of this hospital, to be grateful for. I feel almost guilty that my children are healthy and you, baby, are dead. Why, God, why?

Only God knows. Perhaps, as the good priest who came and prayed for you told me, God has spared you, child, from much of the pain we grownups feel. You have known only love. You will be spared the agony of hatred and loneliness. I must feel something positive about your death, baby. I am your nurse.

My philosophy is to be able to nurture you and all those that I care for back to an optimal level of health.

My philosophy is to do it whether you can pay me or not.

My philosophy is to care for you with respect, scientific and technical expertise, and a heightened sense of observation and ongoing awareness of what problems may next challenge your drive to live.

My philosophy is to care for your whole being—body, soul, family, culture—whatever makes *you* unique.

My philosophy is to make you as comfortable as possible, even if I can't make you better.

My philosophy is to be there to hold your Mom and Dad as your spirit passes on, no matter how difficult that may be, if it is not meant for you to be healthy again.

Institutional rules and regulations, poor staffing, physical exhaustion, and heavy workloads sometimes get in the way of my practicing the art, or philosophy, of nursing the way I feel it should be done. I have to strive for "safe" care knowing there aren't enough bodies to give "good" care. I say things I really don't mean out of anger and frustration. I get so tired.

But not this time, little baby. We must not let any of those bad things hinder the care I must give now. This time, your dear Mom and Dad need that "art" of nursing too much. They will be back early tomorrow morning, you know. They will want to know the brain flow final results. I will kiss you goodnight now and go home. But I will be back early tomorrow morning, too. There may be some terrible moments ahead. But those are the very moments in which I, your nurse, can make a real difference. I wouldn't miss that. It's what nursing is all about . . . for me.

Sleep, baby, sleep.

JEANNE HENNING, R.N.
Pediatric Surgery and
Critical Care Nurse

Contributors

Richard J. Andrassy, M.D.
A. G. McNeese Professor of Surgery, The University of Texas Health Science Center; Interim Chairman, Department of Surgery, and Chief of Pediatric Surgery, The University of Texas Health Science Center, Houston, Texas
Hyperbaric Oxygen Therapy for Childhood Injury

Keith W. Ashcraft, M.D.
Professor of Surgery, University of Missouri—Kansas City School of Medicine; Chief of Urologic Surgery, Department of Surgery, Children's Mercy Hospital, Kansas City, Missouri
Cardiac and Major Thoracic Vascular Injuries

Melinda K. Bailey, M.D.
Associate Professor of Anesthesiology, Medical University of South Carolina, Charleston, South Carolina
Hemostasis, Coagulopathy, and the Use of Blood Products

Gary Wickens Barone, M.D.
Assistant Professor, Vascular and Transplant Surgery, College of Medicine, University of Arkansas for Medical Sciences; Staff Physician, University of Arkansas for Medical Sciences and John L. McClellan Veterans Administration Hospital, Little Rock, Arkansas
Farm Injuries

Sterling H. Blocker, M.D.
Pediatric Surgery Consultants, Springfield, Missouri
Genital and Perineal Injuries

William L. Buntain, M.D.
Professor of Surgery and Chief, Section of Pediatric Surgery, University of Kansas Medical Center, Kansas City, Kansas
Developing Trauma Centers and Standards of Care; Expectations for the Future; Initial Evaluation and Management, Mechanisms and Biomechanics of Traffic Injuries; Spleen Injuries

Edward Buonocore, M.D.
Professor and Chairman, Department of Radiology, University of Tennessee Graduate School of Medicine; Staff Physician, Department of Radiology, University of Tennessee Medical Center, Knoxville, Tennessee
Radiologic Evaluation of the Injured Child

Walter S. Cain, M.D.
Professor of Surgery and Pediatrics, University of Alabama School of Medicine, University of Alabama at Birmingham; Attending Surgeon, Children's Hospital of Alabama and University of Alabama Hospital, Birmingham, Alabama
Chemical Injuries to the Upper Alimentary Tract

Donald Craig Chase, D.D.S.
Director of Dental Affairs, Associate Dean, and Professor and Chairman of Department of Oral and Maxillofacial Surgery, College of Dentistry, University of Tennessee Medical Center, Knoxville, Tennessee
Maxillofacial Injuries

Arnold G. Coran, M.D.
Professor of Surgery, University of Michigan School of Medicine; Director of Pediatric Surgery, University of Michigan School of Medicine; Surgeon-in-Chief, Mott Children's Hospital, Ann Arbor, Michigan
Nutritional Management in Pediatric Trauma

R. Bruce Davey, M.B.B.S., F.R.C.S. (Edinburgh), F.R.A.C.S.
Clinical Lecturer in Paediatric Surgery, Flinders Medical Centre; Clinical Lecturer in Paediatric Surgery, University of Adelaide; Senior Visiting Paediatric Surgeon, Women's and Children's Hospital and Flinders Medical Centre, Adelaide, Australia
Thermal and Electrical Injuries

J. Michael Dean, M.D.
Associate Professor of Pediatrics, University of Utah School of Medicine; Chief, Division of Pediatric Critical Care, and Director, Pediatric Intensive Care Unit, Primary Children's Hospital, Salt Lake City, Utah
Submersion Injuries

Edward J. Doolin, M.D.
Associate Professor of Clinical Surgery, University of Medicine and Dentistry of New Jersey, Robert Wood Johnson Medical School at Camden; Staff Physician, Division of Pediatric Surgery, Department of Surgery, Cooper Hospital—University Medical Center, Camden, New Jersey
Birth Injuries

Jeffrey J. DuBois, M.D., F.A.C.S., F.A.A.P.
Assistant Clinical Professor of Surgery, F. Edward Hebert School of Medicine, Uniformed Services University of the Health Sciences, Bethesda, Maryland; Chief, Pediatric Surgery, David Grant Medical Center, Travis Air Force Base, California
Trauma Protocols for Evaluation and Management

Robert W. Feldtman, M.D.
Clinical Assistant Professor of Surgery, Memorial Hospital, Houston, Texas
Hyperbaric Oxygen Therapy for Childhood Injury

Carol L. Fowler, M.D.

Assistant Professor of Surgery, Division of Pediatric Surgery, University of Kentucky Medical Center, Lexington, Kentucky

Nonaccidental Injuries: The Physically Abused Child

William Edmond Fowler, M.D.

Director, Child and Adolescent Psychology, Methodist Psychiatric Pavilion, New Orleans, Louisiana

Nonaccidental Injuries: The Physically Abused Child

Bruce M. Gans, M.D.

Professor and Chairman, Department of Physical Medicine and Rehabilitation, School of Medicine, Wayne State University; President, Rehabilitation Institute of Michigan, Detroit, Michigan

Rehabilitation Support for the Injured Child

Michael W. L. Gauderer, M.D.

Professor of Pediatric Surgery and Pediatrics, Case Western Reserve University School of Medicine; Chief, Division of Pediatric Surgery, Rainbow Babies and Children's Hospital, Cleveland, Ohio

Colonic and Rectal Injuries

Mitchell H. Goldman, M.D.

Professor of Surgery, University of Tennessee Graduate School of Medicine; Director and Chief, Sections of Vascular and Transplant Surgery, University of Tennessee Medical Center, Knoxville, Tennessee

Organ Procurement in the Fatally Injured Child

Eustace Stevers Golladay, M.D.

Professor of Surgery and Pediatrics, Louisiana State University School of Medicine in New Orleans; Chairman of Trauma, Children's Hospital, Attending Pediatric Surgeon, Medical Center of Louisiana at New Orleans, Tulane Medical Center Hospital and Clinics, and Baptist Mercy Medical Center, New Orleans, Louisiana

Animal, Snake, and Spider Bites and Insect Stings

Dennis C. Gore, M.D., F.A.C.S.

Assistant Professor, Medical College of Virginia, School of Medicine, Virginia Commonwealth University; Director, Surgical Critical Care, Director, Burn Unit, Director, Surgical Trauma ICU, and Director, Surgical Nutrition, Medical College of Virginia Hospitals, Richmond, Virginia

Urinary Tract Injuries

Howard R. Gould, M.D.

Professor of Radiology, University of Tennessee Graduate School of Medicine; Director of Diagnostic Radiology, Department of Radiology, University of Tennessee Medical Center, Knoxville, Tennessee

Radiologic Evaluation of the Injured Child

Jay L. Grosfeld, M.D.

Professor and Chairman, Department of Surgery, and Director, Section of Pediatric Surgery, Indiana University School of Medicine; Surgeon-in-Chief, James Whitcomb Riley Hospital for Children, Indianapolis, Indiana

Ventilatory and Respiratory Support for the Injured Child

Gerald S. Gussack, M.D.

Associate Professor of Surgery, Emory University School of Medicine, Atlanta, Georgia

Ear, Nose, and Throat Injuries

J. Alex Haller, Jr., M.D.

Professor of Pediatric Surgery, Pediatrics, and Emergency Medicine, Johns Hopkins University School of Medicine, Baltimore, Maryland

Submersion Injuries

William D. Hardin, Jr., M.D., F.A.C.S., F.A.A.P.

Associate Professor of Surgery and Pediatrics, University of Alabama School of Medicine, University of Alabama at Birmingham; Attending Surgeon, Children's Hospital of Alabama and University of Alabama Hospital, Birmingham, Alabama

Injury Prevention and Control in the United States

Burton H. Harris, M.D.

Professor of Pediatric Surgery, Tufts University School of Medicine; Chief of Pediatric Surgery, Boston Floating Hospital, and Director, Kiwanis Pediatric Trauma Institute, Boston, Massachusetts

The History of Pediatric Trauma Care; Long-Term Disability and Morbidity after Childhood Injuries

Jeanne Henning, R.N., C.

Nurse Clinician for Pediatric Surgery, University of Kansas Medical Center, Kansas City, Kansas

Initial Evaluation and Management, Mechanisms and Biomechanics of Traffic Injuries

R. Kelly Hill, Jr., M.D.

Medical Director of Hyperbarics, Our Lady of the Lake Regional Medical Center, Baton Rouge, Louisiana

Hyperbaric Oxygen Therapy for Childhood Injury

Thomas M. Holder, M.D.

Emeritus Professor of Surgery, University of Missouri—Kansas City School of Medicine, Kansas City, Missouri

Cardiac and Major Thoracic Vascular Injuries

Thomas L. Hurt, M.D.

Clinical Assistant Professor, University of Washington School of Medicine, Seattle; Attending Physician, Department of Pediatric Emergency and Critical Care Medicine, Mary Bridge Children's Hospital, Tacoma, Washington

Vascular Access and Monitoring of the Critically Injured Child

Elaine K. Jeter, M.D.

Associate Professor, Department of Pathology/Laboratory Medicine, Medical University of South Carolina College of Medicine; Staff Physician, Medical University of South Carolina Medical Center, Roper Hospital, and Charleston Memorial Hospital, Charleston, South Carolina

Hemostasis, Coagulopathy, and the Use of Blood Products

Amie C. Jew, M.D.

Private practice, Menorah Medical Center, Kansas City, Missouri; formerly Chief Resident in General Surgery, University of Kansas Medical Center, Kansas City, Kansas

Initial Evaluation and Management

Philip B. Kellett, M.D.
Director of Anesthesia, East Tennessee Children's Hospital, Knoxville, Tennessee
Anesthesia for the Critically Injured Child

Denis R. King, M.D.
Clinical Associate Professor of Surgery, Division of Pediatric Surgery, Ohio State University College of Medicine and Children's Hospital, Columbus, Ohio
Vascular Injuries

William D. King, R.Ph., M.P.H., Ph.D.
Associate Professor of Pediatrics, University of Alabama School of Medicine, University of Alabama at Birmingham; Divisional Director, Southeast Child Safety Institute of Children's Hospital of Alabama, Birmingham, Alabama
Chemical Injuries to the Upper Alimentary Tract; Injury Prevention and Control in the United States

Ann M. Kosloske, M.D., M.P.H.
Professor of Surgery and Pediatrics, Ohio State University College of Medicine; Chief, Section of General Pediatric Surgery, Children's Hospital, Columbus, Ohio
Foreign Bodies

Peter K. Kottmeier, M.D.
Emeritus Professor of Surgery, College of Medicine, State University of New York Health Science Center at Brooklyn, Brooklyn, New York
Falls from Heights

Don Larossa, M.D.
Professor of Surgery, University of Pennsylvania School of Medicine, Staff Physician, Hospital of the University of Pennsylvania and Children's Hospital of Philadelphia
Wound Healing and Traumatic Soft Tissue Defects

Joseph Laver, M.D.
Associate Professor of Pediatrics, Medical University of South Carolina College of Medicine; Director, Division of Pediatric Hematology/Oncology, Medical University of South Carolina Hospitals and Children's Hospital, Charleston, South Carolina
Hemostasis, Coagulopathy, and the Use of Blood Products

Thom E. Lobe, M.D.
Associate Professor of Surgery and Pediatrics, and Chairman, Section of Pediatric Surgery, University of Tennessee, Memphis, College of Medicine; Chairman, Section of Pediatric Surgery, LeBonheur Children's Medical Center and Saint Jude's Children's Research Hospital; General Surgery Medical Staff, Germantown Community Hospital-Methodist East, Saint Francis Hospital, Regional Medical Center at Memphis, Baptist Memorial Hospital, and Methodist Hospital; Medical Staff, Saint Joseph Hospital, Memphis, Tennessee
Metabolic Response to Major Injury and Shock; Urinary Tract Injuries

Julie A. Long, M.D.
Staff Physician, Broward General Medical Center, Ft. Lauderdale, Plantation General Hospital, Plantation, and Coral Springs Medical Center, Coral Springs, Florida
Penetrating Injuries

Sandra Loucks, Ph.D., A.B.P.P.
Professor of Pediatrics, University of Tennessee Graduate School of Medicine; Director of Behavioral Pediatrics and Pediatric Continuing Medical Education, University of Tennessee Medical Center, Knoxville, Tennessee
Psychological Consequences of Trauma

Thomas G. Luerssen, M.D.
Associate Professor of Surgery, Indiana University School of Medicine; Director of Pediatric Neurosurgery, James Whitcomb Riley Hospital for Children, Indianapolis, Indiana
Spinal Cord Injuries

Frank P. Lynch III, M.D.
Chief, Pediatric Surgery, University of California, San Diego, School of Medicine, LaJolla; Attending Physician, Children's Hospital and Health Center, University of California, San Diego, Medical Center, and Mercy Hospital and Medical Center, San Diego, California
Liver Injuries

Michael B. Marchildon, M.D.
Professor of Surgery and Pediatrics, University of Medicine and Dentistry of New Jersey, Robert Wood Johnson Medical School—Camden; Head, Division of Pediatric Surgery, Cooper Hospital—University Medical Center, Camden, New Jersey
Birth Injuries

Kim Massey, A.R.N.P., C., M.S.N., C.C.R.N.
Courtesy Faculty Position, College of Nursing, University of South Florida College of Medicine, Tampa; Trauma Coordinator, Bayfront Medical Center, Inc., St. Petersburg, Florida
Nursing Care for the Critically Injured Child

Daniel L. Mollitt, M.D.
Professor of Surgery, Department of Surgery, University of Florida Health Science Center, Jacksonville; Active Medical Staff, University Medical Center and Wolfson Children's Hospital, Jacksonville, Florida
Immunologic and Infectious Consequences of Childhood Injuries

Brad W. Olney, M.D.
Associate Professor of Orthopedic Surgery and Associate Professor of Anatomy and Cell Biology, University of Kansas Medical Center, Kansas City; Staff Physician, University of Kansas Medical Center, Kansas City, and Mid America Rehabilitation Hospital, Overland Park, Kansas
Musculoskeletal Injuries

James A. O'Neill, Jr., M.D.
C. E. Koop Professor of Surgery, University of Pennsylvania School of Medicine; Surgeon-in-Chief, Children's Hospital of Philadelphia, Philadelphia, Pennsylvania
Trauma Care Organization for Children

H. Biemann Othersen, Jr., M.D.
Professor of Surgery and Pediatrics, Medical University of South Carolina College of Medicine; Chief, Pediatric Surgery, and Medical Director, Children's Hospital, Medical Center of the Medical University of South Carolina, Charleston, South Carolina
Hemostasis, Coagulopathy, and the Use of Blood Products

Michael A. Pautler, M.D.

Chief Resident, Department of Pediatrics, University of Kansas Medical Center, Kansas City, Kansas; Fellow, Pediatric Critical Care, Children's Hospital and Health Center, San Diego, California

Mechanisms and Biomechanics of Traffic Injuries

K. Perkins, AUA Dep Physio.

Retired Senior Physiotherapist, Women's and Children's Hospital, North Adelaide, South Australia

Thermal and Electrical Injuries

Bradley M. Peterson, M.D.

Associate Clinical Professor in Pediatrics and Anesthesia, University of California, San Diego, School of Medicine, La Jolla; Director, Division of Critical Care, and Senior Staff, Pediatrics and Anesthesia, Children's Hospital and Health Center, San Diego, California

Vascular Access and Monitoring of the Critically Injured Child

Arvin I. Philippart, M.D.

Professor of Surgery, Wayne State University School of Medicine; Surgeon-in-Chief, Children's Hospital of Michigan, Detroit, Michigan

Penetrating Injuries

William J. Pokorny, M.D.

Professor of Surgery and Pediatrics, Baylor College of Medicine; Chief, General Surgery Service, Texas Children's Hospital, Houston, Texas

Nonaccidental Injuries: The Physically Abused Child; Pancreatic Injuries; Trauma Protocols for Evaluation and Management

David B. Reath, M.D., F.A.C.S.

Assistant Professor, Division of Plastic and Reconstructive Surgery, University of Tennessee Graduate School of Medicine; Attending Physician, University of Tennessee Medical Center, Knoxville, Tennessee

Wound Healing and Traumatic Soft Tissue Defects

John F. Redman, M.D.

Professor and Chairman, Department of Urology, and Professor of Pediatrics, University of Arkansas College of Medicine; Chief, Urology Section, University Hospital, and Chief, Pediatric Urology Section, Arkansas Children's Hospital, Little Rock, Arkansas

Genital and Perineal Injuries

Hernan M. Reyes, M.D.

Professor of Surgery and Clinical Pediatrics, University of Illinois College of Medicine; Chairman, Department of Surgery, Cook County Hospital, Chicago, Illinois

Retroperitoneal and Pelvic Injuries

Marleta Reynolds, M.D.

Associate Professor of Surgery, Northwestern University Medical School; Attending Surgeon, Associate Director of Intensive Care Unit, Trauma Director, and Director of ECMO Program, Children's Memorial Hospital, Chicago, Illinois

Pulmonary, Esophageal, and Diaphragmatic Injuries

Richard R. Ricketts, M.D.

Associate Professor of Surgery, Emory University School of Medicine; Staff Physician, Egleston Hospital for Children at Emory and Grady Memorial Hospital, Atlanta, Georgia

Duodenal and Biliary Tract Injuries

Michael J. Rieder, M.D.

Department of Pediatrics, Children's Hospital of Western Ontario, London, Ontario, Canada

Sports and Recreation Injuries

Shauna R. Roberts, M.D.

Pediatric Surgery, Drs. Early, Roberts & Associates, St. Joseph, Missouri

Cardiac and Major Thoracic Vascular Injuries

Bradley M. Rodgers, M.D.

Professor of Surgery and Pediatrics, and Chief, Division of Pediatric Surgery, University of Virginia School of Medicine; Chief, Children's Medical Center, University of Virginia Health Sciences Center, Charlottesville, Virginia

Farm Injuries

David A. Rogers, M.D.

Assistant Professor of Pediatric Surgery, Medical College of Georgia School of Medicine, Augusta, Georgia

Metabolic Response to Major Injury and Shock

Marshall Z. Schwartz, M.D.

Professor of Surgery and Pediatrics, George Washington University School of Medicine; Surgeon in Chief, Children's National Medical Center, Washington, D.C.

Organ System Failure in the Injured Child

Thomas B. Scully, M.D.

Senior Resident, Neurological Surgery, Indiana University School of Medicine, Indianapolis, Indiana

Spinal Cord Injuries

Neil J. Sherman, M.D.

Associate Clinical Professor of Surgery (Pediatric), University of Southern California School of Medicine, Los Angeles; Attending Surgeon, Children's Hospital of Los Angeles and Presbyterian Intercommunity Hospital, Los Angeles; Queen of the Valley Hospital, Napa; Pomona Valley Hospital Medical Center, Pomona, California

Traumatic Injuries to the Stomach and Small Bowel

L. Clark Simpson, M.D.

Otolaryngologist, Brookwood ENT Associates, Brookwood Medical Center, Birmingham, Alabama

Ear, Nose, and Throat Injuries

Laura J. Spence, BSc.N.

Clinical Nurse Specialist, Pediatric Surgery, Hospital For Sick Children, Toronto, Ontario, Canada

Sports and Recreation Injuries

Thomas A. Stellato, M.D.

Professor of Surgery, Case Western Reserve University School of Medicine; Chief, Division of General Surgery, University Hospitals of Cleveland, Cleveland, Ohio

Colonic and Rectal Injuries

Steven Stylianos, M.D.

Assistant Professor of Surgery, Columbia University College of Physicians and Surgeons; Attending Pediatric Surgeon, Babies' and Children's Hospital of New York, New York, New York

The History of Pediatric Trauma Care; Long-term Disability and Morbidity after Childhood Injuries

Leonard E. Swischuk, M.D.

Professor of Radiology and Pediatrics, University of Texas Medical Branch, University of Texas Medical School at Galveston; Director, Pediatric Radiology, Children's Hospital, University of Texas Medical Branch Hospitals, Galveston, Texas

Urinary Tract Injuries

R. Thomas Temes, M.D.

Assistant Professor, Department of Surgery, University of New Mexico School of Medicine; Staff Physician, University Hospital, Veterans Administration Medical Center, Lovelace Medical Center, Albuquerque, New Mexico

Organ System Failure in the Injured Child

John M. Templeton, Jr., M.D.

Associate Professor, Pediatric Surgery, University of Pennsylvania School of Medicine; Associate Surgeon, Children's Hospital of Philadelphia, Philadelphia, Pennsylvania

Expectations for the Future

Joseph J. Tepas III, M.D.

Professor of Surgery and Associate Chairman, Department of Surgery, University of Florida College of Medicine, Gainesville; Chairman, Department of Surgery, University of Florida Health Science Center, Jacksonville, Florida

Triage, Trauma Scores, and Transport

M. Tingay, M.B.B.S., F.F.A.R.A.C.S.

Senior Staff Anaesthetist, Flinders Medical Centre, Bedford Park, Adelaide, Australia

Thermal and Electrical Injuries

E. Bruce Toby, M.D.

Assistant Professor, Section of Orthopedic Surgery, University of Kansas Medical Center, Kansas City, Kansas

Musculoskeletal Injuries

Dennis W. Vane, M.D., F.A.C.S., F.A.A.P.

Associate Professor of Surgery and Pediatrics, University of Vermont College of Medicine, Burlington; Attending in Surgery, Medical Center Hospital of Vermont, Burlington; Fanny Allen Hospital, Colchester; and Southwestern Vermont Medical Center, Bennington, Vermont

Ventilatory and Respiratory Support for the Injured Child

K. A. Wallis, M.B.B.S., F.R.A.C.S.

Senior Visiting Plastic Surgeon, Women's and Children Hospital and Royal Adelaide Hospital, Adelaide, Australia

Thermal and Electrical Injuries

John D. Ward, M.D.

Professor of Neurosurgery, Medical College of Virginia, Virginia Commonwealth University; Chief, Pediatric Neurosurgery, and Director, Neuroscience Intensive Care Unit, Medical College of Virginia Hospitals, Richmond, Virginia

Craniocerebral Injuries

John R. Wesley, M.D.

Clinical Professor, Department of Surgery, University of California at Davis Medical Center; Section Head, Pediatric Surgery, University of California at Davis Medical Center, Sacramento, California

Nutritional Management in Pediatric Trauma

David E. Wesson, M.D.

Head, Division of General Surgery, and Attending Pediatric Surgeon, Hospital for Sick Children, Toronto, Ontario, Canada

Sports and Recreation Injuries

William E. Wise, Jr., M.D.

Clinical Assistant Professor of Surgery, Ohio State University College of Medicine; Head, Section of Colon and Rectal Surgery, Department of Surgery, Riverside Methodist Hospitals, Columbus, Ohio

Vascular Injuries

Foreword

Traumatic injuries and their sequelae kill far more children than any disease state. Although most trauma-related events in children are associated with blunt injuries, penetrating injury has become more frequently encountered in children, particularly in larger metropolitan communities, with the trend toward increased violence in our society and the rapid rise in the use of handguns and other weapons. Parents are increasingly concerned about the welfare and safety of their children as violence has extended from the streets to the playgrounds and schools and has unfortunately become a part of the daily way of life for some young people in the United States. Violence in other parts of the world including the Balkans, the Middle East, and Africa has also resulted in injury to numerous children who are often innocent bystanders in a conflict. Modern satellite media communications have made the viewing of such events as a child on a bicycle being struck by a vehicle driven by a drunk driver, an infant severely injured by an abusing parent, or a youngster shot in a schoolyard available to every household and community. A great deal of interest has been stimulated among both a more informed lay population and the medical community regarding injury prevention and the management of children with severe and often life-threatening injuries.

Management of Pediatric Trauma, edited by Dr. William Buntain, is a very timely publication. Dr. Buntain has recruited a number of experts in the field of pediatric trauma as contributors to this important effort. The text contains contemporary material presented in an orderly and easily readable format. The text appropriately leads off with a history of pediatric trauma care and gives the reader insight into the mechanisms and biomechanics of childhood injuries. One of the frustrating facts associated with pediatric trauma care is that so many of the injuries sustained by children are preventable. A key chapter in the text and a topic of vital interest to both parents and those who care for children is injury prevention. Although establishing trauma centers for adults has received a high priority, the development of trauma centers specifically designated for the care of children has received little attention until recently. This text devotes two chapters to the methodology required to organize trauma care for children, to develop pediatric trauma centers (as more are needed), and to establish standards of care.

The second section of the book contains chapters dedicated to the resuscitation and stabilization phase of pediatric trauma care, including patient triage, transportation of the seriously injured child, use of pediatric trauma scores to predict outcome, and development of trauma protocols. Two exceptionally good chapters that should give the reader an enhanced understanding of the nuances associated with the care of the injured child are those concerning the metabolic response to major injury and the evaluation of hemostasis, coagulopathy, and the use of blood products in children. Other useful chapters in this section include a general approach to the initial management of trauma, starting with the ABCs of trauma care and acquainting the reader with special advances in radiologic investigation and anesthetic management of the injured child.

The third section of the text includes 18 chapters that update the reader in depth regarding injury to specific sites or organ systems, including the management of head and spinal cord injuries; maxillofacial trauma; neck injuries; cardiac, pulmonary, and diaphragmatic trauma; vascular injuries; solid organ (liver, spleen, pancreas) trauma; injuries to the gastrointestinal tract, genitourinary tract, pelvis, and perineum; musculoskeletal trauma; and thermal injuries.

The editor has included a section on unique and special considerations in pediatric trauma, which is an attractive addition to the book. These topics cover situations that are confined to special circumstances, such as falls from heights, ranging from trees in the suburbs to high-rise apartments in the inner city; the management of snake bites, which are usually most prevalent in the South and Southwest; birth injuries; and the management of aspirated foreign bodies and caustic ingestion. Other chapters cover topics that are rarely given much consideration but continue to be areas of growing concern, such as recreational injuries and submersion injuries related to the use of all-terrain vehicles, skateboards, and surfboards; drownings in swimming pools; diving into quarries or shallow "swimming holes"; boating and water-skiing accidents; falls through ice; and the like. Of special interest is a chapter on farm-related injuries that points to an important consideration: access to care for children living in rural areas. It has become alarmingly clear when comparing the outcome of comparable injuries in rural and inner-city children that injured children in rural settings, have a higher risk of dying than inner-city children, who have better access to a pediatric-oriented trauma center.

The fifth section of the book covers the fine points of critical care, including intensive care nursing, ventilator management, vascular access, immunology, nutrition, and organ system failure as it applies to the injured child. The final section is also of interest as it calls attention to the aftermath of injury, or more candidly, the price of survival for the many children who live but are permanently maimed or impaired by the injurious event. The chapters concerning morbidity, rehabilitation, long-term outcome, psychological impact, and obtaining permission for organ donation are important contributions and make this text somewhat different from other previous publications regarding pediatric trauma. The final chapter leaves the reader some thoughtful ideas for the future of pediatric trauma care.

Dr. Buntain and his contributors have produced a quality textbook on pediatric trauma care that is worth reading.

JAY L. GROSFELD, M.D.
Professor and Chairman, Department of Surgery
Indiana University School of Medicine

Foreword

Trauma is the single most important health and social problem in the United States today, accounting for more working years of life lost than cancer and heart disease combined. It is the number one cause of death of persons between ages 1 and 44, and for every death there are three permanent disabilities.

The tragedy of trauma strikes hardest in the very young. In the United States, a white male aged 15 years in 1985 has a 1 in 110 estimated risk of dying of a motor vehicle–related injury by the time he is 30 years old. In contrast, a black male aged 20 years in 1985 has a 1 in 50 estimated risk of dying of homicide by the time he is 35 years of age. Of all white females aged 10 years in 1985 who die during the next 15 years, more than half will die from accidents. Similarly, white males and black males aged 10 years in 1985 who die during the next 15 years, 79% and 74%, respectively, will probably die of injuries.

Many of these deaths and disabilities could be prevented if there were better prevention and treatment programs, including appropriately oriented trauma centers and rehabilitation units. Dr. Buntain has put together a timely and comprehensive text addressing all of these issues. It is a book I strongly recommend to all health care professionals who care for the injured child and teenager.

DONALD TRUNKEY, M.D.
Professor and Chairman
Department of Surgery
Oregon Health Sciences University

The Carnage of Our Children

Webster's dictionary defines *carnage* as "a great and bloody slaughter as in battle." What better description for our current problem with pediatric trauma? Twenty-one years ago Izant and Hubay described pediatric trauma as "one of the poorest understood and most serious social, economic, and medical phenomena of current times." Unfortunately, this problem remains misunderstood and mismanaged and continues to rob society of one of its most precious assets, our children. This state of affairs is truly incredible if we consider the battles won with polio, other infectious diseases, congenital heart diseases, and a multitude of other pediatric problems, most of which have produced far less havoc in our society.

Injuries have remained the leading cause of death in children for the past 20 years, with at least half of childhood deaths annually resulting from the consequences of a traumatic incident. In understanding the problem with morbidity and mortality in pediatric trauma, it is important to consider that at least 75% or more injured children sustain blunt trauma, in sharp contrast to adults, in whom penetrating trauma plays a much bigger role. Motor vehicles remain the most common external force in producing these injuries, including the motor vehicle versus the pedestrian or bicycle rider, an even greater problem for the young child. Such injuries may also involve the motor vehicle occupants; however, this is more often a problem for the older or teenaged child.

The vast majority of these young patients are males, and the prevalence of drugs and alcohol in our society, coupled with the never-ending quest of adolescents to indulge themselves, the adolescent psyche and ego, peer pressure, drugs and alcohol, and the automobile, make for lethal combinations. Among other major causes of pediatric injuries are child abuse and falls, and child neglect often underlies the fall. Although the mechanism for managing child abuse in our society is improving, we have not yet reached the point at which health care professionals can recognize every case. It is time for our society to deal rationally with the concept of returning a child to his or her natural parents; this is not always the best solution, and in certain situations may indeed promote further trauma and even death.

Child neglect is a more subtle problem, and proper management requires the same knowledge and insight as that required for the abused patient. The child who ingests poisonous substances from under a kitchen sink, the child who tips over a pot of boiling water on the stove, the child with access to electrical sockets, and the infant home alone or under the care of a 7-year-old sibling are all examples of child neglect. It is time for all of us to stand up and say, "We have had enough."

By far the largest number of pediatric injuries takes place during the months when children are out of school, leading to the obvious conclusion that children, left to their own devices and not engaged in structured programs, are at the greatest risk for injury. We must strive for better control and awareness of our children and their activities. The simple and perhaps trite bumper sticker that reads "Do You Know Where Your Child Is?" expresses an important thought. We must respond to this challenge to appropriately initiate the process of accident prevention. Because children unfortunately cannot abstract to the consequence of committing a potentially dangerous act because their mental processes have not reached the point at which fear and trepidation intervene, our role as health care professionals should be to provide much of the needed guidance.

Another area of major concern in the field of pediatric trauma is the increasing incidence of teenage suicide. The influence of peer pressure, drugs, alcohol, school pressures, and the ever-present need to succeed and be someone or something may drive an adolescent to believe that life no longer has value. The unfortunate increase in teenage suicide has finally directed us to begin the needed programs for prevention and prophylaxis. Perhaps the aforementioned bumper sticker should read, "Do You Know What Your Child Is Thinking Tonight?"

In 1973, the U.S. Congress passed the Emergency Medical Services Systems Act, dictating the creation of emergency medical systems and defining federal funding for them. Since then the development of emergency medical systems has been spectacular, reaching a high level of sophistication in many communities. However, most of these systems are ill prepared to deal with pediatric patients, who make up approximately 10 to 15% of all paramedic calls, 56% of which are trauma related. The mortality rate in the prehospital setting is higher for a traumatized child than for a similarly injured adult, a fact that is of particular significance in areas in which pediatric trauma centers do not exist.

The problem, then, is simple; the solution unfortunately is quite difficult. Prehospital providers are frequently called on to care for critically ill or injured children; however, they are often poorly prepared for the task. Most of the

Emergency Medical Technician curriculum deals with adult problems, and the logic that if pediatric patients make up only 10 to 15% of all emergency medical service calls, the core curriculum should contain only 10 to 15% of pediatric issues poses a major problem. The skills for caring for injured children not only require greater attention to detail but also are more difficult to learn and maintain because of infrequent use. Two such skills, management of the airway and intravenous access, simple and basic procedures performed by all paramedics in the management of adult trauma, may become impossible when needed for a small child. In addition, many Advanced Life Support units carry minimal, if any, pediatric equipment, and the often common feeling of being ill at ease with pediatric patients makes further development of quality pediatric trauma care difficult in these areas.

Efforts to correct these problems are needed. Specific instruction in management of the critically ill child should be a mandatory component of the paramedic curriculum, and development of continuing education programs to maintain this knowledge base should also be mandatory. Those of us involved in the care of the traumatized child must play a major role in curriculum and training development for prehospital providers.

Recent data suggest that with the exception of airway management, few other therapeutic interventions are necessary in the initial emergency management of the traumatized patient, be it adult or child. However, it is quite clear that appropriate management of the airway, with adequate oxygenation and hyperventilation in patients with a significant head injury, is the most important component of prehospital management.

Head trauma exaggerates the problem of airway management in the field because at least two thirds of injured children present with a head injury as the most severely injured body area. This increased incidence of head injuries in multiply traumatized children further complicates patient evaluation in a group already compromised by size, age, and lack of communicative ability.

The urgency of establishing an airway with subsequent oxygenation and hyperventilation is of obvious significance when reviewing survival data in pediatric patients. Children with severe head injuries and multiple trauma do better and with less sequelae in general than their adult counterparts with similar injuries. This generalization is predicated, however, on early intervention and appropriate therapy, as any delay in vigorous management for the head-injured child results in a less than acceptable outcome. Reviews of pediatric prehospital trauma care have shown that in as many as 17% of patients, a delay in the onset of definitive therapy may have precipitated a less than desirable effect, that prolonged on-scene time results in a lower survival rate, and that the needs of children in the prehospital setting may not be being met.

The problems in managing an injured child are further complicated by the variance in physiologic response, including growth and development, when compared with that of adults. This places health care professionals, who spend most of their career dealing with adults, in a precarious position when called on to manage a traumatized child. If the prehospital providers, emergency department staff, and trauma surgeons are not attuned to the labile response of the young child, then the "golden hour" may pass without appropriate interventions. Everyone who has had occasion to care for injured children realizes quickly that their physiologic responses may progress along and appear to be stable and then suddenly unstable. Age, communication skills, and security needs of children further complicate this scenario. Morbidity, and on occasion even mortality, rates are affected adversely by the psychological trauma sustained when an injured child is delivered into the hands of strangers, most of whom continue the process of pain started by the traumatic incident. As care providers, we do not represent their usual means of psychological and physical support. Separation from parents and similar support individuals creates anxieties, which in turn complicate the physiologic response to trauma.

Finally, if we look at the long-term sequelae of injuries in children, the problems loom larger and become more difficult to overcome. More than 100,000 children are permanently crippled in the United States each year by accidents, and another 2,500,000 are temporarily incapacitated by their injuries. It is obvious to anyone with a pocket calculator that the long-term effect of this morbidity has a greater societal effect than comparable adult problems. Crippling injuries are a tragedy for the child, the family, and the society in which that child lives. If one calculates the loss of productive life years when a 5 year old is permanently crippled, the magnitude of the problem is quickly seen.

A study of the literature in the area of trauma care confirms that whenever a study was done in which no system of trauma care existed, unnecessary and needless deaths were found. Implementation of a system in those areas invariably reduced the unnecessary and needless death rate from trauma. Unfortunately, this same statement is not true for pediatric trauma. The reason is quite simple. Until recent years, trauma systems dealt only with components designed for and dedicated to the management of the adult trauma patient. It is obvious that trauma centers more oriented to the injured child need to be established that include the appropriate specialists as well as the necessary equipment and facilities. The systems in which these facilities exist should be integral components of the aforementioned regional emergency medical service systems, systems that can direct the critically injured child to appropriate facilities for definitive treatment and care.

These are not my ideas alone but rather the thoughts of a great many dedicated and committed health care professionals whose time has come. *Management of Pediatric Trauma* addresses all of these issues, not only as a "reference" but also as a "how to" source. It is necessary reading for all health care providers who care for the seriously injured child. It is the right time to end the senseless carnage and return to our society a most wonderful resource: our children.

Frank Ehrlich, M.D.
Clinical Professor of Surgery
University of Pennsylvania
Deputy Chairman, Department of Surgery
Graduate Hospital

Acknowledgments

Anyone who has undertaken the preparation and production of a comprehensive textbook such as this understands the enormity of the project and the necessity for many persons to be working closely together. To the large number of contributors who demonstrated immense patience in this production and in me, my heartfelt thanks and sincere appreciation. You were wonderful; your efforts will be recognized as such; and the success of *Management of Pediatric Trauma* will largely be because of you. I am also indebted to my editor at W. B. Saunders, Avé McCracken, and to Jacqui Brownstein, production manager, for their continuous encouragement, understanding, direction, professionalism, and competence. It was indeed my pleasure to work and learn with them, and I am profoundly grateful.

Those who have participated in an effort such as this realize the enormity of the personal effort required as well as the time and energy necessary to achieve as near excellence as possible—time that is over and above what is required to take care of patients, time that is by necessity taken from those you love, your family. I recognize that words are insufficient to replace time lost, tired impatience, and unavailability, but I hope my children know that I never stopped loving them, and I hope they are as proud of this work and contribution as I am. Their inspiration contributed immensely.

To Charlotte, my wife, my best friend, my gentle and constructive critic, go my sincerest thanks and appreciation for her immense help. I was fortunate indeed to have her excellence with the word processor for hours, days, evenings, and vacations, which we spent together transcribing, editing, revising, and striving for the excellence necessary to complete this book. We did it, despite the distractions and my impatience; she was persistent and consistent and a very major contributor.

Finally, I thank my secretary, Sondra Montiel, whose extra effort, consistent excellence in transcribing, hours spent at the library confirming and correcting references, calm and reassuring interactions with the contributors and the editors, and ability to get important things to and from the correct persons were all greatly appreciated and considerably important in accomplishing our commitment to excellence. Thank you.

Preface

This worthwhile project, begun some 6½ years ago, has finally reached fruition, an exciting and extremely satisfying realization personally. More important, it has resulted in a contribution that should enhance the care of the injured child considerably. This text is as necessary now as it was when the idea was first conceived, perhaps even more so, because no other single effort is as comprehensive in embracing the management of injured children. Indeed, the impetus for this book was the desire to make available to those involved and interested in the care of injured children a comprehensive text to which they could consistently turn for detailed instruction and information.

Similar such efforts were intended as references and have been received and accepted as such. They largely espouse the views of eminently successful and recognized pediatric surgeons who, for the most part, view trauma as a part, albeit an important one, of their overall practice. These "how I do it" texts have been and will continue to be valuable and useful, and their contributions are commendable. They have partially filled the void of what our effort is intended to accomplish and have done so seemingly without generating much controversy. Trauma surgeons, who are inclined to manage the dynamic or changing situation aggressively yet who are somewhat cautiously apprehensive at applying that proven aggressiveness to the care of children, have deferred to the pediatric surgeon.

This text is also intended as a reference and a "how I do it" book but with a decidedly *how to do it* and *why* flavor. More important, each topic is approached from a *trauma management first* perspective, actively combining the trauma surgeon's aggressive approach with the pediatric surgeon's knowledge and experience in managing children, emphatically addressing controversy as it arises, and presenting the reader with both sides of the argument.

An example of such controversy is the management of the injured spleen (see Chapter 21). Pediatric surgeons have championed the nonoperative approach, usually successfully but sometimes seemingly "at all cost" and often without selection or stratification of injury severity. Trauma surgeons, initially skeptical, have accepted this approach, and although they are more selective and usually stratify injury severity when possible, this practice is not universal and results in unnecessary splenectomies. The objective of management of splenic injury—the overall purpose, it is hoped—is splenic salvage, and patient salvage is not secondary. Whether one achieves this operatively or nonoperatively requires adequate information so that appropriate de-

cisions can be made. We must be willing to use every means at our disposal to accomplish this as well as to educate our less experienced colleagues at the same time.

This is what *Management of Pediatric Trauma* is about, not necessarily consensus but education and elucidation as to how and why an approach is favored. In addition, it is a resource for all physicians who care for injured children, with a perspective from both the pediatric and the trauma surgeon's approach. To this end there are three Forewords to our text. Dr. Jay Grosfeld, Professor and Chairman of the Department of Surgery at the University of Indiana School of Medicine, is an eminently known and widely respected pediatric surgeon. His judgment and opinions reflect those of most pediatric surgeons. Dr. Donald Trunkey, Professor and Chairman of the Department of Surgery at the University of Oregon School of Health Sciences, is an eminently known and widely respected trauma surgeon. His judgment and opinions reflect those of most trauma surgeons. Dr. Frank Ehrlich, Clinical Professor of Surgery at the University of Pennsylvania and Deputy Chairman of the Department of Surgery at Graduate Hospital in Philadelphia, is a trained pediatric surgeon whose interests in the subject matter moved him to become a full-time trauma surgeon. His judgment and opinions reflect the views of most of us with a deep and abiding interest in the injured child.

To obtain this perspective, I have drawn from the experience of more than 80 health care practitioners, all of whom are actively involved in the care of injured children. Because of this multiauthorship, varied perspectives are presented, and there is some repetition and overlap in the subject matter as the authors describe their approaches. We believe this to be healthy; there is more than one way to accomplish or achieve a successful result.

Six separate sections take the reader through 53 chapters covering General Considerations (the history of pediatric trauma, mechanisms and biomechanics of childhood injury, injury prevention, trauma care organizations, and development of standards), Resuscitation and Stabilization (triage, transport, trauma scores, trauma protocols, hemostasis, coagulopathy, blood and the use of blood products, metabolic response to injury, initial evaluation and management, radiologic evaluation, and anesthetic management), Specific Systems Considerations (injuries to the central nervous system, solid viscera, hollow viscera), Unique and Special Considerations (falls, foreign bodies, animal and snake bites, birth injuries, nonaccidental trauma, farm injuries, recreational injuries, submersion injuries, caustic injuries, penetrating injuries, and soft tissue injuries), Critical Care Considerations (vascular access and monitoring, organ system failure, immunologic and infectious consequences of injury, nutritional support, ventilatory and respiratory support, barotrauma and hyperbaric therapy, and nursing care), and then The Aftermath of Childhood Injuries (rehabilitation, long-term disability and morbidity, psychological consequences, organ procurement, and expectations for the future).

Management of Pediatric Trauma is a resource for all who participate in the care of injured children and a call to consider the approach to injured children from the broad perspective of pediatric and trauma-oriented surgeons as an integrated and comprehensive evaluation and management process, patterned after the American College of Surgeons' Advanced Trauma Life Support course, as the common bond that unites all such endeavors. Our intent is to update the information and add new chapters on fledgling areas of interest as needed, every 3 to 5 years, to make available and accessible the information needed by those both intimately and peripherally involved in the management of injuries to children.

WILLIAM L. BUNTAIN

Contents

SECTION THREE
SPECIFIC SYSTEMS CONSIDERATIONS

SECTION FOUR
UNIQUE AND SPECIAL CONSIDERATIONS

SECTION FIVE
CRITICAL CARE CONSIDERATIONS

SECTION SIX
THE AFTERMATH OF CHILDHOOD INJURIES

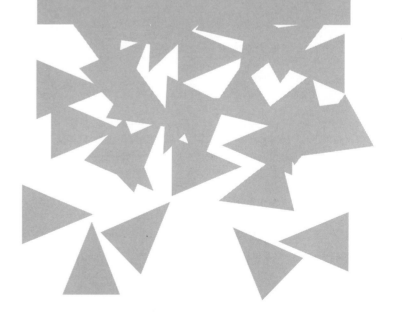

General Considerations

Steven Stylianos
Burton H. Harris

The History of Pediatric Trauma Care

The energy and interest of pediatric surgeons in the care of injured children is nearly as old as the specialty of pediatric surgery itself. In 1917, a collision between a French munitions ship and a Norwegian freighter caused an enormous explosion at a narrow point in the harbor in a densely populated area of Halifax, Nova Scotia, leaving 2000 killed, 9000 injured, and 31,000 homeless. Pleas for medical help were issued throughout the United States and Canada, and a Boston team led by Dr. William E. Ladd responded to the disaster. Dr. Ladd was so moved by the special medical needs of the injured children that he decided on his return to devote himself exclusively to the surgical care of infants and children (Fig. 1–1).[27]

In Dr. Ladd's time, infectious diseases were the most lethal childhood illnesses.[19] Tuberculosis and infections with gram-positive organisms, especially the pneumococcus and the meningococcus, killed thousands of children each year. The situation began to change when sulfa drugs became available in 1932, penicillin became available in the 1940s, and smallpox and polio vaccines were developed. By 1947 the death rate from these illnesses had begun to fall. Sometime in the mid 1940s, trauma became the leading cause of death in children.[20, 26, 61]

1955 TO 1970

The experience of the surgical generation of the late 1930s to the early 1950s, exposed to the military casualties of World War II and the Korean War, spawned a group of physicians who realized that concentration of medical talent and resources could greatly reduce morbidity and mortality from injuries. When these battlefield surgeons returned home, they began the application of their experience to the civilian setting, and adult trauma care, originally developed by orthopedic surgeons, became a recognizable interest within the field of general surgery. Although those responsible for the adult trauma movement were not at first concerned with pediatric patients, the evolution of pediatric trauma care would have been impossible without their efforts. Ironically, applications for new boards of trauma surgery and pediatric surgery were both denied by the Advisory Board for Medical Specialties on the same afternoon in February 1957.[42]

The involvement of pediatric surgeons in trauma care was paralleled by advances in allied specialties and by the recognition of trauma as a syndrome. Within pediatric surgery, the importance of trauma care was noted as early as 1966 when Izant and Hubay[41] called attention to the large numbers of children being killed and injured in accidents, stimulating the beginning of appreciation of the scope of the trauma problem in children. Trauma had become the most important child health issue in North America. Soon Haller described his studies on the mechanism of pediatric abdominal trauma, and Tank and colleagues reported on a group of children with blunt abdominal trauma.[30, 77] The publication of a landmark paper in 1969, *Accidental Death and Disability: The Neglected Disease of Modern Society,* led to the gradual acceptance by the medical profession of trauma as a predictable, treatable illness.[1]

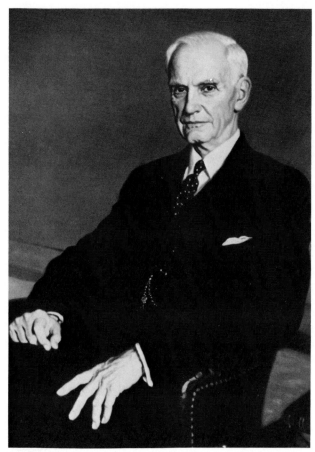

FIGURE 1–1

William E. Ladd, M.D. (From the Library of the Division of Pediatric Surgery, Boston Floating Hospital, div. of New England Medical Center, Boston, Mass.)

1970 TO 1985

Organized pediatric trauma care became recognizable as progress in the care of injured adults led to parallel efforts for children. The most important developments during this period were the emerging concepts of trauma centers and trauma systems, advances in medical treatment that contributed to better outcomes and to the recognition of improved results from regionalization of care. Cowley introduced the concept of the *golden hour,*[16] and trauma center directors increasingly concentrated on the provision and quality of prehospital care and transport.

The trauma center movement advanced significantly when the American College of Surgeons Committee on Trauma (ACS-COT) published the first version of "Optimal Hospital Resources for Care of the Seriously Injured" in 1976.[2] Derived from a previous manual of fracture treatment, this document was the first attempt to outline specifically the services necessary for organized trauma centers, and the ACS-COT supported its suggestions by providing "site-visit teams" to verify compliance of hospitals with national guidelines. The first ACS-COT statement contained the most quoted description of the most universal truth in the trauma literature: "Commitment is the essential ingredient of a trauma center."

These developments led to the formation of the American Association for the Surgery of Trauma, the academic forum for accumulating clinical experience and original research with regard to the science of care of injured persons. As trauma center designation became part of community, regional, and national plans, attention turned to organized systems of care, and the American Pediatric Surgical Association organized its first Trauma Committee in 1972. Three textbooks specifically dealing with injured children became available in the late 1970s.[64, 67, 79]

The federal Emergency Medical Services Systems Act of 1973 stimulated model municipal emergency medical services (EMS) programs by provisions for grant support.[62] The ''9–1–1'' notification system made its first appearance. David Boyd, a Chicago trauma surgeon whose work categorizing the trauma capabilities of Illinois hospitals had received considerable public notice,[10] became director of the Office of Emergency Medical Services in the United States Department of Health, Education, and Welfare. Several prehospital paramedic programs were created, and the success of the earliest of these—Seattle, Washington; Columbus, Ohio; Jacksonville, Florida; and Baltimore, Maryland—encouraged duplication elsewhere. Cities began to compete for the title of ''the safest place to have a heart attack,'' and soon enthusiasm and new resources were applied to effective prehospital care of trauma patients.

Beginning trauma centers and EMS programs were based in cities and metropolitan areas. Transportation of trauma patients from rural sites, although frequently necessary, was usually done by a funeral director whose hearse was also the town ambulance. This type of transport was outside any medical system, although an occasional nurse or doctor was hastily conscripted into service. Helicopters offered a theoretic solution to this problem, but suggestions for aeromedical transport were viewed as science fiction by city councils and hospital boards.

In 1970 and 1971, two demonstration projects revealed the practicality of helicopter transport of acutely sick and injured patients to regional centers. Harris and colleagues[36] and Roberts and associates,[66] working with the Ohio Army National Guard, demonstrated that a paramedic and a doctor staffing a medically outfitted helicopter could function as both a flying rescue squad for trauma patients and a flying intensive care unit for interhospital transfer. In the same year Malone organized the Southeast Mississippi Air Ambulance District, using public funds for a medical helicopter at a regional referral hospital. Cleveland and co-workers in Denver devised a private, leased-aircraft, hospital-based helicopter system that has remained the national yardstick.[13, 14]

Today more than 150 hospitals operate 180 rotary wing aircraft in the United States, and many other aeromedical programs involving fixed-wing aircraft or proprietary or government sponsorship also exist.[15] The growth of civilian aeromedicine could not have been predicted in the early 1970s, but the concept of those pioneers remains intact: to make the accident scene the portal of entry to the health care system, to institute prompt treatment to attempt to shorten the period of hypoxic cell damage, and to provide skilled medical treatment on the scene and in transit while moving the patient rapidly to the most appropriate hospital.[37] Air transport of trauma patients is now a daily event.

During the 1970s, a small group of pediatric surgeons began calling their colleagues' attention to the syndromes of pediatric trauma and the special needs of child accident victims. Kottmeier and Shaftan opened the first trauma service dedicated to pediatrics. Haller and colleagues extended this concept to include referred patients from a statewide network who would be dispatched from a regional center and would arrive by air and ground transport.[31, 32] These efforts generated renewed interest in trauma centers for children. Even before the first pediatric trauma center opened, Morse spoke of the need for organized trauma care in a 1972 address to the American Pediatric Surgical Association.[56] Skivolocki and associates,[75] O'Neill and co-workers,[59] and Smith[76] wrote of their experiences with burn care and prevention in pediatric patients. Harris and Morse began experimental research on blunt injuries,[70] Welch[83] published an analysis of a large series of pediatric trauma patients, and Harris and colleagues[35] described new diagnostic methods specifically for injured children.

The first half of the 1980s was a period of consolidation and rapid growth. The Kiwanis Pediatric Trauma Institute opened in Boston in 1981, combining transportation and referral care for a geographic macroregion with a complete educational program, a research laboratory, and public information and prevention strategies all aimed exclusively at preventing and caring for childhood injuries. The added importance of this venture has been the willingness of community public service organizations to support pediatric trauma centers. The Trauma Committee of the American Pediatric Surgical Association published guidelines parallel to those for adults,[63] and a national pediatric trauma registry was begun. Baker and associates[3] and Champion and co-workers[12] devised indices to quantify injury severity, and Tepas and colleagues described a pediatric trauma score.[78]

Funded pediatric trauma programs now exist in Boston, Baltimore, Buffalo, Washington, D.C., Philadelphia, Pittsburgh, Chicago, Oklahoma City, Charlotte, Fargo, Indianapolis, Dallas, Salt Lake City, New York, and Seattle in the United States and in Toronto in Canada, and there is developing interest in many other locations. Community involvement is an important component in each of these centers.

CLINICAL ADVANCES

Trauma care from 1900 to 1930 was primarily observational with a reluctance to take operative intervention. In 1929, at a time when morbidity and mortality from any operation were considerable, Beekman recorded ''no significant findings'' in 40% of celiotomies in patients explored because they had been in severe accidents.[5] Of 59 injured children who underwent celiotomy, only 28 survived. Beekman urged ''intelligent conservatism in the treatment of intra-abdominal injuries in childhood'' and predicted that it would save lives.

The aggressive surgical approach to abdominal trauma prevalent in midcentury was brought into question in 1959 after the observation by Shaftan that negative celiotomies were often followed by needless mortality and complications.[71] The modern era of selective conservatism in the treatment of abdominal trauma started when diagnosis was based on paracentesis, later by peritoneal lavage, and then by quantitative peritoneal lavage.[29, 60] Because angiography had always been impractical in pediatric trauma patients, a variety of isotopic techniques were adapted for pediatric injuries in the mid 1970s.[35] Used to examine the kidney, liver, and spleen, the radionuclides filled an important gap before modern imaging techniques came into use. Although they served many child accident victims well, these scans are now obsolete.

The first generation of computed tomography (CT) scans added little to the diagnosis of abdominal injury because resolution of air-filled structures was imprecise. With improved technology and enhanced by intraluminal and intravascular contrast agents, double-contrast truncal CT is now the standard by which all other techniques are judged.[49]

The two major influences on the postoperative management of pediatric trauma patients have been the availability of potent antibiotics and the development of techniques for total parenteral nutrition (TPN). The first use of TPN by Wilmore and Dudrick in 1968 involved the care of an infant with midgut volvulus.[85] The 22-month survival period of this unfortunate patient demonstrated that complete nutrition could be provided solely by intravenous feeding and that normal growth and development of a child could progress under such circumstances. Total parenteral nutrition has completely changed the approach to many abdominal injuries, and nutritional care of multiply-injured patients has significantly improved survival and altered surgical strategies after serious injuries.

Other new techniques have become milestones in the quest for improved outcome. Although sepsis and multiple organ failure are far less common in children than in adults after trauma, the ability to tailor antibiotic combinations to mixed flora has been effective in treating wounds of the head and neck, soft tissue injuries, and intestinal perforation. The development of intensive care units, the evolution of pediatric intensive care, improved ventilators, bedside determination of cardiac output and peripheral resistance, and other triumphs of ingenuity and technology all have incrementally improved care.

TREATMENT OF SPECIFIC INJURIES

Spleen

Blood transfusion, intravenous fluid therapy, and rapid diagnosis were unknown and unimagined when the twentieth century began. Any operation had a prohibitive mortality. Splenic injuries were managed nonoperatively but with a 90 to 100% mortality.[54] Reports of successful splenectomy and splenorrhaphy for blunt trauma first appeared at this time; in one instance the spleen was sutured directly, and in the other an iodoform tampon was used.[24, 39, 51] Hilar injuries were considered to be near fatal except in rare circumstances of spontaneous vasoconstriction.[6]

As surgeons became more adventurous, operations on the spleen became more frequent and larger series were published. In 1930, splenectomy had "only" a 27% mortality,[52] and hemoperitoneum frequently became the indication for abdominal exploration. As surgical techniques im-

proved, enthusiasm for splenectomy increased and splenectomy became the standard treatment for such injuries.[45, 47, 73] Fear of death from hemorrhage, delayed rupture, pseudocyst formation, and splenosis were cited as reasons for splenectomy.

In 1911 Kocher stated that "injuries to the spleen demand immediate excision of the gland. No evil effects follow its removal while the danger of hemorrhage is effectively stopped."[48] This approach went unquestioned until the landmark paper of King and Schumacher in 1952, which reported five instances of overwhelming infection in infants who had undergone splenectomy before reaching 6 months of age.[46] Initially, it appeared that children whose splenectomy was performed before the age of 2 years were the only group at risk, but eventually the papers of Diamond,[18] West and Grosfeld,[84] and Singer[74] established the universal application of King and Schumacher's findings. Singer's review showed that asplenic children were 200 times more likely than the normal population to develop sepsis.

The dangers of splenectomy led to attempts at splenic salvage. In 1971, Douglas and Simpson[21] published a report of their precedent-shattering 20-year experience with the nonoperative management of splenic injuries at the Hospital for Sick Children in Toronto. This protocol had been initiated in the 1940s by Wansbrough, and Douglas and Simpson described only one death and six splenectomies in 32 patients. Their series was updated by Shandling[72] in 1986, and now a total of 91 children have been treated nonoperatively at the Hospital for Sick Children without a single death related to nonoperative management. Despite early disbelief and intense criticism, these findings have been consistently confirmed, and in selected patients, conservatism in the treatment of splenic injury is now universally practiced by pediatric surgeons.

Liver

The second most commonly injured abdominal organ is the liver.[58] A marked improvement in the management of penetrating liver injuries was documented in the first half of the century. In 1956, Mikeskey and associates reported that mortality in penetrating injuries had fallen to 15% but that 66% of patients with blunt injury died.[53] Children younger than 10 years of age had a 40% mortality, the highest of all patients with liver injuries.

Lobar resection for major hepatic trauma was advocated as early as 1905 to avoid hematoma, hemobilia, late sepsis, and hemorrhagic complications, and by 1965 Hawkes[38] and Longmire[50] demonstrated that resection had improved outcome after blunt hepatic trauma by reducing mortality. Tank and associates confirmed a 33% mortality of isolated blunt hepatic trauma in children and emphasized the need for prompt diagnosis, large volume transfusion, and rapid control of hemorrhage in the care of major injuries.[77] During this period the usefulness of hypothermia in pediatric liver trauma was controversial. Howland and colleagues[40] suggested using warm fluid and blood to prevent the systemic effects of hypothermia, particularly ventricular fibrillation and platelet inactivation, whereas Welch[82] advocated controlled hypothermia with added quinidine to protect against arrhythmia, allowing prolonged clamping of the hepatic blood supply but avoiding hepatic necrosis. Recent experience shows that the Pringle maneuver can be performed safely in previously normal livers for up to 1 hour if postoperative carbohydrate loading is administered.[22]

Continued improvement in the treatment of hepatic trauma was reported by Defore and co-workers, who described results of the treatment of 1590 liver injuries that were seen consecutively from 1939 to 1974.[17] They illustrated a progressive decrease in mortality from blunt and penetrating injuries from 68% and 20% in the 1940s to 27% and 9%, respectively, in the 1970s. The use of modern techniques with pediatric trauma patients was reported in the late 1970s when Jona described the first successful hepatic arterial ligation to prevent exsanguination in a child with a major liver injury.[43]

The use of CT to document severity of injury began to be applied to the management of hepatic injuries in children in the 1980s,[4] and in 1983 Karp and colleagues reported on 17 children with CT-documented blunt liver injuries, all of whom had been treated nonoperatively with minimal complications and no deaths.[44] Patients in this series had transfusions of a mean of only 8 ml per kg body weight. Oldham and associates detailed the largest series of liver injuries in children, in which only four of 53 patients were operated on for continuing bleeding.[58] Two of the four died of hepatic vein lacerations, and the other two survived right hepatic lobectomies. The remaining 49 patients, in each of whom the diagnosis was known, were managed nonoperatively. One patient had hemobilia and two others had late bile peritonitis, and each had a successful delayed operation.

Pancreas

In 1956, Blumenstock and co-workers reported that 7% of 36 cases of pancreatitis in children were secondary to trauma.[8] Welch described 34 instances of pediatric pancreatic injuries among a total of 627 children with abdominal injuries treated from 1954 to 1977.[81] The mortality rate for traumatic pancreatitis, regardless of associated injuries, was 20%. In Welch's series, 23 patients underwent celiotomy, with four resections and 19 drainage procedures. Pseudocysts developed in 10 children. In 1978, Graham and colleagues reported on a group of 51 children with pancreatic injuries.[28] They found no initial elevation in serum amylase level in penetrating pancreatic injuries, although associated injuries were common. Three patients had pseudocysts that were treated by excision or internal drainage, and 10 patients had pancreatic fistulas, nine of which closed spontaneously. The deaths were caused by massive multiple injuries. In addition to overt trauma, the increasing awareness of child abuse as a subtle cause of unexplained pancreatitis in small children is now receiving appropriate attention.[9]

Duodenum

The most frequent duodenal injury in children is the intramural hematoma of the duodenum. Classically caused by trauma from a bicycle handbar, this injury results when an intrusive object compresses the duodenum against the vertebral bodies.[7] The barium contrast roentgenographic appearances was described in 1954 as the "coiled spring" sign.[23] Surgical management was removal of the obstructing clot and control of the torn submucosal vessels, and it was widely practiced until TPN became available in the early 1970s.[25, 85] Since then, Touloukian[80] and Resnicoff and Morton[65] described successful nonsurgical management using TPN and nasogastric suction until the clot spontaneously resolves. Surgical therapy now should be limited to the occasional instance in which duodenal rupture or another abdominal injury is suspected.

Kidney

Beekman noted the hazards of operating on renal injuries in 1929.[5] Before the introduction of intravenous pyelography, the lack of a diagnostic test often led to renal exploration in instances of gross hematuria or oliguria. Diagnostic capability improved when Harris and Harris[34] and Schencker[69] recommended infusion intravenous pyelography instead of standard pyelography in 1964. Two years later Morse reported excellent results with the same technique in children who had sustained trauma to the upper urinary tract and demonstrated that improved renal salvage depended on early and accurate knowledge of the injuries to identify those patients actually in need of operation.[55] His approach resulted in a 23% operation rate for documented injuries.

In 1968 Samuels and Smith reported the first use of scintillation scanning in pediatric trauma, demonstrating that radionuclide techniques allowed rapid and effective evaluation of renal trauma.[68] This was a major diagnostic advance because of the limitations of selective arteriography in small children. Experimental pediatric renal injuries were studied in 1972 by Schiller and colleagues, who compared infusion pyelography, renal scanning, and arteriography and found the latter two equally diagnostic of renal vascular injuries.[70] Morse and Harris recommended that renal injuries in children first be evaluated by infusion pyelography, followed by an immediate isotopic scan if the kidneys were not visualized.[57] Using the combined approach of prompt diagnosis and conservative management, the exploration rate for genitourinary tract injuries identified by hematuria is now less than 10%.[11]

The current diagnostic recommendation in major blunt abdominal trauma in children is double-contrast CT, the single best test for all of the solid viscera. Excellent visualization of the genitourinary tract is obtained. Infusion pyelography should be obtained when CT is not indicated.[33]

THE FUTURE

Pediatric trauma care has become an art form practiced by many pediatric surgeons who regard it as their field of special interest. The emotional and physiologic differences of young patients and the need to cope with pediatric trauma as a syndrome are now acknowledged to require special techniques and organization best provided by pediatric trauma centers. Improved outcome has been documented beyond reasonable doubt, and the trauma center movement has matured to the point at which legislative and regulatory bodies and insurance carriers are directing seriously injured patients to specialized facilities.

Considerable media and public attention is now being directed toward less common pediatric disorders, and this attention is well deserved. However, it is still possible to forget that injuries kill more children annually than all other childhood diseases combined. Seventy-five years after Dr. Ladd's vision, we are perhaps finally approaching the time in which every pediatric hospital and children's service commits to a special effort to provide advanced pediatric trauma care. The essential ingredient of this care is "commitment to the special needs of injured children—personal, institutional, and community."

References

1. Accidental Death and Disability: The Neglected Disease of Modern Society. Washington, DC, National Academy of Sciences National Research Council, April 1969.
2. American College of Surgeons Committee on Trauma: Optimal hospital resources for care of the seriously injured. Bull Am Coll Surgeons 61:15, 1976.
3. Baker SP, O'Neill B, Haddon WJ, et al: The injury severity score: A method for describing patients with multiple injuries and evaluating emergency care. J Trauma 14:187, 1974.
4. Bass BL, Eichelberger MR, Schisgall R, Randolph JG: Hazards of nonoperative therapy of hepatic injury in children. J Trauma 24:978, 1984.
5. Beekman F: Abdominal injuries in children. Ann Surg 90:206, 1929.
6. Berger E: The injuries to the spleen and their treatment. Arch Klin Chir 68:865, 1902.
7. Bertelsen S, Suhr P: Intramural haematoma of the duodenum. Acta Chir Scand 128:556, 1964.
8. Blumenstock DA, Mithoefer J, Santulli TV: Acute pancreatitis in children. Pediatrics 19:1002, 1957.
9. Bongiovi JJ, Logosso RD: Pancreatic pseudocyst occurring in the battered child syndrome. J Pediatr Surg 4:220, 1986.
10. Boyd DR, Pizzano WA, Silverstone PA, et al: Categorization of hospital emergency medical capabilities in Illinois: A statewide experience. Illinois Med J 146:33, 1974.
11. Cass AS: Renal trauma in the multiple-injured child. Urology 21:487, 1983.
12. Champion HR, Sacco WJ, Carnazzo A, et al: Trauma Score. Crit Care Med 9:672, 1981.
13. Cleveland HC, Bigelow D, Boyd D, et al: An air emergency service: The extension of the emergency department. EMT December:56, 1978.
14. Cleveland HC, Bigelow DB, Dracon D, et al: A civilian air emergency service: A report of its development, technical aspects and experience. J Trauma 16:452, 1976.
15. Collett HM: The 1987 forecast. Hosp Aviation 5:5, 1986.
16. Cowley RA: Maryland Institute for Emergency Medical Services: Foreword. Am Surg 45:77, 1979.
17. Defore WW, Mattox KL, Jordan GL, et al: Management of 1,590 consecutive cases of liver trauma. Arch Surg 111:493, 1976.
18. Diamond LK: Splenectomy in childhood and the hazard of overwhelming infection. Pediatrics 43:889, 1969.
19. Dietrich HF: Accidents, childhood's greatest physical threat, are preventable. JAMA 144:1175, 1950.
20. Dietrich HF: Prevention of childhood accidents. JAMA 156:929, 1954.
21. Douglas GJ, Simpson JS: The conservative management of splenic trauma. J Pediatr Surg 6:565, 1971.
22. Feliciano DV: Personal communication.
23. Felson B, Levin EJ: Intramural hematoma of the duodenum. Radiology 63:823, 1954.
24. Fischer H: Rupture of spleen. Ann Surg 84:124, 1926.
25. Freeark RJ, Corely Rd, Norcross WJ, et al: Intramural hematoma of the duodenum. Arch Surg 93:463, 1966.
26. Godfrey ES: The role of health departments in the prevention of accidents. Am J Public Health 27:151, 1937.
27. Goldbloom RB: Halifax and the precipitate birth of pediatric trauma. Pediatrics 77:764, 1986.
28. Graham JM, Pokorny WJ, Mattox KL, et al: Surgical management of pancreatic injuries in children. J Pediatr Surg 13:693, 1978.
29. Gumbert JL, Froderman SE, Merch JP: Diagnostic peritoneal lavage in blunt abdominal trauma. Ann Surg 165:70, 1967.
30. Haller JA: Injuries of the gastrointestinal tract in children. Clin Pediatr 5:476, 1966.
31. Haller JA Jr: Problems in children's trauma. J Trauma 10:269, 1970.
32. Haller JA, Shorter N, Miller D, et al: Organization and function of a regional pediatric trauma center: Does a system of management improve outcome? J Trauma 23:691, 1983.
33. Harris BH: Management of multiple trauma. Pediatr Clin North Am 32:175, 1985.
34. Harris JH, Harris JH Jr: Infusion pyelography. AJR 92:1391, 1964.
35. Harris BH, Morse TS, Weidenmeier CH, et al: Radioisotope diagnosis of splenic trauma. J Pediatr Surg 12:385, 1977.
36. Harris BH, Orr RE, Boles ET: Aeromedical transportation for infants and children. J Pediatr Surg 10:719, 1975.
37. Harris BH, Schwaitzberg SD, Collett HM: Progress in US Aeromedical Systems. In: Buhler C (ed): Airmed. Zurich, Springer-Verlag, 1986.
38. Hawkes F: Rupture of the pleura and liver. Ann Surg 41:138, 1905.
39. Hitzrot JM: Splenectomy for traumatic rupture of the spleen. Ann Surg 59:757, 1914.
40. Howland WS, Schweizer O, Boyan CP, et al: Physiologic alterations with massive blood replacement. Surg Gynecol Obstet 99:478, 1955.
41. Izant RJ, Hubay CA: The annual injury of 15,000,000 children: A limited study of accidental injury and death. J Trauma 9:292, 1969.
42. Johnson DG: Excellence in search of recognition. J Pediatr Surg 21:1019, 1986.
43. Jona JZ: Ligation of the main hepatic artery for exsanguinating liver laceration in an adolescent. J Trauma 18:225, 1978.
44. Karp MP, Cooney DL, Pras GA, et al: The nonoperative management of pediatric hepatic trauma. J Pediatr Surg 14:512, 1983.
45. Khanna HL, Hayes BR, McKeown KC: Delayed rupture of the spleen. Ann Surg 165:477, 1967.
46. King H, Schumacher HB: Splenic studies. 1. Susceptibility to infection after splenectomy performed in childhood. Ann Surg 136:239, 1952.
47. Knopp LM, Harkins HN: Traumatic rupture of the normal spleen: Analysis of 28 cases. Surgery 35:493, 1954.
48. Kocher ET (quoted by Sherman R): Perspective in the management of trauma to the spleen. J Trauma 20:1, 1980.
49. Kuhn JP, Berger PE: Computed tomography in the evaluation of blunt abdominal trauma in children. Radiol Clin North Am 19:503, 1981.
50. Longmire WP Jr: Hepatic surgery: Trauma, tumors and cysts. Ann Surg 161:1, 1965.
51. Ludlow AI: Suture of the spleen. Ann Surg 41:939, 1905.
52. McIndoe AH: Delayed hemorrhage following traumatic rupture of the spleen. Br J Surg 20:249, 1932.
53. Mikeskey WE, Howard JM, DeBakey ME: Collective review: Injuries of the liver in 300 consecutive cases. Surg Gynecol Obstet 103:323, 1956.
54. Mishalany H: Repair of the ruptured spleen. J Pediatr Surg 9:175, 1974.
55. Morse TS: Infusion pyelography in the evaluation of renal injuries in children. J Trauma 6:693, 1966.
56. Morse TS: Trauma: A call to action. Address to the American Pediatric Surgical Association, 1972.
57. Morse TS, Harris BH: Non-penetrating renal vascular injuries. J Trauma 13:497, 1973.
58. Oldham KT, Guice KS, Ryckman F, et al: Blunt liver injury in childhood: Evolution of therapy and current perspective. Surgery 100:542, 1986.
59. O'Neill JA, Grosfeld JL, Boles ET: A new technique for obtaining fetal skin for homografting. J Pediatr Surg 1:256, 1966.
60. Perry JF, DeMules JE, Root HD: Diagnostic peritoneal lavage in blunt abdominal trauma in children. Surg Gynecol Obstet 131:742, 1970.

61. Press E: The accident problem. JAMA 135:824, 1947.
62. Public Law 93–154: Emergency Medical Services Act of 1973. 93rd Congress, 5.2410, 1973.
63. Ramenofsky ML, Morse TS: Standards of care for the critically injured pediatric patients. J Trauma 22:921, 1983.
64. Randolph JG (ed): The Injured Child. Chicago, Year Book Medical Publishers, 1979.
65. Resnicoff SA, Morton JH: Changing concepts concerning intramural hematoma. J Trauma 9:561, 1969.
66. Roberts S, Bailey C, Vandermade JP, et al: Medicopter: An airborne intensive care unit. Ann Surg 172:325, 1970.
67. Salter RB (ed): Care for the Injured Child. Baltimore, Williams & Wilkins, 1975.
68. Samuels LD, Smith JP: Kidney scanning in pediatric renal trauma. J Trauma 8:583, 1968.
69. Schencker B: Drip infusion pyelography: Indications and applications in urologic roentgen diagnosis. Radiology 83:12, 1964.
70. Schiller M, Harris BH, Samuels LD, et al: Diagnosis of experimental renal trauma. J Pediatr Surg 7:187, 1972.
71. Shaftan GW: Indications for operation in abdominal trauma. Am J Surg 99:657, 1960.
72. Shandling B: Nonoperative management of splenic trauma. Contemp Surg 29:50, 1986.
73. Shires GT (ed): Care of the Trauma Patient. New York, McGraw-Hill, 1966, pp 397–398.
74. Singer DB: Postsplenectomy sepsis. Perspect Pediatr Pathol 1:285, 1985.
75. Skivolocki WP, Harris BH, Boles ET: A new method for skin grafting in a burn patient with epidermolysis bullosa. J Plast Reconstr Surg 53:355, 1974.
76. Smith EI: The epidemiology of burns. The cause and control of burns in children. Pediatrics 44 (suppl):821, 1969.
77. Tank ES, Eraklis AJ, Gross RE: Blunt abdominal trauma in infancy and childhood. J Trauma 8:439, 1968.
78. Tepas JJ, Ramenofsky ML, Mollitt DL, et al: The pediatric trauma score as a predictor of injury severity: An objective assessment. J Trauma 28(4):425–429, 1988.
79. Touloukian RJ (ed): Pediatric Trauma. New York, John Wiley, 1978.
80. Touloukian RJ: Protocol for the nonoperative treatment of obstructing intramural duodenal hematoma during childhood. Am J Surg 145:330, 1983.
81. Welch KJ: Traumatic pancreatitis in childhood. Newton-Wellesley Med Bull 11:22, 1959.
82. Welch KJ: Right hepatic lobectomy for blunt trauma with adjunct hypothermia. Paper presented at the American Association for the Surgery of Trauma, San Diego, California, October 5, 1960.
83. Welch KJ: Abdominal and thoracic injuries. In: Mustard WT, et al. (eds): Pediatric Surgery. Chicago, Year Book Medical Publishers, 1969, pp 708–739.
84. West KW, Grosfeld JL: Postsplenectomy sepsis: Historical background and current concepts. World J Surg 9:477, 1985.
85. Wilmore DW, Dudrick SJ: Growth and development of an infant receiving all nutrients exclusively by vein. JAMA 203:140, 1968.

Michael A. Pautler
Jeanne Henning
William L. Buntain

CHAPTER TWO

Mechanisms and Biomechanics of Traffic Injuries

TRAUMA AS A DISEASE

Henry H. Bliss, a New York real estate agent, innocently stepped off the streetcar he had been riding and was struck by a passing automobile and killed. Thus on September 13, 1899, the first motor vehicle fatality was recorded. In 1992, the United States Department of Transportation estimated that 2,734,000 others have lost their lives in traffic-related accidents since that time, and at current rates, the three millionth victim will be claimed before the one hundredth anniversary of that date.[41]

Worldwide, 500,000 people lose their lives every year in motor vehicle accidents.[9] If a world leader, a natural disaster, or even a virus had been responsible for 3 million deaths, a united world effort would be mobilized to solve the problem as quickly and as efficiently as possible. Yet a fraction of the effort devoted to less threatening, less pervasive problems is expended on this silent epidemic.

Motor vehicle accidents are the third leading cause of death for the U.S. population and are the leading killer of persons between 1 and 35 years old.[9, 52] Yet per year of lives lost, only $29 was spent in 1989 by federally funded agencies on research toward prevention and safety. This amount can be compared with $297 spent for research on cardiovascular disease, $587 for cancer research, and $1092 to combat the acquired immunodeficiency syndrome (AIDS).[9] The disparity in funding exists despite the fact that two to three times as many life-years are lost to injury than to either cardiovascular disease or cancer.[55] There is clearly an inequality present when the leading killer of our nation's children and young adults receives less than 2% of the fiscal attention given to AIDS and less than 10% of that directed toward coronary illness.

A study of the role of motor vehicle accidents in the spectrum of pediatric trauma requires an understanding of the epidemiology of these accidents; the nature of injury itself; the factors that predispose children to accidents; and the differences in physiology, anatomy, and behavior that make children more susceptible to the effects of injury. The mechanism of vehicular injuries, both in general and in relation to specific organs, can then be examined. As always, prevention is preferred over treatment, and a variety of strategies are necessary to continue to reduce the impact of this epidemic on both our society and our patients.

EPIDEMIOLOGY: THE EXTENT OF THE PROBLEM

Motor Vehicle Accidents

According to the National Safety Council, 169 million registered drivers and 194 million registered vehicles are traversing American roads each year.[49] Every year one in 10 of these vehicles or drivers will be involved in an accident that results in either injury or property damage. Analysis of the records of police, insurance agencies, emergency departments, and research offices indicate that an estimated 11.3 million such accidents occurred in 1990.

The carnage wrought by this "wasteful, needless epidemic" is tremendous.[52] Nearly 38,400 accidents involving 57,800 vehicles claimed the lives of 43,500 people in the United States in 1991. In general, improvements in traffic safety have been fairly consistent, but still the problem remains overwhelming, as evidenced by the National Highway and Traffic Safety Administration estimate that 44,529 Americans were killed in 1992, a 2.4% increase.[41]

The 43,500 traffic-related fatalities of 1991 are of course merely the tip of the iceberg. One million six hundred thousand people were injured, 520,000 were hospitalized, and 100,000 were permanently disabled in some way.[49, 50, 55] Cost estimates vary widely, but motor vehicle accidents cost U.S. citizens an estimated $96,100,000,000 in direct costs, such as property damage, hospital bills, insurance adjustments, lost work time, funeral expenses, and the like.[49] If the fact that many of the victims are young, valuable, and productive members of our society is accurate, the true cost yearly has been estimated as high as $334 billion. Even this estimate, as high as it might seem, may actually be low.

Motor vehicle accidents are particularly tragic because they are indiscriminate and destroy previously normal lives, especially those of young persons. More than 41% of those killed each year are younger than 25 years old. Young drivers 16 to 24 years old make up nearly a third of the casualties, as 13,839 of these young men and women lose their lives yearly.

The Children Involved

The biggest tragedy remains the number of children who are killed each year. Children do not drive, and others are responsible for their safety. Yet in 1991, 4210 children, just short of 10% of all traffic-related fatalities, were killed. There is no way to measure accurately the impact of this loss on our society.

The Rate of Improvement

That there has been improvement is undeniable. Since 1981, the number of fatalities has decreased 15%. In fact, 1991 figures have shown the lowest number of fatalities since 1962 (Fig. 2–1). Since the number of fatalities does not reflect population growth or, perhaps more important, the continued industrialization of our society, the absolute fatality rate (number of fatalities per 100,000 population) and the fatality per mile ratio (fatalities per million miles driven) more accurately reflect the safety of our infrastructure. In 1991, 17.2 people per 100,000 were killed in traffic-related fatalities, a 23% reduction over the last 10 years and the lowest rate since 1923. For every million miles driven, 2.01 people were killed, the lowest rate ever recorded, and a 39% reduction since 1981.

Is this rate of improvement acceptable? At first glance, it is somewhat impressive. Unfortunately, anytime morbidity and mortality are at historic lows, proponents of maintaining the status quo can be found. Because one fifth of the total number of fatalities are 18 years old or younger (Fig. 2–2) and because nearly 30% of all children 18 and under that die will die as statistics—victims of this silent epi-

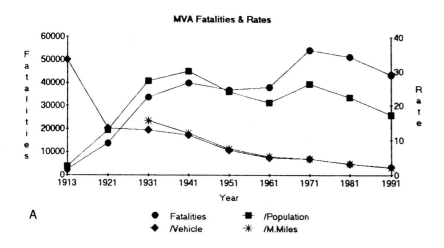

MVA Fatalities & Rates

A

● Fatalities   ■ /Population
◆ /Vehicle   ✻ /M.Miles

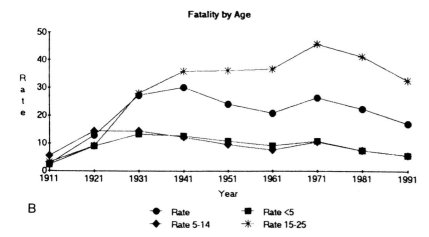

Fatality by Age

B

● Rate   ■ Rate <5
◆ Rate 5-14   ✻ Rate 15-25

FIGURE 2-1

Motor vehicle accident (MVA) fatality characteristics over the last 8 decades. *A* depicts the number of fatalities over this time, as well as the fatalities per 100,000 population, the fatalities per vehicle, and the fatalities per million miles driven. Note that the fatalities per vehicle *and* those per million miles driven have decreased consistently since 1931, whereas the fatalities alone and the fatalities per 100,000 population have remained about the same. *B* depicts the fatalities per 100,000 population by age group. Note that the fatality rate of the 15- to 25-year-old age group has far exceeded that of the rest of the population consistently, particularly the pediatric population.

demic—more effort and diligence in controlling this problem are well worth the effort.

Although the death rate has dropped to 17.2 per 100,000 overall, it is unacceptable high in the 15- to 24-year-old age group, 2.5 times higher than that of the general population, as 40.4 of every 100,000 of these young adults are killed in traffic accidents. The chances that a young adult will die in an accident are three times that of the second leading cause of death[49] (Fig. 2–3). Motor vehicle accidents have been continually identified as the single most prevalent cause of morbidity and mortality of U.S. youth. As long as this is the case, reducing the number of injuries and fatalities due to motor vehicle accidents should receive the same attention as that devoted to any other serious medical condition or disease.

As the population, rate of motorization, and utilization of motor vehicles continues to increase, this issue will remain a major public health concern. The chances of an individual fatality are slight; at two fatalities per million miles, with an average per driver mileage of 11,000 miles per year it would take nearly 4000 miles to develop a single statistical fatality.[9] There is no reason that these numbers cannot be reduced by half yet again. Three-point seat belts (lap-shoulder belts) are known to decrease fatalities by 45 to 55%, and major injuries are decreased as well by nearly 50%.[49] If a fatality occurs in an accident, restrained occupants have a 27% chance of being killed, but unrestrained passengers have a 51% chance.[47] Still, seat belt use continues to be lower than desired. In a 19-city observational survey completed in November 1991, seat belt use was only 51%.[48] Restraint use is considered in detail in the discussion of prevention.

The Effects of Alcohol

Of more concern, however, is the persistence of alcohol intoxication as perhaps the single greatest factor influencing risk. In 1990, alcohol was cited as a contributing factor in 22,084 traffic fatalities.[43] In 50% of the accidents in which

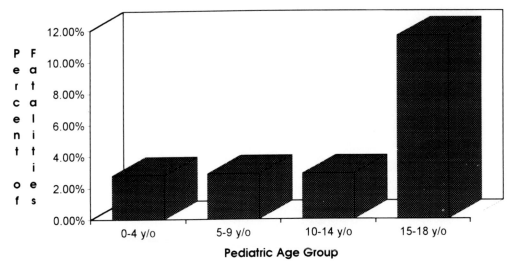

FIGURE 2–2

Percentage of all motor vehicle accident deaths by age group for children. Children younger than 19 represent more than 20% of all deaths due to motor vehicle accidents. The 15- to 18-year-old age group is at the highest risk. (From National Highway Traffic Administration Fatal Accident Reporting System, 1990.)

someone was killed, a driver was legally intoxicated.[53] In one Chicago emergency department, 56% of adults injured in motor vehicle accidents were legally drunk and had a blood alcohol content (BAC) higher than 0.1.[19]

These figures are indeed intolerable, especially considering that one third of those killed by drunk drivers are innocent victims who were not with the driver and that 29% of the children aged 4 and younger are murdered by drunk drivers.[53, 61] Alcohol-related accidents are the number one cause of death in young adults aged 16 to 24.[34]

PEDIATRIC CONSIDERATIONS: CHILDREN ARE NOT SMALL ADULTS

It would be difficult to receive medical training today without hearing the cliché "Children are not small adults." This represents a standard within the medical community, that children are unique in their anatomic, physiologic, and biochemical composition and that efforts to meet their needs are altered accordingly. This is particularly true in terms of automobile safety.

The interaction between an occupant or a pedestrian and an automobile is admittedly complex. The number of variables involved in a collision seems endless and makes specific injury prediction nearly impossible. Velocity, acceleration, contact area, stopping distance, cushioning, restraint systems, and secondary collisions represent only a few of the environmental factors that are studied. Automobile safety researchers would obviously like to minimize the number of variables involved.

Unfortunately, most research on automobile accidents has focused on adult occupants. Adults are, with relatively minor differences, the same in terms of susceptibility to injury and risk factors involved. The crash dummy, a standard within the automotive industry, has been developed to model the interaction of the adult occupant with the automobile environment in a collision situation.

It would be difficult to develop an accurate model for children. Growth is a series of anatomic and physiologic changes, not merely the addition of more material to increase mass. It is also combined with development, the increasing ability to interact with the child's environment. Children are obviously dynamic in their growth and development, and as they reach developmental landmarks in growth, behavior, and skill acquisition, their interaction with the environment changes.

Human development is an astounding process. From conception until birth, a fetus undergoes a 5000-fold increase in length and a billionfold increase in mass as an ovum 50 microns in diameter becomes a newborn weighing an average of 3.5 kg and measuring 50 cm in length.[63] Prenatal growth is based on cellular division and differentiation. After birth, the emphasis shifts to development of the intracellular matrix and functional development as the child grows and adapts to the environment.

Physical Changes after Birth

A term newborn whose growth is appropriate for gestational age should be roughly 50 cm (± 5 cm) in length.[46] A child following the mean growth curve grows 25 cm the first year, adding 50% to initial height. Birth length doubles at 4 years of age, when the child reaches 100 cm. Growth is fairly linear from 2 years of age until the pubescent growth spurt, adding 5 to 6 cm per year. Adult stature is 177 cm on average for males, 165 cm for females.

A normal newborn weighs 3.3 kg (± 0.7 kg) at birth. There is a larger variation in birth weight than birth length, as weight tends to be more reflective of the maternal environment provided for the fetus. This weight doubles by 5 months, triples by 1 year, and quadruples by 2 years.[67] A child typically reaches 10 kg at 1 year, 20 kg at 5 years, and 30 kg at 10 years before the onset of puberty, before reaching the final adult mass of approximately 70 kg for

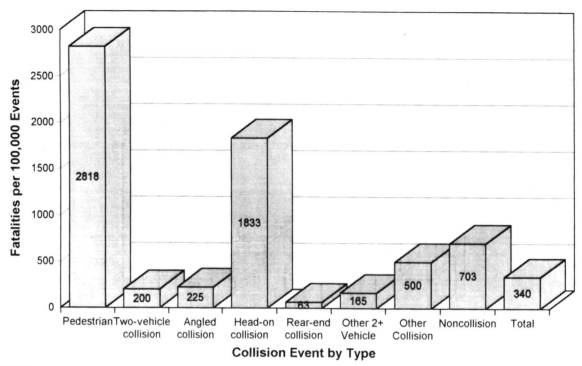

FIGURE 2–3

An evaluation of the relative fatality risk of various mechanisms of motor vehicle accidents reveals that pedestrian accidents are associated with the highest mortality by far. Head-on collisions are the second most deadly mechanism of motor vehicle fatality, and one should note the high fatality rate for "noncollision" events as well. (From National Highway Traffic Administration Fatal Accident Reporting System, 1990.)

males and 67 kg for females. These represent means only, and there is substantial variation.

That weight increases more rapidly than height is a reflection of volume. Individual variation of weight to height can be interpreted using the "ponderal index," or 100 times the cube root of the weight divided by the height, or the "body mass index," which represents the weight divided by the height squared.

Although growth can be evaluated by height and weight, it by no means gives the complete picture. As a child grows, weight distribution is constantly changing as the child changes shape and proportion as well. At birth the ratio of trunk height is roughly 70% of the body height, and this ratio falls as the child grows. The trunk height is 57% of the body at 3 years of age and only 50% as an adult.[8] Likewise, the head is one fourth of the total height of the newborn, declining to one seventh at adulthood.[63]

This shift in weight distribution becomes significant in two ways. First, the center of gravity of the body shifts as the child grows. It is at vertebrae level T-11 to T-12 in the infant and drops until it reaches L-4 to L-5 in the adult. This means that at birth, the newborn's center of gravity is slightly above the umbilicus, is at the umbilicus at 1 year, and continues to descend until it is closer to the pubic symphysis or iliac crests in the adult (Fig. 2–4).

Weight distribution is evident in the way that a toddler "toddles"; because the center of gravity is high and the musculoskeletal support system is still developing, the child walks in a way that artificially keeps the body's weight centered above the hips (Fig. 2–5). As a result, the trunk is

more straight, upright, and rigid, giving rise in part to the unique method of locomotion. It also makes it more difficult for toddlers to keep their balance, as they are essentially top-heavy.

Second, the child's head is large compared with the body. It is also relatively heavier, yet the neck and shoulder support for it is less well developed. When these two factors are combined, the child's motion in a collision is often logical. Unrestrained, the child is light, and a transfer of forward energy in a collision may send the child flying forward, often head first, with enough force to eject the child through a windshield.

Friction with the seat, however, retards the forward acceleration of the lower half of the body. As a result, the head and upper torso are the first to make contact. If the child is restrained in a two-point or lap belt over the iliac crests, the center of gravity is still above the restraint. A forward collision can lead to a jackknife effect as the top-heavy trunk and head continue forward until impact. This is often the mechanism of injury for intestinal and spinal cord injuries. For this reason, lap belts, and even three-point lap-shoulder belts are unacceptable for children under 4 years of age.

The head of the infant is relatively large, mainly because it is the first organ system to fully mature. The newborn's head circumference is around 34 cm, approximately the same as the chest circumference. By 4 years of age, it is nearly 50 cm or 80% of adult size. By age 8, head circumference is 95% of final adult size.[7] The rapidity of neural development in relationship to a pubertal growth spurt is

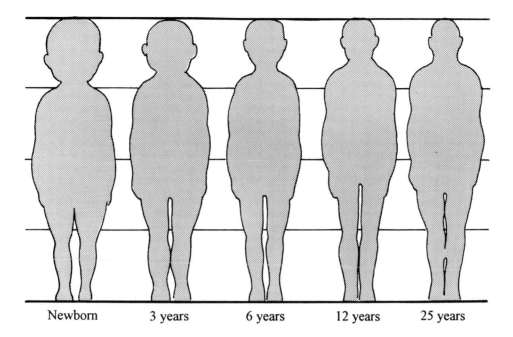

FIGURE 2–4

Pictoral depiction of changing body habitus with age. Note the changing center of gravity, which becomes lower on the body as the child grows and develops. Also note the decreasing percentage of head size. (Adapted by permission of Oxford University Press from Sinclair D: Human Growth after Birth. 4th ed. New York, Oxford University Press, 1985.)

unique to humans. It is interesting that there is a long "prepubertal quiescence" when growth is predictable while neural maturation is complete.[67] This is thought to allow ample time for socialization and development of learned behavior necessary for human survival.

Internally, a dominant feature of growth is muscle development. The lower limbs of the adult contain 55% of the body's muscle weight and make up one half of the body's height. In the infant, lower limb length is one third of the

total length, and the majority of the muscular system is in the neck and trunk. The typical adult has roughly 40% of the total body weight invested in muscle mass, and the organ weight (liver, heart, kidney, and brain) comprises only 5% of body weight. This distribution is drastically different in the infant, who has only 20% muscle mass and 18% organ mass[28] (Table 2–1).

With so much body weight invested in visceral organs, the abdomen is soft and protuberant. Until 2 years of age,

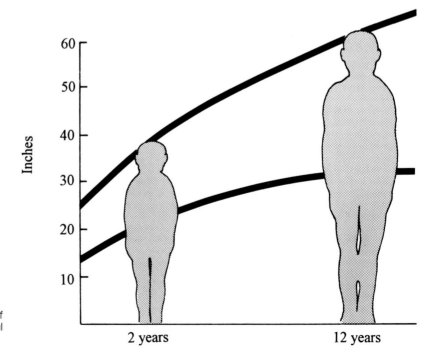

FIGURE 2–5

Graphic depiction of the differing slope of the center of gravity in relation to the total body height.

Table 2-1
Changing Body Composition with Age

| Age | Weight (kg) | Percent Body Weight | |
		Organs	Muscle
Newborn	3.5	18	20
3 mo	5.5	15	22
18 mo	11.0	14	23
5 yr	19.0	10	35
10 yr	31.0	8.4	37
14 yr (male)	50.0	5.7	42
Adult (male)	70.0	5.2	40
14 yr (female)	45.0	4.8	39
Adult (female)	55.0	4.4	35

abdominal girth is the body's equator, having the largest circumference. Muscle development of the abdomen and chest takes time, and the pelvis is small. As a result, the abdominal contents are poorly protected. As the child grows, the strengthened musculature, bony pelvis, and lower ribcage provide increased protection.

The musculoskeletal system and the skin provide the majority of physical protection from injury. With less muscle mass, there is less tissue available to absorb energy, as a greater percentage of body weight is devoted to critical systems. The bones and rib cage are more compliant, and although less likely to fracture, they provide less of a barrier to internal injury, especially contusions. The chest wall, for example, is more likely to compress and squeeze or impinge with force in response to externally applied energy.

The child's skin is thinner and more pliable also. It represents 4% of the total body weight, with a surface area to cover of 800 cm^2 per kg compared with 6% of body weight in the adult with only 300 cm^2 per kg surface area to cover. In other words, the adult has more skin to cover less area than the child. The adult's skin is believed to be stronger as well.

Behavioral Aspects of Development

There are a number of unique characteristics of the psychosocial development of children that also need to be considered to fully attempt to understand the mechanism of injury in this age group. Children may indeed be more likely to be injured once a collision has occurred, but there are also developmental considerations that may increase their risk for involvement in vehicle-related accidents. Most researchers agree that children have less ability to negotiate traffic safely, and because they are impulsive and easily distracted, children are less likely to remember how to be safe pedestrians.

There is no question that children are impulsive, with a nearly constant need for motion or interaction with their environment. Skill acquisition takes time and is not necessarily sequential. Hence, it is society's responsibility to protect its children, and the physician's responsibility to educate society. For example, humans learn to walk before they can speak. The rapid development of the ability to ambulate before the development of the awareness of danger has caused many parents a great deal of worry and concern.

Children have limited ability to assess speed or distance or to localize sound.[4] Visual and auditory perception are skills that need to be developed. Their field of vision tends to be oriented toward a single object and limited by height.[18] In one study, 30% of 6 year olds were found to misjudge the source of an approaching sound.[18] Adults displayed a greater ability to compensate and react when they could not identify the source.

A child's perception of danger and ability to react to it may be limited as well. The child development psychologist Piaget referred to this as the "concrete operations stage" of development, during which the child has limited ability to handle multiple environmental variables, for example, the velocity and distance of approaching cars.[14]

Some cognitive differences have been established. Children are less likely to interpret road signs and vehicle approach times properly.[18, 30] Even the differentiation of right from left may contribute to traffic behavior. The same study found that in their population, the ability of 6, 7, and 9 year olds to distinguish right from left consistently was 58%, 72%, and 92%, respectively.

These results are somewhat surprising but raise a valid question: Do we expect too much from our children? Dunn and colleagues compared children's performance on road-crossing tests and vocabulary tests to parental expectations of performance in children from 5 to 10.[18] In all cases, parents overestimated their children's vocabulary. In another study, parents of 5- to 8-year-old children overestimated their ability to safely cross roads.[60]

Attempts at pedestrian simulations do give some insights into children's behavior. Demetra and associates established a "pretend road," where children cross a road without traffic based on activity on a parallel road bearing traffic.[14] Crossing attempts were appropriate, a "missed opportunity" (not crossing when the traffic gap was adequate), or a "tight fit" (a dangerous crossing attempt). Five-year-old children had roughly the same number of tight fits as adults but 4.5-fold more missed opportunities. Perhaps children set wider margins of safety for themselves to compensate.

Any simulation study fails to observe children in their natural environment, and education is effective only if it overrides instinct and impulse. Sandels trained 9- to 12-year-old children to look behind before making left turns on their bicycles rather than relying on hearing and "feel." Before training, only 10% of 9 year olds and 20% of 10 to 12 year olds would take this precaution. Still, after training and during hidden observation, only 59% and 80% looked before turning across traffic.[60] Education is useful but limited in effectiveness.

As one child expressed it, "First I look to the right, and then to the left and then to the right again. Then I stand there trembling—and then I run."[54] This child eloquently describes the limitations of education. To use knowledge, you must think of the knowledge, and even then, it might not help.

Education helps, but because we "cannot change the sequence of development," education must be carefully targeted and must be combined with the modification of the environment and the education and behavior modification of caregivers.[2]

MECHANISMS OF INJURY—A LESSON IN PHYSICS

The automobile has become such a staple of industrialized culture that it is easy to forget what an artificial environment it provides when we travel. A daily commute is a ritual for most Americans. When we drive, lost in thought, listening to music, or engaged in conversation, we are oblivious to the fact that as the car speeds along at 65 miles per hour (mph), our bodies are also traveling at 65 mph. If the car were to suddenly stop, our bodies would still be traveling at 65 mph. Automobile collisions themselves rarely kill. Rather, people are killed when their bodies, moving at high speeds, hurtle into the stationary interior of an automobile.

One Accident: Four Collisions

An automobile accident can be viewed as a series of four accidents, each with the capability of causing serious, even fatal, injury.[37] First, the initial collision event is when the vehicle strikes, or is struck by, an object. There is then an abrupt change in velocity, direction, or both or in vector motion of the vehicle. During this period there may be direct intrusion or deformation of the vehicle, leading to direct injury of the driver or occupants. If the change in vector motion is immediately transferred to the occupant by a restraint system, the occupant will continue traveling with the original velocity and in the direction the vehicle was traveling before the accident. The second potential collision may then occur as the occupant strikes the interior of the vehicle. This is the most common form of injury from automobile accidents and the area most successfully targeted for prevention through the use of belt restraint systems, car safety seats, and airbags.

The human body is triphasic, with solid, liquid, and gaseous systems combining to provide function and protection.[36] For example, the brain is continually bathed in cerebrospinal fluid, not only to provide nutrition, but also to provide an aqueous layer to dampen energy transmission and provide a shock absorber for the brain. If the cranium undergoes a sudden change in velocity—by striking the windshield during a collision, for example—the change in vector motion is not immediately transferred to the brain, which continues forward until it strikes the anterior aspect of the cranial vault, possibly causing a concussion. This is the third potential collision, as solid organs strike the limits of their confining spaces (Fig. 2–6).

Finally, other objects such as groceries, toys, and automobile parts and tools may be present unrestrained within the interior compartment of the vehicle. These may become projectiles as they continue their original vector motion after a collision, potentially striking an occupant and causing injury (Fig. 2–7).

The Time-Motion-Force Relationship

A moving vehicle and all the occupants and objects in the vehicle have a kinetic energy that allows them to travel at

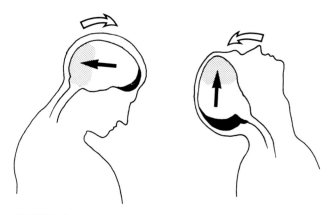

FIGURE 2–6

"Coup-contre-coup" mechanism of injury. The brain strikes the occipital aspect of the skull as the head accelerates; when the head then reflects in the opposite direction, the brain strikes the frontal aspect of the cranium, the so-called third collision.

that speed. The kinetic energy (KE) is the product of the mass (M) of the vehicle multiplied by the velocity (V) squared, or $KE = MV^2$. Because the KE depends on the velocity squared, increasing velocity from 55 to 65 mph leads to a 40% increase in the kinetic energy of the vehicle.

To stop the vehicle, the kinetic energy must be dissipated. This is usually accomplished by the addition of friction, dissipating the energy, by application of the brakes. The car decelerates, and a force (F) is then present equivalent to the product of the mass and acceleration, or $F = MA$.

Because the acceleration is the rate of change in velocity, dV/dT, the greater the magnitude in acceleration, the greater the force. The same kinetic energy must be dissipated, no matter how quickly it is done.

Thus, as a driver approaches a stop sign, an occupant might hardly notice the force applied through the brakes if the deceleration occurs over a long enough period of time. But if the deceleration occurs over a short period of time,

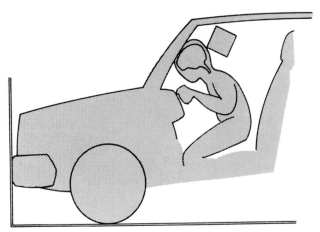

FIGURE 2–7

The "fourth collision," a silent but significant risk. Unrestrained objects—occasionally small children—can act as projectiles in a collision with sudden deceleration.

such as the 0.01 second typical of a frontal vehicle and object collision, a much greater force is applied.[51]

These forces are usually described using the force of gravity for unit comparison, and as it is impractical to measure time, the stopping distance (SD) is used instead. The deceleration force used to dissipate the kinetic energy can then be calculated as $G = V^2 / 30 \times SD$. Stopping a car from 30 mph over 20 feet would then require a deceleration of 1.5 G forces. Stopping the same car in 2 inches would lead to a 180 G force deceleration.

Brakes do not stop the occupant, only the car; therefore, the kinetic energy of the occupant must also be dissipated. In a normal stop, friction with the seat, with or without "holding on," is usually enough. If a 180 G force is applied to an occupant, the energy must be dissipated by other means. The restrained occupant transfers much of this energy to the seat belt; otherwise, it is transferred to interior collision sites, and injury occurs.

Force alone does not produce injury. Force must be applied to the body for an injury to occur. This is better described in terms of stress and strain. Stress is a force applied over a surface area and represents resistance to an externally applied pressure and it has the units of pressure. For example, a 200-pound force placed over 4 square inches gives a strain of 50 pounds per square inch (psi). The same force applied over ¼ square inch applies a strain of 100 psi. Strain represents the deformation of an object under a strain and describes physical characteristics of the object.

Three types of force have the potential to lead to injury, and these represent the methods used to apply force. Compressive strain is from a mechanical load applied directly, as in a crush injury. Tensile strain comes from pulling forces and tests the elasticity of an object. Shearing strain results from forces applied in opposite directions. In reality, all of these stresses may occur simultaneously (Fig. 2–8).

A collision then is a rapid, uncontrolled deceleration that leads to a dynamic transfer of energy to its occupants. If the energy is not absorbed by restraints, inertia forces the occupant to collide with the interior of the automobile. The occupant undergoes stress and strain, which cause injury if tissue tolerance is exceeded.

MECHANISMS OF INJURY IN MOTOR VEHICLE ACCIDENTS

Precise language is used to provide a semblance of order to automotive safety research, but in essence an accident is a chaotic uncontrolled event or incident. Continued study has managed to provide some aspects of predictability. Although the variables in any single collision appear infinite, patterns of events and injuries do emerge. These patterns can be analyzed, and risk factors can be identified, providing a framework for prevention. More practically, from a trauma perspective, knowledge of collision events may provide a high index of suspicion for particular injuries that might otherwise remain undetected.

Frontal Collisions

Without question the greatest risk occurs when an automobile is brought to a sudden stop in a frontal impact, either with another vehicle in a head-on collision or with a stationary object. A head-on collision with another vehicle resulted in 1833 deaths per 100,000 events in 1992.[49] Luckily, only 240,000 of 8.1 million (or 3%) two-vehicle accidents were head-on collisions, reflecting a national effort to physically separate oncoming traffic over the last 50 years.

However, frontal collisions with stationary objects remain a problem. Although two-vehicle collisions outnumber single-vehicle collisions more than 3.6 to 1, the numbers of fatalities are comparable. The fatality rate of a single-vehicle collision is nearly 2.5 times higher than that of a two-vehicle collision.

Between the bumper and the dashboard is a minimum of 2 feet of unoccupied space that is crushed when an automobile strikes an object at 30 mph.[52] This serves to increase the stopping distance of the vehicle by at least 2 feet. Thus, in a 30 mph frontal collision with a stationary barrier, a standard experimental design for automobile safety, a force of 15 G is transmitted to the interior of the automobile (30 mph / 2 feet). In reality the forces are higher than this, from 18 to 28 G.

This deceleration is transmitted to the occupants of the vehicle, but the forces of impact are much higher, particularly for the unrestrained occupant. The entire body is thrown forward, and a fairly predictable set of secondary collisions occur as different parts of the body strike the various parts of the interior. Because they are the closest to an impact site, the knees generally collide first, striking the inferior aspect of the dashboard. However, during this time the automobile has not yet reached a complete stop and is still moving forward. As the impact has already occurred by the time the collision has completed, the knees then are deflected and ride down the remainder of the collision. In addition, the body receives maximal friction resistance on the posterior thigh and gluteal area, further slowing the impact speed. The impact speed is then equal to or less than the 15 G force imposed on the occupant.

The hips act as a hinge point during collision, because nearly all the friction from the car to the body acts on the lower extremities (see Fig. 2–4). This hinging action is exaggerated if a two-point lap belt is the sole restraint. When collision occurs, the upper body and head then advance at a faster rate than the lower body. Higher velocities, further distance until impact, and shorter stopping distances increase the forces exerted during impact and the likelihood of injury.

Chest contact obviously is influenced by position in the car. The driver's side is associated with an increased frequency and severity of chest injury owing to impact with the steering wheel. This is a difficult collision to evaluate because the wheel itself is often angled, which provides a variable impact surface on the chest and abdomen. Depending on the angle and the distance of the driver from the wheel, a variety of injury patterns occur, usually associated with compression of the sternum with or without rib fractures.

The head is the most distal point from the hinge. Because the head of a front seat occupant is usually at least 2 feet from the windshield unit, the collision has ended by the time the head hits the windshield. Thus, the head sustains the full extent of the deceleration at the time of impact. In

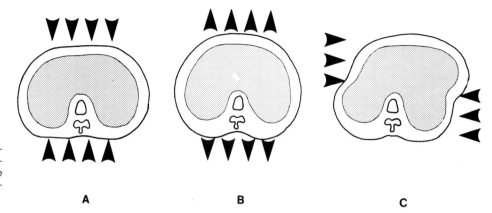

FIGURE 2–8

Different types of forces encountered in a motor vehicle accident. *A,* Compressive force; *B,* tensile force (stretching); *C,* shearing force.

A   B   C

addition, injury depends substantially on the characteristics of the surface that is struck. If the head strikes ordinary glass, as in older cars, very little resistance is met. The glass provides a minimal resistance of impact leading to little deceleration. Ejections frequently resulted as the front seat passenger passed through the windshield frame. If the occupant strikes a contemporary laminated windshield, the glass may deform to the surface of impact as much as 6 inches rather than shattering. If such is the situation, the head experiences a deceleration of 50 G at 30 mph. Compare this figure with that of an impact on the frame or another solid part of the car at which the stopping distance is from 0 to 2 inches: The head decelerates from 30 mph over 0.06 feet, and decelerations of 500 G are encountered.

For the most part, there is little angular momentum in a frontal collision, and the forces are in a single horizontal plane. However, the violence of the decelerations can strain joint spaces, often enough to cause fracture or nerve damage. The internal organ collisions with their encasement can also provide a significant mechanism of injury. These mechanisms are particularly important in head and spine injuries and are examined in a subsequent section.

Angled Collisions

The most common type of automobile accident—the angled collision—represents approximately one third of all reported accidents, and the fatality rate is approximately 225 deaths per 100,000 events.[49] Additional variables are involved in the analysis of an angled collision. Velocity, angle of collision, area of impact, and occupant position all contribute to the risk of injury. Occupants move toward the collision site in general; hence, an occupant migrates toward the front left corner of the car if struck at a 45-degree angle from the left.

The effect on the occupant depends on the occupant's position within the car. The driver hits the side window apparatus and the left side of the steering column. The risk of head injury may be higher because the distance to impact is shorter, and the driver is more likely to strike an unyielding surface, which means a short stopping distance. The front seat passenger may benefit, however, in relation to a full frontal collision, because there are fewer intervening structures and the distance until impact is longer, allowing a greater total stopping distance (Fig. 2–9).

In general, however, angled collisions introduce an even higher level of chaos. Angular momentum is now a variable, and the chance of multivehicle or stationary object collision increases. In addition to the angular momentum, rotational acceleration can occur as well, particularly if the impact occurs off center.

Lateral incursion represents an additional risk in angled collisions. For the most part, injury occurs when occupants strike the interior of the vehicle. However, when the doors are struck directly, the collision occurs at the weakest point of the automobile frame. If velocity is sufficient, the door frame will give, and the door will intrude, striking the occupant directly. In such collisions, because of the combination of multiple vector forces, neck injury becomes distinctly more possible. Neck rests are no longer effective, and high-velocity vector forces may expose the cervical spine to unusual angles, frequently intolerable ones.

Rear-End Collisions

Although rear-end collisions are quite common, nearly one third of two-car collisions, they carry the least risk, with 63 fatalities per 100,000 events.[49] Presumably a significant portion of precrash velocity is lost with brake application before impact. The struck vehicle undergoes a net acceleration rather than the deceleration encountered with frontal collisions.

The occupant then strikes the rear aspect of the interior, in general, the headrest and seat back. Injury may occur secondary to the acceleration itself, that is, whiplash injury, in which the back is restrained by the seat, but the head is not. The neck then is hyperextended, and tension is generated. Muscle and ligamentous strains are common, but severity can include cervical fracture or direct nerve or spinal cord injury. If the occupant is unrestrained, the seats are often elastic enough to provide rebound, and collisions with the frontal aspect of the interior are possible.

Tertiary injuries with this mechanism are common as well. For example, concussions are possible from the intracranial coup-contrecoup mechanism. When the vehicle is struck, the head is rapidly accelerated toward the rear of the vehicle. The brain is protected from the acceleration by the cerebrospinal fluid. It then is struck by the frontal aspect of the cranium, and the brain is accelerated toward the rear. Head acceleration, however, has stopped and is possibly

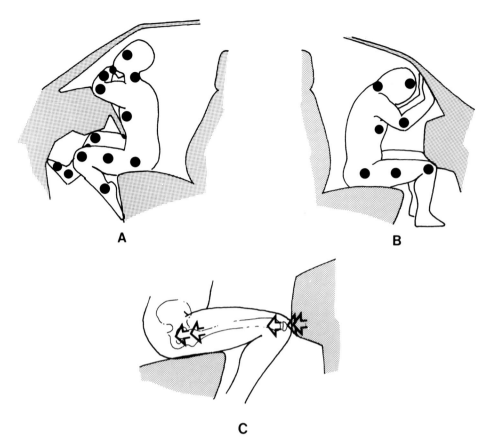

A

B

C

FIGURE 2–9

Common anatomic sites of impact in motor vehicle accidents for drivers (*A*) and passengers (*B*). *C* represents a common mechanism for hip dislocation and femoral fracture in passengers. (Adapted from Daffner RH, Deeb ZL, Lupetin AR, et al: Patterns of high-speed impact injuries in motor vehicle accidents. J Trauma 28(4):498–501, 1988.)

even reversed, so the brain then strikes the occipital aspect of the cranium. Thus, either a frontal or occipital concussion or bleed may be present (see Fig. 2–6). This mechanism of injury is not unique to rear-end collisions.

Vehicle Rollovers

Perhaps the most terrifying and definitely the most chaotic of all collisions is one in which a rollover occurs. Ninety percent of such events occur as the vehicle leaves the road, either through driver error or as a result of external impact. Resulting events are impossible to predict, as angular and rotational momentum is constantly changing; however, any surface of the automobile may be struck by any part of the body. The energy of collision, however, is greatly absorbed by the car itself, and occupants may be surprisingly free of injury compared with the level of damage to the vehicle.

Noncrash Events

Injuries often result from secondary collision with the vehicle interior; hence, a collision from without is not always necessary to provide sufficient change in velocity that results in significant impact. Sudden stops or swerves and ejections from vehicles are also significant causes of morbidity and mortality. In 1991, 640,000 injuries and 4500 deaths were attributed to noncrash events. The risk of fatality is actually higher than that for collisions (except frontal, two-vehicle), with 703 deaths per 100,000 events.[49, 52]

This is of particular concern for children. Agran and co-workers found that 15% of children who had vehicle-related injuries were involved in noncrash events.[3] Nearly 45% of these had been ejected or had fallen from the car. Also, 63% of these children were younger than 4 years old. Although use of restraints was not statistically significant, the nature of the injuries, particularly ejection, suggests that for the most part, these are preventable injuries.

The Rear Seat

Unfortunately, because the rear seat is deemed to be safer in general, safety concern appears to be less of an issue. Although it is true that there are no steering wheels, windshields, or dashboards in the back seat, fatality rates are comparable to those for front seat occupants, and the risk of injury in rear-end collisions is four times as high for rear seat occupants as for front seat occupants.[66] What is even more disconcerting is that the fact that restraint use among rear seat passengers is typically one fifth that of front seat occupants.[66]

Where are children in the car? Often in the back seat. The average age of rear seat occupants presenting to an emergency department after collision is 19 years old, 14 years younger than the average age of 33 years for front seat passengers. If restraint use is only 5%, what are the other 95% of children doing? Unfortunately, many of them are playing or standing by the front seat, thus increasing the risk of serious injury.

MECHANISMS OF INJURY IN BICYCLE ACCIDENTS

Bicycle accidents are a common cause of traumatic injury in children and adolescents. Such accidents resulted in more than 400,000 emergency department visits and 500 to 600 deaths in the United States in 1986.[10] Children are the most frequent victims of such incidents and unfortunately account for a large portion of the more serious injuries that occur.[71] In 1982, 70% of all bicycle-related injuries or fatalities occurred in children younger than 15 years of age, most as a result of head injury.[20, 22, 35, 64] The majority of fatalities result from collision with a motor vehicle, and event incidence peaks between May and September.[22]

The incidence of injury for boys is three times that for girls in several studies, the group between 10 and 14 years being particularly vulnerable and having the highest fatality rates.[22, 35] Members of this high-risk group are also the least likely to be wearing bicycle helmets and the most likely to engage in risk-taking behaviors while cycling, which puts them at an even greater risk.[64] The higher incidence of injury to males parallels that of other types of childhood trauma, such as pedestrian, motorcycle, and firearms injuries, in which boys are consistently involved at a higher rate than girls.[20, 22, 50] Bikers attempting to overtake motorists account for another common mechanism of collision that results in fatality for the cyclist. Crashes most frequently occur between 3 PM and 9 PM and are not strongly associated with adverse weather conditions or darkness.[20]

In the majority of bicycle versus motor vehicle crashes, the vehicle's front end is the initial point of contact with the cyclist.[20] However, cyclists under the age of 12 are more likely to be hit from the left side, as these young children frequently dart out into the street and are struck by a vehicle coming from the left.[20]

Head injury prevails as the major cause of mortality in bicycle accidents and also occurs most frequently in bike accidents that are not fatal.[24, 35, 71] Head injuries accounted for two thirds of hospital admissions related to bike accidents, with skull fractures and concussions being the common nonfatal injuries sustained.[20, 31, 64] Subdural hematomas account for a high number of the deaths.[20, 24] Indeed, it has been estimated that 20% of all significant brain injuries in children aged 14 or younger may be bicycle related.[35] Fife and colleagues reported that nearly all bicycle-related fatal head injuries analyzed were found to be secondary to blunt trauma, not penetrating trauma, and that the majority were not accompanied by serious neck or spinal injury.[20] This strongly suggests that if the head were better protected, thus making head injuries more preventable, many persons who receive potentially fatal injuries would have an improved chance of survival with good neurologic outcome.[20]

Serious associated pulmonary injuries were found to be present in the majority of cyclists with fatal head injuries studied by Fife and colleagues, and liver, spleen, and intestinal disruptions were also frequent, as were fractures, which account for a large portion of hospital admissions in nonfatal accidents.[20, 22]

Because head injuries account for such a large portion of the morbidity and mortality involved in bicycle accidents, considerable attention has been given to evaluating the effect that bicycle helmets worn by cyclists have in preventing serious injury.[56] Bicycle helmets are designed to protect the brain from compression by slowing deceleration and thereby protecting the skull from fracture.[22] Helmets in other sports, such as football and hockey, have significantly reduced the incidence of serious head injury.[71] In a study by Spaite and colleagues, not wearing a helmet in a crash was strongly associated with major head injury in 22% of all patients evaluated, whereas only 1 of 116 patients wearing a helmet during a crash had a major head injury. The question to be answered, however, is do cyclists who choose to wear a helmet also happen to be cyclists who practice safer biking practices overall.[64] Because bicycle helmets do appear to protect the head from injury, their use is strongly promoted for all cyclists, particularly children, throughout the United States and indeed worldwide.[15, 16, 23, 59, 62]

In Victoria, Australia, where bike helmet use was made mandatory in July 1992, there was a significant reduction in bike-related head injuries compared with the rate from the previous year.[59] This mandatory helmet use was encouraged by the Royal Australian College of Surgeons and the Road Traffic Authority, and enactment of the law was preceded by educational and publicity campaigns designed to make people aware of the risk of bike injuries and the protective effect of the helmet.[38, 70]

Use of helmets is actively promoted throughout the United States.[23] Many parents are unaware of the need for bike helmet use or are concerned about the cost.[15, 23] Children and adolescents are often under considerable peer pressure not to wear helmets, and less than 2% of those under 15 years of age wear them.[23, 71] Pediatricians, nurses, and health care personnel who routinely care for children must actively educate parents and children about the importance of helmet use. Nakayama and associates reported that even after a significant bicycle accident requiring hospitalization or emergency department care, helmet use did not increase significantly. However, when a bike safety program was subsequently given during hospitalization, an increased use in helmets after discharge resulted.[45] Consequently, at the time of such an incident, the opportunity to teach safe biking practices should be seized and the child and parents educated. In a study by Illingworth and coworkers of 150 children who had such accidents, 32% of them had experienced previous bike incidents.[31] Hence, teaching directed at the injured child and the child's family can be time well used.

Identification of children who have not yet had an accident yet are known demographically to be at high risk is important so that aggressive educational efforts and peer support can be targeted at them. Boys between the ages of 10 and 14 years are a prime risk group. Just as helmet use has become the norm for sports such as football, bike helmet use must become acceptable and routinely practiced by the cyclist as a means of preventing serious injury during a potentially dangerous activity.[56]

MECHANISMS OF INJURY IN PEDESTRIAN ACCIDENTS

Pedestrian injuries are an important component of traffic-related deaths in children ages 1 to 14 years. Fatal pedestrian injuries are more common than fatal passenger injuries in preschool and school-aged children, especially in cities.[57, 68] As child protective devices are used more frequently for young passengers in automobiles, passenger deaths and injuries will decline. There will then be an increase in the contribution of pedestrian injuries to motor vehicle morbidity and mortality unless it too is addressed by prevention strategies.[68]

Demographically, most fatal and nonfatal pedestrian injuries to children occur between the ages of 4 and 9 years, and there is another peak period for fatal injuries among 18 to 19 year olds.[26] Once again, several studies have demonstrated that boys are much more likely than girls to be involved in pedestrian injuries in all age groups.[26, 57, 65] Sex-related differences in behavior appear to influence this injury experience, as such children have often been noted to be very active, daring, impulsive, and extroverted.[68] They are thus more likely to be involved in dangerous situations, but because of adjustment problems and attention deficits are less able to cope with the impending situation.[40, 68] A child's behavior is a major determinant of actual pedestrian injury when the child is exposed to the risk of traffic.

Studies have also shown that children in poor urban areas are more likely to be injured as pedestrians.[57, 65] Physical characteristics of the neighborhoods, such as lack of safe play areas, contribute to the child's risk of exposure to traffic. Children are more likely to be injured while darting out into the street, as occurs frequently for children who play games in the street, than by crossing at intersections. It is not uncommon for the young child to be hit by a neighbor, a family friend, or a family member while playing in the area near the home. Lack of proper adult supervision may also play a key role in the child's risk. Toddlers and preschoolers are very mobile yet do not comprehend the dangers of traffic. They cannot be taught safe pedestrian skills, so they must be adequately supervised.

Driver negligence has also been shown to be a key element in these injuries, independent of the behavior of pedestrians in many cases.[6] Drivers who are involved in fatal pedestrian crashes often have poor driving records, and many also have behavior problems. Alcohol use by drivers has been implicated as a factor in pedestrian injuries.[6, 72]

The majority of pedestrian injuries involving children occur during daylight hours, particularly during the late afternoon on weekdays.[26, 65] This represents the time that children frequently get out of school and engage in spontaneous activities and behaviors after being inside the school for most of the day. For example, the outgoing, active 5- to 9-year-old boy who has had to sit in school all day finally gets dismissed, is ready to play with his friends, and easily forgets any lessons he may have been given about traffic safety. This is also a busy time of day for traffic, and thus the stage is set for perhaps a tragic encounter.

The most frequent type of pedestrian injury is when the pedestrian is struck by the front of the car, and contact is made with the bumper and then the hood of the car.[39] The exact location of contact with the body depends on the height of the child pedestrian, who then rotates around the leading edge of contact until the head, shoulders, and chest strike the windshield or car frame (Fig. 2–10). The victim is moving at about the same speed as the car by now, and

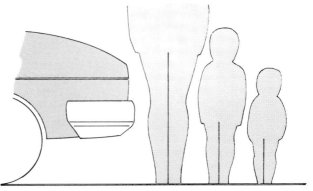

FIGURE 2–10

Bumper height versus pedestrian height. The anatomic site of impact drops as the child grows, changing the body dynamics after impact as well as the pattern of injuries seen. Smaller children obviously will feel the impact higher in the body and roll under the vehicle, whereas older children and adults will go over the vehicle after being struck by it.

if the vehicle brakes, as is usually the case, the car slows down faster than the pedestrian, who continues to move forward and lands on the road, sliding and rolling.[39] There are therefore two phases in a pedestrian collision: the first being multiple contacts with the car, and the second the rolling and sliding impact that occurs with the street.[39] Injury severity is strongly associated with speed during the first phase of such injury but not for the ground contact phase.[39]

The approach to the prevention of child pedestrian trauma in the future must be multifaceted. Separation of children's play areas from traffic has had a positive effect in some countries on reducing pedestrian injuries.[26] Attempts through educational programs to modify the behaviors of children in traffic have not proved very successful in outcome.[57, 68] The normal impulsiveness of young children plus their inability to assess adequately the speed of a vehicle and its distance from themselves result in unsafe behavior in traffic. Considerable research is being done on the overall relationship between vehicle shape and severity of pedestrian trauma, as evidence exists that different car profiles present different risks of injury.[39] Quantitative tests for alcohol for the drivers involved and more stringent and timely punishment in terms of license revocation for those who are shown to be negligent drivers are also recommended.[6]

ANATOMIC PATTERNS OF INJURY

The ultimate goal of injury research is twofold: prevention and prediction. Although the idealistic goal is to eliminate motor vehicle accidents entirely, realistically we know that this will not happen. Hence, once an accident occurs, knowledge of patterns of injury may allow improved detection, diagnosis, and treatment of previously unsuspected injuries. The fact that many injuries occur in patterns has been understood for decades. Literature, both lay and professional, is replete with anecdotal descriptions of common traffic injuries, and because of improved safety inno-

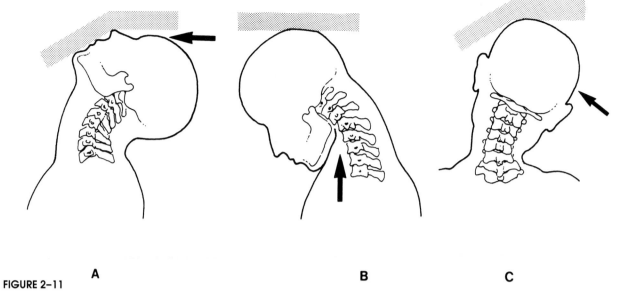

A   **B**   **C**

FIGURE 2-11

Differing mechanisms of cervical spine injuries. *A*, Extension; *B*, flexion-compression; and *C*, lateral bend. (Adapted from Viano DC: Causes and control of spinal cord injury in automobile crashes. World J Surg 16:410–419, 1992.)

vations, the incidence of many of these injuries has been reduced, if not eliminated. For example, traffic fracture of the elbow occurred when the arm that was resting on the open window frame was struck by oncoming traffic. The presence of rounded side panels that serve to distance the upper door frame from oncoming traffic has made these fractures considerably less common.

Head and Neck Injuries

There is little question of the significance of head and neck injuries in children. More than 63% of the mortality in infants and children up to 4 years of age and 73% of that in children 4 to 15 is due to neurotrauma.[62] In the series by Simpson and colleagues, none of these children was properly restrained. Injuries to the cervical spine occur with an incidence that is 1% of brain injuries, but the case-fatality rate is nearly 10 times higher, 57% for cervical spine injuries compared with 7% for head injuries.[33]

Head injuries occur through the application of both contact and inertial forces. Contact occurs with an interior structure, usually the steering wheel (42%) in adults, but impact may occur with any structure. Surprisingly, the windshield is struck directly only 7% of the time.[73] This contact depresses the cranium and can lead to direct contact injury to the brain.

Clinically significant head injuries may or may not be associated with skull fractures, and in one study as few as 30% of head injuries had associated fractures.[32] Direct contact does not need to occur for there to be significant, even fatal, head injury. Inertial injuries occur as a result of the angular and rotational forces incurred during a collision, as the brain can move in relationship to fixed structures.[59]

A subdural hematoma is an example of a displacement injury from inertial forces. The brain moves in relation to the surrounding dura, shearing the bridging veins that con-

nect to the draining sinus. These are always a result of serious trauma and rarely occur in association with retinal hemorrhages even in automobile and pedestrian injuries.[17] Epidural hematomas occur as a result of contact injuries.

Cervical spine injuries occur with a variety of mechanisms (Fig. 2–11). Flexion-compression injuries are the most common, comprising nearly two thirds of cervical spine injuries in this age group. Force is applied abruptly to the occipital area, which leads to acute flexion of the neck. This is particularly common in older children and adults, and injuries to C5–C7 are common.[69]

Thirty percent of cervical spine injuries in motor vehicle accidents are the extension type. These are more common in children as the frontal bones or maxilla strikes an object, leading to direct extension injuries. These are similar to the classic hangman's fracture and occur higher on the cervical spine.[69] This mechanism may also lead to atlanto-occipital disruption, which is 250 times more common in children than in adults.[42]

In addition, lateral collisions may lead to a lateral flexion, and this mechanism accounts for approximately 10% of cervical spine injuries, which generally occur at the C4–C5 level. This often results in further disruption of the tentorial membranes.[42]

Torso Injuries

Blunt injuries to the abdomen and chest (the torso) have more similarities than differences. Generally, direct force applied to the torso and overlying structures is not disruptive, as compliance allows compression, resulting in the force being transmitted to the internal structures.

Compliance is obviously higher in the abdomen, as the abdominal musculature is easily compressed. The bulk of internal organs are viscous, allowing displacement to avoid injury. However, intestinal or gastric rupture is possible and generally occurs with few reliable symptoms except the presence of abdominal tenderness (if the patient is conscious) and the absence of bowel sounds.[11] Traumatic diaphragmatic hernia is another possibility and has been reported as late as 3 years after a motor vehicle accident, almost always on the left and almost always after vehicle-related accidents.[1]

The most common internal abdominal injuries, however, are to the encapsulated organs, particularly the liver and spleen (Fig. 2–12). These injuries are addressed in another chapter (see Chapter 20), but it is important to realize that two- and three-point restraints may actually exacerbate abdominal injuries, both in incidence and severity.[5] This is particularly true for improperly restrained children ages 4 to 9 who may not have enough pelvic development to allow firm anchoring of the iliac crests.[3]

The chest is somewhat protected by the rib cage, but this protection is limited because the rib cage is so compliant, particularly in younger children. If deformation of the chest cage occurs, the deformation itself may relay impact forces to the heart and lungs; if the force exceeds the resilience of the ribs, a fracture may occur. In this instance, the impact force to the underlying structures may increase acutely and a direct injury may occur because of a protruding rib.

Viano studied the relationship between the application of force and internal chest damage and described the nature of the protection offered by the rib cage.[69] For a compression injury to occur, both the amount of load, or percentage of chest compression, and the velocity of compression must be considered. This cross product of velocity and compression was termed the *viscous criteria* or VC. A chest cage may be able to tolerate a heavy crush load if the load is applied slowly enough. In contrast, the lightest load may cause extensive injury if applied with enough velocity. Au-

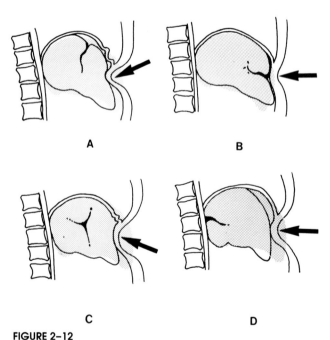

FIGURE 2–12

Examples of the influence of various forces in injuries to encapsulated abdominal organs such as the liver—as depicted here—or the spleen.

tomobiles are damaged by hail because the velocity is so high. Velocity of deformation, load, contact surface area, and compliance are all determinants of injury.

THE EFFECT OF SAFETY SYSTEMS

When we think of automobile safety, we generally think of seat belts, car seats, and airbags. But automobile safety design is an extensive, comprehensive field, and the majority of safety specifications and features remain largely unseen.

The addition of antiburst latches led to a 5% decrease in the number of fatalities.[39] Door latches are now incorporated into the door itself, eliminating a sharp surface as a potential point for a penetrating injury. Knee rests are often sloped and padded to decrease the likelihood of lower extremity injury as the knees are deflected. Steering wheels are collapsible, increasing the stopping distance to the chest. Head rests decrease the incidence of whiplash spinal injuries.

Seat Belts

The impact of seat belts is controversial because seat belts require the cooperation of the occupant. Current use is estimated by the National Highway Safety Administration to be approximately 51%–55% if use is mandatory and 35% if it is not. This estimate is up from an estimated 11% use in 1980.[49] It is estimated that 20 to 25% of drivers with operator-independent belts, that is, automated electric seat belt devices attached to the door, disconnected them. However, there is no question that seat belts are effective. Three-point restraints can decrease the fatality rate of accidents by 40 to 50% and severity of injury by 55 to 60%.[4, 12, 29, 44]

Restraints are designed to minimize contact with the interior. Once deceleration occurs, the restraint system is loaded with the force incurred by the occupant and kinetic energy is dissipated by the restraint system, reducing the velocity of impact with the interior and dampening the forces to tolerable levels.

A two-point system restrains the hips across the iliac crests. Because this type of restraint can actually cause abdominal injury through a jackknife mechanism as well as increase the hinge effect at the hip, these seat belts have been replaced almost universally by a three-point or lap-shoulder belt.

Ideally, the lap belt should fit snugly over the iliac crests, but such a fit is difficult in young children. If the lap belt is too low or too loose, it does not act as a restraint but rather acts as an additional point of impact. If it rides high over the abdomen, then a child can ''submarine'' under the restraint, and direct abdominal injury occurs. The lap belt must also be in the proper place. If it rides too low, it creates a hinge point and increases the risk of hyperflexion injury of the spine (Fig. 2–13). If the shoulder belt is too high, there is a risk for a direct contact injury to the larynx, neck, and face. Booster seats should be employed for children who do not fit the seat belt correctly, as seat belts may

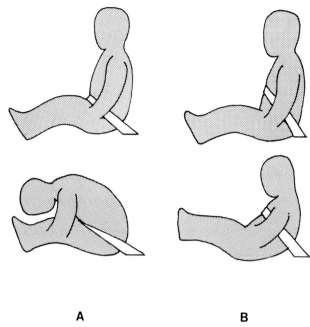

A   **B**

FIGURE 2–13

Mechanisms of injury in improperly restrained children. In *A*, the lap belt is properly applied but the high center of gravity leads to a forced and uncontrolled flexion, a jackknife-like effect, during collision. In *B*, the seat belt rides up over the abdomen, increasing the risk potential for injury, particularly intra-abdominal injury, in smaller children who may be involved in an accident.

not fit snugly across the iliac crests until a child reaches 10 years old.[25]

Car Seats

Car seats, although initially designed for aesthetics and convenience, have become the single greatest automobile safety innovation for children. When used properly with a five-point restraint system and with the child buckled in well, fatality becomes 11 times less likely.[58] The car seat provides excellent torso restraint, as each extremity and the pelvis have their own restraining points. However, cervical spine protection is entirely passive; hence, infants should be placed facing the rear of the car so that rapid deceleration would force the head against the back of the car seat rather than risking hyperflexion. This arrangement is particularly important considering the laxity of the paracervical muscles in the young infant and the relatively large percentage of surface area the head occupies compared with that of the body.

In addition, the seat restraint itself is critical. If the child is properly restrained but the car seat is not, the child may actually be at increased risk of injury because the additional weight of the car seat increases momentum. In a collision or a rapid deceleration event, the child and the car seat would be accelerated as a single unit, possibly striking the interior with an increased force or being ejected as a ''whole'' entity.

Airbags

Airbags are a passive safety system that require no operator intervention yet are controversial because of the additional cost involved. Most other design changes incorporate safety into an otherwise functional system, such as collapsible steering wheels. The steering wheel is obviously a required element; to make it collapsible is simply an alteration to increase safety, one of which the consumer may be unaware. However, airbags add a significant expense, from $220 to $320 per automobile.

Airbags have been shown to reduce mortality by 18% in isolation and by as much as 71% in conjunction with three-point restraints. When the automobile undergoes sudden deceleration or collision, sodium azide is rapidly converted to nitrogen gas, inflating the airbag at roughly 100 miles per hour. Once inflated, the airbag acts as an extremely compliant barrier, increasing stopping distance, preventing impact with a rigid or sharp surface, and providing cushion by distributing the area of impact among a maximal surface area.

Safety is an all-encompassing endeavor. No safety system can eliminate injury or mortality entirely. To maximize progress in motor vehicle safety, a broad-ranged program is necessary, and safety begins before a driver enters the car. Education, attitudes, vehicle design, environmental modification, and emergency system response all combine to characterize the overall safety of our roads.[27]

THE PHYSICIAN'S RESPONSIBILITY

Clearly the prevention of motor vehicle accidents will entail the mobilization of resources in every aspect of our society. From legislation and government intervention to community education to physician involvement, a comprehensive approach to prevention must be undertaken at all levels in an integrated fashion to reduce this public health risk.

Equally clearly, legislation is not enough. Designed to serve as a framework on which to build a policy geared toward changing society-wide behaviors, legislation requires that the law be explained, advertised, and, most important, enforced to be effective. Although all 50 states have child restraint laws, only 10 of these are primary restraint laws, meaning that failure to comply is a violation in and of itself. In other states, violation is an adjunct to other violations.[49] In many cases, proof of ownership of a car seat is all that is required to have citations dismissed.

Law enforcement officials operate at a disadvantage in the fight against driving under the influence of alcohol. In one study, only four arrests were made among 60 injured drunk drivers treated in an emergency department, and none of them was convicted. Accessibility to the patient, cumbersome rules of evidence, conflicts of confidentiality, and officer reluctance were all cited as contributing factors.[19]

For legislation to be effective in behavioral modification on a society-wide basis, negative reinforcement must be consistent and predictable. We must provide support for the police and help advertise both the laws and the purposes behind them.

In essence, however, we are trying to establish new habits and new concepts of socially acceptable behavior, according to Robert Foss, a sociologist at West Virginia University.[21] Like brushing your teeth, quitting smoking, or performing a breast self-examination, a repetitive behavior that is often initially unpleasant and without obvious immediate gain is being constructed. To achieve these changes, we must change the emphasis from compliance because of the consequences of legislation to compliance because these are expected cultural behaviors. Placing a child in a car seat should be "what you do" when you drive with a child. It is part of responsible, effective parenting.

Making such changes is easier said than done. As Foss points out, it is not a coincidence that as a child becomes more assertive and independent, the use of restraints decreases.[21] Parents must be taught that it is their "duty to prevail." Parents must be guided to understand that although it is true that the risk of an accident is minuscule on any given trip, the automobile remains the single biggest threat to their child's life and that their child is at least twice as likely to die without restraint as with it.

Few parents today were forced to use restraints as children. It is a concept that may be foreign to them and will be a learned behavior for them as well. It does little good to attempt to restrain a child if parents do not restrain themselves. A survey in Tennessee showed that if the adults were unrestrained, 42% of the children were unrestrained, but if the adults were restrained, only 9% of the children were unrestrained.[13]

Also, previously appropriate behaviors must be redefined. Many adults were allowed to roam around inside the car as children. As teenagers, they "piled in" as a social ritual. "Let's take my car. We can all fit" was a battle cry for a generation of drivers. The inherent risks in these behaviors are obvious in 1992.

Still, myths pervade our culture, many of which are based on rationalizations. Dr. Foss points out several that influence how children's safety is perceived: "Children tightly held are well protected"; "it's better to be ejected"; "risk increases on long trips"; "seat belts cause injury"; "restraint is inherently cruel"; to name a few. It is the physician's duty to explore these misperceptions and to provide parent education.

At our medical center, parents must bring a certified car seat (or a loaner is provided), watch a safety film, and display proper use of the car seat with the child before a newborn is discharged. Health care workers are encouraged to review child vehicle safety as part of every well child visit. In this way we attempt to provide repeated, positive reinforcement to parents.

References

1. Adeyemi SD, Stephens CA: Traumatic diaphragmatic hernia in children. Can J Surg 24:355–357, 1981.
2. Agran PF: Injuries to children: The relationship of child development to prevention strategies. Public Health Rep 102:609–610, 1987.
3. Agran PF, Dunkle DE, Winn DG: Injuries to a sample of seatbelted children evaluated and treated in a hospital emergency room. J Trauma 27:58–64, 1987.
4. Agran RA, Dunkle DE: Motor vehicle occupant injuries to children in crash and noncrash events. Pediatrics 70:993–996, 1982.
5. Arajarvi E, Santavira S, Tolonen J: Abdominal injuries sustained in severe traffic accidents by seatbelt wearers. J Trauma 27:393–397, 1987.
6. Baker SP, Robertson LS, O'Neill B: Fatal pedestrian collisions, driver negligence. Am J Public Health 64:318–325, 1974.
7. Brook CG: Growth Assessment in Childhood and Adolescence. Boston, Blackwell Scientific, 1982.
8. Burdi AR, Hueller DR, Snyder RG, et al: Infants and children in the adult world of automobile safety design: Pediatric and anatomical considerations of design of child restraints. Biomechanics 2:267, 1969.
9. Campbell BJ: Reducing traffic injury: Size of the problem and lack of research resources. World J Surgery 16:384–388, 1992.
10. Centers for Disease Control: Bicycle-related injuries: Data from the National Electronic Injury Surveillance System. MMWR 36:269–271, 1987.
11. Cobb LM, Vinocur CD, Wagner CW, et al: Intestinal perforation due to blunt trauma in children in an era of increased non-operative treatment. J Trauma 26:461–463, 1986.
12. Daffner RH, Deeb ZL, Lupetin AR, et al: Patterns of high-speed impact injuries in motor vehicle occupants. J Trauma 28(4):498–501, 1988.
13. Decker MD, Dewey MJ, Hutchenson RH, et al: The use and efficacy of child restraint devices. The Tennessee experience, 1982 and 1983. JAMA 252:2571–2575, 1984.
14. Demetra JD, Lee DN, Pitcairn TK, et al: Errors in young children's decisions about traffic gaps: Experiments with roadside situations. Br J Psychol 83:189–202, 1992.
15. DiGuiseppi CG, Rivara FP, Koepsell TD: Attitudes toward bicycle helmet ownership and use by school-age children. Am J Dis Child 144:83–86, 1990.
16. Dorsch MM, Woodard AJ, Somers RL: Do bicycle safety helmets reduce severity of head injury in real crashes? Accid Anal Prev 19:183, 1987.
17. Duhaime AC, Alario AJ, Lewander WJ: Head injury in very young children: Mechanisms, injury types, and ophthalmologic findings in 100 hospitalized patients younger than 2 years of age. Pediatrics 190:179–185, 1992.
18. Dunn RG, Asher KN, Rivera FP: Behavior and Child Expectations of Child Pedestrians. Pediatrics 89(3):486, 1992.
19. Fantus RJ, Zautcke JL, Hickey PA, et al: Driving under the influence—A level I trauma center's experience. J Trauma 31:1517–1520, 1991.
20. Fife D, David J, Tate L, et al: Fatal injuries to bicyclists: The experience of Dade County, Florida. J Trauma 23:745–755, 1983.
21. Foss RD: Sociocultural perspective on child occupant protection. Pediatrics 80:886–892, 1987.
22. Friede AM, Azzara CV, Gallager SS, et al: The epidemiology of injuries to bicycle riders. Pediatr Clin North Am 32:141–151, 1985.
23. Goldsmith MF: Campaigns focus on helmets as safety experts warn bicycle riders to use—and preserve—heads. JAMA 268:308–309, 1992.
24. Guichon DM, Myles ST: Bicycle injuries: One-year sample in Calgary. J Trauma 15:504–506, 1975.
25. Gunby P: Lap seat belts useful but can injure children. JAMA 245:2281–2282, 1981.
26. Guyer B, Talbot AM, Pless IB: Pedestrian injuries to children and youth. Pediatr Clin North Am 32:163–174, 1985.
27. Haddon W: Energy damage and the ten countermeasure strategies. J Trauma 13:321–326, 1973.
28. Hellerstein S: Fluid and electrolyte colon physiology. Pediatr Rev 14(2):70–79, 1993.
29. Hingsen R, Levenson SM, Heeren T, et al: Repeal of the Massachusetts seatbelt laws. Am J Public Health 78:548–552, 1988.
30. Hoffman ER, Payne A, Prescott A: Children's estimates of vehicle approach times. Hum Factors 22:235, 1980.
31. Illingworth CM, Noble D, Bell D, et al: 150 bicycle injuries in children: A comparison with accidents due to other causes. Injury 13:7–9, 1981.
32. Ivan LP, Choo SH, Ventureyra EC: Head injuries in childhood: A 2 year survey. Can Med Assoc J 128:281–284, 1983.
33. Jaffe D, Wesson D: Emergency management of blunt trauma in children. N Engl J Med 324:1477–1482, 1991.
34. Koop CE: Strategy for saving young lives. Washington, DC, US Public Health Service, 1989.

35. Kraus JF, Fife D, Conroy C: Incidence, severity, and outcomes of brain injuries involving bicycles. Am J Public Health 77:76–78, 1987.
36. Kulowski J: Crash Injuries. Springfield, Ill, Charles C Thomas, 1960.
37. Ljungblum BA, Koiter L: Child development and behavior in traffic. In: Marciaux M, Ramaer CJ: (eds): Accidents in Childhood and Adolescence—The Role of Research. Washington, DC, World Health Organization, 1991.
38. McDermott FT: Helmet efficacy in the prevention of bicycle head injuries: Royal Australasian College of Surgeons initiatives in the introduction of compulsory safety helmet wearing in Victoria, Australia. World J Surgery 16:379–383, 1992.
39. MacKay M: Mechanisms of injury and biomechanics: Vehicle design and crash performance. World J Surg 16:420–427, 1992.
40. Manheimer DI, Mellinger GD: Personality characteristics of the child accident repeater. Child Dev 38:491–513, 1967.
41. Marwick C: Traffic death toll may be declining, but experts not ready to celebrate. JAMA 268:301, 1992.
42. Maves DK, Souza A, Prenger EC, et al: Traumatic atlanto-occipital disruption in children. Pediatr Radiol 21:504–507, 1991.
43. Morbidity & Mortality Weekly Report: Trends in alcohol-related traffic fatalities, by sex. MMWR 41(11):189, 1992.
44. Mucci SJ, Eriksen LD, Crist KA, et al: The pattern of injury to rear seat passengers involved in automobile collisions. J Trauma 31:1329–1331, 1991.
45. Nakayama DK, Pasleka KB, Garder MJ: How bicycle-related injuries change bicycling practices in children. Am J Dis Child 144:928–929, 1990.
46. National Center for Health Statistics: Physical growth curves in boys and girls, birth to 36 months of age. Detroit, Ross Laboratories, 1982.
47. National Highway Traffic Safety Administration Fatal Accident Reporting System, Washington, DC, 1990.
48. National Highway Traffic Safety Administration Office of Driver and Pedestrian Research: Occupant Protection Trends in 198 Cities. Washington, DC, November 1991.
49. National Safety Council: Accident Facts. Washington, DC, 1992 Edition.
50. Peclet MH, Newman KD, Eichelberger MR, et al: Patterns of injury in children. J Pediatr Surg 25:85–91, 1990.
51. Perrone N: Biomechanical and structural aspects of design for vehicle impact. Itasca, Ill, Human Body Dynamics.
52. Peterson TD, Royer K: Motor vehicle crash injury: Mechanisms and prevention. Am Fam Physician 44:1307–1312, 1991.
53. Randall T: Driving while under the influence of alcohol. JAMA 268(3):303–305, 1992.
54. Raundalin TS: Every Day Life of Children. Stockholm, Awe/Gebers, 1979.
55. Rice DP, MacKenzie EJ: Cost of injury in the U.S.: A report to congress, 1989. Baltimore, Injury Prevention Center, John Hopkins University, 1989.
56. Rivera FP: Traumatic deaths of children in the United States: Currently available prevention strategies. Pediatrics 75:456–462, 1985.
57. Rivera FP, Barber M: Demographic analysis of childhood pedestrian injuries. Pediatrics 76:375–381, 1985.
58. Roux P, Fisher RM: Chest injuries in children: An analysis of 100 cases of blunt chest trauma from motor vehicle accidents. J Pediatr Surg 27:551–555, 1992.
59. Ryan GA: Improving head protection for cyclists, motorcyclists, and car occupants. World J Surg 16:398–402, 1992.
60. Sandels S: Children in Traffic. London, Elek Press, 1976.
61. Scherz RG: Fatal motor vehicle accidents for child passengers for birth to four years of age in Washington State. Pediatrics 68:572, 1981.
62. Simpson DA, Blumbergs PC, McLean AJ, et al: Head injuries in infants and children: Measures to reduce mortality and morbidity in road accidents. World J Surg 16:403–409, 1992.
63. Sinclair D: Human Growth after Birth. 4th ed. New York, Oxford University Press, 1985.
64. Spaite DW, Murphy M, Criss EA, et al: A prospective analysis of injury severity among helmeted and nonhelmeted bicyclists involved in collisions with motor vehicles. J Trauma 31:1510–1516, 1991.
65. Stevenson MR, Lo SK, Laing BA, et al: Childhood pedestrian injuries in the Perth metropolitan area. Med J Aust 156:234–238, 1992.
66. Still A, Roberts I, Koelmeyer T, et al: Child passenger fatalities and restraints use in Auckland. N Z Med J 105(945):449, 1992.
67. Tanner JM: Physical Growth from Conception to Maturity. Cambridge, Harvard University Press, 1990.
68. Tanz RR, Christoffel KK: Pedestrian injury, the next motor vehicle injury challenge. Am J Dis Child 139:1187–1190, 1985.
69. Viano DC: Causes and control of spinal cord injury in automobile crashes. World J Surg 16:410–419, 1992.
70. Vulcan AP, Mech E, Cameron MH, et al: Mandatory bicycle helmet use: Experience in Victoria, Australia. World J Surg 16:389–397, 1992.
71. Weiss BD: Bicycle helmet use by children. Pediatrics 77:677–679, 1986.
72. Wolfe AC, O'Day J: Pedestrian accidents in the U.S. Health Services Research Institute Res Rev 12:1–16, 1982.
73. Worrall SF: Mechanisms, pattern, and treatment costs of maxillofacial injuries. Injury 22(I):25–28, 1991.

William D. Hardin, Jr.
William D. King

CHAPTER THREE

Injury Prevention and Control in the United States

More children under the age of 15 years die in the United States each year from injury than from all other causes of death combined.[39] The emergence of injury as the leading cause of death in the young is due to a variety of factors. One major factor is the prevention of infectious disease–related death in children. Once a major cause of death in the pediatric population, infectious diseases have been largely brought under control owing to the success of vaccination programs and the widespread use of antibiotics. Prenatal diagnosis of congenital anomalies and modern therapeutic interventions have improved the prognosis of children born with birth defects and those born prematurely. In the past, many children who suffered from gastrointestinal disorders or chronic disease died of malnutrition. Parenteral hyperalimentation has largely overcome that problem. Consequently, over the last 20 years, mortality rates from disease in children have decreased by 56%.[3] During that same period, the rates of death from injury have fallen only 25%. Thus, injury is now the major cause of mortality in children. Rapid urban growth and the ubiquitous presence of the automobile have placed American youth in an increasingly vulnerable position.

From a public health perspective, injury must now be viewed as a national epidemic. More than 150,000 Americans are killed annually by accidents or injury, and another 80,000 sustain permanent disability.[47] One in eight acute care hospitalizations is due to traumatic injury, and the financial cost of all of this to society is estimated at $130 billion annually. Injury is responsible for more years of productive life lost than all other causes, in large measure because the injury problem is so acute in the young, being the leading cause of death in the first 4 decades of life.

C. Everett Koop, former Surgeon General of the United States, once remarked, ''If a disease were killing our children in the proportions accidents are, people would be outraged and demand that this killer be stopped.'' Only recently has coordinated, nationwide attention been focused on the problem. One of the major misconceptions shared by the public, health professionals, and government officials alike is that injuries are accidents. Webster's dictionary defines *accident* as ''an event occurring by chance or arising from unknown causes; an unfortunate event resulting from carelessness, unawareness, ignorance, or a combination of causes; an unexpected happening causing loss or injury which is not due to any fault or misconduct on the part of the person injured.'' In the field of injury prevention, the word *accident* is viewed with disdain, because injuries occur in predictable patterns and thus can be anticipated and prevented. Education, legislation, and community involvement are the antidotes to this epidemic.

CONCEPTS IN INJURY PREVENTION

The field of injury prevention and control is fraught with ambiguous terminology and incomplete data. A basic understanding of commonly used terms and concepts is needed.[51] The classification of injuries as accidents arises from the fact that most such injuries are unintentional. Examples of unintentional injuries include motor vehicle accidents, falls, burns, and drownings. Intentional injuries include homicides, suicides, and other forms of physical assault in which the action causing the injury involves a conscious decision and action on the part of an individual. In the case of homicides and assaults, these actions carry legal implications, because the action is carried out by one party and produces injury to another. Although the concept appears clear, it is frequently difficult to establish intent. Was a self-inflicted gunshot wound unintentional, or was it a suicide attempt? Is asphyxiation in an infant a case of sudden infant death syndrome (SIDS) or an unrecognized homicide?

Another problem with terminology is the distinction between *abuse* and *neglect*. These terms are poorly understood by the lay public and health professionals alike. Abuse and neglect are both perpetrated on children by adults responsible for their care. Abuse may be physical or emotional. Sexual abuse is a form of physical abuse, which also carries a significant emotional or psychological component. Neglect involves a disregard for societal standards of conduct, either through lack of attention or failure to act. In contrast to abuse, assault is most often perpetrated by strangers, peers, or others not responsible for the victim. From a legal standpoint, assault may also be either physical or verbal. *Battery* is the legal term used to describe physical assault.

CHILDHOOD INJURIES—AN OVERVIEW OF THE PROBLEM

The problem of childhood injuries is complex, and the data required to effect change are incomplete. The best data set currently available on pediatric injuries is derived from death certificates. However, deaths are just the tip of the iceberg as a representation of the problem (Fig. 3–1). Quan-

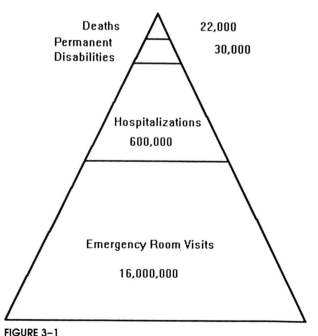

FIGURE 3–1

The injury pyramid in children 1 to 19 years of age.

tification of injuries, disability, and injury costs are estimates based on population sampling and methodologies that may or may not be valid. Death certificates also slant our perspective on the problem because many common injuries cause significant morbidity but do not usually result in death. Burns are a good example; they are among the most costly and devastating of pediatric injuries but result in relatively few deaths. Still, mortality statistics represent a reasonable place to begin in understanding the seriousness of the problem.

Mortality statistics are generally grouped into 5-year increments, which correspond to four general developmental stages: preschool (0–4 years), early school (5–9 years), pre- and early adolescence (10–14 years), and late adolescence (15–19 years). Differences in injury rates and causes of death in these groups make this convention useful in planning and implementing targeted prevention strategies.[27] Overall, 52% of deaths in children 1 to 14 years of age are injury related. In children 1 to 4 years of age, 40% of deaths are caused by injury, and in the group 5 to 19 years, the percentage is approximately 70%.[39] Each year in the United States, approximately 22,000 individuals aged 19 or younger die from injuries.

Another useful way to establish the severity of the problem is to compare death rates in American children with rates in children from other industrialized nations of the world.[21] Noninjury death rates in children are comparable in the United States and other Western countries. U.S. children, however, have the highest death rate from injury among Western nations (Fig. 3–2). The differences are predominantly the result of higher rates of unintentional injury and violence in American youth. The United States leads the Western world in the number of homicides among children, and suicide rates are among the highest. The differences noted are most pronounced in late adolescence and persist through adulthood in many categories.

Available statistics on the morbidity of injuries in children are equally devastating.[23] In 1986, estimates of the injury toll included 30,000 permanently disabled and more than 600,000 hospitalized.[39] Nearly one in five children in the United States requires medical attention for injuries

Table 3–1

Injury Causes of Death in Children 0–19 Years of Age, 1986

Injury Type	Number	% of Total
Motor vehicle	10,535	47.0
Occupant	7412	33.0
Pedestrian	1787	8.0
Other	1336	6.0
Homicide	2877	12.8
Suicide	2151	9.6
Drowning	2062	9.2
Fire and burns	1619	7.2
Other injuries	3157	14.1
TOTAL	22,401	100.0

Adapted from Childhood injuries in the United States. Am J Dis Child 144:627–647, 1990.

each year. The direct cost of medical care for these children approaches $7.5 billion annually, and when indirect costs are factored in, the cost approaches $15 billion.[39] The consequences of pediatric injury extend beyond these children to their parents and families and to society as a whole.

Review of mortality statistics is important in identifying high-risk populations that can be targeted for intervention strategies. Throughout the United States, males are consistently at higher risk for death than females in all injury categories with the exception of motor vehicle occupants.[44] Race has also been identified as a major risk factor, with minorities as much as five times more likely to die from selected injury causes.[39] Interpretation of these data is difficult, as there may be many disconcerting factors involved. With respect to race, it is likely that the socioeconomic status is more important than the racial category. Poor children of all races are at far greater risk of death from injury than more affluent children.

Comparisons of state mortality statistics are also useful in identifying regional or geographic variability in injury mortality risks.[4] Children in Alaska are at greatest risk, whereas children in Massachusetts are at lowest risk. The difference is approximately threefold. On a regional level, children in southern and mountain states are at higher risk, whereas children in the New England, mid-Atlantic, and midwestern states are at less risk. Regional and state variability also extends to the causes of death in children. The risk of death in house fires is greatest in the southeast, and motor vehicle occupant death rates are highest in the south and southwest.

In the United States, the automobile is responsible for more pediatric deaths than all other causes. In 1986, 47% of pediatric deaths were a result of motor vehicle–associated injury[39] (Table 3–1). Nearly 70% of these deaths were in vehicle occupants, with the majority occurring in the older adolescent age group. In younger children, pedestrian and bicycle injuries are the major cause of motor vehicle–related mortality. Approximately one in 12 injury deaths occurs to pediatric pedestrians struck by motor vehicles. The second and third leading causes of death in children in the United States are homicide and suicide. Drownings rank fourth, and burns and house fires rank fifth. Falls account for few deaths but are the leading cause of injury hospitalization and emergency department visits.

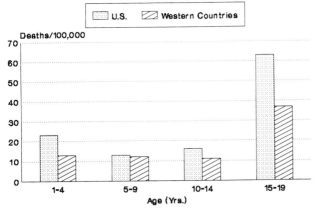

FIGURE 3–2

World pediatric death rates from injury and violence—1985. (Adapted from Trends and current status in childhood mortality. Vital Health Stat 3(26):1–44, 1989.)

Motor Vehicle Occupants

In 1986, 7412 children aged 1 to 19 years died as occupants in motor vehicle accidents.[1, 39] Nearly three fourths of these deaths occurred during late adolescence, with male death rates twice those for females. Children younger than 6 months of age are also at great risk, but there is little difference in death or injury rate by sex. It is estimated that approximately 1600 children younger than 15 years of age die annually in the United States as vehicle occupants.[51] Almost 200,000 children require emergency department care for injuries. Among injury categories, motor vehicle accidents rank third in both rates of emergency department care and hospitalization.

In addition to the automobile, other motorized vehicles present significant risks to children.[51] Nearly 1000 fatalities due to motorcycles are recorded yearly in persons younger than 20 years of age. Approximately 100 children younger than 15 are killed; about half of them are riding as passengers. Estimates on injury are 45,000 in those younger than 20 and 6500 in children younger than 15 years. Deaths are most commonly the result of head or spinal cord injury, whereas leg injuries are the most common nonfatal injury sustained. Many of these injuries, however, cause permanent disability. Mopeds, minibikes, and trailbikes are less of a threat than the more powerful motorcycle but still are the cause of almost 13,000 emergency department admissions each year.[26] Injury rates for these motorized bikes are four times that of the bicycle.

Snowmobiles, all-terrain vehicles, and farm machinery also represent serious threats to our youth.[45] Snowmobiles are associated with approximately 7000 emergency department visits each year, extremity injuries being the most common cause, with deaths primarily attributable to head injuries or drowning while riding over frozen lakes or ponds. All-terrain vehicles result in approximately 30,000 injuries annually. Many of these vehicles are inherently unstable, which led to the 1987 legislation banning three-wheel all-terrain vehicles. Many of these vehicles are unfortunately still in use, but the four-wheel variants also carry risks associated with instability, especially to users under 16 years of age. Farm machinery is the cause of about 70 deaths each year, 70% of which are tractor related.[49] Approximately 4000 injuries each year are due to such equipment, with one of the most severe and disabling injuries being traumatic amputation.[43] Infections from farm-related injuries are especially severe and difficult to treat.[6] Many are the result of anaerobic organisms that contaminate large wounds with devitalized tissue. Osteomyelitis is common. Treatment frequently requires prolonged hospitalization, administration of parenteral antibiotics, and multiple operative procedures for débridement. The highest risk of farm-related injury exists in states like Idaho, South Dakota, Wisconsin, Vermont, Iowa, and Minnesota.

Pedestrians and Motor Vehicles

Pedestrian injury is the leading cause of death in children 4 to 8 years of age, with 6 year olds at greatest risk.[46] Each year in the United States approximately 1100 deaths of children under the age of 15 are classified as traffic-related pedestrian deaths. Another 200 children are killed in non-traffic pedestrian accidents in driveways, parking lots, or off-road areas. Traffic-related pedestrian deaths are the leading cause of injury death among children 5 to 9 years of age, and the rates are highest in urban and low-income areas.[40] Non-traffic–related pedestrian deaths are more common in rural areas. Boys are twice as likely to be injured as girls. Estimates place emergency department visits at almost 80,000 annually for pedestrian injuries. The peak hours for pedestrian injury are the after-school hours of 3:00 PM to 7:00 PM with the hour just past sunset the most vulnerable period.

Children riding bicycles are also at significant risk of injury and death. About 400 children are killed each year, and more than 380,000 require emergency department treatment because of such injuries. More than 90% of children killed are struck by motor vehicles, and boys are four times more likely to be killed than girls. Approximately 80% of the deaths and 70% of the hospitalizations are the result of head injury. In contrast to fatalities, serious, nonfatal injuries are more commonly the result of a fall or an impact with a stationary object.

Homicide

Homicides are the leading cause of injury death in children younger than 1 year of age and the second leading cause next to motor vehicles in all persons younger than 20 years of age.[39] In 1986, 2877 deaths in children 0 to 19 years of age were classified as homicides. The total may underrepresent the problem, because many cases of homicide in the pediatric population may go unrecognized.[19, 34] A review of mortality statistics over the last 4 decades indicates that homicide is the only cause of death in children that has risen in rate over the years since World War II. U.S. children are at higher risk than children in other industrialized nations in the West.[11] Between 1968 and 1985, there was a 44% increase in years of productive life lost as a result of homicides among children.[7]

Review of the data by age group indicates two predominant patterns of homicide: infantile and adolescent.[8] Homicide rates are high in children younger than 3 years of age and in adolescents aged 15 to 19.[33] Overall, 64% of homicides occur in the latter group, although 23% occur in children younger than 5 years of age. Two thirds of the victims are male, and nearly half are black. Rates are five times greater in blacks than in whites, and male-to-female ratios are 2:1 in whites and 3:1 in blacks.[39]

The mechanism of injury in homicides also varies by age. In children younger than 5 years, most homicides are the result of physical assault by an adult; less than 10% are caused by firearms. In the older at-risk cohort, firearms are the predominant cause of death, more than 70% of the deaths among 15 to 19 year olds being caused by firearms. Overall, firearms are involved in half of all homicides in males and one third in females.[9]

Suicide

Suicide is the third leading injury-related cause of death in persons 0 to 19 years of age, accounting for 2151 deaths in

1986.[39] Suicide is rare in children under the age of 10, but suicide rates in the 10- to 19-year-old age group have nearly doubled in the last 30 years.[30] In the adult population during the same period suicide rates have fallen. Unlike rates for other causes of death from injury, suicide rates are highest in whites, approximately twice that for nonwhites. Although males account for approximately 80% of all suicide deaths, females attempt suicide approximately three times more often than males.

Firearms are the proximate cause of death in half of all suicides in children 10 to 14 years of age and in 60% in the 15- to 19-year-old age group. Much of the increase in suicide rates over the last 2 decades is attributable to the use of firearms among females in the 15- to 19-year-old category. Hanging is the method of choice in a third of all suicides in 10 to 14 year olds and in 20% of the older group. Poisoning was the method of choice in 12% of cases in each age group.

Assault and Abuse

Assault and abuse are categories in which data are incomplete and are based on estimates. It is difficult to identify intent accurately, and evidence suggests that many cases of abuse go unreported. An estimated 1.6 million children are abused or neglected each year.[37] Approximately 60% of these cases involve physical abuse, and a large percentage involve sexual abuse, predominantly in girls. For every fatal assault identified an estimated 100 cases of nonfatal assault occur.[41]

Risk factors for the physical abuse of children include young age at maternity, unwanted pregnancy, living in foster care, poverty, and parental history of childhood abuse.[10] Risk factors for sexual abuse include female gender, age 6 to 7 years or 10 to 12 years, parental neglect or discord, and harsh or punitive home environment.[22] Children living in inner city urban settings or environments in which delinquent behavior is common are more susceptible to both physical and sexual abuse.

Drowning

Drownings are the fourth leading injury cause of death and rank second among unintentional injuries.[33] In 1986, drownings accounted for 2062 (9.2%) of pediatric injury deaths. In California, Arizona, and Florida, drowning is the leading cause of death in children younger than 5 years of age.[52] Rates of drowning death are particularly high in the Pacific and gulf coast states. The vast majority of drownings, even in coastal states, occur in fresh water. Nonfatal immersion injuries carry a high morbidity toll, because victims frequently suffer permanent neurologic sequelae. In 1986, estimates of years of productive life lost from drowning were placed at 118,341 years. Drowning deaths occur in a bimodal distribution, with children younger than 5 years representing one peak and children 15 to 19 years the second peak, the highest risk being in children 1 to 3 years of age.

Males are particularly vulnerable to death from drowning

and account for 78% of all drowning deaths and 86% of deaths in those older than 5 years of age. Blacks carry a twofold greater risk of drowning in all age groups except in those 1 to 3 years of age, in which whites are twice as likely to drown. Part of the reason for this disparity may be the association of residential pools with an increased socioeconomic level, creating a higher level of exposure among affluent whites. Children with seizure disorders are at increased risk, and in the adolescent and adult age groups, alcohol is involved in 40 to 50% of drownings.[16]

In children younger than 5 years, 60 to 90% of drownings occur in residential pools. In half of these cases, the children are at home, whereas a third occur at a friend's, relative's, or neighbor's home.[53] In 80% of cases the children are playing in the vicinity of the pool, and most are being supervised, with attention being diverted for only a moment. Immersion times are usually under 5 minutes, although in 60% of cases the initiation of cardiopulmonary resuscitation (CPR) is delayed pending the arrival of the paramedic or emergency medical technician.[42] The morbidity associated with drownings and near drownings is significant. Twenty-five percent of cases require hospitalization, and 15% of those hospitalized die.[48] A study of near-drowning patients admitted to the Children's Hospital of Los Angeles showed that 50% died who required CPR at the initial hospital, 26% survived with permanent neurologic sequelae, and 24% survived neurologically intact.[2] The costs associated with caring for those patients who survive in a permanent vegetative state may exceed $90,000 to $100,000 per year.

Burns and House Fires

Fires and burns are the fifth leading cause of death from injury in children.[39] In 1986, 1619 children were killed from burn and fire-related injuries. It is estimated that more than 23,000 children required hospitalization and more than 440,000 required treatment for burn injuries.[36] In terms of cost, more than 100,000 years of productive life are lost, and the financial cost approaches $3.5 billion annually.

Most deaths from fire are the result of smoke inhalation. Byproducts of combustion include carbon monoxide, cyanide, and hydrogen sulfide. These and the hypoxia that results from combustion are the principal mechanisms by which smoke inhalation produces death. In 1979, 84% of children who died from fire or burns were killed in house fires.[5] Thermal or scald burns are the principal mechanism of burn injury in the infant age group. Other mechanisms of burn injury include electrical, chemical, or radiation exposure.

Accurate data on burns are difficult to obtain, and mortality statistics portray only a part of the problem. The treatment of seriously burned infants and children in burn centers involves lengthy hospitalization, chronic pain, multiple reconstructive procedures, and a lifetime of disfigurement. Unfortunately, the youngest members of our society bear a disproportionate share of these injuries. The Consumer Product Safety Commission conducted an analysis of costs associated with burn wound care and estimated the cost for each hospitalized patient at $40,000 to $70,000;

costs for those treated as outpatients ranged from $2300 to $6800.[31] The most severely burned children are not reflected in these numbers.

All of the statistics available document the prevalence of burn injuries in the youngest children.[17, 39] Infants and toddlers, those younger than 5 years of age, are at greatest risk. Most burns are sustained at home. Scald burns occur in the kitchen or bathroom and, like drownings, may occur with just seconds of inattention. Toddlers are susceptible to electrical burns from chewing on lamp cords and caustic burns from the ingestion of drain cleaners.[50] Preschoolers experimenting with matches or playing around stoves are susceptible to clothing burns, whereas preadolescents and adolescent males are more likely to be burned as a result of the explosion of gasoline or other combustible materials.[12] Electrical burns are seen in the older age group and are often associated with climbing in proximity to high voltage lines.[35] Of note, it is estimated that 5% of burn admissions are the result of child abuse, with most cases clustered in the youngest age group.

PROBLEM ANALYSIS AND SOLUTIONS

The morbidity and mortality of pediatric injuries demand an aggressive approach to both analysis of the problem and appropriate intervention. There are no simple solutions, and significant change requires the persistent efforts of many. One simplistic view is that injuries in children can be reduced if parents take a more active responsibility for their children. The fact is that parents can only do so much. Constant vigilance is an unrealistic expectation of parents and caregivers of children. Safe environments must be provided for children to minimize the risk of injury when supervision fails. The protection of children must be viewed as a community responsibility. Teachers, daycare workers, and babysitters share in the responsibility of supervising children. Police, fire, and emergency personnel have direct responsibility for public safety. The legal system, represented by judges, lawyers, and legislators, plays a vital role in supporting the development and passage of safety legislation; the health care system is responsible for meeting the acute and long-term medical needs of injured patients. The medical needs of the injured begin at the time of injury and end only at the time of death or at the time the child is reintegrated successfully into the home environment. The problem is a societal one, and solutions must be devised that focus on the prevention, treatment, and rehabilitation of injured children.

Data Collection

Central to the effort to control injuries in America is the need for accurate and comprehensive data on which to base resource allocation. Identifying the most serious problems allows targeting of intervention strategies in an attempt to produce the most change. Reliable data are also needed to assess the efficacy of intervention strategies. The issue of data collection is complex. Many sources of injury data are available, but none provides all of the data needs.

One of the most comprehensive data sets available is mortality data, which is derived from death certificates and collected by state and local offices of vital statistics. These data are compiled annually and usually released within a year or two. Most of the data are computerized. The National Center for Health Statistics collects these data and compiles a national summary, which is usually 3 to 4 years old by the time it is available. Death certificates portray mortality data well in demographic terms—age, race, sex, geographic location, and time—but are limited in describing details of injury causation.

A better picture of causation can be gained through a review of individual reports by state or county medical examiners who are charged with the responsibility of investigating sudden, accidental, and violent deaths. These data are usually in narrative form. Rarely are the data available on computers, and tabulation can be a very labor-intensive project. The quality of data is suspect, so it is difficult to compare data collected from different regions using these reports.

Morbidity data are considerably more difficult to come by and in most instances represent only a sampling of the problem. Among the sources used to gain a better understanding of pediatric injuries are trauma registries, analyses of hospital discharge data, small population studies, and focused or sentinel injury databases. Each source adds to an understanding of the problem, but each also suffers from inherent biases. The National Pediatric Trauma Registry was established in 1985 and serves as a central clearinghouse for data submitted voluntarily by contributing member institutions. Compliance is variable, and the data represent the more serious injuries seen by member institutions. The data collected provide a comprehensive picture of the more severe pediatric trauma patients and the correlation between optimal care and outcome.

Hospital discharge data represent a rich source of information to determine which injuries required hospitalization. The demographic data are accurate, and the extent of injuries sustained is well documented. The key link in making these data available is the incorporation of E-coding by the hospital medical records department. E-codes are part of the International Classification of Disease (ICD) coding system and represent the external causes of injury.[32] Hospitals do prepare summaries of discharge data and in some states are required to submit those summaries for compilation into Uniform Hospital Discharge Data Sets. Discharge data sets contain sociodemographic information, E-codes, charges, length of stay, and other vital data. Mandatory E-coding represents the quickest way of making this morbidity data available in the same fashion as mortality data. Reluctance to incorporate mandatory E-coding into hospital record keeping stems from the fact than E-codes are not required for hospital reimbursement.

The true impact of pediatric injuries cannot be established using hospitalization or mortality data alone. Many children with injuries are treated in emergency departments and released or treated in physicians' offices. Less severe injuries may go untreated or may be treated at home. To better understand these aspects of the problem, numerous studies have been performed. The Massachusetts Statewide Comprehensive Injury Prevention Program collected data on more than 87,000 children treated in 28 hospital emergency departments over a 3-year period.[23] The data collected highlighted the problems associated with this data source: data collection is very labor intensive and costly; the data lack specificity on injury causation; and patient confidentiality issues create administrative problems.

Focused or sentinel injury data sets can be alternatives in adding to the understanding of specific problems. The National Highway Traffic Safety Administration maintains two such focused databases, the Fatal Accident Reporting System and the National Accident Sampling System. Both provide comprehensive data on motor vehicle accidents. Poison control centers have also proved effective, both in collecting data on poisoning and in devising strategies to lower morbidity and mortality from ingestions. The introduction of childproof packaging in 1972 is an example of how a focused database can effectively lower the risk of pediatric injury.

The Science of Injury Prevention

Injury prevention is a process in evolution. It is no longer just a well-intentioned goal of a few committed individuals but has acquired the status of a legitimate scientific discipline with a national identity. In 1986, the National Committee on Injury Prevention and Control was formed. The committee was a collaborative group representing the National Highway Traffic Safety Administration, the Bureau of Maternal and Child Health, and the Centers for Disease Control and Prevention. The committee reviewed the state of injury prevention and prepared a summary entitled, *Injury Prevention—Meeting the Challenge.*[38] The work is a landmark in the field of injury prevention.

The history of injury prevention is a remarkable story with some notable milestones. In 1942 Hugh DeHaven published his paper on survival following falls from heights.[15] DeHaven himself was a survivor of an airplane crash and became interested in understanding crash survival. He studied patients who had survived falls of 50 to 150 feet and found that the key to survival was the way in which injury forces were distributed and disbursed at the time of impact. The implications were that vehicle design was an important component of crash survivability.

Another individual who made a major contribution in the field was Dr. John Gordon. In 1949, he pointed out the similarity between injuries and disease processes.[25] Like infectious diseases, injuries occur episodically, with seasonal variation, in susceptible patients grouped by age, sex, and race. The same techniques used to study diseases could therefore be applied to the study of injuries. Also like disease, injuries are the result of an interaction among three important variables: the host, the agent, and the environment.

This concept, which has come to be known as the *epidemiologic model of injury,* was expanded on by psychologist James Gibson and Dr. William Haddon. Gibson noted that "injuries to a living organism can be produced only by some *energy* interchange."[24] He recognized that injuries could be produced by different forms of energy (the "agent" of injury), including mechanical, thermal, chemi-

cal, and radiation energy. He suggested that classifying injuries on the basis of energy source was a more logical way of looking at the problem. Haddon extended the concept to include negative forms of energy, such as the lack of oxygen or heat.[29]

Haddon further extended the concepts first introduced by Gordon and Gibson when he developed the *Haddon matrix.* The matrix, illustrated in Figure 3–3, is a scheme for analyzing ways in which the host, the agent, and the environment interact over time to produce injury. Haddon used the matrix to evaluate both the causes of and the potential prevention strategies for avoiding motor vehicle accidents.[28] Each specific injury type can be analyzed using this process to identify ways in which injuries can be prevented or their morbidity and mortality minimized.

Interventional Strategy Types

Strategies designed for the primary prevention of injury can be classified into one of two categories: active intervention and passive intervention. Active intervention requires education, whereas passive intervention includes legislative or engineering changes that require no action by those to be protected. Educational strategies attempt to influence behavior by providing information. The assumption is that if people are made aware of ways to protect themselves, they will change their behavior. The problem with education as an interventional strategy is that it relies on each person to implement changes that will reduce the risk of injury. The obvious limitation to this strategy is that people do not often follow through each time a preventive action is required.

There are many examples of successful health education campaigns. The American Heart Association has educated the American public on the risks of cigarette smoking, high blood pressure, and cholesterol in the development of heart disease. The American public has responded to the message by quitting cigarette smoking and is far more conscious of high blood pressure and cholesterol than it used to be. Similarly, the public has been educated on the importance of exercise and has responded by becoming far more fitness conscious.

Education also plays a key role in facilitating legislative

Phases	Factors		
	Host	Agent	Environment
Pre-Event			
Event			
Post-Event			

FIGURE 3–3

Skeleton of the Haddon matrix.

and engineering interventions. Mandatory motorcycle helmet and seat belt usage laws are examples of legislative initiatives. Both were vigorously opposed by various groups, and passage occurred only because the public and, consequently, legislators were educated as to their importance in saving lives. Seat belts are an example of an intervention that requires a behavioral change and an active decision by the individual to use the device. Compliance has been influenced by laws that mandate use and punish noncompliance, but the laws are not universally enforced. Air bags represent an engineering intervention, and their use requires no active decision on the part of the individual. Air bags are an example of a passive intervention in which compliance is not an issue; provided they have been engineered correctly, their efficacy is assured.

No single intervention will accomplish the task of reducing morbidity and mortality from injury. Each of the strategy types must be incorporated into a comprehensive injury prevention strategy. Policymakers and the American public must be educated because awareness is the key to preventive action, including safety advocacy. Education requires knowledge that is derived from accurate data. The awareness of risk factors leads to targeting interventions toward specific problems. Legislation is needed to encourage safety-oriented behavior, and engineering changes are needed to provide a safe environment.

The Injury Prevention Program

The American Academy of Pediatrics (AAP) has been committed to reducing the risk of injury during childhood since 1951, when it first formalized its policy statements on the issue.[13] Since that time the AAP has been actively involved in its advocacy of injury prevention initiatives. It has lobbied for legislative changes at the national, state, and local levels. Efforts are coordinated at the national level by the Committee on Accident and Poison Prevention. State chapters of the AAP are also involved in the effort through state accident and poison prevention committees.

Early efforts of the AAP were directed toward the legislative process. Examples include lobbying for passage of the Flammable Fabrics Act of 1953, the Refrigerator Safety Act of 1956, and the Federal Hazardous Substances Act of 1960. Each of these acts was passed in response to tragic episodes that attracted national attention. The Flammable Fabrics Act attempted to address the issue of pediatric burns that occurred as a result of sleepwear catching on fire. The Refrigerator Safety Act followed a series of asphyxiations that occurred as a result of children playing in refrigerators that could not be opened from the inside. The Federal Hazardous Substances Act was initially passed as the Federal Hazardous Labeling Act and was designed to alert parents to potentially toxic substances. The legislation was largely ineffectual, although it did lead to the Child Protection Act of 1966 and to the Poison Prevention Packaging Act of 1972. The effects of these legislative initiatives included limiting the tablet content of baby aspirin containers and requiring child-resistant caps on medicines.

The AAP remains committed and has passed a policy statement that merits reproduction:

▶ **Policy Statement on Injury Prevention Approved by the Executive Board of the American Academy of Pediatrics:**

All children should grow up in a safe environment.
Anticipatory guidance for injury prevention should be an integral part of the medical care provided for all infants and children.
All physicians caring for children should advise parents to provide the following for their children's safety:

1. **Currently approved child car restraints.**
2. **Smoke detectors in the home that would protect the child's sleeping area.**
3. **Safe hot-water temperatures at the tap.**
4. **Window and stairway guards/gates to prevent falls.**
5. **A 30-ml (1 oz.) bottle of syrup of Ipecac.**

In addition, the AAP recommends that all physicians caring for children provide "age-appropriate, season-appropriate, and locality-appropriate prevention strategies." The strategies listed in the policy statement were included because each of these items could be achieved with a single action and together they would address many of the more common causes of pediatric injury.

To assist pediatricians in meeting the goals set forth in the policy statement, the AAP developed The Injury Prevention Program (TIPP). TIPP is an office-based, pediatrician-directed program designed around the developmental stages of early childhood. It is based on surveys designed to assess parents' knowledge of injury risk and provides age-specific handouts for the parents and counseling by the pediatrician. The process can be implemented easily, is relatively time efficient, and is an effective way of delivering injury prevention messages to parents.

The National SAFE KIDS Campaign

In 1987, Dr. Martin Eichelberger and a group from the Washington, D.C., Children's Hospital National Medical Center conducted a study to assess parental knowledge on the prevention of pediatric injuries.[18] The study demonstrated that parents' perceptions of injury risks to children were very low. In addition, parents were not knowledgeable about how to prevent or respond to an injury. As a result, the National SAFE KIDS Campaign was begun. Funding for the effort was provided by Johnson & Johnson. The program is coordinated by the Children's Hospital National Medical Center but relies heavily on the formation of state and local coalitions for implementation of the strategies.[20] Efforts are directed toward promoting education of the public, influencing public policy, and building a grassroots community effort to effect change. Emphasis is placed on arousing the public through use of the mass media.

The National SAFE KIDS Campaign has targeted five areas of unintentional injury risk in children: traffic injuries, fires and burns, drownings, poisonings and chokings, and falls. In the area of traffic injury, efforts have been directed toward motor vehicle occupant, bicycle, and pedestrian injuries. During the first year of the campaign, a major goal was to increase public awareness of the problem through the "SAFE KIDS Are No Accident" campaign.

In 1989, the campaign initiated the Bike Helmet and

Bike Safety Awareness Strategy. Bike rodeos were organized to teach children safe bicycle use, and the importance of helmets in reducing the number of head injuries was stressed. Head injuries are the major cause of death and disability in bicycle riders, and it has been estimated that up to 85% of these could be avoided with the use of safety helmets. Voluntary standards for bike safety helmets have been established by the American National Standards Institute and the Snell Memorial Foundation. A major emphasis of the national campaign is to have the Consumer Product Safety Commission establish mandatory national standards.

In 1990, the campaign launched its Scald Burn Prevention Strategy. Each year more than 4000 children are permanently disabled as a result of scald burns. The problem is particularly acute in children in the lower socioeconomic group. The campaign focused on educating parents, encouraging the use of antiscald devices, developing lower cost and antiscald devices that could be retrofitted to bathtubs and showers, and encouraging the passage of legislation that would incorporate these improvements into plumbing codes.

Project GET ALARMED: A Residential Fire Detection Strategy was initiated to encourage the installation and maintenance of residential smoke detectors. Fires are a major cause of death in children, and one of the most effective intervention strategies is early warning through the use of smoke detectors. State and local coalitions were encouraged to develop programs for distributing and installing smoke detectors. Most smoke detectors are battery operated, and the batteries must be changed annually to keep the devices in working order. The problem is especially acute in lower income areas, and efforts were focused here. At the national level, legislative changes are being encouraged.

Another project sponsored by the National SAFE KIDS Campaign is the SAFE KIDS BUCKLE UP: A Child Occupant Protection Strategy. This campaign focuses on the child as a motor vehicle occupant. It addresses the major cause of injury death in children through encouraging the use of appropriate child restraints. Although mandatory child restraint laws have been passed in all 50 states, compliance and enforcement remain lax. Furthermore, evidence is now accumulating that use is only one aspect of the problem: many children are injured as a result of the improper use of safety seats. Chance fractures to the spine have been associated with the two-point lap belts, and neck injuries have been reported with three-point systems used to restrain small children. This campaign encourages the proper use of car safety seats.

THE FUTURE IN INJURY PREVENTION

It is clear that injury in America is a problem of epidemic proportions. It is also clear that the problem is especially acute in the youngest members of our society: young adults, adolescents, and children. What is less clear is whether society will respond to this scourge with the same intensity of effort it has directed toward other health problems like cancer and heart disease. The groups that bear the brunt of deaths and disability from injury are children, minorities, and the poor, disenfranchised members of our society. They

do not vote, and their economic resources are limited. Until the economic incentives for change are recognized or those empowered are personally touched by tragedy, it is likely that efforts will remain fragmented and the province of selected groups and individuals. A more focused national effort is needed.

One of the most important issues in injury prevention is adequate funding. Funding is needed to maintain accurate data collection, to identify problems, and to assess the efficacy of intervention strategies. It is needed to fund educational initiatives and enforcement efforts. Currently, injuries lead to twice as many years of life lost as from cancer and three times that of heart disease and strokes. Yet, federal funding priorities are heavily weighted toward prevention of cancer and heart disease or stroke. In the 1990 federal budget, cancer received 10 times and heart disease–stroke six times the funding directed toward injuries. National funding priorities need redirection.

Data collection efforts are also critical to long-term success in injury prevention and control. Hospitals should be required to adopt E-coding, and health care providers and health agencies at all levels should be encouraged to maintain ongoing injury surveillance activities. Computerization of data collection is expensive, but over time these costs are mitigated through cost savings that result from injury prevention. It is important to recognize also that injury control is a dynamic process and that success in one area is likely to result in the emergence of new problems. Accurate and timely data collection will allow identification of emerging problems and early intervention.

Evidence suggests that injury prevention and control are becoming recognized nationally. The National Academy of Sciences produced a report entitled *Injury in America,* which details the magnitude of the injury problem.[14] Goals for reducing injury morbidity and mortality have been included in federal agencies like the Centers for Disease Control and Prevention, the Bureau of Maternal and Child Health, and the National Highway Traffic Safety Administration. These agencies are committed to taking leadership roles in the ongoing battle against unnecessary deaths and disability from injury. Advocacy groups like the AAP and the National SAFE KIDS Campaign are important to keep attention focused on the pediatric aspects of the problem. Most important is recruitment of the public, as parents and as concerned citizens, to change a lifestyle and an environment that put so many children at risk.

References

1. Agran P, Castillo D, Winn D: Childhood motor vehicle occupant injuries. Am J Dis Child 144:653–662, 1990.
2. Allman FD, Nelson WD, Pacentine GA, et al: Outcome following cardiopulmonary resuscitation in severe pediatric near-drowning. Am J Dis Child 140:571–575, 1986.
3. Baker SP, O'Neil B, Karpt RS: The Injury Fact Book. Lexington, Mass, Lexington Books, 1984.
4. Baker SP, Waller AE: Childhood Injury: State-by-State Mortality Facts. Baltimore, Md, The Johns Hopkins University School of Public Health, January 1989.
5. Birky MM, Halpin BM, Caplin YJ, et al: Fire fatality study. Fire Materials 3:211–217, 1979.
6. Brennan SR, Rhodes H, Peterson HA: Infection after farm machine-

related injuries in children and adolescents. Am J Dis Child 144:710–713, 1990.

7. Centers for Disease Control, Biometrics Branch and Epidemiology Branch, Division of Injury Epidemiology and Control, Center for Environmental Health and Injury Control: Premature mortality due to homicides: U.S., 1968–1985. MMWR 37:543–545, 1988.

8. Christoffel KK: Homicide in childhood: A public health problem in need of attention. Am J Public Health 74:68–70, 1984.

9. Christoffel KK: The causes, impact, and preventability of childhood injuries in the United States: Childhood assaults in the United States. Am J Dis Child 144:670–676, 1990.

10. Christoffel KK: Violent death and injury in U.S. children and adolescents. Am J Dis Child 144:697–706, 1990.

11. Christoffel KK, Liu K: Homicide death rates in childhood in 23 developed countries: U.S. rates atypically high. Child Abuse Negl 7:339–345, 1983.

12. Cole M, Harndon DN, Desai MH, et al: Gasoline explosions, gasoline sniffing: An epidemic in young adolescents. J Burn Care Rehabil 7:532–534, 1986.

13. Committee on Accident and Poison Prevention: The Injury Control for Children and Youth. Elk Grove Village, Ill, American Academy of Pediatrics, 1987.

14. Committee on Trauma Research: Injury in America. Washington, DC, National Academy Press, 1985.

15. DeHaven H: Mechanical analysis of survival in falls from heights of fifty to one hundred and fifty feet. War Med 2:586–596, 1942.

16. Dietz PE, Baker SP: Drowning: Epidemiology and prevention. Am J Public Health 64:303–312, 1974.

17. East MK, Jones CA, Feller I, et al: Epidemiology of burns in children. In: Carvaljal JF, Parks DH, (eds). Burns in Children: Pediatric Burn Management. Chicago, Ill, Year Book Medical Publishers, 1988, pp 3–10.

18. Eichelberger MR, Gorschall MA, Feely HB, et al: Parental attitudes and knowledge of child safety. A national survey. Am J Dis Child 144:714–720, 1990.

19. Emery JL: Infanticide, filicide, and cot death. Arch Dis Child 60:505–507, 1985.

20. Feely HB, Bhatia E: The National SAFE KIDS Campaign: Cure for the Disease. Unpublished correspondence.

21. Fingerhut L, Kleinman J: Trends and current status in childhood mortality, United States, 1900–1985. Vital Health Stat [3] 26:1–44, 1989.

22. Finkelhor D and Baron L: Risk factors for child sexual abuse. J Interpersonal Viol 1:43–72, 1986.

23. Gallagher SS, Finison K, Guyer B, et al: The incidence of injuries among 87,000 Massachusetts children and adolescents: Results of the 1980–81 Statewide Childhood Injury Prevention Program surveillance system. Am J Public Health 74:1340–1347, 1984.

24. Gibson JJ: The contribution of experimental psychology to the formulation of the problem of safety: A brief for basic research. In: Behavioral Approaches to Accident Research. New York, New York Association for the Aid of Crippled Children, 1961, pp 77–89.

25. Gordon JE: The epidemiology of accidents. Am J Public Health 39:504–515, 1949.

26. Greensher J: Non-automotive vehicle injuries in adolescents. Pediatr Ann 17:114–117, 1988.

27. Guyer B, Ellers B: Childhood injuries in the United States. Mortality, morbidity, and cost. Am J Dis Child 144:649–652, 1990.

28. Haddon W: A logical framework for categorizing highway safety phenomena and activity. J Trauma 12:193–207, 1972.

29. Haddon W: Energy damage and the ten countermeasure strategies. J Trauma 13:321–331, 1973.

30. Holinger PC: The causes, impact, and preventability of childhood

injuries in the United States. Childhood suicide in the United States. Am J Dis Child 144:670–676, 1990.

31. Honton EJ, Richmond CA, Stacey GS: Final Report on Analysis of Burn Costs in the Injury Cost Model. Columbus, Ohio, Battelle, July 1980.

32. International Classification of Diseases. Ninth Revision: Clinical Modification. Ann Arbor, Mich, Commission on Professional and Hospital Activities, 1986.

33. Jason J, Gilliland JC, Tyler CW: Homicide as a cause of pediatric mortality in the United States. Pediatrics 72:191–197, 1983.

34. Kukull WA, Peterson DR: Sudden infant death and infanticide. Am J Epidemiol 10:485–486, 1977.

35. McLoughlin E, Joseph MP, Crawford JD: Epidemiology of high-tension electrical injuries in children. J Pediatr 89:62–65, 1976.

36. McLoughlin E, McGuire A: The causes, impact, and preventability of childhood injuries in the United States: Childhood burn injuries in the United States. Am J Dis Child 144:677–683, 1990.

37. National Center on Child Abuse and Neglect. Study of National Incidence and Prevalence of Child Abuse and Neglect: 1988. Washington, DC, Administration for Children, Youth and Families Children's Bureau, US Department of Health and Human Services, 1988.

38. National Committee for Injury Prevention and Control and Education Development Center, Inc: Injury Prevention: Meeting the Challenge. Report to the Bureau of Maternal and Child Health and Resources Development. The Centers for Disease Control, and The National Highway Traffic Safety Administration. New York, Oxford University Press, 1989.

39. National Safety Council. Accident Facts: 1988. Chicago, National Safety Council, 1988.

40. Neresian WS, Petit MR, Shaper R, et al: Childhood death and poverty: A study of all childhood deaths in Maine, 1976–1980. Pediatrics 75:41–50, 1985.

41. O'Carrol PW: Homicides among black males 15–24 years of age, 1970–1984. MMWR 37(SS-1):53–60, 1988.

42. Present P: Child Drowning Study: A Report on the Epidemiology of Drownings in Residential Pools to Children Under Age Five. Washington, DC, Directorate for Epidemiology, US Consumer Product Safety Commission, 1987.

43. Rhodes KH, Brennan SR, Peterson HA: Machines and microbes. Still serious hazards to youths on the farm. Am J Dis Child 144:707–709, 1990.

44. Rivara FP: Epidemiology of childhood injuries: II. Sex differences in injury rates. Am J Dis Child 136:502–506, 1982.

45. Rivara FP: Fatal and nonfatal farm injuries to children and adolescents in the United States. Pediatrics 76:567–573, 1985.

46. Rivara FP: Child pedestrian injuries in the United States. Current status of the problem, potential interventions, and future research needs. Am J Dis Child 144:692–696, 1990.

47. Rodriguez JG, Brown ST: Childhood injuries in the United States. Am J Dis Child 144:627–646, 1990.

48. Spyker DA: Submersion Injury: Epidemiology, prevention, and management. Pediatr Clin North Am 32:113–125, 1985.

49. Swanson JA: Accidental farm injuries in children. Am J Dis Child 141:1276–1279, 1987.

50. Thompson JC, Ashwal S: Electrical injuries in children. Am J Dis Child 137:231–235, 1983.

51. Wilson MH, Baker SP, Teret SP, et al: The Injury Problem. In: Saving Children: A Guide to Injury Prevention. New York, Oxford University Press, 1991.

52. Wintemute GJ: Childhood drowning and near-drowning in the United States. Am J Dis Child 144:663–669, 1990.

53. Wintemute GJ, Kraus JF, Teret SP, et al: Drowning in childhood and adolescence: A population based study. Am J Public Health 77:830–832, 1987.

CHAPTER FOUR

James A. O'Neill, Jr.

Trauma Care Organization for Children

HISTORICAL BACKGROUND

Emergency medical services (EMS) best function as organized systems capable of providing prompt optimal care to the critically ill or injured of a community or region. The ideal system has yet to be developed, but the elements of what is required are now well defined. With very few exceptions, it was not really until after the Korean conflict that the concepts developed from the experience of treating military casualties were brought back to the United States and used for the civilian population.

Although the American College of Surgeons Committee on Trauma was established in 1922, early efforts focused on the management of fractures. By the late 1950s, however, regional trauma committees of the American Academy of Orthopedic Surgeons also became active in education and in setting standards, and from 1970 on, both these organizations sponsored courses for physicians, emergency department nurses, and the few emergency physicians who existed at that time.[18] The American Medical Association Commission on Emergency Medical Services also contributed by raising the visibility of the problem of injury. However, it was not until a thought-provoking monograph entitled *Accidental Death and Disability: The Neglected Disease of Modern Society* was published by the National Academy of Sciences in 1966, pointing out that accidental death and disability represented a problem of epidemic proportions, that trauma was really recognized as the leading cause of death and disability in individuals under the age of 38 years.[10] It was startling to note that for the young and future adult population of the country a potentially preventable problem was the leading cause of morbidity and mortality.

The Highway Safety Act of 1966 provided an opportunity for all states to develop an EMS program using federal highway construction funds and thus to improve ambulance services from being mere transportation to being remarkably effective instruments of providing effective prehospital care. As the development of EMS programs spread throughout the United States, additional needs became obvious. The American College of Surgeons developed a document establishing the necessary standards for ambulances and minimal equipment.[2] Communication was identified as vital, so that prehospital providers could communicate with emergency department physicians. Also, educational programs for ambulance drivers and emergency medical technicians were necessary. Again, the American College of Surgeons, among others, developed courses for emergency medical technicians (EMTs), which eventually developed into the National Highway Traffic Safety Administration's 81-hour basic EMT course.[23] Since then, more extensive and detailed courses have been devised.

It is fair to say that at least the first 10 years' efforts were placed primarily in the direction of prehospital care, development of emergency medical services, improvement in transportation and communication systems, and education and refresher courses for the continuing education of EMTs. Unfortunately, however, not all regions in all states took advantage of the early enabling legislation that would have permitted the development of uniform systems of trauma care. In 1969, a Conference on EMS was cosponsored by the American College of Surgeons Committee on Trauma and the Committee on Injuries of the American Association of Orthopedic Surgeons.[1] The Division of Emergency Health Services of the Department of Health, Education, and Welfare provided sponsorship for this conference, which was attended by essentially all of the major medical and governmental figures interested in developing an ideal system of EMS. Four task forces were developed for this important Arlie House Conference, including ambulance services, personnel and education, emergency facilities, and administration. This was the first time trauma centers were mentioned in an official document, although the concept was not new. In 1971, the American Medical Association Commission on Emergency Medical Services published the proceedings of an important conference entitled *Categorization of Hospital Emergency Capabilities.*[7] Meant to represent a guideline for hospitals to judge their capabilities in providing a good standard of emergency medical care, this document was used as the basis for the development of standards for trauma centers.

In 1969, the first pediatric surgeon, Dr. James A. O'Neill, was appointed to the Committee on Trauma of the American College of Surgeons. The then chairman of the committee, Dr. Curtis P. Artez, had become aware that trauma was the leading cause of death in childhood, as it is today,[14] and it was his intent that the Committee on Trauma include pediatric considerations in all standard settings and educational programs they would produce and support. These efforts are continuing at the present time.

The value of trauma centers has been well documented. Coles demonstrated that following implementation of a trauma system in Orange County, California, the percentage of potentially preventable deaths from trauma fell from 34% to 15%.[8] In 1985, the first-year assessment of the San Diego trauma system demonstrated a fall in the trauma death rate of 55% after implementation of their new system.[21] Similarly, in Washington, D.C., a 50% reduction in trauma deaths over 5 years was credited to the development of a system of trauma care.[13] It was evident that most of the deaths occurred in patients who were treated in inadequate facilities. These and other studies have proved that centralized care for severely injured patients is capable of reducing mortality and long-term disability provided that the other elements of a trauma system are working in concert.[20, 22]

Although some aspects of EMS systems have been shown to reduce morbidity and mortality for adults, similar results for children were not seen. Even though infants, children, and adolescents also need the EMS systems, their special needs were not generally addressed by EMS agencies, and it was clear that the unique needs of this group required special consideration.[12, 17] Consequently, in recent years, pediatric trauma centers have been developed in regions with pediatric medical centers capable of providing a high level of trauma care. Coinciding with this, interest in pediatric emergency care was increasing, and the American Academy of Pediatrics established a Section on Pediatric Emergency Medicine in 1981. From these interested groups, many of the ideas for the development of Emergency Medical Services for children (EMSC) spawned, grew, and have culminated in grant funding to 20 states between 1985 and 1990 to develop EMSC.

THE SYSTEM

This evolution of concepts of trauma care has identified four components of a trauma system: access to care, prehospital care, inhospital care, and rehabilitation. Each is considered separately; however, variations in systems development may be necessary depending on whether the EMS is located in an urban or a rural area. Transportation is the most obvious variable in the latter case.

Access to Care

Designation of trauma centers requires that institutions that undertake this commitment agree to the concept of serving as a public utility. This means that all injured individuals, without regard to ability to pay, must be accepted by such facilities for the system to function properly. Additionally, all individuals in the region must be made aware of the existence of trauma centers, their location, and how to contact them. The 9-1-1 emergency telephone system is now in existence in all parts of the United States; however, in some rural areas, radio transmitters may be necessary to notify prehospital providers appropriately. Within the same communications system, there must be a mechanism for notification of trauma centers that a patient is on the way, and, ideally, the communication system should permit interaction between the prehospital provider and the hospital.

Similarly, not only must appropriate facilities for children be established, but also must parents and pediatricians be aware of the location and existence of such pediatric centers. Because there is already a well-established EMS system designed for the care of injured individuals, the use of the same system for access to care for children with emergency medical problems is both appropriate and logical. Hence, appropriate systems for children (e.g., EMSC) integrated into the primary EMS system have been developed.

Prehospital Care

Prehospital care involves ambulances, helicopters, and fixed-wing aircraft as well as the EMT personnel who are trained to provide the initial assessment, resuscitation, and care. The American College of Surgeons, in concert with other concerned groups, has developed standards for equipping ambulances and aircraft designed for the transportation of seriously injured patients. In the case of the injured child, appropriate ranges of sizes of endotracheal tubes, medical antishock trousers (MAST), chest tubes, intravenous cannulae, and the like must be available (Table 4–1). Systems for the field categorization of trauma patients have been developed to provide guidance to prehospital providers as to which hospital facility or trauma center the patient should go.[11] Education programs as well as continuing education and advanced courses with modules for pediatric injuries and emergencies exist, but further development and emphasis is needed in other more specific areas (Table 4–2). The EMS grants, sponsored by the federal government,

Table 4–1
Pediatric Equipment Standards for Ambulances

Airway Equipment
Airways in assorted sizes, nasopharyngeal and oropharyngeal
Endotracheal tubes, 3.0 French through adult size
Pediatric laryngoscope and blades 0–3
Small Magill forceps
Multiple oxygen masks
Pediatric Ambu bag
Assorted suction catheters, 8.0–16.0
Suction
Assorted nasogastric tubes, 8–18
Resuscitation Equipment
Intravenous catheters, 24–18 gauge
Scalp vein needles, 21–19 gauge
Intravenous administration sets with volume-control burettes
Ringer lactate in 500-ml bags
Pediatric medical antishock trousers
Various sizes of blood pressure cuffs
Pediatric cervical spine collars
Pediatric dosages of resuscitation drugs
Pediatric extremity splints
Chest tube, 3–24 French

and subsequent knowledge transfer and sharing are helping in this regard.

Triage of pediatric injuries may be performed somewhat along the same guidelines as those used for adults but because most pediatric injuries are blunt in nature, a higher index of suspicion of serious injury must be entertained, particularly when the mechanism of injury has indicated extreme force. The "golden hour," which represents a period of relative stability or safe transportation time for adults, probably should be halved for the small child. Thus, expeditious transportation and constant observation and care are key to ideal prehospital management of the seriously injured child.

Special mention should be made of air transportation of seriously injured children. Appendix D of the Hospital Re-

Table 4–2
Pediatric Trauma Considerations—Emergency Medical Technician Education

Airway
Anatomy
Management of obstruction
Intubation
Breathing
Physiology
Artificial respiration, mask and endotracheal
Circulation
Assessment, monitoring
Basic cardiopulmonary resuscitation
Intravenous, intraosseus access
Methods of defibrillation
Use of medical antishock trousers
Blood volume considerations
Intravenous fluid administration
Use of vasoactive drugs
Chest tube placement
Other
Cervical spine immobilization
Splinting of fractures
Assessment of head injury

Table 4–3
1987 City of Philadelphia Trauma Triage Criteria for Transport to a Trauma Center

1. Vital signs and level of consciousness:
    Glasgow coma score <13 or systolic blood pressure <90 or trauma score ≤12*
2. Anatomy of injury and mechanism of injury:
    Penetrating injury to chest, abdomen, head, neck, or groin†
    Two or more proximal long bone fractures
    Combination with burns of ≥15%, face or airway
    Flail chest
    Amputation above the wrist or ankle or degloving injury
    Multiple amputations (e.g., two fingers, three toes)
    Injury involving two or more body systems (e.g., central nervous system, cardiovascular, pulmonary, gastrointernal,
      genitourinary)
    Unconsciousness with evidence of trauma
    Evidence of high impact:
      Falls of 20 ft or more
      Crash speed of 20 mph or more: 30-inch deformity of automobile
      Extrication required
      Rearward displacement of front axle
      Passenger compartment intrusion 18 inches on patient's side of car and 24 inches on opposite side of car
      Ejection of patient
      Rollover
      Death of same car occupant
      Pedestrian hit at 20 mph or more (includes bicyclist, motorcyclist, mopedist)
      Serious blunt trauma in a child
3. If all above criteria are negative, reevaluate case with medical control as available, especially for patients <5 or >55 or
    those with known cardiac or respiratory disease (lower the threshold of severity resulting in trauma center care); when in
    doubt, transport to trauma center.

*Criteria applicable to the paramedic only.
†Criteria applicable to police.

sources Document published by the Committee on Trauma of the American College of Surgeons outlines these requirements very well.[3] Helicopters or even fixed-wing aircraft may be used to transport a seriously injured patient from the scene of the accident or between hospitals when the patient has been taken to a resuscitation unit first. In most instances it is preferable that helicopters be hospital based and staffed by physicians or nurses especially trained for air transportation and prehospital assessment and intervention. An EMT-paramedic may supplant a physician or nurse. Such air ambulance services must be integrated within the structure of the EMS system for that region and must be subject to the standards established for such services. In addition, there should be an ongoing review of air ambulance services by an appropriate accrediting quality control group. National standards for air ambulance systems exist[3]:

1. More than one crew member is optimal for appropriate transport of critically ill patients. (If only one crew member is present, that person should be a specially trained flight nurse, but if more than one medical crew member is present, the second crew member may be an EMT-A with special training in aeromedical evaluation or beyond.)

2. Three levels of aeromedical crew members have been defined; level II and III members have received additional educational training to enable them to care for critically injured children.

3. All air ambulance systems must have an appropriate medical director experienced in the care of critically ill and injured patients and knowledgeable regarding their aeromedical needs.

4. Equipment and medications appropriate for pediatric

age patients have been defined in Appendix D of the American College of Surgeons Hospital Resources Document.

The EMT-Paramedic or EMT-A is responsible for performing a primary assessment of the injured patient as well as secondary assessment and triage. Appropriate communication with a base communications system with experienced physician input is vital. In the primary assessment, the EMT is responsible for evaluating the adequacy of the airway and breathing, the status of the cardiovascular system, and the state of consciousness; for control of bleeding; and for stabilization of fractures—particularly those of the cervical spine. Following initial assessment, stabilization of airway, and initiation of resuscitation, communication with medical control is achieved so that the trauma center can be alerted to the patient's pending arrival, and appropriate supervision and instructions can be provided to the EMT. The EMT then transports the patient to the closest appropriate trauma center while resuscitation and airway management are continued with proper monitoring.

The EMTs must be capable of providing airway and cervical spine control, appropriate ventilation, stabilization of the chest, management of open pneumothorax, control of bleeding, intravenous access, and infusion of Ringer lactate. They must be able to judge situations in which the application of a MAST garment is appropriate, and they must be capable of providing initial care of critical burn injuries. Triage parameters for direct transport to trauma centers are outlined in Appendix E of the American College of Surgeons Hospital Resources Document.[4] A variation of these criteria has been developed for the Philadelphia EMS system and is outlined in Table 4–3. Ideally, EMTs are capable of field categorization of trauma patients indepen-

Table 4–4
American College of Surgeons Guidelines for Triage of Pediatric Trauma

Pediatric Level I	Pediatric Level II
Patients having serious injury to more than one organ system	Patients with single system injury who will not require intensive care unit management and require a short length of stay
Patients having one system injury who will require pediatric intensive care unit care	Patients with shock who require less than a one blood volume transfusion for stabilization
Patients with signs of shock who require more than a one blood volume transfusion	Patients with a single major long bone fracture
Patients with fractures complicated by suspected neurovascular compartment injury	Patients with stable, not serious, head trauma who will not require ventilation or long-term rehabilitation
Patients with potential for reimplantation of an extremity	
Patients with suspected or actual spinal cord or column injuries	
Patients with head injury having any one of the following:	
Orbital or facial bone fractures	
Cerebral fluid leaks	
Altered states of consciousness	
Changing neurologic signs	
Open head injuries	
Depressed skull fractures	
Required intracranial pressure	
Patients suspected of requiring ventilatory or nutritional support	

From American College of Surgeons: Hospital and Prehospital Resources for Optimal Care of the Injured Patient. Chicago, American College of Surgeons, 1984.

dently, but a triage scheme may also be used under medical control.

Three points in time are critical for trauma deaths: immediately, at the time of the accident; within the next 1 to 4 hours; and several days to weeks later as a result of complications. Thus, ideally patients should be no farther than 30 minutes from a trauma center in urban situations. In rural situations, it may be necessary to treat patients initially at nearby hospitals—those that meet the requirements of a level III trauma center and that have emergency medical staff trained in advanced trauma life support. Under such circumstances air transportation may be appropriate. However, the ideal EMS system has these relationships and times predetermined by protocol so that EMTs know under what circumstances various transportation criteria are to be used. The prime purpose of EMS systems is to provide rapid access to the appropriate level of care for injured patients, particularly for injured children. The prehospital system should be under the same continuing reevaluation and quality control scrutiny as the trauma center itself.

Inhospital Care

Although the inhospital phase of care of the injured patient is the most definitive and perhaps the most critical element in the trauma system, it can function effectively only if prehospital access and response systems are coordinated and working well. In terms of adult trauma care, three levels of hospital facilities have been described to categorize facilities according to their ability to manage various severities of trauma. The level I facility is capable of 24-hour, 7-days-per-week immediate and complete response to the needs of the seriously injured patient. This includes 24-hour emergency department physician coverage; inhouse surgical, physician anesthesia, and operating room nursing

coverage; as well as a full range of diagnostic capabilities that are adequate and appropriate for an intensive care facility. The level I facility is responsible for a broad educational program with both inhouse and outreach programs as well as a trauma research program. Level II adult trauma centers are responsible for having essentially the same medical capabilities as a level I hospital, but a research program is not required and there are a few other minor differences in this respect. A level III hospital designation indicates that the facility is limited in the management of complex trauma, but it is capable of providing appropriate initial resuscitation, airway management, and stabilization if needed when a level I or II center is very distant (that is, farther than 30 minutes away).

With regard to pediatric trauma centers, a two-tiered system is probably more practical and effective. Pediatric trauma constitutes approximately one third of all trauma experience. Appendix J of the Hospital Resources Document of the American College of Surgeons has recommended that the level I pediatric trauma center be located either in a children's hospital or in a large general hospital with a fully capable pediatric unit; in each instance, however, a major interest in and commitment to trauma care is necessary.[5] Although level I and II adult trauma centers are quite similar, the concept is different with regard to pediatric trauma centers. The level II pediatric trauma center is usually located in a general hospital with limited pediatric surgical and medical personnel and facilities. Table 4–4 outlines a categorization of triage for pediatric patients appropriate to level I and II pediatric trauma centers.[6] Pennsylvania was one of the first states to develop standards for pediatric trauma centers, and standards have been developed for level I and level II pediatric trauma center.[15] Table 4–5 lists the criteria for level I pediatric trauma centers developed by the Pennsylvania Trauma Systems Foundation, detailing all elements of personnel and facili-

Table 4–5
Outline of Pennsylvania Trauma Systems Foundation Standards for Pediatric Trauma Centers

General Standards
Commitment of the facility's resources at all times
Adequate volume (150 or more patients per year)
Licensed helipad
Residency in general or pediatric surgery
Trauma program director certified by American Board of Surgery in pediatric surgery
Trauma nurse coordinator
Defined role of trauma nurses
Advanced trauma life support certification of all providers
Council on Medical Education, 50 hours of trauma-related credit over 2 years
Adequate postdischarge follow-up and rehabilitation
Development of pediatric trauma prevention programs
Active involvement in local and regional emergency medical service systems
Trauma registry
Participate in statewide trauma data collection and analysis

Hospital Organization
I. Defined trauma service
II. Pediatric surgical divisions required
    Cardiac Surgery
    General Surgery
    Pediatric Surgery
    Neurologic Surgery
    Ophthalmologic Surgery
    Oral Surgery—Dental
    Orthopedic Surgery
    Otorhinolaryngologic Surgery
    Plastic and Maxillofacial Surgery
    Thoracic Surgery
    Urology
    Obstetrics and gynecology available on consultant basis
III. Emergency Department staffed 24 hours by board-certified physicians trained in emergency care, advanced trauma life support–certified with protocols defining the role of the emergency department physician on the trauma team
IV. 24-hour availability of general surgeon and neurosurgeon and related staff; other pediatric surgical specialty services must be readily available on call
V. Nonsurgical pediatric divisions required
    Inhouse 24 hours
        Emergency medical
        Anesthesia
    On call, promptly available

Cardiology	Neurology
Chest Medicine	Neuroradiology
Gastroenterology	Pathology
Hematology	Pediatrics
Infectious Disease	Physiatry
Internal Medicine	Psychiatry
Nephrology	Radiology

VI. Facilities required
    1. Emergency Department with designated physician director and nurses trained in pediatric trauma care, appropriately equipped to manage all needs of the seriously injured child
    2. Pediatric intensive care unit with inhouse physician staffing and nurses trained in pediatric trauma care and equipped to manage the needs of the injured child
    3. Postanesthesia recovery room staffed by nurses trained in trauma care
    4. Acute hemodialysis capability
    5. Organized burn care or transfer agreement
    6. Acute spinal cord injury management capability
    7. Full radiologic, computed tomography and other diagnostic imaging capability and availability
    8. Social service capabilities
    9. Spiritual counseling
    10. Pediatric medical-surgical units staffed by nurses trained in trauma care and equipped to manage the needs of the injured child
    11. Operating room immediately available and staffed 24 hours a day by nurses trained in trauma care and equipped to manage the needs of the injured child, including cardiopulmonary bypass capability
VII. Clinical laboratories and blood bank with full range of testing available 24 hours a day
VIII. Quality Assurance Program
    1. Audit of trauma deaths
    2. Morbidity and mortality review
    3. Multidisciplinary trauma conference
    4. Medical and nursing quality assessment program, utilization review, and tissue review
    5. Prehospital trip forms
IX. Outreach program for consultation
X. Public education program
XI. Research program
XII. Internal and external Council on Medical Education programs
XIII. Trauma rehabilitation program

From Pennsylvania Trauma Systems Foundation: 1991–1995 Standards for Trauma Center Accreditation—Pediatrics. Mechanicsburg, Pa, Trauma Systems Foundation, 1994.

ties requirements, continuing education requirements, and quality assurance. Designed to parallel and to supplement the hospital resources document for optimal care of the injured patient promoted by the American College of Surgeons, the foundation lists as one of the most important requirements a commitment on the part of the hospital and all of its personnel to the care of the injured child so that the facility's resources are available at all times to all injured children. Qualification for a facility to participate requires the management of at least 150 pediatric trauma

patients per year to maintain skills and expertise. The hospital must be capable of receiving patients by ground ambulance as well as by helicopter. Also, a full range of operating room and intensive care facilities must be available 24 hours a day. All trauma providers, including physicians and nurses, must be specifically trained in trauma and integrated into a single trauma team with a surgeon as trauma director.

Under the hospital organization, there must be a defined trauma service with a designated trauma program director who is certified by the American Board of Surgery in Pediatric Surgery and who has appropriate advanced trauma life support certification. A full range of pediatric surgical and subspecialty surgical capabilities is required as well as pediatric medical subspecialty capabilities. Inhouse coverage is required for pediatric general surgery, neurosurgery, emergency medicine, and anesthesia, and all other specialties must be promptly available on call. There must be a trauma nurse coordinator on the trauma service who works closely with the trauma program director. The trauma nurse coordinator is responsible for coordinating all nursing care and education for the trauma program.

The emergency department must be staffed 24 hours a day by board-certified physicians trained in emergency care. They can be surgeons, emergency physicians, or pediatricians, provided they are appropriately trained in trauma and are familiar with protocols defining the role of the emergency department physician as related to other physicians and surgeons on the trauma team. The intent is to have individuals devoted to the emergency department who do not cross-cover other areas of the hospital. The emergency department must have its own organization with a designated physician director as well as nurses trained in pediatric trauma care.

In addition to a full-scale emergency department, a pediatric intensive care unit must be available 24 hours a day. There must be inhouse physician staffing and nurses trained in pediatric trauma care in the intensive care unit. The intensive care unit equipment standards must meet the needs of the seriously injured child. Similarly, the postanesthesia recovery room must be staffed by nurses trained in trauma care, and the equipment must be appropriate for such patients.

Other requirements are an acute hemodialysis capability, an organized burn care program or transfer agreement, an acute spinal cord injury management capability, a social service capability, spiritual counseling, and related services. Full radiologic, computed tomographic, and other diagnostic imaging capability must be provided. Protocols must be written to demonstrate priority for management of the injured child. Conventional radiographic techniques must be available on an immediate basis, and all other imaging studies must be available within 20 or 30 minutes. This includes not only technical but medical radiologic personnel as well. There must be pediatric medical-surgical units staffed by nurses trained in trauma care and equipped to manage the needs of the injured child.

It is particularly important that an operating room be available at all times and staffed 24 hours a day by nurses trained in trauma care. The operating room should be equipped to manage the needs of the severely injured child, including having cardiopulmonary bypass capability. The latter is particularly important because so many of the serious injuries in children are blunt in nature.

The clinical laboratories and blood bank must provide a full range of testing appropriate for intensive care unit–type patients 24 hours a day. The laboratory must be designed specifically to meet the needs of infants and children, including the ability to make determinations on small quantities of blood.

Quality assurance and improvement in trauma care have been described in detail in Appendix G of the Hospital Resources Document of the American College of Surgeons.[16] This document, as well as the document of the Pennsylvania Trauma Systems Foundation, outlines an ideal quality control program consisting of five elements[15]: (1) all trauma deaths must be specifically audited in detail; (2) at least monthly morbidity and mortality review is done on all patients; (3) daily review of the emergency department activity is required; (4) a multidisciplinary problem-oriented trauma conference including all members of the trauma service team is perhaps the most valuable instrument of quality assessment available as well as being a valuable continuing education instrument; and (5) a combined medical and nursing quality assessment program should be developed for review of all cases, including utilization and tissue review. In addition, it is required that the pediatric trauma center participate in a statewide program of data collection and analysis so that knowledge transfer and utilization may occur.

With regard to education, there must be extensive internal as well as external continuing medical education programs specifically in the area of trauma. The internal programs are designed for physicians, nurses, and other providers on the trauma service team. The external programs are designed for prehospital providers as well as physicians in other units. There also must be a public education program that helps the public learn about appropriate access to trauma centers; in addition, it promotes trauma prevention.

Rehabilitation

Statistics indicate that only one in 10 severely injured patients has access to a rehabilitation service following the acute definitive management. Although the figures may be somewhat better in the childhood age group, the needs are still considerable. Consequently, a broad-based trauma rehabilitation program that begins with admission to the hospital is critical. Inherent in the trauma rehabilitation program is a follow-up program to assess methodology and outcomes. Various models are available ranging from physiatry to orthopedics and rehabilitation, but whichever model is used, the rehabilitation program must begin at the time of admission and continue through discharge. There must be feedback from the rehabilitation physicians to the other providers, particularly those in prehospital areas, to promote better care of the injured child.

Also, there must be a research program that is participated in not only by physicians but also by nurses and other providers to promote better solutions to the currently unsolved problems of the injured child. Epidemiologic studies, physiologic studies, and analysis of outcome are particularly important, but research into EMS systems modification is important as well.

The standards for level II pediatric trauma centers have been developed by the American College of Surgeons and have been modified by other groups or states to fit particular needs. When one analyzes the criteria for referral to level I and II pediatric trauma centers as outlined in Table 4–4, the facility's requirements are related to these standards. Although the level I facility must have a separate pediatric intensive care unit, the level II center may have a generic intensive care unit. Both level I and level II centers must have an operating room that is available at all times, but the level I pediatric trauma center tends to have a wider range of ancillary facilities and personnel specifically and exclusively devoted to pediatric care. The level II pediatric trauma center is not expected to have the full range of pediatric ancillary laboratory and diagnostic services, but the general capabilities must be similar. A level I pediatric trauma center should be directed by a pediatric surgeon, and a full range of pediatric medical and surgical subspecialists should be available. The level I center is expected to be involved in research and a broad-based educational program. The level II facility, however, is not expected to have the full range of pediatric medical and surgical subspecialists; the director of the pediatric trauma service at a level II center might well be a general surgeon with a special interest and experience in pediatric trauma.

CATEGORIZATION AND DESIGNATION

As indicated, the three-tiered system is currently believed to be appropriate for the care of injured adults, and the two-tiered system is probably best for the care of injured children. The categorization of hospital facilities into level I or II pediatric trauma centers is based on the standards that have been outlined previously and listed in Table 4–5. Despite the fact that the American College of Surgeons is recognized as the leader in promoting appropriate standards of care for the categorization of hospital facilities designed for trauma patients, local competitive influences have required that individual regions either accept these standards or develop their own, as have the state of Pennsylvania and others. The establishment of such standards is both a medical and a political process and hence can be difficult, frustrating, and time consuming. However, it is absolutely vital if a system encompassing all aspects of care from the site of injury to the point of rehabilitation is to be established. Unless hospitals are categorized, prehospital providers cannot transport patients to the appropriate facility.

The most difficult step in the entire process, and one that unfortunately has led to legal involvement in many instances, has been the process of designation. Many regions have preferred to follow the process of self-designation, but to a certain extent governmental regulation appears to be needed. In the ideal situation, surgeons experienced in trauma care are involved in the political process in partnership with local and governmental officials so that the appropriate designation can be made. Medical personnel are required for performing site visits to verify that a particular hospital meets the standards and is appropriately categorized, and follow-up assessment is critical. Many of the problems identified at trauma centers require enhancement of the EMS system and thus require the expenditure of public monies and the involvement of governmental authorities. By using outside site reviewers who are not involved in the regional trauma system, an element of impartiality can be introduced into the designation process so that legal challenges are less likely. It appears that most agree that

regionalization of emergency facilities makes sense, so transfer and referral agreements among all the hospitals in these regions are necessary.

ECONOMIC CONSIDERATIONS

The foregoing sections have described ideal and practical elements related to pediatric trauma centers and the EMS systems with which they interact. Although the federal government initially funded the start up of EMS systems in various regions of the country, including the administrative and operating costs, and although a number of regions had outside grants to support additional activities, continuation funding has not been appropriated at an ideal level. Various states have not had the wherewithal to continue adequate funding, although there are certain outstanding exceptions.

Costs related to EMS systems are related to the various aspects of the systems themselves, including prehospital care, hospital care, communications, and management. Transportation systems ordinarily account for approximately one fourth of the total EMS system cost, and, of course, personnel expenses are the largest portion of that. From region to region, these costs vary depending on whether the staff is employed full time or consists of volunteers. Other related costs are equipment, training, and space. If air transportation and helicopters are added to the system, the costs are even greater. Unfortunately, system costs are inversely related to population densities when considered on a per capita basis, so it costs relatively more to fund a prehospital system in a rural region than it does in an urban one. Communication and system administrative management costs constitute approximately 2 to 3% each, although start-up costs are greater than this. The remaining 70% or so of costs related to an EMS system are inhospital costs. Generally speaking, we have depended on the various forms of medical insurance to cover inhospital costs and certain portions of the transportation costs. However, at the very best, collection rates are in the range of 75% or less, so the remainder of the costs related to transportation and hospital care must be made up by other means. Although the hospital may possibly recoup three fourths of its costs from its third-party payers for the patients it treats, the 30% or so of the total cost related to an EMS system in any particular region must be funded by a combination of federal and state funds. Legislative activity must occur throughout the country if the commitment to trauma care is to continue for what amounts to one of the most frequent causes of mortality in the United States. It has been easier to develop funding from federal and state governments and private foundations for start-up needs related to system development, organization, personnel training, and purchase of equipment. However, legislative activity has to occur to provide sufficient operational funds over the long term.

In the last 2 or 3 years, enormous efforts have been expended on the development of prospective payment systems called *diagnosis-related groups* (DRGs) in an attempt to control the rising costs of health care in the United States. Schwab and co-workers published a paper analyzing the inhospital costs related to a level I trauma center in New

Jersey.[19] The startling conclusion was that for the hospital involved, trauma patients accounted for a net loss of $1.86 million in a single year because the DRG system as structured did not support contemporary trauma care as we know it. The investigators concluded that if something were not done to rectify this situation, the trauma system and the concept of trauma centers in voluntary hospitals in the United States would have to be abandoned. Studies such as this should serve as ammunition for governmental groups to address the problem. A similar study of geriatric patients in Rhode Island came to the same conclusions regarding DRG allowances.[9]

Our experience in developing a level I pediatric trauma center at the Children's Hospital of Philadelphia reveals that a good estimation of start-up cost can be made. Standards for ideal level I and other level trauma centers have been developed on a national and statewide basis. Hospitals must then develop the resources and maintain them over time on an operational basis if they are to make a commitment to trauma. The personnel and staffing requirements, educational systems both within and beyond the hospital, equipment requirements, and research programmatic needs, as well as the services that permit an interplay between the hospital and the regional system, approximate $500,000. This presumes that the institution is already a tertiary care center and has many services in place that relate to trauma care. If, for example, the hospital must build a helipad or add new radiographic facilities, the start-up cost may reach $1,000,000. The continuing operational costs are probably in the range of $200,000 to $250,000 per year. At Children's Hospital of Philadelphia we did not have a problem developing the funding for the start-up costs, but the continuing expenses have exceeded the level of reimbursement for the care of pediatric trauma patients by approximately 20%. Legislative action and additional fundraising are going to be required for trauma centers to keep pace with newer developments in trauma care.

References

1. American College of Surgeons, Committee on Trauma, and American Academy of Orthopedic Surgeons, Committee on Injuries: Emergency Medical Services: Recommendations for an Approach to an Urgent Problem. Proceedings of the Arlie Conference on Emergency Medical Services. Chicago, American College of Surgeons and American Academy of Orthopedic Surgeons, 1969.
2. American College of Surgeons: Essential equipment for ambulances. Bull Am Coll Surg 68:36–38, 1983.
3. American College of Surgeons: Hospital and Prehospital Resources for Optimal Care of the Injured Patient, and Appendices A through J. Chicago, American College of Surgeons, 1986, pp 23–28.
4. American College of Surgeons: Hospital and Prehospital Resources for Optimal Care of the Injured Patient, and Appendixes A through J. Chicago, American College of Surgeons, 1986, pp 29–36.
5. American College of Surgeons: Hospital and Prehospital Resources for Optimal Care of the Injured Patient, and Appendixes A through J. Chicago, American College of Surgeons, 1986, pp 53–56.
6. American College of Surgeons: Hospital and Prehospital Resources for Optimal Care of the Injured Patient, and Appendixes A through J. Chicago, American College of Surgeons, 1986, p 54.
7. American Medical Association: Categorization of Hospital Emergency Capabilities. Chicago, American Medical Association, 1971.
8. Coles RH: Trauma mortality in Orange Co: The effect of implementation of a regional trauma system. Ann Emerg Med 13:1–10, 1984.
9. Demaria EJ, Meriam MA, Casanova LA, et al: Do DRG payments adequately reimburse the costs of trauma care in geriatric patients? J Trauma 28:1244–1249, 1988.
10. Division of Medical Sciences: Accidental Death and Disability: The Neglected Disease of Modern Society. Washington, DC, National Academy of Sciences/National Research Council, 1966.
11. Mayer T, Walker ML, Johnson DG, et al: Causes of morbidity and mortality in pediatric trauma. JAMA 245:719–721, 1981.
12. Mullner R, Goldberg J: The Illinois trauma system: Changes in patient survival patterns following vehicular injuries. J Am Coll of Emerg Physicians 6:393–396, 1977.
13. National Highway Traffic Safety Administration: EMS Program and Its Relationship to Highway Safety. Washington, DC, US Department of Transportation, Transport Technical Report, DOT HS 806-832, August 1985.
14. National Safety Council: Accident Facts. Chicago, National Safety Council, 1987.
15. Pennsylvania Trauma Systems Foundation: 1988 Standards for Trauma Center Accreditation—Pediatrics. Mechanicsburg, Pa, Trauma Systems Foundation, 1988.
16. Pennsylvania Trauma Systems Foundation: 1988 Standards for Trauma Center Accreditation—Pediatrics. Mechanicsburg, Pa, Trauma Systems Foundation, 1988, pp 42–47.
17. Ramenofsky M, Luterman QA, et al: Maximum survival in pediatric trauma: The ideal system. J Trauma 24:818–823, 1984.
18. Rockwood CA, Mann CM, Farrington JD, et al: History of emergency medical services in the United States. J Trauma 16:299–308, 1976.
19. Schwab CW, Young G, Camishan RC, et al: Total DRG reimbursement: The demise of the trauma center (The use of ISS grouping as an early predictor of hospital cost). J Trauma 28:939–946, 1988.
20. Seidel JS, Henderson DP: Emergency Medical Services for Children: A Report to the Nation. Washington, DC, National Center for Education in Maternal and Child Health, 1991.
21. Shackford SR, Hollingworth-Fridlund P, Cooper GF, et al: The effect of regionalization upon the quality of trauma care as assessed by concurrent audit before and after institution of a trauma system. J Trauma 26:812–820, 1986.
22. Trunkey DD: The value of trauma centers. Bull Am Coll Surg 67:5–7, 1982.
23. US Department of Transportation: Basic Training Program for Emergency Medical Technicians—Ambulance: Concepts and Recommendations. Washington, DC, National Highway Traffic Safety Administration, 1971.

William L. Buntain

CHAPTER FIVE

Developing Trauma Centers and Standards of Care

HISTORICAL PERSPECTIVES

TRAUMA SYSTEM ORGANIZATION

PROBLEMS IN TRAUMA SYSTEM
DEVELOPMENT
  Political and Economic Influences
  "Turf" Disputes

SUCCEEDING IN SYSTEM DEVELOPMENT
  Establish and Maintain Credibility
  Establish Regular and Ongoing
  Communication
  Be Proactive, Not Reactive
  Don'ts
  Know Your Allies (and Adversaries)

In its 1985 white paper, "Injury In America," the Institute of Medicine's Committee on Trauma Research identified "injury" as the nation's principal public health problem, responsible for the deaths of more Americans up to age 34 than all other diseases combined, the fourth largest killer among all ages, and the nation's most expensive health problem.[19] In the United States, the death rate for teenagers from trauma is nearly twice the worldwide average.[11, 31] Injuries are responsible for more than 60% of all childhood deaths and for 17% of all pediatric hospitalizations. In addition, for every traumatic childhood death, four children are permanently disabled, 10 require trauma center care, and another 100 are temporarily disabled.[13, 22]

There is now incontrovertible evidence that the implementation of trauma care systems reduces trauma-related deaths and disabling injuries to 10% or below, that trauma care as conventionally given at present results in preventable mortality rates of 20 to 55%, and that "appropriate medical care," specifically a trauma system with trauma centers, make a difference.[3, 5, 10, 21, 26, 28, 30] Evidence that a trauma center make a difference in patient outcomes is irrefutable.[30] However, although systems of trauma care have significantly decreased deaths from accidental injury in adults, a similar decrease has been shown in children only where pediatric trauma care systems have been developed.[2, 27]

Provision of optimal emergency care for the critically ill or injured child depends on the development of a comprehensive emergency care system with capabilities designed specifically for the unique needs of the child from the perspective of a consumer whose child's life is threatened. Such a system must facilitate networking among providers to ensure optimal utilization of regional capabilities for each critically injured child. The effects of injury, potential disability, and death due to trauma-related injury are far ranging. Although prevention of trauma through education of the child and the parents is the ultimate goal, the opportunity for rapid medical assessment and intervention is critical to the reduction of this disability and death. Care delivered to the injured child cannot and should not be the focus of a single discipline; rather, the goal should be an integrated multidisciplinary approach that requires constant commitment and reevaluation.

HISTORICAL PERSPECTIVES

The Civil War awakened the American medical profession to the need for improvement in medical care of the injured, and lessons learned in each subsequent war continued to improve the systems concept for trauma care.[6] In 1922 the American College of Surgeons, through its Committee on Fractures, now known as the Committee on Trauma, focused early attention on traumatic injuries and since then has waged a continuous campaign of professional and public education designed to achieve improvements in all phases of the care of the injured.[7] The landmark monograph "Accidental Death and Disability: The Neglected Disease of Modern Society" (1966) prompted a most intense focusing on the trauma issue, pointing out that accidental death and disability, a potentially preventable problem, represented a dilemma of epidemic proportions.[9]

In 1976, the Committee on Trauma of the American College of Surgeons published "Optimal Hospital Resources for Care of the Seriously Injured" and updated it in 1979 and 1983, when it was retitled "Hospital and Prehospital Resources for Optimal Care of the Injured Patient."[17, 18, 24] This document established the need for commitment on the part of surgeons and hospital administrators to the development of trauma centers, and it described the basic personnel and equipment requirements that would be necessary depending on the level of care to be made available. In 1969, Dr. James A. O'Neill was the first pediatric surgeon appointed to the Committee on Trauma of the American College of Surgeons, largely because it was recognized that trauma was the leading cause of death (as it is now) in children.[22] Dr. O'Neill's appointment was intended to ensure significant pediatric input into all "standard setting" and educational programs of the Committee on Trauma with regard to trauma, and these efforts are ongoing.

In 1985, Wolferth surveyed the present status of trauma center designation throughout the United States and found that a large number of the centers were concentrated in just three states (132 of 263). He concluded that the political and professional pressures at the state level have delayed the regionalization process, and a lack of any enabling legislation to correct this was obvious.[32]

TRAUMA SYSTEM ORGANIZATION

A thorough understanding of the systems approach to trauma is imperative if the successful development and implementation of trauma care are to be realized. A trauma care system may be defined as "an organized approach to acutely injured patients that provides personnel, facilities, and equipment for effective and coordinated trauma care in an appropriate geographical area under emergency conditions."[21] An effective, integrated response to the injured patient requires the commitment and participation of many individuals and diverse agencies or institutions, public and private, along with responsible medical professionals (in particular surgeons). All concerned must operate under the principle that people with severe injuries require special medical personnel and care facilities if they are to have their best chance of recovery.[6, 12]

The ideal system is composed of four primary components: (1) a method for system activation at the accident scene, or *access;* (2) patient rescue and evacuation, or *prehospital care;* (3) appropriate triage to a hospital that is organized and prepared to manage a wide variety of injuries, or *inhospital care;* and (4) rehabilitation after initial recovery so that the patient can return to useful activity or *rehabilitation.*[6, 11, 32]

Access. Access to the system involves alerting the appropriate agencies, which respond by dispatching personnel and vehicles to the scene. Technologic elements such as communications equipment, emergency telephone systems, and radio frequencies for emergency medical services communications to permit interaction between the prehospital personnel and the trauma center, as well as public education programs, are needed to ensure prompt and appropriate access to care. All individuals in the region must be aware of the existence of trauma centers, their location, and how to contact them to alert them that a patient is on the way. Appropriate facilities for children must be established, and parents and pediatricians must be aware of the location, existence, and expertise provided by such centers.

Prehospital Care. *Prehospital care* includes the acquisition and maintenance of order at the scene, the provision of specially equipped ambulances and trained emergency medical service personnel to administer life support and provide rapid transport of patients to trauma centers, the evacuation of patients using transport methods that are appropriate for the injuries, and the utilization of medical control when necessary. Triage procedures employed by emergency medical service personnel must be based on community plans that match patient needs with available resources. Because there is already a well-established emergency medical service system designed for the care of injured adults, it seems appropriate to use the same system for access of care for injured children.[23]

Inhospital Care. *Inhospital care* requires the arrangement of health care facilities for the most efficient provision of definitive care. Elaborate and technologically advanced facilities do not guarantee excellence in trauma care.[12] Specialized trauma facilities staffed by experienced and committed surgeons as well as other trained health care personnel, with priority access to sophisticated equipment and services, provide the quality of care needed to ensure that unnecessary death and disability are prevented. The trauma center is the hub of the trauma care system and, as such, must be prepared to meet any reasonable need 24 hours a day, 7 days a week. It must set community and regional standards for prehospital, emergency department, inhospital, and rehabilitative care.[21]

Within the hospital organization for children, there must be a defined trauma program director, certified by the American Board of Surgery with special competence in pediatric surgery and with appropriate certification in advanced trauma life support. The surgeon's role in the organization of the trauma system is crucial. By virtue of training in multisystem disease, the surgeon becomes a catalyst for change, a facilitator of communication, and a spokesperson for health care professionals with an interest in trauma. There is no more demanding task than that required of the trauma surgeon, who must exercise consistent and sensitive judgment in overseeing the continuing care of trauma patients.[12] Commitment is the most important qualification in the selection of surgeons as members of the trauma service. They must take postgraduate courses at a national level on a regular basis and must be willing to participate in teaching programs such as the advanced trauma life support course, preferably as an instructor.

Rehabilitation. Access to rehabilitation services is vital to minimize patient disability and its accompanying costs to society. Statistics indicate that only one in 10 severely injured patients has access to a rehabilitation service following initial treatment.[19] Consequently, a broad-based rehabilitation program that starts at the time of entry into the hospital is most important to the system's success.

Quality Assurance. *Evaluation of results* or *quality assurance* is another important aspect of the system after rescue. Quality assurance includes a comprehensive program that examines and evaluates the broader perspective of trauma system performance, including the specific evaluation of each individual trauma patient's care.[8] This includes much more than an examination of institutional performance; it requires the establishment of trauma system standards that outline the expectations of optimal trauma system performance. Quality assurance must evaluate the structural design and implementation of the system, identify a monitoring mechanism, audit the system and translate that audit into recommendations to the statutory authority for corrective action, if needed; implement further interventions, if needed, and recommend mechanisms to improve the system as identified.[29] Quality assurance, in essence, is the ''closing of the loop'' of trauma care.[25]

Design and Commitment. For any municipality, the design of a trauma care system requires recognition by the community that a need exists. The medical professionals, governmental agencies, and citizenry must share a mutual appreciation that trauma represents a significant public health problem, and all must be willing to address and solve the problem in an atmosphere of mutual respect.[12] The most effective community trauma programs share many characteristics; hence, a plan for trauma system development must use all personnel, equipment, and facilities in the region, and everyone involved must agree on the basic concept of the system. Then a responsible public agency, such as the Board for Licensing Health Care Facilities in Tennessee, usually assumes responsibility for implementation after legislation or proclamations by state government officials mandate the process.[7]

Wisdom and leadership on the part of surgeons and political leaders is necessary, and after the system is in place, continued effort to ensure adequate quality control and communication is essential. Expensive systems are frequently criticized, and the ability to respond to criticism with data and support from the community at large is crucial to maintaining an effective trauma system.[12]

A 1983 survey of emergency medical service directors to establish the extent of state-supported trauma center designation was repeated in 1986 to assess change. In 1983, 23 states had designated centers; in 1986, only 20 states had designated trauma centers, eight having discontinued designation and five new ones having adopted some form of designation. All 20 utilized the American College of Surgeons guidelines, although 10 had modified them, and only 13 were using state agencies to support the process. As of January 1988, there were only 37 level I trauma centers and 107 level II trauma centers in the United States, suggesting that designation as a political process has not been overly successful and may be responsible for the failure of trauma system development nationwide.[1]

PROBLEMS IN TRAUMA SYSTEM DEVELOPMENT

Various influences preclude the development of an ideal, universally effective trauma system.[12] Area geography may impose distances and natural obstacles that make effective evacuation difficult; low population densities may make absolute accident frequency low, resulting in poor maintenance of patient care skills by the health care team; and hospital location and availability of medical personnel may be less than ideal. However, political and economic influences, which lead to intrasystem competition and "turf" disputes, are the major processes that have retarded the development of centers of excellence for care of the trauma patient.

Political and Economic Influences

The development of optimal trauma care criteria and the determination by site review of an institution's compliance are quality care issues, should be developed and determined as such, and are "medical" processes. However, the designation of trauma centers and the implementation of trauma systems is a political process, usually reserved for state governments or agencies responsible for licensing hospital operations and professional personnel.[8, 21] The very nature of the designation and implementation process involves competition among hospitals, as systematization seemingly creates a franchise for a certain category of patients.[8] Problems arise if the designating body lacks the validity or the authority to control the system so that legal challenges and entanglements can stifle the process and thereby divert attention from the primary purpose of designation, which is to improve hospital capabilities to care for the injured.[21] Thus, state statutory and regulatory requirements are essential to ensure system integrity, and it is mandatory that they be articulated precisely by individuals intimately interested and involved in the process from the beginning—primarily the trauma surgeon, pediatric surgeon or otherwise.

Basic to the political problems of trauma center designation is the perception that positive financial incentives accrue to the facilities that achieve designation, whereas those that are not so designated are stigmatized.[21] This is a marketing issue. The establishment of any system becomes worrisome to hospital administrators and physicians alike, because they fear that there will be abuses, that patients who may not need expert trauma care will be "mistriaged" to a trauma center, and that this will have a negative impact on the economics of undesignated hospitals.[30] These economic constraints should not be the overriding issue for effective triage. Lack of information and lack of understanding of the intentions of the proponents of trauma center designation lead to mistrust, suspicion, and delays in the process. For example, terms commonly used and often misunderstood are *overtriage,* which is the incorrect identification of someone as a major trauma patient who is not, and *undertriage,* which is the incorrect identification of a patient who has a serious injury as one who does not.[10] Overtriage is a political problem; it will deliver patients without serious injuries to the trauma center, potentially altering the economic and utilization processes of the facility. Undertriage is a medical problem; it results in deaths that should be preventable. In the design of any trauma system, it is a cardinal principle that the triage method

should err on the side of overtriage and that undertriage should be kept to a minimum.[10] Lack of true understanding of the intent of the system hampers its acceptance.

Modern triage techniques make it possible to achieve relatively accurate triage, but any triage decision is necessarily imprecise because of biologic variability, the short time between injury and evaluation by the paramedic, and the difficulty of diagnosing thoracic and abdominal injuries in the field, particularly in children.[10] The accuracy of a triage method is defined by its *sensitivity,* the fraction of injured patients correctly identified by the triage method adopted, and *specificity,* those patients not seriously injured and correctly identified by the triage method used.[10] A given triage method should maximize both the sensitivity and the specificity and therefore minimize overtriage and undertriage. When correctly applied to the injured child, this would accurately identify the 25% who should be seen at the highest level pediatric trauma center and the 75% who do not require such care.[25]

The concerns have been largely disproved. Cales and colleagues demonstrated that redistribution of a very small patient group of the seriously injured who were indeed triaged to an appropriate trauma center had improved outcome and caused negligible effects on the overall utilization of emergency units and hospitals.[4, 5] Jacobs confirmed that caring for patients with multisystem injuries costs the hospital more than it is reimbursed for by diagnosis-related groups.[20] Despite these findings, hospitals continue to request designation based on interests other than care of the injured, and in some states, efforts have been made to block the process of trauma center designation altogether.

Despite the fact that the American College of Surgeons is recognized as the leader in promoting appropriate standards of care for categorization and designation of hospital facilities designed for trauma patients, many board-certified surgeons and fellows of the American College of Surgeons are and remain unenlightened, uninformed, and therefore inexperienced in modern up-to-date critical trauma care. Consequently, they often are influenced by the busyness of their practices and the perceived threat of the trauma system as promulgated by their hospital administrators. In addition, because of their usually excellent proficiency in most other aspects of their practice they do not appear to recognize possible deficiencies in trauma care in their respective institutions.

Training in trauma care techniques has also been led by the American College of Surgeons through its Committee on Trauma, which has developed a continuing education course that stresses the understanding of trauma pathophysiology and life-saving techniques, the very popular and important advanced trauma life support course (now under the leadership of a pediatric surgeon, Dr. Max Ramenofsky). The effect of these efforts on outcome is not entirely known, but present indications point to a consistent positive influence on results. However, the majority of participants in these courses are emergency physicians, not private general surgeons, whose participation is lacking. Because it is believed that a surgeon should lead the trauma team, improved care, the categorization and designation of trauma centers, and the system of trauma management will likely fail without a concentrated effort to improve the education of practicing surgeons who are now so ably accomplishing other aspects of their professions.

"Turf" Disputes

Another challenge to the development of appropriate trauma systems has come from those who also consider themselves advocates for the welfare of children. As the number of pediatricians has increased, their objectives and interests have been redirected in numerous areas, among which is that of critical care. Pediatricians have long been viewed as advocates for the child, and the critically injured child has benefited from the increased attention, research, and concentrated care that has resulted from these changing interests. Although most recognize the importance of a multidisciplinary approach to the management of these patients whose lives are potentially threatened, some have generated concern and unnecessary conflict among primary care providers for the injured child by promoting themselves as the most appropriate primary caregivers. In an article arguing for improved emergency medical service care for children, an all-inclusive paragraph eliminated all of the usual trained and experienced trauma providers and advocated primary assessment and management by others, many of whom are neither trained nor experienced in trauma or surgery.[2] Haller addressed these conclusions from sound surgical success and emphasized that life-threatening trauma—indeed that 25% referred to earlier—is a surgical disease: "thus, initial surgical evaluation is essential."[14] It is important to note that he addressed *life-threatening* trauma and not simply trauma, because some of the confusion regarding who should treat trauma patients is related to the affirmation that 90% of all pediatric trauma can and should be looked after by pediatricians. This statement probably is accurate if one considers all lacerations, abrasions, contusions, and other minor injuries of children who are seen in private offices and emergency departments and then released. However, this statement does not apply to injured children admitted to hospital who fit into the potential life-threatening category, for whom surgical input and management is mandatory.

Fortunately, wise and more perceptive physicians are prevailing in pediatric emergency medicine and have recognized the importance and ongoing success of the surgeon's role. They are not threatened by it, yet at the same time have carved out an important place for themselves in this area by working closely with surgeons in developing a team approach that is in the best interests of the child. This is commendable, for it is my opinion that there is no place in the care of critically injured children for competition among care providers. Not enough of us can do it the way it should be done without cooperation from our colleagues in pediatric emergency medicine or from our intensivist colleagues in the critical care unit. As surgeons, we should direct the care and lead the team by "informed" consensus and by professional agreement, which is reached hopefully by reasoning and not by imposition.

The public is similarly uninformed as to the costs, dangers, and societal impact of trauma, a fact that is partially attributed to at least two deeply ingrained features of the American personality. Americans are typically guardians of individual liberty and freedom of choice to the unfortunate extreme of protecting the rights of individuals to harm themselves, a fact that is graphically displayed in the mortality records of states that have repealed laws requiring motorcyclists to wear helmets.[12] Also, people view accidents as isolated events that involve only those who are injured. An increased awareness of the costs of trauma to society is essential because the solution to the problem of trauma may require some restrictions on individual freedoms. An integrated system of community awareness, progressive legislation, improved trauma education, and hospital categorization and designation that is pursued vigorously as a national imperative will ameliorate the public's perception of trauma as a health issue.

SUCCEEDING IN SYSTEM DEVELOPMENT

Much can be accomplished through the work of the American College of Surgeons and its Committee on Trauma, the American Pediatric Surgical Association and its Committee on Trauma, the Surgical Section of the American Academy of Pediatrics, and the American College of Emergency Physicians. However, the effectiveness of these groups ultimately rests with their members and their commitment to play an early role in attempting to influence and effect the process of system development, particularly in the critical early stages of development of regional systems of trauma care that can have a positive impact on surgical practice.

It is indeed unfortunate that many politicians and government functionaries believe that physicians are less vocal in regard to political matters than other members of the general community. We have good reasons to become involved in this process, for we should know that health care has become a strategically important socioeconomic matter, both de facto and politically, and that the influence and impact of government on physician practice is important and critical. As physicians and members of the general community, we actually have a built-in role of special importance in governmental health care policy and decisions. We must get involved, at whatever level necessary, to influence the process in a positive manner.

To do this, we must meet the players early, positively, honestly, and—most important—knowledgeably and reasonably. We must establish and maintain credibility, establish regular and ongoing communication, be proactive and not reactive, know our allies and our adversaries, and keep in mind several "don'ts."[15, 16]

Establish and Maintain Credibility

A director's or a potential director's personal viewpoints and recommendations can be most productive in the early developmental stages of the political process. As the process proceeds, it becomes increasingly difficult to effect changes, so early involvement is important. As soon as possible, identify the issue being addressed in an organized and brief manner. Briefness is important in written correspondence, but for the initial contact, be prepared to take whatever time is necessary to educate those you are addressing. Be personal, informative, honest, and, very important, be reasonable. Know the facts, particularly background information, such as where the important national societies like the American Pediatric Surgical Association and the American College of Surgeons Committee on Trauma stand on the issues, what the optimal standards or needs are considered to be, what the specific regions and their problems within your state or area consist of, and what the resources already in place include. One's personal and professional reasons for opinions and advice, which are based on experience, knowledge, understanding, and judgment, are important, and they must be presented objectively.

If possible, know the views and opinions of those being addressed before meeting them, but as this may be difficult, one should certainly have some inclination of where they stand after your meeting. It helps greatly when addressing politicians, or more specifically political appointees and their staffs, to know what has happened in the past, that is, the history of the issue in your state. Most politicians and their appointees and staffs and the public at large may suspect one's intentions, but one's personal opinions and recommendations, if reasonable, receptive, and honestly amenable to the political process of compromise in working toward an acceptable system, will be well received. In Tennessee, the appointment of a Pediatric Task Force to study and develop the system was the initial undertaking, and the state's pediatric surgeons were intimately involved in the process. Individually, a sincere effort was undertaken to present the issues objectively and to avoid recommending specific endpoints but at the same time to discuss all the issues, pro and con. In addition, physicians should openly and honestly indicate a willingness to consider reasonable, negotiable, and alternative recommendations and to work toward an acceptable compromise rather than to become involved in a nonadjustable debate and eventual political defeat.

Know the opposition; there may be more common issues than one thinks, but it is extremely important to understand the opposition's views. Every issue has at least two sides; be prepared to respond to the opposing viewpoint. In expressing opposition and the reasons for it, be tactful to avoid presenting a case that, for the most part, is a series of complaints. This is extremely important when addressing or educating politicians or government appointees; they want to do the right thing for their constituents but will quickly see through self-serving efforts that may significantly downgrade the presenter's personal credibility.

Establish Regular and Ongoing Communication

It is mutually worthwhile and desirable to develop a professional relationship on a personal and friendly basis with the players, particularly with political office holders, their appointees, and their staffs. It is unwise to approach them for the first time when you want something. Develop a rapport

beforehand; as a recognized individual, they will welcome and appreciate your availability, professional knowledge, and expertise relative to specific (perhaps general) health care matters with which they must deal, and your opinions and recommendations on matters of your personal concern will be more carefully and favorably considered. To have more meaningful conversations, educate them by being familiar with the process of developing the system from start to regulation. Maintain communications on matters with which you agree as well as disagree, being as brief as possible yet being complete. Express your views periodically on subjects other than those that are of medical interest. Compliment them sincerely when appropriate, and thank them. Recognized efforts with positive outcomes build relationships, and these are immensely important in the process.

Be Proactive, Not Reactive

Have a position or plan of action with alternative solutions if possible. State your case as positively as possible; if there are special personal reasons for some recommendations, say so, and if they are clear, rational, and merit justification they will be treated favorably. Avoid taking a self-serving position. Keep in mind that politicians and their appointees are looking for political solutions, and they can be found, so be an advocate. Again, be reasonable. Reasonableness often means compromise, but with alternative solutions already considered, acceptable options will be available.

Don'ts

Don't be afraid to defend or to debate an issue, but don't be argumentative or too quick to call attention to, amend, or compromise negative standards or regulations that are already on the books. "Let sleeping dogs lie." People do not appreciate illumination of possible weaknesses; tactfully oppose those with which you do not agree. Don't deliver ultimatums or be threatening, and don't compromise or "make deals" too quickly. Be firm about your convictions.

Don't inform the players about something they already know. Educate them, remember to take the time to be informative and helpful, tell them something they don't know and suggest how they might act to solve their problems, but base what you say on fact and experience and back it up with data. The opposition usually does not have data, just opinion that is often self-serving and can usually be seen for what it is. Don't feel you have to "do something." Sometimes the best approach is to remain neutral; the hardest thing is to do nothing. If your players are well informed and they participate, positive and constructive solutions will develop, but the players must be well informed.

Know Your Allies (and Adversaries)

The most important step in establishing constructive, attainable, and optimal standards that will become regulations is to know the players; without this knowledge you are doomed to frustration and probable failure.

In addition to educated and informed colleagues, particularly those responsible for developing the standards, a most powerful ally is the political person's constituents; the patients and the public. Make the patient and the quality of care top priorities. Educate the regulators regarding the impact of your views on the public: they are most responsive to them. At the same time, communication with local public interest and consumer groups can be helpful as can a relationship with the local media in the hope that appropriate views will be presented to the public fairly. Although the media view their reporting as nonbiased, it frequently is oriented toward sensationalism (particularly the headlines), is incomplete, and does not represent the views of all parties accurately, which can result in misinformation that is confusing to the public and that exacerbates the adversarial relations that already exist with opponents of the system. Experience has shown that if the message is presented accurately, the public *will* understand and will insist on care in the appropriate facility.

The most difficult step in the entire process, one that is seemingly fraught with legal entanglements, has been the political process of designation, also known as ''getting started.'' After 7 years, Tennessee's pediatric trauma center component was accomplished in just over 6 months, a document that addressed level I and level II pediatric trauma centers. This document contained an abridged version or checklist of regulations that is supported by a detailed version modeled after the Pennsylvania standards for pediatric trauma centers but appropriately adapted for Tennessee. No institution in the state that cared for the critically injured child could meet those criteria. However, with the knowledge and consent of the administrative powers in the participating institutions, the recommended regulations purposely included what were believed to be optimal standards, as good as or better than other state and national standards available for comparison, recognizing that all institutions would have to upgrade to meet the criteria. In the 5 years since these criteria were adopted, only one center has succeeded in reaching these standards.

Although the designation process is unquestionably the most difficult step, medical control is the next battle and is also extremely important. However, regardless of the outcome, a true system will be in place only if it includes strict quality assurance in its regulations and closes the loop for trauma care, for then the data generated and contributed to by mandate will expose the deficiencies and point toward correction.

References

1. Aprahamian C, Wolferth CC Jr, Weitzel-DeVeas C, et al: Status of trauma center designation. Presented at Eastern Association for the Surgery of Trauma. Longboat Key, Florida, January 1988. J Trauma 29(5):566–570, 1989.
2. Bushore M: Emergency care of the child. Pediatrics 79:572–576, 1987.
3. Cales RH: Trauma mortality in Orange County: The effect of implementation on a regional trauma system. Ann Emerg Med 13:1–10, 1984.
4. Cales RH, Anderson PG, Heilig RW: Utilization of medical care in Orange County: The effect of implementation of a regional trauma system. Ann Emerg Med 14:853–858, 1985.
5. Cales RH, Trunkey DD: Preventable trauma deaths. A review of trauma care systems development. JAMA 254:1059–1063, 1985.
6. Cleveland HC: Trauma center designation. In: Mattox K, Moore EE, Feliciano D (eds): Trauma. East Norwalk, Conn, Appleton & Lange, 1988, pp 45–52.
7. Committees on Trauma, American College of Surgeons: Blue Book. Chicago, American College of Surgeons, 1982.
8. Cooper GF, Murrin P, Sheridan-McArdle M: Advances in quality assurance. In: Maull KI (ed): Advances in Trauma. Vol. 2. Chicago, Year Book, 1987, pp 1–20.
9. Division of Medical Sciences: Accidental Death and Disability: The Neglected Disease of Modern Society. Washington, DC, National Academy of Sciences / National Research Council, 1966.
10. Eastman AB, Lewis FR, Champion HR, et al: Regional trauma system designation. Am J Surg 154:79–86, 1987.
11. Flint LM, Flint CB: Evolution, design, and implementation of trauma systems. In: Zuidema G, Rutherford R, Ballinger W (eds): The Management of Trauma. Philadelphia, WB Saunders, 1985, pp 787–800.
12. Flint LM, Richardson JD: Organization for trauma care. In: Richardson JD, Polk HC, Flint LM (eds): Trauma: Clinical Care and Pathophysiology. Chicago, Year Book, 1987, pp 5–12.
13. Guyer B, Gallagher SS: An approach to the epidemiology of childhood injuries. Pediatr Clin North Am 32:5–15, 1985.
14. Haller JA: Emergency medical services for children: What is the pediatric surgeon's role? Pediatrics 79:576–581, 1987.
15. Haug JN: Getting involved in the legislative process. Am Coll Surg Bull 73:56, 1988.
16. Hershey SG: Tips on how to write your congressman. Concern, News Magazine of the Society of Critical Care Medicine, Winter 1988, p 10.
17. Hospital and prehospital resources for optimal care of the injured patient. Am Coll Surg Bull 68(10):11, 1983.
18. Hospital resources for optimal care of the injured patient. Am Coll Surg Bull 64(9):8, 1979.
19. Injury in America. A Continuing Public Health Problem. Committee on Trauma Research, Commission on Life Sciences, National Research Council and the Institute of Medicine, Washington, DC, National Academy Press, 1985.
20. Jacobs LM: The effect of prospective reimbursement on trauma patients. Am Coll Surg Bull 70:17–20, 1985.
21. Maull KI, Schwab CW, McHenry SD, et al: Trauma center verification. J Trauma 26:521–524, 1986.
22. National Safety Council: Accident Facts. Chicago, National Safety Council, 1987.
23. O'Neill JA: Trauma care organization for children. In: Buntain W: Management of Pediatric Trauma. Philadelphia, WB Saunders, 1994.
24. Optimal hospital resources for care of the seriously injured. Am Coll Surg Bull 64(9):8, 1976.
25. Ramenofsky ML: Pediatric trauma system components. J Pediatr Surg, in press. (Presented at 19th Annual Meeting of the American Pediatric Surgical Association. Tucson, Arizona, May 11, 1988.)
26. Ramenofsky ML, Luterman A, Quindlen E, et al: Maximum survival in pediatric trauma: The ideal system. J Trauma 24:818–823, 1984.
27. Ramenofsky ML, Morse TS: Standards of care for the critically injured pediatric patient. J Trauma 22:921–933, 1982.
28. Shackford SR, Hollingworth-Fridlund P, Cooper GF, et al: The effect of regionalization upon the quality of trauma care as assessed by concurrent audit before and after institution of a trauma system. J Trauma 26:921–933, 1982.
29. Trunkey DD: Presidential address: On the nature of things that go bang in the night. Surgery 92:123–132, 1982.
30. Trunkey DD: Regionalization of trauma services. In: Hurst J (ed): Common Problems in Trauma. Chicago, Year Book, 1987, pp 23–27.
31. U.S. National Center for Health Statistics: Monthly Vital Statistics Report: Advance Report, Final Mortality Statistics, 1976, Vol. 26, No. 11 Supplement, U.S. Dept. of Health, Education and Welfare. Washington, DC, U.S. Government Printing Office, 1978.
32. Wolferth C: Report, trauma center designation. Dallas, Texas. Committee on Trauma. Am Coll Surg Bull 68(10):11, 1985.

Resuscitation and Stabilization

CHAPTER SIX

Triage, Trauma Scores, and Transport

Triage is a word of French derivation defined as "the sorting and allocation of treatment to patients according to a system of priorities designed to maximize the number of survivors." Nowhere is this concept more appropriate than in the care of the injured child. Approximately one out of every four pediatric trauma victims sustains an injury severe enough to require the specialized care and the unique resources available at a pediatric trauma center.[29] Identifying these patients and transporting them safely and expediently are clearly the keys to improved survival and outcome.

With the evolution of regional trauma systems, increasing emphasis has been placed on the means whereby patients gain access to various levels of care. Specific concern that the most severely injured patients are identified and transported quickly to the most comprehensive facilities and that those with minor injuries do not detract from this function has been one of the most compelling reasons for the development of reliable and efficient mechanisms of triage.[37]

In many respects, triage is the catalyst of a regional trauma system. It not only governs the flow of patients within the system, but also ensures that expensive resources are utilized in a manner than benefits the most patients at the least cost. This should then yield better outcomes, both in decreased mortality and in better quality of life for survivors. Health care dollars will be better spent, and costs will be better controlled. The penalty to a system for overtriage is maldistribution for resources and unacceptably expensive care. The effect of undertriage on a system is limitation of adequate care, unacceptably high mortality, and wastage of human potential.

These problems become even more acute when applied to the pediatric patient. Because children account for approximately one fourth of trauma victims, a regional pediatric trauma referral center must serve a population base approximately three times that of an adult center. With the exception of a very few large urban ares, this expanded service area requires transport considerations that involve significant distances and other geographic factors. Effective triage must then match the proper patient with the appropriate facility, must ensure expeditious transport, and must function with consistent reliability so that patient need and only patient need is the determinant of flow within a regional trauma system.

TRIAGE TECHNIQUE

Proper distribution of patients within a trauma system begins with initial assessment, either at the scene or in a receiving hospital. This assessment should follow a scheme that is simple, reproducible, and reliable, and, most important, one that minimizes the potential for undertriage. Rather than rely on any single factor, it should be the result of an application of multiple considerations that include primarily common sense, critical historical factors, and careful clinical assessment.

Common sense, although apparently self-evident, is the necessary override that allows system access to any patient who has reasonable potential for injury regardless of initial findings or mechanism of injury. It implies the need for occasional special considerations of unusual regional factors such as geography, weather, traffic, or the infrequent need for immediate transfer to regional centers of single specialty care. The majority of injured children, however, can be evaluated according to any one of a number of straightforward protocols that indicate correct disposition most of the time.[36] Consequently a major focus of research in pediatric trauma care has been the development and evaluation of a system that also is the most reliable and reproducible and obviously the most accurate.

TRAUMA SCORES

Trauma scoring as a mechanism of triage is a recent continuum of a longstanding attempt by medical researchers to develop means whereby simple assessment protocols can reliably predict outcome, resource utilization, or other important health care factors.[12–15, 23] The overall goal of scoring for any clinical problem is improved accuracy in stratification of patients for clinical care. In addition, monitoring of patients as they progress through various phases of resuscitation and therapy and prediction of survival and optimization of criteria for utilization of resources are all potential goals of scoring systems.[19] Also the evaluation of quality of care, quantity of care, and outcome are all potential applications for reliable quantification of injury severity or survival potential.[22, 31]

Abbreviated Injury Severity Scale

Scoring systems as applied to trauma patients first began with the development of the *Abbreviated Injury Severity (AIS)* scale by the Committee on Medical Aspects of Automotive Safety in 1971.[11] This particular quantification scheme was an attempt to relate degree of impact injury to a numeric stratification that would be predictive of survival and potentially applicable to the development of standards of care. Although this scaling system was intended to address individual injuries, it has served as the foundation for other methods to evaluate multiply injured patients.

Injury Severity Score

The *Injury Severity Score (ISS)*, developed by Baker, is the most commonly used system of multiple injury assessment and consists of the sum of the squares of the highest AIS codes in each of the three most severely injured body regions.[5] Baker and colleagues evaluated this technique in 2128 multiply injured patients and confirmed a direct relationship between increasing ISS and both mortality and disability. The study group consisted of similar patients from Baltimore, Maryland, and Birmingham, England, and documented the same ISS mortality-disability relationship in both populations.[4] A potential shortcoming of this system is the suggested equivalence of mortality potential for similar AIS scores from different anatomic regions. This problem is especially germane to pediatric injury in which cen-

Table 6-1
Correlation of MISS Neurologic Score with Morbidity and Mortality

MISS Neurologic Score (Glasgow Coma Scale Score)	
5 (≤4)	100% either disabled or dead
4 (5–8)	No mortality—40% disabled
3 (9–12)	No mortality—40% disabled
2 (13–14)	
1 (15)	All normal

MISS, Modified injury severity score.

tral nervous system trauma accounts for two thirds of all deaths.[12, 38]

Modified Injury Severity Score

Mayer and colleagues addressed this problem by developing the *Modified Injury Severity Score* (*MISS*), wherein the AIS score assigned to the head region is related to the initial Glasgow Coma Scale (Table 6–1) rather than the AIS code for the head region.[20, 26] Although this provided an assessment system that was more specific to children, it was still a retrospective score with minimal relevance to triage.[27]

Anatomic Index of Injury Severity and Trauma Score

In 1980, Champion and associates reported their study of a large population of multiply injured patients in which individual injury diagnoses, as coded by the hospital adaptation of the International Classification of Diseases and Accidents (HICDA)-8, were analyzed with regard to the probability of mortality both as single injuries and as factors in combination with other injury factors.[9] This produced the *Anatomic Index of Injury Severity* (*AISS*), which was intended to define retrospectively the severity of injury by objective assessment of the probability of mortality. In an attempt to develop a prospective simple physiologic scoring scheme that would be applicable to field assessment and impact on prehospital triage care, this group developed the *Trauma Score* (*TS*), which consisted of assessment of respiratory rate, respiratory effort, systolic blood pressure, capillary refill, and Glasgow Coma Scale (Table 6–2).[8]

This particular scoring system was intended to be a simple means of initial field assessment that would indicate which patients could be correctly triaged to a trauma center. Morris and co-workers evaluated this scoring system in 1872 patients by comparing the trauma score calculated in

Table 6-2
Trauma Score

Respiratory rate		10–24	4
		25–35	3
		>35	2
		0–9	1 ———
Respiratory effect		Normal	1
		Shallow, reactive	0 ———
Systolic blood pressure		>90	4
		70–90	4
		50–69	3
		<50	2
			1
		No carotid pulse	0 ———
Capillary refill		Normal	2
		Delayed	1
		Absent	0 ———
Glasgow Coma Scale (GCS)			
Eye opening			
Spontaneous	4		
To voice	3		
To pain	2		
None	1		
Verbal response			
Oriented	5		
Confused	4		
Inappropriate words	3		
Incomprehensible words	2		
None	1		
Motor response			
Obeys commands	6		
Localizes	5		
Withdraws	4	Total GCS Points	
Abnormal flexion	3	14–15	5
Abnormal extension	2	11–13	4
None	1	8–10	3
		5–7	2
		3–4	1 ———
Total GCS Points	———		
		TOTAL TRAUMA SCORE	———

Table 6–3

Comparison of Sensitivity and Specificity of Two Levels of Field Trauma Scores (TS₁) as Indicator of Potentially Life-Threatening Injury*

	Number of Patients	
	$TS_1 \leq 14$	$TS_1 \leq 12$
False-negative	66	102
True-positive	114	78
True-negative	812	890
False-positive	107	29
Sensitivity (%)	63.33	43.33
Specificity (%)	88.36	96.84
Accuracy (%)	84.26	88.08

*Defined as Injury Severity Score of 20 or more.

the field by paramedics to that calculated on arrival at the trauma center.[28] Utilizing the ISS as a quantitative indicator of degree of injury, the sensitivity and specificity of the TS was calculated utilizing an ISS of higher than 20 as indicative of severe injury requiring trauma center admission and triage. Table 6–3 summarizes the results of that investigation and indicates that utilization of the TS, although conceptually of significant value, was neither reproducible nor accurate in identifying trauma patients who required triage to trauma centers.[28]

Trauma Injury Severity Score

Despite its limited function as a true prehospital triage tool, the trauma score has been recommended as a component of an assessment scheme designed to evaluate outcome potential. The *Trauma Injury Severity Score* (*TRISS*) was developed as a result of analysis of the relationship between the TS and the ISS.[6, 16] These studies documented a negative correlation between the TS and the ISS and suggested that the survival potential for any patient could be calculated by the application of a logistic regression formula utilizing the TS, the ISS, and the patient's age as the only variables. The cumulative survival potential in any group of patients could then be used for comparison with national norms, thereby providing an evaluation of outcome and a potential assessment of quality of care.

CRAMS Scale

The inconsistent performance of the TS as a true triage tool stimulated the development of the CRAMS scale as a more simple and effective triage protocol.[18] This 10-point scale is the acronym of its five constituent components, which are *C*ardiac, *r*espiratory, *a*bdominal, *m*otor, and *s*ensory functions. Each of these is given a score of 0, 1, or 2 (Table 6–4). This concept was initially evaluated by analysis of 500 paramedic trauma transports during which both the CRAMS scale and the TS were calculated in the field. The patients were then evaluated retrospectively and graded into minor, intermediate, or major injury categories determined on the basis of emergency department disposition. This

study documented a sensitivity for the CRAMS score of 92% and a specificity of 98%. Unfortunately, the criteria for determination of injury gradation were different from those used in Morris's study. Gormican defined major trauma patients as those who required immediate operative intervention by general or neurosurgery and identified a 92% accuracy rate for the CRAMS score compared with a 67% accuracy rate for the TS.

This improvement in function was further documented by Clemmer and colleagues, who analyzed the use of the CRAMS score as a triage tool in the Salt Lake County Trauma System.[10] They modified the scoring protocol by adding a respiratory rate greater than 35 breaths per minute as an extra criterion and confirmed a high degree of accuracy in prediction of severe injury as well as a reliability in the identification of patients that required transport to a level I trauma center.[10] Unfortunately, the improved triage function of the CRAMS score has been offset by generalized criticism of the criteria used for gradation of the abdominal component. Quantification of tenderness can be an extremely subjective process and, therefore, may introduce a wide variance in score accuracy. Nevertheless, the CRAMS concept appears to be a more effective triage tool than the initial TS and is continuing to be evaluated in many regions throughout the county.

Revised Trauma Score

In 1982 the Multiple Trauma Outcome Study was begun through the efforts of Champion and colleagues under the auspices of the Committee on Trauma of the American College of Surgeons.[6] This project has produced a large database oriented specifically to outcome from multiple in-

Table 6–4

Field Categorization of Trauma—CRAMS Scale

Components	Score
Circulation	
Normal capillary refill and systolic blood pressure (BP) >100	2
Delayed capillary refill or BP <85–100	1
No capillary refill or BP <85	0
Respirations	
Normal	2
Abnormal (labored or shallow)	1
Absent	0
Abdomen	
Abdomen and thorax nontender	2
Abdomen or thorax tender	1
Abdomen rigid or flail chest*	0
Motor	
Normal	2
Responds only to pain (other than decerebrate)	1
No response (or decerebrate)	0
Speech	
Normal	2
Confused	1
No intelligible words	0
Score ≤8 = Major Trauma	
Score ≥9 = Minor Trauma	

*"Penetrating wounds to the abdomen or thorax" has been added after the study.

Table 6–5
Revised Trauma Score (RTS)

Glasgow Coma Scale (GCS)	Systolic Blood Pressure (BP) (mm Hg)	Respiratory Rate (RR) (min)	Code Value
13–15	89	10–29	4
9–12	76–89	29	3
6–8	50–75	6–9	2
4–5	1–49	1–5	1
3	0	0	0
Weight: 0.9368	0.7326	0.2908	

Field RTS, Sum of coded value of GCS, BP, and RR (integer 1–12).
Weighted RTS, Sum of coded value × weight − (real number 0–8).

jury. Initial evaluation of the TS of patients entered into this study indicated that revision of the score and elimination of respiratory effort and capillary refill would possibly improve specificity and sensitivity and simplify application. The *Revised Trauma Score* (*RTS*) was thus developed (Table 6–5).[2] It is a more simplified scaling system, which suggests that any patient whose Glasgow Coma Scale, respiratory rate, or systolic blood pressure is categorized as lower than 4 should be triaged to a trauma center. This RTS has likewise been reanalyzed in regard to its function as a component in the TRISS methodology, and a set of normative standards and constants for quantification of survival potential have been developed (Table 6–6). The accuracy of the RTS as a triage tool is presently undergoing evaluation both as a single element of field assessment and as a component of an algorithmic protocol that includes consideration of mechanisms of injury and specific anatomic indices in calculating ultimate triage disposition (Fig. 6–1).[2]

Pediatric Trauma Score

The *Pediatric Trauma Score* (*PTS*) was developed in 1984 in an attempt to improve the accuracy of triage scoring systems' application to the pediatric patient.[36] Most of the trauma scores that had been developed and tested before this time focused primarily on adult trauma patients and were insensitive to many of the unique patterns and characteristics of childhood injury. As a result of this, and as a result of frustrations in applying the adult trauma scores to pediatric patients, a scoring system was devised that considered six components common to the pediatric trauma patient and used them to categorize three degrees of injury (Table 6–7). This system was designed both to segregate the pediatric population by identifying the infant and toddler as a separate group and to focus on initial management

problems by addressing the airway status in a manner that included the results of initial therapeutic intervention. The system was initially evaluated by comparing its scores with patient ISSs calculated retrospectively in a group of injured children treated at a level I trauma center.[35] Further documentation of the relationship between the PTS and the ISS was confirmed in a study of the first 615 children entered into the National Pediatric Trauma Registry.[37] Each of these studies identified a potential cutoff point, suggesting that a PTS of 8 and below was indeed indicative of severe injury and potential for mortality, whereas a PTS of 9 and above identified minor injuries and patients in whom survival was essentially guaranteed. Ramenofsky and co-workers evaluated the predictive validity of the PTS by analyzing 452 injured children transported to trauma centers in South Alabama.[30] They were able to confirm a specificity and sensitivity rate of 98% and 95%, respectively, and more important, to confirm again that children whose PTS fell below 8 were those clearly at risk of dying. Additional studies by Jubelirer and Aprahamian and colleagues have indicated that the PTS does effectively predict which children require trauma center admission and, likewise, can indicate which children should be referred to specific trauma centers after initial stabilization at receiving hospitals.[3, 21] Also, with regard to application of the PTS as a field triage device, Ford and colleagues have reported its use in an urban trauma region and have documented its accuracy both in predicting patients who require trauma center admission and in indicating ultimate level of severity of injury.[17]

Application of the PTS is a very simple process with minimal potential for interrater error. Ramenofsky's group used an interactive computer teaching program to educate and train prehospital personnel and referring physicians within the University of South Alabama trauma region. Their excellent reliability studies clearly document the effect of this effort and emphasize the importance of good educational communication between a trauma center and its prehospital and referring components.

In regard to the specific score components, patient size is self-evident and is primarily intended to identify the injured infant as a patient with a higher potential for mortality as a result of immaturity and small size. Airway assessment is designed to focus on the difficulties of obtaining adequate endotracheal airway control in the pediatric patient. By categorizing all patients who require any type of manipulation intended to provide direct endotracheal intubation into

Table 6–6
Revised Coefficients for New Outcome Norms

	b_0	b_1	b_2	b_3
Blunt	−1.2470	0.9544	−0.0768	−1.9052
Penetrating	−0.6029	1.1430	−0.1516	−2.6676

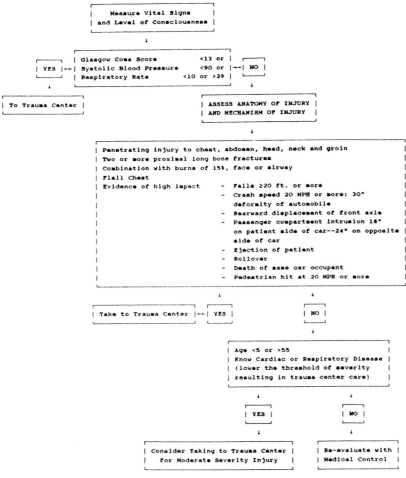

FIGURE 6–1

Table decision scheme.

a category of maximum risk, the potential for difficulties in managing this problem becomes a consideration in patient triage. Furthermore, by identifying those children whose airways are perfectly normal and who require no extraneous support as a separate subgroup, the opposite end of this spectrum becomes a positive consideration in the triage mechanism. Evaluation of level of consciousness instead of the entire Glasgow Coma Scale takes into consideration the problem of accurate assessment of the proverbial child.[24] Because level of consciousness is the primary and most

Table 6–7
Pediatric Trauma Score (PTS)

Component	Category		
	+2	**+1**	**−1**
Size	≥20 kg	10–20 kg	<10 kg
Airway	Normal	Maintainable	Unmaintainable
Systolic blood pressure (BP)	≥90	90–50 mm Hg	<50 mm Hg
Central nervous system	Awake	Obtunded/Loss of consciousness	Coma/Decerebrate
Open wound	None	Minor	Major/Penetrating
Skeletal	None	Closed fracture	Open/Multiple fractures
		Sum_____(PTS)	

If proper-sized BP cuff is not available, BP can be assessed by assigning the following values: +2, Pulse palpable at wrist; +1, pulse palpable at groin; −1, no pulse palpable.
Modified from Tepas JJ III, Alexander RH, Campbell JD, et al: An improved scoring system for assessment of the injured child. J Trauma 25:720–724, 1985.

accurate indicator of potential brain injury, its use as a simple assessment tool is appropriate.[34]

Systolic blood pressure is utilized as the assessment method for cardiovascular function primarily because of the great variation in heart rate that may occur in the pediatric patient. Age, body temperature, stress, and evolving hypovolemia can have a direct effect on heart rate. Systolic blood pressure, however, is an interaction of cardiac function with peripheral resistance and thereby provides a more objective criteria for evaluation. In the absence of an appropriate blood pressure cuff for different-sized patients, the presence of a palpable pulse at either the wrist or the groin can provide an accurate substitute for assessment of this modality.

The presence of a skeletal fracture has been documented to increase significantly the potential for mortality in the child. Because skeletal injury is an extremely common component of pediatric polytrauma, consideration of this in the initial assessment of the patient is paramount. A simple clinical examination is frequently all that is needed to indicate the presence of a fracture that affects immediate and ultimate survival. Accordingly, the assessment scheme is designed to identify this and specifically to segregate children with open or multiple fractures as a category most at increased risk for mortality or potential increased morbidity.[7]

In addition, the consideration of cutaneous injury allows for inclusion of common concomitant penetrating injuries in children whose primary mechanism of trauma is blunt deceleration. It likewise allows consideration of the potentially devastating effect of major tissue loss, avulsion injuries, or deep penetrating injuries caused by assault.

The ability of the PTS to identify severe injury has been assessed by evaluating the National Pediatric Trauma Registry and comparing the specificity and sensitivity of the PTS in its ability to predict ISS. A review of mortality rates for patients cohorted by gradation of ISS demonstrated an increasing mortality that began at zero for an ISS of less than 15 and reached 100% for an ISS of 40. An ISS of more than 15 was thus considered indicative of potentially severe injury and resulted in a PTS specificity of 65% and a sensitivity of 98%. This suggests a potential undertriage rate of below 2% for those children most likely in need of referral to a pediatric trauma facility. A potential overtriage of 35% is a small price to pay for this degree of accuracy and implies that use of the PTS as a triage tool will decrease by two thirds the number of unnecessary trauma center referrals. With regard to simple mortality potential, the survival of children whose PTS is 9 or above continues to be 99.9%, whereas for those whose PTS is 8 or below, a linear increase in mortality exists that suggests a negligible potential for survival for PTS of zero or below.[37]

Compared with the various trauma scores defined for the adult population, the PTS is at least as effective as a triage tool and more specific to the problems of the pediatric patient. Its application in the field is extremely simple, and its use by referring hospitals to determine which children should be transferred to pediatric trauma centers has been documented as valid and accurate.[21] Description of airway management rather than of a single observation of respiratory rate not only provides a better indication of respiratory

status but also allows retrospective analysis of prehospital care. Moreover, the inclusion of skeletal and cutaneous injuries into this system identifies significant anatomic factors that may require care in a specialized pediatric center, despite the presence of normal vital signs. Use of the PTS as a prehospital quality assurance monitor is under investigation at present. The focus of these studies is primarily related to the interaction of airway management and neurologic status. In comparing individuals with similar types of injuries, the outcome achieved can be compared with the initial assessment and management as indicated by the PTS. This comparison may identify trends of care that can be analyzed and improved through educational and feedback programs.

The PTS thus is the most sensitive triage indicator for application to the injured child. Its relationship to the ISS and its potential for determining mortality has been documented in multiple objective studies, and its use as an indicator of system function is currently under investigation.

TRANSPORT OF THE PATIENT

Assuming that effective assessment has produced correct triage, the next most important function of a regional trauma system is transport of the patient. Because of the rapidity with which the injured child may deteriorate, from either a cardiorespiratory or a central nervous system function, transport becomes a major challenge and a potential threat to life. Transport protocols within a regional trauma system must be developed as the system is created. Clearly, the most important feature of these protocols is a means of accurate communication between the referring and receiving institutions and direct physician control of the patient's care during all aspects of actual transport (Fig. 6–2).[2]

As in triage, the most important component of the transport phase of the pediatric trauma care is accurate initial assessment. This must follow a simple scheme that provides a baseline assessment of the patient and allows rapid repetition so that trends in cardiopulmonary and neurologic function can be confirmed. Once the patient has been identified as needing transport, adequate stabilization should be considered if the time in transport is in excess of 30 minutes. If, however, transport to a trauma facility or an adequately staffed receiving facility is a matter of moments, initial stabilization should consist of assessing airway patency and ventilation followed by rapid transfer of the patient to the appropriately equipped facility. It thus becomes obvious that the two variables in determining the appropriate course of action are the level of facility immediately available for assessment and resuscitation and the distance or time required to transport a child to a definitive pediatric trauma center.[25]

The resuscitation capability of hospitals within a trauma region is extraordinarily variable throughout the country. Accordingly, individuals who are charged with developing systems of care for the pediatric trauma patient must carefully assess potential participants in this system and determine which facilities are appropriate initial responders for resuscitation and which facilities should be bypassed in

TraumaOne Resuscitation Record/Flowsheet

NAME			DATE		TRAUMA TEAM:	TIME NOTIFIED:_____

RESUS #	UNIT #	ACCOUNT #

TRAUMA TEAM:
1._____ TIME NOTIFIED:_____
2._____ TIME ARRIVED:_____
3._____ 5._____
4._____ 6._____
7._____

CHIEF COMPLAINT	LEVEL ☐ 1 ☐ 2 ☐ 3

Consultation Service:	Time Called	Time Arrived
Neurosurgery		

ALLERGIES	TETANUS TOXOID

PREHOSPITAL CARE

TRANSPORT
- ☐ Direct from the scene (SIC/SOC)
- ☐ Transferred from _____
- ☐ Auto
- ☐ Ambulance _____
- ☐ Helicopter _____
- ☐ Police
- ☐ Ambulatory   ☐ W/C

MECHANISM OF INJURY
- ☐ Auto   ☐ Driver   ☐ Passenger
- ☐ Motorcycle   ☐ Bicycle   front   back
- ☐ Speed ___ mph   ☐ Crush   ☐ Burn
- ☐ Fall ___ ft   ☐ Stab   ☐ Assault
- ☐ GSW   ☐ Seatbelt Yes☐ No☐
- ☐ Pedestrian vs Auto
- ☐ Other _____

IMMOBILIZATION:
- ☐ C-Collar   ☐ CID
- ☐ LBB/SBB   ☐ KED
- ☐ Blanket-roll
- ☐ MAST:
  - ___ legs ___ Abd
- ☐ Splints: Type _____
- ☐ NONE _____

AIRWAY:
- ☐ ET Tube # _____
- ☐ NT Tube # _____
- ☐ Crico # _____
- ☐ EOA or ☐ PTL
- ☐ 02 @ ___ L/m via _____
- Breath Sounds:
  - Left _____ Right _____

TRAUMA ALERT CRITERIA

YES	NO	
☐	☐	GCS <12
☐	☐	Sys. B/P <90
☐	☐	Resp. Rate <10 >29
☐	☐	Ejection from motor vehicle
☐	☐	Paralysis
☐	☐	Amputation proximal to wrist or ankle

YES	NO	
☐	☐	2nd or 3rd degree burns 15% BSA
☐	☐	Penetrating injury to head, neck, torso or groin

PUPILS
R	L	
☐	☐	Pinpoint
☐	☐	Midposition
☐	☐	Dilated
☐	☐	Fixed
☐	☐	Responding

INITIAL NURSE ASSESSMENT/OBSERVATION

	WNL	ABN	
NEURO	☐	☐	
HEAD	☐	☐	
NECK	☐	☐	
BACK-SPINE	☐	☐	
CHEST	☐	☐	
LUNGS	☐	☐	
ABDOMEN	☐	☐	
PELVIS	☐	☐	
EXTREM	☐	☐	
SKIN	☐	☐	

ADULT VARIABLES
- A. Resp. Rate
- B. Systolic BP
- C. Glasgow Coma Scale

PEDIATRIC VARIABLES
- Size
- Airway
- Open Wd
- Skeletal
- CNS
- Systolic BP

LAB VALUES

Time Results Recieved							
WBC		Na	PT	pH			**DPL**
RBC		K⁺	PTT	PCO₂			RBC
Hgb		Cl	ETOH	PO₂			WBC
Hct		CO₂		HCO₃			Bili
Plt		BUN		TCO₂			Amylase
		Creat		ABE			Gram-stain
		Gluc		SAT			

95029 (REV. 11/91)

FIGURE 6–2

Trauma One resuscitation record/flowsheet. (Courtesy of University Medical Center, Jacksonville, Fla.)

TRAUMA RESUSCITATION ORDERS

TIME	LABORATORY	TIME	X-RAYS	TIME	PROCEDURES
	☐ Type/Cross # U		Lateral C-Spine		O₂ @ L/M VIA
	☐ Type/Hold		Chest ☐ Erect ☐ Supine		ET # By:
	☐ CBC Screen		Pelvis		NT # By:
	☐ Astra 8		Completion C-Spine		Cricothyroidotomy #
	☐ ETOH		☐ T-Spine ☐ L-Spine		Chest Tube Size R /L
	☐ PT/PTT		Extremities		Right Return
	☐ ABG's				Left Return
	☐ Urinalysis		Skull		Auto Transfuser
	☐ UCG		Facial Series		Needle Thoracostomy
	☐ DPL Fluid		Mandible		Thoracotomy
	☐		Esophagram		Pericardiocentesis
	☐		IVP		EKG
	☐		Urethrogram		NG # Return Color
	☐		Cystogram		Rectal Tone: Gualac
	☐		Arteriogram		Foley # Return Color
TIME	MAST Deflation		☐ Other		Urine Dip + -
	ABD BP:				DPL
	R Leg BP:		CT Head		Dextrostick Results:
	L Leg BP:		CT ABD/Pelvis		Restraints: UE LE
			☐ Other		Soft Leather

IV#	VOL./SOLUTION/ADDITIVES	CATH SIZE/SITE	BLOOD PROD.	TIME	RATE	TIME DC	AMT. ABS.	TIME		MEDICATION	DOSE	SITE/RTE	INT.
									1				
									2				
									3				
									4				
									5				
									6				
									7				
									8				
									9				
									10				
									11				
									12				
									13				
									14				
									15				
									16				
									17				
									18				
									19				
									20				
									21				
									22				
									23				
									24				
									25				

TOTAL INPUT		TOTAL OUTPUT			
I.V.		NG		Pastoral Service Notified: Yes ☐ No ☐ NA ☐	
Blood Products		Urine		Social Service Notified: Yes ☐ No ☐ NA ☐	
Oral		C.T.		VALUABLES:	
Disposition: Time Admit Yes ☐ No ☐		Floor		Security #	
Service Physicians		RR		Family/Signature	
Other		OR			
Family Notified: Yes ☐ No ☐		ICU		Clothing Discarded: Yes ☐ No ☐	CCR #
Operative Permit Signed: Yes ☐ No ☐		S/D		Physician's Signature	
		ME			

FIGURE 6–2 *Continued*

Illustration continued on following page

TIME																
CUFF BP																
PULSE																
RHYTHM																
RESP.																
TEMP.																
A-LINE																
OXIMETRY																
CARBOXIMETRY																
CVP																
HOURLY U/O																
GLASGOW COMA SCALE																
1. EYES																
2. BEST VERBAL RESP.																
3. BEST MOTOR RESP.																
TOTAL (1 + 2 + 3)																
SIZE + REACT (L)																
SIZE + REACT (R)																

TIME	NOTES:
	NURSES' SIGNATURE

FIGURE 6–2 *Continued*

favor of transport to a more comprehensive hospital.[2] Once this system is intact and a level of function for the participating centers has been developed utilizing some of the methods mentioned previously, then a series of transport protocols can be developed that focus on initial assessment of the patient, resuscitation that should be initiated, and medical control of the patient until arrival in the trauma center.[1]

The PTS clearly has a role in this initial assessment, as indicated by Jubelirer in initially evaluating injured children presenting to a level II trauma center, specifically comparing those who were referred to a designated pediatric trauma center with those who were managed at the level II center.[21] These children were accurately identified utilizing a PTS of 8 and below. Moreover, the appropriateness of management of a child with a single organ system injury in an adult center was introduced as a potential alternative when transfer to a children's center is impractical. Clearly, all injured children should have the opportunity to be managed in a pediatric trauma center whose staff, equipment, commitment, and personnel are oriented to the special needs of the pediatric population. Unfortunately, this is frequently not possible because of the numbers of injured children and the limited resources that are available for the development and designation of pediatric trauma centers.

Within the actual process of transport, however, a number of considerations must be maintained constantly. All of these focus on the basic life-supporting functions of the cardiorespiratory and neurologic systems. They are specifically intended to prevent the onset of airway obstruction, inadequate ventilation, uncorrected hemorrhage, overhydration, and preventable deterioration of CNS function.[32, 33] The basic principles for management of each of these types of injuries are discussed elsewhere in this text and should be used as reference in designing protocols for transport within regional pediatric trauma systems. As in all phases of trauma care, accurate assessment and concise documentation are essential for safe transport. Figure 6–2 is a suggested transport protocol sheet that provides the receiving facility with an up-to-date summary of the child's status; documents necessary interventional management; and serves as an important reference for subsequent caregivers, system review, and clinical research.

In summary, triage, trauma scoring, and transport of the pediatric trauma patient are in fact a single ingredient that catalyzes the effective provision of care for the injured child. The importance of triage as a governance mechanism within trauma systems is obvious. The use of a reliable trauma score in applying these principles of triage has been well documented and continues to be a significant component of care. Finally, safe transport within this trauma system, once indicated, is indeed the hallmark of an effective regionalized system of trauma care that ultimately not only will improve the potential for survival, but, more important, will affect favorably the quality of life for the injured child.

References

1. American Academy of Pediatrics, Committee on Hospital Care: Guidelines for air and ground transportation of pediatric patients. Pediatrics 78(5):943–949, 1986.
2. American College of Surgeons: Hospital and prehospital resources for optimal care of the injured patient, Chicago, American College of Surgeons, October 1984.
3. Aprahamian C, Cattey R, Walker AP, et al: Pediatric Trauma Score. Predictor of hospital resource use? Arch Surg 125:1128–1131, 1990.
4. Baker SP, O'Neill B: The injury severity score: An update. J Trauma 16:882–885, 1976.
5. Baker SP, O'Neill B, Haddon W, Long WM: The injury severity score: A method for describing patients with multiple injuries and evaluating emergency care. J Trauma 143:187, 1974.
6. Boyd CR, Tolson MA, Copes WS: Evaluating trauma care: The TRISS method. J Trauma 27:370–378, 1987.
7. Champion HR, Sacco WJ: Measurement of injury severity and its practical application. Trauma Quarterly 1:25–36, 1984.
8. Champion HR, Sacco WJ, Carnazzo AJ, et al: Trauma score. Crit Care Med 9:672, 1981.
9. Champion HR, Sacco WJ, Hepper RL, et al: An anatomic index of injury severity. J Trauma 20:197, 1980.
10. Clemmer TP, Orme JF, Thomas F, Brooks KA: Prospective evaluation of the CRAMS scale for triaging major trauma. J Trauma 25:188–190, 1985.
11. Committee on Medical Aspects of Automotive Safety: Rating the severity of tissue damage. The abbreviated scale. JAMA 215:277, 1971.
12. Cullen DJ, Civetta JM, Briggs BA, et al: Therapeutic intervention scoring system: A method for quantitative comparison of patient care. Crit Care Med 2:57, 1974.
13. Cullen DJ, Civetta JM, Briggs BA, et al: Survival, hospitalization charges, and follow up results in critically ill patients. N Engl J Med 249:982, 1976.
14. Cullen DJ, Ferrara LC, Gilbert J, et al: Indicators of intensive care in critically ill patients. Crit Care Med 5:173, 1977.
15. Dionigi R, Cremaschi R, Jemos U, et al: Nutritional assessment and severity of illness classification systems. World J Surg 10:2–11, 1986.
16. Flora JD: A method for comparing survival of burn patients to a standard survival curve. J Trauma 18:701–705, 1978.
17. Ford EG, Jennings LM, Givson AE, Andrassy RJ: The Pediatric Trauma Score: Accuracy of prediction of injury severity in a single large urban pediatric trauma experience. Contemp Orthopedics 16:35–41, 1988.
18. Gormican SP: CRAMS Scale: Field triage of trauma victims. Ann Emerg Med 11:132–135, 1982.
19. Jacobs LM: The effect of prospective reimbursement on trauma patients. Am Col Surg Bull 70:17, 1985.
20. Jonnett B, Teasdale G, Galbraith S, et al: Severe head injuries in three counties. J Neurol Neurosurg Psychiatry 40:291–298, 1977.
21. Jubelirer RA, Agarwal NN, Beyer FC, et al: Pediatric trauma triage: Review of 1307 cases. J Trauma 30:1544–1547, 1990.
22. Knaus WA, Draper EA, Wagner DP, et al: Evaluating outcome from intensive care: A preliminary multihospital comparison. Crit Care Med 10:491, 1982.
23. Knaus WA, Zimmerman JE, Wagner DP, et al: APACHE—Acute physiology and chronic health evaluation: A physiologically based classification system. Crit Care Med 9:591, 1981.
24. Krause JF, Fife D, Cox P, et al: Incidence, severity, and external causes of pediatric brain injury. Am J Dis Child 140:687–693, 1986.
25. Lewis FR, Aprahamian C, Haller JA, et al: Panel: Prehospital trauma care—Stabilize or scoop and run. J Trauma 23:708–711, 1983.
26. Mayer T, Matlack ME, Johnson DG, et al: The modified injury severity scale in pediatric multiple trauma patients. J Pediatr Surg 15:719–726, 1980.
27. Mayer T, Walker ML, Clark P: Further experience with the modified abbreviated injury severity scale. J Trauma 24:31–34, 1984.
28. Morris JA, Auerback PS, Marshall GA, et al: The trauma score as a triage tool in the prehospital setting. JAMA 256:1319–1325, 1986.
29. National Pediatric Registry Annual Report. New England Medical Center, Department of Rehabilitative Medicine, 1988.
30. Ramenofsky ML, Ramenofsky MB, Jurkovich GJ, et al: Predictive validity of the pediatric trauma score. J Trauma 27:830, 1987.
31. Scheffer RM, Knaus WA, Wagner DP, Zimmerman JE: Severity of illness and the relationship between intensive care and survival. Am J Public Health 72:449, 1982.
32. Seidel JS, Hornbein M, Yoshiyama K, et al: Emergency medical services and the pediatric patient: Are the needs being met? Pediatrics 73:769–772, 1984.

33. Seidel JS: Emergency medical services and the pediatric patient: Are the needs being met? II. Training and equipping emergency medical services providers for pediatric emergencies. Pediatrics 78:808–812, 1986.

34. Stablein DM, Miller JD, Choi SC, et al: Statistical methods for determining prognosis in severe head injuries. J Neurosurg 6:243, 1980.

35. Tepas JJ III, Alexander RH, Campbell JD, et al: An improved scoring system for assessment of the injured child. J Trauma 25:720, 1985.

36. Tepas JJ III, Mollitt DL, Talbert JL, Bryant M: The pediatric trauma score as a predictor of surgery severity in the injured child. J Pediatr Surg 22:14–18, 1987.

37. Tepas JJ III, Ramenofsky ML, Mollitt DL: The Pediatric Trauma Score as a predictor of injury severity: An objective assessment. J Trauma 28:425–429, 1988.

38. Young B, Rapp RP, Norton JA, et al: Early predictor of outcome of pediatric injury. J Neurosurg 54:300, 1981.

Jeffrey J. DuBois
William J. Pokorny

CHAPTER SEVEN

Trauma Protocols for Evaluation and Management

In 1917, William Ladd journeyed to Halifax, Nova Scotia, in response to a plea for medical support after a marine munitions explosion. Reportedly, he was so touched by the needs of the injured children that on returning to Boston he dedicated his career to the surgical care of children.[9] It is a curious irony in medical history, then, that the field of pediatric surgery, born on the unique needs of the injured child, should require more than 50 years to develop pediatric trauma centers to care for these patients.

In his review of the development of pediatric trauma care, Harris has described the 15 years from 1970 to 1985 as the ''Age of Progress.''[12] The landmark study by the National Academy of Sciences and the National Research Council in 1966, underscoring the magnitude of death related to accidental injury in the pediatric population, prompted an organized approach to the care of trauma patients overall.[1, 14] Other studies demonstrating that some trauma deaths could have been prevented had an organized, comprehensive approach to trauma care been available led to the Advanced Trauma Life Support (ATLS) training program established by the American College of Surgeons in 1979.[36, 38, 39] This course was later updated with specific attention directed to the particular needs of the traumatized child. The Age of Progress culminated in the development of the pediatric trauma score (PTS) by Tepas and associates, in which the unique characteristics of pediatric trauma patients and their injuries were rated separately and were assigned a score that was different from the system used to determine adult injury severity scores (Table 7–1).[26, 33, 34]

Studies of trauma deaths, by McCoy and Bell and by Ramenofsky and colleagues, identified up to 25% of trauma-related pediatric deaths, unassociated with major neurologic injury, that could have been prevented and that were attributed to ineffective care received in the hospital setting.[17, 25] These studies pointed out not only the need for accurate and effective field treatment and triage to appropriate pediatric trauma centers for the seriously injured child, but also the absolute requirement of an organized and a methodic approach to pediatric trauma at the receiving center.

However, no singular approach to the care of the injured child is necessarily the optimal approach in all centers.

Differences in population densities, available modes of transportation, and availability of institutional resources influence which centers are responsible to the community for pediatric trauma care. Nonetheless, regionalization of trauma care, organization of the receiving institution best equipped to manage the traumatized child, and an algorithmic approach to the assessment and resuscitation of pediatric trauma victims are essential ingredients in the development of such trauma centers.

Responding to a growing demand for pediatric trauma care in Houston outside the already existing level I trauma centers at Ben Taub General Hospital and Hermann Hospital, a third pediatric trauma response team was established at the Texas Children's Hospital in 1990. Although each center provides comprehensive pediatric trauma support, Ben Taub General Hospital's and Texas Children's Hospital's pediatric trauma support is under the auspices of pediatric surgery at Baylor College of Medicine. Each program has evolved a unique approach to the care of the injured child. Although the trauma centers at Ben Taub General Hospital and Hermann Hospital provide for full-time surgical resident coverage in the emergency department, the trauma response team approach adopted at Texas Children's Hospital most closely approximates the availability of pediatric surgical resources at most children's hospitals and metropolitan general hospitals and is the approach outlined in this chapter.

THE PEDIATRIC TRAUMA RESPONSE TEAM

A team approach to the management of pediatric trauma has been advocated by most of those connected with trauma centers.[6, 8, 11, 15] Complex multiple trauma inherently requires an organized approach by a critical group of participants to efficiently and effectively accomplish a series of potentially necessary interventions.

Although most injured children presenting to an emergency department do not have immediate life-threatening injuries, approximately 10% require life-sustaining interventions that are timely and effective.[13] The child with a

Table 7–1
Pediatric Trauma Score

Component	(Check one category for each component) Category		
	+2	**+1**	**−1**
Size	≥20 kg	10–20 kg	<10 kg
Airway	Normal	Maintainable	Unmaintainable
Systolic BP	≥mm Hg	90–50 mm Hg	<50 mm Hg
CNS	Awake	Obtunded/LOC	Coma/decerebrate
Open wound	None	Minor	Major/penetrating
Skeletal	None	Closed fracture	Open/multiple fractures

If proper-sized BP cuff is not available, BP can be assessed by assigning the following values:
   +2, pulse palpable at wrist;
   +1, pulse palpable at groin;
   −1, no pulse palpable.
The Pediatric Trauma Score (PTS) is the sum of grades for each of six categories. It also serves as a rapid assessment checklist. BP, Blood pressure; CNS, central nervous system; LOC, loss of consciousness.

Table 7–2
The ABC's of Resuscitation

Airway (with cervical spine control)
Breathing
Circulation (with hemorrhage control)
Disability (neurologic status)
Exposure (complete disrobement)

closed-head injury, possibly cervical spine injury, and ongoing exsanguinating hemorrhage represents such a challenge, for example. This patient may require intubation with in-line cervical traction, a maneuver that requires a physician; a provider to stabilize the neck; and a respiratory technician to set up the ventilator or provide hand-bagging ventilatory support. In addition, immediate attention must be directed to the source of hemorrhage, whether by direct pressure or another method, to control ongoing blood loss.

As the number and complexity of the injuries increase, the provider support must be capable of accommodating these demands to ensure an optimal outcome. An algorithmic approach is deemed essential to ensure that all details of the evaluation and resuscitation are attended to in an orderly and comprehensive fashion. This approach encompasses not only the management of the ABC's of resuscitation, but also the clear delineation of responsibilities of each member of the team (Table 7–2). These elements are believed crucial to the approach to the child with multiple injuries, and in our center we have adopted a ''two-layered response team'' approach to pediatric trauma (Table 7–3). Activated by prearrival information and triage provided by emergency medical service personnel, the appropriate level of response can be determined and the appropriate personnel notified of the pending arrival of the injured patient.

Primary Trauma Response Team

The Pediatric Trauma Registry has clearly established that patients with a PTS of 8 or less are at substantially greater risk for fatal outcome and therefore are best served by care at a level I trauma center whenever feasible.[26, 34] The primary trauma response team is mandatorily activated whenever a patient with a PTS of 8 or less is en route to Texas Children's Hospital and it consists of the following personnel:

1. The chief resident in pediatric surgery or attending pediatric surgeon, or both
2. The senior surgery resident rotating on pediatric surgery
3. The senior pediatric resident assigned to the emergency center
4. The emergency center nurse in charge
5. An emergency center staff nurse

The chief resident or attending surgeon functions as the team leader, organizing and directing the assessment and resuscitation measures. Should neither the chief resident nor the attending surgeon be immediately available, the senior surgical resident serves as the team leader until their arrival. The other members of the primary trauma response team

assist the team leader in resuscitation efforts, generally following prescribed tasks as well as those directed by the team leader.

Secondary Trauma Response Team

Following initial assessment by the team leader, the secondary trauma response team may be summoned. The secondary trauma response team consists of additional physicians and support personnel who assist in the resuscitation efforts. Their purpose is to function under the direction of the team leader in securing the airway and all catheter devices; obtaining necessary emergency laboratory studies and radiographs; and coordinating disposition and priority with the radiology department, the pediatric critical care unit, and the operating suite personnel before obtaining scans or further radiographic studies, surgical intervention, or critical care monitoring.

The secondary response team consists of the following personnel:

1. The anesthesiologist (attending or resident)
2. The respiratory therapist
3. The pediatric critical care specialist (attending or fellow)
4. A radiology technician
5. A laboratory technician
6. The nursing supervisor responsible for patient admissions

The secondary trauma response team functions less as a discrete team and more as a secondary echelon of support, as individual members may be summoned at the discretion of the team leader. Following this plan, personnel are not involved with the resuscitation unnecessarily, thus improving time utilization and cost effectiveness of these professionals and minimizing congestion in the emergency center.

Assigned Tasks—Primary Trauma Response Team

Team Leader

The team leader's primary responsibilities include making the initial 60-second assessment and establishing the direc-

Table 7–3
Response Team Approach to Pediatric Trauma

Primary Trauma Response Team
Pediatric surgeon (attending or chief resident)
Senior general surgery resident
Senior pediatric resident
Emergency department nurse in charge
Emergency department staff nurse

Secondary Trauma Response Team
Anesthesia (attending or senior resident)
Pediatric critical care (attending or fellow)
Respiratory therapy
Radiology (portable) technician
Laboratory technician
Admitting supervisor

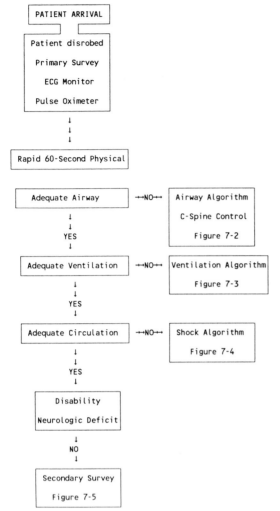

FIGURE 7–1

Algorithm for initial assessment and life-support measures in pediatric trauma. ECG, Electrocardiogram; C-spine, cervical spine.

and for determining appropriate placement of the patient after resuscitation, evaluations, or surgery. It is essential that the team leader assume a proportionately greater role in direct patient care in the initial few minutes of the resuscitation efforts. As stabilization progresses and is achieved, the team leader assumes more of a supervisory role, overseeing other team members' activities during the overall progress of resuscitation.

Senior Surgical Resident

The senior surgical resident stands to the right of the patient assisting the team leader in resuscitation efforts. Responsible for the immediate and complete disrobing of the patient, the senior surgical resident also assists in obtaining vascular access. In the majority of our patients, the emergency department nurse assigned to the resuscitation effort attempts percutaneous intravenous line placement first. If unsuccessful, the surgical resident is immediately available for place-

tion of resuscitation efforts thereafter. He or she ensures patency of the airway and a stable cervical spine (or directs efforts at obtaining these), completes the initial assessment of the nature and extent of the injuries, and directs the immediate resuscitation efforts, generally following guidelines established in conjunction with the American College of Surgeons Advanced Trauma Life Support Course (Figs. 7–1 through 7–5). At any point in the resuscitation, the team leader may engage in technical skills considered beyond the level of expertise of others (e.g., cricothyrotomy, thoracotomy). An erasable board has been developed, adapted from the Kiwanis Pediatric Trauma Institute Trauma Receiving Unit Checklist, that is displayed in a prominent position in the resuscitation room (Table 7–4).[11] All pertinent physical findings and laboratory results are annotated by the team leader as they become available. This aids in ensuring all injuries are addressed and all essential elements of resuscitation have been accomplished. Also, the team leader is responsible for initiating consultation requests; for determining the need for surgical intervention;

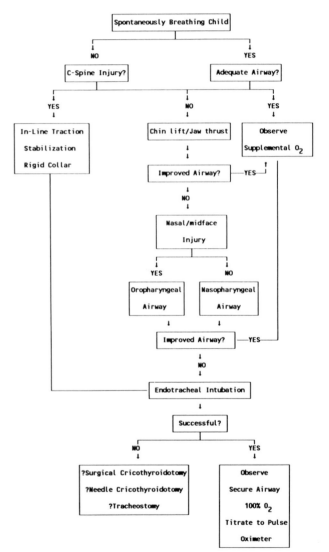

FIGURE 7–2

Algorithm for airway maintenance and cervical spine control for pediatric injuries. C-spine, Cervical spine.

Table 7-4
Trauma Team Checklist

[   ] Perform 60-second examinations (ABC's)
[   ] Immobilize neck
[   ] Stabilize airway
[   ] Provide supplemental oxygen
[   ] Disrobe patient
[   ] Secure intravenous access
[   ] Apply electrocardiogram leads
[   ] Draw blood (T&C, CBC, chemistries, tox screen, coags)
[   ] Insert Foley catheter
[   ] Insert nasogastric or orogastric tube
[   ] Establish arterial line
[   ] Calculate Glasgow Coma Scale and Pediatric Trauma Score
[   ] Complete history and physical examination
[   ] Dress wounds
[   ] Arrange for radiographic studies (e.g., lateral cervical spine, CXR, AP pelvis)
[   ] Supply tetanus prophylaxis, antibiotics, or both
[   ] Consider abuse or neglect
[   ] Contact primary care physician
[   ] List laboratory results on flow sheet
[   ] List all injuries

T&C, Type and crossmatch; CBC, complete blood count; tox, toxicology; coags, coagulation profiles.

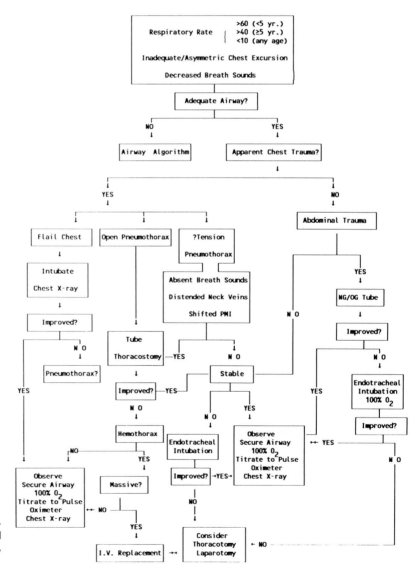

FIGURE 7-3

Algorithm for adequate ventilation in the pediatric trauma patient. PMI, Point of maximal impulse; NG, nasogastric; OG, orogastric; IV, intravenous.

ment of cutdown venous lines or percutaneous central venous access as deemed appropriate. The senior surgical resident also performs tube thoracostomy or pericardiocentesis, or both, as required and may assist in stabilizing the cervical spine during intubation or other assessment maneuvers (e.g., log-rolling the patient), if indicated.

Emergency Department Resident

The senior pediatric resident assigned to the emergency department stands to the left of the patient. This physician assists in the complete disrobing of the patient and in the placement of the peripheral venous or arterial lines (or intraosseous lines, should they be warranted). He or she is then responsible for obtaining appropriate arterial and venous laboratory studies and in ensuring that they are handed to the laboratory technician promptly. Following this, the emergency department resident is then responsible for placement of urethral catheters.

Emergency Department Staff Nurse

The emergency department staff nurse stands to the left of the patient. On complete disrobement of the patient, the staff nurse initiates attempts at percutaneous peripheral intravenous line placement. Often the emergency department physician is examining one extremity while the nurse is examining the other for available peripheral sites. If obtaining peripheral access is unsuccessful, the emergency department nurse contributes by administering supplemental oxygen to patients who do not require intubation and placing electrocardiogram leads, pulse oximetry monitors, and temperature probes. After placement of the monitor leads, the staff nurse then obtains and records vital signs for the duration of the resuscitation, during transport to and while in the radiology suite or the CT scanner, or en route to the operating suite or critical care unit.

Emergency Department Charge Nurse

The emergency department charge nurse stands to the right of the patient and assists the team leader. Initially, the charge nurse is responsible for obtaining the admitting vital signs and for summoning members of the secondary response team if they are not already present. The charge nurse may also assist in obtaining peripheral access and in obtaining valuable historical information and medical background from the family members, the EMS personnel, or both. The acronym AMPLE is a useful mnemonic for obtaining important medical and preoperative information. (Table 7–5).[2] As resuscitation progresses, the charge nurse

Table 7–5
Brief Trauma History

A—Allergies	
M—Medications currently taking	
P—Past medical history (illnesses and previous surgeries)	
L—Last meal	
E—Events immediately preceding the injury	

is responsible for obtaining consultations as directed by the team leader and for communicating with the operating room nurse supervisor, the critical care unit charge nurse, or the admitting supervisor to ensure a smooth transport to the appropriate receiving unit.

Assigned Tasks—Secondary Trauma Response Team

Anesthesia Resident or Staff

The on-call anesthesia resident or staff attending assigned to respond to the trauma are responsible for ensuring a patent airway, intubating as warranted, and maintaining adequate ventilation in coordination with the team leader and neurosurgery department.

Respiratory Therapy Technician

The respiratory therapy technician responding to trauma is responsible for ensuring the availability of supplemental oxygen, assisting in hand-bagging ventilation if so directed, and for managing the proper setup and setting changes for any ventilator needs. In addition, the respiratory technician suctions the endotracheal tube in conjunction with the anesthesiologist or team leader.

Critical Care Fellow or Staff

The critical care fellow assists the team leader as needed and may be responsible for invasive procedures such as the placement of intra-arterial cannulae or central venous catheters or pericardiocentesis in conjunction with the senior surgical resident. The critical care physician is also responsible for relaying care requirements to the critical care or intermediate care units and is available to aid in transport to the critical units if no operative intervention is required immediately.

Radiology Technician

The radiology technician is immediately available on request to obtain chest, cervical, and pelvic radiographs or any other study at the discretion of the team leader.

Laboratory Technician

A technician or phlebotomist is available when the trauma emergency is activated to obtain blood and urine samples and to ensure the expeditious testing and return of results.

Admitting Nurse Supervisor

The nursing admitting supervisor accompanies the trauma team to the resuscitation room and is responsible for keeping family members within the area to be available to the trauma team for pertinent history and medical background.

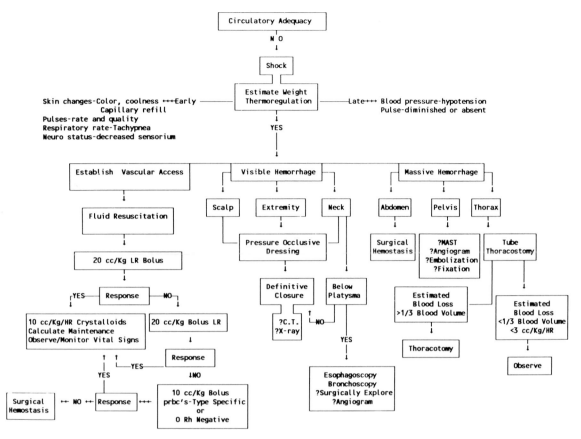

FIGURE 7–4

Algorithm for circulatory assessment and stability. LR, Lactated Ringer; MAST, medical antishock trousers; CT, computed tomography; prbc, patient's red blood cells.

Operating Room Nursing Supervisor

The operating room nurse supervisor is asked by the primary trauma response team to make available the required instrumentation and surgical packs when patients require imminent surgical intervention and to ensure availability of appropriate blood products during the surgical procedure.

PATIENT ADMISSION, STABILIZATION, AND DISPOSITION

As the "golden hour of trauma" suggests, the greater the delay in the administration of definitive therapy from the time of the initial injury, the greater the likelihood of an untoward outcome.[7] Studies involving both adult and pediatric trauma patients have demonstrated that delays in patient care may occur if field resuscitation efforts are prolonged unnecessarily.[24, 31] However, rapid transfer of the injured child does little good if the receiving unit is ill-prepared to accept and treat the patient. In addition to the obvious requirements of a well-trained and equipped trauma team, the orderly approach to patient flow from field treatment through the resuscitation process is equally important.

Field Treatment

The concept of *scoop and run* in the prehospital care of trauma patients has received considerable attention.[4] Indeed, one need only examine the relationship between battle injury mortality and time to definitive care to understand the impact of rapid transport in the management of trauma patients.[35] In World War II, during which the average evacuation time was approximately 18 hours, the hospital mortality of injured soldiers was 18%. By the time of the Korean and Vietnam conflicts, when evacuation times were reduced to less than 2 hours, mortality rates dropped to approximately 2%, a mortality rate similar to today's overall pediatric trauma mortality of 2.9%.[26]

Prehospital stabilization and mode of transport can be a double-edged sword. A review of the treatment of 52 trauma patients compared transport times to the scene and admission blood pressure, amount of intravenous infusion received, and time to establish intravenous access.[31] In all patients, the time to place an intravenous line exceeded the transport time, and nearly 25% of the more seriously injured patients never had access established in the field. Ramenofsky and co-workers showed similar results in pediatric EMS responses: the "in-the-field" times were frequently notably longer than the transport time.[24]

Although the military experience with helicopter trans-

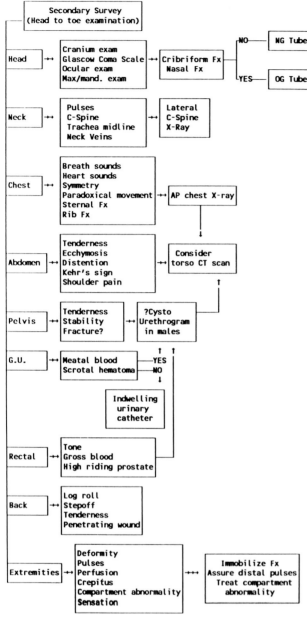

FIGURE 7–5

Algorithm for secondary survey. NG, Nasogastric; OG, orogastric; C-spine, cervical spine; CT, computed tomography; GU, genitourinary; fx, fracture.

port of injured combatants suggests improved survival secondary to this mode of transport, in present-day urban settings, the helicopter may offer no significant survival advantage.[28] For example, repeated attempts at intravenous access before transport may be inappropriate when the receiving institution is within 5 to 10 minutes from the scene. Intravenous lines initiated en route would potentially obviate this dilemma; however, in hypotensive pediatric patients, small vein size and venoconstriction frequently prevent successful line placement at the scene, much less in a moving ambulance.[21] In this regard, the utilization of intraosseous lines may prove to be a safe, effective alternative to intravenous lines without extending transport times, as

such lines placed to pressure bags have shown infusion rates of up to 50 cc per minute, utilizing 13-gauge bone marrow needles.[16, 27, 29]

Coordination and communication with the receiving unit are valuable adjuncts in the prehospital treatment phase. They also provide advance notice to the receiving center as to the severity of injuries and treatment under way, plus the primary trauma response team is alerted and can be available to provide recommendations to the responding EMS personnel over the radio. In addition, the secondary trauma response team, the operating room, and the critical care units can be notified prior to patient arrival, allowing sufficient time to prepare for patient admission, diagnostic evaluation, and surgical intervention.

Patient Admission

Admission of the injured child to the emergency department unfortunately is unpredictable. If all admissions were preceded by an accurate report from EMS personnel clearly delineating the extent of injuries and in sufficient time to summon the required elements of the trauma team, trauma resuscitation might become a more predictable science. However, not infrequently, patients arrive with little or no advance notice or inaccurate injury assessment. This comment is not to admonish the field resuscitation efforts of the EMS personnel, but rather is a reflection of the inherently unpredictable and ever-changing condition of the trauma patient, especially the injured child, and the circumstances under which injuries occur.

With the development of the pediatric trauma score by Tepas, the ability of the responding EMS personnel to accurately triage pediatric trauma patients to appropriate centers and the ability of the receiving unit to summon the necessary trauma team personnel has been greatly improved. When an injured child with a field PTS of 8 or less is en route, the primary trauma response team is alerted and present when the child arrives. As part of the initial assessment and resuscitation effort, an ED-PTS is designated by the team leader, the secondary trauma response team can be summoned, and after completion of the secondary survey (or as indicated by the patient's condition), the appropriate consultants and units can be notified of the patient's condition and required studies or interventions (Fig. 7–6).

Initial Assessment and Resuscitation

On arrival, initial evaluation commences. A rapid primary survey is undertaken, and any immediate life-threatening injury is identified. To facilitate the primary survey and to minimize overlooked injuries, the patient is disrobed and treatment priorities are established by the team leader based on the overall assessment of the patient. Concomitantly, the charge nurse records admission vital signs.

In general, treatment priorities during the primary survey phase follow the ABC's of resuscitation (see Figs. 7–1 through 7–5). The resuscitation phase occurs simultaneously with the primary survey, with measures such as intubation, placement of chest tubes, or venous cutdowns prior-

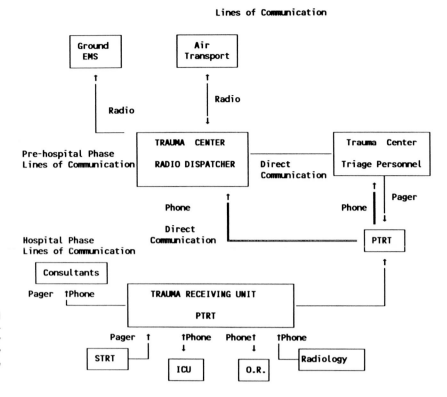

FIGURE 7–6

Algorithm for prehospital and hospital lines of communication. EMS, Emergency medical service; PTRT, primary trauma response team; STRT, secondary trauma response team; ICU, intensive care unit; OR, operating room.

itized by the team leader and relegated to the appropriate assistant.

SPECIFIC ASSESSMENT: THE PRIMARY SURVEY

Airway

The crying child generally attests to a patent airway. Nonetheless, supplemental oxygen should be supplied to all patients, even in the presence of a spontaneously well-maintained airway. However, the quiet but spontaneously breathing child may require assisted airway maneuvers (see Fig. 7–2). Initial maneuvers should include the chin lift or jaw thrust techniques (Fig. 7–7A and B). Because the tongue is relatively large and the oral cavity relatively small, the tongue can fall to the back of the hypopharynx and obstruct the airway when children are lethargic or unconscious. Although oropharyngeal airways come in a variety of sizes and can relieve such an obstruction effectively, a nasopharyngeal airway (in the absence of a cribriform plate fracture) is less likely to precipitate vomiting and may be easier to secure in place (Fig. 7–8).

If endotracheal intubation is required in children younger than 8 years of age, an uncuffed endotracheal tube should be employed. The narrowest portion of the airway in this age group is at the cricoid rather than the true vocal cords, and persistent pressure at this level from cuffed tubes may result in subglottic ulceration and eventual stenosis. The appropriate size for an endotracheal tube varies, as expected, with the age and size of the child. Several tables and formulas exist to assist in determining the proper size

tube (Table 7–6); however, unless such a formula is set to memory or is available for prompt review in the resuscitation room, it is of little use. Alternatively, a simple method for estimating correct endotracheal tube size is to select a tube whose outer diameter approximates the size of the nares or the tip of the child's fifth digit (Fig. 7–9).

Cricothyrotomy is rarely, if ever, indicated in children. In children younger than 8 years of age, cricothyrotomy may be technically unfeasible because of the anatomic restrictions and the risk of developing subglottic stenosis; needle cricothyrotomy with jet insufflation may be a satisfactory temporizing measure until definitive intubation or tracheostomy can be performed.

Breathing

The pediatric chest can transmit breath sounds widely despite pneumothorax, hemothorax, or endotracheal malposition. One cannot rely exclusively on auscultation to exclude these diagnostic possibilities, particularly in a noisy resuscitation room. However, as with adults, any suspicion of a pneumothorax or hemothorax, based on clinical evaluation of mediastinal position, possible penetrating wounds, or unstable chest wall, or a rapid deterioration in breathing with a patent airway should be treated with tube thoracostomy. When the patient is sufficiently stable, a chest radiograph should be obtained. An appropriate tidal volume in intubated children of approximately 7 to 10 cc per kg of body weight should result in symmetric chest wall elevations, but more volume may be required. The appropriate respiratory rate varies with age and representative rates for selected age groups (Table 7–7), but it must be adjusted for

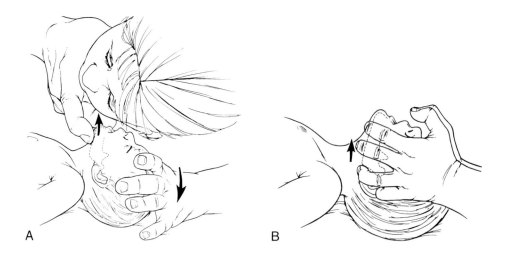

FIGURE 7–7

Initial maneuvers that are potentially helpful in relieving upper airway obstruction. *A,* Head tilt–chin lift; *B,* jaw thrust. (Reproduced with permission from Pediatric Advanced Life Support. Chameides L, Hazinski MF (eds). Dallas, Texas, American Heart Association/American Academy of Pediatrics, 1994, pp 3-4, 3-5. Copyright American Heart Association.)

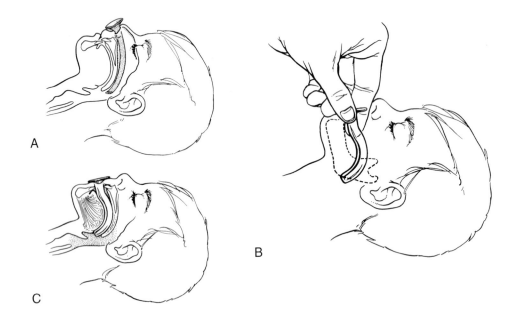

FIGURE 7–8

Additional measures and equipment to help maintain upper airway patency. *A,* Nasopharyngeal airway in place. *B,* Estimating the proper size for an oropharyngeal airway by holding it next to the child's face. *C,* Oropharyngeal airway in place. (Reproduced with permission from Pediatric Advanced Life Support. Chameides L, Hazinski MF (eds). Dallas, Texas, American Heart Association/American Academy of Pediatrics, 1994, pp 4-8, 4-9. Copyright American Heart Association. *B* and *C* adapted from Coté CJ, Todres ID: The pediatric airway. In: Coté CJ, Ryan JF, Todres ID, Groudsouzian NG (eds): A Practice of Anesthesia for Infants and Children. 2nd ed. Philadelphia, WB Saunders, 1993.)

Table 7–6
Endotracheal Tube Formula

16 + age (in years) ÷ 4 = inner diameter in mm

injury specificity as necessary in central nervous system or pulmonary trauma.

Failure to achieve adequate chest wall excursion after intubation and ventilation should prompt a search for possible causes. Hand-bagging with an in-line manometer can identify decreased pulmonary compliance as a potential cause (e.g., massive pulmonary contusion, tension pneumothorax, or open pneumothorax). A methodic search for suspected sources of compromised ventilation is made rapidly. With decreased pulmonary compliance in the presence of an uncuffed endotracheal tube, larger than normal tidal volumes may be required.

Infants ventilate primarily through diaphragmatic movements. Therefore, conditions that limit diaphragmatic excursion, such as direct diaphragmatic injury, intra-abdomi-

Table 7–7
Typical Vital Signs for Three Prototypic Age Groups

	Vital Signs		
	Pulse	Systolic	Respiration
Infant	160	80	40
Preschooler	140	90	30
Adolescent	120	100	20

From American College of Surgeons Committee on Trauma: Advanced Trauma Life Support Course. Ramenofsky ML (ed). Chicago, American College of Surgeons, 1989, p 220.

nal distention, or even gastric distention from aerophagia, can severely impair ventilation. Nasogastric or orogastric decompression should be instituted for all children with severe injuries. For infants, a 10 French Replogle tube is preferred (Fig. 7–10). The sump port of adult sump-type gastric tube may come to lie within the esophagus in a small child, ineffectively decompressing the stomach.[5]

In addition, the mediastinum of infants younger than 6 months of age is particularly mobile. Injuries such as open pneumothoraces may result in abnormal ventilation of the ipsilateral lung and the contralateral side as well. Similarly, tension pneumothoraces, hemothoraces, flail chest, and diaphragmatic incompetence (paralysis or rupture) are poorly tolerated secondary to the to-and-fro motion of the infant's mobile mediastinum.

Circulation—Recognition of Shock

Shock, or developing shock, in the traumatized child must be recognized rapidly and treated vigorously early in the

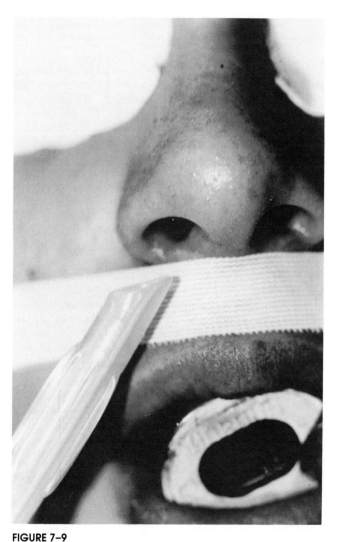

FIGURE 7–9
Choice of endotracheal tubes as related to nares, for size relationship.

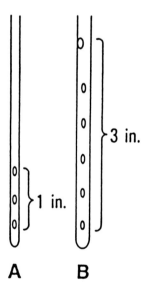

FIGURE 7–10
Comparison of adult and pediatric sump gastric tubes. *A*, Pediatric sump gastric tube (Replogle suction catheter, Argyle, St. Louis, Mo.). *B*, Adult-type sump gastric tube. (From Canty TG: Esophageal atresia and tracheoesophageal fistula. In: Cameron JL (ed): Current Surgical Therapy. Toronto, BC Decker, 1989, p 35.)

Table 7–8
Systemic Responses to Blood Loss in the Pediatric Trauma Patient

	Early		Prehypotensive	Hypotensive
	<25% EBV loss		25–40% EBV loss	≥40% EBV loss
Cardiac	Tachycardia		Tachycardia	Tachycardia to Bradycardia
Blood pressure	Normal ?		+ Tilt test	Frank hypotension
Skin	Cool, clammy		Cold extremities	Pale, cold
Capillary refill	≤2 sec		Prolonged refill	Markedly delayed refill
Central nervous system	Irritable Combative, confused		Changes in level of consciousness	Comatose
Kidneys	Decreased UOP Increased serum globulin		Rising BUN	No UOP

EBV, Estimated blood volume.
Adapted from American College of Surgeons Committee on Trauma: Advanced Trauma Life Support Course. Ramenofsky ML (ed). Chicago, American College of Surgeons, 1989, p 220.

resuscitation process. Tachycardia, although considered the most consistent sign of early hypovolemic shock, may be present in the crying, frightened child in the absence of hypovolemia.[8, 19, 23] However, tachycardia should not be attributed simply to patient anxiety without excluding causes for hypovolemia. Normal blood pressure for children varies (see Table 7–7); however, the lower limit for normal systolic blood pressure in a noncrying child may be estimated by adding 70 plus twice the child's age in years.[23] The expected diastolic blood pressure is approximately two thirds of the systolic pressure.[10] Early in hypovolemia, a small rise in the diastolic pressure without change in the systolic pressure may be observed. The child can compensate for blood losses in excess of 15 to 20% with tachycardia and vasoconstriction in the presence of a normal systolic blood pressure. Hence, in this age group, hypotension can be a late, and often sudden, sign of hypovolemia.[30]

In addition to blood pressure and heart rate changes in hypovolemia, the clinical appearance of the child may reveal signs of decreased tissue perfusion (Table 7–8), with cool, mottled extremities and capillary refill prolonged longer than 2 seconds, strongly suggesting the developing shock. Diminished peripheral pulses and altered sensorium indicate progressively more profound degrees of shock.

In early hemorrhage, up to 25% of the circulating blood volume may have been lost, but in children, clinical signs of blood pressure, capillary refill, and urinary output may be normal. Prehypotensive hemorrhage represents 25 to 35% loss of circulating blood volume. Tachycardia and tachypnea become more readily apparent, and the rise in diastolic blood pressure results in a narrowed pulse pressure, but systolic blood pressure may be within normal ranges. Catecholamine release, responsible for the sustained systolic and elevated diastolic pressure through vasoconstriction, also results in a prolonged capillary refill. Urinary output may be depressed with a concomitant rise in the blood urea nitrogen, and subtle signs of decreased sensorium and a decreased response to pain may become evident.

In patients who have hemorrhaged 40% or more of the circulating blood volume, systolic hypotension is demonstrated consistently.[2] These patients uniformly demonstrate other clinically apparent signs of hypovolemic shock, including tachycardia, diminished or absent urinary output, markedly prolonged capillary refill, and significant changes in mental status progressing to coma.

Circulation—Treatment of Shock

The rapid institution of adequate vascular access and the control of ongoing hemorrhage are the principal elements of treatment during the initial assessment and resuscitation phase of trauma management. Measures to gain vascular access begin almost immediately on arrival in the emergency department, if not already established in the field. Control of hemorrhage, particularly of exposed lacerations, begun during the field resuscitation efforts, is ongoing. Intracavitary hemorrhage, however, requires intervention after arrival at the receiving center in most situations. Medical antishock trousers (MAST), controversial in the treatment of adult patients, have little or no use in pediatric patients. Injured children come in a variety of sizes and shapes, but the MAST are far more limited in sizes. Inappropriately fitted garments may be not only ineffectual in sustaining perfusion to vital organs, but in fact deleterious.[18]

Scalp lacerations can bleed profoundly and can result in shock in the small child. In such children with altered mental status, emergency head CT should not be delayed while definitive wound closures are undertaken. Rather,

Table 7–9
Priorities for Vascular Access

I. Upper Extremity or Major Thoracic Injuries
   A. Percutaneous saphenous vein
   B. Cutdown saphenous vein in ankle
   C. ≤ 3 yr of age—Anterior tibial intraosseous line
      > 3 yr of age—Cutdown saphenofemoral junction or percutaneous femoral line
II. Lower Extremity or Major Abdominal Trauma
   A. Percutaneous cephalic or basilic veins
   B. Cutdown cephalic or basilic vein
   C. Available lower extremity veins (percutaneous or cutdown)
   D. Subclavian vein (last resort)

compressive head dressings should be placed rapidly. Alternatively, a figure-of-eight suture closing a scalp laceration is an effective and rapid hemostatic maneuver. Leaving the tails of the suture long provide for ease in their identification and removal when definitive closure is undertaken.

For gunshot wounds, in which the trajectory of the projectile is important to identify, clipping the entrance site with a radiopaque marker before applying a compressive, hemostatic dressing is also a useful measure.

In the absence of major injuries to the upper extremities, two percutaneous intravenous lines in the upper extremity are the preferred access sites (Table 7–9). The lower extremity is an acceptable alternative, preferably with the lines placed percutaneously, in the absence of major intra-abdominal injuries. Cutdown venous cannulation is occasionally required and is placed using a similar technique as that used with adults (Fig. 7–11). Care should be exercised when cannulating the cephalic vein at the level of the elbow to avoid inadvertent cannulation of the small brachial artery.

Although originally employed in the 1940s for oncologic patients, intraosseous line placement has seen a resurgence of popularity, particularly in the emergency setting. The technique, described well elsewhere, consists of placing a large-bore needle into the marrow space of the upper tibia (Fig. 7–12).[3] Using pressure infusion bags, up to 50 ml per minute may be infused.[29] Concerns for infectious complications have largely not materialized, and, with the exception of hypertonic or strongly alkaline solutions, most resuscitation drugs or fluids can be infused safely.[16, 27]

Central venous catheters have a more limited role in the initial resuscitation. In the absence of suitable peripheral venous sites, a femoral venous line may be useful, and subclavian lines in older children can be placed with little difficulty (Fig. 7–13). However, one should be mindful that most conscious children do not lie still during attempted venous line placement and require restraint; therefore, the risk from central line placement is magnified.

Once intravenous access is established, fluid resuscitation begins with the infusion of crystalloid solutions (Table 7–10). A bolus of 20 ml per kg of lactated Ringer solution

Table 7–10
Resuscitation Fluid Volumes

Product	Volume
Crystalloid	20 ml/kg bolus
Whole blood	20 ml/kg
Plasma	20 ml/kg
5% albumin	20 ml/kg
Packed red blood cells	10 ml/kg
Platelets	1–2 units/5 kg body weight
25% albumin	4 ml/kg

Maintenance Fluid Volumes

< 10 kg body weight	100 ml/kg/day
> 10 kg body weight	100 ml/kg/day for 1st 10 kg + 50 ml/kg/day for 2nd 10 kg + 25 ml/kg/day for each kg > 20 kg
	OR
> 10 kg body weight	1600 ml/M2/day

Table 7–11
Approximate Weight Based on Age

Age	Weight (kg)
Birth	3.5
6 months	6.0
1 year	12.0
4 years	16.0
10 years	35.0

From Eichelberger MR, Randolph JG: Pediatric trauma: An algorithm for diagnosis and therapy. J Trauma 23:91–97, 1983.

infused over several minutes is the preferred initial step in fluid resuscitation. While the child is being assessed for other injuries and for the response to the initial bolus, an infusion rate of 10 ml per kg per hour is safely tolerated for several hours. However, if pressure, pulse, and capillary refill are not improved with the first bolus, a second bolus of 20 ml per kg of lactated Ringer solution is administered. Most children with prehypotensive hemorrhage respond to these measures. Conversely, those with greater degrees of hemorrhage frequently have persistently decreased blood pressure, tachycardia, and poor perfusion after crystalloid infusions. After two consecutive infusions of lactated Ringer solution without significant improvement in clinical parameters, type-specific or type O Rh-negative blood is given at a rate of 10 ml per kg.

Infusion of other blood products should be reserved for specific indications. Fresh-frozen plasma is infused at a rate of 20 ml per kg in the presence of a coagulopathy secondary to the consumption of clotting factors, rather than after an empiric volume of packed cells have been replaced. Platelets, when indicated, are given in volumes of 4 units per M^2 (or 1 unit/5 kg body weight) and should raise the platelet count by approximately 40,000 to 50,000/mm³. Following stabilization, fluids are administered in volumes appropriate for the weight of the child, often utilizing weight estimates based on age (Table 7–11).

Once intravenous access is obtained and fluid resuscitation under way, venous lines should be well secured to prevent inadvertent dislodgement with the anticipated movement of the patient through the radiology suite, the operating room, or the intensive care unit.

Disability—The Brief Neurologic Examination

During the rapid initial assessment and resuscitation, a brief neurologic examination is completed. The purpose of this examination during the primary survey is to identify any immediately life-threatening intracranial lesions or any injury, that if left untreated could result in worsened neurologic impairment. A more complete neurologic examination, including a determination of the Glasgow Coma Scale level of neurologic function, is completed during the secondary survey.

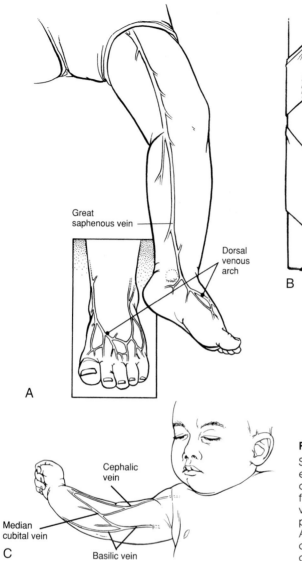

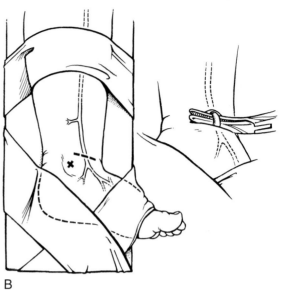

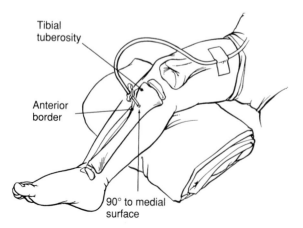

FIGURE 7–11

Selection for "cutdown" venous access, for lower extremity anatomy (A), saphenous venous cutdown access (B), and upper extremity vessels preferred for cutdown if necessary (C). (Reproduced with permission from Pediatric Advanced Life Support. Chameides L, Hazinski MF (eds). Dallas, Texas, American Heart Association/American Academy of Pediatrics, 1994, pp 5-4, 5-13. Copyright American Heart Association.)

FIGURE 7–12

Intraosseous line placement. (Reproduced with permission from Pediatric Advanced Life Support. Chameides L, Hazinski MF (eds). Dallas, Texas, American Heart Association/American Academy of Pediatrics, 1994, p 5-6. Copyright American Heart Association.)

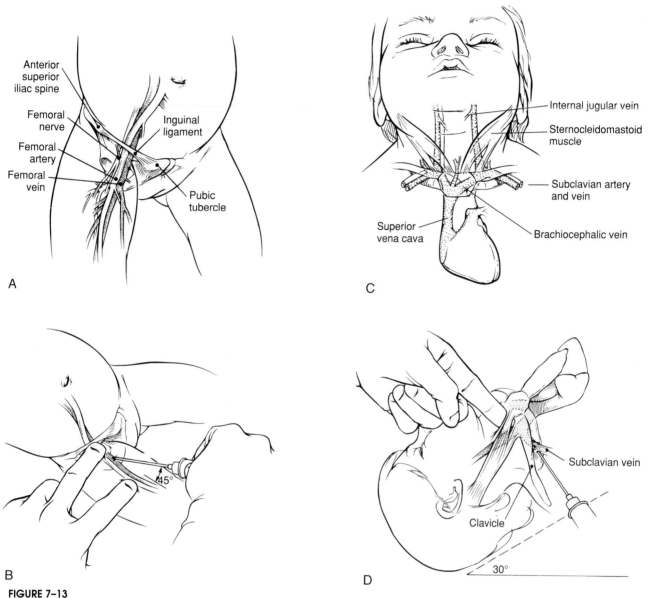

FIGURE 7–13

Central venous access, as needed, with anatomy of the groin (A), percutaneous femoral access (B), anatomy of the major central vein access sites in the neck (C), and percutaneous right subclavian access (D), puncturing the skin approximately one third of the distance along the clavicle from the medial end, directing the needle toward the suprasternal notch with the patient in the Trendelenburg position. (Reproduced with permission from Pediatric Advanced Life Support. Chameides L, Hazinski MF (eds). Dallas, Texas, American Heart Association/American Academy of Pediatrics, 1994, pp 5-9, 5-12. Copyright American Heart Association.)

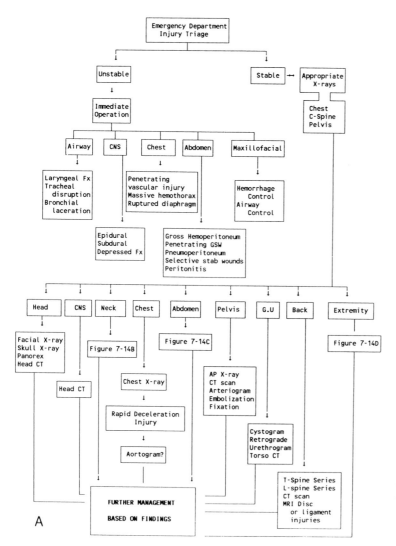

FIGURE 7-14

A–D, Triage algorithm for injury severity in pediatric trauma. C-spine, Cervical spine; CNS, central nervous system; fx, fracture; GSW, gunshot wound; GU, genitourinary; CT, computed tomography; AP, anteroposterior; T-spine, thoracic spine; L-spine, lumbar spine; MRI, magnetic resonance imaging.

Exposure

The final phase of the rapid initial survey is the complete disrobing of the patient to look for other potential injuries. Most patients can be disrobed completely shortly after arrival at the inception of resuscitation efforts. However, for those who have not been disrobed, all remaining clothing is removed (with care to maintain in-line stability of the vertebral column) as part of the primary survey. Examination of the back, particularly in patients with penetrating trauma, is important. In addition, the electrocardiogram leads, pulse oximetry monitor, and nasogastric and bladder catheters are placed at this time.

SECONDARY SURVEY

After completion of the rapid primary assessment and initiation of ongoing resuscitation measures, the patient is sequentially examined in a head-to-toe fashion (see Fig. 7–1). All injuries are recorded as they are noted and priorities for their evaluation and management then determined. It is critical to maintain a constant vigilance over the patient's clinical condition during the resuscitation period. Previously unrecognized injuries may manifest themselves at any time during the primary or secondary surveys and may result in hemodynamic instability. Hemodynamically unstable patients, unresponsive to simple resuscitation maneuvers (e.g., fluid administration, tube thoracostomy, control of visible hemorrhage), generally require prompt operative intervention. However, patients arriving with stable vital signs or those who respond quickly to resuscitation frequently require further evaluation, and at the completion of the secondary survey, the patient is triaged to the operating room or the critical care unit or to the radiology suite for further studies, depending on the severity of the injuries (Figs. 7–14 through 7–17).

Patient Transfer

Patient transfers between the resuscitation room, the radiology suites, the operating rooms, or the critical care units increase exponentially the potential for endotracheal tube dislodgement, disruption of intravenous lines, or the appearance of previously unrecognized but potentially lethal

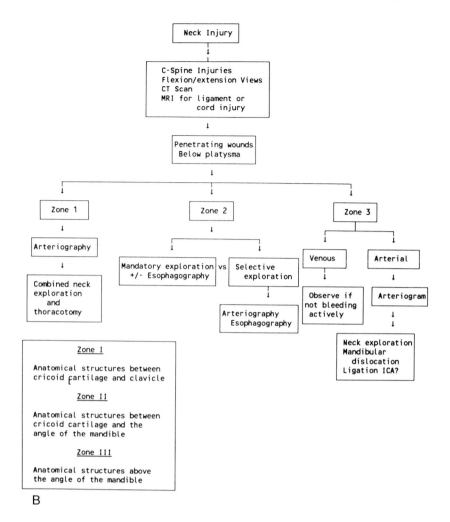

B

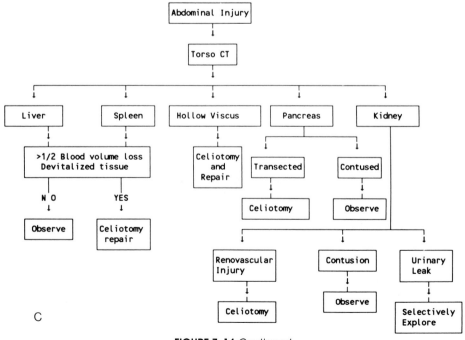

C

FIGURE 7–14 *Continued*

Illustration continued on following page

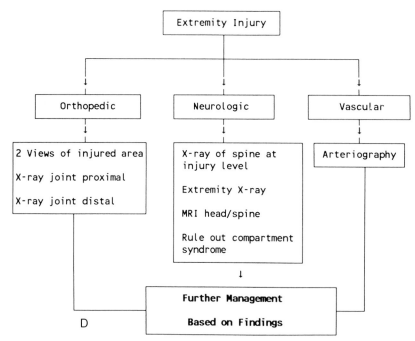

FIGURE 7-14 *Continued*

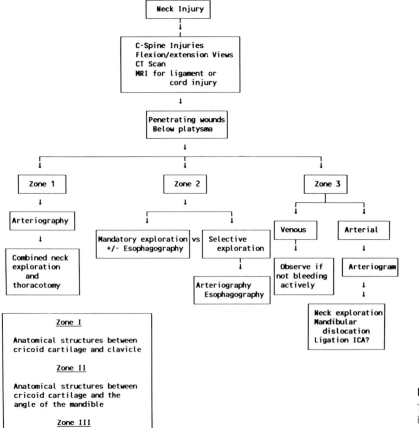

FIGURE 7-15

Triage algorithm for injury severity for neck injuries in children. C-spine, Cervical spine; CT, computed tomography; MRI, magnetic resonance imaging; ICA, internal carotid artery.

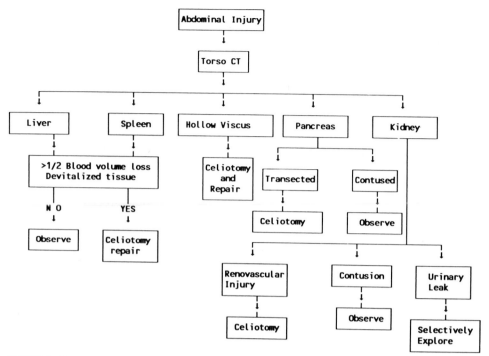

FIGURE 7-16

Triage algorithm for injury severity for abdominal injuries in children.

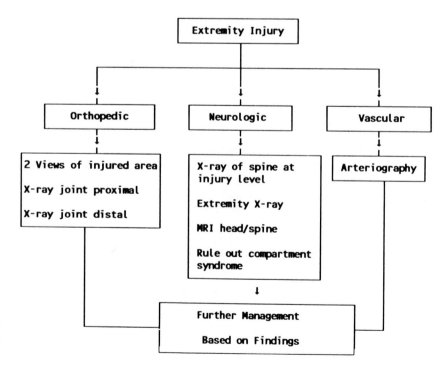

FIGURE 7-17

Triage algorithm for injury severity for extremity injuries in children. MRI, Magnetic resonance imaging.

injuries. An elevator ride to the operating room for a hemodynamically marginal patient can be a source of anxiety to the trauma surgeon and a life-threatening event for the patient.

The ideal solution to patient flow in trauma receiving units would be to place the essential elements of the radiology suite (e.g., fluoroscopy, CT scanner, and film processors) and an operating suite immediately adjacent to the resuscitation room. Although new hospital designs incorporate many of these features into the emergency department construction, older and already established facilities do not. To minimize the development of critical transport situations outside these special care units, patient transports need to occur as seldom and for as limited an amount of time as is necessary. Many radiographic studies can be accomplished satisfactorily in the resuscitation room, in particular, the anteroposterior chest radiograph, the lateral cervical spine films, and the anteroposterior pelvis radiographs, thereby minimizing unnecessary patient movement.

Specialized studies, such as CT, arteriography, retrograde urethrograms, or excretory urograms, are best accomplished in the radiology suite to obtain sufficient detail to be diagnostically valuable. Head trauma is a frequent occurrence in pediatric trauma patients, and hepatic and splenic injuries with resulting hemoperitoneum are also common and not infrequently managed nonoperatively.[20, 22, 37] Yet such injuries need to be assessed carefully and associated injuries that potentially require operative intervention detected to avoid delays in the appropriate management, operative or otherwise, of the multiply injured child. Well-performed, double-contrast (intravenous and intraluminal) CT remains to date the single most sensitive and specific, and therefore frequently employed, study to elucidate these injuries.[32] Hence, transport to CT before definitive disposition of the patient is frequent during the evaluation phase, and appropriate measures should be instituted to ensure continued monitoring and assessment of hemodynamic parameters and stability.

The Transport Team

The transport team is not truly a designated team but rather a concept underlining the need for a prepared and organized approach to patient care during transport from one critical care area to another. Like the team approach to resuscitation, a critical mass of personnel and resources is necessary to deal with any variety of situation as it occurs outside of the special care units. Once a patient is placed in the CT scanner, for example, the ability to monitor and the accessibility to treat should be minimally, if at all, compromised.

The transport team is assembled under the direction of the team leader and is composed of all essential personnel and equipment necessary for monitoring and treating the patient outside the special care unit environment. Intubated patients require a provider capable of reintubating the patient, managing the ventilator, and even treating potential barotrauma to accompany the patient. Frequently, the team leader and the senior surgical resident, in conjunction with an emergency department or critical care unit nurse and a respiratory technician, accomplish this requirement.

In addition to the appropriate personnel, monitors (to include pulse oximetry, automatic blood pressure recorders, and cardiac monitors) and additional supplies (extra liters of lactated Ringer solution, spare intravenous tubing, and intravenous catheters) are selected to accompany the patient during transport. Once the transport team arrives at the patient's next unit, the transport team members (several of whom remain as the surgical and anesthesia teams) assist in the orderly movement of the patient to the radiograph or CT table, the intensive care unit bed, or the operating room table and if necessary relay appropriate vital information to the accepting unit team. Patients in the radiology suite for definitive studies are monitored as if they were still in one of the special care units.

SUMMARY

The management of pediatric trauma requires a carefully orchestrated interplay between the EMS response teams, the emergency department and trauma team personnel, and the accepting units. At each echelon of care, assessment, resuscitation, triage, and reassessment is required. Once in the hospital environment, an efficient, algorithmic approach to the traumatized patient is recommended to facilitate rapid resuscitation, to identify and prioritize each injury, to minimize neurologic sequelae, and to make appropriate management decisions. No singular approach should be considered the only correct approach. Rather, a protocol for trauma care that is attuned to the institution's geographic and urban demographics, the availability of surgical expertise, and the physical limitations of the building itself is appropriate.

References

1. Accidental Death and Disability: The Neglected Disease of Modern Society. Washington, DC, National Academy of Sciences National Research Council, April 1969.
2. Advanced Trauma Life Support Instructor Manual: Initial Assessment and Management. Chicago, American College of Surgeons, 1989, pp 9–30.
3. American Heart Association/American Academy of Pediatrics: Textbook of Pediatric Advanced Life Support. Chameides L (ed). Elk Grove Village, Ill, American Heart Association, 1988, pp 37–46.
4. Border JR, Lewis FR, Aprahamian C, et al: Panel: Prehospital trauma care—Stabilize or scoop and run. J Trauma 23:708–711, 1983.
5. Canty TG: Esophageal atresia and tracheoesophageal fistula. In: Cameron JL (ed): Current Surgical Therapy. Toronto, BC Decker, 1989, pp 33–37.
6. Cleveland HC: Trauma center design. In: Mattox KL, Moore EE, Feliciano DV (eds): Trauma. East Norwalk, Conn, Appleton & Lange, 1988, pp 45–52.
7. Cowley RS, Hudson F, Scanlon E, et al: An economical and proved helicopter program for transporting the emergency critically ill and injured patient in Maryland. J Trauma 13:1029–1038, 1973.
8. Eichelberger MR, Randolph JG: Pediatric trauma: An algorithm for diagnosis and therapy. J Trauma 23:91–97, 1983.
9. Goldbloom RB: Halifax and the precipitate birth of pediatric trauma. Pediatrics 77:764, 1986.
10. Haller AJ, Pokorny WJ: Pediatric trauma. In: Mattox KL, Moore EE, Feliciano DV (eds): Trauma. East Norwalk, Conn, Appleton & Lange, 1988, pp 629–643.
11. Harris BH, Latchaw LA, Murphy RE, et al: A protocol for pediatric trauma receiving units. J Pediatr Surg 24:419–422, 1989.

12. Harris BH, Schwaitzberg SD: Evolution of the care of the injured child. Surg Ann 20:1–15, 1988.
13. Hospital and prehospital resources for optimal care of the injured patient. Bull Am Coll Surg 68:11, 1983.
14. Izant RJ, Hubay CA: The annual injury of 15,000,000 children: A limited study of childhood accidental injury and death. J Trauma 6:65–74, 1966.
15. Joyce M: Initial management of pediatric trauma. In: Marcus RE (ed): Trauma in Children. Rockville, Md, Aspen Publishers, 1986, pp 13–38.
16. Kanter RK, Zimmerman JJ, Strauss RH, et al: Pediatric emergency intravenous access—Evaluation of a protocol. AMJ Dis Child 140:132–134, 1986.
17. McCoy C, Bell MJ: Preventable traumatic deaths in children. J Pediatr Surg 18:505–508, 1983.
18. Mackersie RC, Christensen JM, Lewis FR: The prehospital use of external counterpressure: Does MAST make a difference? J Trauma 24:882–887, 1984.
19. Mattewson JW: Shock in infants and children. J Fam Pract 10:675–703, 1980.
20. Mayer T, Walker ML, Johnson DG, et al: Causes of morbidity and mortality in severe pediatric trauma. JAMA 245:719–721, 1981.
21. O'Gorman M, Trabulsy P, Pilcher DB: Zero-time prehospital IV. J Trauma 29:84–86, 1989.
22. Oldham KT, Guice KS, Ryckman F, et al: Blunt liver injury in childhood: Evolution of therapy and current perspective. Surgery 100:542–549, 1986.
23. Pediatric Advanced Life Support: Recognition of respiratory failure and shock: Anticipating cardiopulmonary arrest. Chameides L (ed). Elk Grove Village, Ill, American Heart Association/American Academy of Pediatrics, 1988, pp 3–9.
24. Ramenofsky ML, Luterman A, Curreri PW, et al: EMS for pediatrics: Optimum treatment or unnecessary delay? J Pediatr Surg 18:498–504, 1983.
25. Ramenofsky ML, Luterman A, Quindlen E, et al: Maximum survival in pediatric trauma: The ideal system. J Trauma 24:818–822, 1984.
26. Ramenofsky ML, Ramenofsky MB, Jurkovich GJ, et al: The predictive value of the Pediatric Trauma Score. J Trauma 28:1038–1041, 1988.
27. Rosetti VA, Thompson BM, Miller J, et al: Intraosseous infusion: An alternative route of pediatric intravascular access. Ann Emerg Med 14:885–887, 1985.
28. Schiller WR, Know R, Zinnecker H, et al: Effect of helicopter transport of trauma victims on survival in an urban center. J Trauma 28:1127–1134, 1988.
29. Schoffstall JM, Spivey WH, Davidheiser S, et al: Intraosseous crystalloid and blood infusion in a swine model. J Trauma 29:384–387, 1989.
30. Schwaitzberg SD, Bergman KS, Harris BH: A pediatric trauma model of continuous hemorrhage. J Pediatr Surg 23:605–609, 1988.
31. Smith JP, Bodai BI, Hill AS, et al: Prehospital stabilization of critically injured patients: A failed concept. J Trauma 25:65–68, 1985.
32. Taylor GA, Fallat ME, Potter BM, et al: The role of computed tomography in blunt abdominal trauma in children. J Trauma 28:1660–1664, 1988.
33. Tepas JJ, Mollitt DL, Talbert JL, et al: The Pediatric Trauma Score as a predictor of injury severity in the injured child. J Pediatr Surg 22:14–18, 1987.
34. Tepas JJ, Ramenofsky ML, Mollitt DL, et al: The Pediatric Trauma Score as a predictor of injury severity: An objective assessment. J Trauma 28:425–429, 1988.
35. Trunkey DD: Trauma. Sci American 249:28–35, 1983.
36. Trunkey DD, Lim RC: Analysis of 425 consecutive trauma fatalities: An autopsy study. JACEP 3:368–371, 1974.
37. Walker ML, Storrs BB, Mayer T: Factors affecting outcome in the pediatric patient with multiple trauma. Child's Brain 11:387–397, 1984.
38. West JG, Cales RH, Gazzaniga AB: Impact of regionalization—the Orange county experience. Arch Surg 118:740–744, 1983.
39. West JG, Trunkey DD, Lim RC: Systems of trauma care: A study of two counties. Arch Surg 114:455–460, 1979.

H. Biemann Othersen, Jr.
Elaine K. Jeter
Melinda K. Bailey
Joseph Laver

CHAPTER EIGHT

Hemostasis, Coagulopathy, and the Use of Blood Products

This chapter deals with a subject that has changed radically within the past few years. Not only has the availability of blood-component therapy increased; also, the philosophy of blood replacement has been reversed. With the specter of blood-borne diseases, pediatric surgeons no longer urge anesthesiologists to infuse blood as it is lost, and innovative methods of avoiding blood transfusions have appeared. With the concern for acquired immunodeficiency syndrome (AIDS) and hepatitis, patients and families are extremely suspicious of any administration of blood. The relative risk of transfusion must be weighed against its benefits. What is more, it is the surgeon's responsibility to minimize blood loss during operative procedures and to maximize the salvage and return of the patient's own blood when bleeding is inevitable.

We present in this chapter the views of a practicing pediatric surgeon, pediatric hematologist, anesthesiologist, and clinical pathologist. An understanding of normal coagulation and of indications for use of blood components is necessary before the development of therapeutic approaches to children who are acutely injured. The principles of evaluation and therapy still apply but must be compressed and abbreviated according to the severity of the injury and the concomitant hemorrhage.

HEMATOLOGIC EVALUATION OF THE INJURED CHILD

Even in acute trauma, a rapid history and evaluation of the child's hematologic status must be performed.

History

A detailed history can be taken quickly, asking specific and direct questions of family or relatives when possible regarding the following:

1. Bleeding in the neonatal period—from the umbilical stump or after circumcision
2. Development of hematomas after intramuscular immunizations
3. Easy bruisability with minor trauma

4. Excessive bleeding after surgical procedures
5. Bleeding into joints
6. Hematuria
7. Gastrointestinal bleeding

Affirmative responses to these questions may be suggestive of a coagulopathy. Nosebleeds are common in children and usually do not require further evaluation unless they have been severe or frequent.[34]

Further questions can be asked regarding other issues:

1. Drugs that might influence hemostasis—e.g., aspirin may cause gastrointestinal hemorrhage and abnormal platelet function[28]
2. Diseases such as nephropathies and collagen diseases are often associated with coagulopathies and prolonged bleeding time
3. Family history of an inherited problem with coagulation
4. Questions concerning thromboses may indicate antithrombin III or protein C or S deficiencies; these abnormalities can result in major intraoperative complications such as massive thrombosis[3, 7]

Physical Examination

Particular attention is paid to skin rashes, petechiae, and the distribution of bruises or hematomas. Hepatosplenomegaly, lymphadenopathy, or joint abnormalities may indicate a primary underlying condition associated with coagulopathy.[36]

Laboratory

Four categories of excessive bleeding require consideration:

1. Defects
2. Disorders in platelet plug formation
3. Abnormalities in fibrin formation
4. Massive trauma (Fig. 8–1)

Few screening tests are needed when there is a negative history of bleeding. Rapid evaluation can be made with a complete blood count (CBC) with platelet count (or the

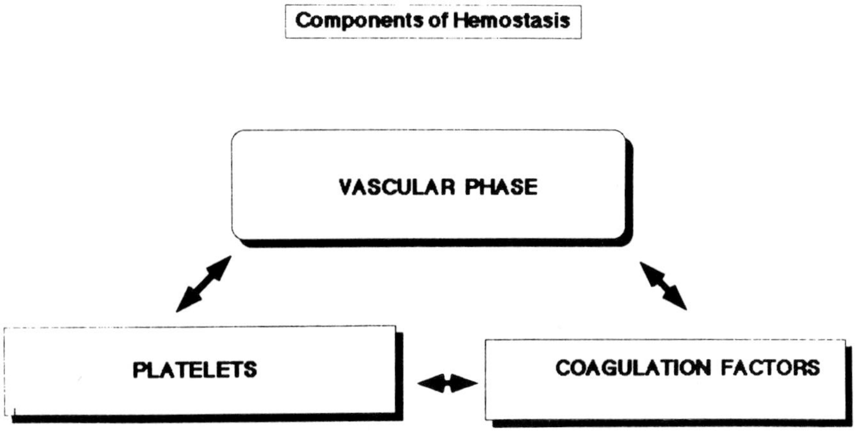

Components of Hemostasis

FIGURE 8–1
The three components of hemostasis.

presence of platelets on the blood smear), activated partial thromboplastin time (APTT), and prothrombin time (PT). A bleeding time test performed by an experienced technologist may detect abnormalities due to platelet dysfunction. If all of these tests are within normal limits, a child may still bleed during or shortly after a surgical procedure, and additional testing may be necessary. Factor XIII deficiency is a rare disorder and can be detected only by specific tests.[18] Mild cases of von Willebrand disease can also be negative on screening and may require special evaluation; usually there is a positive family history of previous coagulopathy.[44]

Preoperative Therapy

Replacement therapy provides the basis for the correction of bleeding disorders, with Factor VIII concentrates available for hemophilia and cryoprecipitate for von Willebrand disease. For other factor deficiencies, fresh frozen plasma (FFP) may be indicated when specific concentrates are not available.

Preoperative Preparation

If there is a positive family history of bleeding or previous hematologic disorders, the family usually is aware of the problem and the possible need for blood transfusion. If the patient's condition permits, consultation can be obtained with a pediatric hematologist and a transfusion medicine physician.

In children with no history of hematologic abnormalities before injury, the family's major concern often is indicated by questions about the necessity for blood transfusions. Parents frequently ask whether any blood needed could be donated by family members. Blood from family members is no safer than blood from a pool of volunteer donors. The risk of transfusions from close family members has been demonstrated by graft-versus-host reactions.[41] This complication has led to the recommendation of irradiation of blood drawn from first-degree relatives (parents, siblings, offspring). Surgeons must be fully informed of the indications and relative risks of treatment with various blood components. Figures 8–2 and 8–3 and Tables 8–1 through 8–4 help clarify the derivation of blood components and their indications and risks.

Pediatric surgeons have been advocates of nonoperative therapy of some visceral injuries such as splenic rupture. In the process of successful therapy of such patients, blood is often administered. Transfusion requirements may increase with the nonoperative approach, whereas operative therapy may arrest hemorrhage earlier with less blood being required; indeed, in some situations, the risk of blood transfusion exceeds that of operative intervention.[20]

NORMAL COAGULATION

The normal mechanism of blood coagulation is demonstrated in Figure 8–4.

OXYGEN TRANSPORT

When considering blood and blood products in the management of injured children, it is important to remember that blood—particularly the red blood cell (RBC) mass—is only a courier with the function of transporting oxygen (O_2) from the lungs to all tissues in the body. On the return trip, RBCs transport wastes (CO_2) from tissues to the lung for elimination.[1] When delivery of oxygen to the organs of the body is inadequate, hypoxia occurs.

TISSUE HYPOXIA

Tissue hypoxia may be defined as "a biochemical state in which there is insufficient intracellular (mitochondrial and extramitochondrial) oxygen to maintain aerobic metabolism."[1] Three subsets of this state may be defined:

1. Ischemic hypoxia (decreased flow)
2. Anemic hypoxia (decreased hemoglobin)
3. Anoxic hypoxia (decreased arterial oxygen)[43]

This chapter is concerned with events, primarily acute hemorrhage, that produce ischemic or anemic hypoxia, or both. It is essential that acutely injured patients have first priority given to the establishment of the airway and oxygen supply so that anoxic hypoxia is not superimposed. Present technology in the form of transcutaneous oxygen monitors ($PtcO_2$) and oxygen saturation monitors in the form of pulse oximetry (SvO_2) allow continuous assessment of oxygenation. It is important to remember that pulse oximetry measures only the saturation of the existing hemoglobin in the circulation. Inadequate hemoglobin and inadequate volume may exist in the presence of 100% saturation with oxygen. Transcutaneous oxygen monitoring, although more difficult to establish and maintain, gives information about the overall adequacy of oxygen delivery and perfusion. Periodic arterial blood gas determinations are necessary for qualitative and quantitative information about oxygen delivery and allow calculation of the transcutaneous oxygen tension index. This index is the transcutaneous oxygen tension divided by the arterial oxygen tension. If oxygen saturation is maintained and intravascular volume restored, as hemoglobin decreases, the viscosity of blood falls and allows better cardiac filling and thus a compensatory increase in cardiac output. This mechanism is the rationale for "isovolemic hemodilution."

BLOOD PRODUCTS

Whole Blood

A unit of whole blood collected from a donor contains approximately 450 ml of blood plus 63 ml of anticoagulant preservative. Two major types of RBC products are available: RBC with CPDA-1 solution consisting of citrate, phosphate, dextrose, and adenine, which gives the cells a 35-day shelf life; and RBC with additive solution (AS-1, AS-3, AS-5), which provides the necessary additional pre-

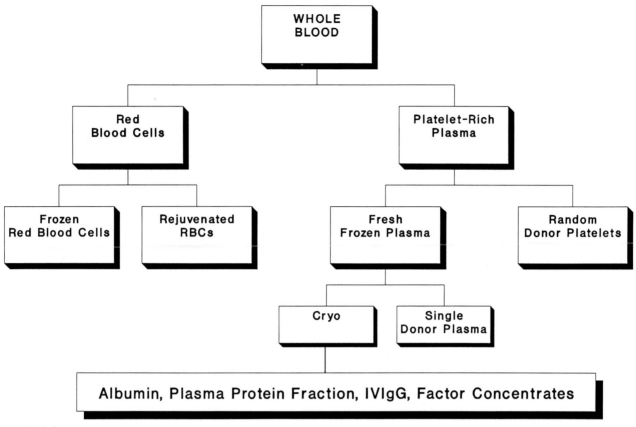

FIGURE 8–2

The derivatives from whole blood. RBCs, Red blood cells; Cryo, cryoprecipitate; IVIgG, intravenous immunoglobulin G.

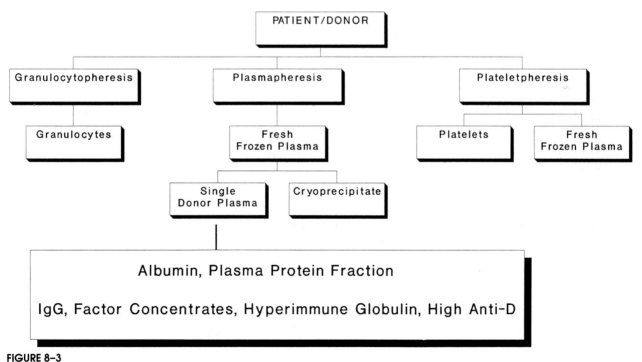

FIGURE 8–3

The derivatives obtained by apheresis.

Table 8–1
Summary of Red Blood Cell Products

Component	Indications	Use
Whole blood (WB)	Symptomatic anemia *and* hypovolemia	To restore O$_2$ carrying capacity To restore blood volume
Red blood cells (RBC)	Symptomatic anemia	To restore O$_2$ carrying capacity
Leukocyte-poor RBC	Symptomatic anemia	To restore O$_2$ carrying capacity
	Febrile transfusion reactions	To decrease human leukocyte antigen (HLA) and platelet alloimmunization To decrease viral transmission
Washed RBC	Symptomatic anemia	To restore O$_2$ carrying capacity
	Febrile or allergic transfusion reactions, or both	To decrease HLA and platelet alloimmunization To decrease viral transmission To decrease metabolic products (K$^+$) of storage
Frozen RBC	Symptomatic anemia	To restore O$_2$ carrying capacity
	Febrile or allergic transfusion reactions, or both	To decrease HLA and platelet alloimmunization
	Sensitized IGA- or IgE-deficient patients	To decrease viral transmission
	Antigen-negative RBCs for patients with unusual RBC alloantibodies	

servative (adenine) to increase the shelf life to 42 days. Phosphate, dextrose, and adenine provide substrate from which RBCs synthesize adenosine triphosphate. The citrate prevents the coagulation cascade. The 100 ml of additive solution allows more than 90 to 95% removal of donor plasma from the RBCs and a lower hematocrit (55–60%) than RBC in CPDA-1 solution (hematocrit 80%). In addition to prolonging storage shelf life, RBC with additive solution obviates the need to dilute RBCs with saline before infusion.

In hospital centers with blood donation facilities, fresh or stored whole blood may be available. Blood less than 24 hours old is rarely available owing to the time required to perform postdonation ABO group testing and Rh typing, to screen for unexpected antibodies, and to complete infectious disease testing. Although whole blood may be utilized when both volume replacement and oxygen-carrying capacity are needed (e.g., in exchange transfusions or in the actively bleeding patients in hemorrhagic shock), there is little scientific justification for its exclusive use.

Whole blood stored for more than 24 hours at 1 to 6°C has few viable platelets and granulocytes. Although the heat-stable coagulation factors (II, VII, IX, X) are main-

tained during storage, the heat-labile factors (V, VIII) decrease to levels not sufficient to correct specific factor deficiencies in the bleeding patient. The use of specific blood components (e.g., RBCs for oxygen-carrying capacity, FFP for coagulation factors, platelets for hemostasis) rather than whole blood provides the optimal method for meeting the specific therapeutic needs of the patient and minimizes the risk of fluid overload and of sensitization to plasma proteins and cellular antigens. In addition, the concept of blood component therapy allows several patients to benefit from a single blood donation, thereby conserving blood resources.

When a unit of whole blood is separated within 8 hours of collection, a unit of RBCs (250–350 ml/unit) and a unit of FFP are produced. The FFP may be stored for 1 year at −18°C or colder. Plasma obtained more than 8 hours after collection is used as single-donor plasma (deficient in factors V and VIII) and may be used in the production of albumin, plasma protein fraction, antihemophilic factor, and other blood derivatives.

Red Blood Cells

To understand and appreciate fully the situations that require transfusion under emergency conditions, a discussion of usual transfusion practices, especially in small children and infants, is necessary.

In the nontraumatized patient, transfusion of RBCs is indicated for anemic patients in whom there is a need to increase the oxygen-carrying capacity without a need for volume expansion. The decision to transfuse RBCs is based on signs and symptoms that include fatigue, pallor, shortness of breath, tachycardia, and orthostatic hypotension. Transfusions of RBCs (autologous, directed, or homologous) are clearly not indicated for volume expansion or in place of a hematinic. It has been shown in normovolemic patients that tissue oxygenation is well maintained at a hemoglobin of 6 to 7 gm per dl.[21] Likewise, it is not uncommon to see patients with 6 to 7 gm per dl of hemoglobin in chronic renal failure or anemia of chronic disease. A single hemoglobin-hematocrit value is not a sufficient criterion on which to base the need for a blood transfusion. At the present time, there is no justification for the administration of RBCs to promote ''well-being'' or to improve wound healing.[39] Wound healing is not impaired until the hematocrit drops below 15%.[25] As indicated in the previous paragraph, maintenance of oxygen saturation and blood volume allows tissue perfusion to be maintained and eliminates the necessity for transfusion of RBCs. Restoration of the RBC mass may be accelerated by the administration of recombinant erythropoietin.[16]

No universally accepted criteria exist for blood transfusion in premature or term infants.[40] Indications for transfusion differ with weight, gestation, circumstances of delivery, bone marrow erythroid function, and respiratory and cardiac function. Red blood cells are administered more aggressively to high-risk newborns in respiratory distress.[30] General indications include restoration of the hematocrit to greater than 40% at birth; maintenance of the hematocrit at greater than 40% in infants requiring ventilators, oxygen

Table 8–2
Summary of Non–Red Blood Cell Products

Component	Indication	Dose	Expected Increment
Random donor platelet	To prevent or treat hemorrhage due to qualitative or quantitative defects	1 unit/10 kg	30,000–60,000/μl
Single donor (apheresis) platelets	To prevent or treat hemorrhage due to qualitative or quantitative defects Minimize donor exposure	1 unit/70 kg	30,000–60,000/μl
HLA matched (apheresis) platelets	To prevent or treat hemorrhage in patients with HLA or antiplatelet antibodies	1 unit/70 kg	30,000–60,000/μl
Granulocytes (apheresis)	To treat infected pediatric patients with severe neutropenia due to bone marrow failure or qualitative neutrophil defects; and neonatal sepsis	15 ml/kg where 15 ml contains 1×10^9 PMNs; daily infusion of 2–3×10^{10} PMNs	Clinical improvement

HLA, Human leukocyte antigen; PMN, polymorphonuclear neutrophil leukocytes.

Table 8–3
Summary of Plasma Products and Plasma Derivatives

Component	Constituents	Indications
Fresh frozen plasma	All coagulant proteins	1. Congenital or acquired 2. Massive blood loss 3. TTP/HUS 4. Coumadin reversal
Cryoprecipitate	Factors VIII and XIII, fibrinogen, fibronectin, von Willebrand factor	Hemophilia A Hypo- or dysfibrinogenemia
Factor VIII concentrates	Factor VIII	Hemophilia A
Prothrombin complex concentrates	Factors II, VII, IX, X	Hemophilia B
5–25% albumin/plasmonate	Plasma proteins; no cellular components	To correct hypotension due to colloid loss and hypoproteinemia
Immunoglobulin preparations Intramuscular Intravenous	90–100 IgG	To provide replacement therapy To provide high-dose immunomodulant therapy (IV only)
Hyperimmune globulin preparations	Tetanus Ig (TIG) Rabies Ig (HRIG) Hepatitis BIg (HBIG) Varicella Ig (VZIG) RhIg (RhIG) Immune Serum Ig (ISG)	

TTP, Thrombotic thrombocytopenic purpura; HUS, hemolytic-uremic syndrome.

Table 8–4
Selection of Blood for Patients with Acute Blood Loss

Blood Product	Use	Availability
Uncrossmatched O red blood cells (RBCs)	Life saving; patient at risk of exsanguination	Immediate; limited number of units often available in emergency department or trauma center
Type-specific RBCs	Urgently required; patient with significant acute blood loss	10–30 min depends on whether prior typing has been performed
Crossmatched RBCs	Blood for O_2 transport required; time to perform crossmatch will not jeopardize patient	45–60 min if no unexpected antibodies; > 1 hr if antibodies are present

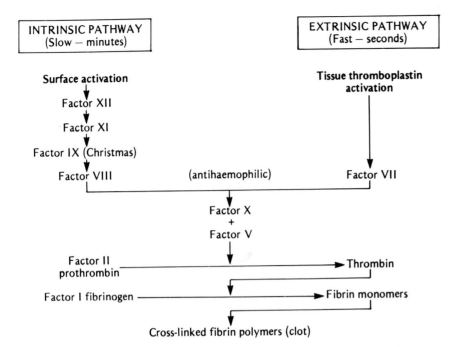

FIGURE 8–4

Normal coagulation diagram. (Reprinted with permission from Marshall V: Clinical Science for Surgeons. 2nd ed. London, Butterworth, 1988.)

support, or both, or in the presence of cyanotic heart disease; maintenance of a hematocrit of greater than 30% during the neonatal period to treat significant problems with tachycardia, tachypnea, apnea, poor weight gain, and diminished vigor; correction of iatrogenic blood loss when more than 5 to 10% of the blood volume is removed for laboratory tests.[19]

The collection of a properly identified and labeled pretransfusion patient sample is critical to safe blood transfusion. The standards for compatibility testing for neonates (younger than 4 months of age) are different from those for other patients because young infants lack a mature immunologic system. Initial testing includes an ABO group and Rh typing of the neonate's RBCs and an antibody screen. The degree of compatibility testing during any one hospitalization is dependent on the presence or absence of maternal antibodies in the neonate's serum and the group and type of any previous RBC transfusions. A 3-ml (red stopper) nonanticoagulated specimen is sufficient for this testing. Cord blood or bullet specimens are not acceptable for compatibility testing. After 4 months of age, routine compatibility testing is mandatory. The volume of patient specimen varies according to the patient's hematocrit and the number of units required for crossmatching. A 7-ml nonanticoagulated specimen is usually sufficient for crossmatching 4 to 6 units of blood. Antibody identification necessitates an additional patient specimen (serum) and should include a EDTA (plasma) anticoagulated blood sample.

Calculating transfusion volumes is not an exact science. The average blood volume in premature infants is approximately 100 ml per kg; full-term infants have 85 ml per kg; children have 75 to 80 ml per kg; and adults average 70 ml per kg. A simple formula for calculating the volume of RBCs to transfuse is the following:

Volume (in ml) of RBC = desired Hgb
      − observed Hgb × weight (kg) × 3

Three ml of RBCs per kg of weight raises the hemoglobin (Hgb) by 1 gm per dl. The average neonatal infusion of RBCs is 10 ml per kg with an infusion rate of 2 to 5 ml per kg per hour.

For routine transfusions, the dose should not exceed 15 ml per kg and is best infused through a mechanical infusion pump. Blood and blood components must be administered through a filter that retains blood clots and other cellular debris.

Constant-rate syringe delivery pumps provide satisfactory RBC transfusion with small-gauge needles.[11, 47] Red blood cells for syringe transfusions may be prefiltered by many transfusion services immediately before issue, thus obviating the need for small-volume RBC filtration at the bedside. For critically ill neonatal patients or massively transfused neonates, RBCs with additive solution (AS-1, AS-3, AS-5) may not be desirable owing to the possible effect of adenine precipitation in the immature kidney.

Although low-temperature storage (1–6°C) retards cellular metabolic functions, the products of biochemical changes accumulate with prolonged storage: glucose, pH, and 2,3-diphosphoglycerate decrease while extracellular lactic acid, ammonia, and K$^+$ increase. These storage changes have little clinical significance in adults or children because most transfusion volumes are relatively small and the recipient's compensatory homeostatic mechanism reverses these changes. However, the byproducts of storage are not tolerated by severely compromised patients or by the very young. When blood is needed urgently and exceeds 7 days of storage, a request for the freshest unit available is indicated.

Leukocyte-Reduced Red Blood Cells

The removal of leukocytes from RBCs ($<5 \times 10^8$) can be accomplished using numerous standard techniques: the removal of buffy coat by centrifugation, the use of washed RBCs or frozen deglycerolized RBCs, and the use of third-generation leukocyte reduction filters. Leukocyte-reduced RBCs are indicated for the prevention of recurrent febrile nonhemolytic transfusion reactions. These reactions occur when donor white blood cell antigen reacts with recipient white blood cell antibody. Washed or deglycerolized RBCs may be used as well to reduce the incidence of urticarial reactions, which are allergic reactions to plasma protein, and anaphylactic reactions in sensitized IgA-deficient patients.

Fresh Frozen Plasma

A unit of FFP consists of approximately 200 to 250 ml of plasma plus anticoagulant. Fresh frozen plasma contains albumin, globulins, antibodies, and all clotting factors (1 unit of factor activity per ml and 200–250 mg of fibrinogen per bag). The posttransfusion increment in coagulation factor levels is limited by the patient's ability to tolerate the infused volume of plasma without developing fluid overload. For this reason, treatment of severe coagulopathies with FFP may be difficult, and when available, patients should receive more concentrated preparations.

Indications for the use of FFP in the injured child include specific coagulation factor replacement for congenital or acquired deficiencies, massive transfusion with coexistent disseminated intravascular coagulation (DIC), antithrombin III deficiency, and thrombotic thrombocytopenic purpura. Plasma is usually not indicated as a volume expander. If only volume expansion is required, crystalloids, colloids, or both are appropriate products of choice. Transfusion using FFP is rarely indicated if the PT and partial thromboplastin time (PTT) are less than 1.5 times normal unless the patient is bleeding or is at risk of central nervous system hemorrhage.

Fresh frozen plasma contains no RBCs; therefore cross-matching or compatibility testing is not required. ABO-compatible FFP should be administered when the patient's blood type is known. When the ABO group is not known, FFP from group AB is preferred. The Rh type is not considered in FFP selection.

Fresh frozen plasma is thawed at 30 to 37°C with agitation. If it is not to be used immediately, it may be stored at 1 to 6°C and must be transfused within 24 hours because rapid loss of factors V and VIII occurs. For factor replacement, 10 to 15 ml per kg of FFP at a rate of 1 to 2 ml per minute is indicated, but for pediatric patients with acute hemorrhage, the dose may be increased to 15 to 30 ml per kg. Fresh frozen plasma is infused through a 170-micron filter. Treatment effectiveness is assessed by cessation of hemorrhage and by monitoring of coagulation function, measured by PT, PTT, or by specific factor assays.

Cryoprecipitate

Cryoprecipitate (cryo), also known as antihemophilic factor, is prepared from a unit of whole blood and contains approximately 80 to 120 units of Factor VIII per bag, 40 to 70% recovery of von Willebrand factor, 150 to 250 mg of fibrinogen, 20 to 30% of Factor XIII, and fibronectin in an average of 10 to 15 ml of plasma. The quantity of Factor VIII in a unit of cryo represents about 50% of the antihemophilic factor originally in the donor unit. Cryo is indicated to correct deficiencies of Factor VIII and congenital and acquired fibrinogen deficiencies. The amount of Factor VIII required for transfusion is calculated as follows:

$$\text{Blood volume (ml)} = \text{weight (kg)} \times 75 \text{ ml/kg}$$
$$\text{Plasma volume (ml)} = \text{blood volume (ml)}$$
$$\times (1.0 - \text{hematocrit})$$
$$\text{Units Factor VIII required} = \text{plasma volume (ml)}$$
$$\times [(\text{desired Factor VIII [U/ml]}$$
$$- \text{initial Factor VIII [U/ml]})]$$
$$\text{Bags of cryo} = \text{units of Factor VIII}/100 \text{ units per bag}$$

For hemophilia A, the minimum recommended Factor VIII levels vary with the magnitude of surgical intervention or the extent of hemorrhage: 20%—treatment of early hemorrhage; 30 to 50%—treatment of established hemorrhage; 50%—major surgery. The initial dose should raise the activity level to two times the minimum level. The initial half-life of Factor VIII is 4 hours owing to equilibration. With subsequent doses, the biologic half-live is 8 to 12 hours. To achieve the desired therapeutic level, the dose may need to be repeated at 8- to 12-hour intervals and monitored by PTT or Factor VIII assay.

Cryoprecipitate contains no RBCs and a small volume of plasma (5–20 ml/bag). Plasma compatibility is preferred but not required. The Rh type is not considered in the random selection of cryo. For ease of administration, single units of cryo are pooled into one container following thawing at 30 to 37°C. Units that are pooled must be transfused within 4 hours of the time they are pooled. Single, non-pooled units of cryo must be transfused within 6 hours of the time they are thawed. The infusion rate is 1 to 2 ml per minute, administered through a blood component set with a standard 170-micron filter.

Platelets

Random donor platelets are obtained by separating platelet-rich plasma from one unit of fresh whole blood. A unit of platelets contains a minimum of 5.5×10^{10} platelets in approximately 50 to 60 ml of plasma. Single-donor pheresis (plateletpheresis) platelets are obtained by automated cell separation devices and contain a minimum of 3.0×10^{11} platelets (equivalent to 6–8 random donor platelets) in approximately 200 ml of plasma. Single-donor platelets decrease the number of donor exposures, thereby reducing the risks of transfusion-transmitted diseases and human leukocyte antigen (HLA) alloimmunization. Whereas HLA-matched platelets play a vital role in patients who are refractory to single- and random-donor platelet transfusions, they have no role in the support of trauma patients.

Although platelet concentrates contain few RBCs, the Rh type of the platelets should be compatible with the patient's Rh type because the quantity of Rh-positive RBCs in platelet concentrate may be sufficient to sensitize an Rh-negative individual.

The goal of platelet transfusion is to prevent or stop bleeding caused by thrombocytopenia. The average pediatric platelet dose is 1 unit of platelets per 7 to 10 kg of body weight. Platelets are infused through a blood component administration set with a 170-micron filter at an infusion rate determined by volume tolerance. In neonates or pediatric patients in whom circulatory overload is a potential problem, plasma-poor (volume-reduced) platelets are indicated. Because of the additional time required by the transfusion service, plasma-poor platelets are not indicated for emergency care. Platelets require gentle agitation and are stored at room temperature for up to 5 days. Pooled platelets must be transfused within 4 hours of preparation.

Platelets are indicated to control or prevent bleeding associated with thrombocytopenia or platelet dysfunction (e.g., congenital, drug). In many medical centers, platelets are recommended prophylactically for patients with platelet counts of 10,000 to 20,000 per μl or for those who show evidence of bleeding with platelet counts of less than 50,000 per μl. It is common practice to maintain the platelet count above 30,000 to 50,000 per μl in patients who are critically ill and in thrombocytopenic patients before initiating invasive procedures.

Factor VIII Concentrates

Factor VIII concentrates are prepared from large pools of donor plasma. To reduce the risk of transmission of viral disease, viral attenuation methods are used in the manufacturing process. These include the use of detergent-solvents, dry heat, pasteurization, monoclonal antibody purification, and suspensions heated in an organic solvent.

Factor VIII (lyophilized) concentrates are indicated to treat moderate to severe hemophilia A (Factor VIII deficiency). The amount of Factor VIII required for transfusion is calculated as follows:

Units of Factor VIII required = plasma volume (ml) ×
(desired Factor VIII − initial Factor VIII)

The concentration of Factor VIII (250–1500 units) is indicated on each vial. It is administered intravenously after reconstitution with sterile diluent. Generally, a level of Factor VIII between 30 to 50% is adequate for hemostasis. However, some physicians recommend more than 50% activity for patients undergoing major surgery. Because the in vivo half-life of Factor VIII is approximately 8 to 12 hours, factor assays should be performed at these intervals and treatment repeated to maintain the desired levels.

Approximately 10 to 15% of hemophilia A patients develop Factor VIII inhibitors. Low-titer Factor VIII inhibitors require individualized therapy, whereas high-titer inhibitors may require the use of large volume of Factor VIII. Plasmapheresis or the use of Factor IX to bypass the extrinsic coagulation cascade may be indicated.

Factor IX Concentrates

Factor IX is prepared from large pools of donor plasma, utilizing either dry heat or heat-organic solvent methods to induce viral inactivation. This concentrate contains the vitamin K–dependent factors (factors II, VII, IX, and X). It is used to treat Factor IX deficiency (Christmas disease), congenital factor VII or X deficiency, and hemophiliacs with potent Factor VIII inhibitors.

Like Factor VIII, Factor IX concentrate is a lyophilized preparation, with the number of factor units indicated on each vial. It is reconstituted with sterile diluent and is administered intravenously.

SELECTION OF BLOOD FOR TRANSFUSION

The ABO Group

The ABO group of a patient is the first criterion in blood selection. Although RBCs from group O may be transfused to all patients, RBCs from a specific ABO group are preferred. Group O individuals can receive *only* group O RBCs. When blood from a patient's own ABO group is unavailable, the next choice is compatible RBCs. For example, when a patient is switched from group B to group O RBCs, the patient continues to receive FFP compatible with the patient's original type (group B or AB FFP). If this patient has been heavily exchanged with group O RBCs, any group of FFP is compatible for use.

The Rh Type

The next consideration in the selection of blood is the Rh type of the patient. Patients who are Rh negative must not, under ordinary circumstances, receive Rh-positive blood. However, a nonsensitized Rh-negative individual can and should be given Rh-positive blood as a life-saving measure when Rh-negative blood is not available. Patients who have Rh-positive blood can be given compatible Rh-negative blood safely. In the sensitized (anti-Rh antibodies) patient, Rh-negative blood must be given. Because group O, Rh-negative blood remains in relatively short supply, some trauma centers and hospital emergency departments have a limited number of uncrossmatched group O, Rh-positive units immediately available. Transfusion of these units before the determination of anti-Rh sensitization in an individual results in extravascular hemolysis. Anti-Rh antibodies are IgG antibodies and do not bind complement. Anti-Rh–coated RBCs are removed predominantly in the spleen.

The Unexpected Red Blood Cell Antibody

The presence of unexpected RBC antibodies is the third consideration in blood transfusion. A positive antibody screen is the first clue to one or more unexpected antibodies. Under normal conditions, the antibody must be identified before blood is available for transfusion. For identification of some antibodies, the delay may be several hours or more. Additional time may be required to screen donor units to obtain antigen-negative units for compatibility testing. An exception may be necessary in clinically urgent situations.

Although group O or type-specific blood should never be withheld from a patient at risk of exsanguination, the patient's physician and transfusion medicine physician should determine whether the critical clinical situation may warrant transfusion of potentially antigen-positive units to a patient with a positive antibody screen.

▶ **Example 1:** A critically injured unidentified patient arrives at a trauma center. A blood sample is obtained with a request for type-specific blood. Transfusion of uncrossmatched group O Rh-negative RBCs is under way. The transfusion service reports a positive antibody screen. Because of the urgent condition, following consultation with the transfusion medicine physician, type-specific blood is infused.

▶ **Example 2:** A surgical patient with a clinically significant antibody who requires massive transfusion intraoperatively may be transfused with antigen-positive RBCs after the equivalent of the patient's blood volume has been transfused. The patient's clinical situation, the blood supply, and the antibody characteristics must be considered. The infusion of antigen-positive units should be limited to minimize the degree of delayed hemolysis once the bleeding begins to come under control.

TRANSFUSION-ASSOCIATED REACTIONS

Like antibiotics, chemotherapy, and other medication, the transfusion of blood or blood components must be prescribed by a physician, has inherent risks and benefits, and is followed by a transfusion effect. In most cases, a favorable effect involves correction of a deficit in the patient. In a small number of cases, 0.5 to 3.0% of transfusions, the recipient may experience an adverse effect that may manifest itself during or immediately following the transfusion or may be delayed for days to months following the infusion.

One of the best methods of avoiding transfusion reactions is attention to pretransfusion care. The order for blood components must be written in light of the patient's clinical condition and the results of laboratory testing. In nonurgent situations, determination of the patient's religious beliefs should be verified, and a court order should be obtained when indicated. The blood sample for compatibility testing should be properly labeled at the bedside after confirming the patient's identification verbally and by arm band. Documentation that the patient or legal guardian understands the benefits and risks of transfusion (informed consent) should be entered in the physician's progress notes. A patient who has been instructed concerning the signs and symptoms of a transfusion reaction is more likely to call medical attention to untoward symptoms of a reaction.

Before initiation of the blood infusion, the blood component and the recipient must be properly identified. Clerical errors in the operating room, at the bedside, and in the blood bank account for most component-recipient mistakes. General guidelines for transfusion include obtaining vital signs before transfusion; starting infusions within 30 minutes of release of blood from the blood bank, not to exceed 4 hours for infusion; inspecting the mechanical infusion pumps and blood warmers for evidence of hemolysis; ensuring that infusion rates are adequate; and repeating tests for vital signs at 10 minutes after initiation of the transfusion. If viscosity must be decreased to promote adequate flow, only 0.9% normal saline or compatible plasma may be used. Drugs should never be mixed with blood components. If medications must be administered during transfusion, they should be given through a separate intravenous line and preferably at a location removed from the blood transfusion.

If at any point during a transfusion signs or symptoms of a transfusion reaction become apparent, the transfusion must be stopped, vital signs obtained, the vein kept open by normal saline, and a clerical check performed. A thorough clinical assessment and treatment of symptoms must be initiated. The blood bag with the attached administration set and tags, along with the completed transfusion reaction form, must be returned to the transfusion service for clerical and serologic workup. Blood and urine samples are submitted to the laboratory. The reaction must also be documented in the physician's progress notes.

Acute Hemolytic Transfusion Reaction

Acute hemolytic transfusion reactions are usually due to ABO incompatibility. Antibodies in the recipient's plasma attach to antigens on the transfused RBCs, activate complement, and cause intravascular hemolysis. The most frequent initial symptom is fever, commonly with chills. Reactions usually occur after only 10 to 15 ml of blood have been transfused. Clinical manifestations include low back pain, flushing, tachycardia, hypotension, hemoglobinemia, hemoglobinuria, acute renal failure, shock, and death. *In the anesthetized or unconscious patient, bleeding at the surgical site (due to disseminated intravascular coagulation), hypotension despite adequate fluids, and hemoglobinuria may be the only manifestations.* The pathophysiology of acute hemolytic transfusion reaction involves activation of three interrelated mechanisms: the neuroendocrine response, with liberation of the kinin system and release of catecholamines; the complement system and intravascular hemolysis; and the coagulation system with resultant disseminated intravascular coagulation.

The investigation of an acute hemolytic transfusion reaction includes an immediate urine sample for hemoglobin. Intact RBCs in the urine are a sign of hemorrhage in the urinary tract and are not caused by hemolytic reactions. However, free hemoglobin in a fresh urine sample is good evidence of intravascular hemolysis. If there has been a delay of several days before urine is obtained or the diagnosis of hemolysis is entertained, hemosiderin in the urinary sediment supports prior hemolysis. Immediate blood samples for total and unconjugated bilirubin, free hemoglobin in the plasma, haptoglobin, PT, APTT, and creatinine provide valuable diagnostic information. A rise in unconjugated bilirubin may be detectable within 1 hour after the transfusion reaction, but it usually peaks at 4 to 6 hours after the reaction. Free hemoglobin in the plasma provides direct evidence of intravascular hemolysis. In the absence of a determination of free hemoglobin in the plasma, pre- and posttransfusion haptoglobin levels may provide indirect evidence of intravascular hemolysis. However, if there is visible hemoglobinemia, there is no need to measure haptoglobins. Haptoglobin levels decrease as haptoglobin-hemoglobin complexes are formed. Creatinine provides evidence of baseline renal function. Prolonged PT and PTT support the diagnosis of disseminated intravascular coagulation.

If a hemolytic transfusion reaction is suspected, repeat ABO and Rh typings are ordered on pre- and posttransfusion patient specimens, as well as on the suspicious blood bag (also any bags immediately preceding the unit in question, if available). Repeat crossmatches are performed on the pre- and posttransfusion specimens. A positive direct antiglobulin test (DAT or direct Coombs test) on a posttransfusion specimen supports in vivo RBC antigen-antibody interaction.

Anaphylactic Reaction

An anaphylactic reaction is an afebrile, nonhemolytic transfusion reaction that occurs after infusion of a few milliliters of blood or plasma-containing products. Symptoms include coughing, bronchospasm, wheezing, and respiratory distress, which may progress to cyanosis, shock, or cardiac arrest. Reactions occur following the infusion of IgA proteins to IgA-deficient recipients who have developed anti-IgA antibody. The diagnosis of IgA deficiency with anti-IgA antibodies is usually made retrospectively. However, for sensitized IgA-deficient patients, RBCs that have been washed extensively or blood from IgA-deficient patients may be used. Washing may require upward of 1 hour per unit, whereas IgA-deficient blood may require more than 24 hours to obtain via rare donor registries. Extensive washing of platelets may be necessary for sensitized IgA-deficient patients who require platelets. IgA-deficient FFP must be obtained from the rare donor registry.

Bacterial Contamination

An acute nonimmunologically mediated reaction occurs following the infusion of blood contaminated by bacteria. Cold-tolerant microorganisms, particularly *Pseudomonas* and *Klebsiella,* have been implicated. Fatal cases of infection from transfusion-associated *Yersinia entercolitica* have been reported to the Centers for Disease Control and Prevention. Symptoms include high fever, chills, circulatory collapse, and death. Treatment of shock is imperative. Cultures of the blood bag and the patient are necessary for identification of the offending organism.

Febrile Transfusion Reaction

Febrile transfusion reactions are the most commonly reported adverse effects of transfusion. By definition, there is a temperature rise of 1°C or more occurring in association with a transfusion and without any other explanation. Patients experience sudden chills and fever, headache, muscle pain, and anxiety. Febrile reactions occur following sensitization to donor white blood cells, platelets, or plasma proteins. Sensitized patients may be pretreated with antipyretics before subsequent transfusions, or they may receive leukocyte-reduced blood products (filtered, washed, or frozen).

Allergic Reaction

Patients with allergic transfusion reactions may experience local or generalized urticaria, flushing, and itching. These reactions result from sensitivity to foreign plasma proteins, such as drugs or food substances. Fever is not a clinical manifestation of allergic (urticarial) transfusion reactions. After antihistamines are administered, a transfusion may be restarted if symptoms have resolved.

Delayed Hemolytic Transfusion Reaction

Delayed hemolytic transfusion reactions may result from primary or secondary (anamnestic) alloimmunization. Clinical manifestations include decreased hematocrit, mild jaundice, and fever that usually occur 7 to 14 days after the transfusion. Transfused RBCs are destroyed by alloantibodies not detectable at the time of crossmatch. When suspected clinically, the diagnosis is confirmed by a positive DAT or a direct Coombs test and identification of the offending serum antibody.

Transfusion-Associated Graft-versus-Host Disease

Transfusion-associated graft-versus-host disease is a rare complication following transfusion of blood components to immunoincompetent patients. Immunocompetent donor lymphocytes engraft and react against tissues of the host-recipient. Patients at risk include those who have congenital immune deficiency syndromes; recipients of autologous and allogeneic bone marrow transplants; premature newborns; and patients with Hodgkin's and non-Hodgkin's lymphomas, hematologic malignancies, and solid tumors. Transfusions from human leukocyte antigen–homozygous blood donors to a recipient sharing the donor's haplotype may predispose to transfusion-associated graft-versus-host disease in immunocompetent patients. It has been documented in recipients of blood from first-degree family members and in homogeneous populations. The only effective method to prevent this disease is gamma irradiation of blood products before transfusion. Doses of 15 to 35 Gy (1500–3500 rads) are capable of inhibiting lymphocyte proliferation.

Infectious Diseases

Transfusion-associated hepatitis is the most frequent serious infectious complication of blood transfusion. Hepatitis transmission has been reduced by mandatory testing of donors, donor self-exclusion, and elimination of paid donors. All blood components carry a risk of transmitting hepatitis except those such as albumin, plasma protein fraction, and serum immune globulin preparations in which the manufacturing process inactivates the virus. New methods of manufacturing coagulation factor concentrates have significantly reduced the risk of transmission of hepatitis B and C (non-A, non-B).

Human immunodeficiency virus (HIV) has been transmitted by whole blood, cellular components, plasma, and clotting factor concentrates, indicating that the virus is present in plasma as well as in the cellular components. There has been no known HIV transmission in albumin and immunoglobulins.

Transfusion-Related Acute Lung Injury

Transfusion-related acute lung injury is an infrequent but serious complication of transfusion attributed to either the passive transfer of donor antibodies against leukocytes or, more rarely, the presence of leukoagglutinins in the recipient serum.[10, 17] Clinical features include fever, chills, tachycardia, cough, and various degrees of respiratory distress. The chest radiograph demonstrates bilateral pulmonary infiltrates in the absence of cardiac enlargement and pulmonary vascular engorgement. The onset of respiratory distress ranges between a few minutes to hours after transfusion.

Circulatory Overload

Circulatory or volume overload, an infrequently reported transfusion reaction, occurs following administration of fluid in excess of the ability of the circulation to accommodate it. Clinical symptoms include cough, rales, dyspnea, tachycardia, and hypertension. Prevention of circulatory overload, particularly in patients with compromised cardiac or respiratory status, may necessitate adjustment in transfusion volume and flow rate, use of RBC concentrates rather than whole blood, or division of units into smaller aliquots.

IN THE OPERATING ROOM

The Anesthesiologist

During major surgical procedures, the anesthesiologist works in close concert with the surgical team in determining the need for transfusion therapy. Vigilance in monitoring blood loss, coagulation status, and hemodynamic parameters is required to avoid unnecessary transfusion in the perioperative period. A growing number of options are also available for blood conservation; these techniques should be considered and customized to meet each individual patient's needs.

Autotransfusion

Perioperative autotransfusion, or the salvage and reinfusion of shed blood, has become a valuable adjunctive technique in solving problems related to blood transfusions.

Three types of autotransfusion have been described: preoperative donation; intraoperative salvage, hemodilution, or both; and postoperative salvage and reinfusion.

Although preoperative donation is obviously not suitable for the initial management of trauma victims, many of these patients do return for follow-up surgery related to the initial injury, and preoperative donation should always be an option in these cases. Preoperative donation has been demonstrated to be effective in children as young as 8 years, who can donate 1 to 5 proportional units of blood before surgery.[37] Guidelines are available, based on weight in kilograms, regarding the amount of blood that can be collected. Oral iron therapy is used simultaneously to increase marrow production, thus resulting in maintenance of hematocrits in the low normal range.

Autotransfusion during the intraoperative period can be accomplished by intentional intraoperative isovolemic hemodilution[12] or, as is more common, by cell salvage directly from the operative field by use of a cell saver system.

Isovolemic hemodilution is based on the principle that bleeding at a lower hematocrit results in less loss of red blood cell mass.[33] It is accomplished by removal of whole blood, usually just after induction of anesthesia, with simultaneous replacement using colloid or crystalloid solution.[32] Blood is collected in bags containing an anticoagulant such as CPDA-1, stored at room temperature for up to 4 hours, and then reinfused at the end of the major blood loss or when the hematocrit reaches a predetermined threshold. This technique has been used successfully for cases of pediatric orthopedic trauma, and it remains the only practical means of obtaining fresh whole blood in the perioperative period. A specialized system that is acceptable to most Jehovah's Witnesses is available.[33]

Intraoperative autotransfusion via cell saver devices such as the Haemonetics Cell Saver IV (Fig. 8–5) has become an established means for decreasing perioperative homologous blood use in elective surgery and is now gaining popularity in busy trauma centers.[14, 27] These devices consist of a collection component that aspirates blood from the operative field and mixes it with an anticoagulant (usually heparin); a reservoir for collection; a blood processing component that spins, concentrates, and washes the RBCs; and finally, a retransfusion component.

Indications for use of the cell saver system in trauma have been reviewed; an initial hematocrit value of less than 35% or more than 2 liters of crystalloid resuscitation in the emergency department have been reported as indicators for a potential role in the use of the cell saver system for trauma surgery.[22] Contraindications include bacterial contamination of the wound or the presence of tumor cells, but even these are controversial.[42] Side effects include hemato-

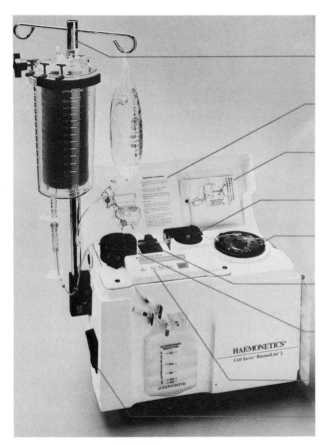

FIGURE 8–5
Cell-saver device. Haemonetics, Cell Saver, HaemoLite 2.

logic alterations, such as thrombocytopenia and decreased clotting factors, and nonhematologic complications, such as air or fat embolus, infusion of cellular debris, and sepsis. Despite these problems, potential benefits are obvious, and blood salvage via the cell saver system should be considered in any surgery in which major blood loss pools in the operative field and is being cleared by suction.

Reinfusion of shed blood collected from mediastinal, pleural, or orthopedic drainage systems has also become accepted practice during the postoperative period. This blood is defibrinated and will not clot; therefore, it does not requires an anticoagulant.

Appropriate Use of Blood and Blood Products

As stated earlier, National Institutes of Health consensus conferences[24–26] have established that the previous thresholds for transfusion therapy (hemoglobin of 10 gm/dl and hematocrit of 30%) are inappropriately high. Many patients do well with hematocrits of 21% or less. Higher values may be necessary, however, in patients who have an increased demand for oxygen or in those who cannot compensate for a reduced delivery of oxygen. Guidelines for transfusion of RBCs must take into account multiple factors, such as the patient's ability to compensate, coexisting medical conditions, and increased requirements due to concomitant trauma such as head injury, pulmonary contusion, and the like.

The ultimate goal of perioperative RBC transfusion is maintenance of adequate oxygen transport and delivery to the various tissue beds of the body. It is important to realize that although hemoglobin level is significant, it is not the only factor that determines oxygen transport. The amount of oxygen available for delivery is dependent on the product of two variables: cardiac output (CO) and oxygen content of arterial blood (CaO_2), such that delivery of O_2 = CO × CaO_2.

The total oxygen content of blood (CaO_2) can be calculated by the following equation:

$$CaO_2 = Hb(SaO_2 \times 1.37) + (PaO_2 \times .003)$$

in which Hb = the hemoglobin concentration in grams per 100 ml of blood; SaO_2 = the percent saturation of hemoglobin in arterial blood; 1.37 = the ml of oxygen that 1 gram of hemoglobin carries when fully saturated; PaO_2 = the partial pressure of oxygen in arterial blood; and .003 = the solubility coefficient of oxygen in blood.

Assuming a 5-liter CO and a normal arterial oxygen content (CaO_2) of 20 volume %, delivery may then be calculated as follows:

$$\text{Delivery} = CO \times CaO_2 = 5 \text{ liters/minute}$$
$$\times\ 200 \text{ ml/liter} = 1000 \text{ ml/minute of oxygen}$$
$$\text{transported to the tissues}$$

Mean oxygen utilization is approximately 2 to 3 ml per kg or 250 ml per minute, such that 750 ml of oxygen returns to the right side of the heart each minute, leading to a mixed venous saturation (SvO_2) of approximately 75%. This represents a mean oxygen extraction ratio of 25%.

It is important to realize, however, that oxygen extraction varies with different tissue beds. The extraction ratio of the coronary bed is highest at 58%, but other organs have lower extraction rates (e.g., 5 to 10%, for the kidney). This fact suggests that the heart may be the organ most vulnerable to injury during normovolemic anemia states.[39] Experimental data in animals have suggested that the heart may be able to compensate up to a critical point corresponding to an overall global extraction ratio of approximately 50% (hematocrit = 10%). The applicability of these studies to the human population is unknown.[39]

Optimization of oxygen delivery requires identification of which factors are submaximal—cardiac output, hemoglobin, or SaO_2. Life-saving measures for the trauma patient may not allow enough time for the placement of invasive monitors capable of measuring variables such as cardiac output and mixed venous oxygen saturation. Once the clinical situation is under control, however, these monitors can provide much data on which to make rational decisions regarding the administration of blood.

Studies have also shown that blood products such as platelets and FFP may be overutilized.[12, 24, 26] Neither of these products has proved beneficial when given prophylactically during massive transfusion. Specific indications for their use have been delineated and discussed previously in this chapter. Once again, laboratory values offer guidance, but clinical correlation is essential. Traditional laboratory testing can produce results that are markedly abnormal in patients with no evidence of clinical coagulopathy.

The thromboelastograph device has been useful for the detection and management of coagulation defects associated with intraoperative blood loss, particularly during hepatic transplantation and after cardiopulmonary bypass surgery. This instrument can provide an on-site assessment of qualitative coagulation kinetics, including platelet function and clot stability, allowing for more rapid interpretation and intervention during progressive blood loss.[45] This device may also be helpful in differentiating disseminated intravascular coagulation from primary fibrinolysis, a diagnosis not easily made by routine coagulation testing.

Pharmacologic Agents to Enhance Blood Clotting

Desmopressin acetate (DDAVP), a synthetic analogue of vasopressin, has been studied in patients undergoing major surgery as an aid to maintenance of hemostasis. This drug works primarily by inducing the release of von Willebrand factor and procoagulants of Factor VIII. Perioperative application of DDAVP stems from its successful use in treating disorders with abnormal platelet function such as uremia. Multiple studies have been published regarding the use of desmopressin in the perioperative period, but proof of efficacy is inconclusive.[31, 35] Currently the perioperative indications for desmopressin remain unclear. It may be useful in conditions with prolonged bleeding times, such as postcardiopulmonary bypass, but further investigation is needed. It should also be noted that the administration of desmopressin is not without side effects, including hypotension secondary to vasodilation if administration is too rapid.

Antifibrinolytics, such as aprotinin, are another class of pharmacologic agents currently under investigation for use in promoting hemostasis during surgery. Prophylactic aprotinin has been used in Europe for decreasing perioperative blood loss during cardiac surgery, and prospective trials for the use of this agent are now in progress in the United States.[12]

Future Trends

Attempts to develop asanguinous oxygen-carrying solutions have produced two alternatives to homologous RBCs: perfluorochemical emulsions and stroma-free hemoglobin solutions. Both sets of these compounds are limited by side effects, and currently neither is licensed for routine use. Perfluorochemicals, such as Fluosol-DA, are limited by their high partial pressure of oxygen (PO_2) requirements (500–600 mm Hg), whereas stroma-free hemoglobin solutions have the disadvantages of elevated oxygen affinity, poor vascular retention, and possible nephrotoxicity. The development of second-generation products, including the production of synthetic erythrocytes or "hemosomes," is presently under way.[2] Perhaps even closer on the horizon is the production of plasma proteins, such as albumin and coagulation factors, using recombinant DNA. Human erythropoietin, a physiologic bone marrow stimulant, is presently

being manufactured via recombinant technology. Preliminary animal investigations indicate that this compound may be useful in the postoperative period as a stimulant for erythropoiesis.[16]

The Pediatric Surgeon

Pediatric surgeons early realized that children had small blood volumes and that each child needed to have "blood units" calculated on an individual basis. The usual unit from the blood bank was 500 ml of whole blood and 250 ml of RBCs. This figure was approximately 10% of an adult's blood volume. For the 3-kg infant, a loss of 50 ml of blood, an inconsequential amount in most adults, represents a 20% loss of blood volume and may be associated with significant pathophysiologic effects. Pediatric surgeons traditionally have urged anesthesiologists to react quickly to this blood loss and to replace lost volume with donor blood. This approach now has been modified because of the risk of transfusion-related infectious diseases being transmitted during the "window" period. The window period is the time a patient is infected with a virus during which the disease can be transmitted but antibodies have not been produced. The lack of antibodies produces a false-negative test result early in the infection. Despite testing for hepatitis and HIV infections, a donor in the window period would escape detection and provide sufficient exposure to infect the recipient.

The anesthesiologist and the surgeon must work together, both to decrease the blood loss during the procedure and to restore blood volume without unnecessary risks. The surgeon must decrease blood loss throughout the operative procedure. In the beginning the surgeon can exert local pressure on skin and can control skin bleeding through the use of electrocoagulation or the Shaw hemostatic scalpel.[9] When peritoneal entry for control of bleeding must be rapid, a midline incision requires less vessel transection than muscle-dividing procedures. The argon beam coagulator works well on raw surfaces such as the liver and spleen.[46] Blood shed during the procedure should be collected via a cell saver and reinfused into the patient. The surgeon's assistants should be in charge of local compression to prevent hemorrhage and should supervise aspiration of blood for reinfusion.

Topical Therapy

Often bleeding is not from large vessels but from diffuse small vessels. Absorbable collagen in the form of sheets[4] with or without topical thrombin[13] may be helpful in controlling this diffuse hemorrhage.

Fibrin glue has been utilized to seal bleeding points in cardiac surgery or at cannulation sites for extracorporeal membrane oxygenation.[15, 23, 29, 38] As with all blood components, the use of fibrin glue, consisting of a mixture of cryo and bovine thrombin, carries a small risk of disease transmission, but its use may decrease transfusion requirements. Fibrin glue is formed by placing in one syringe 10 ml of single-donor cryo and in another syringe 5 ml of 10%

calcium chloride mixed with 5 ml of bovine thrombin (1000 units/ml). The glue is applied topically by simultaneous application of the solution from each syringe much as is epoxy glue with the resin and catalyst.

The surgeon's job is to accomplish hemostasis as quickly and as expeditiously as possible. When the source of hemorrhage is minor, simple techniques should be utilized. When the source of hemorrhage is major, vascular clamps are applied to feeding vessels such as the vessels in the hepatoduodenal ligament (Pringle maneuver) or the splenic artery. Occasionally the aorta may need to be cross-clamped at the diaphragm. Local compression by assistants utilizing lap pads can control continuing hemorrhage and allow mobilization of resources such as extra anesthesia personnel, blood, and additional instruments. The liver is often the site of massive hemorrhage, but only 10% of penetrating and 40% of blunt injuries require complex techniques of hemostasis. Various techniques have been described for control of bleeding in hepatic wounds more than 3 cm in depth. These measures include hepatotomy, resectional débridement, resection, selective hepatic artery ligation, perihepatic packing, and the use of a vascularized patch of omentum placed loosely in a hepatic wound or incision.[8] Various techniques have been described for hemostasis in the spleen, and procedures can be modified according to the injuries that are found.[5, 6]

SUMMARY

The treatment of normal children with massive injuries or of injured children with underlying coagulation defects requires close cooperation among surgeon, anesthesiologist, hematologist, and transfusion medicine physician. The goal is maintenance or restoration of tissue perfusion and oxygenation while minimizing the risks of transfusion of blood and blood components. A knowledge of basic mechanisms of coagulation, indications for blood component therapy, and special techniques in hemostasis are necessary to attain that goal.

References

1. Bernstein DP: Oxygen transport and utilization in trauma. In: Capan LM, Miller SM, Turndorf H: Trauma Anesthesia and Intensive Care. Philadelphia, JB Lippincott, 1991, pp 115–165.
2. Bernstein DP: Transfusion therapy in trauma. In: Capan LM, Miller SM, Turndorf H: Trauma Anesthesia and Intensive Care. Philadelphia, JB Lippincott, 1991, pp 167–205.
3. Broekmans AW, Veltkamp JJ, Bertina RM: Congenital protein c deficiency and venous thromboembolism. N Engl J Med 309(6):340–344, 1983.
4. Browder IW, Litwin MS: Use of absorbable collagen for hemostasis in general surgical patients. Am Surg 52(9):492–494, 1986.
5. Buntain WL, Gould HR: Splenic trauma in children and techniques of splenic salvage. World J Surg 9:398–409, 1985.
6. Buntain WL, Lunn HB: Splenorrhaphy: Changing concepts for the traumatized spleen. Surgery 86(5):748–760, 1979.
7. Comp PC, Dixon RR, Cooper MR, et al: Familial protein s deficiency is associated with recurrent thrombosis. J Clin Invest 74(6):2082–2088, 1984.
8. Feliciano DV: Surgery for liver trauma. Surg Clin North Am 69(2):273–384, 1989.
9. Gallow WJ, Moss M, Gaul JV: The Shaw scalpel: Thermal control of surgical bleeding. Int J Oral Maxillofac Surg 15:588–591, 1986.
10. Gans R, Duurkens VA, van Zundert AA, et al: Transfusion-related acute lung injury. Intensive Care Med 14(6):654–657, 1988.
11. Gibson JS, Leff RD, Roberts RJ: Effects of intravenous delivery systems on infused red blood cells. Am J Hosp Pharm 41:468–472, 1984.
12. Gravlee GP: Blood transfusion and component therapy. ASA Refresher Course Lectures 215:1–7, 1990.
13. Hashemi K, Donaldson LJ, Freeman JW, et al: The use of topical thrombin to reduce wound haematoma in patients receiving low-dose heparin. Curr Med Res Opin 7(7):458–462, 1981.
14. Jacobs LM, Hsieh JW: A clinical review of autotransfusion and its role in trauma. JAMA 251(24):3282–3287, 1984.
15. Kram HB, Ragu CN, Stafford FJ, et al: Fibrin glue achieves hemostasis in patients with coagulation disorders. Arch Surg 124:385–387, 1989.
16. Levine EA, Roen AL, Sehgal LR, et al: Treatment of acute postoperative anemia with recombinant human erythropoietin. J Trauma 29:1134–1139, 1989.
17. Levy GJ, Shabot MM, Hart ME, et al: Transfusion-associated noncardiogenic pulmonary edema. Transfusion 26(3):278–281, 1986.
18. Lorand L, Urayama T, Atencio AC, et al: Inheritance of deficiency of fibrin-stabilizing factor. Am J Hum Genet 22:89–95, 1970.
19. Lubin N: Neonatal anaemia secondary to blood loss. Clin Haematol 7:19–34, 1978.
20. Luna GK, Dellinger EP: Nonoperative observation therapy for splenic injuries: A safe therapeutic option? Am J Surg 153:462–467, 1987.
21. Messmer K, Sunder-Plassman L, Jesch F, et al: Oxygen supply to the tissues during limited normovolemic hemodilution. Res Exp Med 159:152–166, 1973.
22. Moore EE, Medina G: Autotransfusion in trauma. A pragmatic analysis. Am J Surg 148:782–785, 1984.
23. Morton MG, Katz NM, O'Connell J, et al: The use of topical fibrin glue at cannulation sites in neonates. Surg Gynecol Obstet 166(4):358–359, 1988.
24. NIH Consensus Conference: Fresh frozen plasma. Indications and risks. JAMA 253(4):551–553, 1985.
25. NIH Consensus Conference: Perioperative red blood cell transfusion. JAMA 260(18):2700–2703, 1988.
26. NIH Consensus Conference: Platelet transfusion therapy. JAMA 257(13):1777–1780, 1987.
27. Reul GJ, Solis RT, Greenberg SD, et al: Experience with autotransfusion in the surgical management of trauma. Surgery 76(4):546–555, 1974.
28. Roth GJ, Majerus PW: The mechanism of the effect of aspirin on human platelets. J Clin Invest 56:624–632, 1975.
29. Rousou J, Levitsky S, Gonzales-Lavin L, et al: Randomized clinical trial of fibrin sealant in patients undergoing resternotomy or reoperation after cardiac operations. J Thorac Cardiovasc Surg 97:194–203, 1989.
30. Sacher RA, Luban NLC, Strauss RG: Current practice and guidelines for the transfusion of cellular blood components in the newborn. Trans Med Rev 3:39–54, 1989.
31. Salzman EW, Weinstein MJ, Weintraub RM, et al: Treatment with desmopressin acetate to reduce blood loss after cardiac surgery. N Engl J Med 314(22):1402–1406, 1986.
32. Schaller RT, Schaller J, Furman EB: The advantages of hemodilution anesthesia for major liver resection in children. J Pediatr Surg 19(6):705–710, 1984.
33. Schaller RT, Schaller J, Morgan A: Hemodilution anesthesia: A valuable aid to major cancer surgery in children. Am J Surg 146:79–84, 1983.
34. Schulman I: The significance of epistaxis in childhood. Pediatrics 24:489–492, 1959.
35. Seear MD, Wadsworth LD, Rogers PC, et al: The effect of desmopressin acetate (DDAVP) on postoperative blood loss after cardiac operations in children. J Thorac Cardiovasc Surg 98(2):217–219, 1989.
36. Sills RH: Evaluation of a child with a possible bleeding disorder. N Y State J Med 86:143–147, 1986.
37. Silvergleid AJ: Safety and effectiveness of predeposit autologous transfusions in pre-teen and adolescent children. JAMA 257(24):3403–3404, 1987.
38. Spotnitz WD, Dalton MS, Baker JW, et al: Successful use of fibrin

glue during 2 years of surgery at a university medical center. Am Surg 55:166–168, 1989.

39. Stehling L: The safe level of hemoglobin: Is anemia in? ASA Refresher Course Lectures 143:1–7, 1990.

40. Strauss RG: Current issues in neonatal transfusions. Vox Sang 51:1–9, 1986.

41. Thaler M, Shamiss A, Orgad S, et al: The role of blood from HLA-homozygous donors in fetal transfusion-associated graft-versus-host disease after open-heart surgery. N Engl J Med 321(1):25–28, 1989.

42. Timberlake GA, McSwain NE: Autotransfusion of blood contaminated by enteric contents: A potentially life-saving measure in the massively hemorrhaging trauma patient? J Trauma 28(6):855–857, 1988.

43. Tremper KK: The measurement and maintenance of oxygen transport. ASA Refresher Course Lectures 231:1–6, 1990.

44. Triplett DA: Laboratory diagnosis of von Willebrand's disease. Mayo Clin Proc 66:832–840, 1991.

45. Tuman KJ, Spiess BD, McCarthy RJ, et al: Effects of progressive blood loss on coagulation as measured by thromboelastography. Anesth Analg 66(9):856–863, 1987.

46. Ward PH, Castro DJ, Ward S: A significant new contribution to radical head and neck surgery. Arch Otolaryngol Head Neck Surg 115:921, 1989.

47. Wilcox GJ, Barnes A, Modanlou H: Does transfusion using a syringe infusion pump and small-gauge needle cause hemolysis? Transfusion 21:750–751, 1981.

David A. Rogers
Thom E. Lobe

CHAPTER NINE

Metabolic Response to Major Injury and Shock

The more mechanisms of the human response to shock and injury that are understood, the greater the impact of these discoveries on the care of such critically ill patients. Although most of the information obtained thus far has evolved from studies of adult humans and adult animal models, and although this information may be applicable to the injured child, significant age-related differences may exist—particularly in the response of the neonate and infant to trauma.

DEFINITIONS

Injury

Injury may be defined as an event that alters normal function immediately and usually adversely. In its broadest sense, it ranges from the metabolic events associated with elective minor surgery to the derangements that occur with major trauma. In this discussion, injury is a traumatic event. Traumatic injuries are typically divided by mechanism of injury into *penetrating* and *blunt*. Penetrating injury produces alterations specific to the organ or organs involved in addition to the derangements associated with hemorrhage if blood loss is severe. Blunt trauma produces tissue destruction and the release of tissue mediators, with the hemorrhagic shock superimposed if significant blood loss occurs.

Shock

Regardless of the patient's age or the cause of the injury, shock occurs when perfusion of the cell is inadequate. The inadequate provision of substrates, particularly oxygen, and the incomplete removal of the end products of cellular metabolism lead to derangements in cellular physiology and ultimately may lead to disruption of the structure of the cell. This cellular dysfunction affects vital patient functions and may lead to death. The goal of patient management is the prompt recognition of shock and the restoration of normal cellular metabolism.

Shock states typically are divided into different categories based on either etiology or cardiovascular status (Table 9–1).

Neurogenic Shock

Neurogenic shock is characterized by a decrease in peripheral vascular tone and may be seen in the injured child with spinal cord or sometimes cerebral injury. Cardiogenic shock occurs when decreased pump function results from a diminished stroke volume and cardiac output. This form of shock is rare in pediatric trauma patients but may occur if the patient has a preexisting cardiac condition or suffers a cardiac contusion.[125]

Hemorrhagic Shock

Hemorrhagic and septic shock occur more often in the injured child. Hemorrhagic shock typically occurs early in the patient's course, whereas septic shock occurs later. Hemorrhagic shock results in acute anemia and acute hypovolemia. Of these, acute hypovolemia produces the more immediate consequences. Decreased circulating volume results in a decreased preload and a diminished stroke volume and cardiac output. The child compensates by increasing system vascular resistance and heart rate. Both of these mechanisms will maintain a normal blood pressure, but peripheral perfusion will be diminished. As the hypovolemia progresses, the child's ability to compensate is overcome, and blood pressure falls, but only after approximately 30% of the blood volume has been lost.[108]

Acute anemia occurs after trauma as blood loss is replaced with crystalloid solutions. Although the hemoglobin concentration below which significant hemodynamic derangements occur is unknown and varies with each individual patient, experimental evidence suggests that as long as volume can be maintained, hematocrits of as low as 10% can be tolerated without an increased mortality.[94]

Septic Shock

Septic shock in the injured child is usually secondary to the presence of gram-negative bacteria. These organisms release endotoxin, which activates the complement cascade, initiates the release of many inflammatory mediators, directly interferes with cellular metabolism, interacts with the coagulation cascade, and directly alters cardiovascular physiology. The early course may be described as hyperdynamic or compensated because the patient exhibits prominent peripheral pulses and warm extremities. Splanchnic vasodilation occurs, resulting in a relative state of hypovolemia, which is compensated for by an increase in cardiac output. Systemic vascular resistance is diminished, and if the shock remains untreated, the patient deteriorates to a state of decompensated septic shock that is accompanied by a fall in cardiac output and peripheral vasoconstriction.

PHYSIOLOGIC RESPONSES

Neuroendocrine Response

Shock activates the neuroendocrine response via baroreceptors located in the carotid artery and aorta and the stretch receptors in the right atria. Axiation of the tonic inhibition of these receptors produces the release of a number of neuroendocrine mediators.[5]

Cortisol releasing factor is elaborated by the hypothalamus, which induces the release of adrenocorticotropic hor-

Table 9–1
Classification of Shock

Type	Blood Pressure	Cardiac Output	Systemic Vascular Resistance
Hemorrhagic	↓	↓	↑
Neurogenic	↓	↑	↓
Septic (early)	↓	↑	↓
Septic (late)	↓	↓	↑
Cardiogenic	↓	↓	↑

mone (ACTH) from the pituitary gland. ACTH has several important effects, including the release of cortisol and aldosterone from the adrenal cortex. Cortisol functions to promote euglycemia by causing glycogenolysis and gluconeogenesis and decreasing glucose uptake by the peripheral tissues. Also, it has been shown to decrease protein synthesis and to promote proteolysis in somatic muscles while increasing protein uptake and synthesis in the liver.[41] ACTH is a potent stimulus for the release of aldosterone, the effects of which are to enhance the reabsorption of sodium and chloride from the proximal collecting tubule and the exchange of sodium and chloride in the distal tubule. This serves to conserve fluids.

The role of the thyroid hormones is less clear in shock. Triiodothyronine (T_3) and thyroxine (T_4) are decreased after hypovolemic shock. This decrease could contribute to the long-term metabolic effects of shock.

Hemorrhage is a potent stimulus of growth hormone release. Growth hormone has catabolic effects on carbohydrate and fat metabolism that lead to increased serum levels of glucose, fatty acids, and ketones. Unlike the other neuroendocrine mediators, growth hormone has an anabolic effect on peripheral protein utilization.

Endorphins, particularly β-endorphins, are secreted by the pituitary in response to shock. These substances stimulate the release of glucagon and insulin. Their most important effect may be cardiovascular depression.[52]

Vasopressin, or antidiuretic hormone, is released in response to decreased circulating volume. This agent promotes free water absorption by the renal tubule and has a direct vasoconstrictive effect on peripheral blood vessels.

Catecholamines are released by the adrenal medulla in response to shock. Epinephrine and norepinephrine improve cardiac output by increasing heart rate and contractility. They act as an insulin antagonist and so promote an increase in serum glucose by causing glycogenolysis and inhibiting glucose utilization by peripheral tissue.

Increased sympathetic stimulation of the pancreas in shock induces the secretion of glucagon. The actions of this hormone are to promote glycogenolysis, gluconeogenesis, hepatic amino acid uptake, and transamination. Glucagon acts to stimulate peripheral lipolysis and promotes ketogenesis. The actions of most of the neuroendocrine mediators are opposed to the activity of insulin. Insulin concentration is relatively reduced after shock and injury. Insulin normally acts to promote glucose and amino acid uptake and utilization, and it acts on adipose cells to promote storage.

Immune Response

The immune response to shock and injury is a complex process that involves leukocytes, immunoglobulins, and complement. The response has been classically described as serving to identify and to combat foreign materials that invade the patient. It is apparent that the mediators of the immune system modulate the metabolic response to injury. The overall immune response to injury appears at times to be contradictory. Generally, trauma and hemorrhagic and septic shock produce immunosuppression because of the release tactics of mediators of the neuroendocrine

response.[1, 2] However, the initial phase of shock or injury causes an activation of all components of the immune system, which may lead to organ dysfunction, a state recognized as multiple organ system failure.[2, 7]

Leukocytes. The cell-mediated response to injury includes changes in neutrophils and phagocytes. Hemorrhagic shock and trauma reduce leukocyte production.[4, 89] Although production is inhibited, circulating leukocytes are active. In response to injury or release of endotoxin, neutrophils migrate through the vascular endothelium and into the surrounding perivascular space. Phagocytosis is accomplished in conjunction with the C3b complement factor and the immunoglobulins IgG and IgM.[34] Bacterial killing is accomplished through enzymatic and oxidative processes. Evidence suggests that oxygen radicals that cause general and reperfusion injury are produced in this process.[128]

Macrophages include monocytes that circulate in the blood and are found in various organs, for example, the Kupffer cells in the liver. Macrophage activation releases cytokines. These monokines are key mediators of the immune response augmentation.

Shock results in a decrease in the number of T lymphocytes and a reduction of the ratio of T-helper to T-suppressor cells. T lymphocytes produce several cytokines in response to shock states. Their role in the homeostatic response to shock, particularly to septic shock, has been the subject of considerable research.[43] Some of these mediators appear to play a dominant role in the pathophysiologic mechanisms of shock and organ dysfunction.

Of the cytokines, tumor necrosis factor (TNF) appears dominant. Tumor necrosis factor is produced by macrophages, mast cells, endothelial cells, and natural killer cells. In addition to being released after injury, this substance is released in response to lipopolysaccharides and viral particles. This mediator acts to modulate the immune response and has an impact on the metabolic activity of the patient.[29, 41, 43, 61] Tumor necrosis factor is an endogenous pyrogen and activates neutrophil and macrophage production and activity. It acts on the liver and peripheral muscles to produce an increase in acute phase proteins and in peripheral protein catabolism. It also acts on adipose cells to produce lipolysis. The increase in TNF after injury is relatively brief. It activates the neuroendocrine and immune systems, which may explain its role in the prolonged metabolic consequences of injury, and, alternatively, relatively low doses of TNF elicit the metabolic changes that have been described.[29] It may be that TNF concentrations persist at levels that are sufficient to cause metabolic alterations.

Interleukin-1, produced by a number of cell types, is predominantly from macrophages and monocytes. This cytokine stimulates T-cell proliferation, promotes myelopoiesis, acts as an endogenous pyrogen that has many of the same metabolic effects as TNF, and may be the most significant factor in the alteration of hepatic protein synthesis.[43]

Interleukin-6 is secreted by several cells including macrophages. It acts as an endogenous pyrogen and has an impact on the patient's metabolic function, enhancing hepatic acute phase protein production.[51] Interleukin-2 is produced by T lymphocytes and functions to activate lymphocytes for enhanced cytotoxic activities. Levels of this cytokine are reduced after injury.

Gamma interferon is produced by stimulated T lymphocytes. This substance enhances the antimicrobial effects of the macrophages. Colony-stimulating factors are a group of glycoproteins with a diverse set of activities. Among these is the stimulation of the formation of neutrophils, macrophages, and eosinophils.

Immunoglobulins. Another area of the immune response to shock is the response to immunoglobulins. In the normal person, immunoglobulins are produced by B lymphocytes in response to antigenic stimulation. These immunoglobulins then assist in phagocytosis and can activate the remainder of the immune response. Levels of circulating immunoglobulins are depressed after shock and may remain depressed if there is an ongoing process, such as thermal injury.

Complement. The complement system is the last of the three major components of the immune response. Total complement levels are reduced in all phases of shock. This system may be activated via the classical route by an antibody-antigen complex or via the alternate system by components of the bacterial wall. Once activated, amplification occurs. The complement system results in a number of biologically active components that serve as chemoattractants for phagocytes, promote degranulation of mast cells with the release of histamines, and act on platelets to induce clumping and release eicosanoids. Complement C5b is capable of binding to distant cell sites and may be one of the factors responsible for the widespread effects of shock and injury. Complement activation products can directly increase the permeability of vascular endothelium and promote neutrophil adherence to the endothelial cells.[54] In addition, an attack complex, C5 to C9, is involved in cellular disruption of the target cell.

Autacoids

Autacoids are a group of diverse chemical agents that are produced by different cells and that appear to act primarily at their site of origin.[45] They include eicosanoids, kinins, serotonin, and histamine.

The eicosanoids are substances produced by the action of phospholipase A on membrane phospholipids. This action produces arachidonic acid, and, depending on the particular cells involved, arachidonic acid is metabolized to a leukotriene via the lipoxygenase pathway or to a prostaglandin, prostacyclin, or thromboxane via the cyclo-oxygenase pathway.

Prostaglandins have a diverse and sometimes contradictory set of functions. For example, prostaglandin E_1 produces bronchodilation, whereas prostaglandin F_2 produces bronchoconstriction. Among the prostaglandins, prostaglandin E_2 has received considerable attention because of its impact on immune function. Generally, it is regarded as being a regulator of T-cell functions.[67]

Vascular endothelium produces prostacyclin 1, which normally inhibits platelet aggregation and produces vasodilation. Prostacyclin levels are reduced in shock. Platelets produce thromboxanes, which cause vasoconstriction, bronchoconstriction, platelet aggregation, and chemotaxis. The role of platelet aggregation and mediator release is believed to be a central component in the development of adult respiratory distress syndrome, which can occur in children.[139]

Leukotrienes are produced by many cells, including leukocytes, and cause increased capillary permeability. In addition, they cause vasoconstriction, bronchoconstriction, and in some cases are chemotactic for leukocytes.

Platelet-activating factor is produced by neutrophils and macrophages and stimulates exocytosis, aggregation, chemokinesis, chemotaxis of neutrophils, platelets, eosinophils, and macrophages.[6, 69]

The kallikrein-kinin system is another component of the autacoid response to injury. Its activation occurs with both hemorrhagic and septic shock. Prekallikrein is converted to the active form, kallikrein, by the clotting cascade. Kallikrein acts on serum and tissue precursors to produce bradykinin and kallikrein. These activated kinins increase vascular permeability and cause vasodilation and bronchoconstriction.

Serotonin is produced primarily by the enterochromaffin cells of the gastrointestinal tract. It acts primarily on smooth muscle and nerve endings to produce bronchoconstriction, vasodilation, platelet aggregation, and increased cardiac output.

Histamine, released from mast cells and basophils, produces an increase in vascular permeability and induces vasodilation. It may also have a diverse set of actions via the H_1 and H_2 receptors found throughout the body.

Alterations in Energy Substrate

The changes that occur in energy metabolism after severe injury and during sepsis have long been recognized. The postinjury period has been divided into an ebb and a flow phase, with the flow phase being subdivided into an anabolic and a catabolic phase.[45]

During the catabolic phase, persistent hyperglycemia, protein wasting, and lipolysis occurs. Total energy requirements are reduced during the ebb phase and increased during the flow phase. Limited information suggests that the general patterns that have been described for adults are also true for children.[8, 138] If children remain free of complications, they enter an anabolic phase with restoration of protein and, finally, fat stores.

Some generalizations can be made regarding changes that occur after injury. First, considerable controversy remains over the general processes that produce the observed changes. Second, the response of each patient is highly individualistic and is related to the preexisting nutritional status, the nature of the child's injury, and the presence of a secondary infection. Third, the causes of these metabolic disturbances are related to the neuroendocrine changes previously discussed. The precise role of each of these mediators, however, is not clear. Finally, although it is convenient to discuss the changes in carbohydrate, lipid, and protein as separate entities, it is important to recognize that alterations in each of these substrates represent an integrated response.[110]

On a cellular level, metabolic changes that occur during the actual period of hypoperfusion or ebb phase are marked by a shift from aerobic to anaerobic metabolism.[53] This leads to lactic acidosis, which adversely affects oxygen transport. The situation is compounded in sepsis because peripheral tissues have a deficit in their ability to process oxygen. After the ebb phase and the activation of the neuroendocrine and immune responses, alterations occur in the metabolism of carbohydrate, protein, and lipid metabolism.

Carbohydrate Metabolism

The postinjury period is marked by persistent hyperglycemia. Many of the neuroendocrine mediators that are released during this period have an anti-insulin action. Generally, this increases gluconeogenesis and increases glycogenolysis. Uptake by the peripheral tissues is diminished, and oxidation is impaired, but peripheral utilization remains at about the same level as seen in normal controls.[136] Given the increased metabolic demands of the patient, the relative proportion of glucose utilized to meet the total energy requirements falls.

Central gluconeogenesis is driven by the increase in available substrates, including lactate, alanine, and other gluconeogenic amino acids. The hyperglycemia that results may produce several beneficial effects. Initially, hyperosmolarity promotes fluid shifts that help to restore the circulating volume. In the latter stages of the metabolic response, glucose is available for the erythrocytes, the leukocytes, the neural tissues, the renal medulla, and the wound. Although hyperglycemia may serve some useful functions, maintenance of the hyperglycemia has a profoundly negative effect on protein and lipid stores.

Lipid Metabolism

All phases of the postinjury period are marked by lipolysis. This appears to be mediated by the same hormonal milieu that contributes to the hyperglycemia, including the cytokines.[48, 116, 123] Fats serve as the predominate energy source in the postinjury period, and the restoration of stores of body fat is one of the later signs to appear in the anabolic stage. The relatively small amount of fat in younger children may be significant because of the greater degree of protein catabolism required for energy production.[107]

Protein Metabolism

The postinjury period is one of overall negative nitrogen balance. Normally, protein levels are the result of a balance between synthesis and catabolism. In the stress state, catabolism increases with the utilization of amino acids as gluconeogenic substrate or as precursors for acute phase reactants. Hepatic synthesis may be increased or decreased, depending on the magnitude of the injury or the stage of sepsis.[87, 93, 124] The observed effects are due to mediators of the neuroendocrine response and cytokines.[11, 22, 26, 84] Because proteins constitute a structural element of the cell, prolonged catabolism leads to impairment of the organ or muscle involved.

Beyond this total effect on protein stores, shifts occur in the distribution of protein in the body. Generally, protein moves from the peripheral muscles to the visceral organs.[137]

In addition, certain amino acids play unique roles in the overall response to shock and injury. Alanine is the major gluconeogenic amino acid and is involved in the transfer from the periphery to the liver, where it is utilized in the production of glucose. Glutamine functions as an important metabolite in many metabolic pathways.[111] Glutamine is the amino acid found in greatest concentration in the intracellular pool. In addition to performing potentially important regulatory functions, glutamine serves as the primary fuel in rapidly growing cells such as mucosal cells of the intestine and lymphocytes. The gastrointestinal tract is the primary consumer of glutamine in the body.[115] Arginine has been shown to improve cell-mediated immunity.[79]

In shock, the high-branched chained amino acids, isoleucine, leucine, and alanine, appear to be preferentially metabolized by the somatic muscles, although this is controversial.[45]

END ORGAN RESPONSES

Cellular

A cell deprived of adequate metabolites (primarily oxygen) undergoes a gradual morphologic transformation.[127] Early changes in the cell include clumping of nuclear chromatin. As ischemia persists, alterations in the endoplasmic reticulum, the mitochondria, and the cell membrane appear. However, the cell does demonstrate some protective mechanisms. One response to ischemia is the formation of intracellular proteins that may prevent or reverse the changes that occur in the cell.[2] If the injury is not reversed, autodigestion begins and cell membrane integrity is lost, which leads ultimately to cellular death.

Many pathophysiologic processes have been described in the ischemic cell. These relate to ion concentrations across cell membranes and cellular energy metabolism.[86] Early in ischemia there is an influx of sodium and calcium into the cell and a movement of potassium out of the cell. Adenosine diphosphate accumulates and adenosine triphosphate falls as the cell shifts to anaerobic metabolism. The cell demonstrates different responses depending on the degree to which flow is diminished.[66] Paradoxically, the cell receiving no flow survives better than that receiving some perfusion.

Although the previously described changes occur during ischemia, injury continues after blood flow is restored. This phase, reperfusion injury, is believed to be due to free radicals of oxygen.[36, 78] This process is initiated during ischemia and is mediated by calcium influx into the cell. The oxygen radicals that are produced react with the components of the cell, which results in lipid peroxidation that damages cell membranes and disrupts the proteins and nucleic acids. As oxygen radicals accumulate and disrupt the basic mechanisms of the cell, calcium homeostasis is further deranged and the process is amplified.

Another reactive molecule that may play a role in the cellular response to shock is nitric oxide (NO). This molecule is produced by a number of cells, including macrophages, during the oxidation of arginine to citrulline. Its physiologic functions include a possible role in the vasodi-

Table 9–2
Modified Glasgow Coma Scale

Eye Opening Response
Spontaneous
To speech
To pain
None

Verbal Response*
Oriented
Confused conversation
Inappropriate words
Incomprehensible sounds
None

Best Upper Limb Motor Response
Obeys
Localizes
Withdraws
Abnormal flexion
Extensor response
None

***Verbal Response for Young Children and Infants**
Appropriate words or social smiles, fixes and follows
Cries, but consolable
Persistently irritable
Restless, agitated
None

lation, inhibition of platelet aggregation and adherence, inhibition of hepatic protein synthesis, and interference of the growth of some microorganisms.[16, 137]

Nervous System

The brain is composed of neurons, glial cells, and vascular tissues. Neural elements are the most sensitive tissues to perfusion changes.[59] Physiologically, the brain is unique in that it demonstrates a high oxygen and energy consumption with a preference for glucose as its energy substrate. Shock reduces the availability of glucose, which leads to a subsequent decrease in adenosine triphosphate and an elevation of lactic acid.[105] If ischemia persists for at least 5 minutes, then reperfusion injury will occur. Because the neurons have no reparative capacity, cellular death is irreversible.

At the organ level, cerebral perfusion is directly related to the difference between the mean arterial pressure and the intracranial pressure. The initial response to shock involves autoregulation and changes in the systemic cardiovascular system. Autoregulation is remarkably effective in maintaining cerebral perfusion despite systemic hypotension. This mechanism is effective until the mean arterial pressure falls below 60 mm Hg in adults; below this limit, the ability to maintain cerebral perfusion is lost.

Systemic cardiovascular changes occur, which include an increase in cardiac output and a diversion of blood flow from other organs to support the cerebral circulation. Cellular injury results in cerebral edema. Cerebral perfusion is then limited by the increasing intracranial pressure as the swelling brain expands against the bony skull.

In the absence of cerebral trauma, the patient's level of consciousness is directly related to the degree of hypovolemia. The patient's neurologic status will progress from leth-

argy to coma. Other signs may include pupillary dilation, decorticate or decerebrate posturing, and seizures. Systemic signs of neurologic injury may include an altered respiratory pattern or persistent vomiting. These findings may be quantified using a neurologic scale appropriate for the patient's age (Table 9–2).

Pulmonary

Pulmonary insufficiency immediately after injury may be due to a direct mechanical effect or may be secondary to injury of other organs, for example, a closed head injury. The metabolic response to injury activates mediators that may directly injure the lungs. Respiratory insufficiency occurs after many varied insults including trauma and shock.[101, 102] Many stimuli activate the complement system, which results in the migration of neutrophils because of the leukoattractant properties of C5a. Currently, neutrophil activation is believed to be a central element of the mechanism of pulmonary injury, and this injury is accomplished by the neutrophil-mediated release of free radicals of oxygen, arachidonic acid metabolites, and platelet-activating factor. All of these factors function together to produce damage to the alveolar-capillary membrane, and the loss of this endothelial integrity results in the leakage of fluid and proteins into the interstitial space.

Clinically, the first phase of adult respiratory distress syndrome may be mild, consisting of tachypnea, dyspnea, and hypoxemia that is refractory to supplemental oxygen. The chest radiograph is normal during this phase of the pulmonary injury. Depending on the magnitude of the injury, the respiratory insufficiency may resolve, or it may progress to respiratory failure with marked hypoxemia and bilateral infiltrates evident on the chest radiograph. Pathologically, capillary congestion occurs, with interstitial fluid accumulation and filling of the alveolar units with proteinaceous and hemorrhagic fluid.

Because of the increase in interstitial fluid and the loss of surfactant, the alveoli are more prone to collapse, and atelectasis results. The result of this pathologic process is a reduction in the functional residual capacity and an increasingly severe pulmonary shunting. As more alveoli are perfused but not aerated, the hypoxemia becomes increasingly more severe. Hypoxemia, from this inability to oxygenate the blood, results in further anoxic injury.

Adult respiratory distress syndrome is sometimes difficult to diagnose because it can occur in many clinical situations. Although the diagnosis may sometimes be made only as the patient's respiratory insufficiency evolves, it is important that therapy be initiated early.

Endotoxin alone can effect all of the changes that have been described and can impair the phagocytic function of pneumococci in the lung.[92] As the lungs are often infected in the critically ill patient, this impairment would have long-term deleterious effects.

Cardiovascular

Peripheral Vascular

Many changes are evident in the peripheral vascular system during shock. The most commonly discussed changes are those associated with peripheral vasomotor tone. Changes associated with septic shock are different from those from hemorrhagic and other types of shock. In hypovolemic or cardiogenic shock, systemic vascular resistance increases. The patient presents clinically with cool, poorly perfused skin, the systemic vascular resistance serving a valuable function in redistributing the blood flow from the peripheral tissues to the brain and heart. In the early phases of septic shock, the patient is noted to be hyperdynamic, that is, the peripheral vascular resistance is reduced and the extremities are warm and well perfused with bounding pulses.

The second area of alteration is a derangement in the regulatory function of the vascular endothelial cell. Although the mechanism of injury is unclear, it is well recognized that the endothelial cell loses its ability to control fluid movement into the interstitium.[49] Endothelial cells produce several of the cytokines and may represent one of the key modulators of the metabolic response to septic shock.[63]

Cardiac

The heart is a major consumer of the patient's oxygen content, and the myocyte is intolerant of prolonged ischemia. Although the homeostatic response is geared to preserve myocardial function, a number of functional alterations may be seen.

Cardiac output is a product of stroke volume and heart rate. Stroke volume is dependent on preload, afterload, and contractility. Hypovolemic shock produces a reduction in preload by a direct loss in circulating volume. Sepsis produces a relative hypovolemia because of peripheral and splanchnic vasodilation. The cardiac response is related to sympathetic mediators, particularly the catecholamines. This response is characterized by an increase in heart rate and in contractility. The adaptation of increasing heart rate is limited as cardiac output begins to fall with extreme tachycardia. In addition to the relative hypovolemia seen in sepsis, endotoxin has been shown to produce direct negative effects on the left and right ventricle.[113, 122, 141]

Renal

The kidney can maintain perfusion via autoregulation until its perfusion pressure falls below 50 mm Hg.[58] When ischemia occurs, it is tolerated for up to 25 minutes with minimal injury.[130] Once renal vasoconstriction occurs, it does not reverse with restoration of normal blood flow.[118] This reaction extends ischemic injury. After cellular perfusion is restored, reperfusion injury may occur. The kidney plays an important role in preserving circulating volume in shock. Hypotension associated with shock results in decreased renal blood flow, glomerular filtration rate, and, ultimately, urinary output. Besides diminished excretion and changes in free water, alterations in the absorption of solutes occur. Decreased perfusion of the juxtaglomerular apparatus results in activation of the renin-angiotensin system. Angiotensin, besides being a potent vasoconstrictor, causes the release of aldosterone. The major stimulus for aldosterone release, however, is ACTH. Aldosterone acts on renal tu-

bules to promote sodium reabsorption and potassium excretion. Vasopressin also acts on renal tubules to promote free water reabsorption. The end result is the production of small quantities of concentrated urine. If the hypoperfusion is profound, renal tubular damage may occur, and some degree of renal failure will result.

In evaluating the causes of oliguria, the evaluation of serum creatinine determinants may be confusing because they relate to the muscle mass of the patient. The calculation of the fraction excretion (FE) of sodium (Na):

$$\text{FE Na: } \frac{[\text{Urine Na/Serum Na})/}{(\text{Urine Cr/Serum Cr}])} \times 100$$

provides a more accurate assessment of tubular function.[37]

A value of three or greater reflects significant tubular damage. Besides its effects on absorptive and excretory renal functions, shock impairs the gluconeogenic role of the kidney. In late shock, the kidney may become a lactate-producing instead of a lactate-using organ.

In septic shock, endotoxin potentiates many of the changes that occur with hypotension. Its actions result in decreased renal blood flow, increased renal vascular resistance, and decreased glomerular filtration rates. Endotoxin also interferes with the ability of the kidney to utilize its usual metabolic substrates.[9]

Gastrointestinal

The gastrointestinal system has long been ignored in discussions of shock. There is now considerable interest in the role of the gastrointestinal system, particularly in its relationship to multiple organ system failure. Shock has an impact on both the solid viscera and the gut. Of the solid organs, the liver plays a critical role in energy substrate metabolism and phagocytosis.[88, 112] On a cellular level, injury occurs by the mechanisms of direct ischemia and reperfusion.[3, 65, 120] The role of the pancreas in shock is unclear; however, pancreatitis secondary to reperfusion injury has been described.[106, 134]

The vasculature of the gut demonstrates some autoregulatory capabilities.[56] In moderate hypotension, blood flow is maintained to the mucosa, but as hypotension progresses, oxygen supplied to the muscularis and mucosa is diminished.[47] These changes are most marked at the tips of the villi because of short circuiting of the blood through the countercurrent vascular mechanism. Once ischemia occurs, mucosal cell death follows. The mechanism of injury is via the reactive metabolites that are generated during ischemia and reperfusion.[30, 39, 119] Endotoxin present during sepsis and septic shock increases the total metabolic requirements of the gut but decreases its ability to utilize glutamine, its preferred fuel.[114] Mucosal injury is associated with hemorrhagic shock,[10] burns,[35] and sepsis.[81] All result in a derangement of the normal barrier function of the mucosa.[104] This response not only produces a potentially unlimited reservoir for bacterial infection, but also may have a direct immunosuppressive effect.[31]

Clinical evaluation of the effects of shock on the gastrointestinal system are limited. Examination may indicate the return of motility that was lost, but physical findings have not been shown to be a sensitive indicator of activity.[132] Serum liver enzyme elevation may provide evidence of hepatocellular injury. In the future, serum markers may become available to alert the clinician that ischemic damage has occurred.[18] The measurement of intraluminal pH has been shown to be a sensitive indicator of perfusion and may become available as a clinical tool.[56]

Hematologic

The hematologic response to shock involves the leukocytes, erythrocytes, platelets, and clotting cascade.

Leukocytes play a significant role in the immune response to shock and injury. Although neutrophils are activated and participate in the nonspecific response to injury and infection and phagocytes play a role in both host defense and damage to host organs, the overall effect of shock and injury is one of suppression of white blood cell production.[74, 89]

There is relatively little information about the response of erythropoiesis to hemorrhagic shock. It is reasonable to expect, based on leukocytic changes, that severe hemorrhage should be associated with depression of this erythrocyte function.

The clotting system may be activated in the injured patient via the intrinsic pathway by exposed subendothelial collagen and via the extrinsic pathway by tissue thromboplastin. Activation of the system may be beneficial in its role of providing the fibrin that participates in clot formation. Consumptive coagulopathy is a complication of sepsis and as pathologic disseminated intravascular coagulopathy, may lead to active bleeding. The clotting cascade may interact with prekallikrein to activate the kinin autacoid system also.

The platelets serve a variety of functions that may be critical in injury or shock. Platelets adhere to exposed collagen and participate in the formation of the platelet plug. Once activated, they release adenosine diphosphate and serotonin, which attract other platelets and have autacoid effects. Platelets also produce thromboxane A_2, which is a vasoconstrictor and potent platelet aggregator. In addition, platelets participate in the initial stages of clotting.

Somatic Muscle

The muscles are relatively resistant to the hypovolemia of shock.[57] In the late phases of injury, muscles serve as valuable sources of gluconeogenic precursors.

MANAGEMENT

Despite great advances in the understanding of the pathophysiologic consequences of shock and injury, the most effective current therapy remains the reversal of cellular hypoperfusion by the rapid recognition and treatment of shock. For purposes of this discussion, the period of initial trauma management has been divided into four distinct phases: primary survey, resuscitation, secondary survey,

and definitive care.[80] Issues of secondary survey and definitive care are the focus of subsequent chapters. A complete discussion of the management of sepsis is also the focus of another chapter. Here the discussion of sepsis management is limited to issues of resuscitation.

Hemorrhagic Shock

Primary Survey and Resuscitation

The primary survey includes a rapid assessment of airway, breathing, and circulation and a quick assessment of neurologic disability. Evaluation of the patient's airway is performed by listening and looking for evidence of adequate air exchange. If the patient is unconscious, the tongue and its surrounding soft tissue is the usual source of obstruction. In the presence of apparent inadequate air exchange, the first maneuver should be a "jaw lift" or "chin thrust." If this technique is unsuccessful in relieving airway obstruction, an oral airway should be considered, but most likely the child will require endotracheal intubation.

Differences between the airways of the child and the adult are age dependent and have been well documented previously.[97] The appropriate size of the necessary endotracheal tube can be estimated by examining either the diameter of the little finger or the size of the external nares, but a variety of sizes should be available for use. Cervical spine stability should not be jeopardized to obtain airway access. The child's cranium has a relatively large diameter when compared with that of the midface. This causes the supine child's or infant's neck to assume a flexed position, a problem that can be compounded by backboards commonly used by emergency personnel. Some recommend that special backboards be utilized for the transport of children.[60] Stability is best achieved when one member of the team maintains the head in a neutral position for intubation. A lateral cervical spine image should be obtained in the course of the resuscitation; however, it cannot ensure that no injury is present. If intubation is impossible, a needle cricothyrotomy should be performed. However, as with a surgical cricothyrotomy or tracheostomy, such a procedure is rarely necessary and should be avoided in the emergency department setting.

Evaluation of breathing is done by watching for adequate chest or abdominal excursion with respiration. Palpation and observation allow detection of thoracic injuries that may be life threatening, including tension pneumothorax, flail chest, and massive hemothorax. Auscultation is rarely optimal in the resuscitation setting. If these injuries are suspected based on physical findings and clinical course, they must be treated before confirmatory images can be made. Tension pneumothorax can be decompressed rapidly using an angiocatheter followed by the placement of a chest tube. Hemothorax is treated with placement of a chest tube, and flail chest is treated by endotracheal intubation and positive pressure ventilation.

Circulation can be assessed by examining the skin, and capillary refill should be equal to or less than 2 seconds. A normal blood pressure does not ensure that circulating volume is adequate. During initial assessment, management includes obtaining vascular access, administering fluids, and, rarely, pharmacologic support and dysrhythmia management.

When possible, venous access should be obtained with at least two large-bore intravenous catheters. If this is not possible, alternatives such as vascular cutdown over the saphenous or basilic vein or cannulation of the deep venous system using the Seldinger technique via the jugular, subclavian, or femoral venous systems may be done. Although these methods are effective, they must be done by qualified personnel, usually by the surgeon. A third option offers the benefits of speed and performance by a variety of personnel: the technique of intraosseous infusion.[42] A large-bore needle is introduced into the marrow of the tibia inferior and medial to the tibial tuberosity. The procedure can be done quickly, and large volumes of fluid and, if necessary, inotropes may be infused.[15] Complications of this technique are rare. The technique is applicable in children younger than 5 years of age, but it has been used in older children.[117] An obvious contraindication is the presence of a fracture of the proximal tibia, in which case, the contralateral tibia may be used, or the needle may be introduced into the distal femur.

Once access is obtained, fluid resuscitation can be initiated. This portion of management is guided by the knowledge that the blood volume of a child is approximately 80 ml per kg and the principle that minor hypovolemia suggests a loss of 25% of this volume. Hence, a bolus of 20 ml per kg of fluid—usually crystalloid—is given rapidly. If two boluses of 20 ml per kg of crystalloid do not restore peripheral perfusion, then blood replacement should be initiated, with O negative blood if necessary. With modern concerns about the human immunodeficiency virus (HIV), interest in the limits of anemia has been renewed. In nonurgent situations, it is currently recommended that transfusions be held for a hemoglobin greater than or equal to 7 gm per dl.[90] Although this recommendation may not be helpful in the unstable child, it does make the point that continued transfusion to a normal hematocrit in the stable child may be unnecessary.

It is currently believed that in hypovolemia secondary to traumatic injury, crystalloid is at least equivalent to other resuscitation fluids.[90, 129] Hypertonic solutions require less fluid but may result in significant hyperosmolarity. They appear to offer the greatest potential advantage in the battlefield situation in which fluids must be transported manually[33] or in patients with an isolated head injury in which limitation of the volume of fluid utilized is most severe.[133] Another approach has been the use of a fructose 1–6 diphosphate sodium salt for resuscitation. The theoretic advantage of this material is that it provides for improved utilization of carbohydrates in the ischemic cells, but experimental evidence to support this contention is limited.[83] Pressors are not indicated in the resuscitation phase of management of hemorrhagic shock.

Management of dysrhythmia plays a small role in the initial resuscitation of the injured child. Sinus tachycardia is a common rhythm, but its clinical significance is difficult to evaluate in a frightened child. Lethal dysrhythmias are extremely rare in this age group. Cardiac arrest in the injured child is managed according to established protocols

of cardiopulmonary resuscitation with two exceptions. First, the surgeon should consider correctable causes of continued inadequate perfusion, such as pericardial tamponade. Second, emergency department thoracotomy may be required in a patient who has signs of electrical activity but who cannot be resuscitated by standard fluid replacement. Unfortunately, the outcome of children who require this intervention is poor.[13]

If the patient requires resuscitation, routine monitoring measures must be instituted. These consist of electrocardiogram monitors, an oxygen saturation monitor, and a Foley catheter. An arterial catheter and central venous monitoring are indicated in children with severe multiple system injuries. Care must be taken to avoid hypothermia during this period.

Sepsis

The principles of initial airway management and ventilation for septic shock are similar to those outlined for hemorrhagic shock. The cardiovascular derangements that may occur, however, are variable, and the degree of impairment guides the management. Endotoxin results in peripheral vasodilation and functional hypovolemia. As mentioned previously, endotoxin may also depress myocardial function directly. In the patient with only mild hypotension or slightly impaired capillary perfusion, resuscitation may consist of the administration of a fluid bolus only. If the patient fails to respond to a reasonable fluid challenge, then intensive monitoring is indicated, with a pulmonary artery catheter if necessary. Placement of the pulmonary artery catheter and measurement of an arterial and mixed venous blood gas allow for the measurement and calculation of parameters that reflect cardiac performance and oxygen transport and utilization (Table 9–3). The ready availability of microprocessors in most monitor systems obviates the need to make these calculations by hand. Normal values are also provided by most systems. The equations are provided because to make the appropriate clinical manipulation, it is critical to understand the derivation of these parameters.

A decreased pulmonary capillary wedge pressure indicates that the volume for an optimal filling pressure is inadequate. Considerable controversy persists regarding the appropriate resuscitation fluid for septic shock. Several alternatives are available, but essentially they are either colloid or crystalloid fluids. Crystalloids are inexpensive and effective. They distribute rapidly to the extravascular space, and although the potential exists for pulmonary edema to occur from redistribution, we believe that it has been overemphasized. It is true that systemic soft tissue edema occurs with large volumes, but the clinical significance of this is unclear. Colloids are relatively expensive, but smaller volumes are required for resuscitation, and there is more rapid and prolonged expansion of the plasma volume. Although further research with newer products may lead to a clearly superior fluid, we use crystalloids primarily and reserve colloids for situations in which the colloid oncotic pressure falls below the normal ranges.

If the measurement of cardiac performance suggests impaired myocardial function, then inotropes must be added.

Table 9–3
Cardiopulmonary Parameters

Measured Parameter	Equation
Cardiac output	Measured
Mean arterial pressure (MAP)	Measured
Central venous pressure (CVP)	Measured
Heart rate	Measured
Pulmonary capillary wedge pressure	Measured
Cardiac index (CI)	Cardiac output/body surface area
Stroke index	Cardiac index/heart rate
Left ventricular stroke work index	Stroke index × MAP × 0.0136
Systemic vascular resistance index	((MAP − CVP) × 80)/CI
Arterial oxygen content	1.34 × arterial O_2 sat × Hgb + 0.0034 × Pao_2
Venous oxygen content	1.34 × venous O_2 sat × Hgb + 0.0034 × Pvo_2
Oxygen availability	Oxygen content × cardiac index × 10
Oxygen consumption	(Arterial oxygen content − venous oxygen content) × cardiac index × 10
Oxygen extraction rate	(Arterial O_2 content − venous O_2 content)/arterial O_2 content × 10

Sat, Saturation; Hgb, hemoglobin.

Several agents are available[77] and can be compared on the basis of their activity at the different sympathetic receptors (Table 9–4). Alpha$_1$ receptors promote contraction of vascular smooth muscle. Beta$_1$ receptors are present on cardiac muscle, and their stimulation results in increased myocardial performance. Beta$_2$ receptors are present on vascular and bronchial smooth muscle, and their activation results in smooth muscle relaxation.

Because of their relative specificity, dobutamine and dopamine have become the preferred first-line drugs. Norepinephrine and epinephrine are reserved for patients who do not improve with the first-line agents. Dopamine has several additional unique effects based on its activity at dopaminergic receptors. The most useful of these effects is renal artery vasodilation at low doses, an effect lost at higher doses.[14]

All of the information generated by the pulmonary artery catheter is designed to improve the specificity of therapy. Ultimately, the objective is the delivery of adequate oxygen to the cell. In the absence of a direct cellular probe, oxygen delivery and utilization must be estimated. Unfortunately, the deficit may be an impaired ability to utilize oxygen at the cellular level, and there is no effective direct therapy for this.

Beyond prevention and general management, specific therapies are currently under investigation, and some of these will become the standard of care. The discussion that follows outlines some of these therapies that are targeted at alterations in the metabolic response at a cellular or mediator level and new therapies that support individual organ systems.

Cellular

Steroids. Considerable controversy persists as to the value of steroids in the management of shock. Two clinical studies demonstrated no immediate survival advantage when steroids were administered acutely.[17, 131] Steroids should not be prescribed routinely but should be reserved for patients who are not responding to other therapy.

Nonsteroidal Agents. These agents offer an attractive alternative for modifying the systemic response to injury and act by blocking all or part of the arachidonic acid pathway. Experimental evidence indicates that they reduce some of the deleterious changes associated with shock, but currently data to recommend their use are insufficient.[103]

Oxygen Radical Scavengers. The active oxygen metabolites are believed to play a major role in the cellular mechanism of injury. Considerable research has been done to attempt to find a mechanism to neutralize these actions. Such agents are effective if given before or early in the course of ischemia, and there are exciting possibilities for the use of a number of these agents when the period of ischemia and reperfusion can be anticipated, that is, during organ transplantation.[98] The role of this type of agent in hypovolemia due to trauma is less certain.

Neuroendocrine

Naloxone. Naloxone, which blocks the effects of β-endorphins, has been shown to reverse some of the alterations observed in shock models, particularly those in septic shock in which clinical trials have not produced significant differences between placebo and naloxone.[32, 55] Naloxone is not presently indicated; although efficacy may be demonstrated with higher doses, more research is necessary before routine use in these circumstances.[52]

Growth Hormone. Growth hormone, which is unique among mediators of the neuroendocrine response to stress in its anabolic effects on proteins, has been given to septic patients and has been shown to improve the catabolic index slightly and to increase the level of insulin-like growth factor (IGF)-1 without resulting in a significant improvement in the clinical course of the patient.[48] Improvement of the nitrogen balance in other less significantly ill patients, however, suggests that there will be a role for this type of hormonal manipulation in some patients.[82, 96]

Immune

Given the central role of the immune system in activating the patient's response to shock, particularly septic shock, it is not surprising that there have been attempts to modify

Table 9–4
Cardiovascular Inotropes

Agent	Alpha$_1$	Beta$_1$	Beta$_2$
Norepinephrine	4+	4+	0
Epinephrine	4+	4+	2+
Dopamine	4+	4+	2+
Dobutamine	1+	4+	2+

this system with specific immunotherapy. These attempts have included vaccination, but its use is limited by the period of time required for the primary response after the vaccination is given. Vaccines are also limited by the narrowness of the spectrum of protection that they provide and the fact that septic patients may not respond well to this therapy. Another area of immunotherapy is the administration of immunoglobulin, but the use of standard immunoglobulin preparations seems to be limited by their nonspecificity. Some data indicate, however, that they may be helpful in some situations.[40, 44] A more promising area of immunotherapy is the use of monoclonal antibodies in the treatment of septic shock, in which specific antibodies have been generated against bacteria and cytokines.[23]

Interferon. Interferon is normally produced by lymphocytes in response to many different antigens. It acts to improve the processing of antigen by monocytes and augments phagocytosis and intracellular killing by macrophages. In rats subjected to hemorrhagic shock, it restored immune competence and reversed the bone marrow inhibition.[73, 75]

Anti–Tumor Necrosis Factor. If TNF plays a major role in the immune and metabolic response to injury and shock, it is reasonable to expect that treatment with antibodies against the active portion of this molecule should eliminate or at least alter the metabolic response to the insult. In a study that most closely recreates the clinical situation, monoclonal antibody to TNF was administered to baboons after an infusion of *Escherichia coli* was begun.[62] There was a significant improvement in the clinical course and survival in the treated group. Paradoxically, the administration of TNF after hemorrhagic shock in animals appeared to improve immunocompetence.[76]

Neutrophils. Neutrophils play a central role in the metabolic response to injury and shock. Experimental efforts to affect the function of neutrophils include blocking neutrophil adherence and activity.[7] An alternative approach, then, has been to transfuse neutrophils.[40] As the precise role of neutrophils becomes clarified, this area of investigation offers a number of possibilities for clinical manipulation.

Nutrition. There is a growing interest in immunomodulation with different components of nutritional support.[20, 21, 27, 28, 67, 70, 71, 79, 91, 140] This should serve to remind us that many current therapies in the injured patient affect the immune system. Blood must be given to maintain the patient's oxygen-carrying capacity, but it is clearly immunosuppressive.[19, 72, 109] Attempts to modify the immune response may prove to be effective. Surgery, performed in a timely and effective fashion, is a powerful modulator of the immune response.[85]

Cerebral

Many specific therapies have been designed to reduce cerebral injury. These include the use of calcium channel blockers and oxygen radical scavengers.[105] Trials with total body hypothermia have attempted to reduce cerebral metabolism.[126] The best therapy appears to be rapid recognition and management of the source of shock and protection of the brain from further injury by careful attention to electro-lytes, glucose, and acid-base status. The maintenance of mild hypocarbia is recommended.

Pulmonary

Currently, the only effective therapy for adult respiratory distress syndrome is mechanical ventilation with the application of positive pressure. It is best to treat this process before the phase of acute injury has begun. Unfortunately, steroids and anti-inflammatory agents are helpful only if given before injury occurs or in the earliest stages of injury, but these injuries are usually recognized late.

Cardiovascular

Several areas are under investigation that will alter the management of the cardiovascular system of the patient in shock. These include the development of hemoglobin alternatives and improved monitoring techniques, the introduction of new inotropic agents, and a possible role for extracorporeal membrane oxygenation.

The search for hemoglobin alternatives is not new. Currently, available alternatives fall into two categories: stroma-free hemoglobin and fluorocarbons.[68] Stroma-free hemoglobin is readily available, is nonantigenic, and is not nephrotoxic. Its use is limited, however, by an extremely high affinity for oxygen and a short half-life. Fluorocarbons serve as good transporters of oxygen and have a long half-life. Unfortunately, these substances are expensive and may induce depression of the immune response.

The second area of advancement is in the area of monitoring. Although it is possible to place an arterial catheter or a pulmonary artery catheter in an infant, it is technically demanding. Some success has been noted with noninvasive monitoring techniques, and clearly this technology will play an increasing role in the care of small children.[24, 99]

The third area is the introduction of new inotropes. It is reasonable to expect that new agents with greater specificity will continue to be introduced. The phosphodiesterase inhibitors, which provide for both positive inotropic and vasodilating effects, have been introduced, and clinical trials will determine whether these agents have a role in the management of shock in children.[77]

Extracorporeal membrane oxygenation has been used to support neonates with a variety of pathologic conditions. The survival rate for septic neonates, however, is considerably less than that for those with other conditions, as experimental evidence has demonstrated that extracorporeal membrane oxygenation, utilized in an animal model of sepsis, did not improve survival when compared with results from a control group.[50] The introduction and improvement of veno-venous bypass may offer an adjunct in the treatment of these patients.

Renal

Dopamine, used for selective dilation of the renal artery, appears to be useful in the treatment of shock.[46] Experimental evidence indicates that the use of atrial natriuretic hormone with dopamine may also improve renal function in the early postischemic period.[25, 95]

Gastrointestinal

The gastrointestinal tract is the focus of considerable research. It is becoming generally accepted that bacterial translocation in the gut may be the source of multiple system organ failure. Much of this may be preventable through the early application of enteral feeding or the addition of glutamine to parenteral formulations.[4, 12, 115]

Another approach to reducing bacterial translocation is through selective bowel contamination and enteral antibodies. In a rat burn model, the incidence of bacterial translocations was reduced by using this method.[64]

One final area of therapy in the area of gastrointestinal function is the prevention of stress ulceration. Bleeding from stress gastritis is associated with significant morbidity and mortality. The incidence can be decreased by reducing the acidity of the stomach. Although histamine-2 blockers are commonly used for this purpose, they have not proved to be universally effective.[100] Antacids and sucralfate appear more effective.[121] The potential role for proton pump blockers for this purpose has not yet been explored.

SUMMARY

Inadequate cellular perfusion, affecting the cellular level directly, can disrupt cellular function. Injury and shock activate a number of neuroendocrine and immune pathways that affect the patient on a cellular level. The end organ response is a function of the unique characteristics of the cells that comprise the individual organ. All of this constitutes the homeostatic response to shock and injury. In the majority of children, this mechanism promotes survival. In some, the processes can perpetuate organ injury and lead to multiple organ failure.[22, 112, 135] As the current understanding of the mechanisms of injury is challenged, new possibilities for therapeutic intervention will follow.[38]

References

1. Abraham E: Host defense abnormalities after hemorrhage, trauma and burns. Crit Care Med 171:923–939, 1989.
2. Abraham E: Physiologic stress and cellular ischemia: Relationship to immunosuppression and susceptibility to sepsis. Crit Care Med 19:613–619, 1991.
3. Adkison D, Hollwarth ME, Benoit JN, et al: Role of free radicals in ischemia-reperfusion injury to the liver. Acta Physiol Scand 548(suppl):101–107, 1986.
4. Alverdy J, Chi H, Sheldon GF: The effect of parenteral nutrition on gastrointestinal immunity. The importance of enteral stimulation. Ann Surg 202:681–684, 1985.
5. Amaral JF, Caldwell MD: Metabolic response to starvation, stress, and sepsis. In: Miller TA (ed): Physiologic Basis of Modern Surgical Care. St Louis, CV Mosby, 1988, pp 1–35.
6. Anderson BO, Bensard DD, Harken AH: The role of platelet-activating factor and its antagonist in shock, sepsis, and multiple organ failure. Surg Gynecol Obstet 72:416–424, 1991.
7. Anderson BO, Brown JM, Harken AH: Mechanisms of neutrophil-mediated tissue injury. Surg Res 51:170–179, 1991.
8. Andrassy RJ, Dubois T: Modified injury severity scale and concurrent steroid therapy: Independent correlates of negative nitrogen balance in pediatric trauma. J Pediatr Surg 20:799–802, 1985.
9. Ausgten TR, Chen MK, Moore W, et al: Endotoxin and renal glutamine metabolism. Arch Surg 126:23–26, 1991.
10. Baker J, Deitch EA, Li M, et al: Hemorrhagic shock induces bacterial translocation from the gut. J Trauma 28:896–906, 1988.
11. Bankey PE, Mazuski JE, Mariaestela O, et al: Hepatic acute phase protein synthesis is indirectly regulated by tumor necrosis factor. J Trauma 30:1181–1188, 1990.
12. Barber AE, Jones WF II, Minei JP, et al: Glutamine or fiber supplementation of a defined formula diet: Impact on bacterial translocation, tissue composition and response to endotoxin. JPEN 14:335–343, 1990.
13. Baxter BT, Moore EE, Moore JB, et al: Emergency department thoracotomy following injury: Critical determinants for patient salvage. World J Surg 12:671–675, 1988.
14. Bhatt-Mehta V, Nahata MC: Dopamine and dobutamine in pediatric therapy. Pharmacotherapy 9:303–314, 1989.
15. Bilello JF, O'Hair KC, Kirby WC, et al: Intraosseous infusion of dobutamine and isoproterenol. Am J Dis Child 45:165–167, 1991.
16. Billiar TR, Curran RD, Ferrari FK, et al: Kupffer cell: Hepatocyte cocultures release nitric oxide in response to bacterial endotoxin. J Surg Res 48:349–353, 1990.
17. Bone RC, Fisher CJ Jr, Clemmer TP: A controlled clinical trial of high-dose methylprednisolone in the treatment of severe sepsis and septic shock. N Engl J Med 317:653–658, 1989.
18. Bragg LE, Thompson JS, West WW: Intestinal diamine oxide levels reflect ischemic injury. Surg Res 50:22–233, 1991.
19. Brunson ME, Alexander JW: Mechanisms of transfusion-induced immunosuppression. Transfusion 30:651–658, 1990.
20. Carver JD, Cox WI, Barness LA: Dietary nucleotide effects upon murine natural killer cell activity and macrophage activation. JPEN 14:18–22, 1990.
21. Cerra FB: Nutrient modulation of inflammatory and immune functions. Am J Surg 161:230–234, 1991.
22. Cerra FB: The hypermetabolism organ failure complex. World J Surg 11:173–181, 1987.
23. Chmel H: Role of monoclonal antibody therapy in the treatment of infectious disease. Am J Hosp Pharm 47(suppl 3):S6–10, 1990.
24. Claflin KS, Alverson DC, Patrick D, et al: Cardiac determinations in the newborn. Reproducibility of the pulsed Doppler velocity measurement. J Ultrasound Med 7:311–315, 1988.
25. Conger JD, Falk SA, Yuan BH, et al: Atrial natriuretic peptide and dopamine in a rat model of ischemic acute renal failure. Kidney Int 255:1126–1132, 1989.
26. Curran RD, Billiar TR, Stuehr DJ, et al: Multiple cytokines are required to induce hepatocyte nitric oxide production and inhibit total protein synthesis. Ann Surg 212:462–469, 1990.
27. Daly JM, Lieberman M, Goldfine J: Enteral nutrition with supplemental arginine, RNA and omega-3 fatty acids: A prospective clinical trial (abstract). JPEN 15:19S, 1991.
28. Daly JM, Reynolds J, Thom A, et al: Immune and metabolic effects of arginine in the surgical patient. Ann Surg 208:512–523, 1988.
29. Darling G, Goldstein DS, Stull R, et al: Tumor necrosis factor: Immune endocrine interaction. Surgery 106:1155–1160, 1989.
30. Deitch EA, Bridges W, Berg R, et al: Hemorrhaghic shock induced bacterial translocation: The role of neutrophils and hydroxyl radicals. J Trauma 30:942–952, 1990.
31. Deitch EA, Xu D, Qi L, et al: Bacterial translocation from the gut impairs systemic immunity. Surgery 109:269–276, 1991.
32. DeMaria A, Carven DE, Heffernan JJ, et al: Naloxone versus placebo in treatment of septic shock. Lancet 1(8442):1363–1365, 1985.
33. Ducey JP, Mazingo DW, Lamiell JM, et al: A comparison of the cerebral and cardiovascular effects of complete resuscitation with isotonic and hypertonic saline, hetastarch, and whole blood following hemorrhage. J Trauma 29:1510–1518, 1989.
34. Easmon CS: Pathogenesis of septicaemia. J Antimicrob Chemother 25(Suppl C):9–16, 1990.
35. Epstein MD, Tchervenkov JI, Alexander JW, et al: Increased gut permeability following burn trauma. Arch Surg 126:198–200, 1991.
36. Ernster L: Biochemistry of reoxygenation injury. Crit Care Med 16:947–953, 1988.
37. Espinel CH: The FE_{NA} test. Use in the differential diagnosis of acute renal failure. JAMA 236:579–581, 1976.
38. Evans JA, Darlington DN, Gann DS: A circulating factor(s) mediates cell depolarization in hemorrhagic shock. Ann Surg 213:549–555, 1991.
39. Fink MP: Gastrointestinal mucosal injury in experimental models of shock, trauma, and sepsis. Crit Care Med 19:627–641, 1991.

40. Fischer GW, Weisman LE: Therapeutic intervention of clinical sepsis with intravenous immunoglobulin, white blood cells and antibiotics. Scand J Infect Dis 73(suppl):17–71, 1990.

41. Fischer JE, Jasselgren P: Cytokines and glucocorticoids in the regulation of the "hepatoskeletal muscle axis" in sepsis. Am J Surg 161:266–271, 1991.

42. Fiser DH: Intraosseous infusion. N Engl J Med 22:1579–1581, 1990.

43. Fong Y, Moldawer LL, Shires GT, et al: The biologic characteristics of cytokines and their implication in surgical injury. Surg Gynecol Obstet 170:363–378, 1990.

44. Frame JD, Everitt AS, Gordon WN, et al: IgG subclass response to gamma globulin administration in burned children. Burns 16:437–440, 1990.

45. Gann DS, Amaral JF, Caldwell MD: Neuroendocrine response to stress, injury, and sepsis. In: Davis JH (ed): Clinical Surgery. St. Louis, Mosby Year Book, 1987, pp 299–336.

46. Girardin E, Berner M, Rouge JC, et al: Effect of low dose dopamine on hemodynamic and renal function in children. Pediatr Res 26:200–203, 1989.

47. Gosche JR, Garrison RN: Prostaglandins mediate the compensatory responses to hemorrhage in the small intestine of the rat. J Surg Res 50:584–588, 1991.

48. Gottardis M, Benzer A, Koller W, et al: Improvement of septic syndrome after administration of recombinant human growth hormone (rhGH)? J Trauma 31:81–86, 1991.

49. Greenburg AG: Pathophysiology of shock. In: Miller TA (ed): Physiologic Basis of Modern Surgical Care. St. Louis, CV Mosby, 1988, pp 154–172.

50. Griffin MP, Zwischenberger JB, Minifee PK, et al: Extracorporeal membrane oxygenation of gram-negative septic shock in the immature pig. Circ Shock 33:195–199, 1991.

51. Grimble RG: Nutrition and cytokine action. Nutr Res Rev 3:193–210, 1990.

52. Gurll NJ, Reynolds DG, Holaday JW: Evidence for a role of endorphins in the cardiovascular pathophysiology of primate shock. Crit Care Med 16:521–530, 1988.

53. Gutierrez G: Cellular energy metabolism during hypoxia. Crit Care Med 19:619–626, 1991.

54. Hack CE, Nuigens JH, Strack van Schijndel RJM, et al: A model for the interplay of inflammatory mediators in sepsis—A study in 48 patients. Intensive Care Med 16:S187–S191, 1990.

55. Hackshaw KV, Parker GA, Roberts JW: Naloxone in septic shock. Crit Care Med 18:47–51, 1990.

56. Hagland UH, Park PO: Intestinal ischemia. Surg Annu 23:173–186, 1991.

57. Haljamae H: Organ specific metabolic changes in shock. In: Bond RF (ed): Perspectives in Shock Research. New York, Alan R. Liss, 1988, pp 17–26.

58. Hamaji M, Nakamura M, Izukura M, et al: Autoregulation and regional blood flow of the dog during hemorrhagic shock. Circ Shock 19:245–255, 1986.

59. Hamilton GC, Whit BC: The brain in shock. In: Barrett J, Nyhus NM (eds): The Treatment of Shock. Principles and Practice. 2nd ed. Philadelphia, Lea & Febiger, 1986, pp 81–115.

60. Herzenberg JE, Hensinger RN, Dedrick DK, et al: Emergency transport and positioning of young children who have an injury of the cervical spine. The standard backboard may be hazardous. J Bone Joint Surg (Am) 71:15–22, 1989.

61. Hesse DG, Tracey KJ, Fong Y, et al: Cytokine appearance in human endotoxemia and primate bacteremia. Surg Gynecol Obstet 166:147–153, 1988.

62. Hinshaw LB, Tekamp-Olson P, Chang AC, et al: Survival of primates in LD100 septic shock following therapy with antibody to tumor necrosis factor (TNF/alpha). Circ Shock 30:279–292, 1990.

63. Jacobs RF, Tabor DR: The immunology of sepsis and meningitis cytokine biology. Scand J Infect Dis 73(Suppl C):7–15, 1990.

64. Jones WG, Barber AE, Minei JP, et al: Antibiotic prophylaxis diminishes bacterial translocation but not mortality in experimental burn wound sepsis. J Trauma 30:737–740, 1990.

65. Kawasaki T, Marubayashi S: Liver in shock. In: Barrett JC, Nyhus NM (eds): The Treatment of Shock: Principles and Practices. 2nd ed. Philadelphia, Lea & Febiger, 1986, pp 151–162.

66. Kessler M, Hoper J: Mechanisms of cell injury in low-flow and no-flow anoxia. In: Bond RF (ed): Perspectives in Shock Research. New York, Alan R. Liss, 1988, pp 7–16.

67. Kinsella JE, Lokesh B: Dietary lipids, eicosanoids, and the immune system. Crit Care Med 18:S94–S113, 1990.

68. Kramer GC, Walsh JC: Future trends in emergency fluid resuscitation. In: Tuma RF, White JV, Messmer C (eds): The Role of Hemodilution in Optimal Patient Care. Munich, Germany, W Zuckschwerdt Verlag, 1989, pp 89–99.

69. Kucey DS, Kubicki EI, Rotstein O: Platelet-activating factor primes endotoxin-stimulated macrophage procoagulant activity. J Surg Res 50:436–441, 1991.

70. Kulkarni AD, Fanslow WC, Rudolph FB, et al: Effect of dietary nucleotides on response to bacterial infections. JPEN 10:169–171, 1986.

71. Lieberman N, Shou J, Torres A: Effects of nutrient substrates on immune function. Nutrition 6:88–91, 1990.

72. Little AG, Wu HS, Ferguson MK, et al: Perioperative blood transfusion adversely affects prognosis of patients with stage I non–small cell lung cancer. Am J Surg 160:630–632, 1990.

73. Livingston DH: Interferon-gamma reverses bone marrow inhibition following hemorrhagic shock. Arch Surg 126:100–103, 1991.

74. Livingston DH, Gentile PS, Malangoni MA: Bone marrow failure following hemorrhagic shock. Circ Shock 30:255–264, 1990.

75. Livingston DH, Malangoni MA: Interferon-gamma restores immune competence after hemorrhagic shock. J Surg Res 5:37–43, 1988.

76. Livingston DH, Malangoni MA, Sonnenfeld G: Immune enhancement by tumor necrosis factor-alpha improves antibiotic efficacy after hemorrhagic shock. J Trauma 19:967–971, 1989.

77. Lollgen H, Drexler H: Use of inotropes in the critical care setting. Crit Care Med 18:S56–60, 1990.

78. McCord JM: Oxygen-derived free radicals in postischemic tissue injury. NEJM 312:159–163, 1985.

79. Madden HP, Breslin RJ, Wasserkrug HL: Stimulation of T-cell immunity by arginine enhances survival in peritonitis. J Surg Res 44:658–663, 1988.

80. Maier RB: Evaluation and resuscitation. In: Moore EE (ed): Early Care of the Injured Patient. Philadelphia, BC Decker, 1990, pp 56–73.

81. Mainous MR, Tso P, Berg D, et al: Studies of the route, magnitude, and time course of bacterial translocation in a model of systemic infection. Arch Surg 126:33–37, 1991.

82. Manson JM, Smith RJ, Wilmore DW: Positive nitrogen balance with human growth hormone and hypocaloric intravenous feeding. Surgery 100:188–197, 1986.

83. Markov AK, Terry J, White TZ, et al: Increasing survival of dogs subjected to hemorrhagic shock by administration of fructose 1–6 diphosphate. Surgery 102:515–527, 1987.

84. Matthews DE, Pesola G, Campbell RG: Effect of epinephrine on amino acid and energy metabolism in humans. Am J Physiol 258:E948–E956, 1990.

85. Meakins JL: Surgeons, surgery, and immunomodulation. Arch Surg 126:494–498, 1991.

86. Mela-Riiker L: Cellular aspects of shock, sepsis and burns: Mechanisms of cell injury. In: Bond RF (ed): Perspectives in Shock Research. New York, Alan R. Liss, 1988, pp 3–6.

87. Mermel VL, Wolfe BM, Hansen RJ, et al: Comparative effects of thermal and surgical trauma on rat muscle protein metabolism. JPEN 15:128–135, 1991.

88. Moden K, Arii S, Itai S, et al: Enhancement of hepatic macrophages in septic rats and their inhibitory effect on hepatocyte function. J Surg Res 50:72–76, 1991.

89. Moore FA, Peterson VM, Moore EE, et al: Inadequate granulopoiesis after major torso trauma: A hematopoietic regulatory paradox. Surgery 108:667–675, 1990.

90. Moss GS, Rice CL, Lakshman RS, et al: Management of traumatic and hemorrhagic shock. Anesthesiology 17(Suppl 3):25–37, 1990.

91. Murray MJ, Svingen BA, Holman RT, et al: Effects of a fish oil diet on pigs' cardiopulmonary response to bacteremia. JPEN 15:152–158, 1991.

92. Nelson S, Chidiac C, Bagby G, et al: Endotoxin induced suppression of lung host defenses. J Med 21:85–103, 1990.

93. Ohtake Y, Clemens MG: Interrelationship between hepatic ureagenesis and gluconeogenesis in early sepsis. Am J Physiol 260:E453–458, 1991.

94. Pelton JJ, Cheu HW, McAuley CE: The limit of hemodilutional resuscitation in acute hemorrhagic shock. Surg Forum 40:54–57, 1989.

95. Pollack DM, Opgenorth TJ: Beneficial effect of the artrial natriuretic factor analog A68828 in postischemic acute renal failure. J Pharmacol Exp Ther 255:1166–1169, 1990.

96. Ponting GA, Halliday D, Teale JD: Postoperative positive nitrogen balance with intravenous hyponutrition and growth hormone. Lancet 1(8583):483–440, 1988.

97. Ramenofsky L: Pediatric trauma. In: Moore EE (ed): Early Care of the Injured Patient. Philadelphia, BC Decker, 1990, pp 317–327.

98. Reilly PM, Schiller JH, Bulkley GB. Pharmacologic approach to tissue injury mediated by free radicals and other reactive oxygen metabolites. Am J Surg 161:488–503, 1991.

99. Rein AJ, Hsieh KS, Elixson M, et al: Cardiac output estimates in the pediatric intensive care unit using a continuous-wave Doppler computer: Validation and limitations of the technique. Am Heart J 112:97–103, 1986.

100. Reines HD: Do we need stress ulcer prophylaxis? (editorial). Crit Care Med 18:344, 1990.

101. Richardson JD: Common pulmonary derangements and respiratory failure. In: Miller TA (ed): Physiologic Basis of Modern Surgical Care. St. Louis, CV Mosby, 1988, pp 589–610.

102. Royall JA, Levin DL: Adult respiratory distress syndrome in pediatric patients. I. Clinical apsects, pathophysiology, pathology and mechanisms of lung injury. J Pediatr 112:169–175, 1988.

103. Royall J, Levin DL: Adult respiratory distress syndrome in pediatric patients. II. Management. J Pediatr 112:335–347, 1988.

104. Saadia R, Schein M, Macfarlane C, et al: Gut barrier function and the surgeon. Br J Surg 77:487–492, 1990.

105. Safer P: Resuscitation from clinical death: Pathophysiologic limits and therapeutic potentials. Crit Care Med 16:923–941, 1988.

106. Sanfey H, Sarr MG, Bulkley GB, et al: Oxygen derived free radicals and acute pancreatitis: A review. Acta Physiol Scand Suppl 548:109–118, 1986.

107. Schemeling IH, Coran AJ: Hormonal and metabolic response to operative stress in the neonate. JPEN 15:215–238, 1991.

108. Schwaitzberg SD, Bergman KS, Harris BH: A pediatric trauma model of continuous hemorrhage. J Pediatr Surg 23:605–609, 1988.

109. Scorza LB, Waymack JP, Pruitt BA: The effect of transfusions on the incidence of bacterial infection. Mil Med 155:337–339, 1990.

110. Shaw JH, Wolfe RR: An integrated analysis of glucose, fat and protein metabolism in severely traumatized patients. Ann Surg 209:63–72, 1989.

111. Smith RJ: Glutamine metabolism and its physiologic importance. JPEN 14:40–43S, 1990.

112. Smith SD, Tagge EP, Hannakan C, et al: Characterization of neonatal multisystem organ failure in the surgical newborn. J Pediatr Surg 26:494–499, 1991.

113. Snow TR, Dickey DT, Tapp T, et al: Early myocardial dysfunction induced with endotoxin in rhesus monkeys. Can J Cardiol 6:130–136, 1990.

114. Souba WW, Herskowitz K, Klimberg S, et al: The effects of sepsis and endotoxemia on gut glutamine metabolism. Ann Surg 211:543–551, 1990.

115. Souba WW, Herskowitz K, Sallowum RM, Chen MK: Gut glutamine metabolism. JPEN 4:45S–50S, 1990.

116. Spitzer JA: Altered Ca²⁺ homeostasis and functional correlates in hepatocytes and adipocytes in endotoxemia and sepsis. J Trauma 30:S192–197, 1990.

117. Spivey WH: Intraosseous infusions. J Pediatr 111:639–643, 1987.

118. Stahl WM: Kidney in shock. In: Barrett J, Nyhus LM (eds): The Treatment of Shock. Principles and Practice. 2nd ed. Philadelphia, Lea & Febiger, 1986, pp 137–149.

119. Stein HJ, Hinder RA, Oostnuizen MM: Gastric mucosal injury caused by hemorrhagic shock and reperfusion: Protective role of antioxidant glutathione. Surgery 108:467–474, 1990.

120. Stein HJ, Oostnuizen MM, Hinder RA, et al: Oxygen free radicals and glutathione in hepatic ischemia/reperfusion injury. J Surg Res 50:398–402, 1991.

121. Stress ulcer prophylaxis in critically ill patients (editorial). Lancet 2(8674):1255–1256, 1989.

122. Suffredini AF, Fromm RE, Parker MM, et al: The cardiovascular response of normal humans to the administration of endotoxin. N Engl J Med 321:280–287, 1989.

123. Takeyama N, Itoh V, Kitazawa Y, et al: Altered heptic mitochondrial fatty acid oxidation and ketogenesis in endotoxic rats. Am J Physiol 259:E498–505, 1990.

124. Tashiro T, Mashima V, Yamamori H, et al: Alteration of whole-body protein kinetics according to severity of surgical trauma in patients receiving total parenteral nutrition. JPEN 5:169–172, 1991.

125. Tellez DW, Hardin WD, Takahashi M, et al: Blunt cardiac injury in children. J Pediatr Surg 22:1123–1128, 1987.

126. Tisherman SA, Safar P, Radovsky A, et al: Deep hypothermic circulatory arrest induced during hemorrhagic shock in dogs: Preliminary systemic and cerebral metabolism studies. Curr Surg 47:327–330, 1990.

127. Trump BJ, Berezesky IK, Cowley RA: The cellular and subcellular characteristics of acute and chronic injury with emphasis on the role of calcium. In: Cowley RA, Trump BJ (eds): Pathophysiology of Shock, Anoxia and Ischemia. Baltimore, Williams & Wilkins, 1982, pp 6–46.

128. Vedder NB, Fouty BW, Winn R, et al: Role of neutrophils in generalized reperfusion injury associated with resuscitation from shock. Surgery 106:509–516, 1989.

129. Velanovich V: Crystalloid versus colloid fluid resuscitation: A meta analysis of mortality. Surgery 105:65–71, 1989.

130. Venkatachalam MA, Rennke HG, Sandstrom DJ: The vascular basis for acute renal failure in the rat. Preglomerular and postglomerular vasoconstriction. Circ Res 38:267–279, 1976.

131. Veterans Administration Systemic Sepsis Cooperative Study Group: Effect of high-dose glucocorticoid therapy on mortality in patients with clinical signs of systemic sepsis. N Engl J Med 317:659–665, 1987.

132. Waldhausen JH, Shaffrey ME, Skandaris BS, et al: Gastrointestinal myoelectric and clinical patterns of recovery after laparotomy. Ann Surg 211:777–784, 1990.

133. Walsh JC, Zhuang J, Shackford SR: A comparison of hypertonic to isotonic fluid in the resuscitation of brain injury and hemorrhagic shock. J Res 50:284–292, 1991.

134. Warshaw AL, O'Hara PJ: Susceptibility of the pancreas to ischemic injury in shock. Ann Surg 188:197–201, 1978.

135. Wilkinson JD, Pollack MM, Ruttimann UE, et al: Outcome of pediatric patients with multiple organ system failure. Crit Care Med 14:271–274, 1986.

136. Wilmore DW: Glucose metabolism following severe injury. J Trauma 21:705–707, 1981.

137. Wilmore DW, Brooks DC, Muhlbacher F, et al: Altered amino acid concentrations and flux following traumatic injury. In: Blackburn GL, Grant JP, Young VR (eds): Amino Acids. Metabolism and Medical Applications. Boston, Wright-PSG, 1983, pp 387–395.

138. Winthrop AL, Wesson DE, Pencahrz PB, et al: Injury severity, whole body protein turnover and energy expenditure in pediatric trauma. J Pediatr Surg 22:534–537, 1987.

139. Yeston NS, Palter M: The lung in shock. In: Barrett JC, Nyhus NM (eds): The Treatment of Shock: Principles and Practice. 2nd ed. Philadelphia, Lea & Febiger, 1986, pp 59–80.

140. Yoshino S, Ellis EF: The effects of fish oil supplemented diet on inflammation and immunological processes in rats. Int Arch Allergy Immunol 84:233–240, 1987.

141. Zellner JL, Spinale FG, Crawford FA, et al: Right ventricular pump dysfunction with acute experimental septic shock. J Surg Res 50:93–99, 1991.

William L. Buntain
Amie C. Jew
Jeanne Henning

CHAPTER TEN

Initial Evaluation and Management

Of the 60 million injuries that occur annually in the United States, 30 million (50%) require medical care, and 3.6 million (12%) require hospitalization. Nine million of the 30 million injuries are disabling injuries, 300,000 of which are permanent and 8,700,000 of which are temporary. The cost to the nation is staggering, for as impressive as the death rate from injury is—approximately 145,000 deaths annually—each year trauma-related costs are in excess of $100 billion, approximately 40% of the health care dollar.[2]

Although injuries have been recognized as the leading cause of death in childhood for nearly 50 years and the death rate in children from natural causes has decreased almost 50% in the last 3 decades, deaths due to injury in this age group have increased and presently account for nearly six of every 10 children who die—four times the number from any other childhood disease. Further, for each child killed, four are permanently disabled.[3, 24, 47, 48, 58]

Data suggest that nearly 25 to 35% of deaths in seriously injured trauma patients could have been prevented by more effective initial management.[13] In an effort to provide more optimal care and improve on this preventable death rate, communities and institutions regionalized and improved transport of the seriously injured to specialized facilities that had experienced physicians committed to trauma.[33] Although progress and improvements in morbidity and mortality rates in adults occurred, such results were not realized in children, and in fact, in one system the morbidity and mortality rates for children actually increased.[1, 46]

The majority of patients who present to the emergency department with an injury do not have an immediately life-threatening problem and may be assessed and managed in an orderly and a less hurried fashion.[15] Only a small proportion of traumatized patients, approximately 10 to 15%, require a precise, rapid, systematic approach to initial management that is crucial to their survival.[30] In these patients assessment and resuscitation must occur simultaneously, not only in the emergency department but in the field as well. To provide this efficient initial management, a detailed knowledge of cardiopulmonary physiology and the kinematics of injury, an ability to perform certain manipulative skills, and the exercise of compassionate wisdom and understanding in dealing with patients and their families must be utilized.[15] Hence, the systems approach to trauma must include the prehospital provider. Physicians who ultimately are responsible for these children are obligated to have an understanding of the prehospital providers' responsibilities, their capabilities, and the expectations the public and the local governing bodies have for these providers as they act as interfaces between the traumatized patient and the medical team.

EMERGENCY MEDICAL SERVICES

History

Emergency Medical Services (EMS) refers to a systematic approach to the delivery of prehospital care to the acutely ill or injured, the provision of ongoing medical support while transporting that patient to a location for definitive care, and the appropriate communication of patient status to the receiving hospital about the emergency so that the physician can give directions for continued care at the scene as well as en route to the hospital. Prehospital providers can and should stabilize fractures before transporting or moving an injured patient and should provide psychological support for the patient and family.[36]

Historically, EMS had its origins during the time of the Napoleonic wars when Jean Larrey, Napoleon's surgeon, realized that many deaths could be prevented by rapid treatment at the site of the injury. Improving the initial management of wounds on the battlefield by the use of trained personnel, Larrey assumed the responsibility for maintaining this treatment en route, and then followed it with rapid evacuation to a more definitive treatment facility.[34]

In the United States, in 1862, Jonathan Letterman, the medical director of the Army of the Potomac, elaborated on this procedure when he organized the Ambulance Corps, a train of horse-drawn ambulances that transported the wounded from the battlefield to hospitals, but the system did not advance much further until the 1940s with the success of the battalion aid stations during World War II.[36] Today, an extremely important aspect of trauma care is the emphasis on the evaluation of the severity of injury by the emergency medical technician (EMT) in the field, the immediate management of the airway, the stabilization of fractures, the control of external hemorrhage and the initial steps taken for shock management, and the rapid transportation from the scene to definitive care.

Although terminology to designate the various educational and patient care skill levels of EMTs varies from state to state, three nationally accepted levels are recognized. Training programs for all three levels include didactic, clinical, and field internship portions, and only if students spend adequate time in all these areas can they be trained to function adequately in the isolated prehospital arena. The Emergency Medical Technician—Ambulance (EMT-A) and the Emergency Medical Technician—Paramedic (EMT-P) levels are well recognized and approximately equivalent, but there are 32 variations of the intermediate level of prehospital providers throughout the 50 states.[36]

Skill Levels of Emergency Medical Technicians

The EMT-A has to complete the 110-hour course of instruction developed by the United States Department of Transportation.[36] After completing the course, the EMT-A takes a written and practical examination provided by either the National Registry of EMTs or the state or both. Skills used by the technician at this level include cardiopulmonary resuscitation, splinting and bandaging, extrication, emergency childbirth, pneumatic antishock garment application, and airway management using an oral or nasal airway and bag-valve mask.

The Emergency Medical Technician—Intermediate (EMT-I) has completed the EMT-A course and has taken additional training of 150 to 200 hours.[55] Additional hours are used to gain more experience in shock management, advanced patient assessment, physiology, management of the critically ill trauma patient, and improving airway management skills. There are approximately 32 different types of EMT-I technicians in the United States because state laws for this category of expertise vary.

The EMT-P is trained in all the skills identified for the EMT-I as well as in endotracheal intubation and the use of epinephrine, bicarbonate, calcium, dopamine, insulin, glucose, naloxone hydrochloride (Narcan), morphine, diazepam (Valium), nitrous oxide, meperidine hydrochloride (Demerol), furosemide (Lasix), and some others.[11, 35, 38, 56] The major impact of the EMT-P is in the resuscitation of cardiac and major medical problems, making EMT-Ps very effective in urban areas in which response times are short.

Emergency medical technician nurses also play an important role as EMTs, instructors, and quality control proctors. Because nurses have a great deal of understanding of patient care and the long-term results of pathophysiologic processes, they can as EMTs integrate the patient's immediate care with long-term needs. However, a registered nurse cannot carry out the EMT nurse's functions without acceptable EMT training.

On the Scene Protocols

On the scene, medical control supervises the EMTs via monitoring of the communications, on-the-scene observations by the medical director, or providing orders to the EMTs, usually by a physician at the base hospital or by the supervising physician who is in constant radio contact. These orders can be given by the physician or relayed on the radio in the name of the physician by a nurse or an EMT. Though often relayed by nonphysician personnel, they are the legal orders of the physician and that physician is medically and legally responsible for them as well as the care rendered in the physician's name.

If a licensed physician on the scene wishes to assume medical control of the care of the patient, that physician is responsible until the patient is delivered to the care of another physician or until medical responsibility is assumed by another physician, as in any other situation involving patient care. Great caution must be exercised here, however, as there are many anecdotal stories about on the scene physicians who, because of their presence, think they must "do something" and they interject themselves into the situation. Unfortunately, too often they are not trained in EMS techniques, they have had no exposure to the advanced trauma life support (ATLS) course, they are almost always unfamiliar with the area's prehospital medical protocols, and they do not recognize the added risks and hazards to which they are exposing the patient, the EMTs on the scene, and themselves.

If the physician on the scene assumes care, he or she can either accompany the patient to the hospital, supervising the medical care en route, or transfer medical care via radio to the physician at medical control. If the physician accompanies the patient, the on the scene and en route medical care must conform to the prehospital protocols that have been developed and approved by the local medical society. The physician assuming on the scene care assumes the medical

consequences of his or her decisions.[36] The quality of the EMS system is the responsibility of an organized medical society, usually the local county medical society.

THE UNIQUENESS OF CHILDHOOD INJURIES

Perhaps no other emergency creates as much anxiety as that of a critically injured child. The notoriously thin margin for error; the smaller total blood volumes; the age variation for pulse, respiratory rates, blood pressure, and medication dosage; and the relative inexperience of many of the primary care providers in caring for injured children account in part for this uneasiness.[11, 38] As a result, children have a greater chance of dying once injured, both at the scene and in the emergency department.[51]

Children differ in mechanism of injury and physiologic response, and resuscitation requires not only an understanding of the pathophysiology of injury but also an appreciation of the problems of trauma peculiar to childhood.[26]

Emotional and Psychological Considerations

The child's primary emotion is fear. Children are afraid of being hurt—*and we do hurt them* (not deliberately, of course); of having their bodies invaded or disfigured, or both; of being separated from their parents and the places they are familiar with; and of never returning home again.[20] They are also afraid of the unknown and often are very disturbed by the general air of panic and confusion that usually surrounds an emergency. Properly educated, prehospital personnel can significantly affect this response and turn a potentially dangerous situation into a positive one.

The necessary interventions must be made, however, and the responder—either the EMT or the receiving physician—must also be compassionate, talking quietly, confidently, and sympathetically to the child and the parents, if present (often they are not). If the child or family members ask questions for which answers are not readily available, it is okay for the EMT to say "I don't know," leaving the responsibility for responding to the physicians at the hospital. If the parent and the child cannot be reassured that the child is all right, reassure them that everything possible is being done.

Young infants, younger than 6 months, need their parents and generally are emotionally tied to them. They cannot understand what is happening to them, and when they experience pain in any part of their body it is expressed as whole body pain. They are also unable to verbalize and when hurt are almost always combative or uncooperative. Therefore, if a seriously injured infant is not combative or uncooperative the provider should be alerted because the infant may be physically compromised to the point of not being able to respond appropriately.

Parents of such infants may be very upset; calm reassurance that everything possible is being done can be very defusing. If possible, let one parent ride in the ambulance;

it may be a good time to get a history of what happened and at the same time may relieve some of their concerns. If the parent is too upset or is interfering with the management of the child, have the parent take a cab or be driven by somebody else, perhaps the police.

Older infants, 6 to 12 months, clearly need their parents or primary care provider and without them are usually distressed and often highly agitated and combative. They calm significantly with parents present, and letting a parent ride in the ambulance may be very helpful.

Toddlers, between 1 and 3 years of age, are the most difficult to examine, even when they are not really injured. However, at their age they are most likely to experience short-term and long-term emotional difficulties as a result of the emergency and should be handled with special care. They are terrified at being without their parents and separated from the familiar, such as their primary care providers, a blanket, or a toy. They do not have the capacity to understand that things are being done for their benefit, and they are not able to understand verbal explanations. These children should be restrained as gently as possible and should be accompanied by a toy or a blanket and quiet talk, and parents should be reassured.[20]

Preschoolers, 3 to 6 years old, usually have the fears of the younger children, particularly if they are separated from their parents or if they suffer further bodily injury, and they are likely to consider the accident or injury, or both, their fault, regardless of whether it is. Although verbal, their ability to understand complex problems is *very* limited. Preschoolers may think they are being punished for something they did, and although they may appear to understand an explanation, very likely they do not and are frightened as well, particularly if the discomfort is significant, if there is blood present, or if they were with their primary care provider who is now not around to comfort or help them. Reassurance, given quietly but confidently and kept simple, and cleansing and dressing the injuries, as gently as possible, help calm the child.

Grade-school children, 6 to 12 years old, are likely to be the easiest to manage; these children usually understand rational explanations. However, they are still children and may be frightened and in pain. They may view such situations as punishment, often perhaps because they were indeed involved in something they were not supposed to be doing. They do not understand technical words, they do not have a clear concept of their internal anatomy, and they are very modest and do not like to be exposed, particularly to strangers. If hemodynamically stable, cover them, reassure them everything is being done, and include them in your conversation, particularly if you are getting a history of the incident. They will be much more cooperative.[20]

Teenagers, 13 to 18 years old, generally understand what is happening to them, and they may be good historians; however, they also may be preoccupied with their own bodies and are very disconcerted when bodily injury occurs because they are aware of the possibility of their own death and they fear permanent disability or disfigurement. Modesty is very important, particularly if the teenager is the opposite sex of that of the medical caregivers. Teenagers are capable of hysterical reactions and often exaggerate their responses. They may respond to quiet reassurance, so even if provoked, do not get angry.

The family of an injured child is dramatically affected. When treating the child, treat the family as well. The child experiences discomfort and pain with injury and resuscitation, and the parents often suffer equally. Those of us who are used to caring for such children expect this; those who are not can be frustrated. The one positive emotion that must be fostered is *trust*. The responder must reassure teenagers that everything possible is being done. Bring the parents to the emergency department if possible. If they cannot or will not come, insist they follow promptly. *Your first priority is to the injured child.* Hence, efficiency, quickness, reassurance, compassion, and calmness is important.[20]

Patterns of Injury

The most important reason for specialized care of children is that they have special needs, and often serious problems arise over and above those relating to the emotional response to their injury.[11] Such diverse considerations as difficulty of vascular access; difficulty of airway access; peculiarities of ventilation in rate, volume, and compromise from abdominal distention; and the need for accuracy in fluid administration are indeed not minor.[46] Size is important; the smaller the size the more technically challenging the procedure. An awareness of these physiologic differences combined with an understanding of the predictable patterns and mechanisms of injury helps considerably in the initial assessment and progression of management. Patterns of injury in children are important and are quite different from those seen in adults, and these differences are primarily related to the mechanism of injury. In this age group blunt trauma accounts for almost 90% of injuries; up to two thirds of the children have isolated head injuries, and at least 15% have multisystem injuries including the head.[40] The San Diego experience, indeed that of most reporting pediatric trauma centers, including our own, confirms that the injured child will have a serious central nervous system injury up to 80% of the time, serious chest injuries 40% of the time, orthopedic injuries 30% of the time, and abdominal injuries 25% of the time.[11]

Physical and Physiologic Considerations

The pediatric airway differs from that of the adult in several important anatomic and physiologic ways[18, 19]: (1) the larynx is relatively cephalad in position, located at the level of the third cervical vertebra; (2) the epiglottis is U shaped and protrudes into the pharynx; (3) the vocal cords are short, concave, cartilaginous, distensible, and easily damaged; (4) in infants and children younger than 8 years of age the narrowest portion of the airway is at the cricoid cartilage below the vocal cords (in older children and adults the narrowest portion is at the vocal cords); (5) the trachea in the child is short, approximately half the length of the adult trachea; and (6) the orocavity is relatively small in children; the tongue is relatively large; the tonsils and adenoids sometimes partially occlude the small space; and with decreased consciousness the tongue may fall back into the hypopharynx and obstruct the airway.

INITIAL ASSESSMENT AND INITIATION OF CARE—THE PREHOSPITAL PHASE

Advanced Trauma Life Support Course

The most successful and recognized method of orderly assessment of the injured patient developed to date continues to be the ATLS course developed by the Committee on Trauma of the American College of Surgeons.[15] The ATLS course provides the physician with a proven acceptable method for the safe immediate institution of care and with the basic knowledge do the following to[2]:

1. Assess the patient's condition rapidly and accurately
2. Resuscitate and stabilize the patient on a priority basis
3. Determine whether the patient's needs are likely to exceed a facility's capabilities
4. Arrange for the patient's interhospital transfer
5. Ensure that optimal care is provided each step of the way

The initial version of the ATLS course was appropriately based on the assumption that early and timely care could improve significantly the outcome of the injured.[2] In 1982, this assumption was proved to be correct with the identification of the "trimodal distribution of death" due to trauma, confirming that death due to injury occurs in one of three time periods.[2]

The *first peak* occurs within seconds to minutes of the injury, usually due to laceration of the brain, brain stem, high spinal cord, heart, aorta, or other large blood vessels. Few of these patients can be saved because of the severity of the injuries, and those that can be are primarily in large urban areas where rapid prehospital care and transport are available. Optimal salvage in this group is best accomplished by effective preventive strategies.

The *second peak* occurs within minutes to several hours after injury. The ATLS course focuses primarily on this peak, because deaths occurring during this period are usually due to subdural or epidural hematomas, hemopneumothorax, ruptured spleens, lacerated livers, pelvic fractures, or other multiple injuries associated with significant blood loss. Early and appropriate intervention should affect the death rate. Hence, the first hour of care following injury is characterized by "rapid assessment" and "resuscitation," which are the fundamental principles of the ATLS program. This first hour of resuscitation following trauma is often referred to as the "golden hour of resuscitation," during which time the prompt reversal of shock and the immediate diagnosis and treatment of life-threatening injuries are of primary importance.[32]

The *third peak* occurs several days to weeks after the initial injury and is most often due to sepsis or multiple organ system failure, or both. Care provided during each of the preceding time periods affects the outcome during this stage; hence, the first and every subsequent responder to

see the injured patient has a direct effect on long-term outcome.

Little has been recorded about outcome in pediatric trauma. Attempts to evaluate it indicate that the majority of deaths do not occur in hospitals but at the scene of the accident or during transport and that the highest death rates occur in children younger than 6 months of age, predominantly those 2 to 3 months of age.[5] Because the vast majority of injuries in children result from blunt impact trauma, multisystem injuries are common and account for more than 50% of all such trauma deaths.[33] A study on the prevention of needless deaths due to trauma in children evaluated more than 900 pediatric deaths and concluded that with proper education and the input of trained pediatric specialists the mortality rate could be decreased by nearly 50%.[57]

The original—and current—target of the ATLS course was the physician who does not manage major trauma on a daily basis.[2] Now ATLS is accepted as the gold standard for the first hour of trauma care by all who provide for the injured, whether the patient is treated in an isolated rural area or a state-of-the-art level I trauma center.

The concept of ATLS was simple and profound but a marked deviation from the usual approach to patient assessment that is taught in medical school: taking an extensive history, doing a physical examination, developing a differential diagnosis, establishing a firm diagnosis, and then managing the problem.[2] The ATLS approach is different, a very important conceptual approach that directs "treatment of the greatest threat to life first." It teaches that "the lack of a definitive diagnosis should never impede the application of an indicated treatment" and that a detailed history is not the essential prerequisite to begin the evaluation of an acutely injured patient.[2] This new approach led to the development of the "ABCs" approach to evaluation and treatment of the injured.

In addition, the ATLS course teaches that life-threatening injuries kill and maim in certain reproducible time frames; for example, the loss of an airway kills more quickly than the loss of circulating blood volume, and the presence of an expanding intracranial mass lesion is the next most lethal problem. The ATLS course emphasizes the importance of first hour of initial assessment and primary management of the injured patient, starting at the point in time of injury and continuing through initial assessment, life-saving intervention, reevaluation, stabilization, and, when needed, transfer to a trauma center.[2]

Prehospital Trauma Life Support

A parallel type of course is the prehospital trauma life support course, sponsored by the National Association of Emergency Medical Technicians and developed in cooperation with the American College of Surgeons Committee on Trauma. The PHTLS course is based on the concepts of the American College of Surgeons ATLS program and is conducted for emergency medical technicians, paramedics, and nurses—the providers of prehospital care. Similar trauma courses for nurses have also been developed with similar concepts and philosophies.

Initial Assessment

The treatment of seriously injured patients requires the rapid assessment of injuries and the institution of life-preserving therapy. Because time is of the essence, a systematic approach that can be reviewed and practiced is desirable. This process is termed *initial assessment* and includes the following:

1. Prehospital assessment
2. Triage
3. Primary survey (ABCs)
4. Resuscitation
5. Secondary survey
6. Continued postresuscitation monitoring and reevaluation
7. Definitive care

The primary and secondary surveys are repeated frequently to ascertain any deterioration in the patient's status, and necessary treatment is instituted at the time an adverse change is identified.[2] Although theoretically one progresses in the evaluation of the patient as an ongoing longitudinal progression, in fact many of these activities occur in parallel or simultaneously.

Preparation for the trauma patient occurs in two different clinical settings. First, the *prehospital phase,* from which all events must be coordinated with the physicians at the receiving hospital. Second, the *inhospital phase,* during which preparations must be made to facilitate the rapid progression of resuscitating the trauma patient.

Prehospital Assessment

Coordination with the prehospital agency greatly expedites patient management in the field. The prehospital personnel who respond should always notify the receiving hospital before transporting the patient from the scene. At the scene, emphasis should be placed on airway maintenance, control of external bleeding and shock, immobilization of the patient, and immediate transport to the closest appropriate facility, preferably a certified trauma center.

Every effort should be made to minimize time spent at the site of injury. Unlike care of adults, therapy for an injured child or infant cannot be initiated as readily in the field, technical interventions may be time consuming and challenging, and intravenous access can be fraught with difficulty and frustration. Less experienced field personnel in particular, but even experienced field responders, may not have much experience with trauma care of small children, and time wasted fruitlessly may affect the outcome adversely. Hence, the initial responder must weigh the time and value of on the scene treatment against the benefit of rapid transport to the nearest pediatric-oriented trauma facility—the "load and go" or "scoop and run" approach. The injured child who is apparently stable at the scene, has no apparent life-threatening injuries, and is less than 10 to 15 minutes from an appropriate facility should not be treated in the field. For the child whose condition is unstable, rapid transport is even more urgent.

Although a major advance in the emergency care of injured patients during the past decade has been the extension of life-saving maneuvers from the emergency department to the prehospital arena, controversy exists over the amount of time paramedics spend in the stabilization of injured persons at the scene, particularly older children and adults. The ability of first responders to execute procedures in a timely fashion has been strongly challenged; some advocate little or no paramedic intervention at the scene, and others have found airway control and the initiation of volume resuscitation to be life saving.[17]

Cwinn and colleagues reviewed the care of critically injured blunt trauma victims to analyze the field time expended in the prehospital arena when physician medical control was strongly emphasized. Care provided at the scene included safe extrication, obtaining vital signs and surveying the patient for injuries, immobilization of the cervical and lumbar spines, securing an airway, establishing an intravenous (IV) line and obtaining blood in vacuum tubes for type and cross-match and routine tests, administration of oxygen, continuous electrocardiographic monitoring, stabilization of obvious long bone fractures, restraining limbs of combative patients, and loading the patient into the ambulance. Further IV access may be established in the ambulance en route. Closed-chest cardiopulmonary resuscitation was also performed in cases of traumatic cardiac arrest. One hundred and fourteen victims of blunt trauma were evaluated, and the mean on the scene time was 13.9 minutes, despite the addition of increasing numbers of ATLS procedures; in fact, for the 13 patients who had such procedures, the mean on the scene time was 12.4 minutes. The investigators concluded that when the field performance is provided efficiently, time spent on these procedures in the field saves time in the emergency department.[17]

Our experience with capable and competent paramedics at the University of Tennessee in Knoxville as well as at the University of Kansas in Kansas City is that even the seriously injured children consistently arrive with one or two IV lines in place. Indeed, often attempts at establishing a second or third access line in the receiving emergency department are unsuccessful or unusually prolonged. We believe this is representative of the physiologic "time" difference with regard to blood loss and the body's response to the injury between the time when the prehospital persons established access and the arrival of the patient in the emergency department, if resuscitation is not initiated at the same time. Hence, the ability to establish IV access in the field, at least in our practice, is both important and critical to success for the injured patient, and, as the Denver group points out, the patient receives the benefit of the procedures earlier. Cwinn and colleagues concluded that paramedic ATLS intervention can be performed expeditiously and that the high procedure success rates and brief on the scene times reported were a reflection of effective strategies for a direct medical control in that system.[17]

We believe this to be extremely important: it is not enough just to obtain access; resuscitation should be initiated as well. Other studies have reported the initiation of resuscitation in the field, comparing 272 injured patients and evaluating trauma scores from the field to the emergency department.[31] Patients who had ATLS intervention in the field showed a significantly greater improvement in trauma scores than did the patients who had only basic life-support interventions. Several other studies have confirmed this, demonstrating a threefold increase in survival following a 50-meter fall if paramedics responded and initiated resuscitation, a significant improvement in perfusion as indicated by increased blood pressure after volume resuscitation in the field, and a 23.9% decrease in mortality following institution of prehospital ATLS by paramedics. A Wisconsin study showed that hemodynamic stability and patient survival were significantly better if paramedics had initiated ATLS resuscitation in the field.[4, 16, 23, 41]

Emphasis also should be placed on obtaining and reporting pertinent information needed for triage at the hospital: the time of the injury; the events related to the injury; and the patient's history, which should be as complete as possible given the circumstances.[2] The mechanism of injury can also suggest the degree of injury severity as well as the specific injuries for which the patient must be evaluated, which is helpful information for the receiving medical team.

Triage

Sorting patients based on the need for therapy and the treatment rendered is based on the ABCs of trauma care and pertains to sorting patients in the field as well as at the referring and receiving facilities. It is the responsibility of the prehospital personnel and their medical director to see that the appropriate patients arrive at the appropriate facility. Unfortunately, sometimes this is a political decision, but it should not overrule the medical decisions regarding care.

Injury severity scores, methods to characterize each patient with reference to an anatomic-physiologic index, offer a helpful representation of injury seriousness and also allow reliable prediction and comparison of survival rates.[22] A more detailed discussion of these scores can be found in Chapter 6. The purpose of such scoring systems is to categorize a similar group of trauma patients so that, as nearly as possible, a single expression indicates the severity of injury, estimates the probability of survival, and can be used in the prehospital triage phase of trauma care.[45] However, such scoring systems, clinical or anatomic, have been the topic of considerable controversy, particularly in regard to adequately discriminating serious injuries in children.

The Trauma Score (TS), an analysis system developed by Champion and Sacco and others, is a numerical grading system for the estimation of *severity* of injury and is a combination of the Glasgow Coma Scale score and measurements of cardiac and pulmonary function.[14] Initially, no allowance was made for the different pediatric age groups, particularly with regard to the neurologic parameter in the Glasgow Coma score; recent modifications have attempted to correct this, however.

Perhaps a more acceptable system for injured children, applicable for triage and for prediction of injury severity, is the Pediatric Trauma Score (PTS), an arithmetic sum of three variables in each of six parameters, developed by Tepas[53, 54] (see Chapter 6). Each parameter is evaluated as normal ($+2$), abnormal (1), or life threatening (-1). The

scores from all six parameters are totaled, and a trauma score is derived.[22]

Scores range from -6 to $+12$ and have provided an excellent method of triage and survival prediction. Data suggest that an injured child with a PTS of 6 or less should be sent to a trauma center with a strong pediatric component.

Accurate determination of the prognostic value of the PTS necessitates an accepted standard for comparison. The Injury Severity Score (ISS) is an established and effective tool in the analysis of trauma care; the documented relationship between the ISS and the mortality rate provides a valid basis for evaluating the utility of the PTS as a method of predicting injury severity and subsequent outcome in the injured child.[54] A PTS of 6 or less has an ISS of 30 or greater and therefore a likelihood of mortality of 25% or more. Patients with a PTS of 6 or greater have an ISS of 6 or less and a likelihood of mortality of less than 1%. A comparison of the PTS and ISS in terms of dead versus alive patients reveals that the mean PTS for the group of children dying was 2.9 ± 2.9. The mean PTS for injured children who survive their injuries was 9.09 ± 1.1.[11] This is important information for both the prehospital responder and the receiving physician because it provides some accurate appreciation of the severity of the injuries that have been sustained and what to expect on arrival.

Protocols for the management of patients with critical injuries are designed to direct systematic efforts aimed at decreasing death and disability secondary to injury. They have had a positive effect on the outcome for injured children by improving recognition of injury and influencing therapy in a beneficial way.[21, 22, 27]

As with inhospital care, field or on the scene management is either resuscitative or definitive. *Resuscitative care* begins with the initial assessment and initiation of care, including the establishment of a patent airway and the replenishment of the circulation by achieving adequate vascular access and providing appropriate fluids. The overall objective of resuscitation is stabilization, which usually occurs in the emergency department for seriously injured patients and is the preparation for definitive care. *Definitive care* invariably occurs in the hospital and includes the operative, postresuscitative nonoperative, and critical care unit management of the patient.

The *initiation of stabilization* begins in the prehospital arena with the initial assessment and institution of resuscitation by the primary responders.[11] The communication between the hospital and the prehospital EMS is an important part of the regional triage protocols, which define the pediatric trauma patient's injuries that require transport to a designated pediatric-oriented trauma center within the shortest travel time. Also known as "destination guidelines," these criteria are based on published experience, the assumption being that the mechanism of injury and the resultant anatomic and physiologic derangements provide important information in sorting critically injured patients at the scene. These criteria are as follows:

1. Mechanism of blunt injury: Essentially, this means evidence of high impact and includes falls of 20 feet or more, crash speeds of 20 miles per hour or more, a 30-inch deformity of the crash vehicle, a rearward displacement of

the front axle with impact, a passenger compartment intrusion of 18 inches on the patient's side of the car and 24 inches on the opposite side, an ejection of the patient or a rollover, a pedestrian hit at 20 mph or more, and a death of an occupant in the same car.

2. Gross location of injuries: Historically, these have been associated with a high-energy transmission of force as a cause of injury: open fractures; uncontrolled traumatic hemorrhage; severe maxillofacial injuries; tracheal and laryngeal injuries; unstable chest injuries; major pelvic fractures; blunt abdominal injuries with traumatic hypotension; penetrating wounds to the head, neck, chest, abdomen, pelvis, or groin; neurologic injuries such as loss of consciousness, posturing, lateralizing signs, or paralysis; two or more proximal long bone fractures; or a combination of any of these.

3. Physiologic distress indicative of a serious or major injury, as evidenced by shock or respiratory distress after injury or hemorrhage; a TS of 12 or less, a PTS of 6 or less, a Glasgow Coma score of 13 or less, a systolic blood pressure of less than 90 (in the small child, normal systolic blood pressure is $80 + 2 \times$ age in years; hence, any discernible reading for systolic blood pressure that is 10% less than what is expected should prompt immediate response as if hypotensive), or a respiratory rate of less than 10 or greater than 29.

Controversy about the validity of these criteria for triage or destination guidelines is considerable, and unfortunately, most of it is *politically motivated.* Whatever one's view of the validity of these criteria, their presence should immediately prompt the first responder to consider that *such injuries or characteristics of the accident are indicators of a serious injury.* The responder should act accordingly at the scene and during transport.

The Primary Survey

In the primary survey, injured patients are assessed and treatment priorities are established based on the severity of the injuries, the stability of the patient's vital signs, and the injury mechanisms. In the severely injured patient, logical sequential treatment priorities must be established based on overall patient assessment. Management must consist of rapid primary evaluation, resuscitation of vital functions, more detailed secondary assessment, and, finally, initiation of definitive care. This process constitutes the ABCs of trauma care and identifies the life-threatening conditions.

   A. *Airway* maintenance with cervical spine control
   B. *Breathing* and ventilation
   C. *Circulation* with hemorrhage control
   D. *Disability,* neurologic status
   E. *Exposure* or environmental control: completely undress the patient but prevent hypothermia.

During the primary survey, life-threatening conditions are identified and management is begun *simultaneously.* The prioritized assessment and management procedures are basically the same for children as for adults, although the specified quantities of blood, fluids, and medications and

the size of the child, the degree of heat loss, and the injury patterns may differ.[2]

The Secondary Survey

The secondary survey is a more complete physical examination during which any other injuries are identified and the response to the therapy that was initiated during the resuscitation phase is evaluated. During this period, more sophisticated tests are done at the receiving facility, such as diagnostic peritoneal lavage, computed tomography (CT), or angiography, to prepare the patient for the definitive care phase. The definitive care phase of initial assessment is the period of the patient's management that is carried out in the operating room, the intensive care unit, or another area of the hospital that has sophisticated facilities suitable for management of these serious injuries. Proper management of the patient during this last, final phase is imperative to avoid adding to the patient's injuries.

In addition, the continued reassessment of trauma patients throughout their hospitalization is important to avoid missing occult injuries that may not have been evident at the time of initial assessment.

The Trauma Team

At our institution, the pediatric trauma team is directed by a pediatric surgeon or the surgeon's representative, such as a senior surgical resident, in whom the pediatric trauma surgeon has designated as being capable of such response. The team encompasses persons with very specific skills. Because airway patency and maintenance is of primary importance, the team most often includes an anesthesiologist, a critical care specialist, or both who along with the pediatric surgeon coordinates resuscitation, including the establishment of vascular access (if not already achieved in the field) and the initiation of diagnostic workup. Experienced pediatric-oriented registered nurses, respiratory therapists, and laboratory and radiologic technicians are important members of the team, as is the social worker who serves as a very effective interface with the family during this difficult time.

THE INITIATION OF CARE—THE INHOSPITAL PHASE

Patient Arrival

On arrival from the field, preferably in a designated trauma room, an adequate airway is ensured and the child is transferred from the transport gurney to another gurney, ideally one that is designed specifically to allow ongoing resuscitation and complete diagnostic evaluation without having to move the patient again.

A systematic approach to the assessment and resuscitation is then undertaken, with prompt, efficient evaluation occurring simultaneously with appropriate treatment of potentially life-threatening conditions, the team recognizing that failure to institute needed therapy rapidly may preclude survival.[11] The goal is optimal oxygenation and ventilation with protection of the cervical spine. Constant reevaluation is necessary to allow modification of treatment plans according to the dynamic state of the child.[49]

The Airway and the Presence of Multiple or Neurologic Injuries

Although this initial evaluation and initiation of resuscitation requires prompt attention to potential life-threatening abdominothoracic (torso) and neurologic injuries with the establishment of normal cardiopulmonary function, *the establishment of an unobstructed airway receives top priority* along with the prompt diagnosis and management of any clinical conditions that may produce profound systemic hypoxia.[11, 33, 49] Airway compromise may be sudden and complete, insidious and partial, progressive, or recurrent, and maintaining oxygenation and preventing hypercarbia are critical, especially if the patient has sustained a head injury.[2] It is for these reasons that we are *very aggressive* in our approach to the initial management of the injured child's airway.

An important major concept of pediatric craniocerebral injury and resuscitation to the trauma surgeon is the pathophysiology of *primary* and *secondary* brain injury. Primary injuries occur at the time of initial trauma—a direct injury to the brain from the initial impact—and are caused by cerebral contusions, lacerations, and cranial fractures that result from acceleration-deceleration and shearing forces. Definitive management of these injuries is the responsibility of the neurosurgeon.[33, 59] Secondary brain injury occurs from the sequence of physiologic events that follow the primary trauma and may occur as a result of hypoxia, hypotension, hypercarbia, intracranial hypertension related to overhydration and edema, or infection. Protection of the patient from these phenomena and potential disability is the responsibility of the trauma surgeon.[11]

The airway can be physiologically compromised by massive head injury or chest injury with resultant hypoxia or venous return abnormalities and potential or impending low cardiac output. In addition, a state of reduced consciousness; severe, direct maxillofacial injury; regurgitated secretions; foreign bodies; or vomitus can cause relaxation, distortion, and upper airway obstruction, which is also lethal unless corrected promptly. Aggressive resuscitation and management to avoid secondary brain injury plus intensive therapy to counter intracranial hypertension have dramatically altered morbidity and mortality in pediatric head trauma.

Nine percent of pediatric patients with head injuries die.[6] Note that 50% of the deaths from head trauma are the result of a secondary injury, from hypoxia possibly related to other injuries or ongoing borderline stability. Recognition is the key, of course, to preventing these catastrophes, but what of the subtle barely unrecognizable yet potentially lethal neurologic injuries that may indeed worsen without intervention, particularly in the uncooperative child who may be resisting efforts to help because of pain or fear and

may be in addition hypoxic and mentally agitated. It is our belief that left to themselves, such situations can go from bad to worse.

Control of intracranial pressure, maintenance of adequate cerebral perfusion, and prevention of hypoxia are mandatory. Prevention of cerebral edema is most rapidly achieved by hyperventilation because destructive increases in intracerebral pressure occur with hypercarbia and hypoventilation. Most children hyperventilate spontaneously and correct beginning hypercarbia with the correction of airway obstruction.[59] However, because head injury is frequent and is the major cause of death in injured children, the prevention of secondary brain injury from increase in intracranial pressure requires early airway control.[7, 19, 39]

In our practice, with ongoing resuscitation and perhaps even stabilization, *we paralyze the child and place an endotracheal tube,* often very early following arrival in the emergency department, particularly if the child has a Glasgow Coma score of 8 or less or a PTS of −1 and unless the child is acutely alert, appropriately responsive, and properly aware of surroundings and self. Among other positive benefits, this allows a more relaxed approach by all the responders without the concern of ''fighting'' the child and it enables us to *find and evaluate all the injuries* in a prompt and expeditious manner.

Once the airway is secured, the child is hyperventilated to a Pco_2 of between 20 and 30 mm Hg, and paralysis and sedation are maintained. Initially this is done to help prevent bucking and combativeness in the emergency department and the radiology department for procedures such as CT scans, but it is also helpful in the critical care unit if operative intervention is not initially necessary or after operative intervention to enable controlled ventilation, monitoring, and general management. Supplemental oxygen with the ventilation to keep the Pao_2 between 95 and 100 mm Hg is maintained. We have found this to be superior physiologically as well as for patient management. Patients can receive more appropriate medication to control pain and discomfort, lines and invasive tubes are much more stable and less apt to be dislodged inadvertently; hence, medications, fluids, and other possible IV interventions are better controlled. We have also found that the families are much more relaxed and the nurses much more confident in monitoring the child accurately because they are not having to fight with them emotionally or physically to avoid loss of lines or tubes. We have found the clinical course to be smoother, with less oxygen use and less nutrition burned up by excessive nonpurposeful movement, which results in a more stable healing process with the chances of increased intracranial pressure secondary to agitation and hypertension being better controlled.

Although our neurosurgeons have sometimes objected, it is important to note that nearly all other more serious neurosurgical injuries require intubation and hyperventilation with serial CT scans to evaluate for a change in status of the injury. The approach advocated here simply extends that management to the multiply injured child seriously at risk for secondary neurologic compromise.

Another important consideration is that the lower airway in infants and smaller children is smaller and has less supporting cartilage. Hence, it can become obstructed much more easily by mucus, blood, pus, edema, and reactive constriction, resulting in increased airway resistance and compromise.[44] Gaining access to these secretions for tracheal toilet rather than depending on the child to mobilize them and thus risking progressive ventilatory compromise represents another reason to aggressively intubate severely injured children. Even a minor reduction in the small diameter of the pediatric airway results in a large reduction of the cross-sectional area (Fig. 10–1).

Yet another reason for early direct endotracheal access in the critically injured child is that we caretakers make the assumption that, except for the current trauma, these children are for the most part healthy. In fact, however, ongoing respiratory infections are not uncommon, and even the child's primary care providers may not be aware of an illness just beginning that may further compromise an already at-risk airway. Such an event exacerbates hypoxemia and promotes hypercarbia; may indeed decrease lung compliance; increase the work of breathing and therefore oxygen consumption, which directly interferes with the exchange of oxygen and carbon dioxide; or produce mismatching of ventilation and pulmonary perfusion, which leads to shunting, hypoxemia, and hypercapnia. Aggressive, early endotracheal access, as described previously, with careful close monitoring of oxygenation and ventilation counteracts the possible insidious onset of these complications, placing the caretakers in an optimal position to adjust and manage such problems quickly and without having to respond at an inopportune time, such as in the middle of the night.

In addition, a well-known axiom among pediatric critical care responders is that "the stomach is always full." Hence, in the critical situation, unexpected emesis can threaten airway patency and parenchymal integrity, requiring turning of the head and usually log rolling in the re-

strained child with possible cervical spine injury. Endotracheal intubation offers protection from this problem plus immediate access to suction possible debris from the trachea should this occur with associated potential aspiration around the tube.

In essence, the endotracheal tube has the following advantages[44]: (1) it isolates the larynx and trachea from the pharynx, preventing gastric distention and minimizing the risk of aspiration; (2) it permits suctioning of airway secretions, blood, mucus, or previously aspirated debris; (3) it can provide a means to administer medications—rare in the trauma setting in our experience; and (4) if needed later, such as with pulmonary contusions and subsequent less than optimal oxygenation, it permits the application of positive end-expiratory pressure (PEEP).

Endotracheal Intubation

Recognition of Airway Compromise

To manage the airway effectively and efficiently, recognition of existing or potential airway compromise is mandatory with the initial assessment, and the following must be considered[33]: (1) Is the patient breathing adequately, or are respiratory efforts labored or stridulous? (2) Is the trachea in proper midline position, the thorax expanding equally bilaterally, and are the heart sounds normal in intensity and position? (3) Are the neck veins distended, and is the patient in circulatory collapse? (4) Is the patient cyanotic or comatose? Answers to these questions must be obtained as the provider scans the upper body and maintains immobility of the cervical spine.

Initially, the simplest methods of maintaining airway patency may be utilized, particularly in the prehospital phase. To understand the maneuvers that are required to establish and maintain airway patency, an understanding of the basic anatomy of the airway is mandatory (Fig. 10–2). The upper airway extends anatomically from the oral or nasal orifices to the vocal cords and the lower airway from the vocal cords distally. Upper airway obstruction is the most frequent source of ventilatory insufficiency in the injured child and fortunately is often the easiest to treat. Manual positioning—the chin lift or jaw thrust maneuvers—carefully avoiding overextension of the cervical spine, and manual removal or suctioning of secretions or debris from the oropharynx may suffice in an uncomplicated case of upper airway obstruction (Fig. 10–3). If obstruction continues despite proper manual positioning or removal of secretions or if ventilation is inadequate, direct examination of the oropharynx for foreign bodies and for access to the lower airway is necessary.

In an obtunded or otherwise unresponsive child, some recommend an oral or nasal airway to bypass the upper airway obstruction and maintain a patent airway. In our experience, particularly with younger children, these devices are very poorly tolerated, and if the child is semicomatose or somewhat combative, attempts to place them may indeed stimulate vomiting and further add to an already compromised airway. Our preference, as indicated earlier, is to intubate these children promptly, with or without pa-

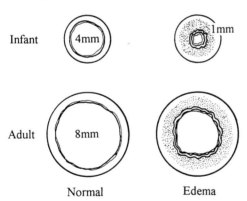

FIGURE 10–1

Normal airways represented on the left. A reactive edematous or constrictive response to disease, aspiration, or manipulation results in a 75% decrease in cross-sectional lumen opening with a 16-fold increase in resistance in the infant compared with a 44% decrease in lumen opening and a three-fold increase in resistance in the older child or adult (right). (Reproduced with permission from Pediatric Advanced Life Support. Chameides L, Hazinski MF (eds). Dallas, Texas, American Heart Association/American Academy of Pediatrics, 1994, p 4-3. Copyright American Heart Association. From: Coté CJ, Todres ID: The pediatric airway. In: Ryan JF, Todres ID, Coté CJ, Goudsouzian N (eds): A Practice of Anesthesia for Infants and Children. 2nd ed. Philadelphia, WB Saunders, 1993, p 62.)

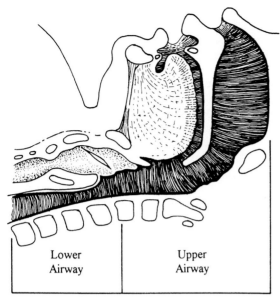

FIGURE 10-2

The upper airway extends from the oral or nasal orifices to the glottis—the vocal cords. Maneuvers such as the chin lift and the jaw thrust as well as the use of oral and nasal airways are intended to bypass obstruction in this section of the airway. Such obstruction is usually secondary to a conscious or semi-conscious state with partial or complete obstruction as the soft tissues of the mandible, tongue, and structures anterior to the upper airway fall against the posterior wall.

The lower airway extends distally from the glottis or vocal cords. Failure to relieve airway obstruction with the maneuvers outlined for the upper airway should usually prompt endotracheal intubation for definitive airway control.

ralysis depending on need, and to stabilize and maintain the airway definitively. Again, hypoxia should always be suspected in the agitated or combative child who may also be dyspneic or tachypneic.[11]

Blunt or penetrating trauma to the larynx or trachea is unusual in children but can occur with "clothesline" injuries or when a child strikes a sharp edge, such as the dashboard of an automobile.[42] Laryngeal edema and obstruction can also result from inhalation injury from burns.[19] Disruption of the trachea, bronchus, or esophagus is probable when initial examination demonstrates subcutaneous emphysema of the neck.

We believe that under such circumstances, direct endotracheal intubation is indicated, particularly if a glottic injury or severe maxillofacial trauma is present or suspected. This is done nasotracheally if elective and if the expertise is available, because nasotracheal tubes are more stable and better tolerated in the child and the nursing care is easier. However, intubation is performed expeditiously, orotracheally at first if not elective and nasotracheally later under more controlled circumstances, if desired.

Induced Paralysis, Sedation, and Intubation

Intubation, when done by surgeons, is accomplished with either pancuronium bromide (Pavulon) or vecuronium bromide, 0.05 to 0.1 mg per kg IV slow push (60 to 90 seconds), and then maintained with bolus doses of one half

of this while the injured child goes through the system: radiographs and CT scans taken, possible (but rarely) diagnostic peritoneal lavage performed, and then on to more specific procedures, such as would be handled in the critical care unit or the operating room. In the critical care unit, following surgery if necessary, a continuous narcuron drip, at 0.05 to 0.1 mg per kg per hour, is infused and adjusted to control movement.

Appropriate sedation always accompanies the induced paralysis, and we usually use fentanyl, 0.5 to 1.0 μg per kg, as an initial dose. This is boluced with half of the initial dose, as needed in the emergency department or in special procedures areas, and then an infusion of continuous drip fentanyl at 1.0 to 1.5 μg per kg per hour in the critical care area. In the grade schoolers and particularly the teenagers, and indeed occasionally in the preschoolers and toddlers, we also add a continuous infusion of midazolam HCl (Versed) at 0.05 to 0.1 mg per kg per hour. The amnestic effect of this, particularly on the older children, is both remarkable and rewarding, because while they stabilize and start to heal, they go through the otherwise emotionally traumatic period of hurting and induced discomfort of seemingly endless tests and procedures with little or no recollection of its happening. This has been referred to by our critical care nurses as "bagesthesia" (Table 10-1).

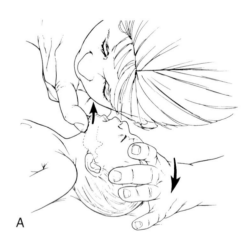

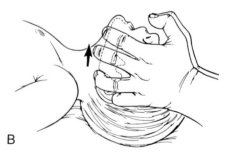

FIGURE 10-3

The head tilt–chin lift (A) and the jaw thrust (B) are the initial maneuvers to relieve upper airway obstruction. (These have been discussed previously in Chapter 7.) (Reproduced with permission from Pediatric Advanced Life Support. Chameides L, Hazinski MF (eds). Dallas, Texas, American Heart Association/American Academy of Pediatrics, 1994, pp 3-4, 3-5. Copyright American Heart Association.)

CASE 1

A 15-year-old boy, struck by an out-of-control race car as he was working on his father's car in the pit, arrived unconscious, with multiple fractures of the upper extremities, a nearly avulsed left lower extremity, fractures of his right lower extremity, a moderately severe pulmonary contusion, and a closed-head injury. He remained on continuous drip vecuronium bromide, fentanyl, and midazolam HCl for 11 days, during which time he underwent multiple trips for CT scans; multiple formal surgeries, initially to attempt revascularization of his left lower extremity but eventually for amputation; as well as multiple procedures to splint and stabilize his other fractures. On discontinuance of first the vecuronium bromide, then gradually the fentanyl, and finally the midazolam HCl, he was neurologically intact and is now neurologically normal, with very little recollection of those first 11 days. He has essentially recovered completely despite ongoing rehabilitation for prosthesis fitting and occupational therapy for his orthopedic injuries.

The use of this technique requires multiple IV lines, usually accomplished by using a double- or triple-lumen central catheter plus an arterial line, which is almost always placed in a peripheral artery of the upper or lower extremity but occasionally in a femoral vessel.

If intubation is not done by the surgeons, succinylcholine has been the preferred paralyzing agent, "because it is short acting and if children cannot be promptly intubated it will rapidly wear off and they will breath on their own." The supposition is often made that these children are able to breathe adequately on their own. We have no such confidence that they can; we are indeed concerned that the altered physiology and potential neurologic and ventilatory compromise will delay or obviate entirely the normal breathing reflex. In addition, we want the children to be still and comfortable to allow us to stabilize them promptly, to allow our necessary interventions to be accomplished quickly and with less discomfort, and to study them definitively during special procedures without artifactual movement.

Technique of Endotracheal Intubation

Endotracheal tube size is most often determined by the size of the patient's nares; it is the part of the external anatomy

Table 10–1
Bagesthesia

I.	Initial or induction bolus dose
	Pancuronium bromide 0.05 to 0.1 mg/kg (slow IV) (Pavulon)
	Vecuronium bromide 0.05 to 0.1 mg/kg (slow IV)
II.	Intermittent (as needed) bolus dose during workup and evaluation
	Pancuronium bromide One-half initial dose—draw up (Pavulon) as initial dose and give half. Vecuronium bromide
III.	Drip infusions for maintenance or control in critical care unit after the injury or operation
	Vecuronium bromide 0.05 to 0.1 mg/kg/hr Fentanyl 0.5 to 1.0 μg/kg/hr Midazolam 0.05 to 0.1 mg/kg/hr HCl (Versed)

that best or most closely approximates the size of the cricoid cartilage in children, the circumferential ring that represents the smallest diameter of the pediatric airway.

There are several methods of establishing appropriate endotracheal tube size. The size of the nares or the fifth finger both estimate or approximate the relative size of the appropriate endotracheal tube for use in a child. An alternate method is to estimate the size using the formula age (in years) plus 16, divided by 4. Using this method, premature infants require a size 2.5 endotracheal tube and normal-sized newborns a size 3.5. An assortment of sizes, one size larger and one size smaller than the estimated tube size should always be available when preparing to intubate an injured child. The responder delegated to intubate should remember that the smallest portion of the childhood trachea is the cricoid ring, so the size of the endotracheal tube to be used should be based on this, rather than the glottic opening.

Once it has been established from the guidelines discussed earlier that endotracheal intubation is necessary, we have found the following technique to be consistently successful. A ventilation face mask enables the rescuer to ventilate and oxygenate the patient with the child's head in the so-called sniffing position, that is, neutrally situated with the neck slightly flexed and then brought forward with the hand and an appropriate-sized mask (this may require trying a few for fit). As mentioned earlier, we give the child pancuronium bromide and fentanyl (or morphine, whichever is available, usually morphine in the emergency department), and with evidence of activity of the drugs, the chest almost always rises with appropriate positioning and squeezing of the bag and mask (Fig. 10–4). During mask ventilation, the degree of extension to open the airway varies, and great care should be taken to avoid stressing the cervical spine.

Sometimes with this assisted ventilation, inflation of the stomach occurs. This should be avoided if at all possible, and a previously placed nasogastric tube, on suction, helps considerably. Gastric distention predisposes to regurgitation and aspiration and may also prevent adequate ventilation by limiting downward displacement of the diaphragm.[44] The Sellick maneuver also helps. If the child is small enough, the small finger of the hand holding the mask can drop down and gently push on the cricoid posteriorly, effectively occluding the esophagus. If the child is too large for this to be done comfortably, an assistant can perform the task (Fig. 10–5).[50, 52]

An appropriate-sized endotracheal tube is selected, cuffed or uncuffed; we use both depending on the size of the child and the anticipated ventilation requirements and considering the possible injuries. If a cuffed tube is used, it is almost always in children older than 2 or 3 years of age, and the cuff itself is positioned beyond the cricoid to avoid any chance of compression injury to the cricoid mucosa. Usually, at this time, we do not inflate it. Only later if required in the course of management is it inflated and then only until the audible air leak disappears and the frequent routine assessment for minimal occlusive volume is carried out.

Several sizes of laryngoscopes are available, but we prefer a straight Miller-type blade for the infants and toddlers

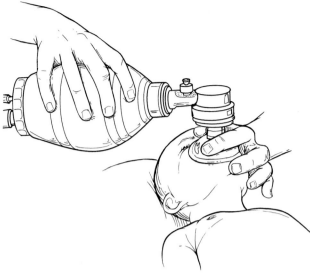

FIGURE 10–4

After selection of an appropriate-sized mask for the child, the mask is held firmly and snugly against the face covering the nasal and oral orifices. The mask is held primarily with the thumb and first finger, the second or middle finger gently wrapping around the prominent point of the jaw and very gently elevating and lifting the jaw and attached soft tissues anteriorly and tilting the head to initiate alignment of the axes of the mouth, pharynx, and trachea (see Fig. 10–6). In-line traction on the cervical spine is recommended, and great care taken to avoid unnecessary movement here. (Reproduced with permission from Pediatric Advanced Life Support. Chameides L, Hazinski MF (eds). Dallas, Texas, American Heart Association/American Academy of Pediatrics, 1994, p 4-10. Copyright American Heart Association.)

and a curved blade for the larger and older children. Other instruments helpful to have close by at the bedside within easy reach are a Magill forceps (two sizes—small and smaller), a stylet (rarely necessary), and an oxygen saturation monitor to help correlate optimal access time. An end-tidal carbon dioxide monitor to help determine proper placement is a luxury and is usually not available in the emergency department. A working and adequate suction apparatus is mandatory.

Using 100% oxygen through the mask and striving for 100% oxygen saturation on the saturation monitor, one must keep in mind that attempted intubation interrupts ongoing ventilation. Hence, attempts to intubate should be limited to 30 seconds or less, monitoring heart rate and oxygen saturation during the procedure. A useful rule of thumb is that when the procedure is started, the person intubating should take a breath; when the intubator has to breathe again, so does the child. Also, we firmly believe that intubation in any injured child *is not the job for a novice or a first or second timer*. Intubation in a child should always be done by the most experienced person available.

After selecting the appropriate laryngoscope and blade and checking that its light is working and adequate and that the previously mentioned monitoring and instruments are present and in place, the head is preferred in the neutral or sniffing position, with an assistant providing in-line cervical traction. The laryngoscope is inserted gently into the mouth

and along the right side of the tongue down to the area of the epiglottis and glottis. To achieve unimpeded direct visualization, the axes of the mouth, pharynx, and trachea must be aligned (Fig. 10–6). No manipulation should be necessary. Usually the child is paralyzed and flaccid at this point, and simply by *lifting the tongue and attached mandibular structures away from the posterior pharynx at a 45-degree angle* (Fig. 10–7), the rescuer can look directly down at the glottis with the cords prominently displayed. It is neither necessary nor appropriate to rock the laryngoscope back on the maxillary ridge or the upper teeth and gums; indeed, this is considered *poor technique*.

With the vocal cords thus displayed, the endotracheal tube is simply passed through and on past the cricoid to position the tip of the tube in the mid-to-distal trachea. Observation of condensation in the tube after placement and bilateral chest expansion and careful auscultation of bilateral breath sounds, both before and after intubation, confirm an appropriate placement. The absence of breath sounds over the stomach adds to this confirmation.

Some blindly pass the tube into a main bronchus once it is in the trachea (usually the right side) and listen for breath sounds, withdrawing the tube back slowly until the breath sounds are bilateral and positioning the tip just above the carina. Accurate placement, regardless of technique, is confirmed by anteroposterior chest radiograph, and we prefer the tip of the tube approximately 1.0 cm above the carina.

Essentially the same technique is utilized for positioning when performing nasotracheal intubation. With a well-lubricated endotracheal tube passed through the nares and visualized in the posterior pharynx and with the laryngoscope in the left hand and in place as described earlier, the

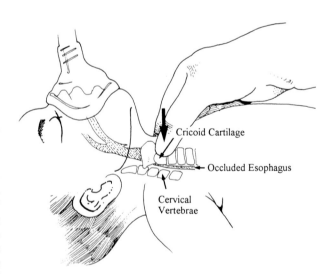

FIGURE 10–5

The Sellick maneuver helps to prevent the inadvertent escape of air generated by masking down the esophagus and the subsequent stomach distention, as well as the inadvertent escape of regurgitated gastric contents up into the upper airway and the subsequent possible aspiration. In infants this can be done by simply curling the small finger of the hand holding the mask down and compressing the cricoid against the vertebral column. In larger or possibly combative children, an assistant can perform this maneuver, as is illustrated.

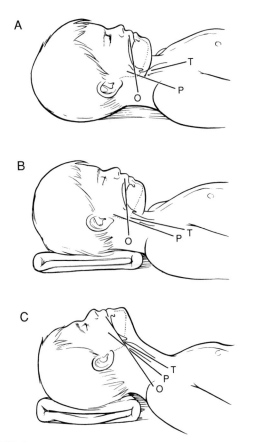

FIGURE 10–6

Correct positioning of the child older than 2 years of age for ventilation and tracheal intubation. *A,* With the patient on a flat surface, the oral (O), pharyngeal (P), and tracheal (T) axes pass through three divergent planes. *B,* A folded sheet or towel placed under the occiput of the head aligns the pharyngeal and tracheal axes. *C,* Extension of the atlanto-occipital joint results in alignment of the oral, pharyngeal, and tracheal axes. (Reproduced with permission from Pediatric Advanced Life Support. Chameides L, Hazinski MF (eds). Dallas, Texas, American Heart Association/American Academy of Pediatrics, 1994, p 4-11. Copyright American Heart Association. Adapted from Coté CJ, Todres ID: The pediatric airway. In: Coté CJ, Ryan JF, Todres ID, Groudsouzian NG (eds): A Practice of Anesthesia for Infants and Children. 2nd ed. Philadelphia, WB Saunders, 1993.)

tube is gently advanced forward to the glottis in position to directly advance between the vocal cords and on down the airway. Most often, after advancing the tip of the tube to the visualized area of the glottis, it is gently lifted with Magill forceps in the right hand and guided between the cords and on into the airway. Confirmation of position is checked as described previously.

Once intubation is confirmed, all patients are hyperventilated to a P_{CO_2} of 28 to 32 mm Hg until the evaluation is complete. The blood gases are then adjusted to near normal, depending on the extent of injuries identified and the anticipated needs.

Important errors in intubation include mainstem bronchus intubation, esophageal intubation, bronchopleural fistula, or pharyngeal laceration. Unsuccessful urgent endotracheal intubation rarely occurs. When it does, however, surgical access to the lower airway via cricothyroidotomy

is indicated. Access is best accomplished via the cricothyroid membrane by either needle cricothyroidotomy or by a direct surgical approach.

The first step in needle cricothyroidotomy is the identification of the cricothyroid membrane. The landmark is the thyroid cartilage, the so-called Adam's apple. Remaining in the midline and palpating 1 to 2 cm inferiorly, a "step-off" is appreciated, which is the cricothyroid membrane.[29] While an assistant provides in-line cervical traction, the cricoid and thyroid cartilages are stabilized between the forefinger and the thumb of the left hand and a number 12 or 14 plastic cannula-over-needle intravenous catheter attached to a syringe under suction is advanced through the cricoid membrane into the trachea. A soft "pop" is perceived as this happens, and air can be aspirated via the syringe. With the aspiration of air, the cannula is advanced over the needle into the trachea, and oxygen is provided via a Y or a three-way stopcock connector. Oxygen is then provided at 10 to 15 liters per minute, and by occluding the Y connector or one end of the three-way stopcock with a finger at a normal ventilatory rate for the patient, one can gain several minutes of time to obtain more permanent surgical access or expertise.[11, 49] Alveolar hypoventilation eventually occurs, but in children below the age of 5 years acceptable levels of arterial oxygen and carbon dioxide can be maintained for up to 15 minutes.[28]

In our practice, the adequacy of ventilation is closely monitored by placement of a percutaneous peripheral arterial line, usually at the wrist. We do not follow capillary blood gases, and if percutaneous arterial access is not expeditiously obtained after appropriate attempts, cutdown visualization of the pulsating arterial vessel is accomplished, with direct vision access then obtained. We do not encircle or tie off the vessel, surgical access being used primarily for finding the elusive artery.

Once the airway has been established and secured, pulmonary compliance is assessed by the ventilating physician. Significant reduction in compliance with apparent compromise of ventilation prompts an immediate search for an open or tension pneumothorax.[11] Because penetrating injuries to children occur in less than 10% of injuries, an open pneumothorax is rare in this age group and is usually quickly excluded. A tension pneumothorax is recognized by a sucking sound at the site with inspiration and bubbling or frothing with expiration, accompanied by hyperresonance to percussion and decreased breath sounds over the involved hemithorax.[33] In this situation the uninvolved lung can be compromised rapidly, particularly in the younger child because of the mobility of the mediastinum; hence, prompt and appropriate intervention is necessary. This is accomplished by converting the open pneumothorax to a simple pneumothorax by placing an air-tight seal (usually Vaseline gauze) over the wound and providing drainage of the residual intrapleural air with tube thoracostomy.

Pneumothorax and Chest Tube Placement

Pneumothorax is an often silent but frighteningly lethal abnormality that requires consistent suspicion on the part of the managing physicians until they are convinced it is not a factor or they make a prompt diagnosis and then attempt

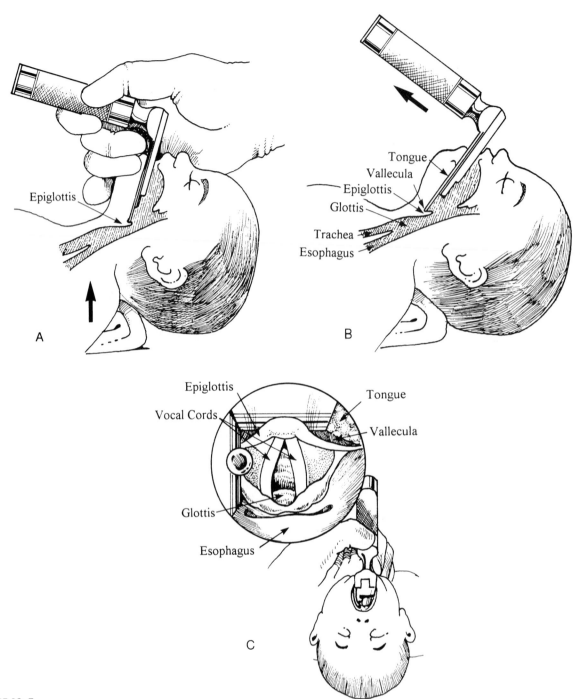

FIGURE 10–7

A, With in-line external cervical traction or stabilization of the head and neck in a similarly effective manner, we prefer to use a straight Miller-type blade and insert its tip along the right side of the mouth, gently manipulating the tongue to the left, until the tip of the blade reaches the vallecula just anterior to the epiglottis. *B*, Lifting the mandibular soft tissue block away at a 45-degree angle from the flat surface of the stretcher, the structures flatten out and move anteriorly; the epiglottis flips up anteriorly as well; and because the axes of the mouth, pharynx, and trachea are now aligned and the head has not moved, the operator is looking directly at the glottis and vocal cords with their surrounding structures (*C*). The endotracheal tube can now be inserted (see text).

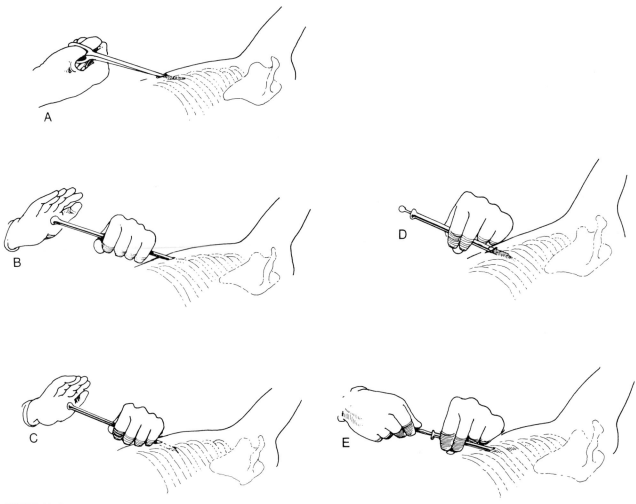

FIGURE 10–8

Trocar chest tube placement is preferred, but such placement requires experience. *A,* Once the incision-entrance site is selected, usually in the anterior axillary line at the fifth intercostal space, a tunnel is developed with a hemostat up over at least one and preferable two ribs. *B,* The rigid catheter and trocar unit is threaded through the incision and along the tunnel, then grasped firmly with the first and second fingers of the left hand at a distance of 2 to 5 cm (depending on the size of the child) from its leading sharp tip in such a manner that when the tip of the catheter penetrates the pleura it does not penetrate farther than this distance. *C,* With the unit at a 45-degree angle to the patient, a sharp blow is applied to the blunt end of the trocar-catheter unit with the right hand so that the catheter enters the pleural space but advances no farther than the previously exposed sharp tip—when the firmly grasping left hand touches the chest wall. *D,* The grasping left hand is then released, the angle of insertion dropped to approximately 10 to 15 degrees, and the catheter advanced another 2 to 5 cm. *E,* The catheter is then advanced over the trocar to its intended position.

rapid proper intervention. When a tension pneumothorax is present with rapidly deteriorating vital signs, a large catheter-over-needle vascular access needle promptly inserted in the second intercostal space anteriorly, on the appropriate side, provides instantaneous but partial relief; it is almost always necessary to follow this with an appropriate-sized chest tube. Temporizing time can be gained by attaching a three-way stopcock to the catheter-needle and drawing off large volumes of air with a syringe while awaiting chest tube placement.

Chest tube placement is accomplished through a mid or anterior axillary line approach at the fifth or sixth intercostal space, tunneling cephalad at least over one rib. The usual insertion method recommended by the ATLS course that utilizes a hemostat for tunneling, pleural puncture, and

chest tube catheter positioning is recommended for those with minimal or no experience, indeed even for those with considerable experience who are most comfortable with this technique. We prefer the trocar chest tube catheter, using a size 10 to 24 depending on the size of the child, and using the same landmarks noted previously (Fig. 10–8). Once the incision site is located or marked, a small incision large enough to accept only the catheter is made and a tunnel is developed with a hemostat up over at least one rib space, two in the smaller children. The rigid catheter and trocar unit is firmly grasped with the first and second fingers of the left hand at a distance of 2 to 5 cm from its leading sharp tip (depending on the size of the child) in such a manner that with penetration of the pleura the tip does not penetrate farther than this distance. With the end of the tube and trocar then inserted along the tunnel and up over the rib or ribs, the unit is raised at a 45-degree angle, and a sharp blow is applied to the blunt distal end so that the catheter enters the pleural space but advances no farther than the previously exposed proximal end. Forward movement of the catheter stops when the firmly grasping hand touches the chest wall (see Fig. 10–8). The grasping hand is then released, the angle of catheter insertion is dropped to 10 to 15 degrees, the catheter is advanced over the trocar a further 2 to 5 cm, the position determined by movement of the trocar, and then the catheter is fixed in the usual manner.

This technique is faster and as efficient and effective as the hemostat technique, *in experienced hands,* a condition that cannot be emphasized enough. Reluctance to use this approach has been largely because the pulmonary parenchyma and other intrathoracic structures have been inadvertently lacerated or impaled in inexperienced hands, indeed even in some experienced hands. Mishaps have occurred with the hemostat-Kelly technique as well, so no one technique is the perfect answer. It must be emphasized, however, that *experience is a prerequisite.* The procedure is being done to remove air or blood or both from within the pleural cavity, and by definition the pulmonary parenchyma must be pushed away from the chest wall. Controlled placement of the chest tube accesses these abnormal substances first; hence, added injury to intrathoracic structures should be virtually nonexistent.

CLOSED-CHEST INJURIES REQUIRING PROMPT ATTENTION

Closed-chest injuries secondary to blunt trauma are not uncommon in children. Once the airway is secure, the mechanics of breathing depend on the integrity of the thorax. Up to 30% of traumatized children have chest injuries. The mortality rate ranges from 7 to 14% in older children to 25% in those younger than 5 years of age, and the addition of two major extrathoracic injuries raises the mortality rate for all children to 58%.[19] Successful treatment of life-threatening thoracic injuries depends on early recognition. A detailed discussion of thoracic injuries is given in Chapters 17 and 18 of this text. However, because these injuries may require prompt intervention during the initial phase of resuscitation and management, a brief discussion is warranted here.

Pulmonary Parenchymal Lacerations and Contusions

Lacerations and contusions of the pulmonary parenchyma frequently accompany rib fractures and may result in a ball-valve mechanism that leads to the progressive accumulation of air within the pleural space without exit, the so-called tension pneumothorax. Ventilation is rapidly compromised as the lung collapses, the diaphragm is pushed downward, and the mediastinum shifts away from the midline, compromising the uninvolved lung and further reducing effective

ventilation and cardiac output by decreasing venous return.[11] Cyanosis and distended neck veins may be present, but the diagnosis is made on clinical suspicion with decreased breath sounds and hyperresonance on the involved side and displacement of the trachea and heart sounds away from the injury. Prompt needle or tube thoracostomy is indicated.

Hemothorax

Hemothorax is rare in children as blood loss from parenchymal pulmonary injuries is rare and is usually pressure related, and intravascular pulmonary pressure is low. When present, however, it is a space-occupying lesion that can contribute to both circulatory collapse and ventilatory insufficiency. Pallor, tachycardia, and hypotension accompany decreased breath sounds and dullness to percussion, and with progressive expansion, mediastinal shift occurs. Central venous distention is uncommon because of the associated hypovolemia. Management includes aggressive volume replacement and fluid resuscitation along with tube thoracostomy.[33]

Flail Chest

Flail chest is unusual in children, particularly in smaller ones; however, because of the marked flexibility of the chest wall, it can occur whenever multiple rib fractures are sustained and even if the ribs are broken only at one site. Once present, respiratory efforts, greatly compromised by the paradoxical chest wall motion, are further aggravated by the pain and splinting secondary to the rib fractures.[11] Progressively severe respiratory insufficiency occurs. Diagnosis is easily made by visualization of the paradoxical movement, subcutaneous emphysema, and usually palpable rib fractures. Prompt stabilization of the mobile section provides almost immediate improvement; however, endotracheal intubation and mechanical ventilation are usually required to stabilize the patient and ensure adequate ventilation and oxygenation. In our practice, children with flail chest would be paralyzed and sedated promptly.

The magnitude of trauma necessary to produce flail segments in children is substantial, and associated intrathoracic injury is common. Pulmonary or myocardial contusions, then, must be considered as well as aortic arch injuries, and appropriate radiographs, electrocardiographs, echocardiograms, and myocardial enzyme determinations must be obtained and torso CT scans adjusted to include the aortic arch with the contrast phase.

Cardiac Tamponade

Cardiac tamponade is usually the result of penetrating injury and is relatively uncommon in children. The triad of Beck, elevated venous pressure, decreased arterial pressure, and muffled or distant heart sounds may occur, however, and pulsus paradoxus can be seen.[11] Needle aspiration of the pericardium using a subxyphoid approach with accompanying cardiac monitoring is the definitive diagnostic and usually therapeutic maneuver. A 16- to 18-gauge cannula-over-needle intravenous catheter with an attached 20-ml syringe on a T connector under suction is directed toward the tip of the left scapula from a subxyphoid approach and is technically straightforward and safe. Aspiration of blood that does not clot, even in small amounts, particularly in the smaller children, may be life saving because the pericardial sac is a small, semirigid organ that is easily compromised by an abnormal amount of accumulated fluid. Removing the needle once any abnormal amount of accumulated fluid is aspirated, we leave the catheter in the pericardial sac and flush the T connecter and catheter with a small amount of heparinized solution (just enough to fill the connector and catheter) and then fix it to the torso, periodically aspirating and again flushing to make certain this problem is not ongoing.

Cervical Spine Injury

Any injured child, particularly those with torso or head injuries, should be presumed to have a cervical spine injury and treated accordingly, with in-line traction of the head in the neutral position, and should be stabilized there by a cervical collar, sandbags and tape, or manually applied traction. A lateral radiograph of the cervical spine is then obtained as part of the initial radiographic evaluation, and all seven cervical vertebrae as well as T_1 must be demonstrated. (Chapter 14 deals with spinal cord injuries including injuries to the cervical spine in detail.)

CIRCULATORY INSUFFICIENCY

Sudden, continuing hemorrhage is the phenomenon that makes trauma so different from the other emergency conditions of childhood.[29] Once a patent airway and adequate ventilation have been established, circulatory insufficiency or shock becomes the highest priority. *Successful management requires simultaneous treatment and diagnosis* with the reconstitution of normal circulating blood volume and tissue perfusion. Because trauma patients may suffer hidden loss of blood, inadequate restoration of cardiac output may produce or exacerbate ongoing tissue injury with significant hemodynamic embarrassment during diagnostic or therapeutic interventions.[11] Diminished cardiac output results in the nonspecific clinical picture of tachycardia, tachypnea, altered mental status (often restlessness), oliguria, and cool to cold extremities. The clinician must determine the cause of the inadequate circulation and the magnitude of the insult and must initiate appropriate therapy. (The basic pathophysiology of hemorrhagic shock is beyond the scope of detail here; see Chapter 9.)

The assessment of adequate circulation and tissue perfusion is complicated by the variability of normal heart rate and blood pressure among infants and children. The variability of normal circulating blood volume depending on size must be considered also. Blood pressure also varies with age and can be estimated as follows: Systolic blood pressure is 80 plus twice the age in years; diastolic blood pressure is two thirds of the systolic blood pressure. Normal circulating blood volume is 80 to 90 ml per kg in an infant and more closely approximates the 70 ml per kg of adults in older children and adolescents.

Assessment and Initial Management

Although the treatment of internal hemorrhage usually requires surgical hemostasis, control of external hemorrhage is an emergency procedure requiring prompt attention.[29] Direct pressure stops almost all external hemorrhage, but the temptation to use a hemostat should be resisted, particularly with large vessels in the proximal areas of extremities, because the tissue crushed by such instruments may be the critical length in subsequent surgical repair and important nerves, often uninjured, course anatomically with these vessels. Injury to these may be irreparable. When the external hemorrhage is controlled, access to the circulation becomes the next priority.

Acute loss of 10 to 15% of circulating blood volume is well tolerated in the healthy child and easily compensated for. Dynamic changes in the child's vasomotor tone allow rapid compensation with peripheral vasoconstriction, decreased stroke volume, and compensatory mild tachycardia as a result of baroreceptor stimulation of catecholamine release, and systolic blood pressure is maintained. However, diastolic pressure rises initially, indicative of diminished peripheral perfusion, and produces the typical cool, mottled extremities with the thready pulse. Diminished peripheral perfusion leads to systemic acidosis and mild compensatory tachypnea. These mechanisms allow the mean blood pressure to be maintained in spite of as much as a 20% blood volume loss.[33, 49] These clinical signs and symptoms of mild compensated shock are easily monitored at the bedside. Hypotension, a systolic blood pressure less than 80 mm Hg, results *after* 20% of the blood volume is lost and is a late clinical sign of shock in children.[22] An acute hemorrhage of 25% or more of the circulating blood volume almost certainly results in a clinically apparent hypovolemic state in a child and requires aggressive intervention. The most reliable clinical indicators of early hypovolemia in children are persistent tachycardia, cutaneous vasoconstriction, and diminished pulse pressure. As this occurs, stroke volume decreases, cardiac output falls, and hypotension ensues. (Many physicians would add here that capillary refill is prolonged. However, because we have personally observed nearly normal, if not normal, capillary refill in a child who expired from sepsis, we have placed minimal importance on this diagnostic criteria, and recent literature has confirmed this concern.[25]) Circulatory insufficiency at the cellular level produces metabolic acidosis, renal blood flow is compromised, and urine output is diminished. Hemorrhage in excess of one half the blood volume produces profound hypotension that can be fatal.

Definitive Interventions, Vascular Access, and Management

It is usually assumed that pediatric trauma patients who present clinically with hypovolemia and signs of circulatory insufficiency have lost between 25 and 50% of their total blood volume. Management of uncomplicated hemorrhagic shock is the restoration of effective circulating blood volume with improved tissue perfusion, best reflected by the restoration of a normal pulse, adequate urine output, and normal acid-base balance. A urinary catheter is indispensable for this and should be placed early in the course of resuscitation, following a normal genital and rectal examination.

Therefore, once the airway is secure and adequate ventilation is achieved, if not already present, two large-bore intravenous access lines are established and secured. We prefer to establish such access in one or both upper extremities, thereby ensuring adequate venous return to the heart, particularly if abdominal, pelvic, or retroperitoneal injuries are suspected. If unsuccessful, subclavian catheterization—usually from the left side—is placed, depending on age, with an appropriate adult-sized large-bore cannula-over-needle catheter that can be changed out later over a wire to one containing two or three lumens. Although some disapprove of this method, other physicians have found that such catheters expeditiously placed in small children or infants provide outstanding access for the necessary resuscitation and stabilization period. In our hands, these catheters have been extremely useful and have been accompanied by an exceeding low failure or complication rate. In the exsanguinating patient, femoral cutdowns can be done, although reconstruction of these vessels may be required later, particularly in the smaller child.[11]

Another option, rarely necessary in our experience but certainly available in selected situations of profound shock, is intraosseous (IO) infusion.[37] First described in the early 1920s, bone marrow is utilized as a route for infusion of virtually any type of regular IV fluid normally used for resuscitation purposes as well as medications of numerous types. The bone marrow sinusoids communicate with large medullary venous channels that drain via nutrient emissary veins into the systemic circulation. Circulation times for IV and IO injections are nearly identical.[43]

The advantages of IO infusion are threefold. First, it is an extremely accessible route of vascular access, because the tibia, sternum, ileum, or femur can be used. Second, very little skill is necessary to perform the procedure. The easiest site for access is the flat, anterior portion of the tibia, 1 to 2 cm distal and slightly medial to the tibial tuberosity. A traditional bone marrow needle functions very well—we prefer the Illinois length–adjustable needle—but a 16- to 20-gauge spinal needle with a trocar can be used. Placing the needle over the selected site at a 90-degree angle to the bone and advancing it firmly through the cortex of the bone into the marrow, a soft pop indicates penetration into the marrow, confirmed by the lack of resistance to aspiration of bone marrow into the syringe, as well as the free flow of fluid into the marrow without evidence of subcutaneous infiltration (Fig. 10–9). The needle can then be attached to standard IV tubing, usually with a T-connector adapter, and fluid, blood, or drugs may be infused. The extremity selected for IO infusion should be injury free. The third advantage is the remarkable lack of complications with the procedure, the most common being mild subcutaneous infiltration with needle removal.

Intraosseous infusion can be very useful in the nonurgent situation when percutaneous venous cannulation has failed but the child is apparently hemodynamically stable. In these rare situations, IO infusions can help replenish intravascular volume to make venous access easier and allow better peripheral access. However, the serious hypovolemic trauma situation with apparent brisk ongoing blood loss does not seem to us to be the scenario applicable to IO infusions. Hence, we use subclavian or femoral lines in situations of inadequate peripheral access. Unfortunately, the limitations of IO infusions are related to the rate of volume allowed by this technique, which is less that 40 ml per minute under pressure, and in exsanguination circumstances this is not sufficient. In such dire circumstances in which IV access cannot be achieved, we perform a left thoracotomy that can be extended across the sternum for better access as necessary. The aorta can then be cross-clamped and direct cardiac access initiated if needed.

External and internal jugular vein access (percutaneous or cutdown) in urgent posttraumatic situations is not appropriate initially because of the need for manipulation of the head or neck, or both, in a patient with a possible cervical spine injury. These sites are very useful later during the definitive care and rehabilitation phases of management, however. Although peripheral cutdowns of the saphenous or antecubital veins have been advocated by many, we rarely use them simply because of the better access provided as outlined earlier.

Fluid Resuscitation

Once appropriate vascular access has been established, fluid resuscitation for circulatory insufficiency in injured children begins with the rapid infusion, over 5 to 10 minutes in bolus volumes, of a balanced salt solution, usually Ringer lactate. Children in shock are assumed to have an acute blood loss of between 25 and 50% of their blood volume; hence, the immediate volume to be replaced is 20 to 40 ml per kg. The hemodynamic response to the bolus infusion determines further therapy. Reestablishment and stabilization of normal vital signs and perfusion, with slowing of the heart rate, increase in pulse pressure, decrease in skin mottling, increase in the warmth of the extremities, clearing of the sensorium, increase in the urinary output to 1.0+ ml per kg per hour, and increase in systolic blood pressure suggest further fluids can be given at usually acceptable maintenance rates. If the physiologic response is inadequate, a repeat bolus is administered and the child is crossmatched for blood. If circulatory insufficiency persists, 10 ml per kg of packed red blood cells or 20 ml per kg of whole blood, O negative, or type specific if necessary, is given. Once the volume deficit is replaced, complete fluid resuscitation proceeds at a 1.0 to 1.5 maintenance level. Resuscitation using crystalloid usually requires the administration of three times the volume of shed blood to completely restore the circulating blood volume.[2, 22, 33, 49]

This technique is time honored and works well in the *nonexsanguinating patient* when blood loss is in the 20 to 25% range and when a rapid response to resuscitation can be anticipated. In children with greater losses, that is, up to

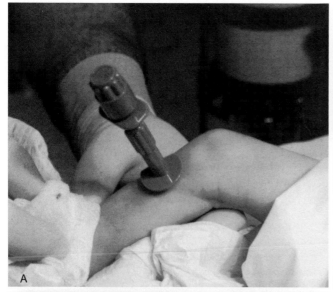

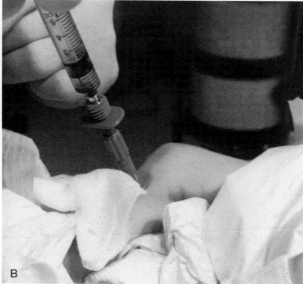

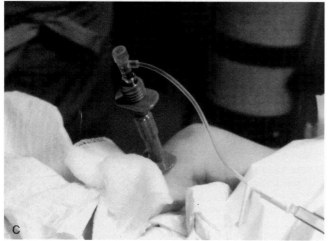

FIGURE 10–9

The preferred site for intraosseous access is an uninjured lower extremity, accessed most easily in the upper tibia, 1 to 2 cm distally and slightly medial to the tibial tuberosity using an appropriate bone marrow needle. *B*, With entrance into the marrow, a soft ''pop'' is perceived, and marrow can be aspirated freely into a syringe. *C*, Free flow of fluid into the marrow without evidence of subcutaneous infiltration confirms proper placement, and the needle can be attached to standard intravenous tubing and fluid, blood, or drugs infused.

50% or even more, it works less well, requires precious time to await the physiologic response to therapy during which ongoing metabolic disruption may be further compounded, and requires a relatively accurate estimate of blood loss as well as the child's weight. Weight estimation is relatively easy; however, in our opinion, an attempt to calculate blood loss mentally based on information obtained from paramedics that may be second hand or estimated in the dark and to compare it with calculated blood volume based on the estimated weight to reconstitute that loss at best results in inaccurate numbers and at worst can threaten a child's life. In the stressful confusion around a seriously injured child who may be exsanguinating, such an attempt is also wasted time and energy, and we simply achieve vascular access and aggressively resuscitate to hemodynamic stability and normal tissue perfusion, continuously monitoring the usual physiologic parameters, as both underresuscitation and overresuscitation can be harmful.

Low-titer, O-negative blood should be available continuously in the emergency department for the exsanguinating patient, with type-specific blood available within 10 minutes.[11] Constant reevaluation and readjustment of fluid or-

ders is essential. Highly stressed children rapidly deplete glycogen stores, and all maintenance fluids should include 5% dextrose. Forty-eight hours after injury, once major hemodynamic changes have stabilized and reached equilibrium, we begin intravenous nutrition.

Pneumatic Antishock Garment

Persistent hypotension despite apparent adequate volume replacement means either massive initial hemorrhage or persistent active ongoing blood loss, and occult intrathoracic or intra-abdominal bleeding must be considered.[33] The use of a pneumatic antishock garment with a systolic blood pressure of less than 60 mm Hg has been recommended in such situations, as it can increase peripheral systemic vascular resistance and translocate some blood from the extremities into the intravascular space.[11] Application of the abdominal portion of the garment may be particularly helpful for tamponading retroperitoneal bleeding such as with pelvic fractures; however, frequently garment size does not correspond to patient size, particularly in the smaller children, and some of the important contraindications must also be considered: (1) it further compromises respiratory insufficiency by limiting diaphragmatic excursion; (2) it eliminates the use of lower extremity vascular access; (3) pulmonary edema may occur if afterload is increased too extensively; (4) in the presence of diaphragmatic injury, such as disruption, it produces rapid and severe deterioration and possibly death. Hence, controversy regarding such interventions in children is justifiable, and valuable on the scene time should not be wasted considering the use of this garment.

Persistent failure of the patient to respond suggests massive intracavitary bleeding and may require left thoracotomy and supradiaphragmatic occlusion of the aorta as a life-saving procedure.

While the airway is being secured, breathing established, and adequate circulation ensured, a nasogastric tube and urinary catheter are placed. A well-resuscitated patient should demonstrate normotension, slight if any tachycardia, slight if any tachypnea, good mentation, well-perfused extremities, and good urine output. It must be remembered, however, that inadequate resuscitation is common when blood pressure and urine output are the only measures of circulatory adequacy.[12] Mindful of this, late in the resuscitative phase and on through the postresuscitative or support phase, we monitor transcutaneous oxygenation, the transcutaneous PO_2, and compare it with arterial oxygen, the PaO_2, as a ratio, the so-called transcutaneous to arterial oxygen index. We have found this to be an extremely sensitive and accurate measurement of peripheral perfusion and resuscitation status, reflecting pulse pressure alterations well before they are identified by routine monitoring.[11]

SECONDARY SURVEY AND DIAGNOSTIC WORKUP

Decisions must now be made regarding further disposition: immediate operative therapy, further diagnostic evaluation—primarily radiographic—or admission to the critical care unit for continued support, observation, and monitoring.[58] In this phase, pertinent other screening radiographic studies are carried out, needed additional vascular access is accomplished, and a complete head-to-toe examination performed as an ongoing part of the continuum of care concept, adding or updating evaluations, decisions, and new requirements to existing care.[9, 11]

Secondary Survey

The secondary survey includes all organ systems, beginning with the head. Careful examination for contusions, lacerations, abrasions, open or closed fractures, blood behind the ear drums, draining cerebrospinal fluid or bleeding, and oral injuries is all done with the cervical spine immobilized or under traction until cleared radiographically.

The torso is similarly palpated and examined for open or closed soft tissue or bony injury, and the thorax, mediastinal, and intra-abdominal structures are ausculated and checked for position, distortion, and quality of sound. The abdomen is examined for pain and peritoneal signs, but these are difficult to elicit and interpret in injured children, particularly when they are uncooperative or combative or when they are paralyzed, sedated, and intubated.

The integrity of the pelvis is assessed and the genitalia carefully examined, checking for blood at the urethral meatus, evidence of extravasation of blood into the scrotum or labia, blood in the rectum, position of the prostate, and sphincter tone. Extremities are similarly examined for soft or bony tissue injury or deformity, and all peripheral pulses are palpated, particularly those in which fractures are present. Examination of the back is usually deferred until screening radiographs have cleared potential neurologic injury, but when necessary the child can be log rolled and this area examined definitively.

If the clinical presentation is indicative of exsanguination with an intra-abdominal or intrathoracic catastrophe and existing or impending hemodynamic instability, the essential preoperative measures—cervical spine, chest, and pelvic radiographs; complete blood count; blood typing for crossmatch purposes; and continuation of resuscitation—are carried out while the patient is managed through the emergency department and to the operating suite.[8]

If an unstable pelvic fracture is confirmed by radiograph and the child is hemodynamically unstable possibly because of this, the child is moved to the radiology suite for arteriography and selective vessel embolization if indicated, while maintaining continuous monitoring and resuscitation and stabilization in keeping with the continuum of care concept. Should the pelvic radiograph show normal findings and the abdominal origin of the instability be questionable, diagnostic peritoneal lavage is done in the emergency department or on the operating table.

We perform diagnostic peritoneal lavage as follows: a small infraumbilical skin and fascial puncture wound is made with a number 11 scalpel blade in an area previously locally infiltrated with 1% lidocaine (Xylocaine) with epinephrine. A pediatric dialysis catheter with a trocar guide is inserted into this wound, "hooking" the tip of the catheter-sheathed trocar in the fascial "nick" and lifting perpendicularly away from the abdomen while at the same time gently inserting the catheter cephalad into the peritoneal cavity. The trocar is then withdrawn. In some cases, the immediate appearance of frank blood terminates the procedure, and expeditious operative intervention is undertaken. An absence of bloody return prompts the infusion of 0.9% sodium chloride solution at 20 ml per kg total, and returned fluid is sent to the lab for Gram staining (for bacteria), a white blood cell count (normal being less than 800/mm³), a red blood cell count (normal being less than 80,000/mm³), and an amylase content (normal below the normal serum amylase). Abnormal results contribute significantly to management in some centers. We do not accept as important or significant the ability or inability to read printed material through the drainage tubing. Such urgent and needed diagnostic peritoneal lavages are fortunately very rare but can and do occur. As a routine, however, we do not do diagnostic peritoneal lavage because we believe CT scanning of the abdomen to be much superior in the determination of injury and its severity. In addition, the presence of blood in the peritoneal cavity by diagnostic peritoneal lavage is not necessarily an indication for surgery in the pediatric patient; hence, except for the urgent indication in the nonstable patient as described earlier we do not do diagnostic peritoneal lavage.

Radiologic Assessment

During the careful and thorough secondary survey, pertinent screening radiographs are obtained while the examination is temporarily interrupted. Examination and resuscitation gurneys should allow a complete head-to-toe radiologic examination, preferably with a fixed, overhead roentgen tube in the trauma resuscitation room but certainly within the emergency department. This allows rapid high-quality films.

The most important radiograph is that of the lateral cervical spine. With combined axial traction on the head and downward traction on both arms to lower the shoulders, seven cervical vertebrae and the first thoracic vertebra must be visualized clearly and the presence or absence of abnormality noted. The absence of fractures on the lateral cervical spine film does not absolutely rule out spinal cord injury in children, and in the comatose patient, we leave the firm cervical collar in place until somatosensory responses can be obtained. In children whom we purposely paralyze, intubate, and maintain with paralysis and sedation, we do the same.

Chest films are also necessary, looking for pneumothorax; hemothorax; rib fractures, particularly the first, second, or third; mediastinal shifting, widening, or the presence of air; and pulmonary contusions or traumatic air cysts. One must remember that, particularly in smaller children, the pediatric mediastinum flattens out in the supine position and may falsely appear to be widened.

Radiographs of the pelvis are obtained in nearly all circumstances and can include abdominal films and anteroposterior and cross-table lateral films (rarely done in our practice because of our preference for CT). Pneumoperitoneum may or may not be seen (depending on severity), and fractures are noted carefully. In such instances, the gastric air shadow is inspected carefully for distention, position of gastric tubes, and border continuity; intra-abdominal bleeding such as from the spleen can extend into the supporting structures, particularly the gastrosplenic ligament and be visualized as indentations or displacement of the stomach shadow.

Long-bone extremity radiographs are also obtained but only if indicated by evidence of injury.

During this early postresuscitation-stabilization phase, arterial lines are placed (if not already present) for monitoring and sampling purposes, usually accomplished by cannulating the radial artery after an Allen test. Nasogastric tubes and urethral catheters are also placed if not already present.

At this point, critical decisions regarding triage must be made: immediate operative therapy (e.g., the exsanguinating unstable patient), admission to the critical care unit for observation and monitoring, or further diagnostic evaluation.

Computed Tomography

Routinely, the majority of our patients go to the radiology suite for further diagnostic evaluation, particularly the patients with multiple trauma or injuries involving the head, chest, abdomen, or pelvis. Because it is generally well accepted that the severity of injury greatly influences patient outcome and a delay in diagnosis is closely related to morbidity and mortality (e.g., unsuspected retroperitoneal injuries account for 40% of initial deaths in children with combined blunt abdominal trauma and head injuries,[58] we have consistently utilized CT as the definitive diagnostic mechanism for determination of management direction.[10] This is done primarily for three reasons: (1) it is diagnostic, both qualitatively and quantitatively, for major injury in most; (2) it finds unsuspected minor injuries that have previously gone unrecognized; and (3) it consistently reduces diagnostic confusion later for some clinical situations. For example, a child with a primary head injury later develops a fallen hematocrit and a distended abdomen. It is very helpful to know already from the time of resuscitation that there is no major intra-abdominal solid viscus injury and to repeat the CT scan, utilizing the initial one as a base line.

Also, in our opinion, the application of CT scanning to the evaluation of traumatized patients reduces the number of ancillary tests required for diagnosis, provides more accurate information regarding the extent and severity of injury, and results in more appropriate decisions regarding the need for operative versus nonoperative management. A clear, understandable presentation of findings in the third dimension, including assessment of the retroperitoneum, and the ability to do this in a short time are other important advantages. Intravenous contrast for vascular and renal assessment as well as contrast opacification of the small intestine is important. Computed tomography scanning of the head and torso can readily be accomplished with concomitant evaluation of organ structure and function.[11]

With ongoing resuscitation and stabilization, monitoring equipment, and support personnel, the child is moved to the CT area following the continuum of care concept alluded to earlier. We consider transportation and care in the radiology suite of extreme importance. With new improvements in portable monitoring equipment this is relatively easy. Intubated patients are hand ventilated during transport, but in all other ways their level of care remains as it was in the resuscitation and critical care area of the emergency department. Patients are monitored continuously during their study, and should any deterioration occur the scan can be interrupted and the child again stabilized. It is important that the patient's level of care not change during the diagnostic phase of the workup. Patients who have significant, apparently treatable or survivable head injuries are transported to the radiology suite for CT scanning of the head. Those with operable intracranial lesions immediately go to the operating room for craniotomy. However, before anesthesia is administered, abdominal paracentesis is performed as noted earlier. Because the majority of patients do not have intracranial lesions that require intervention, their assessment is benefited by CT evaluation of the torso.

References

1. Aaler JA: Organization and management of pediatric emergency care: Organization of a regional pediatric trauma and emergency center. In: Mayer TA (ed): Emergency Management of Pediatric Trauma. Philadelphia, WB Saunders, 1985, pp 501–507.

2. Advanced Trauma Life Support Course. American College of Surgeons, Committee on Trauma, 1993.

3. Alpert JJ, Guyer B: Forword. Symposium on injuries and injury prevention. Pediatr Clin North Am 32:1–4, 1985.

4. Aprahamian C, Thompson BM, Towne JB, et al: The effect of a paramedic system on mortality of major open intra-abdominal vascular trauma. J Trauma 23:687–690, 1983.

5. Baker SP: Motor vehicle occupant deaths in young children. Pediatrics 64:860–861, 1979.

6. Bruce DA, Schut L: Management of acute craniocerebral trauma in children. In: Tindall GP, Long DM (eds): Contemporary Neurosurgery. Vol. 1. Baltimore, Williams & Wilkins, 1979, pp 1–17.

7. Bruce DA, Schut L, Bruno LA, et al: Outcome following severe head injury in children. J Neurosurg 48:679–688, 1978.

8. Buntain WL: Splenic trauma. In: Hurst J (ed): Common Problems in Trauma. Chicago, Year Book Medical Publishers, 1987, pp 78–89.

9. Buntain WL, Conner E, Emrico J, et al: Transcutaneous oxygen (TcPo₂) measurements as an aid to fluid therapy in necrotizing neterocolitis. J Pediatr Surg 14:728–732, 1979.

10. Buntain WL, Gould HR: Splenic trauma in children and techniques of splenic salvage. World J Surg 9:398–409, 1985.

11. Buntain WL, Lynch FP, Ramenofsky ML: Management of the acutely injured child. In: Maull, KI (ed): Advances in Trauma. Vol. 2. Chicago, Year Book Medical Publishers, 1987, pp 43–86.

12. Burchard KW: Clinical and hemodynamic assessment of fluid and volume status. Trauma Quarterly 2:7–17, 1986.

13. Cales RH, Trunckey DD: Preventable trauma deaths. A review of trauma care systems development. JAMA 254:1059, 1985.

14. Champion HR, Sacco WJ, Carnazzo AJ, et al: Trauma score. Crit Care Med 9:672–676, 1981.

15. Collicut PE: Initial assessment of the trauma patient. In: Moore EE, Mattox KL, Feliciano DV (eds): Trauma. 2nd ed. East Norwalk, Conn, Appleton & Lange, 1991, pp 109–127.

16. Copass MK, Oreskovich MR, Baldergroen MR, et al: Prehospital cardiopulmonary resuscitation of the critically injured patient. Am J Surg 148:20–26, 1984.

17. Cwinn AA, Pons PT, Moore EE, et al: Prehospital advanced trauma life support for critical blunt trauma victims. Ann Emerg Med 16:399–403, 1987.

18. Eckenhoff JE: Some anatomic considerations of the infant larynx influencing endotracheal anesthesia. Anesthesiology 12:401, 1951.

19. Eichelberger ML: Trauma of the airway and thorax. Pediatr Ann 16:307–316, 1987.

20. Eichelberger ML, Mize MG, Runion E: Pediatric Emergencies—EMS Training Program. 2nd ed. Washington, DC, Department of Health and Human Services and Department of Transportation, 1986.

21. Eichelberger ML, Randolph JG: Pediatric trauma: An algorithm for diagnosis and therapy. J Trauma 23:91–97, 1983.

22. Eichelberger ML, Randolph JG: Progress in pediatric trauma. World J Surg 9:222–235, 1985.

23. Fortner GS, Oreskovich MR, Copass MK, et al: The effects of prehospital trauma care on the survival from a 50 meter fall. J Trauma 23:976–980, 1983.

24. Gallaher SS, Finison K, Guyer B, et al: The incidence of injuries among 87,000 Massachusetts children and adolescents: Results of the 1980–81 statewide childhood injury prevention program surveillance system. Am J Public Health 74:1340–1347, 1984.

25. Gorelick MH, Shaw KN, Baker MD: Effect of ambient temperature on capillary refill in healthy children. Pediatrics 92:699–702, 1993.

26. Haller JA Jr; Pediatric trauma; The number 1 killer of children. JAMA 249:47, 1983.

27. Haller JA Jr, Shorter N, Miller D, et al: Organization and function of a regional pediatric trauma center: Does a system of management improve outcome? J Trauma 23:691–696, 1983.

28. Harris BH: Priorities of treatment—The 20 minute drill. In: Harris BH (ed): Progress in Pediatric Trauma. Boston, Nobb Hill, 1985.

29. Harris BH, Latchaw LA, Murphy RE, et al: The crucial hour. Pediatr Ann 16:301–304, 1987.

30. Hospital and prehospital resources for optimal care of the injured patient. Bull Am Coll Surg 68:11, 1983.

31. Jacobs LM, Sinclair A, Beiser A, et al: Prehospital advanced life support: Benefits in trauma. J Trauma 24:8–12, 1984.

32. Joyce M: Initial management of pediatric trauma. In: Marcus RE (ed): Trauma in Children. Rockville, Md, Aspen Publishers, 1986, pp 13–38.

33. King DR: Trauma in infancy and childhood: Initial evaluation and management. Pediatr Clin North Am 32:1299–1310, 1985.

34. Larrey DJ: Memoirs of a Military Surgeon (Willmott R, translator). Classics of Surgery Library. Birmingham, Ala, Joseph Cushing. As quoted by McSwain NE. In: Moore EE, Mattox KL, Feliciano DV (eds): Trauma. East Norwalk, Conn, Appleton & Lange, 1991, pp 99–107.

35. McSwain NE (ed): Prehospital Trauma Life Support. Akron, Ohio, Educational Directions, 1990.

36. McSwain NE Jr: Prehospital emergency medical systems and cardiopulmonary resuscitation. In: Moore EE, Mattox KL, Feliciano DV (eds): Trauma. East Norwalk, Conn, Appleton & Lange, 1991, pp 99–107.

37. Mayer TA: Evaluation and general management of the injured child. In: Mayer TA (ed): Emergency Management of Pediatric Trauma. Philadelphia, WB Saunders, 1985, pp 10–12.

38. Mayer TA: Preface. In: Mayer TA (ed): Emergency Management of Pediatric Trauma. Philadelphia, WB Saunders, 1985, pp xi–xiii.

39. Mayer TA, Matlak M, Johnson D, et al: The modified injury severity scale in pediatric multiple trauma patients. J Pediatr Surg 15:719, 1980.

40. Mayer TA, Walker ML, Johnson DG, et al: Causes of morbidity and mortality in severe pediatric trauma. JAMA 245:719–721, 1981.

41. Ornato JP, Craren EJ, Nelson NM, et al: Impact of improved emergency medical services and emergency trauma care on the reduction in mortality from trauma. J Trauma 25:575–579, 1985.

42. Otherson HB: Cardiothoracic injuries. In: Touloukian RJ (ed): Pediatric Trauma. New York, John Wiley and Sons, 1978.

43. Papper EM: The bone marrow route for injecting fluids and drugs into the general circulation. Anesthesiology 3:307–313, 1942.

44. Pediatric Advanced Life Support. Dallas, Texas, American Heart Association/American Academy of Pediatrics, 1988.

45. Ramenofsky ML: Trauma scores and outcome studies. Presented at the first national conference on pediatric trauma. Sponsored by New England Medical Center and Kiwanis Pediatric Trauma Institute, Boston, September 16–17, 1985.

46. Ramenofsky ML, Luterman A, Quindlen E, et al: Maximum survival in pediatric trauma: The ideal system. J Trauma 24:818–823, 1984.

47. Ramenofsky ML, Morse TS: Standards of care for the critically injured pediatric patient. J Trauma 22:921–933, 1982.

48. Rivara FP: Traumatic deaths of children in the United States: Currently available prevention strategies. Pediatrics 75:456–462, 1985.

49. Ryckman FC, Noseworthy J: Multisystem trauma. Surg Clin North Am 65:1287–1302, 1985.

50. Salem MR, Wong AY, Mani M, Sellick BA: Efficacy of cricoid pressure in preventing gastric inflation during bag-mask ventilation in pediatric patients. Anesthesiology 40:96, 1974.

51. Seidel JS, Hornbein M, Yoshiyama K, et al: Emergency medical services and the pediatric patient: Are the needs being met? Pediatrics 73:769–772, 1984.

52. Sellick BA: Cricoid pressure to control regurgitation of stomach contents during induction of anaesthesia. Lancet 2:404, 1961.

53. Tepas JJ, Alexander RH, Campbell JD, et al: An improved scoring system for assessment of the injured child. J Trauma 25:720–722, 1985.

54. Tepas JJ, Mollitt DL, Talbert JL, et al: The pediatric trauma score as a predictor of injury severity in the injured child. J Pediatr Surg 22:14–18, 1987.

55. United States Department of Transportation: National Standard EMT—Intermediate Curriculum. Washington, DC, US Government Printing Office, 1986.

56. United States Department of Transportation: National Standard EMT—Paramedic Curriculum. Washington, DC, US Government Printing Office, 1986.

57. Velcek FT, Weiss A, DiMaio D, et al: Traumatic death in urban children. J Pediatr Surg 12:375–384, 1977.

58. West KW, Grosfeld JL, Weber TR: Multiple trauma. In: Zimmerman SS, Gilda JH (eds): Critical Care Pediatrics. Philadelphia, WB Saunders, 1985, pp 484–490.

59. Wisoff JH, Epstein FJ: Management of pediatric head trauma. In: Zimmerman SS, Gildea JH (eds): Critical Care Pediatrics. Philadelphia, WB Saunders, 1985, pp 368–374.

Howard R. Gould
Edward Buonocore

CHAPTER ELEVEN

Radiologic Evaluation of the Injured Child

METHODS OF EVALUATION

The prime consideration in the initial imaging evaluation of the injured child is to obtain the greatest amount of information in the shortest possible time without compromising the patient's condition. Initial clinical evaluation and, if necessary, resuscitation, proceed concurrently. Localized extremity injuries require conventional radiographs and, rarely, angiography if vascular compromise is suspected.

In the critically injured child with neurologic or multisystem injuries, prompt and judicious selection of the proper imaging procedure is most important. Preliminary routine radiographic films include a supine chest, a lateral cervical spine, and an anteroposterior (AP) pelvis. Supine chest radiographs are obtained to determine the presence of hemothorax or pneumothorax, fractures of the chest wall, and mediastinal and cardiac abnormalities (Fig. 11–1). Abnormalities in the contour of the aortic arch, displacement of the trachea and esophagus (nasogastric tube), and depression of the left main stem bronchus all suggest the possibility of an aortic injury and are an indication for immediate aortography (Fig. 11–2). An apparently elevated or indistinct diaphragm or an unusually high position of the stomach raises the possibility of a diaphragmatic injury.

The lateral view of the cervical spine should include all of the cervical vertebrae and the top of T1. Depending on the gravity of the patient's condition, AP and, if necessary, modified oblique views are obtained. If adequate visualization is not achieved or if a cervical spine injury is still suspected, the patient is maintained in a collar and protected as if an injury were present until the spine is determined to be normal by computed tomography (CT) or tomography. The AP pelvis radiograph is made to rule out fractures that may be unsuspected because of the patient's other injuries. Pelvic fractures can be a source of significant extraperitoneal pelvic and retroperitoneal hemorrhage.

In our original protocol,[14] patients with clinical signs of a spinal injury would have crosstable lateral views taken of the entire spine, followed by AP views. Further experience has generated a high level of suspicion for these injuries, and most patients with significant blunt trauma, and especially those with a seat belt injury (Fig. 11–3), have the entire spine radiographed (Fig. 11–4). In a series of 63 spinal injuries, Pal and colleagues found that 27% were cervical, 27% thoracic, 38% lumbar, and 8% in multiple areas.[24] Of the cervical, thoracic, and lumbar fracture patients, 41%, 40%, and 17%, respectively, had associated closed-head injuries or skull fractures. The researchers accordingly recommended that the entire spine be radiographed in patients who have multiple injuries with a skull fracture or altered state of consciousness. Intra-abdominal[1] as well as spinal injuries can occur with the use of lap seat belts in children as in adults.

Head injury patients are best evaluated by CT scans, allowing a rapid and accurate determination of the type and magnitude of injury and whether it requires operative or nonoperative therapy (Figs. 11–5, 11–6). Magnetic resonance (MR) scanners give superb neuroradiologic images but are usually not available on an emergency basis, because they require a longer examination time and it is difficult to monitor the patient physiologically in the elon-

gated MR scanner. Magnetic resonance imaging is the procedure of choice for traumatic spinal cord lesions. The ability of MR to do direct sagittal scans of the entire spine (Fig. 11–7) gives it a distinct advantage over other techniques of imaging.

Angiography is used at our institution for suspected thoracic injury (see Fig. 11–2) and only rarely for other injuries in children. The paucity of mediastinal fat in children makes interpretation of the mediastinum difficult. Although a hematoma, especially in adults, can be diagnosed using CT, angiography remains the gold standard for the evaluation of thoracic aortic trauma. Therapeutic embolization may be necessary to control hemorrhage in various solid organs and in association with pelvic fractures. Traumatic arteriovenous fistulae can also be treated by using this method.

In our hands, orally administered contrast studies of the gastrointestinal tract are rarely used in the evaluation of the acutely injured patient. An esophagogram is performed to rule out perforation in patients with unexplained pneumomediastinum and a duodenogram to rule out duodenal hematoma or perforation in those patients with a history that arouses suspicion or a questionable CT scan. Water-soluble contrast is used in both instances.

Excretory urography has been a frequently used tool in confirming suspected renal trauma. A study that yields normal results virtually excludes significant upper urinary tract

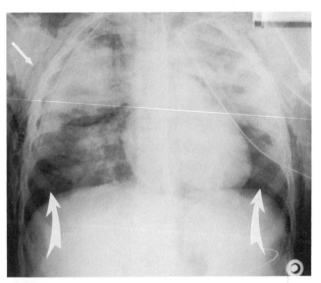

FIGURE 11–1

Evidence of bronchial avulsion. An 8-year-old boy was thrown from a jeep in a motor vehicle accident and was supposedly impaled on the tail light of another vehicle. Two open chest wounds were treated with chest tubes at another emergency department, and the patient was transferred by helicopter to our facility. On physical examination, extensive subcutaneous emphysema from the maxilla to the scrotum was present. A chest radiograph showed the extensive subcutaneous emphysema (*arrow*), pneumomediastinum, bilateral areas of lung opacification, and bilateral chest tubes with basal pneumothoraces (*curved arrows*). Bronchoscopy revealed a distal tracheal and right main bronchus injury. At surgery the right main stem bronchus was partially avulsed from the trachea with extension of the tear proximally up the trachea. A pneumonectomy was performed.

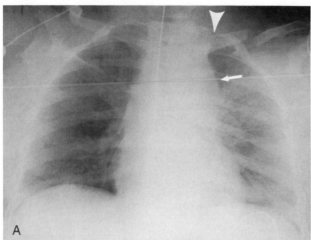

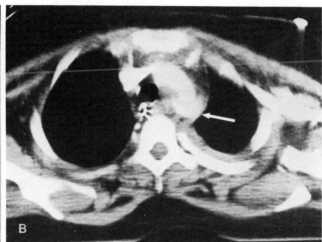

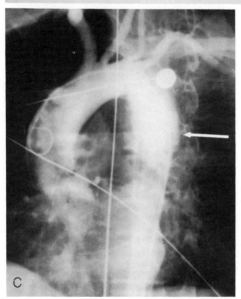

FIGURE 11–2

Traumatic aortic pseudoaneurysm. A 12-year-old girl who was an unrestrained passenger in a motor vehicle accident was transferred by helicopter to our facility. The patient sustained a mild closed-head injury, laceration of the right eyebrow, and fractures of the pelvis, right femur, tibia, and fibula. The chest radiograph *(A)* showed a fracture of the left clavicle, a small left apical cap *(arrowhead)*, a wide left superior mediastinum *(arrow)*, a minimal irregularity of the contour of the aortic arch, and some depression of the left main stem bronchus. The trachea and esophagus (nasogastric tube) are slightly to the right of the midline. A few cuts of the chest *(B)* were done during the torso computed tomography scan. These showed mediastinal hemorrhage and an extraluminal collection of contrast *(arrow)*. An aortogram *(C)* confirmed a traumatic aortic pseudoaneurysm *(arrow)*, which was repaired surgically without complications.

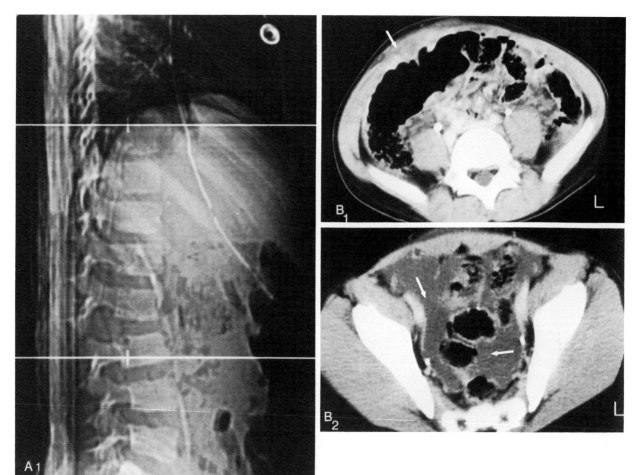

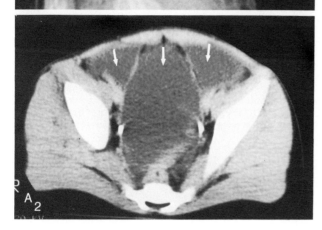

FIGURE 11-3

Lap seat belt injuries. Three male siblings, ages 6, 7, and 12, were restrained by lap belts in the back seat of a vehicle involved in a motor vehicle accident. The passenger in the right front seat was killed. All were transferred by helicopter, one from the scene and the others following an initial evaluation at another emergency department. *A (1),* Lateral scout film of a computed tomography (CT) scan of a 6-year-old boy showing a hyperflexion injury at L2–3 and a distraction dislocation of posterior elements, resulting in paraplegia, *(2)* a hemoperitoneum *(arrows)* secondary to mesenteric laceration, and multiple areas of contusion and lacerations in an 18-inch segment of jejunum. *B,* CT scans of a 7-year-old boy showing *(1)* hematoma and contusion of the anterior abdominal wall *(arrow)* and *(2)* hemoperitoneum *(arrows)* secondary to multiple serosal tears of the sigmoid colon and caecum, laceration of the ileum, and a 4-cm actively bleeding laceration of the mesentery.

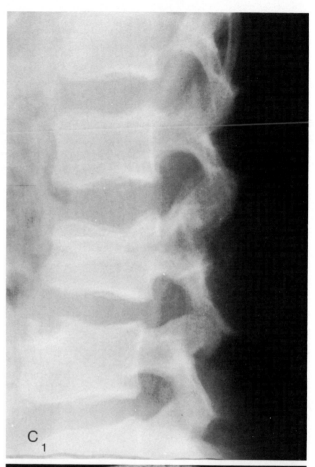

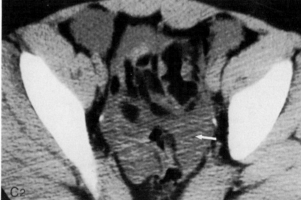

FIGURE 11–3 *Continued*

C, Lateral lumbar spine film and CT scan of a 12-year-old boy with *(1)* a Chance fracture at L3 and *(2)* a hemoperitoneum *(arrow)* secondary to sigmoid colon avulsion from mesentery, avulsion of midjejunum from mesentery, mesenteric injury of the terminal ileum, and a tear in a branch of the superior mesenteric vein.

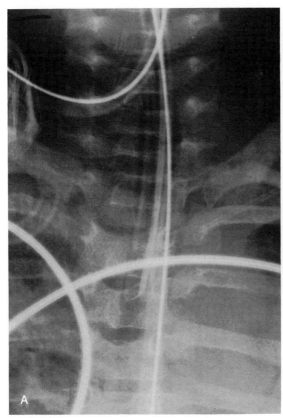
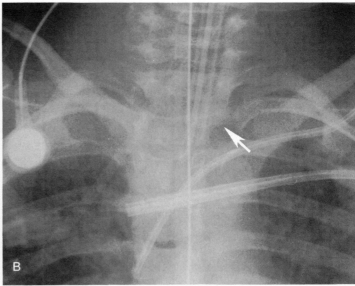

FIGURE 11–4

Spinal injury. A 5-year-old boy was transferred by helicopter from another hospital after a motor vehicle accident. The child was comatose with no history of movement in his lower extremities since the accident. A computed tomography (CT) scan of the head showed a frontal skull fracture, a pneumocephalus, an intra- and extra-axial frontal hemorrhage, and a midline shift. The extra-axial collection was subsequently drained. A computed tomography scan showed a hemoperitoneum with no definite solid organ injury. Diagnostic peritoneal lavage confirmed the hemoperitoneum. At celiotomy the patient had a contusion of the mid ileum and an 8- to 10-cm serosal denuding of the sigmoid colon but with intact mucosa. A sigmoid colectomy was performed. The initial spine films (A) were normal, but a follow-up study of the chest several days later (B) showed a lateral dislocation of T1 on T2 (arrow). A subsequent myelogram at this level showed a complete block with a pseudomeningocele.

injury,[5, 25] although an excretory urogram may be unreliable in cases of penetrating trauma.[4] There is no correlation between the degree of renal injury and the amount of hematuria,[6, 13, 16] and an excretory urogram may be inaccurate in staging the degree of renal injury.[6] For these reasons, and the fact that 20 to 34%[17, 21] of children with renal injuries have multiple organ injuries, we rarely use the excretory urogram as a primary imaging modality. However, operative excretory urograms may be used just before or during emergency surgery to determine whether two kidneys are present and functioning.

Radionuclide imaging of the solid viscera has been reported to be as good as or nearly as accurate as CT in imaging the liver, spleen, and kidney by some investigators.[3, 11, 20, 21] However, staging of a solid organ injury by demonstration of a perfusion abnormality is difficult. Furthermore, radionuclide imaging does not identify or quantify the amount of intraperitoneal or retroperitoneal hemorrhage and gives no information about the pancreas or other abdominal viscera, intraperitoneal or retroperitoneal. A major disadvantage of radionuclide scanning is the requirement for multiple injections of different tracers to study each organ system.

The ability to use portable equipment is a distinct advantage of both radionuclide and sonographic examinations. Radionuclide imaging of bile duct leaks,[28] which can provide an estimation of the amount of leak versus that entering the gut,[26] can be of great clinical value. Highly sensitive bone scanning for a demonstration of occult fractures in suspected child abuse[26] is another valuable application of radionuclide imaging.

Sonography has several advantages as an imaging method. It does not involve ionizing radiation, is usually less expensive than other modalities, and, as mentioned previously, can be performed at the bedside. Sonography is accurate in detecting free intra-abdominal fluid and injuries to the liver and kidney[3] but can have a false negative rate as high as 50%[20] in detecting splenic injuries. Excessive gas with paralytic ileus is detrimental to the adequate imaging of the peritoneal cavity by sonography.[21]

Both radionuclide imaging and sonography are of value in the serial monitoring of known solid organ injuries until they have healed.[2, 21] Sonography is also useful in following posttraumatic pancreatitis, fluid collections, and secondary infection.[19] However, our experience and that of others[2, 16, 19, 21, 22] has shown that CT should be the primary imaging modality in the severely injured child. One examination can be used to evaluate multiple organ systems and anatomic

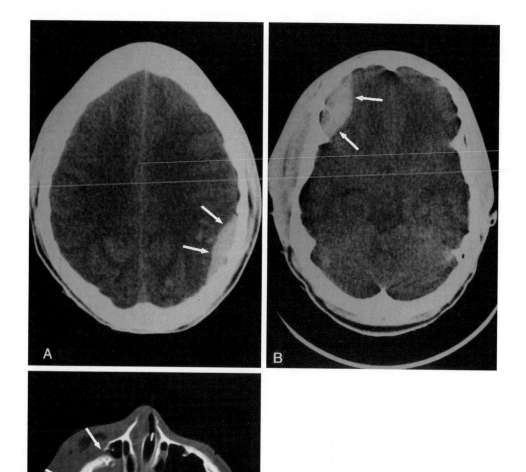

FIGURE 11–5

Epidural hematoma and facial fractures. A 16-year-old male was transferred intubated by helicopter from another facility after a motor vehicle accident. *A and B,* A computed tomography (CT) scan showed bilateral epidural hematomas *(arrows). (C),* Multiple facial fractures *(arrows)* were identified on scans through the facial bones. A CT scan of the abdomen showed a fractured liver with 1+ hemoperitoneum. This was treated without surgery. The patient never recovered from his head injuries and died on the seventh day in the hospital.

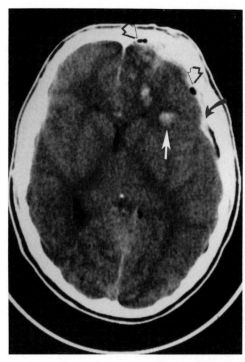

FIGURE 11–6

Pneumocephalus, subdural hematoma, and intracerebral hemorrhage. A 16-year-old male was transferred by helicopter from another facility after a motorcycle accident. A computed tomography scan of the head showed a left frontal parietal skull fracture with extension into the left temporal bone and orbital rim. A pneumocephalus (open arrows) was present with a small left subdural hematoma (curved black arrow). There was extensive left frontal hemorrhage and contusion (white arrow), with a midline shift from left to right. A type 2 splenic injury without a significant hemoperitoneum was identified on the body scan. The patient was treated without abdominal surgery and was transferred to a rehabilitation center on the fifty-sixth hospital day.

areas, and, most important, CT can be done early in the postinjury period with consistent accuracy and in three dimension. Our initial indications for CT were as follows[14]:

1. Evidence of blunt abdominal trauma with possible multisystem injuries in
2. Hemodynamically stable or easily resuscitated patients with
3. Equivocal or unreliable physical examination due to
   a. Altered level of consciousness secondary to head injury, alcohol, or drugs;
   b. Pelvic and spinal injuries;
   c. Age, that is, in small or younger uncooperative children;
4. Hematuria.

With continuing experience, we have developed a high level of suspicion and now tend to scan children who have been in a motor vehicle accident that involved a fatality and those who are at risk for a lap belt injury.

Follow-up scans are performed on those who might have an equivocal bowel injury on the initial scan and on those who have an unexplained falling hematocrit.

TECHNIQUE

In our experience, injured children rarely require sedation or anesthesia for the examination. When necessary, we do not hesitate to use sedation and analgesia as required and even paralysis if the patient has been intubated because of lack of cooperation or belligerence, which is usually related to age or injury or both.

Oral contrast is not used routinely. Our experience in the large majority of children is that there is significant retained food and fluid in the stomach at the time of examination. In those patients to whom we have given oral contrast medium, bowel opacification has usually been inadequate due to dilution and ileus. If there is any question of a duodenal abnormality on the scan, however, a fluoroscopic study with full strength aqueous contrast is obtained immediately after the CT scan. All patients who have a follow-up do receive oral contrast for bowel lumen opacification.

Preliminary precontrast scans of the upper abdomen are usually performed before the main study. These use a low-dose technique with a widely spaced interval (e.g., a 10-mm slice every 25 mm or a 5-mm slice every 15 mm in the smaller child). These precontrast scans (usually five or six in number) do not cause a significant delay and are valuable in setting up the upper and lower limits of the dynamic scan run. Occasionally they have been invaluable in interpreting the contrast scan, for example, in differentiating preexisting dense hematoma from extravasation of contrast and in providing an estimation that both kidneys are normal. An obvious serious renal abnormality might change the dose of contrast used for the dynamic scan. Rarely, a large hemoperitoneum negates the requirement for the contrast scans, and the patient is taken to surgery immediately.

Our dynamic scan technique includes the use of 60% intravenous contrast medium, usually at a dose of 2 ml per kg up to a maximum of 90 to 100 ml. A dose of approximately 5 ml is injected several minutes before the main scan, or even before the "noncontrast" studies, to ensure that opacification of the renal collecting systems and ureters is adequate. The main contrast injection is timed so that approximately one third to one half of the volume is administered before the first scan is started and the remainder is injected during the initial two thirds of the dynamic scan. A power injector is used for larger children. Smaller children and infants usually receive a hand injection. Because only an estimation, rather than actual weight, is usually available on these children, the use of nonionic contrast may offer a greater margin of safety in addition to decreasing the chance of vomiting during the procedure.

The initial dynamic scan sequence extends from the dome of the diaphragms to the lower pole of the kidneys with contiguous 10-mm slices every 10 mm in the larger child and 5-mm slices every 8 or 5 mm in the smaller child and infant. In children who are old enough to cooperate, an interscan delay of 6 seconds allows time for one respiration between each slice. A minimum interscan delay of 3.5 seconds is used with uncooperative or small children and those on a ventilator.

Depending on the number of slices (usually 14–20) and the interscan delay, the initial dynamic run is accomplished in about 1 minute 30 seconds to 2 minutes 40 seconds. A

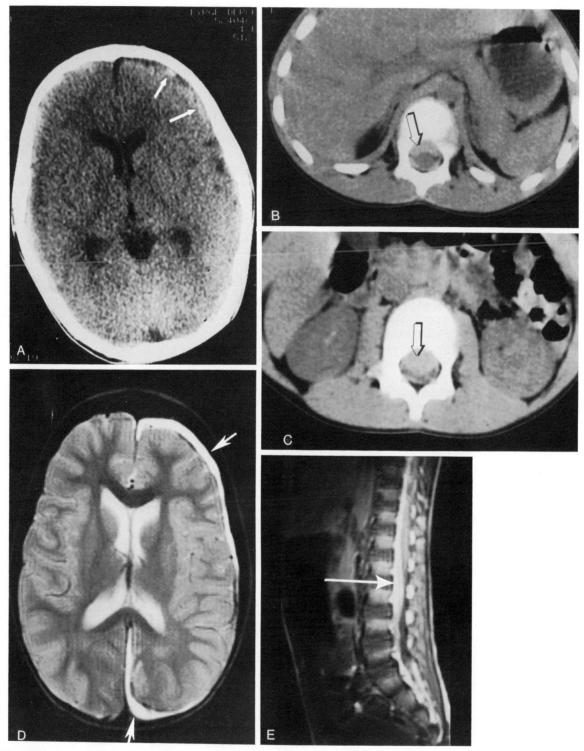

FIGURE 11-7

Cerebral subdural hematoma and spinal epidural hematoma. A 4-year-old boy allegedly fell from a bunk bed on the evening before hospital admission; he had a history of having been ''paddled'' on the buttocks 2 to 3 days previously. Examination showed numerous bruises of varying age. The child had a left hemiparesis, left third and seventh cranial nerve paresis, and bilateral lower extremity rigidity. *A,* Cranial computed tomography (CT) examination showed a small left frontal subdural hemorrhage *(arrows). B and C,* Abdominal CT showed no intra-abdominal abnormality but a dense extra-axial intraspinal collection *(open arrow)* compatible with an epidural hematoma. The patient remained clinically stable. *D,* A follow-up magnetic resonance (MR) scan of the head 4 days later showed a subacute subdural hematoma *(arrows)* encasing the left cerebrum. *E,* An MR scan of the spine showed a ventral extra-axial hematoma *(arrow)* in the thoracic and lumbar region. The child slowly, but steadily improved and was eventually transferred to a rehabilitation center with a diagnosis of presumed nonaccidental injuries.

second dynamic sequence, with no additional contrast medium, is immediately made of the lower abdomen, from the lower pole of the kidneys to the ischiopubic ring. A gap between slices is allowed, that is, a 10-mm slice every 20 mm or a 5-mm slice every 15 mm in smaller children and infants. If the patient has a urinary catheter in place, it should be clamped before the start of scanning.*

The scans are performed under the direct supervision of an attending radiologist and are interpreted immediately. We believe this is of the utmost importance if the clinical management of the patient will be based largely on the CT findings. "Diagnoses rendered the following day are of little help when rapid and often life saving decisions must be made in the middle of the night."[14]

EXPERIENCE

Over a 3-year period from September 1, 1984, to August 31, 1987, 1979 CT examinations were performed on 1443 patients; 601 abdominal CT examinations were done, and of these, 103 were on children aged 16 years or younger, with the youngest being 11 days old. The age distribution is shown in Figure 11–8. Fifty-six patients also had head injuries, and 22 had skull fractures.

Motor vehicle accidents (Table 11–1) accounted for the majority of the cases. Forty-six of the patients were brought to our hospital by helicopter, and of these, 83% were transferred from another hospital. The median time from injury to arrival at our hospital was estimated to be 2 hours 23 minutes. On arrival and after stabilization, an initial assess-

---

*With the advent of modern helical scanners, we have modified the previously described technique.

Table 11–1
Type of Trauma

Motor vehicle accident	55%
Pedestrian	16%
Motorcycle accident	8%
Fall	9%
Other	12%

ment, which included taking plain films, and a determination of the need for CT scanning were made. Of the patients who underwent torso CT, the median time from hospital arrival to CT scan was 58 minutes. Eighty-two percent of these children were in the scanner in less than 2 hours from arrival. The time of day of the CT examinations, as shown in Table 11–2, was between 11 PM and 7 AM in 32% of the examinations and after 7 PM or on weekends in 68% of the examinations.

An abnormality was demonstrated in 59% of the abdominal examinations. Twenty-two patients had proof of positive or negative findings, 19 at celiotomy, two at autopsy, and one at organ donation. A total of 39 solid organ injuries were identified (Table 11–3).

Spleen Injuries

There were 23 splenic injuries in the 130 pediatric patients (Table 11–4). Splenic injuries were classified[7, 8] using a system previously reported from our institution and abbreviated as follows:

1. Type 1: capsular or subcapsular hematoma
2. Type 2: lacerations that do not involve the hilum or major vessels (Fig. 11–9)

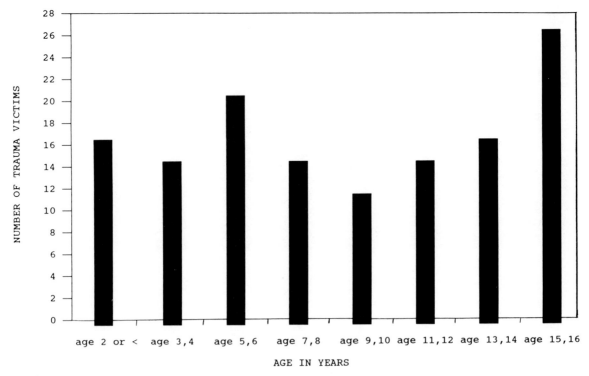

FIGURE 11–8

Computed tomography scans performed on trauma patients ages 16 and under, University of Tennessee Medical Center, 1984–1987.

Table 11–2
Time of Computed Tomography in Abdominal Trauma

Day	Time	Percentage	
Monday–Friday	0700–1900	32	
Monday–Saturday	1900–0700	35	} 68
Saturday–Monday	0700–0700	32	

Table 11–3
Computed Tomography (CT) Scanning in Blunt Abdominal Trauma

Injuries	No.	Positive Diagnosis on CT	Explored	False +/−
Spleen	23	23	12	1/1*
Liver	11	10	3	0/1†
Kidney	5	5	3	0/0

*At a celiotomy performed 6 months later for another reason a posttraumatic scar was seen in the lower pole of the spleen.
†Four capsular tears and a single 12-mm deep tear between the right lobe and the caudate found at autopsy.

3. Type 3: deep lacerations involving the hilum or major vessels (Fig. 11–10)
4. Type 4: totally shattered or avulsed spleen

In addition to the one false positive and the one false negative results (Fig. 11–11), three cases were misstaged. Two type 3 cases were understaged, and one type 2 case was overstaged. Twelve of the 23 injured spleens underwent celiotomy with two splenectomies, one partial splenectomy, and eight splenorrhaphies. The splenectomies and partial splenectomy were all in patients with type 3 or 4 injury.

Difficulties in interpretation of splenic injuries may be caused by motion or inadequate contrast. A unique artifact in the spleen is the inhomogeneous perfusion that may occur during a dynamic scan.[12] These defects simulate lacerations (Fig. 11–12) but are not associated with perisplenic hematoma or hemorrhage. They are observed in the cephalic aspect of the spleen on the early contrast slices. Immediate rescanning of the area in question shows homogeneous perfusion in the normal spleen. This artifact occurs when the scanning sequence is initiated before an adequate contrast bolus has reached the upper abdomen and is not a common occurrence in children because of their rapid circulation time. It is seen more often in the elderly with low cardiac output.

Congenital splenic clefts (Fig. 11–13) are not uncommon and simulate laceration. Again, there is no surrounding hemorrhage or hematoma, and, if large enough, fat can be identified in the cleft.

Liver Injuries

Eleven patients had liver injuries. There were no false positive cases. There was one false negative result. This patient died of other injuries. At autopsy this patient had multiple

capsular tears and a single 12-mm deep tear between the right and caudate lobes, none of which had caused significant hemorrhage. Three of the eleven had surgery. One of these patients required a nephrectomy for an avulsed renal pedicle, a hepatorrhaphy, and a subsequent hepatic artery embolization for continued hemorrhage. A second hepatorrhaphy was necessary before hemorrhage control was achieved. The second (see Fig. 11–10) had surgery primarily because of her splenic injury, and the third (Fig. 11–14) was the only patient who had surgery for a solitary liver lesion. The eight remaining cases were treated without surgery, and all recovered. Liver injuries are sometimes limited to the parenchyma with an intact capsule (Fig. 11–15) and with no intraperitoneal hemorrhage. Follow-up CT scans, sonography, or nuclear scintigraphy may be used to confirm healing.

Oldham and associates have used an elevation of hepatic enzymes, serum glutamic-oxaloacetic transaminase (SGOT) and serum glutamate pyruvate transaminase (SGPT), as an indicator for CT scanning after trauma.[23] In their series of 44 children, 19 (43%) with an elevated SGOT and SGPT were found to have liver injuries.

Urinary Tract Injuries

Five patients had renal injuries. One had a nephrectomy for an avulsed renal pedicle, and two others had celiotomies for intra-abdominal injuries but no treatment of the renal injuries. The remainder (Fig. 11–16) were treated without surgery.

Table 11–4
Splenic Injuries

	Radiographic Diagnosis (true positives)	Surgery	Surgical Diagnosis	Type Operation
Type 1	2	0		
Type 2	11	3	Type 2: 1	Splenorrhaphy: 2
			Type 3: 2	Splenectomy: 1
Type 3	8	8	Type 2: 1	Splenorrhaphy: 6
			Type 3: 7	Splenectomy: 1
				Partial splenectomy: 1
Type 4	1	1	Type 4: 1	Splenectomy: 1

False positive 1—patient had 3 + hemoperitoneum from a fractured liver.
False negative 1—patient did not undergo surgery. At a celiotomy performed 6 months later for another reason, a posttraumatic scar was noted in the lower pole of the spleen.

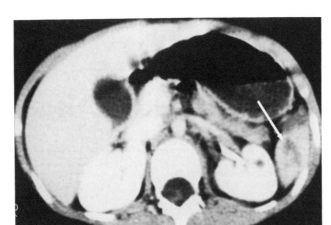

FIGURE 11-9

Type 2 splenic injury. A 4-year-old boy run over by a car across the chest and abdomen sustained abrasions of the entire upper abdomen and lower chest. A computed tomography (CT) scan revealed a contusion of the left lung, a small left pneumothorax, a type 2 splenic injury *(arrow)*, and a minimal pelvic hemoperitoneum. The patient remained stable and was treated nonoperatively and discharged on the tenth day. A follow-up CT scan of the spleen approximately 6 weeks after the injury showed normal findings.

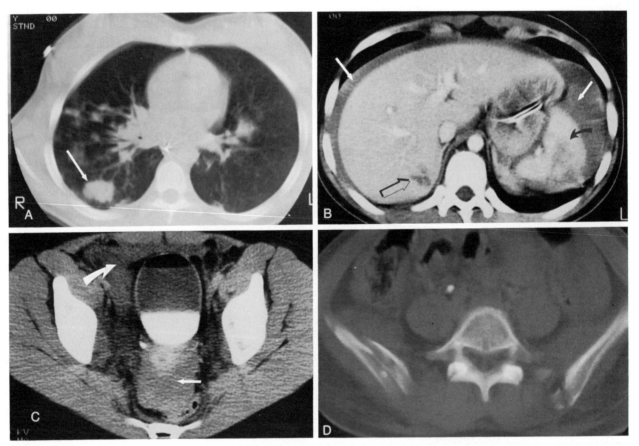

FIGURE 11-10

Pulmonary contusion, type 3 splenic injury, liver injury, and fractured pelvis. A 14-year-old girl, an unrestrained motor vehicle accident victim, was transferred by helicopter from another emergency department with a closed-head injury. Computed tomography (CT) scans showed *(A)* pulmonary contusions *(arrow)*; *(B)* type 3 splenic injury *(curved black arrow)*, intrahepatic liver laceration *(open arrow)*, hemoperitoneum *(white arrow)*; *(C)* pelvic hemoperitoneum *(arrow)*, extraperitoneal pelvic hemorrhage *(curved arrow)*; and *(D)* bilateral pelvic fractures. At celiotomy the patient had several fractures into the hilum of the spleen, with active hemorrhage and about 400 ml of blood in the peritoneal cavity. Splenorrhaphy was successful in controlling the hemorrhage. External fixation of the pelvis was achieved with a Hoffman device. A follow-up CT scan in 5 weeks showed healing of the liver injury and a residual nonenhancing area in the superior pole of the spleen due to either residual hematoma or infarction. The patient showed gradual neurologic improvement and was transferred to a rehabilitation center on the forty-sixth hospital day.

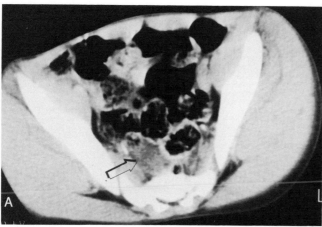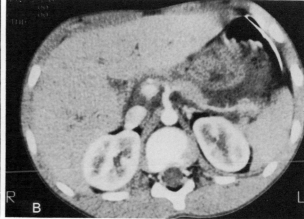

FIGURE 11-11

Missed splenic injury. An 11-year-old male pedestrian struck by an automobile was unresponsive at the scene and was transferred by ambulance from another facility after resuscitation and the administration of intravenous fluids. The child had a closed-head injury, an intraventricular hemorrhage with a midline shift, and a fracture of the femur. *A,* A computed tomography (CT) scan showed a small amount of fluid in the right pelvis *(arrow),* which was thought to represent a minimal hemoperitoneum. No solid organ injury was demonstrated, and the spleen *(B)* was thought to be normal. A repeat CT scan with enteric contrast the following day showed no evidence of a bowel injury, and there was no longer evidence of a hemoperitoneum. The patient was transferred comatose, with a left hemispheric infarction, to a rehabilitation institution on the seventy-second hospital day. At celiotomy, 6 months later for a feeding gastrostomy, he was found to have a small scar in the lower pole of his spleen, indicating a prior injury.

FIGURE 11-12

Variations in splenic perfusion that simulate a fracture. An 8-year-old girl who was an unrestrained passenger in a motor vehicle accident was transferred from the scene by ambulance. The child sustained facial and scalp lacerations. A torso computed tomography scan was performed because of the high degree of suspicion of intra-abdominal injury with this mechanism of injury. A dynamic scan (2-second scans with a 6-second interscan delay and table incrementation) was performed. On the early scans through the upper portions of the spleen, there is nonhomogeneous perfusion *(arrows),* which simulates multiple fractures. There is no perisplenic hematoma and no evidence of hemoperitoneum. Immediate rescanning of these areas in the spleen showed that enhancement was uniform. The patient was discharged on the following day.

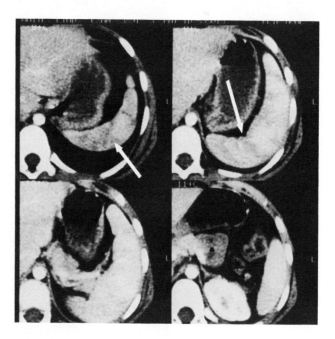

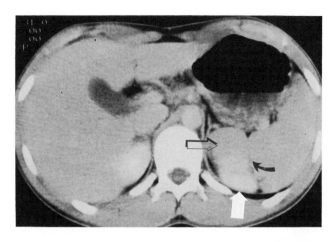

FIGURE 11–13

Splenic lobule and cleft. A 15-year-old boy fell from a haywagon, and a wheel ran over his chest. An oval mass *(open arrow)* behind the stomach was interpreted as a splenic lobule overlying the left kidney *(white arrow)*. The lobule is separated from the remainder of the spleen by a cleft *(curved black arrow)*. Sonography was normal. The patient had a closed-head injury, abrasions of the left chest, and a fractured metatarsal. He was discharged on the eighth day without surgical intervention.

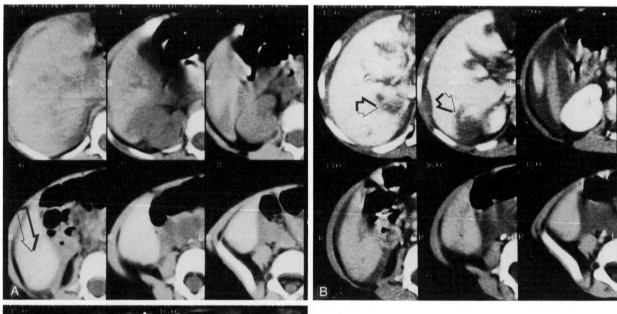

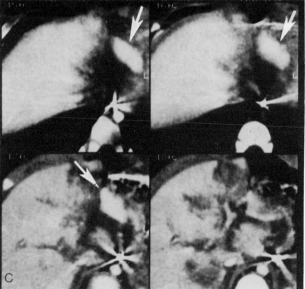

FIGURE 11–14

Liver injury with hemoperitoneum. An 18-month-old girl was playing in her driveway behind a car that backed over her lower chest. She was transferred to our facility by helicopter from another hospital. Physical examination revealed grunting respirations and a diagonal contusion across her anterior chest. A chest radiograph showed a poorly defined left upper lobe contusion. *A,* A computed tomography scan without contrast showed a dense, smooth mass in the right lower quadrant *(open arrow)*. *B,* Following a contrast injection, there was evidence of fractures in the right and caudate lobes of the liver *(open arrow)* and a nonenhancement of the right lower quadrant mass. *C,* Extravasation was contrast *(arrows)*, indicating active hemorrhage from a jagged irregular edge of the left lobe of the liver. The multiple liver injuries were controlled, as was an intraoperative cardiac arrest. The patient recovered, with a slight foot drop as the only neurologic deficit and was discharged on the twenty-sixth hospital day.

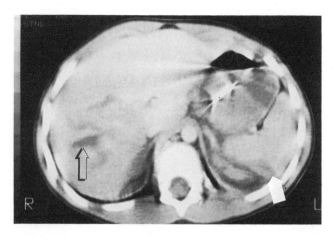

FIGURE 11–15

Liver and splenic injuries. A 7-year-old boy was transferred from another emergency department after a motor vehicle accident because of altered mental status. He had a fractured femur and fractures of the left zygoma and frontal bone with pneumocephalus but no intracerebral hemorrhage. A computed tomography (CT) scan of the torso showed multiple intrahepatic fractures of the liver *(open arrow)* and a small type 2 fracture of the spleen *(solid arrow)* with no significant hemoperitoneum. The facial and femoral fractures were treated surgically, but the abdominal injuries were treated nonoperatively. A follow-up CT scan on the twelfth day showed partial resolution of the liver lesions and a normal spleen. He was discharged on the twenty-fourth day.

One of the pitfalls of the dynamic scanning technique is the fact that there may not be any contrast in the renal pelvis and ureter when the upper abdominal scans are performed. An error in diagnosis occurred when a perinephric and retroperitoneal fluid collection (Fig. 11–17) was assumed to be a hematoma. If there is no contrast in the collecting system and there is fluid around the kidney, delayed scans should be done to rule out urinary extravasation. A small amount of contrast medium injected (about 5 ml) a few minutes before the main injection ensures that the renal pelvis is filled and prevents a recurrence of this error.

Intestinal and Mesenteric Injuries

The CT findings of intestinal and mesenteric injuries[9] include thick bowel walls (Fig. 11–18), peritoneal fluid, free intraperitoneal air, and thick mesentery. Bowel wall thickening is difficult to diagnose when no oral contrast is used but may be visualized if enhancement of the bowel wall occurs with intravenous contrast.

Five bowel and mesenteric injuries occurred in the 130 patients in the series. One of these was a perineal and rectal injury requiring a colostomy. There were no missed bowel injuries. Unexplained fluid or blood in the peritoneal cavity

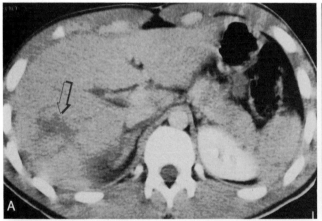

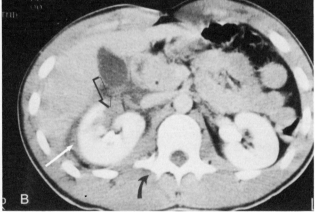

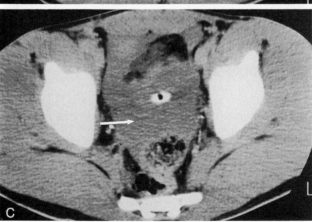

FIGURE 11–16

Liver and kidney injury with intraperitoneal hemorrhage. A 15-year-old male, apparently thrown from a vehicle after a motor vehicle accident, was transferred from another emergency department intubated en route. The patient was unresponsive with gross hematuria. A computed tomography (CT) scan of head showed bifrontal intracerebral hemorrhage and contusion. A CT scan of the torso showed *(A)* a laceration of the right lobe of the liver *(arrow)*, *(B)* a laceration of the right kidney *(open arrow)* with perinephric hemorrhage *(white arrow)*, fracture of a transverse process *(curved black arrow)*, and *(C)* a pelvic hemoperitoneum *(arrow)*. Other scans showed fractures of the right transverse processes of L1, 2, 3, and 4 and the left transverse process of L12. His abdominal injuries were treated without surgery, and after some neurologic improvement, he was transferred on the fifteenth day to another facility for rehabilitation.

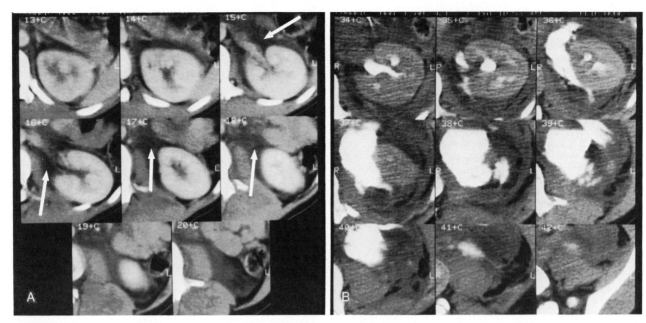

FIGURE 11-17

Ureteral injury. A 9-year-old boy struck by a car was unresponsive at the scene and was transferred to our facility by ambulance. The initial computed tomography (CT) scan of the head was normal. Routine films showed an upper lobe contusion in the chest, fractures of the left humerus, and several transverse fractures of the lumbar spine. *A,* A CT scan showed transverse process fractures, left perinephric and retroperitoneal fluid interpreted as blood *(arrows),* normal enhancement of the left kidney, no other solid organ injury, and no intraperitoneal fluid. There was no contrast in the left renal collecting system or left ureter. The scan was repeated 4 days later because of a falling hematocrit. Again the left kidney was normal, but because the collecting system and ureter were not filled, delayed scans *(B)* were made. These revealed massive contrast extravasation from the urinary system with no visualization of the left ureter distally. A diagnosis of ureteral disruption was made. At surgery the left ureter was completely avulsed from the left renal pelvis with no other injury to the kidney. This was repaired without complication.

is considered suspicious for bowel injury, and further evaluation is done by follow-up scan with oral contrast, diagnostic peritoneal lavage, or even celiotomy. Additional cases (see Fig. 11–3) since the close of this series have reinforced this regimen, especially in those instances with lap belt injuries.

Pancreatic Injuries

No pancreatic injuries, even in retrospect, were found in this group of children. Early CT signs of pancreatic injury include pancreatic swelling, patchy parenchymal hypodensity and inhomogeneity on contrast-enhanced scans, pancreatic or parapancreatic hematoma, low-density fracture planes in the gland, and thickening of the left anterior penal fascia.[14, 15, 18] Pancreatic lacerations may be extremely subtle soon after the injury, and early scans may lead to a false negative diagnosis.[15] Follow-up scans may be necessary to show the later signs of pancreatitis.

Pneumothorax and Lung Injury

All of the patients with severe injury have their initial chest radiograph performed in the supine position. Because a pneumothorax rises to the highest portion of the thoracic cavity, it may be missed on radiographs in the supine pa-

tient. Wall and co-workers in their review of more than 500 cases showed that of 35 cases of pneumothorax seen on CT scans, only 25 were demonstrated on chest radiograph, a miss rate of 28%.[27] Our own data in the general population, including more than 300 cases of trauma, show an even higher miss rate of 59% (19 of 32 patients).[14] In the present series, after eliminating patients who already had a chest tube in place, pneumothorax (Fig. 11–19) was not seen on the chest radiograph in four of seven patients on which it could be identified on the CT scan. Patients with pneumothorax have chest tubes inserted before general anesthesia or mechanical ventilation. Pulmonary hemorrhage, contusion, and pneumatoceles can usually be evaluated better as to extent and location on CT scans rather than routine chest radiographs.

Retroperitoneal Hemorrhage

Retroperitoneal hemorrhage is readily identified, and even small amounts of blood can be visualized; however right-sided retroperitoneal hemorrhage is sometimes difficult to differentiate from intraperitoneal blood in Morison's pouch. Retroperitoneal hemorrhage around the second or third portions of the duodenum is an indication for a peroral or a tube-injected water-soluble contrast study to exclude a duodenal leak. Although sometimes unexplained (Fig. 11–20), retroperitoneal hemorrhage is most frequently associated

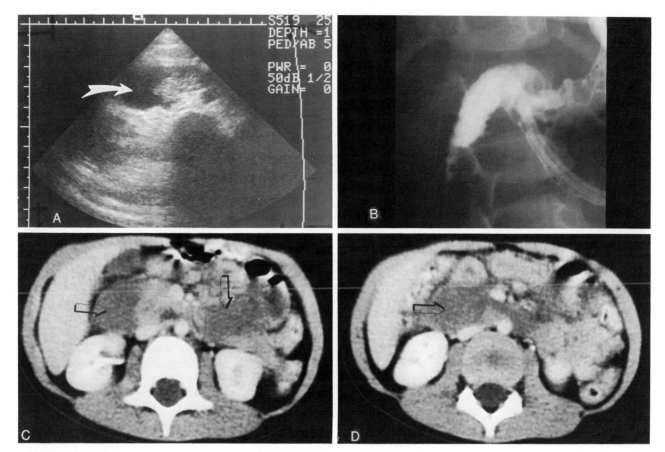

FIGURE 11-18

Intramural hematoma of the duodenum. A 3-year-old boy was transferred from another emergency department with a diagnosis of suspected child abuse. The child had experienced nausea, vomiting, and abdominal pain. *A,* Sonography demonstrated a fluid collection *(arrow)* in the expected location of the duodenum, compatible with a diagnosis of duodenal hematoma. *B,* A gastrointestinal (GI) series confirmed the diagnosis. Because of the possibility of other injuries, a computed tomography scan (*C and D*) was performed. This revealed complete obstruction to passage of the previous GI contrast and a 3-cm nonenhancing mass in the duodenum extending from the second portion of the duodenum into the proximal jejunum *(arrow)*. In addition there was a focal thickening in the medial wall of the right colon that was also thought to represent a hematoma. Only a minimal amount of intraperitoneal fluid was present. Because of increasing abdominal tenderness, the patient was rescanned the following day, revealing a significant increase in the amount of intraperitoneal fluid. Celiotomy was performed, the hematomas of the duodenum and right colon were confirmed, and the duodenal hematoma was evacuated. The patient was discharged with no symptoms on the eighteenth hospital day.

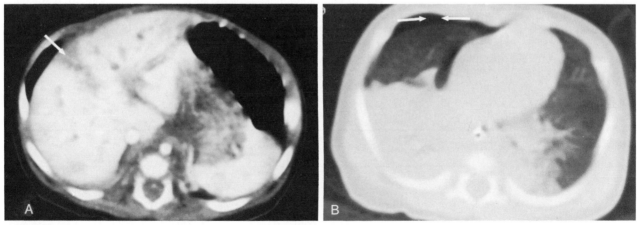

FIGURE 11-19

Pneumothorax and liver injury. A 5-week-old girl was transferred from another emergency department with a possible history of abuse. The child was comatose, intubated, and had bilateral pulmonary contusions. No pneumothorax was seen, even in retrospect, on the admission chest radiograph. *A,* A computed tomography scan revealed consolidation of the right lower lobe, a right pneumothorax *(arrows)*, and some consolidation in the left lower lobe. *B,* A scan through the liver showed a wedge-shaped laceration *(arrow)* in the anterolateral aspect of the liver. The child was managed without surgery and was declared brain dead approximately 3 weeks later.

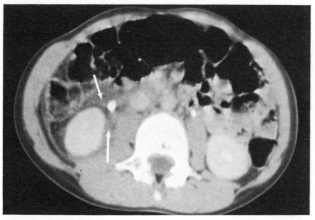

FIGURE 11-20

Retroperitoneal hemorrhage. A 7-year-old boy was transferred from the scene of a bicycle–motor vehicle accident by helicopter. He had multiple contusions, including a large abrasion across the left anterolateral chest. There were puncture wounds in the left thigh, with a fracture of the left femur. Urinalysis was normal with 0 to 3 red blood cells per high power field. A computed tomography scan showed a right retroperitoneal and perinephric hematoma *(arrows)* with no evidence of a renal injury or urinary extravasation. A duodenogram with water soluble contrast excluded a duodenal injury. The patient recovered without operation and was discharged on the tenth hospital day.

with renal injuries or vertebral and pelvic fractures. There were seven vertebral and 15 pelvic fractures in this series, an incidence of 5% and 12%, respectively.

Hemoperitoneum

Federle and Jeffrey described the CT findings of hemoperitoneum and a system of quantification.[10] We have used a modified quantification system that arbitrarily divides the peritoneal cavity into three sections: (1) upper, surrounding the liver or spleen or in Morison's pouch; (2) mid, in the flanks or around the mesentery; and (3) pelvis.[14] Hemorrhage in one of these areas is staged as 1+, in two areas as 2+, and in three areas as 3+. The correlation between higher numbers in this quantification system and subse-

quent need for celiotomy is high (Table 11–5). Thirty-three patients had hemorrhage or dense fluid in the peritoneal cavity that was demonstrated on CT scan. Scanning after diagnostic peritoneal lavage makes the diagnosis and quantification of hemoperitoneum difficult. Occasionally one can see a hematocrit effect in the flanks or in the pelvis after an unsuccessful lavage if hemorrhage is present.

The one type 3 hemoperitoneum patient who did not have surgery had a concomitant severe head injury and eventually died as a result of it. At autopsy the patient had primarily retroperitoneal hemorrhage as well as some intraperitoneal fluid.

Diagnostic Peritoneal Lavage

Peritoneal taps or diagnostic peritoneal lavage (DPL) were obtained on eight patients. Four of these were negative, two of which had been performed at another hospital before transfer. Both of these had negative results on CT scans. Of the other two cases, one had a retroperitoneal hemorrhage, and the last, with a red blood cell count per millimeter of 50,000 on DPL, had a liver injury and a 1+ hemoperitoneum. None of these four patients underwent celiotomy.

Four patients had a positive DPL or peritoneal tap. Three of these had surgery, two for bowel injuries, and the third for a splenic injury. The fourth patient, a 1-year-old girl, had a liver injury and 2+ hemoperitoneum on CT. A peritoneal tap showed gross blood and no evidence of intestinal compromise; she was treated without surgery and discharged on the fifth day without complications.

SUMMARY

Computed tomography scanning fulfills our requirement to obtain the greatest amount of information in the shortest amount of time with the least detrimental effect on the patient's condition. Effective imaging requires close cooperation between the surgeon and the radiologist, particularly during the imaging procedure. The presence and degree of hemoperitoneum and the positive diagnosis and staging of organ injuries can be used as an indicator for operative versus nonoperative management.

Table 11-5
Hemoperitoneum and Celiotomy

Computed Tomography Grade of Hemorrhage	Number of Patients	Celiotomy (%)	Type of Surgery
1+	14	1 (7)	Hepatorrhaphy-nephrectomy
2+	9	7 (78)	Splenorrhaphy: 5
			Splenectomy: 1
			Sigmoid resection: 2
3+	10	9 (90)	Splenorrhaphy: 3
			Splenectomy: 2
			Partial splenectomy: 1
			Hepatorrhaphy-partial hepatectomy: 1
			Repair superior mesenteric vein: 1
			Repair jejunal laceration: 1

References

1. Agran PF, Dunkle DE, Winn DG: Injuries to a sample of seatbelted children evaluated and treated in a hospital emergency room. J Trauma 27:58–64, 1987.
2. Alder DD, Blane CE, Coran AG, Silver TM: Splenic trauma in the pediatric patient: The integrated roles of ultrasound and computed tomography. Pediatrics 76:576–580, 1986.
3. Babcock DS, Kaufman RA: Ultrasonography and computed tomography in the evaluation of the acutely ill pediatric patient. Radiol Clin North Am 21:527–550, 1983.
4. Bergren CT, Chan FN, Bodzin JH: Intravenous pyelogram results in association with renal pathology and therapy in trauma patients. J Trauma 27:515–518, 1987.
5. Bresler MJ: Computed tomography of the abdomen. Ann Emerg Med 15:280–285, 1986.
6. Bretan PN, McAninch JW, Federle MP, Jeffrey RB Jr: Computerized tomographic staging of renal trauma: 85 consecutive cases. J Urol 136:561–565, 1986.
7. Buntain WL, Gould HR: Splenic trauma in children and techniques of splenic salvage. World J Surg 9:398–409, 1985.
8. Buntain WL, Gould HR, Maull KI: Predictability of splenic salvage by computed tomography. J Trauma 28:24–31, 1988.
9. Donahue JH, Federle MP, Griffiths BG, Trunkey DD: Computed tomography in the diagnosis of blunt intestinal and mesenteric injuries. J Trauma 27:11–17, 1987.
10. Federle MP, Jeffrey RB: Hemoperitoneum studies by computed tomography. Radiology 148:187–192, 1983.
11. Gelfand MJ: Scintigraphy in upper abdominal trauma. Semin Roentgenol 19:308–320, 1984.
12. Glazer GM, Azel L, Goldberg HI, Moss AA: Dynamic CT of the normal spleen. AJR 137:343–346, 1981.
13. Godec CJ: Genitourinary trauma. Urol Radiol 7:185–191, 1985.
14. Gould HR, Buntain WL, Maull KI: Imaging in blunt abdominal trauma. Adv Trauma 3:53–100, 1988.
15. Jeffrey RB Jr, Federle MP, Crass RA: Computed tomography of pancreatic trauma. Radiology 147:491–494, 1983.
16. Karp MP, Cooney DR, Berger PE, et al: Role of CT in the evaluation of blunt abdominal trauma in children. J Pediatr Surg 16:316–323, 1981.
17. Karp MP, Jewett TC Jr, Kuhn JP, et al: The impact of computed tomography scanning on the child with renal trauma. J Pediatr Surg 21:617–623, 1986.
18. Kaufman R: CT of blunt abdominal trauma in children: A five year experience. In: Siegel MJ (ed): Pediatric Body CT—Contemporary Issues in Computed Tomography. New York, Churchill Livingstone, 1988, pp 313–347.
19. Kaufman RA, Babcock DS: An approach to imaging the upper abdomen in the injured child. Semin Roentgenol 19:308–320, 1984.
20. Kaufman RA, Towbin R, Babcock DS, et al: Upper abdominal trauma in children: Imaging evaluation. AJR 142:449–460, 1984.
21. Kuhn JP: Diagnostic imaging for the evaluation of abdominal trauma in children. Pediatr Clin North Am 32:1427–1447, 1985.
22. Mohamed G, Reyes HA, Fantus R, et al: Computed tomography in the assessment of pediatric abdominal trauma. Arch Surg 121:703–707, 1986.
23. Oldham KT, Guice KS, Kaufman RA, et al: Blunt hepatic injury and elevated hepatic enzymes: A clinical correlation in children. J Pediatr Surg 19:457–461, 1984.
24. Pal JM, Mulder DS, Brown RA, Fleiszer DM: Assessing multiple trauma: Is the cervical spine enough? J Trauma 28:1282–1284, 1988.
25. Sandler CM, Raval B, David CL: Computed tomography of the kidney. Urol Clin North Am 12:657–675, 1985.
26. Sty JR, Starshak RJ, Hubbard AM: Radionuclide evaluation in childhood injuries. Semin Nucl Med 8:258–282, 1983.
27. Wall SD, Federle MP, Jeffrey RD, Brett CM: CT diagnosis of unsuspected pneumothorax after blunt abdominal trauma. AJR 141:919–291, 1983.
28. Weissmann HS, Byun KJC, Freeman LM: Role of Tc-ggm IDA scintigraphy in the evaluation of hepatobiliary trauma. Semin Nucl Med 13:199–222, 1983.

CHAPTER TWELVE

Philip B. Kellett

Anesthesia for the Critically Injured Child

This chapter is meant to provide a practical guide to anesthesia for the critically injured child for both the practicing anesthesiologist and the other trauma team members. In many ways pediatric anesthesia is more an art form than a science, but the management of pediatric trauma is an equipment-intensive endeavor best done with a thorough knowledge of the pathophysiology involved. The key to handling severe pediatric trauma is preparation. The anesthesia team, the surgeon, the operating room personnel, the operating room, and the equipment must be ready at all times.

In this chapter we advocate a systematic approach to treatment of the child. This is to facilitate assessment and treatment of the child from the emergency department to the operating room to the critical care units.

PREPARATION AND EQUIPMENT

Trauma patients are usually transported to the hospital by rescue squad or trauma service helicopter, and advance radio communications convey the approximate size and age of the patient, as well as an estimate of the extent of injury, before the patient arrives. This procedure allows awaiting teams to be appropriately prepared for the patient's arrival

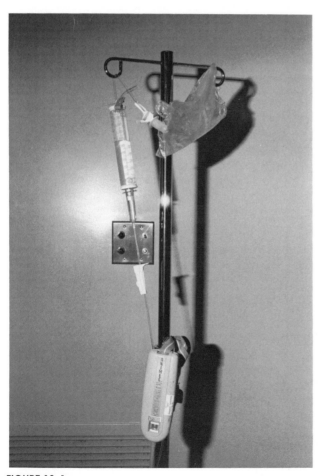

FIGURE 12–1
Animec infuser warmer.

so that necessary studies and interventions can be undertaken, and, if necessary, the child can go immediately to the operating room.

Anesthesia, an equipment-intensive specialty especially for trauma anesthesia, is an integral and extremely important contributor to the care of the injured child. It is imperative that proper pediatric equipment be kept well maintained and ready and that the anesthesia department be ready at a moment's notice to participate in any pediatric trauma case.

Operating Room

The largest piece of equipment is the trauma operating room, which should be reserved for trauma use only. It should be supplied at all times with the necessary equipment for dealing with trauma cases so that the anesthesia personnel do not have to leave the room repeatedly to obtain it.

It is imperative that all trauma patients be maintained as closely as possible to a normal temperature. Hypothermia can contribute significantly to morbidity and mortality both intraoperatively and postoperatively.[59] The injured child can be warmed using heating blankets, blood warmers, heated humidifiers, and direct radiating heating lamps. In addition to keeping the room warm, trauma team members can wrap the child in blankets, foil, or plastic wrap and can keep warming blankets on the operating table, plugged in and operating.

Fluid-Warming Devices

In major injury cases, the child cools rapidly unless all intravenous fluids and blood products are warmed. A pediatric trauma victim might weigh from 3 to 50 kg; hence, the amount of blood transfused in identical injuries, such as a lacerated liver, might vary from 500 ml to 25 liters. It is therefore essential that blood warmers in different sizes be available. Three types are kept in our trauma room with effective flow rates varying from 12 ml per minute to 1500 ml per minute.

To warm fluids and blood products for infants, we use the Animec infusion warmer (Figs. 12–1, 12–2), which has an effective flow rate of 3 to 12 ml per minute. Figure 12–1 shows the warmer being used to heat maintenance fluids, and Figure 12–2 shows the configuration we use to warm blood products. The syringe is attached to a Hemo-nate 18-micron blood filter, which allows warmed, filtered blood to be given in 5- to 10-ml increments.

The American MedicaSystems Model DW 1000 D blood warmer (Fig. 12–3) has an effective flow rate of 270 ml per minute which is suitable for large children or for very rapid transfusions in infants. For major or severe trauma in large children, a Level One Company infusion device with an effective flow rate of 1500 ml per minute is used (Fig. 12–4). However, this device is useful primarily for major or severe injuries, such as liver lacerations.

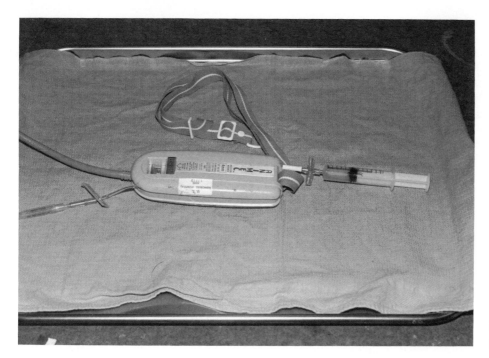

FIGURE 12–2
Animec infuser warmer.

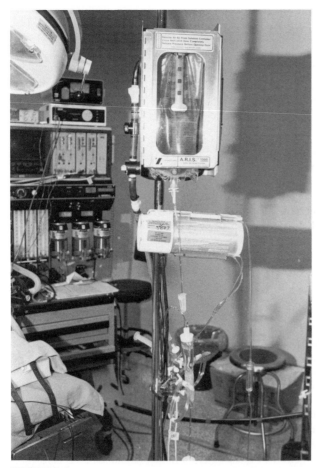

FIGURE 12–3
American MedicaSystems Model DW 1000 D blood warmer.

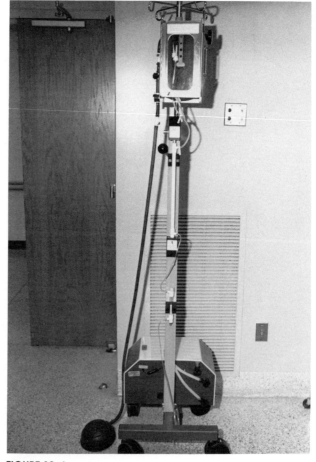

FIGURE 12–4
Level One Company infusion device.

Anesthesia Equipment

The child with multisystem injuries may require separate procedures by the trauma surgeons, the neurosurgeons, the reconstructive surgeons, and the orthopedic surgeons, and the anesthesiologist may be called on to manage the child's physiologic needs for many hours, ranging from providing anesthetic needs to being a short-term intensivist. In patients with chest trauma and lung contusions, the traditional anesthesia equipment and ventilator may not be sufficient to ventilate the patient adequately. We use the Siemens Servo 900C anesthesia machine (Fig. 12–5). To our knowledge, this is the only anesthesia machine that is capable of ventilating the smallest neonate at high frequency to the largest adult with severe respiratory distress syndrome. It is equipped with an end-tidal carbon dioxide monitor and oximeter as well as a three-channel cardiac monitor and other standard anesthesia equipment.

To respond to pediatric emergencies throughout our institution, we utilize a pediatric equipment box (Fig. 12–6). This essential box permits immediate access to all the equipment needed for anesthetizing and resuscitating pediatric patients, including drugs such as ketamine and muscle relaxants that are not kept on the regular resuscitation carts. The boxes are checked for completeness daily.

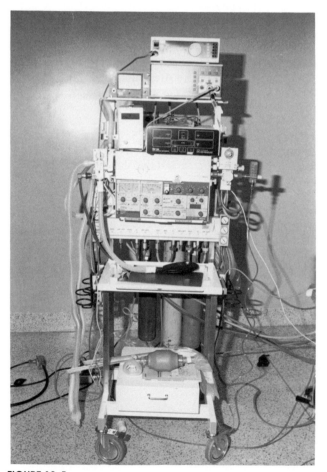

FIGURE 12–5
Siemens Servo 900C anesthesia machine.

INITIAL EVALUATION AND TREATMENT

Predictable patterns occur in pediatric and adult trauma. The approach to initial assessment and treatment of the pediatric patient should follow well-established guidelines for the injured child.[2]

In emergency trauma situations, anesthesia personnel must evaluate and treat the patient's abnormalities simultaneously according to priority, utilizing a "head to toe" approach. This allows the anesthesia personnel to recognize and treat the problems systematically as well as to develop an intelligent plan of action for the patient's hospital course.

Head and Airway

Head injuries occur in 70 to 80% of children with multiple injuries.[42] Initial assessment involves quick evaluation of the color of the skin (e.g., pale, dusky, oxygenated) and the neurologic status (e.g., fully awake and conscious, obtunded, unconscious, or seizing). All of these potential states of consciousness affect how the clinician deals with the first priority—the airway.

Assessment and establishment of a clear airway is accomplished first. An obstructed upper airway might be due to the relatively larger tongue of an obtunded or unconscious child falling back and occluding the airway. This problem can be treated initially by forward displacement of the mandible with the "chin lift" or "jaw thrust" maneuver or, in some instances, by removal of foreign bodies. Foreign bodies in the upper airway must be checked for and removed before any attempt is made to assist the ventilation. Attempts at relieving the airway should be performed rapidly. If no improvement occurs in 15 seconds, one should proceed with the definitive control of the airway with an endotracheal tube, a surgical airway if necessary. The protocol we use for airway management is listed in Figure 12–7. Throughout the initial assessment and treatment of the airway, the patient should receive 100% oxygen by mask.

During attempts at endotracheal intubation, the cervical spine must be protected. The easiest method of protecting the neck is to have an assistant maintain traction on the neck by pulling cephalad on the hair while the intubation is carried out.

There are several techniques for determining proper endotracheal tube sizes. The diameter of the fifth finger or the external nares correlates well with the size of endotracheal tube needed. In children older than 1 year of age, the formula "age (years) + 18 ÷ 4" gives the approximate size in millimeters needed. Owing to the natural subglottic narrowing in children younger than 10 years of age, uncuffed tubes are used. Using the correct size should result in a small air leak.

The method chosen for the establishment of a definitive airway depends on several factors that must be determined during the initial assessment. Facial trauma or evidence of a frontal skull fracture precludes any attempt at a nasal intubation. Severe facial trauma, especially to the mandible, might require an immediate tracheostomy. If it is decided to intubate the patient orally, sedation, and often paralysis,

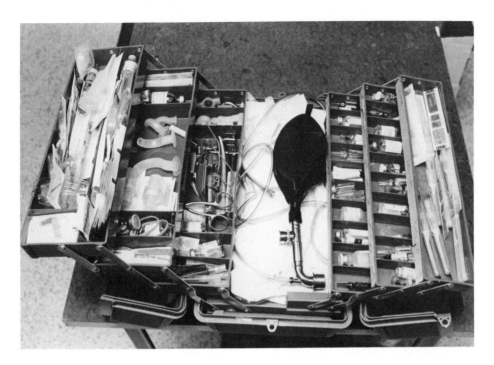

FIGURE 12–6
Pediatric equipment box with equipment for anesthetizing and resuscitating pediatric patients.

is used. Traditionally, the muscle relaxant of choice has been succinylcholine, a 1 mg per kg intravenous (IV) dose or a 5 mg per kg intramuscular (IM) dose, but it is contraindicated in open eye injuries, severe crush injuries, and burns, and some evidence indicates that it can be associated with increased intracranial pressure. The fast-acting, nondepolarizing muscle relaxant vecuronium is a better choice. If rapid relaxation is required, an IV dose of 0.2 mg per kg is given. Although cricoid pressure to prevent aspiration of gastric contents is helpful, care must be taken to avoid airway compression in small children.[37]

Endotracheal intubation must be accomplished within 20 seconds. If initial attempts fail, an oral airway can be

AIRWAY MANAGEMENT

1. Deliver 100% oxygen at airway.
2. Maintain inline traction of the neck or use a Philadelphia collar if the child is older than 4 years.
3. Suction secretions with a large-bore suction; remove foreign bodies.
4. Employ the chin lift or jaw thrust.
5. Ventilate with 100% oxygen by mask.
6. Insert an oral or a nasal airway if needed to maintain the airway.
7. If there is a significant anterior neck injury, *do not* attempt intubation.
8. Employ cricoid pressure if the patient is comatose before inserting an endotracheal tube.
9. Perform endotracheal intubation.
10. Make 30-second attempts at intubation with the oxygen source at the mouth.
11. Ensure 100% oxygen mask–assisted ventilation between attempts.
12. After several unsuccessful attempts at intubation or in cases of an anterior neck injury, perform a cricoidthyroidotomy or tracheostomy.

FIGURE 12–7
Protocol for airway management.

placed, and the patient can be ventilated by mask while cricoid pressure is maintained. If endotracheal intubation cannot be accomplished because of damage to the upper airway or the trachea, the team must proceed to emergency tracheostomy. Tracheal damage can often be predicted if signs of external impact to the neck are visible. If the patient is in a protective neck collar, remember to check beneath it for injury before attempting intubation. The presence of severe impact to the neck in rare instances might necessitate an immediate tracheostomy rather than oral intubation.

Once a definitive airway is established, it is necessary to ensure that the patient is being ventilated, that bilateral breath sounds are present, and that the endotracheal tube is not in the esophagus. In more relaxed situations, the fiberoptic bronchoscope can be an invaluable tool for evaluating neck and facial injuries and for establishing a difficult airway (Fig. 12–8). The endoscope depicted has a 4-mm outer diameter, allowing it to pass through an endotracheal tube with a 4.5-mm inside diameter. For small children, we use the wire guide method when necessary. When the vocal cords are visualized, a soft-tipped Seldinger wire (0.038 inch or 0.09 cm or less) is passed through the cords via the suction port. The scope can be carefully removed, leaving the wire. An endotracheal tube can then be passed over the wire into the trachea.

Thorax

The bony thorax in children is more elastic than that in adults, allowing more compression with less external evidence of trauma and fewer fractures. However, significant pulmonary and myocardial injury can occur, with little or no external signs of injury. Such blunt trauma accounts for 90% of all life-threatening chest injuries in children.[66] Pul-

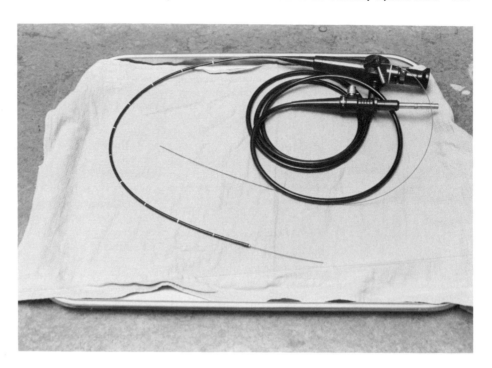

FIGURE 12–8

Fiberoptic bronchoscope with a 4-mm outer diameter.

monary contusions occur in 31 to 76% of all blunt trauma injuries to the chest,[30] with death occurring in 7 to 14% of children older than 5 years of age and 20% of children younger than 5 years of age.[24]

If after the establishment of a definitive airway lung expansion is absent or poor, a cause must be determined and alleviation must be effected promptly. The differential diagnosis includes esophageal intubation, placement of the endotracheal tube or the tracheostomy between tissue planes, foreign body in the trachea, blockage of the endotracheal tube by blood or mucus, tracheal rupture, pneumothorax, hemothorax, severe contusion, or aspiration of blood or stomach contents. The establishment of the correct diagnosis should be done by clinical examination and should be followed by rapid and effective treatment. There is rarely time to wait for a chest radiograph, even though one must be done rapidly as part of the initial workup.

Once ventilation is established the next priority is to ensure that blood is circulating adequately. During the initial auscultation of the chest, the clinician should also listen for heart tones, noting the approximate rate, the quality of the tones, the presence or absence of murmurs, and the position of the apical beat. The majority of cases of hypotension, poor perfusion, or cardiac arrest are due to blood loss or hypoxia. However, direct trauma to the heart must not be overlooked.

Myocardial injury occurs in children and ranges from contusion to myocardial rupture. Contusion results in extravasation of red blood cells into and between myocardial muscle fibers, causing muscle necrosis.[62] More severe trauma can cause rupture of chambers or valves. The right ventricle is the most vulnerable to contusion owing to its proximity to the sternum. A reduction in cardiac output is the most immediate consequence of myocardial contusion, and its incidence has been underestimated.[31, 36, 62] This diagnosis is best made with serial electrocardiogram, two-

dimensional echocardiography, and creatine phosphokinase (CPK)–myocardial band (MB) enzymes.[62]

At this point, we should be ventilating the child and are more than 1 minute into the assessment process. The determination of heart rate, blood pressure, and volume status must be made at the same time as the establishment of intravenous access. The process of obtaining intravenous access can be frustrating and time consuming, particularly in the hypovolemic child. Protocols evaluated for establishing intravenous access showed that effective lines can be placed using a combination of percutaneous peripheral, femoral, saphenous cutdown, and intraosseous infusion if all else fails.[35] Femoral vein catheter insertions were successful in 86% of the children studied but resulted in arterial punctures in 14% and documented thrombi in 11%.[34] Anesthesia personnel usually are more experienced at internal and external jugular catheterization and prefer these over the more hazardous subclavian approach once the cervical spine has been cleared.

As the clinician places intravenous lines, the patient's volume status is being assessed simultaneously. Clinical signs of hypovolemic shock, tachycardia, hypotension, poor peripheral perfusion, and a weak, thready pulse are noted, and appropriate interventions are initiated. Absolute numbers of heart rate and blood pressure that are abnormal are difficult to remember, because the normal heart rate and blood pressure change significantly with the age of the child (Tables 12–1, 12–2), but trends in these numbers are important. These data correlated better with the Advanced Trauma Life Support classification of severity of injury (Table 12–3).

Initial fluid resuscitation in the operating room begins with crystalloid at a dose of 10 to 20 ml per kg and albumin at a dose of 5 to 10 gm per kg of body weight. These doses are repeated until normovolemia is achieved or blood is available. The clinical assessment of volume status is diffi-

Table 12-1
Average Pulse Rates at Different Ages

Age	Lower Limits of Normal	Average	Upper Limits of Normal
Newborn	70	120	170
1–22 mo	80	120	160
2 yr	80	110	130
4 yr	80	100	120
6 yr	75	100	115
8 yr	70	90	110
10 yr	70	90	110

From Kaplan S: The cardiovascular system. In: Nelson, WB (ed): Textbook of Pediatrics. 14th ed. Philadelphia, WB Saunders, 1992, p 1127.

cult, but the insertion of a central venous pressure (CVP) line, an arterial line, and a urinary catheter are all helpful in this regard. Insertion of a central line should have high priority, because a line of adequate size allows not only assessment of volume status, but also rapid administration of large volumes, if needed. It is usually safe to give sufficient crystalloid and albumin to raise the CVP to 10 cm of water.

Abdomen and Extremities

Traumatic disruption of the liver, spleen, kidneys, bladder, or other intra-abdominal structures must also be considered. These potential problems are especially important if the child has other obvious injuries, such as orthopedic trauma. Intraoperative hypotension during an orthopedic case, secondary to a missed splenic rupture, can be a very serious event. Almost all of our children with serious multiple injuries undergo head and torso (nipples to knees) computed tomography (CT) before any operative intervention to identify such injuries and determine severity and need for intervention.

The last area of assessment is the extremities. Fractures, soft tissue injuries, and vascular injuries are sought as they might be missed because of an initial concentration on more lethal or life-threatening injuries. All peripheral intravenous lines are checked to ensure that they are in the correct place to prevent fluids from being infused into the subcutaneous tissues.

Spinal Cord

Acute spinal cord injury can often be diagnosed in severe trauma by careful attention to cardiovascular abnormalities. A study primarily with adults demonstrated persistent bradycardia in all severe cervical cord injuries, along with hypotension, supraventricular arrhythmia, and often cardiac arrest.[38] Mild cervical cord injury or thoracolumbar injury resulted in fewer of these abnormalities. The mechanism is believed to involve acute autonomic imbalance created by the disruption of sympathetic pathways in the cervical cord. Such hypotension often responds to fluid replacement and vasoconstrictor drugs like phenylephrine and dopamine.

Isoproterenol infusion as low as 0.07 mg per minute was found to eliminate sinus pauses and sinus arrest.[38]

In the absence of evidence of spinal cord injury, the anesthesia personnel must always assume injury and protect the back and neck from potential added injury during transport.

TRANSPORT FOR DIAGNOSTIC TESTS

The use of CT has revolutionized the rapid diagnosis and management of injuries for the injured child. Once used primarily for assessment of head trauma, it is now consistently used in the management of chest and abdominal injuries.[13, 51] A serious issue associated with the use of CT scanning is transport of the critically injured child to the radiology suite. If careful monitoring is not used, deterioration of the patient during transport and while away from the critical care environment may occur.[11] Monitors now available have battery-powered electrocardiographs with two pressure channels for use in transport. These monitors, along with portable pulse oximetry, provide excellent monitoring of the patient during this critical interval.

Portable ventilators are also available and can provide continuous ventilation for children with such a need. These ventilators provide, along with appropriate humidity, better control of secretions, carbon dioxide, and oxygenation. Use of complete monitoring and support systems is not new.[18]

A disadvantage of the CT scan is that it requires a motionless patient. For patients not already intubated, this presents a dilemma. Because many injured children are uncooperative and sometimes combative, we often administer pancuronium bromide (Pavulon) and intubate these children to protect their airways and allow more aggressive management of their discomfort while at the same time enabling optimal utilization of CT, which is so helpful in diagnosing the presence and the severity of all injuries. Equipment and

Table 12-2
Normal Blood Pressure for Various Ages
(Adapted from data in the literature. Figures have been rounded off to nearest decimal place.)

Age	Mean Systolic ± S.D.	Mean Diastolic ± S.D.
Newborn	80 ± 16	46 ± 16
6 mo–1 yr	89 ± 29	60 ± 10*
1 yr	96 ± 30	66 ± 25*
2 yr	99 ± 25	64 ± 25*
3 yr	100 ± 25	67 ± 23*
4 yr	99 ± 20	65 ± 20*
5–6 yr	94 ± 14	55 ± 9
6–7 yr	100 ± 15	56 ± 8
7–8 yr	102 ± 15	56 ± 8
8–9 yr	105 ± 16	57 ± 9
9–10 yr	107 ± 16	57 ± 9
10–11 yr	111 ± 17	58 ± 10
11–12 yr	113 ± 18	59 ± 10
12–13 yr	115 ± 19	59 ± 10
13–14 yr	118 ± 19	60 ± 10

*In this study the point of muffling was taken as the diastolic pressure.
From Nadas AS, Fyler DC: Pediatric Cardiology. 3rd ed. Philadelphia, WB Saunders, 1972.

Table 12-3
Advanced Trauma Life Support Classification of Shock

Class I	Class II	Class III	Class IV
15% acute blood volume loss or less Blood pressure normal Pulse 10–20% No change in capillary refill	20–25% loss of blood volume Tachycardia >150 beats per minute Tachypnea 35–40 breaths per minute Capillary refill prolonged Systolic blood pressure decreased Pulse pressure decreased Orthostatic hypotension >10–15 mm Hg Urine output >1 ml/kg/hr	30–35% blood volume loss All of the above signs Urine output <1 ml/kg/hr Lethargic, clammy, vomiting	40–50% blood volume loss Nonpalpable pulses Obtunded

trained personnel must be available in the CT suite for such management as necessary.

SECONDARY EVALUATION

Once the initial evaluation and treatment are accomplished, we perform a secondary survey to assess damage to organ systems that might alter plans for anesthesia. Evaluation is best done in a head to toe fashion, with decisions made at each organ system as to what effect such injury may have on the intraoperative as well as the postoperative course.

Scalp lacerations, usually of low priority in major multiple injuries, can result in significant blood loss. Unless controlled, they may continue to bleed for several hours while more urgent problems are managed, despite the initiation of temporary measures that are usually limited to the application of pressure dressings. Definitive control may be necessary to avoid this problem.

During surgery an avulsed tooth can be forgotten while major organ systems are treated. Teeth found during the preoperative period can be reinserted slowly but firmly back into an irrigated socket with light compression for several minutes.[14] An oral surgeon can then place splints to ensure reimplantation, if necessary.

Head injuries occur in 70 to 80% of children with multiple injuries.[42] Many factors are responsible for this increased susceptibility of the child. The head is larger in relation to body size than that of the adult, the brain has less myelination, and the cranium is thinner and less developed. A neurologic exam needs to be done by the anesthesiologist during evaluation using the Glasgow Coma Scale and pupillary findings. Changes in pupils may be the only signs of cerebral deterioration during surgery and should be done frequently.

Early signs of pulmonary contusion include blood suctioned from the endotracheal tube and subcutaneous emphysema. Fluffy exudates on chest radiographs and arterial hypoxemia in suspected chest injuries suggest pulmonary contusion. This injury results in edema, hemorrhage, and atelectasis of the pulmonary parenchyma and can result in serious and immediate hypoxemia and respiratory distress if it is not considered and measures are not undertaken to manage it.

The anesthesiologist must be careful in the management of head and pulmonary injuries to avoid overhydration and excessive fluid in the damaged lung. A pulmonary artery catheter for measuring the pulmonary artery occlusion pressure can be helpful in minimizing this overload while optimizing oxygen delivery to the tissues.

In severe cases, ventilatory support with positive end-expiratory pressure (PEEP) may be necessary and must be available for transport and in the operating room. Therapy for children is similar to that for adults, with support being determined by severity of hypoxemia and respiratory parameters. Serial arterial blood gases and serial chest radiographs need to be monitored carefully.[57]

INDUCTION OF ANESTHESIA

The procedure for induction of anesthesia in the child should be the same whatever the location. If definitive airway control is needed in combative head injury patients to allow CT scanning, the procedure, equipment, and drugs used should be the same as those for inducing anesthesia in the operating room.

The airway in the injured child requires diligent consideration for many reasons. The trachea and pharynx are small, but the tongue is large for body weight.[25] The larynx is more cephalad and anterior than in adults, lying at the level of the third cervical vertebral body. The vocal cords are cartilaginous, distensible, and easily damaged. In addition, the trachea is one half the length of an adult's, leading to more frequent endobronchial intubations.

In our judgment, blind nasotracheal intubation in the presence of facial trauma is contraindicated. Introduction of foreign material (blood, bone, teeth) into the trachea can occur without direct visualization, and damage to the airway by passing a tube through injured tissue can also occur. Passage of any tube such as a nasogastric tube can lead to intracranial placement in the presence of basilar skull fracture.[29] Also nasal intubations in children even without facial trauma are complicated by the presence of adenoid tissue large enough to obstruct the endotracheal tube.

Oral endotracheal tubes are placed in less time, require less skill to place than nasal tubes, and are preferred in emergency airway control. If postoperative ventilation is required, a nasotracheal tube can then be placed under more controlled conditions, allowing better fixation of the tube for the care providers as well as greater comfort for the child.

The goal for induction of anesthesia is to render patients amnestic and insensible to pain. Although a study in adults documents an incidence of recall of 43% during surgery in the trauma patient,[9] no induction agent is ideal, and the selection of drugs for induction is dependent on the hemodynamic stability of the child. The incidence of recall must be balanced against the decreasing sympathetic tone induced by these drugs.

Ketamine, a "dissociative anesthetic," in IV doses of 1 to 2 mg per kg can provide a rapid onset of amnesia and analgesia for most pediatric trauma patients. Wide variations exist in the dose and dosage of ketamine needed to prevent movement during surgery.[40] There is still controversy regarding the use of this drug in the hypovolemic patient. Cardiovascular changes may be identical to those produced by thiopental and sometimes even worse, at least in animals.[64] In shock models, ketamine is associated with greater survival rates than the use of halothane.[41] Blood pressures are better maintained with this drug but at the expense of tissue perfusion.[65] We believe that ketamine is a useful drug for the induction of anesthesia, although it does have the potential for increasing both intracranial and intraocular pressure.[16]

If thiopental is used as an induction agent, the available data confirm that children generally need more drug than adults.[33] The thiopental dose necessary for fast, reliable induction in healthy children older than 1 year of age was found to be 5 to 6 mg per kg; in infants younger than 1 year, 7 to 8 mg per kg were needed. These doses are reduced in the hypovolemic child.

Narcotic induction using fentanyl is the method we use most often in patients that we believe will need postoperative assisted ventilation. Given at an IV dose of 10 to 20 µg per kg, fentanyl provides analgesia but does not produce unconsciousness and amnesia. It can be used in combination with reduced doses of thiopental or ketamine. Fentanyl at 20 to 50 µg per kg can produce unconsciousness, although not consistently. Amnestic drugs still must be used at this dose.

Midazolam is a water-soluble benzodiazepine, which, when used as an induction agent, provides amnesia during the maintenance phase. Shown to be an effective induction agent in high-risk adults, it still has the hypotensive effects of the other intravenous induction drugs.[1, 50] More studies are needed to confirm its reliability in pediatric trauma situations because recent data reveal that the drug does not produce consistent loss of eyelid reflex in healthy children.[54]

If the child's blood pressure is normal and intubation and ventilation for head or pulmonary injury are required, a rapid sequence induction technique is recommended. Intravenous thiopental, 4 to 5 mg per kg, and intravenous lidocaine, 1.5 mg per kg, along with a muscle relaxant, serve to accomplish this while controlling intracranial pressures.

Anesthesiologists have long considered succinylcholine as the muscle relaxant of choice for the rapid sequence induction technique frequently necessary in the trauma pa-

tient. Although newer relaxant drugs and techniques offer some advantages over succinylcholine, the latter still produces the fastest onset of intubation conditions, usually 60 seconds or less. If succinylcholine is used, the IV dose should be 1 mg per kg.

Complications of succinylcholine administration fall into three groups. The most dangerous is the hyperkalemic response secondary to the exaggerated release of potassium during muscle fasiculations. Conditions that can produce this response in an acute trauma situation are preexisting neuromuscular disease, renal failure, crush injuries, and burns. Although rare, this release of potassium can occur in closed-head injury patients or even in healthy children, causing hyperkalemic cardiac arrest.[20] Succinylcholine administration is also associated with significant increases in intraocular pressure.[21, 44] Despite this, a large number of patients with open eye injuries were studied using succinylcholine for paralysis. When nondepolarizing pretreatment was used, no significant expulsion of global contents occurred.[39] Lastly, succinylcholine produces increased intragastric pressures in adults; however, it does not appear to do this in children.[53]

The intermediate-duration nondepolarizing relaxants, vecuronium and datracurim, are rapidly replacing succinylcholine and even pancuronium for rapid sequence intubations. The use of these drugs avoids the side effects of succinylcholine while achieving almost equal intubation time.

We believe the drug of choice when succinylcholine is contraindicated is vecuronium. Rapid onset can be achieved with the use of the "priming principle." Vecuronium in doses of 0.02 mg per kg, followed in 2 to 3 minutes by 0.08 mg per kg, can provide intubating conditions in 90 seconds or less while maintaining cardiovascular stability.[45]

An alternative drug is atracurium besylate, given as a priming dose of 0.05 mg per kg followed in 2 to 3 minutes by 0.4 mg per kg. An advantage is its unique metabolism via the Hoffman reaction making it especially suitable in patients with renal failure.[61] Its disadvantages are the hypotension caused by histamine release and the possible increases in intraocular pressure.[19]

Using the priming dose of these drugs may induce significant muscular weakness, increasing the time that the airway is at risk. This may be avoided by giving large single doses of vercuronium of 0.2 to 0.4 mg per kg, which results in intubating "conditions" in less than 90 seconds but longer duration of action.

For rapid reversal of neuromuscular blockade edrophonium chloride is the drug of choice. Atropine, 10 to 15 µg per kg, followed 30 seconds later by 1.0 mg per kg of edrophonium generally results in the return of muscle function in 2 minutes.[27] An alternative drug choice is neostigmine, 70 µg per kg. The best assessment of return of neuromuscular function is sustained tetanic response; this should always be measured regardless of relaxant and antagonist use.

MAINTENANCE OF ANESTHESIA

Once anesthesia is induced and an airway established, anesthesia is best maintained with narcotics, nondepolarizing muscle relaxants, and low concentrations of inhalation anesthetics.

If the patient is cardiovascularly stable, morphine, fentanyl, and sufentanil are all acceptable narcotics. In the unstable patient, we prefer fentanyl in doses of 1 to 3 μg per kg per hour because it has more stable cardiovascular effects. We find vecuronium to be an excellent relaxant for maintenance because of the cardiovascular stability it affords and its relatively short duration of action. Maintenance requirements are in the range of 0.05 to 0.1 mg per kg per hour. Our choice of inhalation agents is isoflurane because of its apparent lack of toxic side effects.

Nitrous oxide should be avoided initially in all trauma cases. One hundred percent oxygen should be used until adequate arterial oxygen levels are documented. The use of nitrous oxide is harmful in the presence of a pneumothorax. The administration of a 75% nitrous oxide mixture can double the volume of a pneumothorax in thirty minutes.[23] The impact of a rapidly expanding pneumothorax may be difficult to detect in a hemodynamically unstable trauma patient.

MANAGEMENT OF FLUIDS

During the initial assessment of the pediatric trauma patient, the clinician not only must assess the patient's volume and fluid status, but also must act rapidly to correct any deficiencies. The clinical signs of hypovolemic shock, tachycardia, hypotension, poor peripheral perfusion, and thready peripheral pulses are all well known to the experienced physician. Clinical symptoms are listed in Table 12–3 to help in the assessment of blood loss.

The immediate priority is, of course, the placement of intravenous lines and the administration of crystalloid—lacerated Ringer solution or normal saline—to initiate the correction of the intravascular deficits. In the previously healthy injured child, the immediate administration of 10 to 20% of the child's blood volume in the form of crystalloid is a safe initial procedure.

It is then important to obtain further invasive cardiovascular monitors that allow the clinician to assess the degree of hypovolemia, including an arterial line, a CVP line, and a urinary catheter. The CVP line gives the best initial measuring of the patient's blood volume.

In the initial resuscitation, the hematocrit is of limited value, because acute blood loss does not lower the hematocrit until blood volume is restored. After the initial resuscitation, the clinician can assess accurately the total blood loss, the acceptable blood loss, and the patient's requirements for the administration of blood.

Clinically, anesthesiologists have tended to use a hematocrit of 30% and a hemoglobin of 10 gm per 100 ml as levels that suggest the need for blood. The objective of fluid resuscitation should be the restoration of normal blood volume with an adequate mass of red blood cells. Clinically, this state will be evidenced by near normal heart rates, blood pressure, and CVP, with a urine output of a minimum of 1 ml per kg per hour. In this context, a urinary catheter is as valuable, if not more valuable, than a CVP line, especially after the initial resuscitation.

Formulas that list predetermined volumes of crystalloid to be given in set circumstances are difficult to follow. We recommend estimating accurately the maintenance fluids necessary for each child and then giving sufficient extra fluid for the child to produce 1 to 2 ml of urine per kg per hour (Table 12–4). Fluid requirements may be as high as 10 to 20 ml per kg per hour in severe abdominal trauma.

Although the crystalloid versus colloid controversy continues, we replace extracellular fluid losses with either 0.9% saline or Ringer lactated solution. Enough glucose, usually 4 to 6 mg per kg per minute, should be given to keep blood glucose levels in the normal range. The glucose can be given via a separate line, using 5% dextrose and water, or can be mixed with the crystalloid solutions.

Blood loss must be replaced with three times its volume of crystalloid until allowable blood loss is exceeded. Class III or IV patients should have blood loss replaced with blood. The best way to determine volume of blood present and amount of crystalloid needed is by frequent assessment of volume status and hematocrit level.

TRANSFUSION

Anesthesiologists are responsible for more than 50% of the blood transfused in the country.[60] The rapid infusion of cold, packed red blood cells is facilitated by the use of warm crystalloids as a diluent. Solutions that contain calcium, such as lactated Ringer, may cause the formation of small clots because the amount of calcium exceeds that of the citrate anticoagulant.[52] This is especially likely to happen because of the slow rate necessary for infusing small children. Hypotonic solutions are contraindicated because they cause clumping of cells or hemolysis.

Large-volume infusions of normal saline can result in a hyperchloremic nonanion gap metabolic acidosis from dilutional loss of bicarbonate with chloride replacement.[6] A more appropriate diluent for large volumes may be Plasma-Lyte or Normosol-R. These are solutions that contain no calcium but do contain acetate that a functioning liver can convert to bicarbonate.

A still somewhat controversial practice is using filters with a pore size of 170 μm for the administration of red blood cell products, platelets and granulocyte concentration, fresh frozen plasma, and cryoprecipitate. The use of microaggregate (20–40 μm) filters has not been shown to

Table 12–4
Fluid Requirements

Maintenance		
Weight	Fluids	Totals
1–10 kg	4 ml/kg/hr	4–40 ml
11–20 kg	2 ml/kg/hr	40 + ml
≥21 kg	1 ml/kg/hr	60 + ml

Trauma Requirement (in addition to maintenance)

Mild (e.g., craniotomy): 2 ml/kg/hr
Moderate (e.g., thoracotomy): 4 ml/kg/hr
Severe (e.g., abdominal surgery): 6 ml/kg/hr

reduce the incidence of respiratory distress syndrome after multiple transfusions but does appear to reduce febrile reactions.[60] The recommended starting volume for transfusion in the child is 20 ml per kg for whole blood and 10 ml per kg for packed red blood cells.[26]

The most common coagulopathy following massive transfusions is dilutional thrombocytopenia. Significant bleeding from thrombocytopenia in massive transfusion is unlikely unless 1 to 2 blood volumes are replaced.[49]

Platelet counts lower than 50,000 per ml or significant bleeding that is believed to be secondary to a platelet disorder should be treated with platelet transfusions.[15] The pediatric dose of platelets is 1 unit per 10 kg of body weight. Each unit of platelets also contains 50 to 70 ml of plasma, so ABO blood type–compatible platelets are used if possible.

Fresh frozen plasma should be reserved for patients with multiple transfusions or patients who have documented coagulation defects.[63] There is no evidence to support the prophylactic administration of fresh frozen plasma to trauma patients.[60] If given, fresh frozen plasma should be infused in volumes of 20 ml per kg.

Posttransfusion hepatitis is estimated to occur in 7 to 10% of transfused patients, and 87% of these have non-A, non-B hepatitis.[10] The transmission of acquired immunodeficiency syndrome (AIDS) occurs in 1 in 100,000 to 1 in 1,000,000 units transfused.[28] Although children account for 12% of these transfusion-related transmissions, they are primarily in the population with congenital bleeding disorders. Owing to the reduced number of total units of blood transfused in the pediatric populations, this incidence is lower for a given patient. Despite widespread testing, the risk probably never will be eliminated.[43]

The use of the new erythrocyte preservative AS-1 in many hospitals has led to a longer shelf-life for blood of up to 42 days. Although the hematocrit of 59 plus or minus 5% is less than that obtained with other preservatives, it does allow for infusion rates equal to that of whole blood.[47]

METABOLIC RESPONSE TO SURGERY

A series of articles demonstrated the functional integrity of the autonomic nervous system and the stress response of neonates undergoing surgery.[3, 5, 32, 48] However, there is little knowledge about the metabolic and endocrine response of the injured child to trauma.

In noncardiac surgery there is a marked release of the catabolic hormones, catecholamines, glucagon, and growth hormone. The main anabolic hormone, insulin, shows inhibition during surgery.[3] These hormonal responses to surgery and trauma may lead to altered substrate mobilization and increased catabolism in the postoperative period. In adults, some evidence indicates that this may lead to increased morbidity and mortality.[4] The data concerning neonates and infants are unclear, but these hormonal releases may be particularly harmful owing to the poor metabolic reserves of infants and the increased metabolic demands.[3] The anesthesia used and its ability to block these effects may determine the postoperative course in the trauma patient.

POSTOPERATIVE MANAGEMENT

In most institutions the operating room and the pediatric intensive care units are not in close to each other. The transition from the operating room to the pediatric intensive care unit can be very hazardous unless appropriate equipment is used and correct protocols followed. The following checks should be made:

1. Ensure that the unit is ready with the ventilator set up and the transducers calibrated.
2. Ensure that the elevator is ready.
3. Ensure that the child is stable and has an adequate blood volume.
4. Ensure that the child is moved with the appropriate monitoring, oximetry, electrocardiogram, and blood pressure equipment necessary.

In severe injuries, continuing resuscitation may need to be done in the pediatric intensive care unit, with the administration of large volumes of blood, blood products, and fluids. In such situations, the critical care unit must be properly equipped with blood warmers and other appropriate equipment, as well as with the staffing to continue the care that is provided intraoperatively. The anesthesia team should not leave the unit until the patient is stable or is under the care of the receiving physician.

Pain control in the postoperative period is a seldom discussed topic in regard to the pediatric patient. Information is sparse, but occasionally physicians have surgery and report the inadequacy and horror of postoperative analgesia.[12] Reports have indicated that the problem is worse in children.[8, 55, 56] Common beliefs are that children tolerate pain better than adults and need medication less often. However, there is limited support in the literature for neurologic differences between adults and children.[56] If an injury causes pain in an adult, it causes pain in a child, yet physicians are less likely to order narcotics for infants and young children, and when they do, it is at half the frequency.[55] Infants cannot verbalize their need for pain medications, and older children may not know appropriate ways to verbalize their distress and fear of ''needles,'' so they often remain silent. We believe that the comfort of and pain control for injured children in the postoperative—indeed the postinjury—period is extremely important. Frequently, we leave these infants and children paralyzed and intubated to allow maximum pharmacologic control of pain or discomfort and anxiety.

Physiologic clues to such pain, such as increased heart and respiratory rate and increased blood pressure, are helpful indications to provide this relief safely.[8] Unrelieved pain can start a cycle of anxiety, sleep deprivation, fear, and helplessness, which is often difficult to control.[46]

Excellent discussions are available for pain control in the injured child.[7] New treatment options such as the use of intercostal nerve blocks[58] and lumbar and thoracic epidural anesthesia[17, 22] are now being used more frequently.

References

1. Adams P, Gelman S, Reves JG: Midazolam pharmacodynamics and pharmacokinetics during acute hypovolemia. Anesthesiology 63(2):140–146, 1985.

2. American College of Surgeons, Committee on Trauma: Advanced Trauma Life Support Course. Chicago, 1985, pp 1–78.

3. Anand KJS: Hormonal and metabolic functions of neonates and infants undergoing surgery. Curr Opin Cardiol 1:681–689, 1986.

4. Anand KJS: The stress response to surgical trauma: From physiological basis to therapeutic implications. Prog Food Nutr Sci 10:67–132, 1986.

5. Anand KJS, Sippell WG, Azinsley GA: Randomized trial of fentanyl anaesthesia in pre-term babies undergoing surgery—Effects on the stress response. Lancet 1(8524):62–66, 1987.

6. Appel GB, Chase HS: Diagnosis and treatment of acid base disorders. In: Askanazi J, Stoaker PM, Weissman C (eds): Fluid and Electrolyte Management in Critical Care. Boston, Butterworths, 1986, pp 145–170.

7. Bean JP, Rogers MC: Anesthetic considerations and pain management in the pediatric intensive care units. In: Rogers MC (ed): Textbook of Pediatric Intensive Care. Baltimore, Williams & Wilkins, 1987, pp 1347–1381.

8. Beyer JE, DeGood DE, Ashley LC, et al: Patterns of postoperative analgesic use with adults and children following cardiac surgery. Pain 17(1):71–81, 1983.

9. Bogetz MS, Katz JA: Recall of surgery for major trauma. Anesthesiology 61:6–9, 1984.

10. Bove JR: Transfusion-associated hepatitis and AIDS—What is the risk. N Engl J Med 317(4):242–245, 1985.

11. Braman SS, Dunn SM, Arnico CA, et al: Complications of intrahospital transport in critically ill patients. Ann Intern Med 107:469–473, 1987.

12. Bryan-Brown CW: Development of pain management in critical care. In: Cousin MJ, Phillips GD (eds): Acute Pain Management. New York, Churchill Livingstone, 1986, pp 1–20.

13. Buntain WL: Splenic trauma. In: Hurst JM (ed): Common Problems in Trauma. Chicago, Year Book, 1987, pp 78–89.

14. Cleary P, Spolnik K, Barton PJ: The avulsed tooth: A treatment rationale. J Irish Dent Ass 32:7–10, 1986.

15. Consensus Conference: Platelet transfusion therapy. JAMA 257:1777–1780, 1987.

16. Cunningham AJ, Barry P: Intraocular pressure—Physiology and implication for anaesthetic management. Can Anaesth Soc J 33(2):195–208, 1986.

17. Dalens B, Haberer JP: Epidural anesthesia in children (letter). Anesthesiology 66(5):714–715, 1987.

18. Dawson ADG, Babington PCB: An intensive care trolley—An economical and versatile alternative to the mobile intensive care unit. Anaesth Intensive Care 15:229–233, 1987.

19. Dear GL, Hammerton DJ, Hatch TD: Anaesthesia and intraocular pressure in young children. Anaesthesia 42:259–265, 1987.

20. Delphin E, Jackson D, Rothstein P: Use of succinylcholine during elective pediatric anesthesia should be reevaluated. Anesth Analg 66(11):1190–1192, 1987.

21. Eakins KE, Katz RL: The action of succinylcholine on the tension of extraocular muscle. Br J Pharmacol 26:205–211, 1966.

22. Ecoffet C, Dubousset AM, Samii K: Lumbar and thoracic epidural anaesthesia for urologic and upper abdominal surgery in infants and children. Anesthesiology 65:87–90, 1986.

23. Eger EI: Pharmacokinetics. In: Eger EI (ed): Nitrous Oxide. New York, Elsevier, 1985, pp 81–107.

24. Erchelberger MR: Airway and thorax trauma. Pediatr Ann 16(4):307–316, 1984.

25. Eichelbarger MR: Airway management. Proceedings of the Pediatric Trauma Conference. Pediatr Emerg Care 2(2):131–135, 1983.

26. Eichelberger MR, Randolph JG: Pediatric trauma—An algorithm for diagnoses and therapy. J Trauma 23(2):551–553, 1985.

27. Fisher DM, Cronnelly RS, Shauna M, et al: Clinical pharmacology of edrophonium in infants and children. Anesthesiology 61:428–433, 1984.

28. Friedland GH, Klein RS: Transmission of the human immunodeficiency viruses. N Engl J Med 317(18): 1125–1135, 1987.

29. Galloway DC, Grudis J: Inadvertent intracranial placement of a nasogastric tube. South Med J 72(2):240–244, 1975.

30. Haller JA Jr, Buck J: Does a trauma-management system improve outcome for children with life-threatening injuries? Can J Surg 28(6):477, 1985.

31. Harley DP, Mena IM, Miranda R, et al: Myocardial dysfunction following blunt chest trauma. Arch Surg 118:1384–1387, 1983.

32. Harris BH: Pediatric trauma (editorial). J Pediatr Surg 22(1):1–2, 1987.

33. Jonmarker CW, Westring PL, Sylvia A, et al: Thiopental requirements for induction of anesthesia in children. Anesthesiology 67(1):104–107, 1987.

34. Kanter RK, Zimmerman JJ, Strauss RH, et al: Central venous catheter insertion by femoral vein: Safety and effectiveness for the pediatric patient. Pediatrics 77(6):842–847, 1986.

35. Kanter RK, Zimmerman JJ, Strauss RH, et al: Pediatric emergency intravenous access. Am J Dis Child 140:132–136, 1986.

36. Kron IL, Cox PM: Cardiac injury after chest trauma. Crit Care Med 11(7):524–526, 1983.

37. Lawes EG, Campbell I, Mercer D: Inflation pressure, gastric insufflation and rapid sequence induction. Br J Anaesth 59(3):315–318, 1987.

38. Lehman KG, Lane JG, Piepmeier JM, et al: Cardiovascular abnormalities accompanying acute spinal cord injury in humans: Incidence, time course and severity. J Am Coll Cardiol 10(1):46–52, 1987.

39. Libernati MM, Leahy JJ, Ellison N: The use of succinylcholine in open eye surgery. Anesthesiology 62:637–640, 1985.

40. Lockhart CH, Nelson WL: The relationship of ketamine requirements to age in pediatric patients. Anesthesiology 40:507–511, 1974.

41. Longnecker DE, Sturgill BC: Influence of anesthetic agents on survival following hemorrhagic shock. Anesthesiology 45:516–521, 1976.

42. Marion WL, Stors BB, Mayer TA: Spinal cord injury. In: Mayer TA (ed): Emergency Management of Pediatric Trauma. Philadelphia, WB Saunders, 1985, pp 249–253.

43. Napier JAF: AIDS and blood transfusion (editorial). Br J Anaesth 59(6):669–671, 1987.

44. Pandy K, Gudda RP, Sumer S: Time course of intraocular hypertension produced by suxamethonium. Br J Anaesth 44:191–194, 1972.

45. Payne JP: Atracurium. In: Katz RL (ed): Muscle Relaxants. Orlando, Grune & Stratton, 1985, pp 87–101.

46. Phillip GD, Cousins MJ: Neurological mechanism of pain and the relationship of pain, anxiety and sleep. In: Cousins MJ, Phillips GD (eds): Clinics in Critical Care Medicine—Acute Pain Management. New York, Churchill Livingstone, 1986, pp 21–48.

47. Pineda AA, Rypiteau ND, Claire DE, et al: Infusion flow rates of whole blood and AS-1 preserved erythrocytes—A comparison. Mayo Clin Proc 62:199–202, 1987.

48. Poland RL, Roberts RJ, Gutierrez-Mazorra JF, et al: Neonatal anesthesia. Pediatrics 80(3):446, 1987.

49. Reed RL, Cavarella D, Heinback DM, et al: Prophylactic platelet administration during massive transfusion. Ann Surg 203:40–48, 1986.

50. Reitan JA, Scliman IE: A comparison of midazolam and diazepam for induction of anesthesia in high-risk patients. Anaesth Intensive Care 15(2):175–178, 1987.

51. Reyes HM, Fantus R: Computed tomography in the assessment of pediatric abdominal trauma. Arch Surg 121:703–707, 1986.

52. Ryder SE, Oberman HA: Compatibility of common intravenous solutions with CPD blood. Transfusion 15:250–255, 1975.

53. Salem MR, Wong AY, Lin JH: The effects of suxamethonium on the intragastric pressure in infants and children. Br J Anaesth 44:166–170, 1972.

54. Salomen M, Kanto J, Iisalo E, et al: Midazolam as an induction agent in children: A pharmacokinetic and clinical study. Anesth Analg 66(7):625–628, 1987.

55. Schechter NL: Pain and pain control in children. Curr Probl Pediatr 15(5):1–67, 1985.

56. Schechter NL, Allen DA, Hansen K: Status of pediatric pain control: A comparison of hospital analgesic usage in children and adults. Pediatrics 77(1):11–15, 1986.

57. Shackford SR, Virgilio RW, Peters RM: Selective use of ventilator therapy in flail chest injury. J Thorac Cardiovasc Surg 81:194–201, 1981.

58. Shelby MP, Park GD: Intercostal nerve blockade for children. Anaesthesia 42:541–544, 1987.

59. Slotman GJ, JED EH, Burchard KW: Adverse effects of hypothermia in postoperative patients. Am J Surg 149(4):495–501, 1985.

60. Stehling L: Question-answers about transfusion practices. Committee on Blood Products of the American Society of Anesthesiologists. Park Ridge, Ill, American Society of Anesthesiologists, 1987.

61. Stenlake JB, Waigh RP, Urwin J, et al: Atracurium: Conception and inception. Br J Anaesth 55:3S–10S, 1983.

62. Tenzer ML: The spectrum of myocardial contusion: A review. J Trauma 25(7):620–627, 1985.

63. Tullis JL: Fresh frozen plasma. Indication and risk. Consensus conference. JAMA 253:551–553, 1985.

64. Weiskopf RB, Gogetz MS, Roezin MF, et al: Cardiovascular and metabolic sequelae of inducing anesthesia with ketamine or thiopental in hypovolemic swine. Anesthesiology 60:214–219, 1984.

65. Weiskopf RB, Townsley MI, Riordan KK, et al: Comparison of cardiopulmonary response to graded hemorrhage during enflurane, halothane, isoflurane and ketamine anesthesia. Anesth Analg 60:481–492, 1981.

66. Yaster M, Haller JA: Multiple trauma in the pediatric patient. In: Rogers MC (ed): Textbook of Pediatric Intensive Care. Baltimore, Williams & Wilkins, 1987, pp 1265–1322.

Specific Systems Considerations

John D. Ward

Craniocerebral Injuries

Trauma is the leading cause of death in the pediatric age group over the age of 1 year.[61] At least half of these traumatic deaths are due to a head injury. Annegers and colleagues studied head trauma in Olmstead County, Minnesota, from 1935 to 1974 and found a mortality rate from head injury to be 16 per 100,000 for boys under the age of 5 years and 12 per 100,000 for boys between 5 and 14 years of age. The rate for girls was 5 per 100,000 and 6 per 100,000, respectively.[4] These are just the mortality rates. The rate of head injury in general is approximately 200 per 100,000, which makes it a common problem in the pediatric population. If quality survival is to be obtained, these children need to be treated aggressively and appropriately.

The purpose of this chapter is to provide the background, general principles of care, and specific details about pediatric head injuries so that they can be handled appropriately. It should be recognized that what is presented here is one way of dealing with the difficult problem of head injury in children. There are certainly other ways to care for the variety of problems that arise. Significant controversy over a particular aspect of care is indicated with the presentation of opposing views, which, it is hoped, will lead to a balanced approach to the difficult yet common problem of pediatric head injury.

UNIQUE FEATURES OF THE IMMATURE BRAIN

One of the most striking differences between the pediatric and the adult brain is that of size. This is true in terms of the absolute size of the brain and its size relative to the rest of the body. At birth, the brain comprises 15% of the body's weight, an amount that decreases steadily to 3% in the adult. Relative to the rest of the body, the brain grows fairly rapidly and reaches 75% of its adult weight by the second year of life and more than 90% of its adult weight by the sixth year of life.[20] When these facts are coupled with the facts that the neck musculature of the child is not strong at birth and its head control is poor, it is clear that the brain in the younger child (up to 2–3 years) is at risk for acceleration and deceleration injuries that are uncommon in older children and adults. This combination of factors led Caffey to postulate the concept of the *shaken baby*.[13] Although current studies have thrown portions of this concept into question, it can still be appreciated that the infant and early toddler are at a mechanical disadvantage compared with the adult.

In the young child, the skull is also different from that of the older child and adult. Up to approximately 3 years of age, the skull of the child has unfused sutures. In addition, it is thinner and more pliable. Direct blows to the skull, therefore, tend to cause more local deformation and, to a limited extent, to absorb some of the force of the impact and convey less force of the blow to areas of the brain remote from the area of impact. This applies only when velocity and force are low. In addition to differences in the container properties of the skull in the young child and the adult, there are structural and physiologic differences in the brain itself. The cortical neurons are formed at about 10 to 25 weeks of gestation, with a peak at 14 weeks, and once

developed are unable to form new elements.[43] The one exception to this are the neurons in the cerebellum, which continue to form until about 2 years of age. Dendritic process formation and differentiation is gradual and begins at about 14 weeks of gestation and continues up to 6 years of age.[57] Finally, there is a gradual process of myelination of fibers, which in some areas can continue into the second decade of life. It is believed that the timing of myelination of a fiber system correlates well with its onset of function.[75] The earliest areas to undergo myelination are the cranial nerves and the spinal roots, which are completed by term. The pyramidal tracts are completed after the second year of life, and the reticular system myelination continues on into adult life. Little work has been done on the actual elastic properties of brain tissue in the young, but it seems that the unmyelinated brain tissue of the infant and young child is more susceptible to shearing injuries than that of the older child or adult.

Certain physiologic differences may make the young child more susceptible to injury. As will be shown later, the ability of the brain to maintain normal cerebral blood flow (CBF) is quite important. Some studies indicate that autoregulation in newborns is not well developed.[44] However, other investigators have shown that the neonate may handle anoxia and hypoxia better than the adult.[16]

One of the more popularized concepts regarding the differences between the child and the adult brain is that the concept of the plasticity of the central nervous system. This idea is based on the observation that young children are able to sustain injuries and recover function whereas their older counterparts are not. The best examples are injuries to the left hemisphere of children who, if under the age of 5 years, may recover quite well.[43]

In summary, therefore, the skull and brain of children and adults differ significantly, with the differences being most marked early in life and less so as the child approaches maturity. It is important to realize that whenever a child suffers a head injury, there damage is done not only to the current structures but also to the process by which the immature nervous system progresses to a mature state. Recovery, therefore, means regaining not only what was present at the time of the accident but also the ability to mature beyond the incident to a normal functioning adult central nervous system. When caring for a young child, it is important to keep in mind the significant differences between the young brain and its response to injury and that of the adult.

MECHANISM OF INJURY

The mechanism of injury or cause is an important factor in determining the extent of injury and, therefore, the outcome for the injured child. The incidence of different injuries varies depending on the severity of injury under consideration, the age group, the economic situation, and the geographic location. However, some general statements can be made. If pediatric head injuries are considered as a whole, regardless of the severity of the neurologic injury, then falls are the most common cause of head injury in the pediatric age group and occur in approximately 35% of patients.[36] In this group, motor vehicle injuries account for around 25%. If, however, only patients with severe injuries are considered, then motor vehicles account for about 75 to 80% of the injuries. Falls drop to about 15%.[16, 27, 52] Superimposed on these statistics is an age factor. In a series of patients from Norway who had all types of head injury, Lundar and Nestvold looked at children from 0 to 4 years, 5 to 9 years, 10 to 14 years, and 15 to 19 years. He found motor vehicle accidents as the cause of the head injury in 23%, 47%, 65%, and 82%, respectively.[45] Clearly in the older age groups, the automobile is the major cause of head injury, both moderate and severe. Other causes are peculiar to the pediatric age group. The walker or stroller has been implicated in causing significant injury to the face and head, especially when the child falls downstairs.[60, 74] Recreational vehicles, such as the all-terrain vehicle, have been the frequent subject of articles on head injury in the pediatric age group.[37, 68] Clearly, these mechanisms of injury have characteristics that suggest steps to be taken in the future to decrease the number of preventable head injuries in children. The final significant cause for head injury in children is child abuse. This is discussed in a separate section of this chapter (see also Chapter 35).

PATHOLOGY AND PATHOPHYSIOLOGY OF HEAD INJURY

It is useful to divide the types of injury that the brain sustains into primary—that which occurs at the moment of impact—and secondary—that which occurs as the result of hypoxic or ischemic insult to an already damaged brain.

Fractures of the skull are sustained as a primary injury. The degree of tissue damage to the brain is more severe in the more severely damaged child. The main injuries that the tissue sustains are contusions and lacerations. Contusions usually occur over the poles of the frontal and temporal lobes and on the orbital surface of the frontal lobe and the undersurface of the temporal lobe. This is where the brain comes into contact with the wall or bony protuberances of the skull.[2] Initially, there is extravasation of blood into the tissues, which, over time, becomes small scars of gliosis. In the young infant, the typical surface contusion does not appear as often. More common are tears in the white matter parallel to the surface and tears in the superficial cortical layers.[46] In addition, the incidence of contrecoup lesion is quite small in the infant. This difference exists until about 5 months of age.[42]

In addition to the more localized injury, a more diffuse type of injury occurs in severe head trauma. *Diffuse axonal injury* consists of diffuse injuries to the axons, lesions in the corpus callosum, lesions in the dorsal brain stem, and lesions in the cerebellar peduncles.[1] Pathologically, diffuse injury is seen initially as retraction bulbs in the white matter. Later, there is an aggregation of microglia and eventually wallerian degeneration.[2] The duration of coma and the degree of diffuse axonal injury seem to be related.[25] It is believed that this diffuse axonal injury occurs at the moment of impact and not as a result of some secondary insult. This type of injury has also occurred to a less severe degree in experimental models of mild to moderate head injury.[56]

Other structures sustain primary damage during a head injury; the cranial nerves, especially the second, sixth, third, and seventh, are either contused or stretched at the moment of impact. The hypothalamus and pituitary stalk may also be damaged, resulting in signs of deficiency of hormones located in these areas (i.e., diabetes insipidus).

After the brain has sustained primary damage, several complications can occur that, if left untreated, result in the secondary insults of hypoxia and ischemia. These are diffuse cerebral swelling and intracranial bleeding (e.g., epidural, subdural, and intracerebral hematoma) and are discussed in the section on specific problems.

Secondary injuries are those that occur to the brain as a result of hypoxia, ischemia, or direct compressive damage from shift. The brain is dependent on receiving an adequate supply of nutrients to sustain cellular function; as a whole, it has little capacity to store these essential nutrients to draw on if they become scarce. If the supply of oxygen is insufficient, which can occur in up to 30% of adult patients, the brain can undergo hypoxic damage that will be added onto the primary damage that has already occurred.

Ischemia to the brain can occur in one of two ways. First, the blood pressure can drop from some systemic injury such that perfusion to the brain is compromised. If this is allowed to continue, ischemia and infarction of brain tissue occur. Second, blood pressure may be adequate, but owing to cerebral swelling or an intracranial hematoma, intracranial pressure may rise. The result is compromised blood flow to the brain, from which ischemic damage results.

Similarly, if the patient is allowed to get hypoglycemia or develop a severe intracranial infection, further damage can occur after the original injury has taken place. All efforts after the initial head injury has occurred are aimed at preventing, if possible, and treating, if necessary, all secondary injuries so that the brain can recover whatever cellular function is salvageable after the initial injury.

BASIC PRINCIPLES AND PHYSIOLOGY

Several basic principles should be kept in mind when caring for a child with a severe head injury. The first is that the central nervous system has a very difficult time regenerating itself. Although some evidence indicates that some regeneration can take place, it is difficult for significant damage to be repaired. It is, therefore, better to prevent damage than to try and recoup lost function. The second principle is that a damaged nervous system is less able to protect itself from secondary insults. Therefore, it is the job of the physician to assume that any change in neurologic status is organic and needs to be investigated. It may be that a child is less responsive because he or she is tired, but this should not be assumed unless appropriate tests have been carried out. The third principle is that a child in a coma from trauma is an emergency and should be evaluated and investigated as if a space-occupying lesion were present.

Several basic physiologic principles are also important in the understanding of central nervous system trauma management. Much of what is applied to the care of pediatric patients was learned from the care of adult patients. This is true of cerebral homeostasis. In the infant and toddler, some of the concepts have yet to be proven. However, in the school-aged child through the adolescent age group, much of what has been shown for the adult can be applied.

In general terms, the brain must have sufficient CBF to meet its metabolic needs. Cerebral blood flow is felt to be about 50 ml per 100 gm of brain tissue per minute in the older child and adult.[34] It is probably lower in the newborn and infant. What constitutes adequate flow to the brain is a difficult question. The answer depends on the age of the patient, the current metabolic activity, and other factors. Most believe that ischemic damage can occur when CBF falls below 18 to 20 ml per 100 gm of brain tissue per minute.[35] It should be remembered that flow may vary from region to region of the body; hence, it may be adequate in some areas and insufficient in others. The bottom line is that CBF must be adequate to supply nutrients to meet the metabolic needs of the entire brain.

At least four variables have a significant effect on CBF: (1) systemic blood pressure; (2) arterial blood gases; (3) metabolic demands of the brain; and (4) intracranial pressure (ICP). It is useful to think of the relationship of blood pressure to CBF in terms of the formula $CPP = MAP - ICP$[30]: cerebral perfusion pressure (CPP) is equal to mean arterial pressure (MAP) minus ICP. If accurate, and it is believed to be, it implies that high flows exist in patients while they are having seizures[8] and low flows when metabolism has been suppressed, such as because of high doses of barbiturates. To understand the relationship between flow and metabolism, the formula $CMRO_2 = CBF \times AVDO_2$ is helpful. This says that the metabolic rate of the brain (in this case that for oxygen) is equal to the blood flowing through the brain times the amount of oxygen that is extracted from the blood as it flows through the tissue. When there is a mismatch between flow and metabolic need, metabolic uncoupling is said to have occurred. As is discussed later, this is seen when blood flow is high (hyperemia) through a brain that is badly damaged with a low metabolic rate.

Having looked at the complexities of CBF, it is necessary to examine the concept of ICP: what are its causes, its relationship to CBF, and its importance in the understanding and care of the child with a head injury? Intracranial pressure is the pressure measured in the ventricle, subarachnoid, subdural, or epidural space. Under many circumstances, these pressures are similar, so people have come to equate them all with ICP. As is shown later, this may not always be accurate. When discussing ICP, it is necessary to know where it is being measured. Ventricular pressure is the usual standard against which other measurement techniques are compared.

It is important to the understanding of ICP that it be seen as a pressure that is the result of a constantly changing interplay of several systems: (1) the cerebrospinal fluid (CSF) system; (2) the cerebral blood volume, both venous and arterial; and (3) the brain tissue with both intra- and extracellular fluid. Each of these systems exerts a pressure, the cumulative end result of which is termed ICP.

Another important concept to grasp is that for practical purposes, the volume of the craniospinal contents is constant and incompressible and that any added volume or enlargement of an existing volume must be balanced by an equal loss of an existing volume or ICP will rise.[38] This can be seen in Figure 13–1, in which ICP is plotted against a volume that is added to the intracranial contents and the compartments of the intracranial cavity are represented schematically by boxes. The boxes representing blood volume and CSF change size if there is an added mass in the head (e.g., an epidural or a subdural hematoma) and there is no immediate rise in ICP. However, if the mass reaches a size that can no longer be compensated for, the ICP rises rapidly. This accounts for the lucid period that can sometimes be seen in a patient with an epidural hematoma. It can also be seen that the situation at the initial portion of the curve is quite different from that at the portion of the curve just before it rises.

In the first situation, the patient is able to compensate if some additional mass is added, such as an expansion of a clot or a transient increase in the blood volume compartment as seen with a high arterial carbon dioxide tension ($PaCO_2$). However, if the patient is in the second situation with all compensatory mechanisms exhausted, then any small increase in volume results in a precipitous rise in ICP with resultant possible compromise in CPP and CBF. It is, therefore, useful to visualize each patient as being on this curve. It is the task of the patient's caregivers to see that the patient remains on the initial portion of this curve. If this is not possible and ICP rises, then the various compartments (e.g., CSF, blood volume) are manipulated to lower the patient's ICP and to return the patient to the initial portion of the curve. This, in short, is the way ICP is controlled in the patient with a head injury.

The methods of ICP monitoring and indication of ICP control are discussed later. However, a brief account of how ICP is controlled is appropriate at this point. As was mentioned earlier, control of ICP is accomplished by acting on the various systems that contribute to its maintenance. The CSF compartment can be decreased in size by the introduction of a ventriculostomy and with subsequent periodic drainage. Cerebrospinal fluid is formed at the rate of 0.33

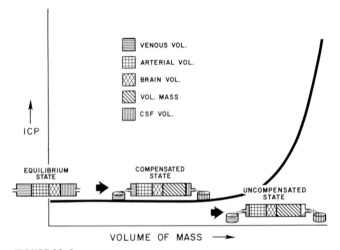

FIGURE 13–1

Pressure volume curve with the various compartments illustrated with boxes. Note that when mass increases in size, some compartments decrease in size to compensate. CSF, Cerebrospinal fluid.

ml per minute, 20 ml per hour, or about 400 to 500 ml per day.[15] Probably the rate of CSF production is a bit lower for newborns and infants.[73] By removing this fluid, a considerable amount of compensation can be achieved. The blood volume compartment is manipulated in several ways. First, care is taken not to impede veins in the neck so pressure does not build up in the cerebral veins. To some extent, this is the rationale for elevation of the head in these patients. As was mentioned earlier, the size of the blood volume compartment can be quickly and significantly affected by altering the $PaCO_2$. With hyperventilation of the patient to a $PaCO_2$ of 25 to 30 mm Hg, a significant drop in ICP can be achieved.[28] This is, in fact, the first level of treatment for a patient with an ICP problem.

Another method of ICP control is controversial. It involves accepting the concept that if the patient is autoregulating and if the blood pressure is raised, the patient should vasoconstrict because additional CBF is not needed and there will be a resultant drop in ICP.[26] Obviously, this technique should be performed cautiously because if the patient is not autoregulating, the ICP will rise as the blood pressure is elevated. In addition, some work indicates that one of the mechanisms by which mannitol exerts its effect is vasoconstriction secondary to increased CBF because of decreased viscosity when mannitol is administered.[51]

The brain can be manipulated directly only by removal. This is not currently recommended unless there is contused, necrotic brain tissue present and it is exerting a mass effect. The removal of edematous but otherwise normal brain is not usually a reasonable option. Osmotic and loop diuretics are used quite frequently. The presumed site of effect is on extracellular water in normal brains. This, however, continues to be a controversial issue. However, ICP can be lowered quite effectively by the use of mannitol, usually in doses of 0.25 to 2.0 gm per kg. The amount is governed by the rapidity and extent of rise in ICP and the current serum osmolality. Furosemide can also be used to control ICP. Its onset of action is not quite as rapid as that of mannitol, and it does not lower the ICP quite as much.[55, 63] Glycerol and urea are used much less and have only a restricted indication.

If ICP is to be treated, it is important to know when to start and at what level. Normal ICP is felt to be up to 10 mm Hg. From 10 to 20 mm Hg, pressure is felt to be elevated but is probably not detrimental per se. However, for pressures higher than 20 mm Hg, many people recommend treatment, and almost all believe ICP should be kept under 25 mm Hg if possible.

Ideally, the decision on what level of ICP to treat is based on an exact knowledge of what the current ICP is doing to brain function, electrical activity, the reserve of the brain, CBF, and metabolism. Because in most circumstances this information is not available, the following guidelines seem reasonable. If any clinical deterioration occurs at any ICP, then treatment will be given until a cause is determined and the neurologic deterioration is altered. If there is no change in a patient's neurologic function, then ICP should be kept under at least 25 mm Hg. The reasons for this are several. First, the ICP may go higher before treatment can be effective. Second, CPP should be kept in the normal range of around 60 mm Hg. If mean blood pressure is running about 70 to 80 mm Hg, then an ICP of 20 would accomplish this. Third, if ICP is kept in this range, the patient may better tolerate other insults that may occur. It can be seen that much of this is empirical, although there is some evidence for a tighter control of ICP at these suggested levels in patients with head injuries.[64]

The final topic of ICP has to do with the monitoring device. Many times the device with which the neurosurgeon is most familiar and comfortable is the one used. However, the ventricular catheter is the device that is most accurate and provides for CSF drainage. It can be difficult to insert in the presence of small ventricles and is associated with a certain risk of infection.[48] The subarachnoid or Richmond bolt and all its variants are easier to insert, have a lower incidence of infection, usually do not afford the possibility of drainage, and can be inaccurate at higher pressures. The epidural devices are easier to insert, have almost no infection rate, allow no drainage, are probably the least accurate owing to drift, have problems with dural tension if not inserted correctly, and have no means of calibration. The most recent device is the Camino catheter. It is a fiberoptic cable; is easy to insert either in the subdural, subarachnoid, or ventricular space; and has little drift; but does not afford the possibility of CSF drainage unless used in a ventricular catheter.[53]

Regardless of the device used, several things should be remembered. There should be familiarity with the device, its proper insertion, when it is accurate, and when it is malfunctioning. If ICP monitoring is to be employed, the numbered output should be able to be used and interpreted appropriately. The nursing staff should be well trained in ICP monitoring. Also, it should be remembered that ICP is a number and is only one variable that indicates how the patient is doing. Knowing a patient's ICP is not a substitute for examining the patient and should not take precedence over a careful and complete assessment of the patient's clinical condition.

EVALUATION AND CARE

The care of a child with a head injury begins at the moment of injury and continues until the child has reached as full a recovery as possible. It is important to realize that many events that occur early in the patient's course can have a profound effect on recovery. A child who has a potentially nondisabling injury can, with improper care, be left with a profound disability. It is therefore imperative to keep in mind the basic principles and ideas that have been covered in the earlier sections of this chapter when considering the evaluation and care of the child with a head injury.

At the scene it is important to remember the basic tenets of critical care: attention to the airway and circulatory status of the patient. Someone at the scene should not try to determine the extent of neurologic injury but rather be sure that the patient has an adequate airway and a pulse and blood pressure. Care should then be exercised to prevent further injury to the patient. Any movement of the child should be done with careful support of the neck and head.

The exact incidence of cervical spine fracture in patients with severe head injury is not known. However, it has been estimated at about 7 to 10%. Therefore, any patient with a head injury should be considered to have a cervical spine injury until proven otherwise. If the expertise is available, all patients who are unconscious should be intubated. If intubation is not possible and if a skilled specialist is available, the patient should have a cricothyrotomy. It should be stressed that this procedure is for the older child and adolescent. These types of maneuvers can be quite difficult in the young child and infant and should be performed only by those specifically trained in these skills.

The child should be taken from the field to the nearest trauma center where there are neurosurgeons and a 24-hour operating room capability. This usually means to the nearest level I trauma center. Even if other hospitals are a little closer, time is saved and definitive care can be given more quickly if the child with a significant head injury is taken to a level I center.[69] If a level I center is not within a reasonable travel time and distance, then these children should be taken to the next level center.

In the emergency department, attention is focused initially on vital signs. As was mentioned, all patients who are unconscious should be intubated, if possible, or have a cricothyrotomy or tracheostomy. It has been well shown, at least in the adult, that patients with a severe head injury have a significant incidence of respiratory compromise and that patients who are hypoxic after their injury do worse than those who are not.[21, 49] Thus, providing an adequate airway prevents the secondary insult of hypoxia to an already injured brain. Care should be exercised in the insertion of the airway. If the patient is to be intubated, it should be done by those skilled in intubating children, and the patient probably should be paralyzed before intubation to avoid coughing and bucking that would elevate the ICP, which could be detrimental in the presence of a mass lesion. Obviously, the patient needs a quick neurologic assessment before the administration of any paralyzing agents. Concurrent with airway placement, adequate intravenous access should be instituted. Fluids and blood should be administered as indicated to maintain a normal circulating vascular volume. Fluids should not be restricted in the patient with a head injury unless there is a problem in another body system. Much more damage can be done if the patient has a marginal vascular volume and becomes hypotensive. If balanced isotonic solutions are used, the risk of brain edema being promoted by the administration of fluid is low.

After vital functions are stabilized, an adequate neurologic examination should be performed. The neurologic examination does not need to be exhaustive. It should answer the following questions: (1) How badly is the brain damaged?, (2) Are there any focal signs?, and (3) is the patient getting better, worse, or staying the same? To answer these questions, the following components of the neurologic examination are necessary: an assessment of level of consciousness, pupillary function, brain stem function, and motor function. Each of these is examined in a little more detail.

Level of Consciousness. The level of consciousness is best evaluated by the Glasgow Coma Scale (GCS).[70] This score is also being used with increasing frequency by rescue squads and emergency personnel so the patient's clinical progress can be assessed. Basically it consists of an assessment that is based on a patient's motor response ranging from obeying commands to flaccid, eye opening response ranging from spontaneous to none, and speech response ranging from answering appropriately to mute. A number is assigned for each level of functioning in each category. The numbers are then summed, and a total score is assigned (Fig. 13–2). The normal patient has a GCS of 15, whereas the brain dead patient scores 3. A severe head injury is indicated by a GCS of 8 or less. The advantage of this scoring method is that it can be used by persons with dissimilar backgrounds and yield reproducible and similar results.

Pupillary and Brain Stem Function. The GCS is not sufficient to assess brain injury, so an evaluation of pupillary function and oculovestibular (brain stem) function is also added. In checking the pupils, a sufficiently strong light must be used. Both the direct and consensual response should be elicited. The oculovestibular response can be assessed by using either the doll's eye response or the caloric response with iced saline. If the caloric test is done, care should be taken that the tympanic membrane is intact. If the doll's eye maneuver is chosen, then the cervical spine should be cleared for the presence of a cervical fracture. Each of these two tests checks the integrity of the vestibular pathway, starting at the inner ear, along the eighth cranial nerve, and into the pons and the vestibular nuclei. From there the impulses travel up the brain stem via the medial longitudinal fasciculus to the third and sixth cranial nerve nuclei. Impulses then travel via the respective nerves to the muscles of the eyes, causing them to move appropriately. If this reflex is intact, then a significant portion of the brain stem is functioning. However, if impairment of this response has occurred and the peripheral components of the system (i.e., third nerve) are intact, there has been brain stem damage and the outcome is worse.

Motor Function. The ability of the limbs to move as well as their asymmetry of movement is evaluated. It

GLASGOW COMA SCALE

Eye opening	E	4
spontaneous		3
to speech		2
to pain		1
nil		
Best motor response	M	6
obeys		5
localizes		4
withdraws		3
abnormal flexion		2
extensor response		1
nil		
Verbal response	V	5
oriented		4
confused conversation		3
inappropriate words		2
incomprehensible sounds		1
nil		

Coma score (E + M + V) = 3 to 15

FIGURE 13–2

Glasgow Coma Scale. (Adapted from Teasdale G, Jennett B: Assessment of coma and impaired consciousness. Lancet 2:81–84, 1974. © The Lancet, 1974.)

should be noted that it is unusual for a patient with a head injury not to have any movement. If a patient is unable to move the limbs, then the evaluator should think of the possibility of abnormal vital signs, spinal cord injury, alcohol or drug intoxication, the use of paralyzing agents by another treating facility, or brain death. Otherwise, the patient should show some sort of movement, even if it is abnormal.

Other parts of the neurologic exam can be done but often are not necessary. An assessment of the fundi is usually unproductive. The reflexes are often increased in a severe brain injury, and, in addition, it is not unusual for the patient to have the Babinski reflex as well. If the neurologic examination demonstrates focal signs that may suggest a mass lesion, then the measure discussed earlier for the control of ICP should be done. The child is hyperventilated, mannitol is started, blood pressure is maintained, and steps to diagnose a mass lesion are carried out as quickly as possible.

The laboratory that is needed for the patient with a severe head injury is similar to that for any trauma patient. It is useful for an ethanol level and a toxic screen to be sent because these substances can alter the neurologic examination. If the patient might need surgery, sufficient blood should be typed and cross matched, because surgery will have to be done expeditiously. Coagulation studies should be sent because there is a high incidence of the results of at least one of them being abnormal and a 40% chance of the results of at least three studies being abnormal.[50] If abnormalities are recorded, the patient should be treated with fresh frozen plasma and platelets as indicated. It is not appropriate to wait for bleeding to occur.

The radiographic procedure of choice in a patient with a severe head injury is a computed tomography (CT) scan,[11, 71] and any child who is not normal after a head injury should have a CT scan. To wait until a child who is lethargic shows focal signs or progressive neurologic deterioration is not appropriate, as there is a 25% incidence of mass lesions in children who are admitted and unable to obey commands or worse.[72] Because these children can deteriorate, rapid diagnosis is imperative before significant neurologic damage can occur. If the child is too unstable to take to the CT suite and must go immediately to the operating room, then an air ventriculogram can be performed, looking for an operative mass lesion.[5] A good rule of thumb when dealing with children who have had any type of head injury is to get a CT scan if you have any doubts about the diagnosis. Even if the initial CT scan is normal, a repeat CT scan is indicated at any point the child shows a change for the worse neurologically because delayed hematoma, cerebral swelling, or edema around a contusion can occur as a late development.[9, 29] If the patient is deteriorating rapidly, there may not be sufficient time for a CT scan, in which case the child is taken to the operating room where burr holes, a craniotomy, or both are performed on the side indicated by the focal signs. Fortunately, this is a rare occurrence, and usually sufficient time is available to make an adequate diagnosis. The role of magnetic resonance imaging (MRI) in head trauma is still being developed. Currently, it has no routine place in the acute workup of the severely injured patient. However, MRI is able to show

lesions and edema better than the CT when used in the patient with a milder head injury and in the evaluation and follow-up of the more stable patient with a severe injury.[24, 40]

If a mass lesion is diagnosed, proper steps should be initiated to control elevated ICP, and then the child should be taken immediately to the operating room and the mass managed. Afterward the child should be moved to an intensive care setting where appropriate care and monitoring are given. There is not sufficient space to discuss in detail the intensive care of the child with a head injury. However, a few important points should be stressed.

I believe that the ICP of all children who were unconscious from a head injury before surgery or who had no mass lesion but are in coma should be monitored and that this monitoring should continue until they are awake or until their ICP has been at a normal $PaCO_2$ for at least 24 hours. In addition, any child who worsens and becomes unconscious should be monitored very closely in the critical care unit.[10] The aim of intensive care of the patient with a head injury is to maintain a normal physiologic environment to allow whatever recovery is possible.

The decision to admit the child with a severe injury is not difficult. However, the choice between admission and observation and discharge can be difficult when evaluating the child with a mild or moderate head injury. Table 13–1 is a list of criteria used at the Medical College of Virginia to determine whether a child should be admitted. Some of the items such as seizures and the presence of a deficit are obvious. Others such as length of unconsciousness are not. In the final analysis, the physician should feel fairly comfortable that the child is stable neurologically before the time of discharge. If there is any uncertainty, the child should undergo further tests or periods of observation.

SPECIFIC PROBLEMS

Specific problems are discussed in this section. The basic principles that have been covered are operative in all these conditions. Even though these problems are discussed separately, it should be recognized that in many patients several of these conditions can occur at the same time. Often, one condition may predominate, such as an acute subdural hematoma, while another coexisting lesion, such as a skull fracture, seems to require less immediate attention. However, they will have interacting influences, and therefore each problem should be recognized, investigated, watched, and managed as indicated.

Table 13–1
Criteria for Admission

Any neurologic deficit
Seizure
Vomiting
Severe headache
Fever
Skull fracture
Prolonged unconsciousness
Altered mental status
Any unexplained injury (child abuse)

Skull Fractures

The overall incidence of skull fractures in patients who present to the emergency department with head trauma is approximately 27%.[31] However, this number rises to about 40% if only the children with a GCS of 8 or less are considered. Skull fractures are linear (Fig. 13–3) if there is no malalignment of the two tables of the skull. A skull fracture is considered to be depressed if either the inner or outer table (usually both) are driven below the surface of the skull. This usually happens when a large amount of force is exerted over a small area of the skull. Linear fractures are usually of no clinical consequence other than as evidence that sufficient trauma has occurred to fracture the skull and that other possible intracranial lesions should be considered and watched for. There is some controversy over whether the presence of a linear skull fracture in the absence of any neurologic abnormality or loss of consciousness changes the course of treatment. However, some physicians admit a child if an acute linear skull fracture is found. Admission is probably not indicated for children who arrive in the emergency department 24 hours or more after trauma with a linear skull fracture but no evidence of neurologic abnormalities. If a child has just received a skull fracture, the development of an intracranial hematoma or other neurologic problem is probably more dependent on other factors such as the loss of consciousness and the presence of neurologic abnormalities. However, it has been our policy to admit all children who have been shown to have a linear skull fracture and observe them for a 24-hour period. If the linear fracture occurs in one of the sutures, it is termed a *diastatic fracture*. The most common suture when this occurs is the lambdoid suture. When diastatic fracture occurs, a careful watch for epidural hematomas is appropriate. One of the uncommon complications of a linear skull fracture is that of a leptomeningeal cyst or growing skull fracture. This problem usually occurs only in children under the age of 3 years. It appears as a nontender pulsatile growing mass in the same location as the fracture. Its treatment is usually surgical.[39] Therefore, it seems rea-

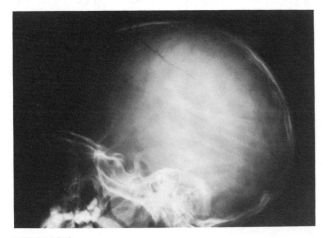

FIGURE 13–3
Linear skull fracture. Note the dark linear density at the top of the skull.

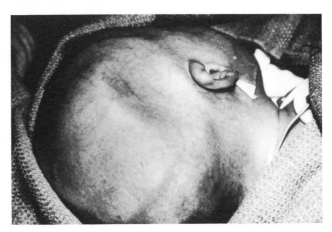

FIGURE 13–4
Depressed skull fracture in tempoparietal area.

sonable to obtain a follow-up skull radiograph in all children under the age of 3 years who have had a linear skull fracture.

Depressed fractures are those in which the tables of the skull are no longer at the same level (Fig. 13–4). A depressed fracture is not usually considered to be different from a linear fracture until it is depressed at least the thickness of the skull. If there is no break of the skin over the depressed fracture, it is termed a *simple fracture*. If there is a laceration, then it is called a *compound depressed skull fracture*. The treatment of depressed fractures depends on the location of the fracture, the extent of the depression, and whether there is an opening in the scalp. All depressed fractures that are compound and have an obvious penetration of the dura as manifested by CSF leak, intracranial air, or obvious brain tissue are operated on. Depressed fractures that are below the thickness of the skull and over the motor strip are elevated. The rest are evaluated on an individual basis. Antibiotics are usually started in a compound skull fracture that is to be operated on.

Basilar fractures are through the base of the skull, usually through the anterior fossa floor or through the temporal bone. The incidence in pediatric head injury is about 3 to 4%.[17] Associated clinical signs include CSF leaking through the nose (rhinorrhea) or ear (otorrhea); bruising of the skin over the mastoid bone (Battle sign); injury to the olfactory nerve, facial nerve, or eighth nerve; and meningitis. Thus, the importance in the diagnosis of a basilar skull fracture lies not in the fracture itself but in the associated complications. The controversy about the use of prophylactic antibiotics is long and involved. The bottom line is that antibiotics are probably not indicated in the presence of a basilar skull fracture, with or without a CSF leak.[17, 32, 33] Patients with a basilar skull fracture are admitted and observed for at least 48 hours to determine if they will develop any of the complications mentioned previously.

It is perhaps appropriate to conclude the section on skull fractures with a brief discussion of their radiographic diagnosis. There has long been a controversy regarding the method that is used to decide whether to obtain skull radiographs. Some argue that skull radiographs should be taken routinely so that a patient with a skull fracture is not missed. The opposing view is that the too frequent use of skull films is not economically responsible and that criteria should be used to maximize the yield of positive skull radiographs. This argument may never be resolved; however, a prospective study involving a number of institutions and 7035 patients has shed some light on the controversy. The patients were divided into low-, medium-, and high-risk groups. Those in the low-risk group had trivial head injuries, headaches, or a little dizziness, no other symptoms but could have a scalp hematoma, laceration, or contusion. No one in the low-risk group had an intracranial injury, and no injury would have been missed had skull radiographs been omitted in this group.[47]

Brain Swelling

Diffuse brain swelling occurs in both the adult and the pediatric age group. Bruce and colleagues originally reported that as many as 29% of conscious and 40% of unconscious children with head injuries develop this problem.[9] Obrist and associates have shown that this may be a rather frequent condition in the adult patient as well, although the patients tended to be the younger adults.[52] The appearance of this condition on CT is manifested by small ventricles and compressed or absent cisterns. The cause of this cerebral swelling is believed, in some cases, to be hyperemia with metabolic uncoupling.[52] The course may be subtle, with the child initially doing satisfactorily and then becoming obtunded with headache, nausea, and vomiting that progresses to coma. The treatment is first to monitor ICP to determine its level and then to institute hyperventilation, initially starting at a $PaCO_2$ of 25 to 30 mm Hg. This level can be lowered further to 20 to 25 mm Hg as needed. If this treatment is not effective along with paralysis and sedation, the use of mannitol is indicated, although mannitol may not be effective if the mechanism is removal of brain water. However, if the mechanism suggested by Muizelaar and co-workers is correct in that it works at least in part by vasoconstriction, then it may be effective.[51] If these measures do not hold ICP below a reasonable level (i.e., 25 to 30 mm Hg for most of the time), the use of barbiturates is indicated.[9]

Epidural Hematoma

The overall occurrence of epidural hematomas in the pediatric head injury population is about 2.6%,[14] with a somewhat higher incidence in the more severely injured patient of about 6 to 7%.[10] It is a lesion that tends to occur in the younger patient population, with 60% occurring in those under the age of 20 years.[23] It is quite clear that these lesions can occur with or without a skull fracture. It is believed that they originate from a tear in a vessel in the dura, usually a branch of the meningeal artery. Because they are arterial in origin, these lesions can expand quite quickly. These hematomas usually occur supratentorially, although they can also occur in the posterior fossa.[3] When they do, deterioration can progress quite rapidly. The diagnostic procedure of choice is CT scanning. On CT, an

epidural hematoma has a lens-shaped appearance (Fig. 13–5).

The clinical presentation can occur in one of several ways. The first is the more classical way, with the child sustaining an injury with a period of consciousness, which is then followed by a gradual decline in the level of functioning, followed by the classic signs of herniation, and leading to irreversible brain damage if untreated. The second is the patient who has suffered significant brain damage in association with the extradural hematoma. The patient presents in coma with a certain picture of neurologic damage and then deteriorates further as the expanding clot causes further compromise. The third clinical presentation is the patient who has a head injury but is neurologically intact. The CT scan shows a small epidural hematoma without shift or compromise of the cisterns. These patients do quite well and usually do not require surgery.

The treatment for the other two groups of patients is surgical. The result is dependent on the clinical condition of the patient at the time of surgery. It is, therefore, mandatory that the diagnosis and treatment of these lesions be carried out as soon as possible. These patients can deteriorate quite rapidly, and treatment should not be postponed. The only time it is proper to observe a patient with an epidural hematoma is if the patient is normal and alert, the CT does not show significant shift, and the cisterns are normal. The patient who qualifies for observation is followed in the intensive care unit and taken immediately to the operating room if any sign of deterioration occurs.

It has been suggested that an emergency burr hole be placed if a neurosurgeon is not available immediately. If the patient is in a remote place and cannot be transported to an appropriate facility within an hour or so, this might be a reasonable alternative. However, in the majority of circumstances, the patient can be stabilized and improved with intubation, hyperventilation, and mannitol such that those treating the patient can "buy time" until the patient

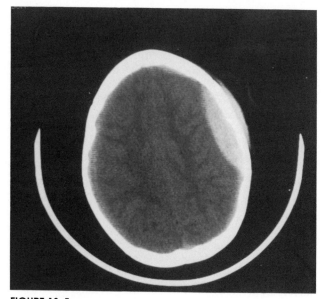

FIGURE 13–5

Epidural hematoma. Note the high-density lens-shaped clot.

can be transported to an appropriate facility. In addition, it is very difficult to remove clotted blood through a small hole.

Overall, the mortality for patients with an epidural hematoma is about 18%.[58] However, if the comatose patients are analyzed, the mortality jumps to 41% with half of these patients having an associated cerebral contusion.[65] It is, therefore, reemphasized that the better the patient's condition before surgery, the better the outcome, pointing to the need for prompt transportation, appropriate stabilization, aggressive diagnosis, and rapid treatment.

Subdural Hematoma

It is useful in the pediatric age group to separate the subdural hematomas into two groups: acute and chronic. Subacute subdural hematomas occur but are not common. The acute subdural hematoma in the newborn is most likely due to tearing of a bridging vein from the sagittal sinus. As a result, a large number of acute subdural hematomas occur in the interhemispheric fissure. Other possible mechanisms that could cause these hematomas include tearing of the dura, direct trauma to the brain with tearing of a cortical vein, and tearing of a sinus.

Birth trauma is a cause of subdural hematoma in 23.5% of newborns with a head injury from birth.[62] It usually occurs as a result of birth trauma to the head secondary to a fetal head–maternal birth canal disparity. The incidence of breech delivery in these infants is high. The location of the subdural hematoma may be supratentorial or, less commonly, in the posterior fossa. These infants present with a globally depressed state with decreased motor activity, a poor cry, and diminished reflexes. Seizures may be present, and if the ICP increases, the fontanelle will be tense and bulging. The most reliable method of diagnosis is the CT scan (Fig. 13–6). Subdural taps were recommended in the past. However, to do a tap without obtaining a CT scan is not appropriate unless the situation is desperate. The treatment of this lesion is somewhat controversial. The two methods currently in use are subdural tapping with aspiration[62] and craniotomy with evacuation of the clot.[54] It seems reasonable to try to do as little as possible to these children and yet still treat the problem adequately. A subdural tap can be done initially to see if a significant portion of the clot is liquid. If, however, the majority of the clot is solid, a craniotomy is warranted.[54]

Acute subdural hematoma in the older infant is usually due to trauma and occurs in approximately 8% of children with a severe head injury, usually in the older child and adolescent. The symptoms of these children are a result of both the clot and the associated parenchymal damage. As in the newborn, the diagnosis is made with a CT scan (see Fig. 13–6). The treatment is dependent on the clinical condition of the child as well as the contribution of the clot to the clinical picture. If it is thought that the hematoma is contributing to or is directly responsible for the clinical picture, it is removed via a craniotomy that is performed as rapidly as possible. If, however, the CT shows only a very thin rim of hematoma and a markedly swollen brain, the best treatment may be to try and control ICP with medical

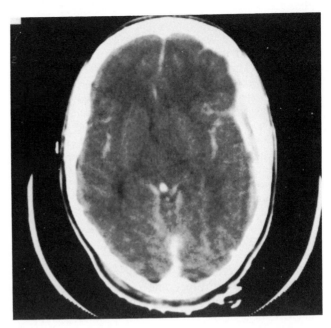

FIGURE 13–6

Acute subdural hematoma. Note the diffuse high-density, extra-axial clot and the shift of the ventricular system.

means because it is unlikely that removing a few milliliters of clot will have a significant effect.

A chronic subdural hematoma is different from an acute hematoma. It occurs more commonly and is usually seen in children under the age of 2 years. These children present with macrocrania irritability, failure to thrive, anemia, and, in 40% of patients, seizures. The head is enlarged, usually in the biparietal diameter. Again, the diagnostic procedure of choice is the CT scan. In the chronic subdural hematoma, the initial treatment consists of subdural taps. If after multiple taps, there seems to be no decrease in the size of the collections, then a subdural peritoneal shunt may be needed. However, this usually is not necessary if taps are done carefully and the child is followed closely.

Child Abuse

Head injury is the leading cause of death in children who are injured from child abuse.[67] In one series, child abuse accounted for 64% of head injuries in children under 1 year of age, exclusive of an isolated skull fracture, and 95% of severe head injuries in this age group.[7] The mechanism of injury in many cases is similar to any case of assault. However, Caffey was the first to propose the possibility of injuring an infant by shaking it.[13] This proposition has been questioned, and the belief is that in addition to the acceleration and deceleration, an impact against something must also occur. Regardless, the concept of the shaken baby helped to focus attention on this difficult problem in infants. The pathology of injury is similar to that of other head injuries with subarachnoid hemorrhage, intracranial hematomas, and diffuse axonal injury having been reported. One of the distinctive combinations is a child who presents with an acute subdural hematoma and retinal hemorrhages.[59] The

Table 13-2
Facts That Should Alert Physicians about Possible Child Abuse

1. Unexplained cause of injury
2. Significant delay in obtaining treatment
3. Injuries in various parts of extremities associated with mild or moderate head injury
4. Radiographs showing injuries of various ages
5. Child reported to ``suddenly'' become limp

care of these children is similar to that of children with other head injuries. What should be emphasized is the need to recognize that a child may be a victim of child abuse and to take proper steps to ensure that it does not occur again. Several clues can alert the physician that child abuse may be the cause of a head injury (Table 13–2). Chief among these is an injury whose severity is out of proportion to the description of the accident. Other warning signs include multiple injuries of different ages and delay in seeking attention when a child is obviously injured. It is imperative that individuals who care for children recognize the signs of child abuse and be willing to take the proper steps to prevent it from recurring.

OUTCOME

As a general statement, children do better than adults in terms of outcome after a severe head injury. The exact reason for this difference is unclear but is probably multifactorial. Age, ICP, GCS on admission, presence of mass lesions, presence of hypoxia or hypotension or both, mechanism of injury, duration of coma, and presence of multiple injuries all have been implicated as having an effect on the outcome in the patient with a head injury.[18] The mortality for children with severe head injuries (GCS 8 or less) ranges from 6 to 32%, with the most serious reporting 14 to 24%.[6, 12, 19, 21, 66, 72] It is interesting to note that the outcome figures were not obtained at the expense of a large number of vegetative patients. This was true in the majority of the series. Mortality was also dependent on the lesion: children with epidural lesions had better outcomes than children with acute subdural hematomas. In one series, children with mass lesions had worse outcomes than those without mass lesions.[72] This points to the importance of prompt transport and care of these children at appropriate centers.

Besides mortality, significant behavioral and neuropsychological deficits follow a head injury, whether it is moderate or severe. Although the space for a detailed discussion is insufficient, it is appropriate to outline a few of the major areas of difficulty. Language,[41] memory,[22] visual spatial cues, motor speed, and ability to consolidate information are all, to some extent, impaired in the child with a severe head injury. These problems should be recognized and anticipated so that when children recover sufficiently to return home and to school these problems become less of a barrier to a good functional recovery.

It should be emphasized that although the mortality in children with a severe head injury is significant, the majority of children will achieve a functional recovery. However, these results are obtained only with an aggressive approach to the diagnosis and treatment of the growing problem of head injury. It is imperative that these children have access to the technology of modern intensive care, including appropriate monitoring, if they are to have the potential to achieve a functional recovery. Although the bulk of this chapter has discussed the care of the child after a head injury has occurred, it would be remiss not to mention that the best cure for head injuries is to prevent them in the first place. Until there is strong, realistic commitment by all segments of our society to accident prevention trauma, head injury will continue to be a killer and producer of disability in our young.

References

1. Adams JH, Graham DI, Murry LS, Scott G: Diffuse axonal injury due to non-missile head injury in humans: An analysis of 45 cases. Ann Neurol 12:557–563, 1982.
2. Adams JH, Graham DI, Scott G, et al: Brain damage in non-missile head injury. J Clin Pathol 33:1132–1145, 1980.
3. Ammirayi M, Tomita T: Posterior fossa epidural hematoma during childhood. Neurosurgery 14:541–544, 1984.
4. Annegers JF, Grawbow JD, Kurland LT, Vaws ER: The incidence, causes and secular trends of head trauma in Olmstead County, Minnesota 1935–1974. Neurology 30:912–919, 1980.
5. Becker DP, Miller JD, Butterworth JF, et al: The outcome from severe head injury with early diagnosis and intensive management. J Neurosurg 47:491–502, 1977.
6. Berger MS, Pitts LH, Lovely M, et al: Outcome from severe head injury in children and adolescents. J Neurosurg 62:194–199, 1985.
7. Billmire ME, Myers PD: Serious head injury in infants: Accident or abuse? Pediatrics 75:340–342, 1985.
8. Brodersen P, Paulson OB, Bolwig TB, et al: Cerebral hyperemia in electrically induced epileptic seizures. Arch Neurol 28:334–338, 1973.
9. Bruce DA, Alavi A, Bilaniuk L, et al: Diffuse cerebral swelling following head injuries in children: The syndrome of malignant brain edema. J Neurosurg 54:170–178, 1981.
10. Bruce DA, Raphaely RC, Goldberg AI, et al: Pathophysiology, treatment and outcome following severe head injury in children. Child's Brain 5:174–191, 1979.
11. Bruce DA, Schut L: The value of CAT scanning following pediatric head injury. Clin Pediatr 19:719–725, 1980.
12. Bruce DA, Schut L, Bruno LA, et al: Outcome following severe head injury in children. J Neurosurg 48:679–688, 1978.
13. Caffey J: On the theory and practice of shaking infants. Am J Dis Child 124:161, 1972.
14. Choux M, Grisoli F, Peragut JC: Extradural hematoma in children. Child's Brain 1:269–290, 1975.
15. Cutler RWP, Page LK, Gralicick J, Watters GV: Formation and absorption of cerebrospinal fluid in man. Brain 91:707–720, 1968.
16. Duffy TE, Vannucci RC: Metabolic aspects of cerebral anoxia in the fetus and newborn. In: Berenberd SR (ed): Brain, Fetal and Infant. The Hague, Martinus Nijhoff Medical Division, 1977, pp 316–323.
17. Einhorn A, Mizzrahi EM: Basilar skull fractures in children. The incidence of CNS infection and the use of antibiotics. Am J Dis Child 132:1121–1124, 1978.
18. Eisenberg HM: Outcome after head injury: General considerations and neurobehavioral recovery. Part I: General consideration. In: Becker DP, Povlishock JT (eds): Central Nervous System Trauma Status Report, National Institute of Neurological and Communicative Disorders and Stroke. National Institute of Health, Bethesda, Md, 1985, pp 271–280.
19. Esparza J, M-Portillo JM, Sarabia M, et al: Outcome in children with severe head injury. Childs Nerv Syst 1:109–114, 1985.
20. Friede RL: Developmental Neuropathology. New York, Springer Verlag, 1975.
21. Frost EAM, Arancibia CU, Shulman K: Pulmonary shunt as a prognostic indicator in head injury. J Neurosurg 50:768–772, 1979.

22. Fuld PA, Fisher P: Recovery of intellectual ability after closed head injury. Dev Med Child Neurol 19:495–502, 1977.

23. Galbraith SL: Age distribution of extradural hemorrhage without skull fracture. Lancet 2:1217, 1973.

24. Gandy SE, Snow PB, Zimmerman RD, Deck MDF: Cranial nuclear magnetic resonance imaging in head trauma. Ann Neurol 16:254–257, 1984.

25. Gennarelli TA: Head injury in men and experimental animals—Clinical aspects. Acta Neurochir 32(suppl):1–13, 1983.

26. Gray WJ, Rosner MJ: Pressure volume index as a function of cerebral perfusion pressure. Part 2: The effect of low cerebral perfusion pressure and autoregulation. J Neurosurg 67:377–380, 1987.

27. Gross CR, Wolf C, Kunitz SC, Jane JA: Pilot traumatic coma data bank: A profile of head injuries in children. In: Dacey RG Jr, Winn HR, Rimel RW, Jane JA (eds): Trauma of the Central Nervous System. New York, Raven Press, 1985, pp 19–26.

28. Grubb RL, Raichle MI, Eichling JO, Ter-Pogossian MM: The effects of changes in PaCO$_2$ on cerebral blood volume, blood flow and vascular mean transit time. Stroke 5:630–639, 1974.

29. Gudeman SK, Kishore PRS, Miller JD, et al: The genesis and significance of delayed traumatic intracerebral hematoma. Neurosurgery 5:309–313, 1979.

30. Harper AM: Autoregulation of cerebral blood flow: Influence of arterial blood pressure on the blood flow through the cerebral cortex. J Neurol Neurosurg Psychiatry 29:398–403, 1966.

31. Harwood-Mash DC, Hendrick EB, Hudson AR: The significance of skull fracture in children. A study of 1,187 patients. Radiology 101:151–155, 1971.

32. Hoff JT, Brewin UHS: Antibiotics for basilar skull fracture (letter). J Neurosurg 44:649, 1976.

33. Ignelzi RJ, Vanderark GD: Analysis of treatment of basilar skull fractures with and without antibiotics. J Neurosurg 43:721–726, 1975.

34. Ingvar DH, Croquist S, Ekberg R, et al: Normal values of regional cerebral blood flow in man including flow and weight measurements of gray and white matter. Acta Neurologica Scand 41(suppl 14):72–78, 1965.

35. Jones TH, Morawetz RB, Crowell RM, et al: Threshold of focal cerebral ischemia in awake monkeys. J Neurosurg 54:773–782, 1981.

36. Kraus JF, Fife D, Cox P, et al: Incidence, severity and external causes of pediatric brain injury. Am J Dis Child 140:687–693, 1986.

37. Kriel RL, Sheehan M, Krach LE, et al: Pediatric head injury resulting from all terrain vehicle accidents. Pediatrics 78:933–935, 1986.

38. Langfitt TW: Increased intracranial pressure. Clin Neurosurg 16:436–471, 1971.

39. Lende RA, Erickson TC: Growing skull fractures of childhood. J Neurosurg 18:479–489, 1961.

40. Levin HS, Ampalo E, Eisenberg HM, et al: Magnetic resonance imaging and computerized tomography in relation to the neurobehavioral sequelae of mild and moderate head injuries. J Neurosurg 66:706–713, 1987.

41. Levin HS, Eisenberg HM: Neuropsychological outcome of closed head injury in children and adolescents. Child's Brain 5:281–292, 1975.

42. Lindenberg R, Freytag E: Morphology of brain lesions from blunt trauma in early infancy. Arch Pathol 87:298–305, 1969.

43. Lou HC: Developmental Neurology. New York, Raven Press, 1982, pp 1–80.

44. Lou HC, Lassen NA, Fris-Hansen B: Impaired autoregulation of cerebral blood flow in the distressed newborn infant. J Pediatr 94:118–121, 1979.

45. Lundar T, Nestvold K: Pediatric head injuries caused by traffic accidents. A prospective study with 5-year follow-up. Childs Nerv Syst 1:24–28, 1985.

46. McLaurin RL, Towbin R: Cerebral damage in head injuries in the newborn and infant. In: Raimondi AJ, Choux M, Dirocco C (eds): The Pediatric Spine. New York, Berlin, Heidelberg, Springer-Verlag, 1986, pp 183–201.

47. Masters SJ, McClean PM, Arcarese JS, et al: Skull x-ray examinations after head trauma: Recommendations by a multi-disciplinary panel and validation study. N Engl J Med 316:84–91, 1987.

48. Mayhall CG, Archer NH, Jamb VA, et al: Ventriculostomy-related infections: A prospective epidemiologic study. N Engl J Med 310:553–559, 1984.

49. Miller JD, Sweet RC, Narayan R, et al: Early insult to the injured brain. JAMA 240:439–442, 1978.

50. Miner ME, Kaufman HH, Graham SH, et al: Disseminated intravascular coagulation and fibrinolysis following severe head trauma in children. In: Grossman RG, Gildenberg PL (eds): Head Injury: Basic and Clinical Aspects. New York, Raven Press, 1982, pp 251–258.

51. Muizelaar JP, Wei EP, Kontos HA, Becker DP: Mannitol causes compensatory cerebral vasoconstriction and vasodilation in response to blood viscosity changes. J Neurosurg 59:822–828, 1983.

52. Obrist W, Langfitt TW, Jaggi JL, et al: Cerebral blood flow and metabolism in comatose patients with acute head injury. J Neurosurg 61:241–253, 1984.

53. Ostrup RC, Luerssen TG, Marshall LF, Zornow MH: Continuous monitoring of intracranial pressure with a miniaturized fiberoptic device. J Neurosurg 47:206–209, 1987.

54. Pierre-Kahn A, Renier D, Sainte-Rose C: Acute subdural hematomas in term neonates. Childs Nerv Syst 2:191–194, 1986.

55. Pollay M, Fullenwider C, Roberts PA, Stevens FA: Effect of mannitol and furosemide on blood-brain osmotic gradient and intracranial pressure. J Neurosurg 59:945–950, 1983.

56. Povlishock JT, Becker DP, Cheng CLY, Vaughan CW: Axonal change in minor head injury. J Neuropathol Exp Neurol 42:225–242, 1983.

57. Pupura DP: Dendritic differentiation in human cortex: Normal and aberrant developmental patterns. In: Kreutenberg GU (ed): Advances in Neurology. Vol. 12. New York, Raven Press, 1975.

58. Reale F, Delfoni R, Mencattini G: Epidural hematomas. J Neurosurg Sci 28:9–16, 1984.

59. Rekate HL, McClelland CW, Rekate MW: The neurosurgical implications of child abuse. In: Shapiro K (ed): Pediatric Head Trauma. New York, Raven Press, 1983, pp 195–212.

60. Rieder MJ, Schwartz C, Newman J: Patterns of walker use and walker injury. Pediatrics 78:408–493, 1986.

61. Rivara FP: Epidemiology of violent deaths in children and adolescents in the United States. Pediatrician 12(1):3–10, 1983–1985.

62. Romodava AP, Brosky YUS: Subdural hematomas in the newborn. Surgical treatment and results. Surg Neurol 28:253–258, 1978.

63. Sampson P, Beyer CW Jr: Furosemide in the intraoperative reduction of intracranial pressure in patients with subarachnoid hemorrhage. Neurosurgery 10:167–169, 1982.

64. Saul TG, Ducker TB: Effect of intracranial pressure monitoring and aggressive treatment on mortality in severe head injury. J Neurosurg 56:498–503, 1982.

65. Seelig JM, Marshall LF, Toutant SM, et al: Traumatic acute epidural hematoma: Unrecognized high lethality in comatose patients. Neurosurgery 15:617–620, 1984.

66. Shapiro K, Marmarou A: Clinical applications of the pressure volume index in treatment of pediatric head injuries. J Neurosurg 56:819–825, 1982.

67. Showers J, Apolo J, Thomas J, Beavers S: Fatal child abuse: A two-decade review. Pediatr Emerg Care 1:66–70, 1985.

68. Stevens WS, Rodgers BM, Newman BM: Pediatric trauma associated with all terrain vehicles. J Pediatr 109:25–29, 1986.

69. Stone JL, Lowe RJ, Jonasson O, et al: Acute subdural hematoma: Direct admission to a trauma center yields improved results. J Trauma 26:445–450, 1986.

70. Teasdale G, Jennett B: Assessment of coma and impaired consciousness—A practical scale. Lancet 2:81–84, 1974.

71. Walker ML, Storrs BB, Mayer T: Factors affecting outcome in the pediatric patient with multiple trauma. Further experience with the modified injury severity scale. Child's Brain 11:387–397, 1984.

72. Ward JD, Alberico AM: Paediatric head injuries. Brain Inj 1:21–25, 1987.

73. Welch K: The intracranial pressure in infants. J Neurosurg 52:693–699, 1980.

74. Wellman S, Paulson JA: Baby walker related injuries. Clin Pediatr 23:98–99, 1984.

75. Yakovlev PJ, Lecours AP: The myelogenetic cycle of regional maturation of the brain. In: Muakowski A (ed): Regional Development of the Brain in Early Life. Oxford, Blackwell, 1967, pp 3–70.

Thomas B. Scully
Thomas G. Luerssen

Spinal Cord Injuries

The incidence of spinal cord injury in the pediatric age group is variably reported as 0.65% to just over 9% of all spinal cord injuries.[1-5, 10, 11, 20, 31, 34, 35, 47] The incidence of vertebral injury is approximately 2 to 3% of all children's injuries.[4, 5, 27] Although spinal column and spinal cord injuries are uncommon in the pediatric age group, the clinical consequences of these injuries can be devastating. Furthermore, failure to diagnose a vertebral column injury in a child may result in a delayed spinal cord injury or may aggravate a potentially reversible incomplete injury. Modern neuroimaging has added much to our knowledge regarding traumatic myelopathy and its management. Despite this, the major therapeutic efforts for patients of all ages with spinal cord injuries continue to be aimed at preventing reinjury to the spinal cord and ameliorating as much as possible the secondary injuries of hypoxia and ischemia and the subsequent biochemical processes associated with traumatic spinal cord injury.

In general, the early diagnostic and therapeutic algorithms for children with injured spines are similar to those for adults. However, specific and substantial differences in anatomy, clinical presentation, radiographic findings, and indications for surgery are characteristic of children. This chapter focuses on these basic elements. As with injuries to other systems in the pediatric age group, the best outcomes are obtained through a cooperative effort of specialists, beginning at the time of evaluation of the initial injury and resuscitation and carried through the long-term rehabilitation process.

ANATOMIC AND RADIOLOGIC CORRELATES OF SPINAL INJURY

A general knowledge of the normal anatomic development of the spinal column is necessary to interpret correctly the radiographic studies routinely obtained in the evaluation of patients with such injuries. So informed, the physician can usually separate a traumatic disruption of the bony elements from an array of normal synchondroses and epiphyses routinely visualized on plain spine radiographs and computed tomography (CT) scans. These anatomic differences have been outlined in numerous previous reviews.[5, 6, 10, 13, 24, 31, 32, 36]

The infant's vertebral column consists mostly of cartilage, and therefore the intervertebral disk space appears wide in relation to the vertebral bodies (Fig. 14–1). As the child matures, the vertebral bodies ossify and the proportion of bone to cartilage increases. However, the vertebral bodies maintain a wedge shape and appear more narrow anteriorly. This pattern persists until about the age of 7 years, at which time the vertebral bodies assume the more square shape of the adult spine.[6, 13, 52]

The atlas originates from two ossification centers, one for the neural arches and one for the body. The body is not ossified at birth but becomes radiographically apparent during the first year of life.[4-6] Hence, the anterior arch of the atlas is not usually seen on plain spine radiographs in this age group. The neural arches of the atlas are separated by the neurocentral synchondroses, which fuse around the age of 7 years.[6, 13, 52] These synchondroses can usually be distinguished from fractures because they are bilateral symmetric lucencies. However, occasionally the arch of the first cervical vertebra develops from asymmetric centers and can mimic a traumatic lesion (Fig. 14–2).

Four ossification centers are present in the axis at the time of birth.[6, 13, 52] There is one center for each neural arch, one for the body, and one for the odontoid process. These synchondroses begin to fuse by the age of 3 years and are almost universally fused by the age of 7.[13] Therefore, a radiolucent line traversing the odontoid process in a child over the age of 7 years is probably traumatic in origin.

The remaining cervical vertebrae are each derived from three ossification centers, one for the body and one for each neural arch. The neural arches close in the second to third years, and the synchondroses that fuse the arches to the vertebral bodies close between the third and sixth years.[6] In most cases, a child's cervical spine has reached a radiographic appearance similar to an adult's by the age of 10 years.

The pediatric spine is much more mobile than the adult spine for several reasons.[44, 47, 49, 52] The cervical musculature does not become completely supportive until puberty. A young child has very lax intraspinal ligaments and joint capsules, and the intervertebral facet joints are oriented in the horizontal plane in children, allowing for more forward displacement during flexion maneuvers.[32] The facets assume the more vertical adult alignment at about 5 years of age.[13] These features account for the well-described "pseudosubluxation" of the cervical spine in children[3, 5, 13, 22, 27, 31, 32, 49] (Fig. 14–3). Most pseudosubluxation occurs between the second and third vertebral bodies. This apparent anterior subluxation can measure up to 4 mm in as many as 40% of normal children between the ages of 1 to 7 years.[13, 49] Less frequently, one can see pseudosubluxation at the third and fourth interspaces. Furthermore, the increased mobility of the pediatric spine can affect the appearance of the first and second vertebral bodies whereby the distance between the anterior arch of the atlas and the dens can be up to 3 mm during flexion.[49] This gap can be misinterpreted as ligamentous injury on the spine films.

The increased mobility of the cervical spine in childhood explains some of the clinical features of the injuries that occur, and the overall rarity of spinal cord injury in young children may be related to this increased mobility. This mobility seems to be protective by distributing injury forces over several vertebral levels; however, increased mobility may also account for the syndrome of "spinal cord injury without radiographic abnormality," which is essentially an injury of childhood.[15, 16, 42, 46, 47] Postmortem examinations of children killed by violent injuries have revealed unstable cervical fractures through the cartilage and disruption of the spinal ligaments, with apparent anatomic alignment of the bony structures.[4]

All large series reported of spinal injuries in children demonstrate a bimodal age distribution.[2, 27] Children under 8 years of age suffer injuries to the cervical spine almost exclusively, whereas older children suffer spinal injuries in a distribution similar to that of adults.[22] This bimodal age distribution is explainable by the anatomic differences of the cervical spine and not by a dissimilarity of injury mechanism.[6] The previously described anatomic characteristics and their related biomechanical properties combine with the

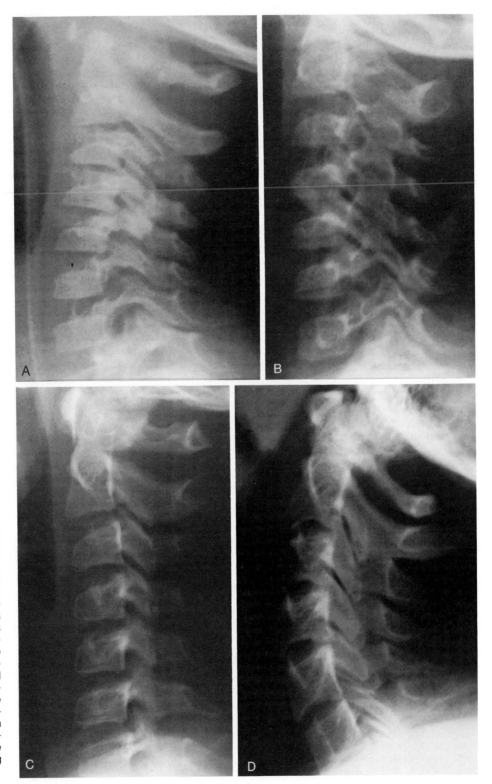

FIGURE 14–1

The radiographic appearance of a normal lateral cervical spine in a 2 year old (*A*), a 4 year old (*B*), a 12 year old (*C*), and an 18 year old (*D*). The studies have been photographed in a comparable scale to highlight the changes in appearance as the child's spine assumes the adult configuration. Note the progressive loss of the wedge-shaped appearance of the vertebral bodies, the decrease in the relative size of the disk space separating the vertebral bodies, the progressive angulation of the facet joints, and the decrease in the relative size of the spinal canal with increasing age.

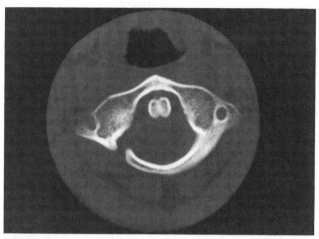

FIGURE 14–2

Incomplete formation of the arch of the atlas. This congenital malformation of the spine might be misinterpreted as a traumatic lesion.[21] The smooth edges and the lack of soft tissue injury suggest a congenital process.

relative disproportion of the child's head with his torso and increase the likelihood of a cervical spine injury.[2–4, 8] Younger children tend to have extremely rostral cervical injuries, and this tendency is lost with increasing age.[3] The thoracolumbar spine of the child also differs from that of the adult by virtue of the ossification centers, increased mobility, and presence of the ring apophysis. However, because the thoracolumbar spine of the child assumes the biomechanical properties of the adult by the age of 10 years, adolescents with injuries in this region of the spine appear clinically and radiographically similar to adults.[5, 6]

CLINICAL EVALUATION

Because vertebral and spinal cord injuries are extremely rare in childhood, it is possible that some patients harboring a vertebral injury or a partial cord injury could be overlooked, especially if more overt injuries are present. The initial clinical evaluation of any injured child should allow the physician to develop an index of suspicion regarding vertebral or neurologic injury.

Certain mechanisms are associated with spinal cord injury in younger children, with motor vehicle accidents, either as a pedestrian or a passenger, and falls from heights being the major mechanisms of injury.[24, 35, 47] Occasionally, infants may suffer a spinal cord injury as the result of abuse.[23, 50] In older children, recreational activities and sports account for a large percentage of these injuries.[8] The tandem occurrence of a head injury and a vertebral or spinal cord injury is possible in the pediatric age group, although this circumstance is much less frequent than that reported for adults.[48] Nevertheless, all comatose children, especially those injured by an appropriate mechanism, must be considered to have suffered a vertebral or spinal cord injury until proven otherwise.

Any complaints of neck, back, or radicular pain or numbness in this age group must be considered related to verte-bral or spinal cord injury until proven otherwise. Acute painful torticollis may also be an indicator of atlantoaxial rotatory luxation. Hyperflexion injuries due to the use of a lap belt may be suggested by the presence of abdominal bruising, and such a finding requires detailed evaluation for neurologic injury.

The physical examination is extremely important in the frequently uncommunicative young child. Spinous processes should be palpated for alignment, gaps, and tenderness. The skin should be observed for signs of changes in sympathetic tone. The cornerstone of the examination is a careful assessment of neurologic function, both to diagnose the presence of any dysfunction and to serve as a baseline for future examinations. The motor examination is of particular interest, because a young child will not cooperate with a critical examination of the sensory modalities. In older children and adolescents, a critical assessment of sensory modalities, including those mediated through the dorsal columns, is necessary. Muscle tendon reflexes and superficial cutaneous reflexes must be studied. Finally, an examination of the sacral area for sensation, rectal tone, and the bulbocavernosus reflex is essential. Sensation or reflexes in this area may be the only indicator of a partial spinal cord injury in a patient who seems otherwise paralyzed.

RADIOLOGIC EVALUATION

The plain spine radiograph is still an essential part of the early evaluation of the child with an injured spine. When multisystem trauma is being evaluated, the entire spine must be visualized. Cervical spine radiographs must demonstrate clearly the entire cervical spine to the cervical-thoracic junction. As previously described, interpretation of the plain spine radiographs must be performed in view of the patient's age and the presence of torticollis and muscle spasm. Loss of normal cervical lordosis on the lateral view is suggestive of cervical injury in adults; however, in the pediatric age group, 20% of children have either a straight or a kyphotic appearance of the cervical spine in the neutral position. With depression of the chin 1 inch, the incidence of this finding increases to 70%.[52]

Flexion and extension views of the cervical spine can aid in the determination of spinal instability and can resolve the question of subluxation, but they are not indicated in the presence of clear vertebral or ligamentous disruption or neurologic deficit. However, if the issue of normal ligamentous laxity versus injury is raised and if the child is awake and can cooperate, flexion and extension studies can provide very useful information.[5, 6, 10, 12, 13] These studies are best performed under the guidance of the physician; no child should be forced to move the neck past the range of comfort for any acute study.

Compression fractures due to hyperflexion injuries are the most common type of thoracic spine fractures seen in the pediatric age group.[20, 28] The radiographic studies will demonstrate flattening or compression of the end plate or vertebral body. A number of compressed vertebrae may be seen because the elastic, resilient intervertebral disks transmit the injury forces to adjacent vertebrae.[26] True fracture

FIGURE 14-3

Pseudosubluxation of the cervical spine in a 7-year-old girl. A, Note the appearance of movement at the interspace between the second and third cervical segments during flexion. The true alignment of the posterior elements and the spinal canal does not change. B, Extension. The pseudosubluxation is "reduced." Children with neck pain tend to hold the spine in mild flexion, giving the appearance of subluxation.

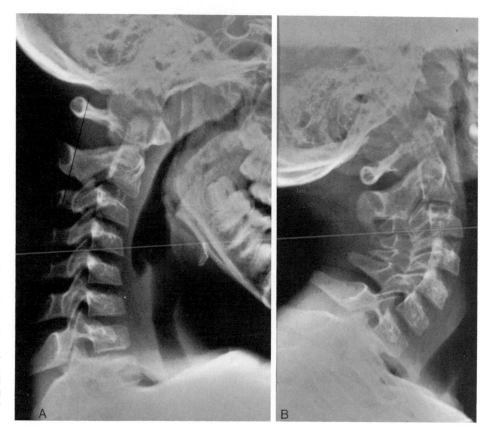

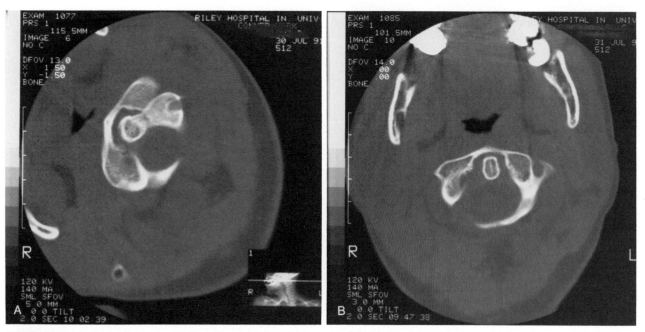

FIGURE 14-4

A computed tomography (CT) scan of a 12-year-old boy who is asthmatic and who awoke with a coughing spell and developed a painful fixed torticollis. A, The initial CT scan of the spine shows rotatory luxation of the atlas on the axis that measures about 45 degrees. B, Immediately following closed reduction under general anesthesia, the relationship of the two segments is now normal. He was treated with immobilization for 6 weeks.

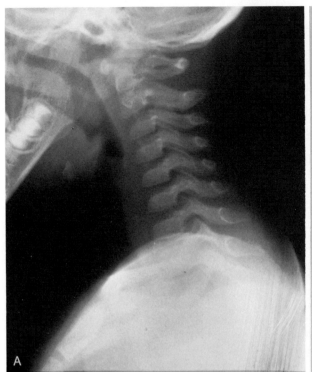

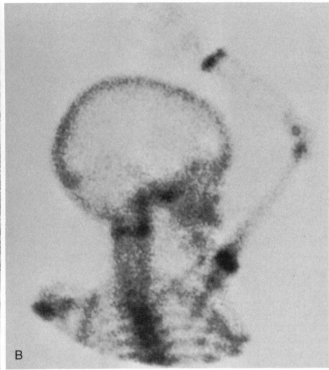

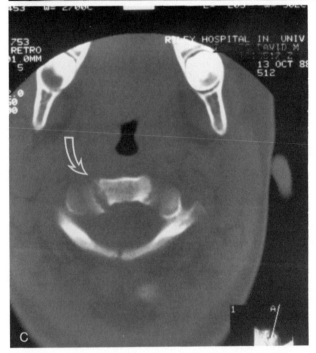

FIGURE 14–5

This 3-year-old child presented with a prolonged history of irritability and nuchal rigidity that had been ascribed to meningitis. There was a history of a fall off a playground structure. *A*, Plain cervical spine radiography was normal, including flexion and extension studies. *B*, Radionuclide bone scan shows uptake in cervical spine. *C*, The computed tomography scan demonstrates a fracture of the vertebral body through the synchondrosis. This child was successfully treated with immobilization.

dislocations, the Chance fracture,[14] and ligamentous ruptures of the thoracolumbar spine are rare, but they can occur, especially in adolescents. These injuries are, by definition, unstable. Furthermore, unstable fractures can occur through the unossified apophyses, and the natural elasticity of the paraspinal tissues may realign the vertebral elements such that they are not radiographically evident on initial films.[33] A strong index of suspicion is necessary, and further studies should be performed if there is any question of injury at this level.

Computed tomography of the spine is extremely helpful for elucidating areas of injury, rotatory luxation (Fig. 14–4), and subtle fractures (Fig. 14–5).[19] Furthermore, soft tissue swelling and areas of major hemorrhage can be visualized. Computed tomography is the best way to visualize the capacity of the neural canal and foramina after traumatic injury.

Magnetic resonance imaging (MRI) has virtually supplanted the use of myelography for spinal cord injury. With the exception of gunshot wounds or other penetrating injuries that might result in metallic artifacts in the region of the potential spinal cord injury, most clinically relevant information about the anatomy of the spinal cord can be obtained noninvasively with MRI.[39, 51] Frequently, the only radiographic abnormalities detectable are on the MRI.

COMMON SPINAL INJURIES OF CHILDHOOD

Because of the biomechanical properties of the flexible cervical spine and the relatively large head of the child, most vertebral and spinal cord injuries in this age group occur in the cervical region, the pattern of injury usually being mechanism dependent.

Craniocervical Dislocation

This injury usually occurs in younger children and is due to a sudden and forceful deceleration. The mechanism places the disproportionately large head anterior to the atlas.[4, 24, 27] This injury is usually lethal owing to brain stem or high cervical cord injury, but occasional survivors have been reported.[41] The spinal injury is extremely unstable, and skeletal fixation and craniocervical fusion is required.

Atlantoaxial Injuries

A variety of injuries occur at this level because of the complex mechanical relationships of these two spinal segments. The common injuries of childhood include rotatory subluxation, ligamentous disruption, odontoid process injury, and ring fracture.[5, 9, 10, 12, 17] Children generally suffer a different type of injury at this level from that suffered by adults. In older children and adults, the odontoid process fractures before the ligamentous complex disrupts. In the younger age group, the increased ligamentous laxity protects against this. This laxity is frequently amplified by inflammatory processes in the oropharynx and upper respiratory tracts that are common in childhood. Thus, rotatory or anterior luxations are more often seen in children, and if the rotation is greater than 40 degrees, the facets are involved.[17]

Anterior Luxations

Transverse atlantal ligament damage results in a separation of the anterior ring of the atlas from the dens of more than 5 mm. This finding is best seen on the lateral spine film. The capacious spinal canal at this level usually protects against neurologic injury.[27] These injuries usually heal with immobilization, but an occasional persistent instability requires arthrodesis.[45]

Rotatory Luxations

An injury at this level frequently results in acute painful torticollis. There may be a history of minor trauma or a sensation of a snap or crack in the posterior neck, followed immediately by pain and stiffness. The head is generally carried in a fixed position of slight flexion, the chin is downward and the head is rotated and flexed laterally. This position has been described as the "cock robin" posture. The patients are neurologically normal. Although the plain spine films are suggestive, the views are compromised by the torticollis. As shown in Figure 14–4, the CT scan is characteristic. This injury may reduce spontaneously or with careful manipulation and can be treated initially with immobilization. Recurrent rotatory luxations require operative fusion.

Odontoid Process Injuries

Childhood odontoid fractures occur through the base of the odontoid synchondrosis where it attaches to the vertebral body. Children with this injury are somewhat older and present with neck pain and muscle spasm.[2, 5, 9, 21, 24, 32] The trauma may be minor and may be overshadowed by a head injury. Neurologic signs are infrequent. The odontoid is found to be anteriorly displaced and easily reduces in extension. These injuries heal readily with immobilization.

Os odontoideum is a smooth round ossicle located in the region of the odontoid and is associated with atlantoaxial instability. It is likely that the etiology of this disorder is an unrecognized injury to the odontoid in early childhood.[18, 25] Although the children are neurologically normal, they are at risk because the spine is unstable (Fig. 14–6). Operative fusion is required.

Ring and Arch Fractures

The Jefferson fracture, a fracture of the arch of the atlas, is extremely rare in childhood. The mechanism is usually vertex compression, and therefore the spinal injury may be masked by a concurrent head injury. The CT scan is diagnostic. The few children with this fracture that have been reported in the literature have been treated with immobilization.[37] The "hangman fracture," a fracture of the posterior arch of the axis, can occur in older children and responds well to immobilization.

Other Cervical Injuries

Injuries involving the second and third cervical segments are frequently due to ligamentous disruption and may be difficult to differentiate from the normal ligamentous laxity at this level.[13, 22, 27, 31, 43, 45, 49] No universal clinical or radiographic sign can be relied on to detect a true ligamentous disruption. The presence or history of a neurologic deficit, even a transient one, or the presence of direct spinous process tenderness should alert one to this injury. Most patients respond well to immobilization. However, as with other ligamentous injuries, persistent instability requires operative fusion.

Injuries below the third segment are unusual. Serious injuries are associated with ligamentous disruption and car-

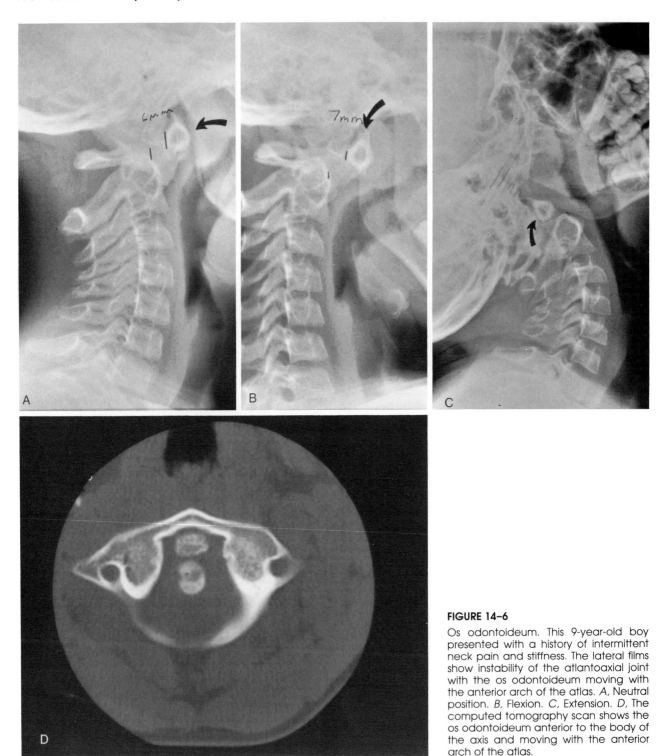

FIGURE 14–6

Os odontoideum. This 9-year-old boy presented with a history of intermittent neck pain and stiffness. The lateral films show instability of the atlantoaxial joint with the os odontoideum moving with the anterior arch of the atlas. *A,* Neutral position. *B,* Flexion. *C,* Extension. *D,* The computed tomography scan shows the os odontoideum anterior to the body of the axis and moving with the anterior arch of the atlas.

tilaginous end plate fractures. These injuries may not be readily apparent on plain spine radiographs and at the time of study may have reduced spontaneously. Repeating the studies frequently, especially if any symptoms persist, may demonstrate the injury. Treatment is dictated by the magnitude of the instability.

Thoracolumbar Injuries

Compression fractures are the most common spinal injury at these levels. These fractures are associated with hyperflexion injuries and frequently occur at multiple levels.[28, 32] Children complain of back pain that is aggravated by sitting

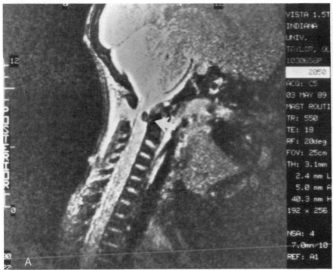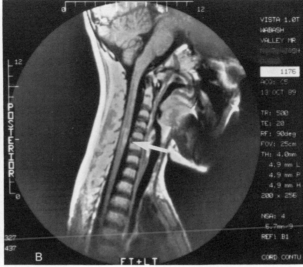

FIGURE 14–7

Magnetic resonance imaging (MRI) scans of two children with the so-called spinal cord injury without radiographic abnormality (SCIWORA). *A*, This 4-year-old boy was struck by an automobile and suffered the rapid onset of a flaccid quadriparesis and respiratory distress. Findings on the plain spine films and computed tomography (CT) scan of the spine were normal. The MRI scan (TR = 550 msec, TE = 18 msec) showed a hemorrhagic lesion at the cervicomedullary junction. He was treated with immobilization and progressively improved. He can now ambulate freely but has a mild spastic hemiparesis. *B*, This 8-year-old boy fell off a trampoline. He continued to play. Several hours later he developed neck pain and subsequently developed a mild quadriparesis. Results on the plain radiographs and the spinal CT scan were normal. The MRI scan (TR = 500 msec, TE = 20 msec) showed increased signal intensity in the cervical cord. The boy improved to normal over several weeks.

and exhibit local tenderness to spinal palpation. Treatment with bed rest and immobilization usually suffices. Other stable injuries include burst fractures, which are related to axial loading, and fractures of the posterior arch, facets, and transverse processes that frequently are due to direct blows to the spine.[29]

Fracture dislocations in the thoracic and lumbar spine occur rarely but have devastating neurologic sequelae. The common mechanism of injury is motor vehicular accidents. Lap belt injuries can cause a tension fracture that is unstable because of the disruption of the posterior ligaments.[30] The presence of this particular injury is suggested by a characteristic seat belt bruise on the abdominal wall and may be associated with life-threatening visceral injury.

Spinal Cord Injuries without Radiographic Abnormality

Children seem predisposed to this particular type of spinal cord injury, with some investigators reporting an incidence of two thirds of all spinal cord injuries in the pediatric age group.[15, 16, 40, 42, 46, 47] By definition, plain spine radiographs, CT scans, and tomograms are normal. These injuries seem to occur by any mechanism and can occur at any level of the spinal axis. Most investigators have concluded that the increased mobility of the pediatric spine is involved, but other causes, including transient disk herniations, vascular occlusions, and vasospasm, have been proposed.[42] Unfortunately, the neurologic character of the spinal cord lesions does not fit with any one cause.

This syndrome is complicated by the very frequent oc-currence of delayed symptoms. In about half of the cases reported, the onset of symptoms occurred hours to days after the traumatic event. Younger children tend to have more severe neurologic involvement, and the lesions occur more rostrally in the spinal neuraxis.[42, 46, 52] The neurologic injuries include complete transection, the hemisection syndrome of Brown-Séquard, central cord syndromes similar to those seen in adults with spondylogenic traumatic myelopathies, and a variety of partial spinal cord syndromes that do not fit any specific pattern. The majority of lesions are severe or complete, and the prospects for recovery are relatively poor compared with those for other partial spinal cord injuries in children.

With the advent of MRI, the descriptive appellation of spinal cord injuries without radiographic abnormality loses some accuracy. Swelling of the spinal cord or intramedullary hemorrhage is frequently seen on MRI, and these abnormalities correspond to the level of spinal cord injury (Fig. 14–7). Furthermore, dynamic studies of the spine in the area of concern may demonstrate hypermobility of the spinal segment. Immediate and prolonged immobilization is necessary to avoid further injury to the spinal cord.

MANAGEMENT

The basic principles of management for children with spinal injuries are not significantly different from those for adults. Proper immobilization of the patient at the scene of the injury is essential. The head should be immobilized in the neutral position. This becomes important when dealing with younger children who have cranial somatic disproportion.

These children should have additional support under their bodies so that the head may fall back into the true neutral position.

If the spinal canal is compromised by fracture or dislocation, the area of injury should be reduced by skeletal traction. For young children, we have found that a halo ring secured with six to eight pins at low torque provides safe and effective cranial traction and external fixation. Older children are treated with the standard Gardner-Wells device. With adequate reduction and immobilization of acute spinal fractures or dislocations, surgical decompression is rarely needed.

The medical management of the patient requires attention to maintaining adequate systemic circulation and preventing respiratory compromise from either neurologic involvement or gastric dilation. Neurogenic hypotension can accompany cervical or thoracic spinal cord injuries, and careful attention to maintaining the systemic blood pressure with vasopressors and avoiding volume overload by managing fluid administrations is essential.[36]

The pharmacotherapy of spinal cord injury is an area of extremely active basic and clinical research. At the time of this writing, the results obtained from the Second National Acute Spinal Cord Injury Study indicate that early therapy with high doses of methylprednisolone improves the outcome from traumatic spinal cord injury.[7] This study did not involve pediatric patients; however, it seems reasonable to assume that the biochemical processes are similar and that this therapy should be beneficial in children also. We have been administering the recommended doses of 30 mg per kg as a loading dose followed by 5.4 mg per kg per hour infusion for a total of 24 hours.

OUTCOME

With the exception of the patients who have spinal cord injuries without radiographic abnormalities, most recent series reporting the outcomes of children suffering spinal cord injuries indicate that in the absence of complete physiologic transection, most patients show some neurologic improvement over time. The mortality from spinal cord injury in children is very low and seems to occur almost exclusively in patients with complete injuries.[20] Children with spinal injuries who survive present very specific long-term orthopedic, urologic, and growth problems as well as a major challenge for rehabilitation professionals.[38]

References

1. Ahmann PA, Smith SA, Schwartz JF: Spinal cord infarction due to minor trauma in children. Neurosurgery 25:301–307, 1975.
2. Anderson JM, Schutt AH: Spinal injury in children. A review of 156 cases seen from 1950 through 1978. Mayo Clin Proc 55:499–504, 1980.
3. Apple JS, Kirks DR, Merten DF, Martinez S: Cervical spine fractures and dislocations in children. Pediatr Radiol 17:45–49, 1987.
4. Aufdermaur M: Spinal injuries in juveniles. Necropsy findings in twelve cases. J Bone Joint Surg (Br) 56:513–519, 1974.
5. Babcock JL: Spinal injuries in children. Pediatr Clin North Am 22:487–500, 1975.
6. Bailey DK: The normal cervical spine in infants and children. Radiology 59:712–719, 1952.
7. Bracken MB, Shepard MJ, Collins WF, et al: A randomized, controlled trial of methylprednisolone or naloxone in the treatment of acute spinal cord injury. Results of the Second National Acute Spinal Cord Injury Study. N Engl J Med 322:1405–1411, 1990.
8. Bruce DA, Schut L, Sutton L: Brain and cervical spine injuries occurring during organized sports activities in children and adolescents. Prim Care 11:175–194, 1984.
9. Bucholz RD, Cheung KC: Halo vest versus spinal fusion for cervical injury: Evidence from an outcome study. J Neurosurg 70:884–892, 1989.
10. Burke DC: Spinal cord trauma in children. Paraplegia 9:4–14, 1971.
11. Burke DC: Traumatic spinal paralysis in children. Paraplegia 11:268–276, 1974.
12. Campbell J, Bonnett C: Spinal cord injury in children. Clin Orthop 112:114–123, 1975.
13. Cattell HS, Filtzer DL: Pseudosubluxation and other normal variations in the cervical spine in children. J Bone Joint Surg 47:1295–1309, 1965.
14. Chance CQ: Note on a type of flexion fracture of the spine. Br J Radiol 21:452, 1948.
15. Chen LS, Blaw ME: Acute central cervical cord syndrome caused by minor trauma. J Pediatr 108:96–97, 1986.
16. Cheshire DJE: The pediatric syndrome of traumatic myelopathy without demonstrable vertebral injury. Paraplegia 15:74–85, 1977.
17. Fielding JW, Hawkins RJ: Atlanto-axial rotatory fixation. J Bone Joint Surg (Am) 59:37–44, 1977.
18. Fielding JW, Hensinger RN, Hawkins RJ: Os odontoideum. J Bone Joint Surg 62-A:376–383, 1980.
19. Fielding JW, Stillwell WT, Chynn KY, et al: Use of computed tomography for the diagnosis of atlanto-axial rotary fixation. A case report. J Bone Joint Surg (Am) 60:1102, 1978.
20. Gaufin LM, Goodman SJ: Cervical spine injuries in infants. Problems in management. J Neurosurg 42:179–184, 1975.
21. Gehweiler JA, Daffner RH, Roberts L: Malformations of the atlas vertebra simulating the Jefferson fracture. AJR 140:1083–1086, 1983.
22. Hachen HJ: Spinal cord injury in children and adolescents: Diagnostic pitfalls and therapeutic considerations in the acute stage. Paraplegia 15:55–64, 1977.
23. Hadley MN, Sonntag VKG, Rekate HL, Murphy A: The infant whiplash-shake injury syndrome: A clinical and pathological study. Neurosurgery 24:536–540, 1989.
24. Hadley MN, Zabramski JM, Browner CM, et al: Pediatric spinal trauma. Review of 122 cases of spinal cord and vertebral column injuries. J Neurosurg 68:18–24, 1988.
25. Hawkins RJ, Fielding JW, Thompson WJ: Os odontoideum: Congenital or acquired. J Bone Joint Surg (Am) 58:413, 1976.
26. Hegenbarth R, Ebel KD: Roentgen findings in fractures of the vertebral column in childhood: Examination of 35 patients and its results. Pediatric Radiology 5:34–39, 1976.
27. Hill SA, Miller CA, Kosnik EJ, Hunt WE: Pediatric neck injuries. A clinical study. J Neurosurg 60:700–706, 1984.
28. Hubbard DD: Injuries of the spine in children and adolescents. Clin Orthop 100:56–65, 1974.
29. Hubbard DD: Fractures of the dorsal and lumbar spine. Orthop Clin North Am 7:605–614, 1976.
30. Johnson DL, Falci S: The diagnosis and treatment of pediatric lumbar spine injuries caused by rear seat lap belts. Neurosurgery 26:434–441, 1990.
31. Kewalramani LS, Kraus JF, Sterling HM: Acute spinal cord lesions in a pediatric population: Epidemiological and clinical features. Paraplegia 18:206, 1980.
32. Kewalramani LS, Tori JA: Spinal cord trauma in children: Neurologic patterns, radiologic features, and pathomechanics of injury. Spine 5:11–18, 1980.
33. Kling TF: Spine injury in the multiply injured child. In: RE Marcus (ed): Trauma in Children. Rockville, Md, Aspen Publishers, 1986, pp 175–197.
34. Kraus JF, Franti CE, Riggins RS, et al: Incidence of traumatic spinal cord lesions. J Chron Dis 28:471–492, 1975.
35. LeBlanc JH, Nadell J: Spinal cord injuries in children. Surg Neurol 2:411, 1974.
36. Luce JM: Medical management of spinal cord injury. Crit Care Med 13:126–132, 1985.

37. Marlin AE, Williams GR, Lee JF: Jefferson fractures in children: Case report. J Neurosurg 58:277–279, 1983.
38. Mayfield JK, Evkkila JC, Winter RB: Spine deformity subsequent to acquired childhood spinal cord injury. Orthop Trans 3:281–282, 1979.
39. Mirvis SE, Geisler FH, Jelinek JJ, et al: Acute cervical spine trauma: Evaluation with 1.5 T MR imaging. Radiology 166:807–816, 1988.
40. Osenback RK, Menezes AH: Spinal cord injury without radiographic abnormality in children. Pediatr Neurosci 15:168–175, 1989.
41. Pang D, Wilberger JE: Traumatic atlanto-occipital dislocation with survival: Case report and review. Neurosurgery 7:503–508, 1980.
42. Pang D, Wilberger JE: Spinal cord injury without radiographic abnormalities in children. J Neurosurg 57:114–129, 1982.
43. Papavasiliou V: Traumatic subluxation of the cervical spine during childhood. Orthop Clin North Am 9:945–954, 1978.
44. Pennecot GF, Gouraud D, Hardy JR, Pouliquen JC: Roentgenographical study of the stability of the cervical spine in children. J Pediatr Orthop 4:346–352, 1984.
45. Pennecot GF, Leonard P, Peyrot Des Gachons S, et al: Traumatic ligamentous instability of the cervical spine in children. J Pediatr Orthop 4:339–345, 1984.
46. Pollack IF, Pang D, Sclabassi R: Recurrent spinal cord injury without radiographic abnormalities in children. J Neurosurg 69:177–182, 1988.
47. Ruge JR, Sinson GP, McLone DG, Cerullo LJ: Pediatric spinal injury: The very young. J Neurosurg 68:25–30, 1988.
48. Sneed RC, Stover SL: Undiagnosed spinal cord injuries in brain injured children. Am J Dis Child 142:965–967, 1988.
49. Sullivan CR, Brewer AJ, Harris LE: Hypermobility of the cervical spine in children. A pitfall in the diagnosis of cervical dislocation. Am J Surg 95:636, 1958.
50. Swischuck LE: Spine and spinal cord trauma in the battered child syndrome. Radiology 92:733–738, 1969.
51. Tracy PT, Wright RM, Hanigan WC: Magnetic resonance imaging of spinal injury. Spine 14:292–299, 1989.
52. Wilberger JE Jr: Spinal Cord Injury in Children. Mount Kisco, NY, Futura, 1986.

Maxillofacial Injuries

EPIDEMIOLOGY AND CHARACTER OF INJURY

Gussack and colleagues reported that pediatric maxillofacial trauma constitutes 15% of the population sustaining such injuries.[8] In their series of pediatric injuries, the higher predominance of male patients as seen in the adult population was not seen in the pediatric age group. The pediatric population, however, is at greater risk in motor vehicle-versus-pedestrian injuries and has a significantly higher risk of multiple system injuries, particularly cranial and orthopedic. In terms of distribution of anatomic sites of injury, the reduced incidence of midface or maxillary injury is believed to be a reflection of the more flexible maxillofacial structure system in the child. The mandible, however, from an epidemiologic standpoint, was found to be equally susceptible in both age groups to these types of injuries.[1]

DIAGNOSIS

From a diagnostic standpoint, Gussack and associates also reported that conventional tomograms were required more often for characterization of pediatric mandibular fractures when compared with a matched sample of adults.[8] Increased use of enhanced imaging techniques such as computed tomography (CT) in the pediatric population enabled a better understanding of the complex anatomy of the maxillofacial structures of children, that is, multiple tooth buds, a lower percentage of cortical bone, and a higher incidence of greenstick fractures of cortical bone. Interestingly, CT was used more often to characterize midface orbital fractures, whereas tomography was considered the diagnostic method of choice for mandibular fractures.

PRINCIPLES OF MANAGEMENT

Management of pediatric maxillofacial trauma in many cases mimics adult treatment.[2, 12] This is especially true when considering the anatomic sites for fixation, surgical access to cortical bone, or anatomic reduction. Derivatives of adult management protocols for the treatment of children may be appropriate, but growth and development significantly influence the choice of treatment guidelines for the child. For example, adult dentition has always been the keystone for reconstruction of the anatomic form and subsequent function or rehabilitation of the maxillomandibular structures. Some physicians believe that the integrity of the mandible and the anatomic intermaxillary fixation of the teeth in a correct fashion take precedence over the anatomic positioning of severely comminuted or displaced midface structures. Corroboration of treatment has been promoted through the retrospective use of the cephalometric radiograph from the lateral as well as the posteroanterior position.

This theory of management of maxillofacial injuries in adults may be valid. However, the application of these protocols in the child requires particular diligence. For example, in the child, the physician must consider the variability in occlusion between the primary and permanent dentitions. This wide range of variability is not necessarily a reflection of a functional or anatomic constraint but is more a reflection of the growth and development that occurs, enabling the face to grow in three planes during the remaining childhood and adolescent periods of life. Because of this variability, Gussack and associates reported that "observation only" occurs more often in pediatric patients than in adults with similar injuries.[8] This observation-only therapy not only is a reflection of the higher incidence of greenstick injury to the cortical bone of the maxilla and mandible in children, but also is to be considered in nondisplaced fractures of the body and ramus of the mandible, unilateral condylar fractures, and occasionally bilateral condylar fractures that have normal reproducible occlusion. Gussack and colleagues presumed correctly that if such fractures exist, and occlusion form is not displaced during normal motion between the mandible and skeletal attachments, the physician should treat the patient and not the radiographic findings.[8]

Furthermore, when teeth of the pediatric patient are used for intermaxillary fixation, a number of considerations must be made. Root resorption of the primary dentition after 5 years of age with incomplete root formation of newly erupted permanent teeth compromises the dentition as a means of sustaining intermaxillary fixation. If indiscriminate dental fixation is used without appropriate splinting of teeth, avulsion of primary or newly erupted permanent teeth can result. Therefore, the dentition of a child between the ages of 5 and 9 years should be used for intermaxillary fixation with the application of appropriate splinting and circumferential wiring to ensure that skeletal fixation does occur and that the teeth do not move indiscriminately.[1–3]

The older pediatric patient also differs from the adult patient in the rate of osteogenic potential. As soon as occlusion is reproducible, the pediatric patient should be released from intermaxillary fixation. The full range of motion must be ensured by the surgical team during the immediate as well as the long-term follow up of the patient. If the rapid response of the osteogenic potential shortens the time of healing for the pediatric patient and subsequently shortens the intermaxillary fixation time, it is important that delay in the reduction of displaced fractures does not extend beyond 4 days.

Nasal fractures in children also differ from those in adults; this difference is directly related to the growth potential of the nasal septal cartilage. Evacuation of septal hematomas with subsequent management by repositioning of the nasal bones and septum should be undertaken early and monitored carefully so that growth is not impaired. Nasal reconstruction in the child is probably not indicated and may in fact be harmful to a child's subsequent nasal and nasal-maxillary development.[1]

APPLIED SURGICAL ANATOMY

Anatomy of Teeth and Supporting Structures

Injuries to the hard tissues of the head and neck region of children in most cases involve teeth as a part of the maxillomandibular skeleton. If the child is injured at a young age, only the primary dentition may be injured. If the injury displaces or avulses the primary dentition, injury can be sustained to the underlying follicles in which the developing permanent teeth lie. Assessment of the injury should determine whether all teeth are present.

Vascular and Supporting Structures of Teeth

In primary and permanent dentition, the teeth are attached to the alveolar bone of the maxilla and mandible by means of periodontal ligaments (Figs. 15–1 and 15–2). One side of the periodontal ligament gives rise to the precursor cells that produce cementum, the tooth root covering matrix, and the opposite side of the periodontal ligament gives rise to the precursors of the osteoprogenitor cells, which contribute to the lamina dura or the interior cortical plate of the mandible. Injury to the tooth itself that exposes the root or the vital pulp structures must be assessed and prioritized for treatment. If the injury involves the periodontal ligament or the attachment of the tooth to the alveolus, early identification and subsequent reduction or restoration of proper anatomy minimizes the long-term sequelae, which may include loss of the tooth, loss of bone, or malposition of the structure.

Traumatic injuries to the underlying developing perma-

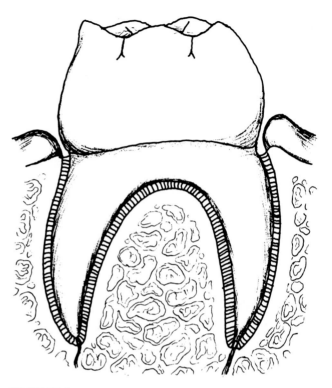

FIGURE 15–2
Lateral view of tooth with periodontal ligament.

nent tooth follicles may occur but in most cases are rare. The permanent tooth follicle (see Fig. 15–1), in its early stages, is a well-vascularized organ and is rarely susceptible to the long-term sequelae of traumatic injuries. If tooth follicles are exposed and teeth avulsed, anatomic repositioning of the erupting tooth into its appropriate site should be undertaken if possible (Table 15–1).

Anatomy of the Developing Permanent Tooth

The most serious damage to the developing dentition may occur in the permanent tooth that has a partially developed root (see Fig. 15–2). When the tooth has erupted into the oral cavity, approximately two thirds of the root has completed development (Figs. 15–3 through 15–5). The strength and integrity of the attachment, however, is immature and makes the individual permanent teeth susceptible to injury before the root has completely formed. If permanent teeth are avulsed, they should be placed immediately in a surgically clean container, moistened with sterile saline, and cooled until they can be reimplanted. Reimplantation must take place within 1 hour.

The presence of teeth and developing follicles in the mandible and maxilla necessitates many anatomic considerations that must be contemplated with injury. The occlusion of the teeth is a delicately balanced mechanism, and any disturbance resulting from the malunion of fragments that bear teeth reduces or impairs the masticatory efficiency. Conversely, the presence of a malocclusion may predispose

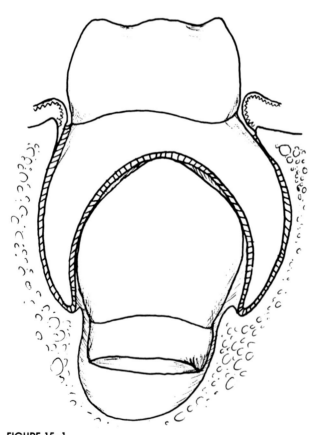

FIGURE 15–1
Primary molar with succeeding permanent tooth and follicle.

Table 15–1
Guidelines for Treatment of the Avulsed Tooth

I. Extraoral time
   A. One of the most critical factors affecting prognosis
   B. If possible, replant the tooth immediately at the site of the injury
      1. If notified by phone, instruct patient, parent, or caller on replantation technique
      2. Stress importance of seeing dentist immediately for follow-up splinting and treatment
II. Storage media
   A. Preferably in the socket
   B. Oral fluids (buccal vestibule, but must be conscious of the possibility of aspiration, especially in the young child)
   C. Milk
   D. Water
III. Management of the socket
   A. Leave alone or gently aspirate without entering and use light irrigation if a blood clot is present
   B. Do not curette the socket
   C. Do not vent the socket
   D. Do not make a surgical flap unless bony fragments prevent replantation
   E. After replantation spread apart
IV. Management of the root surface
   A. Do not handle the root surface; hold tooth by the crown
   B. Do not scrape or brush the root surface or remove any of the root
   C. If the root appears clean, replant as is
   D. If the root surface is dirty, rinse with tap water or saline solution; if persistent debris remains on the root, use cotton pliers to gently pick away any debris, or use a wet sponge to gently brush off debris
   E. No medicaments, disinfectants, or chemicals are applied to the root surface
V. When to do endodontic treatment
   A. Tooth with an open apex
      1. Replant and try for revitalization of the pulp

      2. Follow closely every 2 weeks for signs of pathology
      3. If pathology noted, extirpate pulp and fill canals with calcium hydroxide (i.e., apexification)
   B. Tooth with a fully formed apex
      1. Pulp must be removed between 7 to 14 days postinjury
      2. The canal is then filled with calcium hydroxide
      3. Reclean the canal and repack the calcium hydroxide every 3 mo for a minimum of 6 to 24 mo
      4. Following the above, reclean the canal and fill with a permanent root canal filler
   C. Endodontic treatment is performed in the mouth in all situations
VI. Filling materials
   A. Treatment filling of calcium hydroxide for a minimum of 6 to 24 mo
   B. At completion of calcium hydroxide treatment, permanent obturation with gutta-percha
VII. Splinting
   A. Use acid etch resin alone or with soft arch wire, orthodontic brackets with arch wire or large monofilament fishing line, or as a last resort, suture in position
   B. Splint is left in place for 7 to 10 days
   C. Major bony fractures may require longer splinting times
   D. Diet during splinting
      1. No biting on splinted teeth
      2. Soft foods high in protein
      3. Increase fluid intake
VIII. Adjunctive drug therapy
   A. Refer to physician for tetanus consultation within first 48 h postinjury
   B. Antibiotic therapy not recommended unless medically indicated or in cases of contaminated avulsion

the jaw to more serious injury by creating aberrant forces or a loss of structural integrity. In impacted teeth that are undiagnosed or embedded in the maxilla or mandible, a structural weakness is often created and found many times to rest in conjunction with a fracture produced by the traumatic injury. During diagnosis of maxillary and mandibular fractures, it is important to note the position of tooth-bearing fragments of the mandible and maxilla to determine deviation from their pretraumatic relations.

The anatomy of the mandible in the child varies according to age. The site of embryologic development is the first branchial arch and the cartilage of the first branchial arch gives rise to the site of intermembranous bone development. As the components of the mandible grow, the mus-

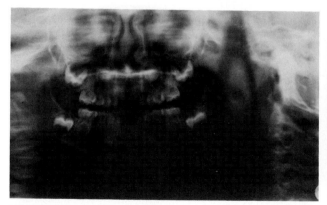

FIGURE 15–3
Pediatric mandible and maxilla.

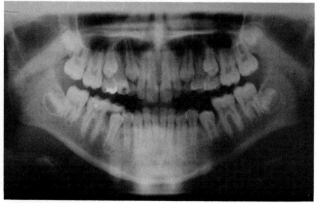

FIGURE 15–4
Adolescent mandible and maxilla.

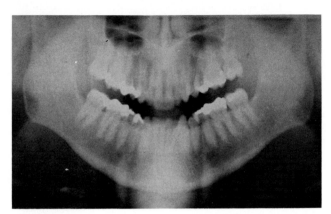

FIGURE 15–5
Adult mandible and maxilla.

cular processes of the gonial angle and the coronoid process becomes more mature and distinct. At the same time, the condyle becomes more mature and increases in size with increasing age of the patient (Fig. 15–6).

The mandible is able to sustain a considerable amount of compressive and tensile loading. There is some degree of flexibility in the adult mandible, and most physicians believe there is more flexibility in the pediatric mandible; because of this, greenstick or partial fractures involving only one cortical plate are more commonly found in pediatric injuries. The sites of injury of the pediatric mandible are specific and correspond for the most part to the sites of adult injury, with some deviation based on age-determining characteristics.

The soft tissue of the mandible appears to play only a small role in influencing the site of mandibular fractures or subsequent displacement. However, the attachment of the periosteum plays an important role in the viability of cortical fragments in the severely injured or comminuted mandible. The inferior alveolar artery is the primary central vascular channel to the mandible. Along with the inferior alveolar artery rests the neural component to the mandible, the mandibular division of the trigeminal nerve. This neu-rovascular bundle provides sensation to the teeth, mucosa, chin, and lip area after the nerve exits the mental foramen. Damage to the inferior alveolar artery and veins may predispose the mandible to ischemia but only in cases in which periosteal attachment has also been separated.

CLASSIFICATION OF INJURIES

Fractures of the Mandible

The zygomatic arch of the child gives some measure of protection to the condyle from direct trauma. However, the condyle may be injured at one of three levels. An intracapsular fracture may take place at the high articular surface area (Fig. 15–7). The impact transmitted to the neck of the condyle determines the extent of the injury. Injury may also occur without a fracture of the calcified component of the mandible; this is known as a subcondylar fracture (Fig. 15–8). This injury may produce hemarthrosis or avulsion of the temporomandibular ligament or joint capsule and result in fracture dislocation (Fig. 15–9).

The ramus and cornoid processes are the muscular or calcified processes for attachment of the temporalis muscle in the jaw. The muscles of mastication, in addition to the force of trauma, dictate the degree of displacement of anatomic injuries. For purposes of treatment, a fracture can be classified as *favorable* or *unfavorable* from either the *lateral, horizontal,* or *vertical* perspective. In fractures of the body of the mandible, in which the mylohyoid produces a medial pull on a proximal fracture, the fracture may be classified as medially displaced or unfavorable. If the fracture line has a relation or direction that prevents displacement when the normal forces of the temporalis, medial pterygoid, masseter, and mylohyoid muscles close the jaw, the fracture may have a horizontal, favorable component (Fig. 15–10). Care should be taken in defining the planes or directions of net muscle pull on each of the separate fractures of the mandible. After definition of muscle pull has been considered in context with the direction of fracture, appropriate classification of the injury can be made.

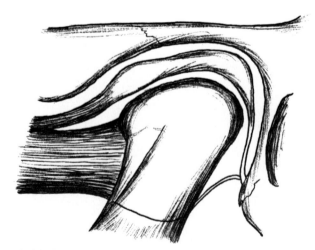

FIGURE 15–6
Temporomandibular joint.

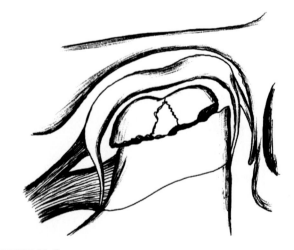

FIGURE 15–7
Intracapsular condylar fracture.

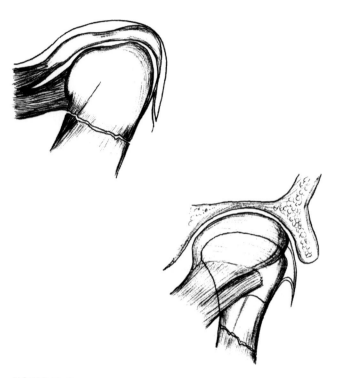

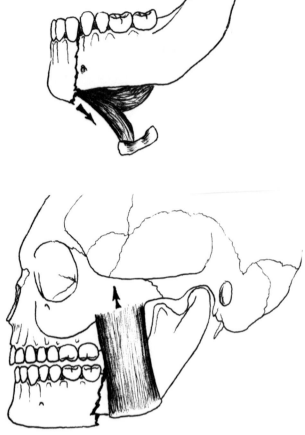

FIGURE 15–8
Subcondylar fracture. The lateral view is upper left; the antero-posterior view is lower right.

Further classifications involve fractures of the tooth-bearing area of the mandible. When the tooth-bearing area of the mandible is fractured, and the periodontal ligaments have been disturbed, an open or compound classification should be applied. The only exception is when the fracture area is near that of the unerupted wisdom tooth or the unerupted molar follicle that does not have a preceding primary tooth. This type of fracture is classified as an open or compound injury, and appropriate antibiotics are prescribed to prevent mandible and temporomandibular joint infection.

FIGURE 15–10
Fracture classification of the mandible: favorable, unfavorable of angle, body, symphysis, and dentoalveolar. Arrows indicate direction of displacement due to muscle pull.

Fractures of the mandible can be classified according to the location of the break as (A) condylar, (B) angle, (C) symphysis, (D) dentoalveolar, or (E) body fracture. Fractures may also occur in a wide variety of combinations (Fig. 15–11). Displacement of the fracture by the actual force of injury or subsequent displacement by the muscle attached to the fragment and determination of the favorability or unfavorability of the fracture provide a means of classifying and grouping these injuries. Although the diagrams in Figure 15–11 are simple in this classification system, some concern must always be directed at the degree of disruption of the condylar capsule. In some instances when a fracture does not occur, malocclusion may be reported or noted by the patient and is a reflection of a hemarthrosis and subsequent edema of the joint. The envelope of motion for the mandible is also compromised if the net contraction of the lateral pterygoid displaces the fracture. A caveat worth remembering states: "The mandible deviates to the side of the injury if a fracture dislocation of the mandibular condyle exists." This is understandable if the physician considers the attachment of the lateral pterygoid and the integration of its relation to the functioning muscles of mastication.

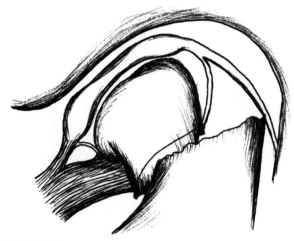

FIGURE 15–9
Condylar fracture with displacement and deviation.

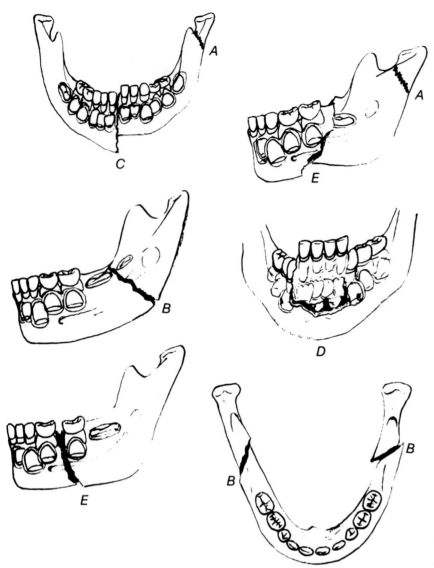

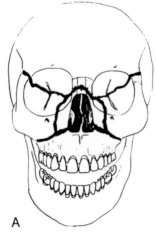

FIGURE 15–11

Mandibular fractures demonstrating displacement due to pull of muscles of mastication (including mylohyoid and suprahyoid).

Anatomy of the Middle Third of the Face

The maxillofacial skeleton is composed of the maxilla, zygomatic bone, zygomatic process of the temporal bone, and zygomatic process of the frontal bone. The nasal and ethmoid bones contribute to the nasal orbital component of the maxillofacial skeleton. The palatine bone constitutes the most posterior margin of the palate, and the pterygoid plates of the sphenoid bone provide the buttress systems for the posterior maxilla.

The classification of midface fractures was developed and defined by Le Fort (Fig. 15–12). A Le Fort I fracture is a horizontal fracture of the maxilla above the alveolar process and horizontal plate of the palatine and palatal process of the maxilla. A Le Fort II fracture is a pyramidal fracture involving the orbital floors, the lamina papyracea of the ethmoids, and separation of the frontal nasal suture. A Le Fort III fracture involves craniofacial disarticulation with separation of the facial bones from the cranial buttress

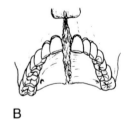

FIGURE 15–12

A, Le Fort maxillary fractures. See text for classification and description. *B* shows a view of a palatal split.

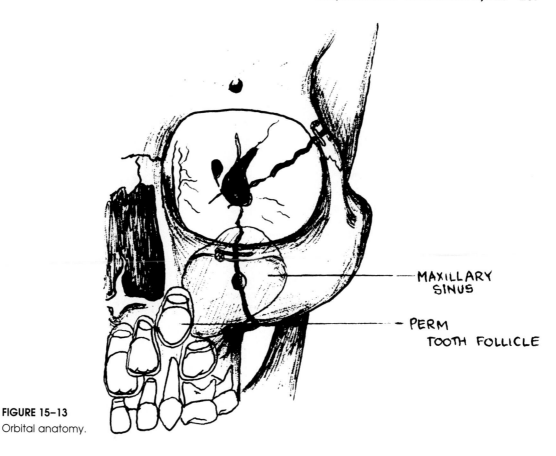

FIGURE 15–13
Orbital anatomy.

systems. Separation normally occurs at or near the fronto-zygomatic suture at the lateral orbital wall.

Anatomy of the Zygomaticomaxillary Complex

The anatomy of the orbit is illustrated in Figure 15–13. The optic nerve enters through the optic canal of the sphenoid bone. Through a fissure between the greater and lesser wing of the sphenoid, the nerve passes through the superior orbital fissure to the lateral rectus muscle, the superior oblique muscle, the ocular motor nerve, and the other extraocular muscles. Arteries enter the orbit centrally and pass to the optic nerve and the other orbital structures through the superior orbital fissure (Fig. 15–14). The contents of the superior orbital fissure are important in terms of compression or scissor-type injuries in instances of significant or marked displacement of the zygoma. If this type of injury occurs, ophthalmoplegia, proptosis, and chemosis may be present as external findings, and dilation of the pupil may occur due to sympathetic predominance in the control of the ciliary muscles. Ischemic changes or injury to the optic nerve should be of the utmost concern in characterizing or classifying injuries to the zygomatic or nasal orbital complexes.

Along the medial aspect of the inferior orbital rim is the lacrimal fossa, which opens into the nasal passage below the inferior concha through the lacrimal duct system. The soft tissues of the eye are supported by suspensory liga-

ments attached medially to the lacrimal crest and laterally to the frontal process of the zygoma. This suspensory ligament system is a part of the periorbital periosteum and is also the attachment of the origin of the orbicularis oculi muscles. The physician must take these normal anatomic landmarks into consideration during the diagnosis of fractures in the zygomatic area.

An anatomic depression exists on the anterior surface of

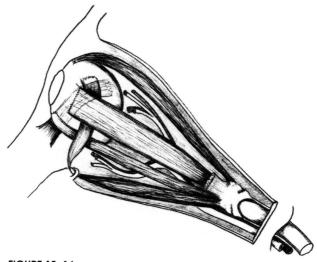

FIGURE 15–14
View of orbital contents and extraocular muscles.

the zygomatic process of the frontal bone. This anatomic depression is known as the lacrimal fossa, and it results in structural weakness in the buttress system of the orbit in the midface and may be the location of a frontozygomatic separation with severe trauma. This angular process fracture is significant because of the relation of the lacrimal fossa to the extension of the anterior cranial fossa in or near the zygomatic process of the frontal bone.

Radiographic Examination

Although radiation exposure should be minimized, critical views of anatomic structure should be attained in at least two planes. Traditionally, the following radiographs have been used for mandibular or maxillofacial injuries: right and left lateral oblique views, posteroanterior view of the mandible, Towne view for assessment of condylar neck regions of the mandible, and Water sinus view for evaluation of midfacial structures and sinuses and orbital injury assessment. For more refined treatment of the teeth and dentoalveolar structure, a panoramic radiograph or individual dental periapical films, or occlusal views of the maxilla or mandible can be obtained after the critical care phase of management.

Classification of Fractures of the Maxillofacial Skeleton

Structural weakness exists in the maxillofacial area of the adult skeleton at three distinct anatomic levels. These levels or areas, described by Le Fort and discussed previously, are listed as follows: Le Fort I, horizontal fracture of the maxilla (see Fig. 15–12); Le Fort II, pyramidal fracture of the maxilla; Le Fort III, cranial facial disarticulation. A Le Fort I or horizontal fracture of the maxilla in the child's skeleton is a rare occurrence because of the incomplete development of the maxillary sinus. Le Fort II and Le Fort III injuries in

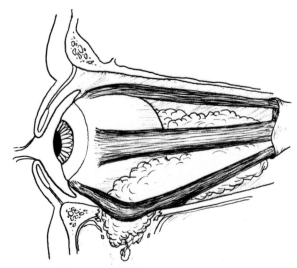

FIGURE 15–15
Orbital blowout fracture.

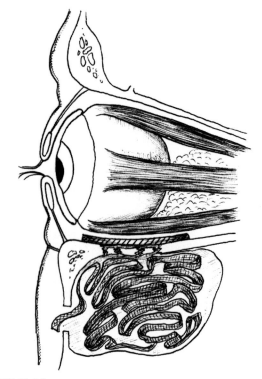

FIGURE 15–16
Orbital floor implant with antral packing.

the pediatric patient are also extremely rare because of the pliable nature of the midface structures in this age group.

Another unusual injury that occurs more often in the adult than in the child or adolescent is the orbital floor fracture (Fig. 15–15). As the orbit increases in size and the antrum pneumatizes the body of the maxilla and zygoma, a thin bone separates the orbit from the maxillary sinus. The orbital blowout is rarely seen before the maxillary sinus is near its adult size. This fracture is caused by hydrostatic forces transmitted through the orbital contents to the area of structural weakness between the orbital floor and the maxillary sinus, and it is easily treated by antral packing of the orbital floor after an implant is placed (Fig. 15–16).

Zygomatic injuries can occur in an isolated fashion with separation of the frontozygomatic suture of the infraorbital rim, the temporal process of the zygoma, or the zygomaticomaxillary buttress. Zygomatic fractures can occur in conjunction with a Le Fort II or Le Fort III injury or in an isolated fashion.

TREATMENT CONSIDERATIONS

Reduction of Dentoalveolar Fractures

Dental wiring[5] or fixation of alveolar fractures has traditionally been performed by using Erich arch bars (Fig. 15–17), stainless steel wiring (Fig. 15–18), or cold cured acrylic to stabilize individual or groups of teeth (Fig. 15–19). On occasion, cold cured acrylic splints can be used to stabilize teeth, and suture type splints (Fig. 15–20) can be used for partially erupted teeth. The acrylic splints can be fashioned

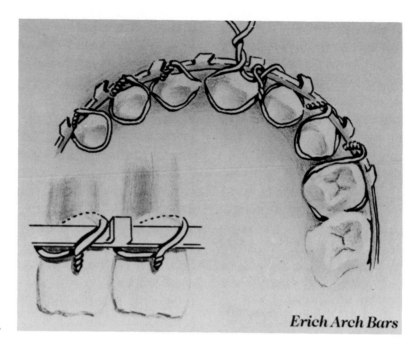

FIGURE 15–17
Erich arch bars.

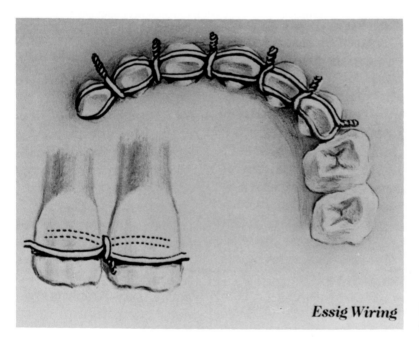

FIGURE 15–18
Continuous dental wiring.

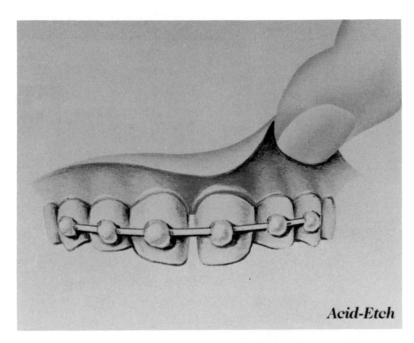

FIGURE 15-19
Cold-cured acrylic fixation with orthodontic wire.

after plaster molds are made of the injured teeth and the teeth are reapproximated to the original position. After dentoalveolar stability has been achieved, injury of the supporting bone of the maxilla and mandible can be addressed. If edentulous segments are present, the patient's partial or complete dentures can be used to stabilize the fragments, and the denture can be used for intermaxillary reduction of the injury.

Dislocation of the Mandibular Condyles

If radiographic assessment of the mandibular condyles shows that they are anatomically positioned near the gle-

noid fossa, the mandible can be positioned in intermaxillary fixation and then assessed for fragments that are not properly reduced or will be affected by muscle pull. Fixation should include the following steps, based on the complexity of the injury: (1) stainless-steel ligature interosseus wiring, which consists of stainless-steel mesh fixations with compatible wire or screws and rigid fixation using stainless steel or other biocompatible alloys; or (2) application of the Joe Hall Morris external fixation system (Fig. 15–21) to the proper location sites of the mandible, condylar-neck region, external oblique region, and inferior border, demonstrating close coupling of forces with a minimum of two pins per segment. If the transverse dimension of the mandible cannot be reduced effectively, a lingual splint should be fabricated (Fig. 15–22).

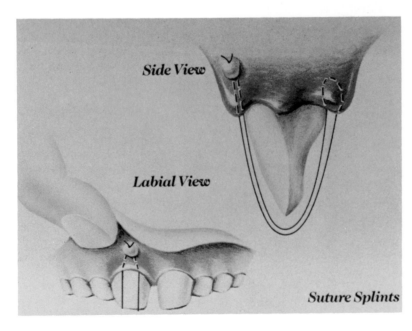

Suture Splints **FIGURE 15-20**
Suture-type splints.

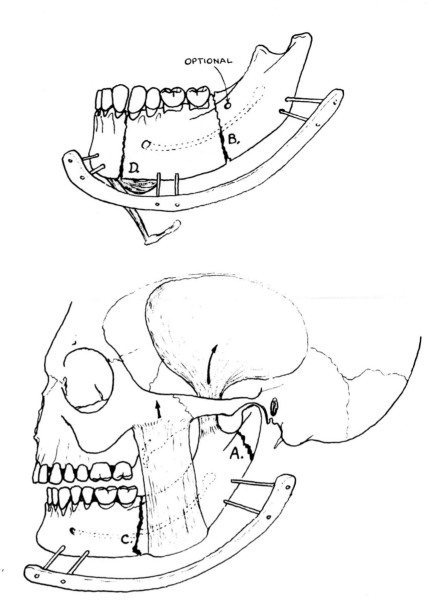

FIGURE 15–21
Mandibular fracture with ''Joe Hall Morris''
external pin fixation.

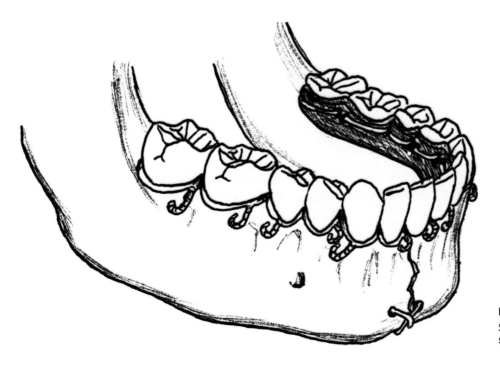

FIGURE 15–22
Symphysis fracture with lingual
splint and inferior border wiring.

Open Reduction and Internal Fixation of Angle and Body Fractures

Open reduction and internal fixation of unfavorable angle and body fractures may require consideration. Internal fixation is traditionally achieved through a Risdon incision (Fig. 15–23). The incision for this approach is located approximately 1 cm below the angle of the mandible, below the marginal mandibular branch of the facial nerve. The dissection is performed by sharp division of the platysma muscle and blunt dissection through the superficial layers of the deep cervical fascia to the angle of the mandible. The periosteum is incised and reflected to identify the fracture line. Preoperative radiographs are used to determine the location of the fracture in relation to the unerupted tooth follicles. The location of these tooth follicles and the nearby neurovascular bundle should be considered when determining placement of interosseous wires or rigid fixation devices.

If the mandibular growth is nearly complete and the fracture occurs through the unerupted third molar, an intraoral approach for open reduction and internal fixation can be considered.[7] The developing third molar tooth and follicle can be removed through an incision along the crest of the ridge into the lateral aspect of the mucosal buccal surface. Stainless steel wire fixation can then be used to reduce the fracture. The parts of fixation should be located in the area of the external oblique ridge for optimum strength.

Open reduction and internal wire fixation of maxillofacial structures is often complicated by bacterial contamination.[8] Appropriate broad-spectrum antibiotics should be included as part of the treatment regimen, because open fractures are exposed to the nosocomial bacteria of the oral cavity.[9]

Fractures located more anteriorly in the body of the mandible can also be treated by open reduction and internal fixation from an extraoral approach. This is especially helpful if the fragment is forced medially by the muscle pull of the mylohyoid and the medial pterygoid muscles and control cannot be effected by arch bars ligated to the teeth located in the proximal fragment.

Condylar Fractures

If a condylar fracture occurs in association with other mandibular or maxillary fractures, the condylar fracture may need to be reduced and internally stabilized to provide vertical facial stability. A Dingman and Constant preauricular approach or a Risdon approach below and behind the angle of the mandible to the condylar region provides the surgeon with two options. If fixation is required in the high condylar head or neck area, a preauricular incision made 0.5 cm in front of the tragus of the ear can be used (Fig. 15–24). If the fracture is subcondylar, a submandibular or Risdon approach, as previously described, can be used. The surgeon has a variety of options for fixation of condylar fractures after they are exposed. A two-dimensional Vitallium screen with either wire or Vitallium screw fixation is illustrated in Figure 15–25.

MIDFACIAL FRACTURES

Because optimal management of maxillofacial fractures is best considered from a three-dimensional perspective, efforts to establish mandibular continuity have proven to be the most consistent initial step. After completion and stabilization of injuries to the mandible, intermaxillary fixation and subsequent zygomatic or craniofacial suspension is undertaken in the majority of midfacial fractures.[10] A retrospective analysis of Le Fort fractures[11] emphasized the importance of suspension in Le Fort I, II, and III midfacial injuries to the most proximate superior stable abutment. The surgeon has three options for such fixation or suspension (Fig. 15–26).

More complex or comminuted fractures of the midfacial skeleton may require a combination of interosseous stainless steel ligatures in the buttresses of the maxilla and zygomatic areas. Modifications of stainless steel, Vitallium, and titanium bone plates provide the surgeon with a variety of options for internal fixation if required (Fig. 15–27).

The Role of the Caldwell-Luc Operation in Open Reduction and Fixation of Midface Fractures

Identification and repair of midface structural injuries can be accomplished through a Caldwell-Luc incision to approach the maxillary sinus (Fig. 15–28).[4, 13–16] The surgeon can inspect for comminution of the anterior buttresses, the nasal piriform buttress, and the zygomatic buttress and with minimal extension, examine the maxillary sinus with an aperture large enough to palpate or inspect the infraorbital

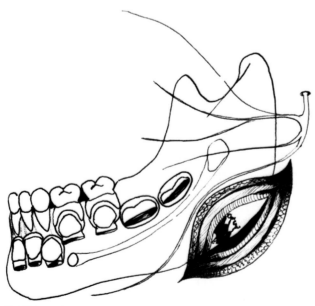

FIGURE 15–23
Open reduction and internal fixation of angle fractures.

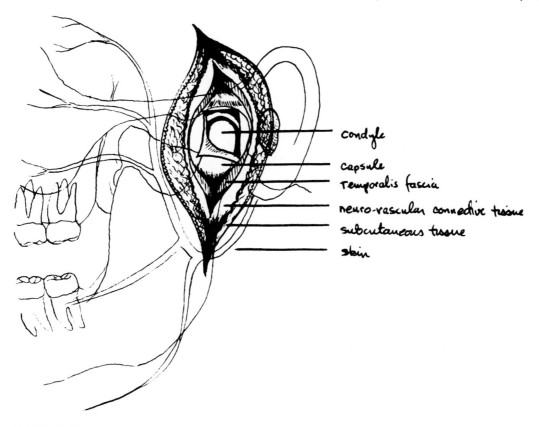

condyle
capsule
temporalis fascia
neuro-vascular connective tissue
subcutaneous tissue
skin

FIGURE 15-24
Open reduction and fixation of condylar fracture (preauricular approach).

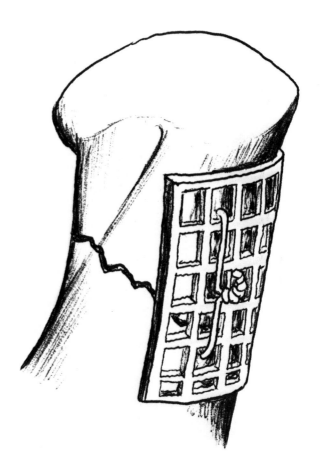

FIGURE 15-25
Vitallium screen fixation of condylar fracture.

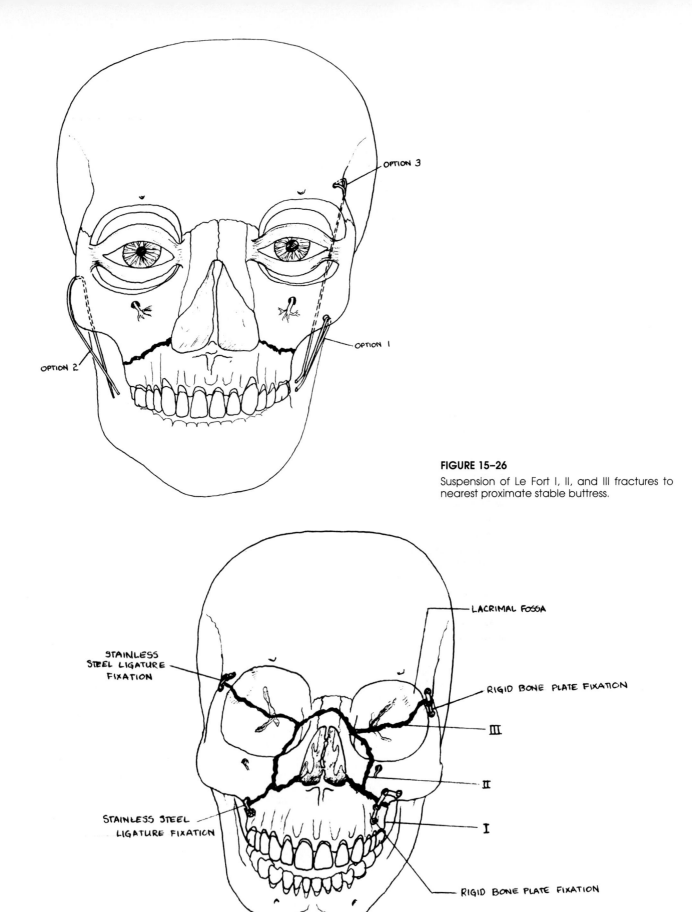

FIGURE 15-26
Suspension of Le Fort I, II, and III fractures to nearest proximate stable buttress.

FIGURE 15-27
Internal fixation option for Le Fort I, II, and III fractures.

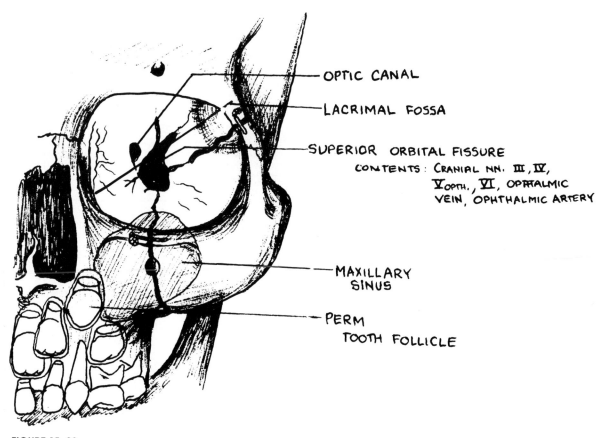

OPTIC CANAL

LACRIMAL FOSSA

SUPERIOR ORBITAL FISSURE
CONTENTS: CRANIAL NN. III, IV,
V opth., VI, OPHTALMIC
VEIN, OPHTHALMIC ARTERY

MAXILLARY SINUS

PERM TOOTH FOLLICLE

FIGURE 15–28
Structures approachable through a Caldwell-Luc incision.

floor. If displacement of the zygomatic arch has occurred, a large Kelly clamp or urethral sound can be used to elevate the zygoma and reestablish integrity of the zygomaticomaxillary buttress at the arch. Interosseous wiring, rigid fixation, or packing of the sinus can then be accomplished to reduce and stabilize the zygoma. Maxillary packing, if also accomplished, should be gentle so as not to compress structures or displace comminuted fragments into the orbit.[17, 18] If comminution of the orbital floor has occurred and no deficit exists in extraocular movement, a traction test or forced duction test, in which forceps are used to grasp the ocular globe at the insertion of the inferior rectus muscle approximately 7 mm from the limbus, to examine the inferior rectus muscle can also be performed during the operation. A few drops of local anesthetic instilled into the conjunctival sac allows the eyeball to be grasped. This test provides a means of differentiating entrapment of the inferior rectus muscle from weakness or paralysis of the superior rectus muscle, and it is pathognomonic for a blowout fracture of the floor of the orbit. Additional management of the comminuted orbital floor may be required, including an organic implant with packing (see Fig. 15–16). In the pediatric patient, care should be taken to enter the maxillary sinus only after radiographic confirmation that an orbital fracture exists, and such an approach should be performed at a level high enough to avoid damaging the follicles of the maxillary cuspid and premolar teeth.

If the frontozygomatic suture is intact, and midface sta-

bility cannot be effected by interosseous fixation of the zygomatic buttress, circum zygomatic wires may be attached after being passed through and over the intact zygomatic arch (see Fig. 15–27, Option II). However, if the frontozygomatic suture is not intact, it may be the next most superior buttress to require vertical facial suspension. This procedure is best approached through a brow incision slightly medial to the eyebrow and overlying the frontozygomatic suture. The frontozygomatic suture is identified, and an interosseous stainless-steel ligature is placed.

After assessment of facial symmetry, treatment is customized to the nature of the midface fractures, with attention given to appropriate anatomic reduction of the orbital floor as necessary. Loss of orbital integrity requires a subciliary or skin fold incision that allows a stair-stepped approach through the skin, subcutaneous tissue, and periosteum of the infraorbital rim. This type of incision reduces scar formation and subsequent lymphedema, which can produce ectropion of the lower lid (i.e., an outward turning or eversion of the eyelid margin).

After the infraorbital rim is reduced and fixed, if the infraorbital rim is also fractured, the fragments are realigned and fixation maintained by interosseous ligature fixation. Restoration of the continuity of the orbital floor is required in all orbital floor fractures. An iliac bone graft or plate is usually preferable and well able to resist infection. In comminution and loss of integrity of the infraorbital floor, similar autografted or allografted bone or inorganic implants such as Dacron mesh or Silastic sheets can be used (see Fig. 15–16), obviating the need for bone harvesting. The purpose of the orbital floor insert is to reestablish continuity of the floor, seal off the orbit from the maxillary sinus, and restore the volume of the orbital cavity.

With fractures of the medial orbital wall, or nasal-orbital-ethmoid injuries, definition of the injury should include intercanthal measurements. If loss of integrity of the nasal bridge and nasal-orbital area exists, the intercanthal dimension should be palpated to note whether the medial canthal ligament is attached to any of the comminuted fragments. If the medial canthal ligament is indeed attached to comminuted bone, a transnasal suture is passed posterior and superior to the lacrimal crest, through the ethmoids and the nasal septum below the cribriform plate, and out the contralateral side. A similar suture is then placed below the medial canthal ligaments through the comminuted fracture to the contralateral side (Fig. 15–29; see Figs. 15–13 and 15–28). A dental cotton roll or malleable metal splint can then be secured, ensuring that the proper intercanthal dimension is restored when the wire or suture is tightened.

After completion of this procedure, care should be taken to inspect the nasal bones and septum for displacement or deviation. In the event of cerebral spinal fluid rhinorrhea, no nasal packing should be performed, but the nasal bone and septal reduction should be observed and revised at a later date if necessary.

Isolated Zygomatic Fractures

The Knight and North system[13] continues to be the standard classification for zygomatic fractures. This system of classification helps to predict the clinical features of the fracture and plan treatment (Table 15–2). This classification is useful also because of its predictability of stability. Arch fractures and lateral rotated body fractures all appear to be stable and require little treatment other than reduction of the displacement. Medially rotated body fractures are unstable and require antral packing or fixation at the buttresses. Unrotated body fractures that are unstable are satisfactorily treated by antral packing alone. Complex fractures that are unstable require either direct wiring or fixation by some

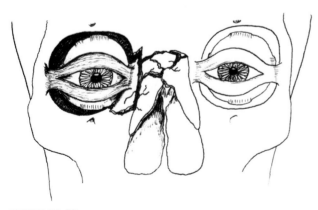

FIGURE 15–29
Naso-orbital ethmoid fractures.

Table 15–2
Knight and North Classification of Zygomatic Fractures

Class I: No significant displacement—fracture visible by roentgenogram but fragments aligned
Class II: Arch fractures with inward buckling of the arch and no orbital or antral involvement
Class III: Unrotated body fractures—downward and inward displacement but no rotation
Class IV: Medially rotated body fractures—downward or inward and backward displacement with medial rotation
Class V: Laterally rotated body fractures—downward, backward and medial displacement with lateral rotation
Class VI: Complex fractures—all classes, with additional fracture lines crossing the main fragment

Adapted from Knight JS, North JF, Chir B: The classification of malar fractures: An analysis of displacement as a guide to treatment. Br J Plast Surg 13:325–339, 1961.

other mechanism. Diplopia, as a component of isolated zygomatic fractures, usually reflects displacement of the orbital floor with possible entrapment of the inferior rectus muscle.

GENERAL CONSIDERATIONS IN MANAGEMENT OF ZYGOMATIC FRACTURES

The initial evaluation phase of management of these injuries should include gentle irrigation with removal of foreign bodies, bridges, dentures, and tooth and bone fragments from the wounds, oral cavity, and upper airway. In the semiconscious or unconscious individual, assessment and management of the airway by either oropharyngeal, nasopharyngeal, or endotracheal intubation, or if necessary, a tracheostomy, must be considered. Control of intraoral and extraoral bleeding should be accomplished by either direct pressure or subsequent individual ligation of bleeding vessels, if necessary.

Temporary stabilization of fractures, particularly in the mandible with dental wiring, is helpful and may concurrently control bleeding and provide some improved comfort to the patient while more critical injuries or management problems are being attended. If severe bleeding is encountered from either nasal or nasopharyngeal injuries, care should be taken in assessment of the bleeding to ensure that cerebrospinal fluid rhinorrhea is not a contraindication to anterior nasal packing, because the cribriform plate is superior to the pressure imposed by such packing.[6, 14] Rarely is posterior nasal packing required; however, it can be accomplished in the presence of severe bleeding from injuries to the nasal orbital ethmoid or upper midface areas.

Intubation via the nasal endotracheal route is not contraindicated in the case of severe nasal or nasal orbital ethmoid injuries, because the nasal endotracheal tube should traverse the lower portion of the nasal cavity and should not impinge on a cribriform plate injury.

A thorough eye examination should be done on all patients, particularly those suspected of zygomatic or maxillary injury. Teeth in the line of fractures should be examined, and if they are highly mobile, removed to prevent aspiration. Further efforts should be directed at diagnosis to determine evidence of root fracture or severe crown injury.

GROWTH ABNORMALITIES SECONDARY TO TRAUMATIC INJURIES

Maxillofacial growth abnormalities secondary to facial trauma can be primary or secondary to the injury. If the hard tissue skeleton is not returned to its original anatomic position, the primary deformity or asymmetry in the midfacial bone will be apparent on resolution of the swelling and edema. Secondary growth abnormalities are observed much later in the sequence of healing and are a reflection of impaired function.

Ankylosis of the Temporomandibular Joint

Damage of the growth center by an intracapsular condylar injury (see Fig. 15–7) results in the most dramatic or severe secondary growth abnormalities and is a reflection of failure to correctly diagnose the extent of the injury, with subsequent undermanagement of problems related to function of the mandible. An example of this type of injury is an intracapsular condylar fracture in the child or adolescent. Often, this injury does not produce anatomic deformity or malocclusion, and the initial symptoms may be only pain or swelling with restriction of motion of the ipsilateral temporomandibular joint. If there is pain or limitation in the range of motion but no abnormality in the malocclusion, the patient's range of motion should be supervised at weekly intervals and normal motion encouraged by either forced vertical opening or appropriate physical therapy to return the jaw to a full range of motion.

An impaired or incomplete range of motion with either deviation to the injured side or limited opening results in ankylosis of the temporomandibular joint, development of intracapsular adhesions, and possibly subsequent bony ankylosis. During the period of time between the first observable reproducible occlusion of the teeth without intermaxillary fixation or guidance, supervised forced vertical opening should be instituted by either the patient, parent, or surgeon. The range of motion must be restored to prevent ankylosis and subsequent growth deformity (Fig. 15–30), which is a reflection of incomplete expression of the growth potential from the temporomandibular joint and vertical ramus. Ankylosis of the temporomandibular joint can be classified as follows:

1. True ankylosis: fibrous adhesions (i.e., syndesmosis) or bony ankylosis of the temporomandibular joint that restricts the translation of the condyle and limits vertical opening.

2. False ankylosis: restricted range of motion secondary to fibromyositis or muscle spasm.

Ankylosis of the temporomandibular joint should be suspected, diagnosis made, and management instituted at the earliest possible time to minimize these consequences of growth impairment.

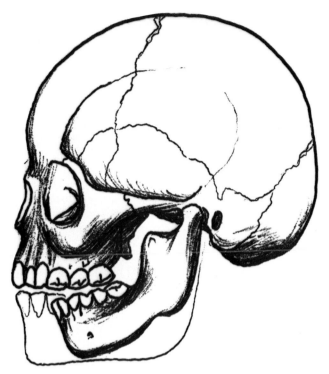

FIGURE 15–30
Retrognathic mandible due to condylar fracture with ankylosis.

Zygomaticomaxillary Deficiency Secondary to Facial Trauma

The growth of the zygomaticomaxillary complex is due to appositional growth on the surface and at the sutures separating the bones of the maxillofacial skeleton. The cartilaginous nasal septum and cartilages increase their size through interstitial growth and are believed to play a role in coordinating the nasal profile and directing the vertical and anteroposterior dimensions to the maxilla. The importance of approximation of mucosal covering by packing in nasal fractures requires emphasis, because the perichondrium must be appropriately reapproximated to achieve integrity of the nasal septum. Because the perichondrium is the primary source of nutrients for cartilage viability, appropriate treatment in this area is extremely important. If viable cartilage is not maintained in the child, liquefactive necrosis and scar formation causes deviation of the nasal septum and possible disfiguring alteration of the nasal profile and related maxillary structures. Prevention of this deformity is important and certainly produces a more successful outcome than rehabilitation during the postoperative period of growth.

Skeletal growth of the zygomaticomaxillary and nasal regions appears to be somewhat refractory to interosseous rigid fixation. Little is known about the impaired growth potential of the midfacial structures due to rigid fixation. Stress shielding may occur with some of the more rigid bone-plating systems, impairing growth and surface apposition of the midfacial bones. Bone plates should probably be removed after healing of the facial fractures has taken place to minimize these consequences of asymmetric or impaired growth.

SUMMARY

Maxillofacial injuries in the child provide special challenges to the trauma team and trauma surgeon. The early identification and removal of foreign bodies, denture fragments, tooth fragments, and bone fragments from the oral cavity should be the highest initial priority; this is especially the case in the obtunded, semiconscious, or unconscious patient. After the restoration or establishment of airway patency, control of intraoral and extraoral bleeding and temporary stabilization of gross or displaced fractures should be considered. If severe bleeding occurs from the nasal maxillary area, appropriate control with packing should be accomplished. Teeth in the line of fracture should be examined for looseness to prevent subsequent loss and aspiration.

Diagnostic considerations for the adolescent patient are not substantially different from those for the adult other than the smaller anatomic size and a special consideration for unerupted teeth and preservation of tissue, because the related growth potential is important. The objective of treatment of pediatric maxillofacial injuries should be to return or restore the original position at the earliest, safest time to diminish subsequent deformity and impaired function.

References

1. Adams WM: Internal wiring fixation of facial fractures. Surgery 12:523–540, 1942.
2. Behrman SJ, Behrman DA: Facial injuries. In: Wade PA (ed): Surgical Treatment of Trauma. New York, Grune & Stratton, 1960, pp 402–448.
3. Camp JH: Recommended guidelines for treatment of the avulsed tooth. J Am Dent Assoc 107:706, 1983.
4. Dingman RO, Alling CC: Open reduction and internal wire fixation of maxillofacial fractures. J Maxillofac Surg 12:140–156, 1954.
5. Donoff RB: Manual of oral and maxillofacial surgery. St Louis, CV Mosby 1987.
6. Finizio TA: Dentoalveolar trauma. American Association of Oral and Maxillofacial Surgeons, Clinical Update, Winter 1987/1988, pp 2–6.
7. Finley PM, Ward-Booth RP, Moos KF: Morbidity associated with the use of antral packs in external pins in the treatment of the unstable fracture of the zygomatic complex. Br J Oral Maxillofac Surg 22:18–23, 1984.
8. Gussack GS, Luterman A, Powell RW, et al: Pediatric maxillofacial trauma: Unique features in diagnosis and treatment. Laryngoscope 97:925–930, 1987.
9. Heimgartner-Candinas B, Heimgartner M: Results of treatment of midfacial fractures. J Maxillofac Surg 6:293–301, 1978.
10. James DR: Maxillofacial injuries in children. In: Rowe NL, Williams JL (eds): Maxillofacial Injuries. Vol. 1. New York, Churchill Livingstone, 1985, pp 538–558.
11. James RB, Fredrickson C, Kent JN: Prospective study of mandibular fractures. J Oral Surg 39:275–281, 1981.
12. Kaban LB, Mulliken JB, Murray JE: Facial fractures in children: An analysis of 122 fractures in 109 patients. Plast Reconstr Surg 59:15–20, 1977.
13. Knight JS, North JF, Chir B: The classification of malar fractures: An analysis of displacement as a guide to treatment. Br J Plast Surg 13:325–339, 1961.
14. Kreutziger KL: Complex maxillofacial fractures: Management and surgical procedures. South Med J 75:783–793, 1982.
15. Paul JK, Acevedo A: Intraoral open reduction. J Oral Surg 26:516–522, 1968.
16. Reynolds JR: Late complications vs. method of treatment in a large series of mid-facial fractures. Plast Reconstr Surg 61:871–875, 1978.
17. Shira RB: Open reduction of mandibular fractures. J Oral Maxillofac Surg 12:95–111, 1954.
18. Steidler NE, Cook RM, Reade PC: Residual complications in patients with major middle third facial fractures. Int J Oral Maxillofac Surg 9:259–266, 1980.

Gerald S. Gussack
L. Clark Simpson

CHAPTER SIXTEEN

Ear, Nose, and Throat Injuries

The management of injuries to the ears, nose, and throat in patients in the pediatric population begins by following the basic axioms of all trauma management; early establishment and maintenance of an adequate airway, arrest of hemorrhage, and assurance of adequate circulation. Factors unique to the injured pediatric patient, such as smaller circulating blood volume, smaller airway, and relatively late appearance of clinical signs of hypovolemic shock, must be considered.[45] The initial workup and evaluation also includes, if possible, a careful history of the mechanism of the injury along with a brief but concise medical history of the patient. A tetanus history should be specifically sought and appropriate immunizations given if they are inadequate. A careful physical examination and assessment, appropriate for the patient, should also be undertaken to look for associated injuries.[2] A review of 30 children with head and neck injuries at the University of South Alabama trauma center noted a 66% incidence of major associated injuries, the majority of which were orthopedic or neurologic in nature, or both.[22]

NASAL TRAUMA

Etiology

Nasal trauma is a frequent childhood occurrence and accounts for the majority of facial fractures in most reviews of pediatric maxillofacial injuries.[24, 31] The etiology of these is multiple and includes trauma occurring during delivery in the neonate, falls and household accidents in the toddler age group, sports and recreational injuries in the older child, and major trauma from high impact injuries such as motor vehicle accidents in the adolescent group.

Physical Examination

Nasal injuries can result in fractures of the bony pyramid, the cartilaginous nasal vault, the septum, or a combination of all three. Hence, examination of the nose, with inspection of the internal and external airways, is essential. Initially, swelling and edema secondary to ecchymosis may mask the deformity, and reexamination may be required 3 to 4 days following the injury.[63] A small pediatric nasal speculum and good illumination are important, and careful evaluation for evidence of a septal hematoma is undertaken. This would appear as a soft fluctuant area by both visual examination and palpation.[49] A topical vasoconstrictor sprayed in the nose, such as phenylephrine hydrochloride (Neo-Synephrine) 0.25%, is helpful. A septal hematoma, if not recognized early, may develop into an abscess and cause destruction of the septal cartilage that can lead to a saddle nose deformity later in life.[20]

A septal hematoma should be drained through an incision of the mucoperichondrium in the inferior dependent portion of the septum. When the hematoma involves both sides of the septum, bilateral incisions should be made. Prophylactic antibiotics are also indicated along with a basting suture through the nasal septum or nasal packing for a short period of time.

Palpation of the bridge and dorsum of the nose is helpful to clinically define any fractures or dislocations. An "open book" type of fracture is very common in children when the midline nasal suture is not fused. The upper lateral cartilages are loosely attached to the nasal bones and may be disrupted easily.

Radiographs

Routine radiographs are probably not necessary in the diagnosis and treatment of these injuries. However, plain films may be utilized to document a fracture that has been diagnosed clinically. A negative radiographic report should never be used as a substitute for a complete intranasal examination in any child with nasal trauma because some confusion exists in the everyday interpretation of such films that is related to the common appearance of vascular markings that run longitudinally over the dorsum of the nasal bones.[49] True nasal fractures are seen as lines that run transversely or perpendicular to these vascular markings.

Treatment

Treatment of nasal fractures may be undertaken in the immediate postinjury period or delayed for 3 to 4 days. Closed reduction under general anesthesia is the most efficacious approach with younger children and allows a more complete examination of the septum. Local anesthesia combined with topical cocaine application and intravenous sedation may be utilized in older children.

The question of how extensive a nasal operation to perform in children remains a source of controversy.[19, 49] Grymer and colleagues reviewed 57 children 0 to 16 years of age who sustained fractures of the nose. They noted a significant percentage of these patients had osseous and cartilaginous deformities along with deviated septums, nasal spine abnormalities, and saddle nose deformities.[20] A follow-up study of those patients who were treated with closed reduction during different periods of nasal development revealed no significant differences among groups.[19] These findings, plus our own experience with more than 30 children with severe nasal injuries, have prompted the adoption of a policy of early surgical repair of any nasal bony pyramid or septal deformity in this age group. Operation is aimed at repairing the specific deformity with very limited or conservative resection of the cartilage of the nasal septum; an effort to restore all of the appropriate structures to the midline is the goal. This approach nicely preserves the growth center within the nasovomerine complex, and significant deformities of the nose have not resulted.

Nasoethmoid Fractures

Complex nasoethmoid fractures with telescoping of the nasal bones posteriorly are uncommon in the pediatric population. When present they are usually caused by a significant force, and one should suspect associated intracranial injury. The evaluation of these injuries is best depicted by a computed tomography (CT) scan[11] (Fig. 16–1). This scan accurately demonstrates fractures to the nasal, ethmoid, and orbital areas in addition to anatomically defining any associated intracranial problem.

Nasoethmoid fractures may result in disruption of the medial canthal ligaments with resulting pseudohypertelorism or traumatic telecanthus. Saddle nose deformities and disorders of the lacrimal apparatus may also result. Definitive treatment of these injuries is best undertaken with open reduction and internal fixation using small 26- and 28-gauge wires. The child in Figure 16–2 sustained such an injury and was managed with open reduction and internal fixation (Fig. 16–2A and B). Lead or acrylic plates may be used externally with through and through wire fixation if lateral support of the nasal bones appears inadequate. The resulting posttraumatic deformity of these injuries can be quite severe, and late reconstructive management is sometimes less than satisfactory.

Soft Tissue Nasal Injuries

Laceration and avulsion type injuries of the nose are seen in children who have also sustained significant blows to the face. An accurate assessment of the degree of tissue disruption and possible soft tissue loss is extremely important. Children with animal bites to the face that involve the nose often present with this form of injury. A history of the rabies vaccination status of the animal should be determined, and appropriate measures for rabies prophylaxis undertaken if this is unable to be obtained. Although the soft tissue damage may appear quite severe at first glance, careful inspection usually reveals all of the components of the external nose to be present (Fig. 16–3). The majority of these injuries involve the alar rim and tear through the lower lateral cartilage.

A methodic layered reapproximation of the tissues beginning with the mucosal layer should be accomplished (Fig. 16–4). Two areas of importance in achieving an acceptable

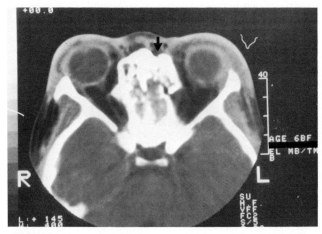

FIGURE 16–1
A computed tomography scan of the nose and paranasal sinuses in the axial plane demonstrating a telescoping nasoethmoid fracture.

cosmetic result depend on anatomic reapproximation of the lower lateral cartilage and exact repair of the alar rim. These sutures should be placed before the closure of the superior portions of the wound. Lacerations that involve the anterior nasal septum can also be seen in more severe cases and may be managed with reapproximation of the cartilage using interrupted 4-0 absorbable sutures and internal nasal splints for support as needed.

Certain soft tissue nasal injuries result in a complete loss of a portion of the alar rim. This situation is best managed with the use of a composite graft of appropriate size and configuration. Such a graft from the helical rim works nicely and should be less than 1 cm in size.[18] Immediate reconstruction at the time of the original repair is believed preferable.

PARANASAL SINUS INJURIES

Incidence

Injuries of the paranasal sinuses are less common in children than in adults. The major reason for this is the lack of pneumatization of the sinuses and their relatively protected environment in the young child. Sinus fractures accounted for less than 20% of such injuries in a review of pediatric maxillofacial trauma from our institution and was noted in only one child below the age of 6 years.[22]

The evaluation of any paranasal sinus injury should include the possibility of orbital involvement. A complete examination of the eye should be undertaken with documentation of the visual acuity and extraocular muscle movements in the older child, specifically looking for restriction of upward gaze. Fundoscopic examination should also be included. These examinations are more difficult in the younger child, and the services of an ophthalmologist may be required. These examinations should also be repeated as indicated if there is any question of an injury to the globe itself or if the initial examination was inadequate. Patience and diligence almost always pay off. Any loss of visual acuity should be documented, and attempts should be made to determine whether it is treatable. This would include the evacuation of a retrobulbar hematoma or the performance of a lateral canthotomy to decompress the globe should ocular hypertension be present.

Maxillary Sinus

Fractures of the maxillary sinuses account for the majority of paranasal sinus injuries in children. This is the first sinus to pneumatize and is the largest of all the paranasal sinuses. Injuries to this sinus are secondary to blunt trauma to the malar area and orbital rim. There is often associated periorbital ecchymosis and swelling of the eyelids. Routine facial radiographs often demonstrate an opacified maxillary sinus and possible displacement of the lateral walls of the maxillary sinus (Fig. 16–5). An associated fracture of the zygomatic arch or trimalar complex may also be present.

In our experience, CT scanning of the face in an axial and possibly a coronal plane provides the best method for

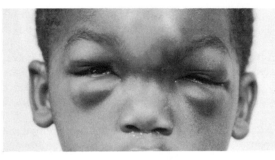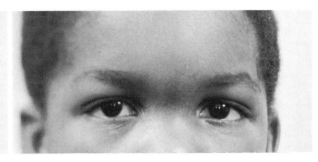

FIGURE 16–2

Preoperative (*A*) and postoperative (*B*) photographs of the child whose computed tomography scan is depicted in Figure 16–1. Struck over the bridge of the nose with a swing, the child underwent open reduction and internal fixation of these fractures.

confirming the anatomy of these fractures. The presence of bilateral maxillary sinus fractures should alert the clinician to the possibility of a Le Fort I or II fracture, which is determined by correlating the CT scan findings with that of careful physical examination of the face.

Management of these injuries depends on the degree of bony disruption of the sinus. Small linear nondisplaced sinus fractures can be treated nonoperatively with a combination of saline nasal irrigations, topical decongestants, and antibiotics. Fractures that cause a moderate degree of opacification of the maxillary sinus may require intranasal antrostomy to evacuate the blood. More severe trauma results in multiple fractures of the anterior and lateral walls of the sinus. These will be depicted accurately on CT scan. The best surgical management for these fractures is an anterior maxillary antrostomy or a Caldwell-Luc procedure, which permits the removal of any loose bone fragments or injured mucosa and the evacuation of blood within the sinus. These injuries, when bilateral, must always be differentiated from the more severe Le Fort I fracture. Le Fort fractures require intermaxillary fixation for 2 to 3 weeks.

Frontal Sinus

Frontal sinus fractures are usually caused by direct blunt forehead trauma, which results in a depression of the ante-

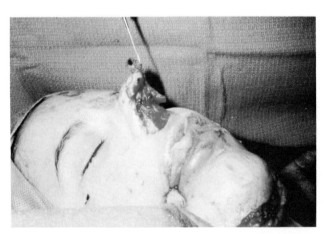

FIGURE 16–3

Eleven-year-old girl who sustained a severe laceration to the nasal tip and columellar area. Operative inspection revealed all of the anatomic components to be present.

rior or posterior table, or both. Frontal sinuses are among the last of the major sinuses to develop and are not usually well developed until the child reaches at least 6 years of age. The degree of displacement and comminution determines the best technique for repair. These injuries can also be associated with a significant percentage of intracranial injuries in the more severe cases.[6] A CT scan provides the most accurate anatomic assessment of both the frontal sinus and the cranial injuries (Fig. 16–6). A trephination through a small incision through the eyebrow and subsequently the floor of the frontal sinus allows reduction of depressed anterior table fractures that are not comminuted. Significant comminution of the anterior table, however, mandates that exposure of the entire sinus be obtained via either a bicoronal incision or a bilateral brow butterfly approach. The individual fractures may then be wired into place.

More extensive frontal sinus injuries, with comminution of the anterior and posterior tables, may require an osteoplastic sinusotomy, removal of all mucosa, and, finally, obliteration of the sinus utilizing a fat graft.[7] When these injuries include a frontal bone depressed skull fracture with involvement of the anterior cranial fossa, cranialization of the frontal sinus should be performed; this is easily undertaken via a bifrontal craniotomy by drilling away the posterior table of the sinus and allowing the brain and dura to fill the dead space.[5] Careful inspection and repair of any defects of the anterior cranial fossa should always be undertaken at this time to avoid the problems of cerebrospinal fluid leakage.

LARYNGEAL AND PHARYNGEAL INJURIES

Airway Management

Injuries to the larynx and pharynx in the pediatric population are uncommon. The relative protection of these structures by the mandible above and the sternum below, along with their elasticity, makes these injuries infrequent. The major cause of pediatric neck injuries remains motor vehicle related, and these injuries are often life-threatening emergencies. Near strangulation and choking types of injuries are also seen, especially in abused children. Appropriate investigations should always be undertaken when child abuse is suspected.[36]

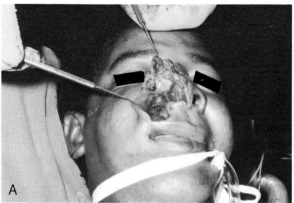 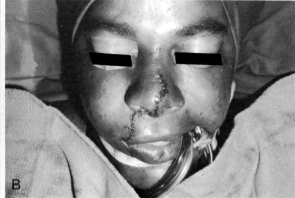

FIGURE 16–4

Preoperative (*A*) and postoperative (*B*) photographs of an extensive nasal tip and septum injury with extension to the upper lip.

Obviously, airway management remains the primary focus in any traumatic injury. When the airway itself is the site of injury, then both quality and preservation of life are threatened. Emergency personnel must be alert to the signs and symptoms of laryngotracheal injury. These may appear as a spectrum, depending on the severity of the trauma, and symptoms may include hoarseness, soft tissue crepitance, subcutaneous emphysema, hemoptysis, stridor, or partial to near-complete upper airway obstruction.[33, 55] Once these injuries are suspected, then a practiced protocol for confirmation and appropriate intervention should be undertaken.

Protocol of Management

An algorithm used in our institution is depicted in Figure 16–7.[21] The keys to the management of all laryngeal injuries are recognition of potential injury, immediate assessment for same, establishment of airway support, and prompt management within 24 hours. Controversy exists as to the best manner of managing emergency airway injuries, some favoring endotracheal intubation and others advocating primary tracheostomy.[33, 55] This decision is dependent on the expertise of the physician managing the airway and the degree of laryngotracheal disruption present. Of primary importance is that the establishment of the airway not further disrupt the injury to the larynx. Severe laryngotracheal

FIGURE 16–5

The Waters view, demonstrating a fracture of the right orbital rim and opacification of the right maxillary sinus in an 18-month-old infant.

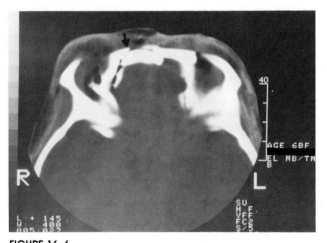

FIGURE 16–6

A computed tomography scan in a 6-year-old child showing a posteriorly displaced fracture of the frontal sinus.

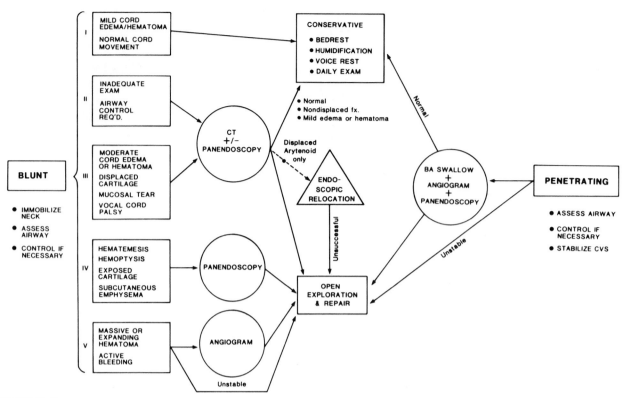

FIGURE 16–7

An algorithm utilized for the evaluation and management of laryngotracheal injuries. (From Gussack GS, Jurkovich GJ, Luterman A, et al: Laryngotracheal trauma: A protocol approach to a rare injury. Laryngoscope 96(6):660–665, 1986.)

separation with a great deal of disrupted mucosa is best managed with a standard tracheostomy. If obstruction is secondary to hematoma formation while the integrity of the laryngeal skeleton is intact, endotracheal intubation may be safely carried out in a more expeditious fashion. Cricothyrotomies in the pediatric population, advocated by many in emergency situations, are not without serious problems as the long-term complication rate and sequelae are significant.[10]

If these injuries are suspected, flexible fiberoptic laryngoscopy provides an excellent means of examining the larynx once the patient is known to have a stable airway. Vocal cord mobility, epiglottic disruption, glottic and supraglottic hematoma formation, and arytenoid displacement may all be assessed. Computed tomographic scanning is also very helpful in determining the degree of laryngeal skeletal injury (Fig. 16–8).[38–41] Calcification of the laryngeal cartilages in younger children is less than that in older children and adults, and the detail is not as well defined; however, these studies still remain helpful, especially in injuries of intermediate severity, and often assist considerably in the determination of the necessity for operative exploration.

With single-system injuries limited to the laryngeal area, conservative (or nonoperative) therapy consisting of voice rest, observation, humidification, and repeat examinations is indicated for isolated glottic hematomas without obstruction, supraglottic hematomas, and nondisplaced fractures of the thyroid cartilage. Children who have these injuries

should be placed in a setting in which they are monitored carefully until the course of their injury can be determined accurately. Pulse oximetry may also be utilized effectively in pediatric airway management as an accurate noninvasive means of determining adequate oxygen saturation.[23]

Operative management of laryngeal trauma is indicated

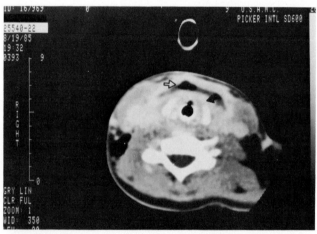

FIGURE 16–8

A computed tomography scan showing blunt trauma that resulted in laryngeal fracture. Note the fracture site (*solid arrow*) along with air in the deep fascial spaces of the neck (*open arrow*).

for injuries resulting in displaced laryngeal fractures, mucosal disruption, arytenoid displacement, subcutaneous emphysema, or laryngotracheal separation. The approach is through a collar-type incision with midline thyrotomy, and then mucosal reapproximation is undertaken with interrupted fine absorbable sutures. Cartilage fractures are first reduced and then held in fixation with 28- or 30-gauge wire, care being exercised when tightening these to avoid cutting through the cartilage and adding to the injury.

The use of indwelling stents for more severe injuries is also controversial.[35] Debate includes the indications, type of stent, and length of time that stenting is required. Personal experience supports the use of this technique, and we have utilized stents made of soft sponge-filled finger cots or rolls of Silastic sheeting in preference to hard acrylic type stents. Two weeks appear to provide an adequate length of stabilization time for the majority of children; however, a longer time may be required for older children or teenagers. Such stents should always be placed in such a fashion that they can be removed endoscopically. In addition, the carbon dioxide laser has provided an excellent means of controlling granulation tissue and keeping the airway clean after stent removal.[21]

The results of surgery for laryngeal injury are dependent on the degree of disruption of the laryngeal skeleton and the adequacy of the repair. The three major functions of the larynx involve speech, respiration, and distal airway protection. Compromise of any one or of all three of these functions may occur. The majority of patients, if treated early and properly, are able to maintain adequate protective functions of the larynx. Subglottic stenoses, glottic abnormalities, and dislocated arytenoids are the most common post-traumatic laryngeal sequelae, and vocal dysfunction characterized by a weak or breathy voice is the usual outcome.

MOUTH AND PHARYNGEAL INJURIES

The majority of injuries to the mouth and anterior pharynx are secondary to falls and blunt trauma. The lips, tongue, and cheek are usually injured from biting the soft tissue. Most of these injuries are self-limited and heal very quickly without formal repair. Larger lacerations of the tongue, soft palate, or buccal mucosa may be closed with single-layer absorbable sutures.

Teeth are frequently affected in blunt trauma and probably represent the most common oral injury. Loosened deciduous teeth may be left alone or removed without significant long-term sequelae. Totally avulsed permanent teeth may be reimplanted with a good chance for viability if replaced within the first hour after injury. Parents or rescue workers at the scene should be instructed to place the tooth in milk and have the child seen by a pediatric dentist as soon as possible.[54]

Penetrating pharyngeal wounds are seen primarily in two major groups of injuries. The first and most common is an impalement of the soft palate, posterior pharyngeal wall, or tonsillar pillars secondary to a child falling with a sharp object, such as a pencil, in the mouth. Although the majority of these injuries are quite benign, the potential for dis-

astrous complications, including possible carotid artery injury, retropharyngeal abscess or hematoma formation, or penetration into the parapharyngeal space, is significant. Evaluation of children with these injuries should include an examination of the posterior pharynx, a careful neurologic examination, and a lateral airway radiograph x-ray to investigate these potential injuries fully. All of these children should be admitted for overnight observation as delayed complications may occur. Arteriography should be employed for any child with evidence of a focal neurologic defect.

The second group of penetrating pharyngeal injuries is gunshot wounds. Children with these injuries should undergo the standard protocols for the management of penetrating neck trauma. The surgeon should be alert to the possibility of airway compromise and not hesitate to establish appropriate airway support.

EAR TRAUMA

Scope of the Problem

Trauma to the ear is common in the pediatric population. Head trauma occurs in 72% of motor vehicle accidents, and when severe cranial injuries occur, the ear is the most frequently affected sensory organ.[28] External ear injuries can result in unsightly cosmetic deformities and multiple corrective procedures for the child, especially if the injury is mismanaged initially. Functional problems can occur from trauma to the temporal bone, such as hearing loss, balance disorders, facial paralysis, and cerebrospinal fluid leakage. The incidence of hearing loss with all head injuries has been cited as approaching 33%. When head trauma is complicated by loss of consciousness, hearing loss is present 50% of the time, with 30 to 80% of these cases being sensorineural in nature. Conductive hearing losses are seen in 15% of these cases and result from hemotympanum, tympanic membrane rupture, or ossicular chain injury.[48] Seventy percent of acute, severe head injury patients have an otologic abnormality (hemotympanum most commonly), and 7 to 14% have a temporal bone fracture.[1, 60] When temporal bone fractures occur, the incidence of facial nerve injury is 30 to 50% in transverse fractures and 10 to 20% in longitudinal fractures.[48] Dizziness is seen in up to 90% of head injury patients.[37]

The pediatric ear is similar to its adult counterpart because embryologically the ear differentiates quite early, and inner ear structures are of adult size at birth. The infant's facial nerve is an exception, occupying a more vulnerable lateral position because the mastoid tip does not finish developing until 12 to 24 months. The external canal and pinna do not reach adult size until age 9.[58]

Anatomically, the ear is divided into three divisions: the external ear, the middle ear, and the inner ear. Trauma, both blunt and penetrating, can affect all three divisions as well as the facial nerve and vascular structures. Other forms of trauma such as thermal and chemical injury typically affect the external ear; barotrauma can affect the middle and inner ear; and acoustic trauma affects primarily the inner ear.

Lightning is also a cause of ear damage to all three divisions.[28]

Evaluation

The evaluation of the ear in major trauma begins only after life-threatening problems are addressed. A good history and physical examination are the cornerstones for accurate evaluation. The single most important assessment to make in any patient with ear trauma is to determine whether inner ear damage has occurred.[46] Inner ear damage may lead to progressive hearing loss if not recognized and treated. Ear symptoms include pain, drainage, hearing loss, tinnitus, fullness, vertigo, facial weakness, or other neurologic symptoms. Awareness of preexisting medical conditions, hearing loss, or previous ear surgery is important.

A methodic examination begins with the pinna, with a check for skin or cartilage loss and hematoma formation. Ear canal involvement is determined by gently cleaning out debris and blood with suction and assessing the tympanic membrane for perforations, color, and mobility. Tuning forks and whisper tests are used for gross assessments of hearing. Examination is then undertaken for postauricular ecchymosis, facial weakness, level of consciousness, cerebrospinal fluid otorrhea, and nystagmus. It is crucial to perform a complete neurologic examination, including cerebellar testing.[46]

Radiographic studies include mastoid films, skull series, or CT scans. Arteriography is performed if vascular injury is suspected. Audiometry is rarely available at the initial evaluation; therefore, tuning fork examinations become important medicolegal documentation. Pure tone audiometry with discrimination should be performed before surgical repair of the hearing mechanism or facial nerve is undertaken. Infants or comatose patients may be evaluated with auditory brain stem response. Vestibular testing using electronystagmography, caloric testing, rotary chair platform testing, or facial nerve testing may be performed electively.

Management

Soft tissue injuries should be managed within 12 hours if possible. Tetanus prophylaxis should be given if needed and appropriate antibiotics administered. Tympanic membrane and ossicular chain problems are not treated as an emergency as a general rule, although an otolaryngologist should see the patient expeditiously. Prompt evaluation should be undertaken if sensorineural hearing loss or dizziness occurs to determine whether an inner ear fistula is present. Profound hearing loss or long-term balance disorders may occur if this injury goes unrecognized. Facial nerve function should be assessed as soon as possible. When recognition of facial paralysis is delayed, the physician is unable to determine whether paralysis was present immediately or is of delayed onset. This information is important, as the former patient would be a surgical candidate and the latter is typically treated with observation. The only life-threatening emergency involving ear trauma is hemorrhage occurring from the carotid artery or from a jugular bulb–sigmoid sinus injury. Packing is the initial step for control of the hemorrhage.

EXTERNAL EAR

Lacerations and Abrasions

Lacerations and abrasions are the most frequently seen external ear injuries. These occur because of the prominent position of the pinna and most often occur in motor vehicle accidents, altercations, and falls. Cartilage involvement must be recognized, as failure to repair it can result in noticeable notching of the ear. The administration of local anesthesia using lidocaine (Xylocaine) with epinephrine is appropriate unless vascularity is in question. Copious irrigation with normal saline and removal of clearly devitalized tissue and foreign debris with a water pick or brush prevents later infection or tattooing.

Every effort is made to save all tissue, and questionably viable tissue may be débrided after further demarcation. Exposed cartilage is débrided below the level of the perichondrium.[64] Cartilage repair is best accomplished by suturing the perichondrium; however, repair using a few absorbable sutures through the cartilage is acceptable.[38] The physician closes the skin with interrupted nonabsorbable sutures, taking care to align known anatomic landmarks during the repair. An ear that appears to be normal can be achieved if tissue loss has not occurred. A systemic antistaphylococcal antibiotic is recommended along with antibacterial ointment and pressure dressing for 1 to 2 days. Should chondritis develop, more aggressive débridement is indicated.

Lacerations of the ear canal and meatus are stented both to promote initial hemostasis and to prevent later stenosis. Circumferential loss of tissue is managed with split or full thickness skin grafts. Packing saturated with otic antibiotic drops is used for 7 to 10 days. Bleeding is managed with adrenaline sponges, silver nitrate sticks, bipolar cautery, and pressure packing.[38]

Another common auricular injury occurs when earrings are ripped from the ear, which results in a tear through the lobule. These may be managed by primary closure with a Z-plasty at the rim to prevent notching.[56] Keloid formation, however, is a complicating factor, occurring more frequently in blacks, and often requires medical or surgical management consisting of steroid injections, excisions, and pressure dressings.[38]

Avulsions

Avulsions are a more severe form of external ear trauma. Partial or complete avulsions of the pinna are frequently seen in persons involved in motor vehicle accidents and in altercations including human and dog bites. Therapy of avulsive injuries is dependent on the size of the avulsed portion and whether any soft tissue attachment is present. Before the repair of any avulsed part, the portion can be cleaned with a povidone-iodine solution (Betadine) and saline, placed in 200 ml of lactated Ringer solution containing

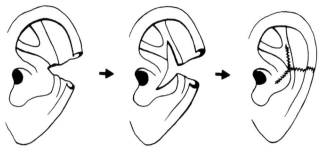

FIGURE 16–9

Traumatic helical rim defect with repair utilizing Burow triangles to avoid buckling of the ear.

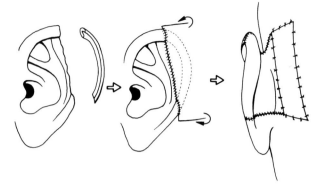

FIGURE 16–10

Partial avulsion of the ear. A postauricular flap utilizing salvaged or autograft cartilage in a two-stage repair. The donor site must be closed with a split thickness skin graft.

gentamicin (80 mg) and heparin (1000 units), and placed on ice. This decreases the metabolic requirements, prevents clotting of the vessels, and diminishes contamination leading to infection.[13] Partial avulsions of the pinna of less than 2 cm may be reattached if the injury is only a laceration. Avulsed segments larger than 2 cm can be managed by débriding and burying the cartilage postauricularly for later repair with a composite flap.[32, 64] Other recommendations include reattaching the avulsed part and following that with aggressive medical therapy, including the administration of intravenous broad-spectrum antibiotics, heparin vasodilators, and low molecular weight dextran (dextran 40, 750 ml daily for 5 days). Performing multiple stab incisions through the skin to avoid lymphatic stasis is undertaken in the initial period.[13] If tissue death becomes imminent, the skin may still be débrided and the cartilage buried for later reconstruction. An adequate blood supply for the entire ear usually remains when any soft tissue attachment is present. The portion should therefore be reattached, and aggressive medical therapy should be instituted.[64]

Ear avulsion with missing tissue is usually managed by reapproximating the remaining tissue as best as possible. Local flaps and composite grafts are best performed at a later operation after primary healing has occurred. Simple wedge excision is used for small helical rim defects of less than 2 cm. Larger defects may be closed by helical rim rotation with Burow triangles (Fig. 16–9). A composite graft from the opposite ear along with pre- or postauricular flaps is another option.[32, 44]

The first stage in reconstruction utilizing buried cartilage involves the creation of a broad base for vascularization by dermabrasion of the skin down to the dermis (Fig. 16–10). The base of the cartilage is then attached along the cut edge of the remaining ear, and the entire segment is buried in a postauricular pocket. Second-stage reconstruction 2 weeks later involves raising this portion, which by now has revascularized. The anterior surface will reepithelialize from the dermal elements, and a full thickness skin graft is placed on the posterior surface.[44] Depending on the site of the defect, an anterior, superior, inferior, or posterior pocket or flap may be used.[32, 44] Microvascular anastomosis has been recommended by some.

When total avulsion occurs and the tissue fails to survive, an artificial ear becomes an easier and probably more cosmetically acceptable alternative than multiple reconstructive procedures.[53] A silicone prosthesis that is anchored in bone

is recommended.[65] Although dog bites can be closed primarily after copious cleaning, human bites should be managed as contaminated wounds and are best treated openly, with secondary closure performed after 4 days. Antibiotics with anaerobic coverage and moist dressings are used during the period of delay.[34]

Hematomas

Hematomas occur with blunt injuries such as those caused by a fist. Blood accumulates between the cartilage and its overlying perichondrium, thereby separating the cartilage from its blood supply and leading to cartilage necrosis and a cauliflower ear deformity. Diagnosis is made by demonstrating areas of fluctuance on the lateral surface of the pinna, with loss of normal landmarks and a typical dull red or blue discoloration (Fig. 16–11). Treatment involves as-

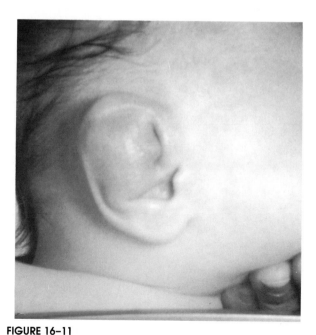

FIGURE 16–11

Hematoma of the auricle in a 10-month-old infant.

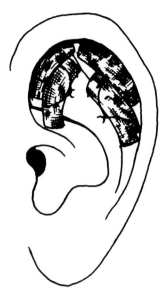

FIGURE 16–12

Treatment of recurrent hematoma with incision and drainage, followed by placement of cotton bolsters.

piration of the blood using an 18-gauge needle and taking care to ensure sterility and application of a pressure dressing. Saline-soaked cotton balls are used as a conforming dressing to fill the contours of the ear, and a bulky mastoid dressing is applied. Reaccumulations in the hematomas are treated with repeat aspiration followed by placement of through and through mattress sutures over cotton bolsters[53] (Fig. 16–12). Further hematoma reaccumulations or organized clots often cannot be aspirated, and incision and drainage are required. Formation of neocartilage requires incision with removal of the overlying perichondrium and neocartilage down to the normal cartilage. Thinning of the remaining skin allows it to settle back onto the normal underlying cartilage, restoring a normal appearance.[15] Antistaphylococcal antibiotic coverage is recommended.

Perichondritis may develop from hematomas and is caused by either *Staphylococcus aureus* or *Pseudomonas aeruginosa*. The ear becomes red, puffy, and tender on movement, though not necessarily fluctuant. Early treatment involves aspiration, followed by appropriate intravenous antibiotics and through and through drains for irrigation of antibiotic solution (Fig. 16–13). Aminoglycosides may be used in this manner with very little risk of systemic absorption with its potential for oto or nephrotoxicity.[27] Any necrotic cartilage, however, must be resected surgically for healing to occur (Fig. 16–14). Extensive involvement may require a bivalving technique to remove dead cartilage and apply topical antibiotic soaks.[32]

Thermal Injuries

Burns

Ears are involved in 90% of all facial burns. It is important to determine the depth of burn. First- and second-degree

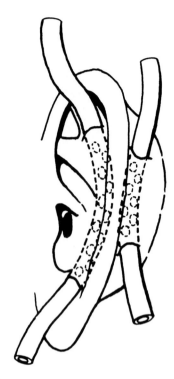

FIGURE 16–13

Perichondritis. Placement of drains for irrigation with antibiotic solution.

burns are kept clean and treated as an abrasion; these burns reepithelialize rapidly. Second-degree burns that become infected and third-degree burns are more difficult problems. Management involves a conservative surgical but aggressive medical approach. Débridement of dead tissue and regular cleaning using topical agents such as silver sulfadiazine, matenide acetate (Sulfamylon), or 0.5% silver nitrate are performed. Tetanus prophylaxis and application of a light gauze dressing are typically used. The administration of antibiotics is reserved for a definite infection. Split thickness skin grafts may be applied after granulation has occurred.[64] Burn center statistics indicate that 80 to 90% of patients admitted have burns of the ear, with up to a 24%

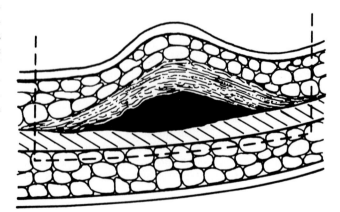

FIGURE 16–14

Perichondritis. Surgical removal of infected soft tissue with necrotic cartilage within the area depicted.

incidence of chondritis and a loss of the pinna in 5%.[27, 53] Avoiding pressure on the ear from the head resting on a pillow and instituting aggressive therapy has avoided the complication of chondritis in our burn unit.

Frostbite

Frostbite is actual freezing of tissue with ice crystal formation that typically occurs in moist cold (lower than $-7°C$ or 19°F). However, with preexisting vascular compromise, such as that due to trauma or radiation therapy or submergence, frostbite may occur at a higher temperature.[64] Involvement may be superficial or may include deep structures. Symptoms include pain, erythema, blisters, and, importantly, loss of sensation. Avoidance of further tissue trauma is essential, and rapid rewarming with sterile, water-soaked towels or cotton at 38 to 44°C (100–108°F) is recommended. Slow warming may result in the re-formation of ice crystals, causing further damage.[57] In contrast to the procedures with burns, tissue that appears to be devitalized is observed and débrided only when clearly demarcated.[53] Rupturing of blebs should be avoided, and topical antibiotics may be used. The area is cleaned gently and regularly following the procedures for open wound therapy. Antibiotics are given if perichondritis develops.[64]

Foreign Bodies

Foreign body injuries are included in this discussion because most occur in small children. The presence of a foreign body as well as attempts at its retrieval may certainly be traumatic to the ear canal and possibly even the tympanic membrane and the middle and inner ear structures. Ears previously instrumented elsewhere are assessed for hearing as a medicolegal prerequisite before removal of foreign bodies deep in the canal, and if the child is uncooperative, removal is best performed under general anesthesia to avoid the risk of further trauma. If the foreign body is vegetable matter, no water should be used, as the object will swell. Alligator or Hartmann forceps are used to remove it. Spheric objects are extracted by using a hook or wax loop placed medial to the object by going into the anterior superior quadrant of the canal. Mineral oil is applied to kill insects, after which they are removed with forceps.[27] Visible trauma is treated by using antibacterial drops, which should also be antifungal if an insect has been present. The tympanic membrane must be visualized to be sure that it is intact. Only experienced personnel should attempt the removal of foreign bodies to avoid iatrogenic injuries.

MIDDLE EAR

Tympanic Membrane Perforations

A perforation of the tympanic membrane may result from a penetrating injury or from blunt blows (e.g., a hand slap, a fall while water skiing, an explosion) (Fig. 16–15). Patients with head injuries may have a tympanic membrane rupture

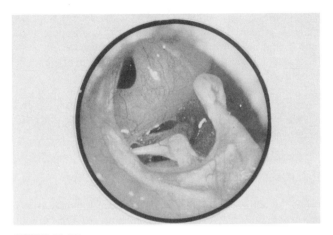

FIGURE 16–15
Large tympanic membrane perforation of right ear, showing the malleus, the incudostapedial joint, and the round window niche.

as the result of a temporal bone fracture. The patient may complain of hearing loss, pain, and bloody otorrhea. Otoscopic examination typically reveals blood in the canal and a variably sized central perforation. The most important point in an evaluation of these injuries is to determine the presence of inner ear damage. Patients with vertigo, nystagmus, evidence of sensorineural hearing loss, or posterior superior perforation in which damage to the ossicles is likely should be admitted for treatment of a possible inner ear fistula; early surgical intervention may be required.[9] Otherwise, initial treatment of a perforation is keeping the ear dry and using drops only if contamination has occurred and the ear begins to drain. The ear should be examined under a microscope within a few days. When the edges of the perforation have curled under, they may be rolled out and stented with a paper patch along with Gelfoam for support within the middle ear.[62] Most perforations treated in this manner heal spontaneously within 3 months. When healing fails to occur, elective tympanoplasty may then be performed.[17] Children who are younger than 8 years of age with uncomplicated perforations may have repair of the perforation delayed until the age of 8, when the period of recurrent otitis media has passed. Normal eustachian tube function improves the success rate of the tympanoplasty. Other factors taken into account include the hearing status of the opposite ear and how well the child is doing in school.

Hot metal (slag) burns, as occur in welding injuries, cause perforations that tend to heal quite poorly. The foreign body causes an inflammatory response within the ear, and the vascularity of the remaining drum may be poor. Treatment involves removal of the foreign body and later repair of the tympanic membrane.[62] Perforations resulting from electrical or lightning bolt injuries also heal poorly.[48]

Occasionally, a marginal perforation occurs that requires earlier surgical intervention to prevent the ingress of squamous epithelium into the middle ear and its resulting bone-eroding cholesteatoma. Over many years, the presence of untreated cholesteatoma can result in a number of complications 5 to 10% of the time. Intratemporal complications include mastoiditis, subperiosteal abscess, lateral semicircular canal fistula, labyrinthitis, facial palsy, and petrositis. Intracranial complications include meningitis; lateral sinus thrombophlebitis; epidural, subdural, or brain abscess; or otitic hydrocephalus. Cholesteatoma requires surgical management in almost every case, with complete removal of the disease and preservation of the normal ear architecture, or externalization of the disease by removal of the posterior canal walls and scutum.[59]

Ossicular Chain Injuries

Problems with the ossicular chain are seen less commonly than perforations of the tympanic membrane. The contour of the external canal tends to deflect penetrating objects toward the anterior part of the drum away from the ossicles. Compressive forces, however, such as a hand slap or a blast, along with some penetrating objects, may result in posterior perforations and damage to the underlying ossicles. Temporal bone fractures may also cause disruption of the ossicular chain, typically in a longitudinal fracture. The most common ossicular damage involves incudostapedial joint separation, followed by massive dislocation of the incus, with stapes injury being third (Fig. 16–16).[26, 48] Typically, a perforation is present as well. The hearing loss in these cases is more severe than in simple perforations. However, unless the hearing loss appears to be sensorineural in nature (tuning fork, audiogram) or dizziness is present, these injuries are not treated as emergencies.

A conductive hearing loss may result from the presence of blood in the middle ear or from a perforation. Monitoring of the patient's hearing over several weeks provides additional information. Exploration should be undertaken if an air-bone gap, indicating disruption of the chain, of greater than 50 decibels initially or of greater than 30 decibels 2 months after the trauma exists.[47] Ossicular chain reconstruction may be performed at the time of tympanic membrane repair.

Incudostapedial joint separation or dislocation may require a realignment and repositioning of the incus and support by Gelfoam or fascia. The incus or malleus head may be sculpted and inserted between the long process of the malleus and stapes as another option. A goblet prosthesis, cartilage, bone, or hydroxyapatite prosthesis may be inserted as another option. A partial ossicular replacement prosthesis (PORP) with overlying cartilage is the standard and may be used quite successfully. Absence of the stapes suprastructure with or without the footplate requires a total ossicular replacement prosthesis (TORP) or repositioned incus.[26]

Barotrauma

Barotrauma to the middle ear can occur from pressure changes such as the rapid descent in airplanes and scuba diving or explosions. This results in a bloody effusion within the middle ear. Barotrauma is often quite painful, with hearing loss, aural fullness, and mild unsteadiness. Inner ear damage must be ruled out. Examination reveals a hemotympanum with a blue or reddish tympanic membrane that has decreased mobility. Tuning forks indicate lateralization to the involved ear (Fig. 16–17). When tuning fork examination lateralizes to the unaffected ear, immediate consultation of an otolaryngologist is necessary as inner ear barotrauma may be present. Management involves the administration of analgesics and decongestants, as well as autoinsufflation using the Valsalva maneuver, or politzerization to introduce air nasally into the middle ear. Myringotomy with or without the tube insertion gives immediate pain relief.[46]

Temporal Bone Fractures

Temporal bone fractures and gunshot wounds can cause damage to the middle ear structures and mastoid, as well as to the inner ear, the seventh and eighth cranial nerves, and major vascular structures.

INNER EAR

Inner ear damage can result from penetrating or blunt trauma, barotrauma, or acoustic trauma. The actual pathophysiology may be inner ear hemorrhage, intralabyrinthine fistula (membranous disruption), perilymphatic leak, or nerve interruption.

Perilymphatic Fistula

Perilymphatic fistula may result in an extensive loss of inner ear fluid and a hearing loss that is complete and irreversible. Occasionally, the loss of fluid is only partial, with a slow, ongoing leak. This condition is considered an

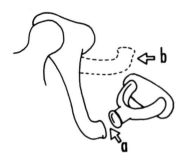

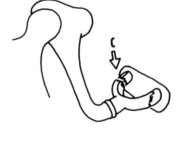

FIGURE 16–16

Ossicular chain injuries: a, incudostapedial joint separation; b, dislocation of the incus (*dashed line*); c, fracture of the stapedial crura.

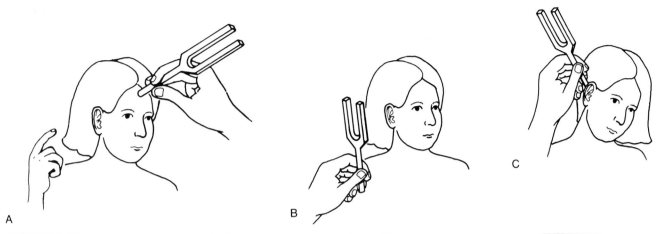

FIGURE 16–17

Tuning fork examination. *A*, Weber test: The fork is louder in the involved ear with a conduction loss or in the good ear with a neurosensory loss. *B and C*, Rinne test: With normal hearing or neurosensory loss, air is louder than bone. With a conduction loss, bone is louder than air.

emergency in that correct management may be able to restore hearing or at least stabilize the loss and in most cases result in vertigo resolution. Blunt or sharp trauma can cause disruption of the annular ligament at the stapes footplate–oval window interface, whereas barotrauma is more likely to result in a round window fistula (Fig. 16–18).

Symptoms include hearing loss and vertigo with audiogram and tuning forks demonstrating a mixed or neurosensory hearing loss pattern. A fistula test involving the application of positive and negative pressure to the tympanic membrane through a pneumatic otoscope may be positive 50% of the time.[3] A positive test result is either a visible deviation of the eyes or the sensation of vertigo or dizziness by the patient. Other tests include an eyes closed turning stagger test and a reverse Dix-Hallpike test.[61] Audiometry typically shows a high-frequency sensorineural hearing loss with decreased discrimination, although any audiometric pattern may be found.[3] Diagnosis ultimately rests with having a high degree of suspicion and an exploration of the ear to demonstrate the leakage of perilymph.

Treatment of a suspected fistula involves admission for bed rest, elevation of the head of the bed, avoidance of straining, and using stool softeners and cough suppressants. Patients who have progressive hearing loss or losses showing no evidence of resolution should have an exploration of the middle ear to rule out a fistula when there is a strong history of trauma.[16] A fistula is closed by denuding the mucosa around the involved window and sealing it with a connective tissue graft. When a fistula is not seen yet the historical features support this diagnosis, a graft is inserted for reinforcement of a presumably healed microfistula.[3, 52]

Examination of the results of fistula closure reveals an almost 100% relief or at least marked improvement of vertigo; however, the chance of hearing improvement is only

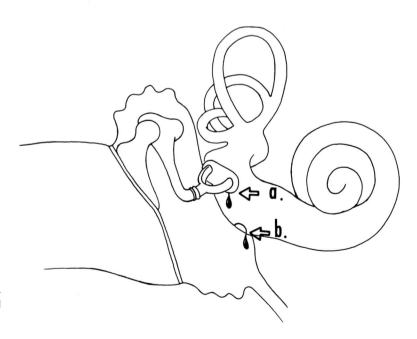

FIGURE 16–18

Perilymphatic fistula: Primary sites are the footplate–oval window region (a) and the round window niche (b).

40%.[16] Recurrent fistulas may occur in up to 30% of patients, and the opposite ear should also be considered as a possible source of fistula.[61] Ultimately, any posttraumatic patient with ongoing inner ear symptoms should be considered for fistula exploration, because vertigo relief is accomplished in almost all and hearing improvement in some even if several months have lapsed.[16]

Labyrinthine Concussion

Hearing loss, vertigo, and tinnitus can occur with blunt head trauma without the presence of a demonstrable temporal bone fracture. Labyrinthine concussion results in a sensorineural hearing loss tending to be primarily at the 4000 hertz frequency as seen in acoustic trauma. There may be high-frequency tinnitus as well as nonspecific vertigo or unsteadiness.[50] Children have difficulty relating or describing a sense of unsteadiness and may have trouble walking, may fall frequently, and may be considered clumsy. However, they have no difficulty with fine motor skills. This condition is generally self-limiting as central compensation occurs.

Cupulolithiasis

A special form of inner ear injury that occurs with blunt trauma is benign paroxysmal positional vertigo, known as *cupulolithiasis*. It is thought that the delicate otolithic membrane is disrupted, allowing the otoconia of the utricular macula to be detached and settle into the posterior semicircular canal. This results in a vertigo that develops in certain positions. The problem may be quite resistant to treatment. Typically, there is intense vertigo that lasts for 10 to 15 seconds with the affected ear down, and the nystagmus it causes has a latency period after assuming the provoking position. The nystagmus is rotatory, fatiguable, and is not evident on repeat positional testing.[48] Labyrinthine dizziness may be managed with positional exercises and vestibular suppressants. Patients with head injuries display headache, personality change, and dizziness. This dizziness may be central in nature and respond to autonomic drugs, or it may be cervical in origin and respond to positional exercises. Head injury patients with persistent vertigo or dizziness should be evaluated by electronystagmography (or computerized rotary chair). After 6 months, electronystagmography is repeated, and further therapy should be undertaken if symptoms persist. Treatment should be medical, with surgical therapies such as vestibular nerve or singular nerve section reserved for refractory disabling cases.[48]

Endolymphatic Hydrops

Another possible long-term sequela is delayed endolymphatic hydrops that develops years after temporal bone trauma from damage to the endolymphatic duct and sac. Initial treatment involves the prescription of diuretics and a low-salt diet. Attempts at surgical therapy should be used only in cases of extreme disability after medical therapy has failed. Should surgery be undertaken, vestibular nerve section is the procedure of choice, as endolymphatic sac drainage procedures are usually unsuccessful if the endolymphatic duct is the site of injury.[48]

Inner Ear Barotrauma

Inner ear barotrauma can be seen in children as both the tympanic membrane and inner ear membranes can rupture in water as shallow as 7 feet.[51] Typically, the round window is the site of involvement, with a perilymphatic fistula.[16] Intralabyrinthine hemorrhage or Reissner membrane tears may also occur, resulting in sensorineural hearing loss. These usually improve or resolve completely with bed rest, elevation of the head of the bed, and avoidance of sneezing or straining for 10 days. The patient may resume full activity in 6 weeks. One theory is that patients who demonstrate persistent loss at one frequency had a break in the Reissner membrane corresponding to that frequency. When coexisting inner and middle ear barotrauma occur, middle ear exploration is risky and should be postponed until the inner ear symptoms have resolved.[51]

Acoustic Trauma

Mention should be made of acoustic trauma because it can occur in blast injuries or concussions. The hearing thresholds in the mid- to high-frequency range (4000–6000 hertz) deteriorate but tend to improve over the next 1 to 3 weeks. Accurate assessment of the permanent hearing loss may be determined by 3 weeks.[46] A head blow resulting in an inward movement of the stapes into the vestibule is more damaging than one causing the stapes to move outward, explaining why a blow to one side of the head can cause more hearing loss in the contralateral ear.[66]

TEMPORAL BONE FRACTURES

Evaluation

Basilar skull fractures invariably involve the temporal bone.[48] Cerebrospinal fluid leakage, appearing as otorrhea or otorhinorrhea, with the resulting risk of meningitis, occurs in 10 to 40% of temporal bone fractures. Temporal bone fractures are classified as longitudinal, transverse, or mixed by their relation to the long axis of the petrous bone (Fig. 16–19). Most are mixed radiographically but can be divided clinically based on whether sensorineural or conductive hearing loss, or both, is present.[28] Eighty percent of the fractures are longitudinal fractures and typically occur with temporoparietal blows. These run parallel to the petrous ridge and involve the squamous portion of the temporal bone, the posterior superior canal wall, and the tympanic ring and result in a step-off at the level of the tympanic membrane. Typically the tympanic segment of the facial nerve near the geniculate ganglion and the greater superficial petrosal nerve are also involved. The ossicular chain is injured in the fracture, which then extends anterior

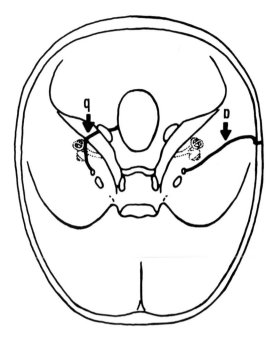

FIGURE 16–19

Temporal bone fracture: a, longitudinal; b, transverse.

to the cochlea to terminate at the foramen lacerum or foramen spinosum. The fracture is anterior and lateral to the otic capsule. Bleeding from the ear is the hallmark of a longitudinal temporal bone fracture. The hearing loss, is typically conductive in nature.[28, 48] There can also be cerebrospinal fluid otorrhea with vertigo or dizziness.

On examination, bloody fluid, a hemotympanus with a tympanic membrane laceration, and a visible break in the bony annular ring are evident. A laceration of the skin of the external auditory canal and a positive Battle sign are also present. Facial paralysis is present in 10 to 20% of the cases, and spontaneous nystagmus should be sought.[28] The fluid in the canal may be tested to ascertain if cerebrospinal fluid is present. Laboratory evaluation for chemistries should include glucose, protein, and beta subunit of transferrin.[25] Testing for the target sign, which is done by placing a drop of the fluid on filter paper, results in a central bloody spot with a clear surrounding halo signifying the more rapidly diffusing cerebrospinal fluid. Audiometry tests reveal a conductive or mixed loss. Bilateral fractures are seen in 8 to 29% of cases.[48]

Twenty percent of temporal bone fractures are classified as transverse and occur with an occipital or frontal blow. These fractures extend from the foramen magnum and cross perpendicularly to the axis of the petrous bone. They involve the otic capsule or the internal auditory canal, as well as the labyrinthine segment of the seventh nerve at or proximal to the geniculate ganglion. The fracture terminates in the area of the foramen lacerum or spinosum. Because the fractures cross the axis of the petrous bone, the tympanic membrane may be intact with or without a hemotympanum. The ear is profoundly deaf. Unconsciousness is the rule, and extensive neurologic injury may be found as extremely severe blows cause this type of fracture. Audiometry shows a profound sensorineural hearing loss. Facial nerve palsy is

present in 40 to 50% of cases.[48] When the tympanic membrane is intact, cerebrospinal fluid leakage results in otorhinorrhea, as the fluid passes through the eustachian tube into the nose. Cerebrospinal fluid rhinorrhea is a sign easily missed if not specifically sought, as patients may think they merely have a runny nose. The diagnosis is made by having the patient lean forward and again testing the resultant clear fluid as previously described.

The diagnosis is confirmed with plain skull films or CT scan, which often demonstrates that the temporal bone fracture is actually a combination of longitudinal and transverse fractures (Fig. 16–20). The diagnosis of basilar skull fracture may be made if the clinical picture is strong even with negative radiographic studies. Repeat films at a later date may confirm the diagnosis. Vestibular testing of the involved ear that shows an absent caloric response typically indicates a transverse fracture.[48]

Management

Temporal bone fractures can affect all three divisions of the ear as well as cause facial nerve injury and vascular injury. Management, therefore, is dependent on the specific injury. Series have shown a lower incidence of permanent sequelae and complications in children with temporal bone fractures compared with the incidence for adults; hence, a conservative approach is recommended.[60] Observation suffices if no specific deficits are present. Neurologic consultation should be obtained on all cases with loss of consciousness and apparent brain injury.[47] Injuries to the pinna and ear canal should be managed as previously described.

Middle Ear or Mastoid Injury

Middle ear injuries that show a conductive hearing loss of more than 50 decibels denote an ossicular chain discontinuity and should be explored. Injuries that demonstrate less than a 50-decibel conductive hearing loss should be monitored. Tympanic membrane perforations should also be

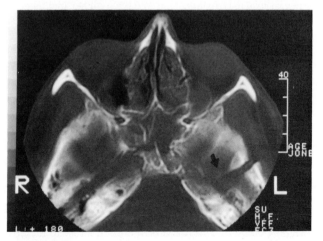

FIGURE 16–20

A computed tomography scan showing a left transverse temporal bone fracture.

managed with observation.[47] One particular problem that may develop with temporal bone fractures is an acquired cholesteatoma. These occur if the tympanic membrane has been torn at a marginal site, thus allowing the ingress of squamous epithelium. Squamous epithelium may enter the mastoid air cells through a longitudinal fracture involving the posterior superior canal wall or may be implanted into the air cells by penetrating trauma. Should this diagnosis be made, aggressive management for removal of squamous epithelium and prevention of further ingrowth is required. The posterior canal wall may be taken down by combining mastoidectomy with tympanoplasty, or the canal wall defect may be repaired using tragal or conchal cartilage.

Sensorineural Hearing Loss

Irreversible, profound sensorineural hearing loss is usually not amenable to therapy and typically occurs with transverse temporal bone fracture. This may be secondary to damage to the labyrinth or the eighth cranial nerve. Stable sensorineural hearing loss should be observed. Children with unilateral losses who are doing well in school may not require hearing amplification. A hearing aid may be employed by children with mild to moderate or moderately severe losses.

In severe to profound hearing losses, a rehabilitative option is the use of a contralateral routing of signals (CROS) aid, in which signals from the deaf ear are routed by FM transmission to a receiver in the good ear. A CROS aid may be combined with a hearing aid for the better ear if there is some loss in this ear as well, allowing the patient the benefit of binaural hearing. This enables children to localize sounds and hear better in a noisy environment.

Other rehabilitative options include implantable hearing aids for patients unable to wear conventional hearing aids and cochlear implants for a select group of bilateral profoundly deaf patients. It must be emphasized that without rehabilitation, the acquisition of normal speech is hindered in a young child with a hearing loss. Patients with a progressive sensorineural hearing loss should be explored for a perilymphatic fistula. Persons with low-frequency sensorineural loss may be expected to have a higher incidence of recovery than those with high-frequency losses. Combined low- and high-frequency losses usually demonstrate no recovery.[48]

Vertigo

Patients experiencing vertigo should be evaluated with electronystagmography. Symptomatic treatment utilizes medications, such as meclizine or droperidol, and positional exercises. The symptoms of disequilibrium should resolve as compensation from labyrinthine damage typically occurs over 3 to 6 weeks. Electronystagmography may be repeated in 6 months if symptoms persist.[47] Dizziness persisting beyond 12 months is typically central and not of labyrinthine origin. Central dizziness can be quite refractory to therapy. Recent endeavors demonstrate that autonomic medications such as propranolol or amitriptyline may benefit this group of patients.

Cerebrospinal Fluid Leakage

Cerebrospinal fluid leaks occur in 6% of basal skull fractures. Otorrhea or otorhinorrhea occurs in 10 to 40% of temporal bone fractures. The patients diagnosed with cerebrospinal fluid otorrhea should not have tympanic membrane or middle ear manipulation for 1 to 2 weeks, as retrograde contamination may occur. Treatment includes bed rest and elevation of the head of the bed. However, the rate of meningitis appears to be about 4% whether antibiotics are used or not.[48] Surgical closure of a cerebrospinal fluid leak is performed for profuse leaks persisting 8 to 10 days or for slower leaks if still present at 2 weeks. Localization of the leak may be aided by the use of intrathecal fluorescein or metrizamide combined with CT scanning. It is important to note that temporal bone fractures heal by fibrous rather than bony union, so a potential pathway for meningeal contamination always exists.[48]

Facial Nerve Injury

Head trauma accounts for 25% of all facial paralysis being second only to Bell's palsy.[48] Injury to the facial nerve may occur anywhere along its route from the facial nucleus through the cerebellopontile angle, near the intratemporal or extratemporal portion of the internal auditory canal. Penetrating injuries of the extratemporal nerve typically sever the nerve, resulting in immediate onset of complete or divisional facial palsy. Such injuries should be explored within 3 days so that the distal segment may be found and the nerve repaired.[30] Contamination of the wound or instability of the patient's condition may make this unfeasible. It is then important to try to identify the cut nerve endings and tag them with silk sutures during the initial 36 hours if at all possible. Nerve injury posterior to a vertical line down from the lateral canthus should be repaired. Paralysis resulting from injuries medial to this line resolve spontaneously.[14] Repair of distal nerve injuries is undertaken with a single epineural suture. Truncal injuries require the epineurium to be retracted and perineural sutures placed using 10.0 nylon. Intrafallopian canal nerve injuries do not require sutures.[30, 43] Penetrating injuries of the temporal bone should demonstrate evidence of progressive denervation on nerve excitability testing before exploration is undertaken.[8]

Blunt injuries can cause the immediate onset of paralysis secondary to intraneural hematoma. Because only 50% of patients with immediate complete palsy recover completely, immediate surgery is recommended by some even if a fracture is not demonstrated.[47] Blunt injuries, however, are more likely to cause swelling of the nerve within the temporal bone, resulting in a delayed onset of facial paralysis. When the onset is delayed, the prognosis for spontaneous return of function is 73% and surgical intervention should be withheld.[48] Steroids may be given and the patient followed with an electrical stimulation test. When facial nerve testing demonstrates a progressive loss of function, that is, greater than 3.5 milliamps by Hilger stimulator or 90% denervation on electroneuronography, in the first 2 weeks after onset, decompression is undertaken.[14] Incomplete facial nerve paralysis usually results in a complete recovery.

The most important aspect in management at this point

is eye protection, as inability to close the eye may result in corneal ulceration and resultant keratopathy. Protection may be accomplished using Lacri-Lube and tape, or a tarsorrhaphy may be performed.[14] Eighty-five percent of patients who eventually recover completely have the onset of recovery within the first 3 weeks.[48]

Management of Intratemporal Injury. Surgical management of an intratemporal facial nerve injury, if indicated, includes decompression of the nerve proximal and distal to the site of injury with incision of the epineurium and removal of any hematoma.[14] A transmastoid-translabyrinthine combined approach is taken for temporal bone fractures with total sensorineural losses. Temporal bone fractures in patients with normal hearing or only a conductive hearing loss are treated with a middle fossa approach followed by a transmastoid exploration to preserve hearing. Penetrating injuries are treated with a transmastoid–middle ear exploration to expose the site of the injury.[4]

Fisch has recommended exploration of the nerve in cases of a temporal bone fracture if denervation of 90% is reached within 6 days after the onset of paralysis. Both the time course and the denervation level are important prognostic signs. This series revealed bony fragment impinging on the nerve in 17%, transection of the nerve in 26%, and intraneural hematoma in 57%.[12] Ninety-three percent of Coker's longitudinal fracture cases had involvement of the labyrinthine segment or geniculate ganglion, so that mastoid exposure alone was not adequate.[4]

Intraneural hematomas require incision of the epineurium and careful evacuation of the clot. Transected nerves are treated by trimming the nerve edges at 45-degree opposing angles to increase the surface area of the neurotubules to promote the ingrowth of fibers. Closure is undertaken without tension, utilizing 10-0 nylon in the epineurium only. Impingement of a bony fragment is treated by careful extraction, along with decompression of the nerve 5 mm proximal and distal to the injury, followed by incision of the epineurium for intraneural hematoma evacuation.[14]

Patients who experience traumatic facial nerve paralysis without return of function within 12 to 18 months after the previously outlined measures may be offered the therapeutic alternative of a hypoglossal to facial nerve anastomosis. This is useful if the facial musculature has not atrophied, which can be demonstrated with electromyography. Other alternatives include dynamic muscle transfers using the temporalis and masseter muscles, static slings, face lift, or insertion of weights or springs in the upper eyelid for eye closure.[30, 42, 43] These measures do not prevent a cosmetic deformity, but successful eye closure with protection of the cornea and with facial symmetry at rest should be deemed a successful outcome.[43]

Facial paralysis may occur in the newborn, with or without forceps delivery, from compression of the nerve by the pelvis during delivery. A temporal bone fracture may also be present. The differential diagnosis of a newborn with facial paralysis should also include congenital absence of the facial nerve or the facial musculature. This may be elucidated with electrical tests. Traumatic facial paralysis in the newborn typically resolves spontaneously.[29]

Vascular Injury

Temporal bone trauma may result in life-threatening hemorrhage if the jugular bulb, sigmoid sinus, other dural sinus, or carotid artery is injured. Initial management should be tamponade of the external auditory canal. Computed tomography scanning may then be used to demonstrate the site of injury along with arteriography for further evaluation. Venous sinus injuries may be managed through a mastoid or craniotomy approach with compression, intraluminal packing, or ligation of the sigmoid sinus and the internal jugular vein. Carotid artery injuries that do not respond to initial pressure must be exposed in the intratemporal course and repaired, ligated, compressed, packed, or occluded with a balloon.[8]

Penetrating Injuries of the Temporal Bone

Gunshot wounds to the temporal bone are addressed as a separate entity because the evaluation and management of these injuries differ from those of other temporal bone injuries. Gunshot wounds to the temporal bone cause 6% of all temporal bone fractures and can cause damage not only from bullet fragmentation, but also from resultant bone comminution. Typically a mixed fracture occurs, resulting in sensorineural hearing loss secondary to cochlear damage or acoustic trauma. Computed tomography scanning and arteriography are performed as 32% of gunshot wounds to the temporal bone result in vascular injury. Conventional tomograms are useful in this situation because scatter from the metal fragments as is seen with CT scans is absent. Gunshot wounds to the temporal bone may result in retained metal fragments in the middle ear and mastoid. Manipulation of such fragments is fraught with possible severe consequences. Damaged inner ear structures are usually nonfunctional, but ossicles and the facial nerve may be intact initially only to be damaged by iatrogenic manipulation. Metal fragments in the mastoid may be left without consequence. Exploration should be performed if there is facial paralysis, impaction of skin elements in the mastoid, vascular injuries, persistent cerebrospinal fluid leakage, conductive hearing loss, chronic infection, or progressive sensorineural hearing loss.[8]

Exploration of Gunshot Injuries. A combined transcanal and transmastoid approach is utilized for temporal bone gunshot wounds. When the posterior canal wall and the stapes are intact, ossicular chain reconstruction and tympanoplasty are performed. Posterior wall defects may be reconstructed or taken down and a modified or radical mastoidectomy performed.[8] Perilymphatic fistulas and cerebrospinal fluid leaks may require obliteration of the middle ear and mastoid. Facial nerve palsies from a gunshot wound may be secondary to edema or intraneural hemorrhage. Decompression usually yields excellent results. However, more commonly, a section of nerve is missing, so primary repair is impossible.[30] Interposition grafting with greater auricular or sural nerve through a middle ear or mastoid approach works well in these cases. On return of function, resultant slight weakness and synkinesis is typical. Geniculate ganglion involvement, as evidenced by absent tearing on a Schirmer test, requires a combined middle fossa-mastoid approach if hearing is preservable. When hearing is already lost, the internal auditory canal may be approached by a translabyrinthine dissection.[8] A hypoglossal facial anastomosis is performed if function does not return and the injury is less than 18 months. Muscle fibrillation potentials should be documented by electromyography. When 18 months have passed, the facial muscles are usually no longer capable of receiving neural input, and options for rehabilitation are those listed earlier. Canal injuries require early local débridement, topical therapy, and packing to prevent stenosis. Should stenosis occur, excision with split thickness skin grafts works well. Cholesteatoma may develop if skin is forced into the mastoid or middle ear. Prolapse of the mandibular condyle may require a condylectomy or canal wall down mastoidectomy to ensure patency of the ear canal.[8]

References

1. Aguilar EA III, Hall JW III, Mackey-Hargadine J: Neuro-otologic evaluation of the patient with acute, severe head injuries: Correlations among physical findings, auditory evoked responses, and computerized tomography. Otolaryngol Head Neck Surg 94:211–219, 1984.
2. Bailey BJ: Management of soft tissue trauma of the head and neck in children. Otolaryngol Clin North Am 10(1):193–203, 1977.
3. Bluestone CD, Supance JS: Perilymph fistula in infants and children. In: Gates GA (ed): Current Therapy in Otolaryngology—Head and Neck Surgery, 1984–1985. Burlington, Ontario, Canada, BC Decker, 1984, pp 68–72.
4. Coker NJ, Kendall KA, Jenkins HA, et al: Traumatic intratemporal facial nerve injury: Management rationale for preservation of function. Otolaryngol Head Neck Surg 97:262–269, 1987.
5. Donald PJ: Frontal sinus ablation by cranialization. Arch Otolaryngol 108:142–146, 1982.
6. Donald PJ, Bernstein L: Compound frontal sinus injuries with intracranial penetration. Laryngoscope 88:225–232, 1978.
7. Donald PJ, Ettin M: The safety of frontal sinus fat obliteration when sinus walls are missing. Laryngoscope 96(2):190–193, 1986.
8. Duncan NO, Coker NJ, Jenkins HA, et al: Gunshot injuries of the temporal bone. Otolaryngol Head Neck Surg 94:47–55, 1986.
9. Emmett JR, Shea JJ: Traumatic perilymph fistula. Laryngoscope 90:1513–1520, 1980.
10. Esses BA, Jafek BW: Cricothyroidotomy: A decade of experience in Denver. Ann Otol Rhinol Laryngol 96:519–524, 1987.
11. Finkle DR, Ringler SL, Luttenton CR, et al: Comparison of the diagnostic methods used in maxillofacial trauma. Plast Reconstr Surg 75(1):32–38, 1985.
12. Fisch U: Prognostic value of electrical tests in acute facial paralysis. Am J Otol 5:497–498, 1984.
13. Fuleihan NS, Natout M, Webster RC, et al: Successful replantation of amputated nose and auricle. Otolaryngol Head Neck Surg 97:18–23, 1987.
14. Gantz BJ: Traumatic facial paralysis. In: Gates GA (ed): Current Therapy in Otolaryngology—Head and Neck Surgery, 1984–1985. Burlington, Ontario, Canada, BC Decker, 1984, pp 112–115.
15. Giffin CS: The wrestler's ear (acute auricular hematoma). Arch Otolaryngol 111:161–164, 1985.
16. Glasscock ME III, McKennan KX, Levine SC: Persistent traumatic perilymph fistulas. Laryngoscope 97:860–864, 1987.
17. Griffin WL: A retrospective study of traumatic tympanic membrane perforations in a clinical practice. Laryngoscope 89:261–282, 1979.
18. Gross CW: Soft tissue injuries of the lip, nose, ears and preauricular area. Otolaryngol Clin North Am 2:265–302, 1969.
19. Grymer LF, Gutierrez C, Stoksted P: The importance of nasal fractures during different growth periods of the nose. J Laryngol Otol 99(8):741–744, 1985.
20. Grymer LF, Gutierrez C, Stoksted P: Nasal fractures in children: Influence on the development of the nose. J Laryngol 99:735–739, 1985.
21. Gussack GS, Jurkovich GJ, Luterman A: Laryngotracheal trauma: A protocol approach to a rare injury. Laryngoscope 96(6):660–665, 1986.
22. Gussack GS, Luterman A, Powell RW, et al: Pediatric maxillofacial trauma: Unique features in diagnosis and treatment. Laryngoscope 97(8):925–930, 1987.
23. Gussack GS, Tacchi E: Pulse oximetry in the management of pediatric airway disorders. South Med J 80:1381–1384, 1987.
24. Hall RK: Injuries of the face and jaws in children. Int J Oral Surg 1:65–75, 1972.
25. Hicks GW, Wright JW Jr, Wright JW III: Cerebrospinal fluid otorrhea. Laryngoscope 90(25):1–25, 1980.
26. Hough JVD: Otologic trauma. In: Paparella MM, Shumrick DA (eds): Otolaryngology, Vol. II. The Ear. Philadelphia, WB Saunders, 1980, pp 1656–1679.
27. Hughes GB, Levine SC: Disorders of the external ear. In: Hughes GB (ed): Textbook of Clinical Otology. New York, Thieme-Stratton, 1985, pp 267–270, 279.
28. Hughes GB, Papsidero JA: Temporal bone trauma. In: Hughes GB (ed): Textbook of Clinical Otology. New York, Thieme-Stratton, 1985, pp 357–362.
29. Hughes GB, Tucker HM, Klein AM: Congenital facial palsy. In: Hughes GB (ed): Textbook of Clinic Otology. New York, Thieme-Stratton, 1985, pp 253–256.
30. Johns ME, Crumley RL: Facial nerve injury, repair, and rehabilitation. Self-Instructional Package. Rochester, NY, American Academy of Otolaryngology, 1984.
31. Kaban LB, Mulliken JB, Murray JE: Facial fractures in children. An analysis of 122 fractures in 109 patients. Plast Reconstruct Surg 59(1):15–20, 1977.
32. Lacher AB, Blitzer A: The traumatized auricle—Care, salvage, and reconstruction. Otolaryngol Clin North Am 15(1):225–239, 1982.
33. Lambert GE Jr, McMurry GT: Laryngotracheal trauma: Recognition and management. JACEP 5(11):883–887, 1976.
34. Lawson W: Management of soft tissue injuries of the face. Otolaryngol Clin North Am 15(1):35–48, 1982.
35. Leopold DA: Laryngeal trauma. A historical perspective. Arch Otolaryngol 109:106–111, 1983.
36. Line WS, Stanley RB, Choi JH: Strangulation: A full spectrum of blunt neck trauma. Ann Otol Rhinol Laryngol 94:542–556, 1985.
37. Linthicum FH, Rand CW: Neuro-otological observations in concussion of the brain. Arch Otolaryngol 13:85, 1931.
38. Liston SL: Injury of the external ear. In: Gates GA (ed): Current Therapy in Otolaryngology—Head and Neck Surgery—3. Burlington, Ontario, Canada, BC Decker, 1987, pp 93–95.
39. Maceri DR, Mancuso AA, Canalis RF: Value of computed axial tomography in severe laryngeal injury. Arch Otolaryngol 108:449–451, 1982.
40. Mancuso AA, Calcaterra TC, Hanafee WN: Computed tomography of the larynx. Radiol Clin North Am 16(2):195–208, 1978.
41. Mancuso AA, Hanafee WN: Computed tomography of the injured larynx. Radiology 133:139–144, 1979.
42. May M: Gold weight and wire spring implants as alternatives to tarsorrhaphy. Arch Otolaryngol Head Neck Surg 113:656–660, 1987.
43. May M: Traumatic facial paralysis. In: Gates GA (ed): Current Therapy in Otolaryngology—Head and Neck Surgery—3. Burlington, Ontario, Canada, BC Decker, 1987, pp 84–88.
44. Mladick RA: Salvage of the ear in acute trauma. Clin Plast Surg 5:427–435, 1978.
45. Morse TS: Step by step with an injured child. Emerg Med Clin North Am 1:175–185, 1983.
46. Nadol JB Jr: Ear emergencies. In: Wilson WR, Nadol JB Jr (eds): Quick Reference to Ear, Nose, and Throat Disorders. Philadelphia, JB Lippincott, 1983, pp 97–111.
47. Olson JE: Temporal bone injury. In: Holt GR, Mattox DE, Gates GA (eds): Decision Making in Otolaryngology. St. Louis, CV Mosby, 1984, pp 156–157.
48. Olson JE, Shagets FW: Blunt trauma of the temporal bone. Self-Instructional Package. Rochester, NY, American Academy of Otolaryngology, 1986.
49. Olsen KD, Carpenter RJ, Kern EB: Nasal septal trauma in children. Pediatrics 64(1):32–35, 1979.
50. Pappas DG: Sensorineural hearing loss associated with trauma. Diag-

nosis and Treatment of Hearing Impairment in Children. San Diego, Calif, College-Hill Press, 1985, pp 147–166.

51. Parell GJ, Becker GD: Conservative management of inner ear baro-trauma resulting from scuba diving. Otolaryngol Head Neck Surg 93:393–397, 1985.

52. Parell GJ, Becker GD: Results of surgical repair of inapparent peri-lymph fistulas. Otolaryngol Head Neck Surg 95:344–346, 1986.

53. Parkin JL: Injuries of the pinna. Current Therapy. In: Gates GA (ed): Current Therapy in Otolaryngology—Head and Neck Surgery, 1982–1983. Trenton, NJ, BC Decker, 1982, pp 96–98.

54. Potsic WP, Handler SD: Primary care. In: Pediatric Otolaryngology. New York, Macmillan Publishing Co, 1986, pp 116–121.

55. Schaefer SD: Primary management of laryngeal trauma. Ann Otol Rhinol Laryngol 91:399–402, 1982.

56. Serafin D, Georgiade N: Pediatric Plastic Surgery. St. Louis, CV Mosby, 1984, p 535.

57. Sessions DG, Stallings JO, Mills WJ Jr, et al: Frostbite of the ear. Laryngoscope 81:1223–1232, 1971.

58. Shambaugh GE Jr: Developmental anatomy of the ear. In: Shambaugh GE Jr, Glasscock ME III (eds): Surgery of the Ear. Philadelphia, WB Saunders, 1980, pp 5–29.

59. Shambaugh GE Jr, Glasscock ME III: Meningeal and nonmeningeal complications of otitis media. In: Shambaugh GE Jr, Glasscock ME III: Surgery of the Ear. Philadelphia, WB Saunders, 1980, pp 289–347.

60. Shapiro RS: Temporal bone fractures in children. Otolaryngol Head Neck Surg 87:323–329, 1979.

61. Singleton GT: Perilymphatic fistula. In: Gates GA (ed): Current Therapy in Otolaryngology—Head and Neck Surgery—3. Burlington, Ontario, Canada, BC Decker, 1987, pp 52–54.

62. Storrs L: Tympanic membrane perforation. In: Gates GA (ed): Current Therapy in Otolaryngology—Head and Neck Surgery, 1982–1983. Trenton, NJ, BC Decker, 1982, pp 11–14.

63. Stucker FJ, Bryarly RC, Shockley WW: Management of nasal trauma in children. Arch Otolaryngol 110:190–192, 1984.

64. Thomas RJ: Auricular trauma. In: Holt GR, Mattox DE, Gates GA (eds): Decision Making in Otolaryngology. St. Louis, CV Mosby, 1984, pp 158–159.

65. Tjellstrom A, Yontcher E, Lindstrom J, et al: Five years experience with bone-anchored auricular prosthesis. Otolaryngol Head Neck Surg 93:366–372, 1985.

66. Ward WD: Noise-induced hearing damage. In: Paparella MM, Shum-rick DA (eds): Otolaryngology, Vol. II. The Ear. Philadelphia, WB Saunders, 1980, pp 1788–1803.

CHAPTER SEVENTEEN

Marleta Reynolds

Pulmonary, Esophageal, and Diaphragmatic Injuries

Most chest injuries in children occur in those who have multiple injuries. Mayer and colleagues reviewed the cases of 110 children with multiple injuries and found thoracic injuries present in 25%.[9] More recently, the Pediatric Trauma Registry from the National Institute of Disability and Rehabilitation Research documented 7850 admissions for trauma.[11] At Children's Memorial Hospital over the same 2½-year period 1118 children were admitted because of injuries; only 4% of these children had chest trauma, and none of the trauma-related deaths was due to a thoracic injury. Welch reported that the hospital mortality rate for isolated chest injuries is indeed low; however, the mortality rate triples when chest injuries occur along with other injuries.[13]

In children, blunt chest trauma continues to be more common than penetrating trauma, especially in the younger age groups. Blunt chest trauma is reported by the Pediatric Trauma Registry to occur 95% of the time in children with chest injuries.[11] At Children's Memorial Hospital we see few children involved in violent crime, and our numbers reflect this population. We have treated only three children with penetrating chest injuries in the last 2½ years. The remaining 42 chest injuries were from blunt trauma.

The circumstances surrounding chest injury in children are different from those in adults. Infants and small children are more often involved in falls; older children are injured as pedestrians or as occupants of motor vehicles; adolescents are more often involved with violent crime and penetrating chest trauma. In addition, some specific thoracic injuries are more common in children. A child's curious and inquisitive nature may lead to the accidental ingestion of corrosive materials or the ingestion or aspiration of foreign objects. Iatrogenic injuries occur frequently in infants and children who are being treated for respiratory insufficiency. Therapeutic instrumentation of the tracheobronchial tree, esophagus, and pleural space can result in significant trauma. Barotrauma produced by aggressive management of respiratory failure in premature infants and neonates has created a new spectrum of pulmonary and tracheobronchial pathologies.[4]

Several physical features of the chest of children differ from those of adults, which affects not only which organ is injured but also how the patient responds to the injury. The soft cartilage and developing bone of the child render the thorax very pliable; thus rib fractures are uncommon and, when present, reflect a powerful force as the mechanism of injury. Children also may sustain significant chest injury and show little or no external evidence of trauma. The mediastinum is easily displaced in a child by air or fluid, and marked mediastinal shifts can compromise venous return and cardiac output as well as reduce lung volume. The mediastinum in an adult does not tend to shift to the same degree, and an adult can usually tolerate a mediastinal shift with cardiovascular compromise better than a child. However, recovery from thoracic injury in children is speeded by the absence of preexisting cardiopulmonary disease and the tobacco habit.

CHEST WALL INJURY

The elasticity and flexibility of a child's thoracic cage often protects the child from serious chest wall injury. Flail seg-

ments are as uncommon as rib fractures but when they occur, they are often associated with severe parenchymal pulmonary injury. A pulmonary contusion may not be visible on the initial chest roentgenogram, thus, roentgenograms should be repeated at 12 and 24 hours or at signs of respiratory deterioration. These delayed roentgenograms often demonstrate a fluffy infiltrate that is characteristic of a pulmonary contusion. The advent of more frequent torso computed tomography has enabled earlier identification of these injuries.

Children with rib fractures usually present with chest pain and varying degrees of respiratory distress. Palpation of the chest wall helps to identify points of tenderness or crepitus. A flail segment results in paradoxical movement of the chest wall with each respiration, is a serious injury regardless of age, and is identified by simple inspection. Flail chest decreases the efficiency of ventilation, increases the work of breathing, and may lead quickly to respiratory failure.[2] Children with multiple rib fractures or a flail segment may be tachypneic or cyanotic. Oxygen is administered by face mask, and a chest roentgenogram is obtained to verify the rib fractures and identify any other associated chest injury (Fig. 17–1).

Simple rib fractures are treated with analgesia and pulmonary toilet to prevent atelectasis.[1] Intercostal nerve blocks can be used to provide prolonged pain relief. Supplemental oxygen is often administered. If adequate ventilation cannot be maintained, endotracheal intubation and positive pressure mechanical ventilation should be instituted. No attempt should be made to externally immobilize the chest wall. In children, remodeling of the chest wall occurs rapidly, leaving no permanent deformity.

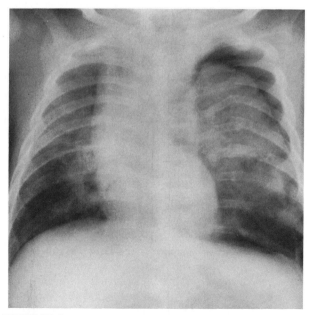

FIGURE 17-1

This chest roentgenogram was obtained on a 2-year-old child who was an unrestrained passenger in a motor vehicle accident. There are five fractured left ribs and a pneumothorax. Oxygen was administered. The pneumothorax resolved with a tube thoracostomy.

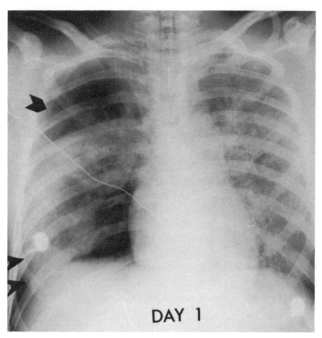

FIGURE 17–2

A 10-year-old boy was accidentally pinned under an automobile. Findings on the original chest roentgenogram were normal. This chest roentgenogram taken the day following admission reveals a small right pneumothorax and bilateral pulmonary contusions. Recovery was uneventful.

TRAUMATIC ASPHYXIA

Traumatic asphyxia is usually associated with blunt chest and abdominal trauma. We have treated three children with traumatic asphyxia in the past 5 years. All were pinned under an automobile. To produce traumatic asphyxia, the glottis must be closed and the thoracoabdominal muscles tensed at the moment of impact. The force of injury is transmitted up the superior vena cava into the head and neck with subsequent disruption of superficial capillaries. Haller and Donahoo's experience with three children supports this combination of superior vena caval obstruction and sudden increase in intratracheal or intrapulmonary pressure.[5]

At presentation the child is usually disoriented and tachypneic. There are petechiae covering the face, neck, and upper chest as well as subconjunctival and retinal hemorrhages. The face and neck are usually blue and swollen. Below the level of impact the skin is normal. A careful search for underlying chest injuries must be undertaken and any respiratory insufficiency treated with oxygen or mechanical ventilation. An injury to the great vessels, a cardiac contusion, a pneumothorax, and a pulmonary contusion may coexist. A chest roentgenogram and electrocardiogram should be obtained (Fig. 17–2). These patients should be observed in the intensive care unit. Although rare, progressive pulmonary insufficiency may develop and may require mechanical ventilation. A follow-up over time (4.4 years) of patients with traumatic asphyxia revealed no long-term disability.[8]

TRACHEOBRONCHIAL INJURY

Tracheobronchial injuries can result from blunt or penetrating trauma. A review by Kelly and associates, who reported on more than 100 patients with penetrating or blunt injuries of the neck or chest, described abnormal shearing forces in blunt trauma that may lead to laceration of the intrathoracic trachea or main bronchi.[7] The laceration is usually circumferential and may result in complete disruption of the trachea or bronchus. The majority of blunt tracheal injuries occur within 2.5 cm of the carina, and vascular and esophageal injuries are commonly associated, particularly with penetrating injuries.

Injury to the tracheobronchial tree should be suspected in any patient with blunt or penetrating trauma to the neck or chest. In the series reported by Kelly and associates all patients presented with signs of airway compromise: tachypnea, dyspnea, cyanosis, subcutaneous emphysema, or an abnormal breathing pattern. A major tracheobronchial disruption is usually suspected with massive subcutaneous emphysema, persistent air leak, failure of the involved lung to reexpand following tube thoracostomy, or persistent anoxia. Other findings may include mediastinal air, hemoptysis, or tension pneumothorax (Fig. 17–3).

Airway management is the first priority in treating patients with suspected tracheobronchial injury. Endotracheal intubation is often necessary, and a tracheostomy may be required. An associated pneumothorax should be treated with tube thoracostomy (Fig. 17–4). Specific treatment of tracheobronchial injuries depends on the location and extent

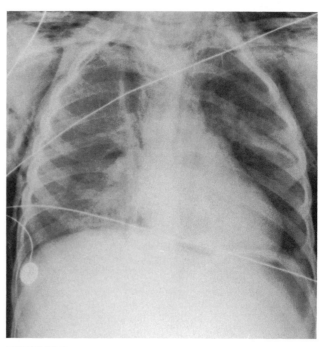

FIGURE 17–3

After endotracheal intubation and an elective hernia repair, this 11-year-old boy developed massive subcutaneous emphysema. Crepitus could be palpated from neck to thighs and is demonstrated in the soft tissue in this chest roentgenogram.

of the injury, information that can often be obtained by bronchoscopy.

The management of a tracheobronchial injury ranges from observation of a small tracheal disruption to thoracotomy. Some tracheal injuries are so small that they cannot be seen at bronchoscopy. These injuries can usually be observed. Larger lacerations of the membranous or cartilaginous portion may be treated with endotracheal intubation and often surgical repair. The cervical trachea can be approached through a transverse neck incision to allow careful evaluation of adjacent vascular structures and the esophagus. Thoracotomy is required for repair of the thoracic trachea and major bronchi, and direct repair is often possible. Segmental tracheal resection or lobar resection may occasionally be necessary. A bronchus may be injured, and the injury may seal immediately. However, the bronchus is held together with only surrounding adventitia, and as healing progresses, granulation tissue and a stricture can develop. The child presents with pneumonia or atelectasis distal to the stricture. If the stricture is accessible through the bronchoscope, it may respond to dilation. However, resection and primary repair may be required. Iatrogenic strictures of the main stem bronchi may develop from overzealous tracheobronchial suctioning in an intubated neonate. The clinical presentation and the management are identical to those for a traumatic stricture (Fig. 17–5A and B).

LUNG INJURY

Pneumothorax

A pneumothorax can result from penetrating or blunt chest trauma and is one of the most common thoracic injuries reported in children. Blunt trauma can produce a pneumothorax if a fractured rib punctures the lung parenchyma or if the force of injury is sufficient to cause rupture of alveoli or of a portion of the tracheobronchial tree. Air leaks into the chest and may dissect into the soft tissues of the chest wall, mediastinum, and neck. The ipsilateral lung usually collapses. Penetrating injuries of the chest that produce a pneumothorax almost always produce a concomitant hemothorax.

A child with a pneumothorax may be asymptomatic or may present with respiratory distress of varying degree. Physical examination of the chest may reveal subcutaneous emphysema and decreased breath sounds. If time allows, a chest roentgenogram can be obtained to confirm the diagnosis (Fig. 17–6). However, sudden or rapid deterioration of a child with a suspected pneumothorax necessitates immediate needle aspiration of the pneumothorax (a no. 20 angiocatheter is used and left in place) until a chest tube can be inserted. All traumatic pneumothoraces should be treated with a tube thoracostomy. The fourth intercostal space in the anterior axillary line is utilized for tube thoracostomy in patients at Children's Memorial Hospital, and the tube is then connected to water seal or underwater suction. The chest tube is removed when the lung is fully expanded, the air leak has ceased, and the chest roentgenogram is unchanged after 24 hours of drainage.

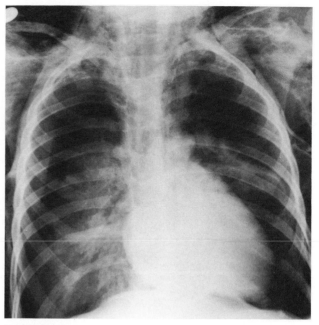

FIGURE 17–4

The same boy (illustrated in Fig. 17–3) with a small tracheal laceration demonstrated at bronchoscopy developed bilateral pneumothoraces as shown on a subsequent chest roentgenogram. Bilateral tube thoracostomies were placed. The injury did not require repair, and the child made a complete recovery.

Infants treated with positive pressure ventilation for respiratory distress risk developing pulmonary interstitial emphysema, pneumomediastinum, and pneumothoraces. Hall and Rhodes suggest that distending airway pressure creates excessive alveolar distention, and intra-alveolar rupture may occur with dissection of air along the perivascular spaces to the mediastinum and eventual rupture into the pleural space.[4] A pneumothorax that develops in this fashion is also treated with tube thoracostomy.

Tension Pneumothorax

A tension pneumothorax usually develops as a result of blunt trauma. Increasing amounts of air in the pleural space result in total collapse of the ipsilateral lung and displacement of the mediastinal structures into the contralateral chest, resulting in an encroachment of the contralateral lung and a decrease in venous return to the heart. Intrapulmonary arteriovenous shunting also occurs.

The diagnosis of tension pneumothorax must be made during the initial survey of the patient. Respiratory and cardiovascular compromise are often present. The child is usually anxious, tachypneic, and often cyanotic. The trachea is shifted toward the contralateral side as are the heart sounds. The involved chest is hyperresonant to percussion and has absent breath sounds. Immediate aspiration of the ipsilateral chest may be life saving; it should be followed by tube thoracostomy. A chest roentgenogram is then obtained to identify other intrathoracic injuries and check chest tube placement (Fig. 17–7A and B).

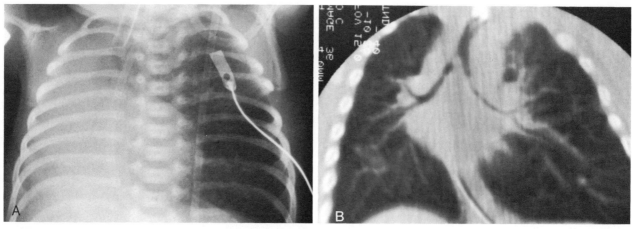

FIGURE 17–5

A, This chest roentgenogram prompted bronchoscopy in a premature infant who had been ventilated for 1 month. Previous chest roentgenograms had shown good aeration bilaterally. At bronchoscopy, granulation tissue and a stricture were identified at the origin of the right main stem bronchus. *B,* Repeated and aggressive dilations have improved the stenosis, as demonstrated on this computed tomogram.

Hemothorax

Severe blunt and penetrating trauma may produce a hemothorax. A concomitant pneumothorax is almost always present. Bullet and knife wounds may injure the lung parenchyma and the intercostal vessels as well as the chest wall, and occasionally the great vessels or pulmonary vessels are also injured. Depending on the amount of blood loss, the patient may be hypotensive. Respiratory insufficiency may

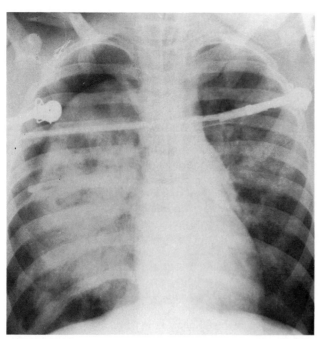

FIGURE 17–6

A pneumothorax should be suspected in any child with blunt chest trauma. This chest roentgenogram of a child who fell out of a tree reveals a fractured clavicle and right pneumothorax.

develop from a coexisting pneumothorax or from collapse of the lung by blood or hematoma. The breath sounds are decreased on the ipsilateral side, and the chest is dull to percussion.

A chest roentgenogram confirms the presence of fluid in the chest (Fig. 17–8). With massive hemorrhage, a tube thoracostomy may need to be placed before obtaining the chest roentgenogram, and volume resuscitation should be started simultaneously. On chest roentgenogram the cardiophrenic angle appears blunted or completely obliterated. All the blood should be removed from the chest by tube thoracostomy to prevent a fibrothorax from developing. A posterior chest tube in the sixth or seventh intercostal space provides optimal drainage.

Indications for operation for a hemothorax include an ongoing hemorrhage of greater than 100 ml per kg per hour or greater than 20% of the child's blood volume being drained immediately. Continuing hemorrhage usually is secondary to injury to the intercostal vessels, internal mammary vessels, or great vessels.

Pulmonary Contusion

A pulmonary contusion is often unrecognized in the initial assessment of an injured child. It is not usually apparent on initial chest roentgenogram, and often, particularly in infants, no external evidence of thoracic trauma is present. The symptoms of a pulmonary contusion usually develop over time, with tachypnea, dyspnea, and hemoptysis signaling worsening pulmonary function. Fluffy infiltrates develop on subsequent chest roentgenograms, and respiratory failure may follow (Fig. 17–9).

A contusion is characterized by edema and hemorrhage with bronchospasm. Treatment is usually symptomatic. All children with suspected chest trauma should receive supplemental oxygen. Endotracheal intubation and positive pressure ventilation may be required to maintain adequate ventilation until the lung recovers.

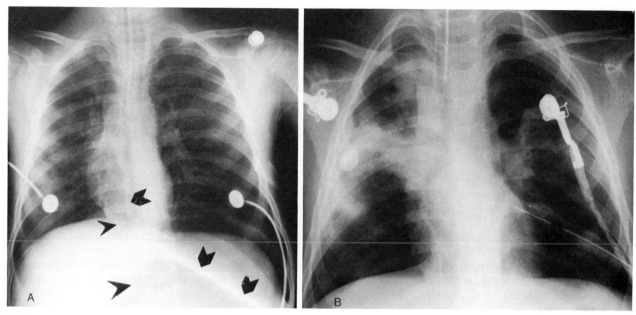

FIGURE 17–7

These two chest roentgenograms were obtained on a 14-year-old boy who was struck by an automobile. *A*, The wide arrows outline a tension pneumothorax. The thin arrows demonstrate a central line placed for monitoring purposes. *B*, Soon after left tube thoracostomy, the lung reexpanded and the mediastinum returned to the midline. The right-sided pulmonary contusion is becoming more obvious on this film.

THORACIC DUCT INJURY

Injury to the thoracic duct is usually a complication of thoracic surgery. It occasionally occurs as a result of a penetrating injury to the chest. Operations associated with the development of a chylothorax include ligation or division of a patent ductus arteriosus, coarctation repair, pulmonary-systemic shunts, and any other operation that involves dissection around the aorta. The operations are usually left sided, but the thoracic duct can be injured through the right chest.

A pleural effusion is identified on chest roentgenogram, and aspiration yields a milky fluid in a child who is on enteral alimentation. Initial treatment includes tube thoracostomy to water seal or suction; abstinence of oral alimentation and peripheral or central hyperalimentation is undertaken. Once the drainage stops, a no-fat diet or a diet with

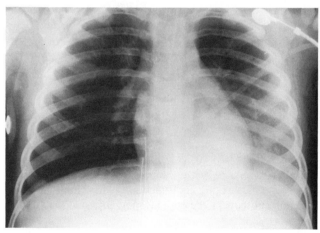

FIGURE 17–8

A 2-year-old boy survived a 10-story fall and presented to our emergency department with tachypnea. This chest roentgenogram revealed fluid in the left chest, and a thoracostomy tube drained 300 ml of blood. The boy recovered without complication.

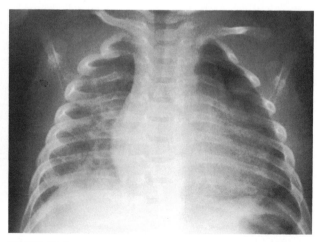

FIGURE 17–9

A chest roentgenogram was obtained because this 5-month-old infant developed tachypnea 8 hours after being admitted for blunt chest trauma. The original chest roentgenogram was normal. New infiltrates are now seen bilaterally. Oxygen was administered, and the infant was observed closely. The infant recovered without incident.

fat restricted to only medium-chain triglycerides can be initiated.

Most chylothoraces resolve spontaneously. If persistent, a left thoracotomy is utilized to identify the thoracic duct just above the diaphragm, and ligation may be facilitated by the instillation of vegetable dye into the distal esophagus.

ESOPHAGEAL INJURY

Because the esophagus lies deep in the mediastinum, is elastic and mobile, and is surrounded by other mediastinal structures, blunt and penetrating injury are uncommon. Accidents resulting in rapid deceleration are usually responsible for blunt trauma to the esophagus. A sudden increase in the esophageal luminal pressure may cause the esophagus to rupture, usually in the distal esophagus on the left side. This portion of the esophagus is not as well supported by the other structures in the mediastinum.

Iatrogenic injuries account for the majority of penetrating injuries of the esophagus in children. Traumatic pseudodiverticulum, perforations, and esophagopleural fistulas may result from the passage of nasogastric tubes; suction catheters; and esophageal stethescopes, endoscopes, and dilators (Fig. 17–10A and B). Other factors that contribute to esophageal perforation in children include ingestion of foreign bodies and caustic agents and anastomotic strictures secondary to the repair of congenital defects. Regardless of whether the injury is blunt or penetrating, esophageal perforations are diagnosed and managed in the same fashion in the adult as in the child.

A hole in the esophagus leads to the spillage of gastric and oral secretions and bacteria into the mediastinum. Air escaping into the mediastinum may dissect into the neck and chest wall. Consequently, patients may present with subcutaneous emphysema in the neck and chest. If the perforation extends into the chest, a pneumothorax, and hydrothorax, or both result. Fever, dyspnea, and shock may be the presenting signs and symptoms. Some patients complain of abdominal or chest pain.

Radiologic evaluation of the esophagus should be considered in any patient in whom an esophageal injury is suspected. Bullets that cross the midline may injure the esophagus at any level and thus warrant evaluation. An esophagogram with a non-ionic water soluble agent should be obtained. Small perforations may not be identified, and persistent contrast material in the mediastinum may obscure further management. If the study does not reveal a major leak, it can be repeated later. Extravasation of contrast material confirms the diagnosis. Esophagoscopy is indicated only if obtaining an esophagogram is not feasible because of the condition of the patient or if the esophagogram appears normal and the index of suspension for injury is very high.

Management of esophageal injury depends on the location and nature of the injury, the history of previous esophageal damage, the presence of an associated pneumothorax or hydrothorax, and the general health of the child. Very small perforations in the neck and chest can be treated with

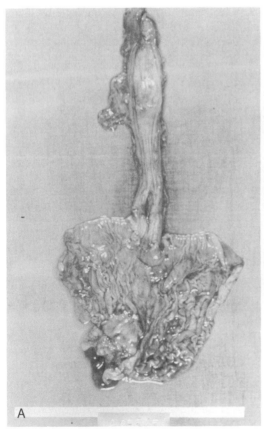

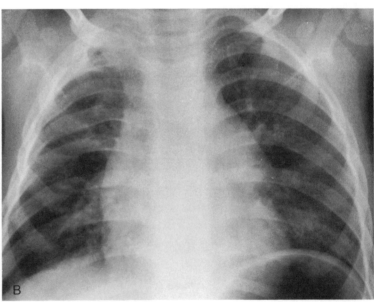

FIGURE 17–10

A, This autopsy specimen shows a large linear tear of the distal esophagus resulting from a dilation for a stricture. *B,* This chest roentgenogram was obtained on the infant following the esophageal dilation. Although no abnormality can be seen, the infant died within 16 hours. If an injury of the esophagus is suspected, a contrast study of the esophagus should be obtained.

the administration of parenteral antibiotics, the cessation of oral alimentation, and the insertion of one or two chest tubes, if appropriate. Large injuries of the upper two thirds of the esophagus should be approached through the right chest. Lower esophageal injuries are approached via a left thoracotomy. The mediastinal pleura is opened, and the edges of the perforation are débrided. A two-layer closure of the esophagus using absorbable suture is performed, reinforced by a pleural or intercostal muscle flap. Drainage is accomplished with large chest tubes for the mediastinum and chest. Proximal and distal diversion with cervical esophagostomy and gastrostomy may be necessary if direct repair is not advisable or possible.

Traumatic tracheoesophageal fistula is rare. An esophagogram may confirm the diagnosis; however, both bronchoscopy and esophagoscopy are indicated to identify the extent of the injury and are believed by some to be the superior diagnostic approach. Direct repair of these injuries is performed through a right thoracotomy, and a pleural flap should be interposed between the suture lines of the trachea and esophagus. If there is major injury to the esophagus or trachea, the esophagus can be diverted with a cervical esophagostomy, the trachea can be repaired, and a gastrostomy can be used for enteral feedings.

Significant morbidity can result from esophageal perforation. Prolonged hospitalization and treatment for sepsis and empyema are sometimes necessary. Mortality figures in the adult population are high. Shepherd and associates reported a 0% mortality in their series of esophageal perforations in 12 children.[12]

DIAPHRAGMATIC INJURY

Traumatic disruption of the diaphragm is usually the result of blunt abdominal trauma. Automobile accidents, falls from great heights, and crush injuries account for the majority of diaphragmatic disruptions. The left side is reported to be involved 95% of the time,[10] but Estrera and associates reported an incidence of 34% right-sided injuries.[3]

Penetrating injuries of the diaphragm are equally distributed between the right and left sides and may be located anywhere on the diaphragmatic surface. However, the majority of blunt injuries occur in the posterolateral area and extend out in a radial direction, and the greater curvature of the stomach may herniate into the chest followed by the omentum, the colon, and the small bowel.

Because the force required to rupture the diaphragm is considerable, the incidence of associated injuries is high. Hood reported a 78% incidence of rib and skeletal fractures, a 35% incidence of splenic injury, an 18% incidence of intracranial injury, and a 9% incidence of liver injury.[6] Orringer and Kirsh reported that associated visceral injury occurred in 9 to 55% of cases.[10] With right-sided injuries, the liver is the most commonly injured organ, with inferior vena cava and hepatic vein avulsion a serious threat.[3]

The patient with traumatic rupture of the diaphragm may be asymptomatic or may have marked cardiorespiratory compromise. The signs and symptoms are related to the associated injuries and the amount of intra-abdominal content that herniates into the chest. Compromise of the lung may be unilateral and may become bilateral if the mediastinum is forced to the opposite side. Most patients with traumatic rupture of the diaphragm present with dyspnea and abdominal or chest pain. Physical examination reveals abdominal tenderness and decreased breath sounds on the ipsilateral chest. Bowel sounds are usually decreased or absent.

An upright chest roentgenogram may be diagnostic. Hood listed findings on the chest roentgenogram that are suggestive of diaphragmatic rupture.[6]

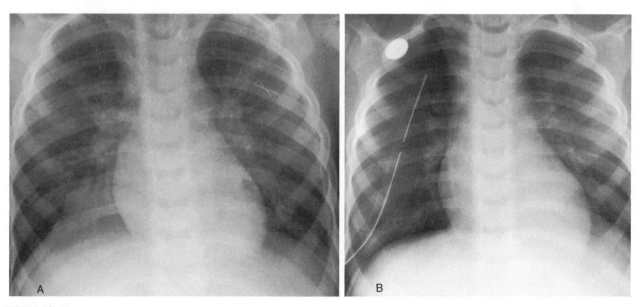

FIGURE 17–11

After being injured in an automobile accident, a 12-year-old boy complained of right-sided upper abdominal pain. *A,* This chest roentgenogram reveals abnormal elevation of the right hemidiaphragm. *B,* Following repair of the diaphragm, the chest roentgenogram reveals the right hemidiaphragm to be normal.

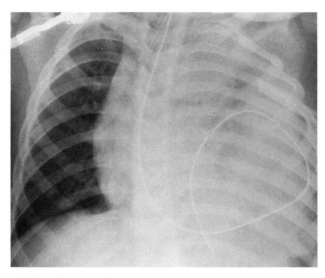

FIGURE 17–12

A nasogastric tube can be seen coiled in the left chest of this 7-year-old boy who was struck by an automobile. The diaphragm was ruptured. The tear extended superiorly and avulsed the phrenic nerve from the pericardium. The boy's recovery was uneventful.

1. An archlike shadow suggesting elevation of the hemidiaphragm (Fig. 17–11A and B)
2. The appearance of obstruction or irregularity of the hemidiaphragm
3. Extraneous shadows above the diaphragm
4. Atelectasis adjacent to the archlike shadow
5. Pleural fluid
6. Air and fluid levels within the hemithorax
7. Mediastinal shift to the contralateral side

A nasogastric tube passed in the stomach may be seen above the expected level of the diaphragm (Fig. 17–12). Water soluble contrast material injected into the stomach can confirm the presence of the stomach in the chest.

All injuries to the diaphragm are managed surgically, and complete preoperative resuscitation is important and usually possible. If cardiovascular collapse occurs, immediate surgery is indicated. The approach to the diaphragmatic rupture must be individualized. The patient with a massive right-sided hemothorax and ongoing bleeding may best be approached through a right thoracotomy. With obvious abdominal distention and ongoing hemorrhage, an abdominal approach might be advocated. For right-sided injuries, an abdominal incision can always be extended into the right chest or into a median sternotomy if the inferior vena cava or hepatic veins are injured. The abdominal approach is preferred for left-sided injuries because the incidence of associated intra-abdominal injury is high. A separate thoracotomy incision can be made to address an intrathoracic injury, or the incision may be extended into the chest. In an autopsy series, Estrera and colleagues reported 16 diaphragmatic ruptures in 307 people who died from thoracoabdominal trauma in a 2-year period. Fifteen of the 16 had an associated thoracic aortic injury.[3] This injury should not be overlooked in the pediatric age group.

Penetrating injuries to the diaphragm occur with gunshot wounds, stab wounds, and wounds from other missiles or instruments. The external landmarks of the diaphragm are crucial in identifying whether the diaphragm could have been injured in any penetrating injury. The resting diaphragm is located at the level of the anterior fourth intercostal space. Any wound around the nipple could involve the diaphragm as it moves up and down with respiration. Any penetrating injury below this level posteriorly could also involve the diaphragm (Fig. 17–13).

At surgery, the abdomen is thoroughly explored to identify any other injuries. The diaphragmatic edges are débrided and the diaphragm sutured with nonabsorbable suture. At Children's Memorial Hospital Dacron pledgets are used to bolster the sutures if there is no associated gastrointestinal injury. Any of the prosthetic materials are acceptable to close the defect. Marlex mesh, proline mesh, and Gore-Tex surgical membrane have been used to close diaphragmatic defects. A large chest tube is placed in the ipsilateral chest to drain blood and serum in the postoperative period.

The early and late mortality associated with diaphragmatic rupture is directly related to the major associated injuries and the acute cardiovascular collapse than can occur with mediastinal shift. Hood reported a mortality of 18% in his series of 429 patients with diaphragmatic rupture.[6] Wiencek and associates reported the highest mortality rates with blunt diaphragmatic injury (27%) and with gunshot wounds (18%).[14]

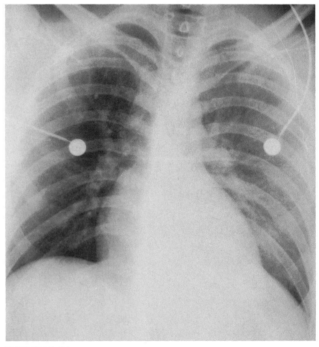

FIGURE 17–13

This seemingly normal chest roentgenogram was obtained because a young man was stabbed in the left chest. At surgery a lacerated diaphragm, spleen, and stomach were repaired. Minimal fluid was found in the chest.

CONCLUSION

Thoracic injury is relatively uncommon in children, and the majority of such injuries are primarily due to blunt trauma. Iatrogenic thoracic injuries are increasing in incidence as modern technology improves our ability to care for the most seriously ill infants and children. Associated injuries are usually responsible for the mortality and morbidity in the multiply injured child with thoracic injury. Thoracic injury must be suspected in any child with multiple injuries, and immediate assessment and management are often life saving.

References

1. Eichelberger MR: Trauma of the airway and thorax. Pediatr Ann 16(4):307–316, 1987.
2. Eichelberger MR, Randolph JG: Thoracic trauma in children. Surg Clin North Am 61(5):1181–1197, 1981.
3. Estrera AS, Landay MJ, McClelland RN: Blunt traumatic rupture of the right hemidiaphragm: Experience in 12 patients. Ann Thorac Surg 39(6):525–530, 1985.
4. Hall RT, Rhodes PG: Pneumothorax and pneumomediastinum in infants with idiopathic respiratory distress syndrome receiving continuous positive airway pressure. Pediatrics 55(4):493–496, 1975.
5. Haller JA, Donahoo JS: Traumatic asphyxia in children: Pathophysiology and management. J Trauma 11(6):453–457, 1971.
6. Hood RM: Traumatic diaphragmatic hernia. Ann Thorac Surg 12:311, 1971.
7. Kelly JP, Webb WR, Moulder PV, et al: Management of airway trauma I: Tracheobronchial injuries. Ann Thorac Surg 40(6):551–555, 1985.
8. Landercasper J, Cogbill TH: Long-term follow-up after traumatic asphyxia. J Trauma 25(9):838–841, 1985.
9. Mayer T, Matlak M, Johnson D, et al: The modified injury severity scale in pediatric multiple trauma patients. J Pediatr Surg 15:719, 1980.
10. Orringer MB, Kirsh MM: Traumatic rupture of the diaphragm. In: Kirsh MM, Sloan H (eds): Blunt Chest Trauma. Boston, Little, Brown & Co, 1977, pp 129–141.
11. Pediatric Trauma Registry, National Institute of Disability and Rehabilitation. Personal communication.
12. Shepherd RL, Raffensperger JG, Goldstein R: Pediatric esophageal perforation. J Thorac Cardiovasc Surg 74(2):261–267, 1977.
13. Welch KJ: Thoracic injuries. In: Randolph JG, et al (eds): The Injured Child. Chicago; Year Book Medical Publishers, 1979, pp 215–231.
14. Wiencek RG, Wilson RF, Steiger Z: Acute injuries of the diaphragm. J Thorac Cardiovasc Surg 92:989–993, 1986.

Shauna R. Roberts
Thomas M. Holder
Keith W. Ashcraft

CHAPTER EIGHTEEN

Cardiac and Major Thoracic Vascular Injuries

HISTORY

Perhaps the earliest case of blunt cardiac injury was reported by Akenside in 1763. A 14-year-old waiter was carrying a plate when he was struck by his master, forcing the plate between his ribs. He became ill immediately and died from his injury 6 months later. Autopsy showed left ventricular transmural necrosis.[74] In 1897, Rehn reported the first successful suture closure of a cardiac wound.[43] In a more modern era, 1943, Blalock and Ravitch recommended pericardiocentesis as definitive therapy for pericardial tamponade.[83] Essentially, most other advances in the care of cardiac and great vessel injuries came after the discovery and refinement of extracorporeal circulation.[43]

CHILDREN ARE DIFFERENT

Cardiac and great vessel injuries are life threatening and require expedient assessment and accurate therapy. Although these injuries occur less frequently in children than in adults, probably because the vessels are more pliable, adults and children suffer the same types of thoracic trauma. The physiology of young children is distinctly different, however, and does not begin to parallel adult physiology until after the age of 13.[74, 83, 101]

Although children are resilient, they are also physiologically labile in that they make much higher metabolic demands on the cardiovascular system and have less respiratory reserve, a more easily obstructed airway system, weaker thoracic musculature, and greater instability of temperature maintenance.[33, 37, 39, 110] Their metabolism and relatively greater body surface area require more fluid per kilogram of body weight.[33]

Injured children should be cared for in an organized manner by a team experienced in pediatric trauma. One person, preferably a pediatric surgeon, should have the primary responsibility for directing the assessment and subsequent management of the injured child to contain and minimize morbidity and mortality.[17, 38, 39, 50, 58, 71] The experienced team with adequate facilities usually achieves the best result for the child with significant thoracic trauma.[39] Although most patients with major cardiovascular injuries die before reaching the hospital, most such pediatric deaths *in hospital* resulting from thoracic trauma are preventable.[38, 87] Elapsed time from injury to hospital care is a major factor in survival.[45, 83]

The ABC's (airway, breathing, circulation) of general trauma care should be instituted promptly on arrival of the child in the emergency department.[101] Airway management may be complicated by aspiration of a foreign body (e.g., gum, candy, or teeth) as well as by emesis, particularly in the child with a head injury.[9, 38, 39, 50] Tracheal deviation may indicate pneumothorax or large hemothorax.[9] Other aspects of the initial evaluation may be made more difficult by the restless or struggling child, particularly the child with shock or head injury.[45, 83, 95]

Clues to cardiac injury present on physical examination may include a bruised precordium, upper body cyanosis, or unexplained hypotension. Dysrhythmias may also be present. Hemopericardium with tamponade, massive or recurrent hemothorax, or pneumopericardium should raise suspicion of major cardiovascular injury.[53] There may be a difference in systolic blood pressure between arms, but patients may also have good pulses despite major arterial injury.[1, 7] Also physical evidence may be absent despite significant vascular injury.[28]

Children have a compliant thorax that transfers kinetic energy to the intrathoracic structure.[60, 74, 93, 101] This energy is somewhat dissipated when the ribs or sternum is fractured.[33, 60] Although fracture of the first and second ribs is often associated with mediastinal injury, high mortality has been reported in children with no thoracic fractures (ribs, sternum).[5, 18, 47, 49, 74] The subtlety of rib fractures in children may decrease the frequency of their recognition.[93] Hence, it is important to remember that there may be no external marks, no thoracic fractures, and few signs or symptoms in children with heart and great vessel injuries due to blunt trauma.[5, 26, 33, 37, 39, 49, 57, 65, 101] A high index of suspicion must be maintained.[33]

Continuous electrocardiogram (ECG) and frequent blood gas determinations are mandatory in any patient with possible serious thoracic injury.[5, 58] Early chest radiographs may be normal despite major mediastinal injury, and therefore repeated roentgenograms should be done, although 92% of patients with aortic disruption have a wide mediastinum on initial chest radiograph.[12, 58]

In small children, a percutaneously placed subclavian central venous line should be used judiciously for massive fluid resuscitation because of the possibility of misplacement, which may produce pneumothorax or free fluid extravasation into the chest.[33, 38, 50] However, in adolescents and older patients, subclavian venous central lines offer less risk and can be very beneficial.[65] It is important to recognize that the central venous pressure (CVP) will be falsely elevated when the patient is straining, shivering, or crying or has abdominal guarding because of peritoneal irritation.[100] In addition, the CVP may be falsely *low* in the presence of tamponade if the patient is profoundly hypovolemic. An abnormally elevated CVP may be appreciated only after volume resuscitation.[10, 83]

Multiple injuries are five times more common in blunt trauma than in penetrating trauma.[92, 93] Thoracic trauma in children is usually associated with other injuries, particularly head injuries.[12, 26, 33, 37–39, 49, 58, 59, 65, 83, 92, 93, 98] This may be due to the greater head-to-body size and weight ratio and the high center of gravity in the small child.[9, 33] Overall, the mortality rate in pediatric trauma patients seems to be more related to the presence or absence of head injuries than to the number of systems involved.[17, 50, 91] The presence of multiple injuries, however, is probably responsible for the longer hospital stay in children who have sustained blunt cardiac injuries rather than penetrating ones.[65]

Thoracic trauma accounts for 25% of deaths due to trauma in adults, but these data are less specific in children.[26, 47] Velcek's autopsy series reported that of those children who died before treatment, 27.7% had thoracic injuries. Overall, cardiovascular trauma is more common than appreciated, but the exact incidence of nonpenetrating injury is unknown.[87, 109] Blunt injuries are more common in young children, most of whom are struck by a vehicle.[4, 33, 37–39, 58] Penetrating injuries are more common in urban settings, especially in adolescents.[65, 92]

Previously corrected disorders may complicate trauma in children.[17, 33, 66, 110] In one such instance, a 7-year-old boy who had undergone closure of an ostium primum atrial septal defect developed an aortoatrial fistula after blunt chest trauma; the fixation from scar tissue was thought to have contributed to the tissue avulsion.[87] Lasky and colleagues reported on the case of a 21-year-old man who, many years after the repair of a tetralogy of Fallot, sustained lacerations of the atrial and ventricular septa, a lacerated aorta, and a tamponade. Again, scar tissue was thought to contribute to the injury.[57]

BLUNT CARDIAC INJURIES

Occupants of a car collision at 60 miles per hour sustain a force of 120 G. Ejected passengers may receive up to 10 times that force on impact.[27] In animal studies, the type and severity of cardiac and great vessel injury sustained was related to the degree of force.[57] When either impact velocity or thoracic compression is increased, the severity of cardiac and great vessel injuries increases.[103]

Three types of physiologic disturbances with major blunt cardiac injuries occurs, tamponade being the most common.[83] Seventy percent of patients with cardiac rupture present with tamponade.[31] Thirty percent of patients with cardiac rupture also have pericardial rupture and exsanguinate into the thorax rather than develop tamponade. The third physiologic disturbance is cardiac failure. This may occur because of contusion, concussion, direct conduction system injury, or coronary artery injury.[83]

Pericardial Tamponade

Pathophysiology

Although pericardial tamponade is not an isolated "injury," its importance as a pathophysiologic event in chest injury cannot be overemphasized. The pericardium is made up of a serosal layer and a fibrous layer. The serosal layer is contiguous with the epicardium at the great vessels, which covers the heart and intrapericardial great vessels. The pericardial cavity is a potential space with the two layers in contact. Some fluid is normally present, but this potential space can accommodate *large* volumes of fluid if it is accumulated over time. In emergency situations, bleeding or accumulation of fluid causes the intrapericardial pressure to rise rapidly as volume is increased and cardiac tamponade occurs.[10, 36, 83]

Tamponade occurs because the pericardium lacks elasticity. Rapid accumulation of pericardial fluid increases ventricular end-diastolic pressure, which restricts and can ultimately prevent cardiac filling. If the ventricle does not fill completely, the stroke volume, cardiac output, and blood pressure decrease.[19, 30, 36, 71, 83] Compensatory tachycardia is a physiologic attempt to maintain cardiac output. Atrial filling is also decreased, resulting in elevation of the CVP. However, if the patient is hypovolemic, the venous pressure may not be elevated until volume is restored.[10] Coronary arterial flow, which occurs during diastole, is also reduced

by the tamponade, further depressing myocardial function.[71] Progressive subendocardial ischemia occurs, and diminished tissue perfusion and acidosis further depress myocardial contractility.[10, 68] The child has a small pericardial volume, and relatively little hemorrhage is needed to cause tamponade.[33]

Pericardial tamponade occurs most frequently with penetrating injury in adults, whereas blunt injury is the most frequent mechanism in children.[10, 11, 50, 87] Tamponade following blunt chest injury usually is caused by chamber rupture or coronary artery laceration.[53, 59] It may also be secondary to great vessel or pericardial bleeding.[45] Cardiopulmonary resuscitation, dissecting aortic disease (e.g., Marfan syndrome), and bleeding diathesis may be complicated by tamponade.[10, 79] Even when the pericardium is lacerated, it frequently seals so that decompression into the mediastinum or pleura does not occur.[10, 79] Although it can be lethal, a tamponade may also allow temporary stabilization and time for the patient to receive help.[71] Therefore, time is a critical factor in survival.[60, 68, 83, 87]

Diagnosis

Other injuries may mask tamponade as a source for decreased blood pressure.[31] Beck's triad (muffled heart sounds, hypotension, and elevated venous pressure) is unreliable and may be difficult to appreciate in the turmoil of the emergency department setting.[10, 31, 33, 53, 100, 108] Only one third of patients have all three components.[10, 37] Neck vein distention is notoriously difficult to evaluate in small children. However, cyanosis of the upper half of the body is a frequent finding in tamponade, particularly when it is secondary to atrial rupture.[53, 59]

Tamponade should be suspected when shock is out of proportion to blood loss, and differential diagnosis should include tension pneumothorax, massive hemothorax, and right ventricular failure from contusion.[53, 71, 87] Tension pneumothorax also produces decreased breath sounds, tympany on percussion, and tracheal deviation in addition to CVP elevation and decreased blood pressure.[10] Hemothorax may produce dullness to percussion and trachea deviation. Acute right heart failure is accompanied by an elevation in the CVP. Chest roentgenogram findings help differentiate tamponade from these other entities but usually do not establish the diagnosis of tamponade.[10, 18, 31, 87, 100] The cardiac silhouette often does not change acutely, although this sign of tamponade has been reported frequently in children with tamponade.[72, 79, 100] The younger, more flexible mediastinum may be responsible for this fact. Echocardiography is an excellent diagnostic tool if patient stability allows time for the examination.[9–11, 14] Electrocardiogram results *may* show S-T and T wave changes as well as low voltage but may not be helpful at all.[10, 71, 100]

Diagnostic Pericardiocentesis

When pericardial tamponade is suspected in the hypotensive patient, a pericardiocentesis should be performed.[10] The surgeon must be aware that the pericardiocentesis needle may injure any organ it touches. For example, pneumothorax, pericardial laceration, myocardial laceration, or coronary artery laceration may occur during the process of pericardiocentesis.[10, 31, 63, 80] As a diagnostic tool, pericardiocentesis has a false negative rate of 20 to 40%.[10, 31, 53] In a collected series, 96% of patients with cardiac stab wounds had a hemopericardium: in 41% of patients, the blood was clotted; in 19% it was liquid; in the remainder, the results were mixed.[72, 108] The assessment of clotting after pericardiocentesis is inconsistent.[10, 31, 53, 83, 100] False positive results may occur when blood is aspirated from the cardiac chambers.[100] Pericardiocentesis can be used as a diagnostic tool or as a temporizing measure only in the dying patient.[10, 14, 30, 33, 36, 37, 59, 75, 87] Emergency therapeutic pericardiocentesis has been shown to decrease the mortality of tamponade from 25 to 11%, hence playing a vital role.[10, 16, 68, 83]

Pericardiocentesis should be performed utilizing aseptic technique. A 15-gauge needle should be inserted just below the xiphoid process at a 45-degree angle from the skin and directed 45 degrees toward the right shoulder.[9, 53] Aspirating 15 to 35 ml of fluid may improve the patient's hemodynamic status markedly.[53]

Definitive Therapy

Alcohol, various anesthetic agents, and positive pressure ventilation decrease tolerance to tamponade.[83] Rapid deterioration during induction of anesthesia is common. If possible, in situations in which cardiac tamponade is strongly suspected, the patient should be prepared and draped in the operating room and pericardiocentesis or a pericardial window performed under local anesthesia before induction; the patient should be allowed to breathe spontaneously, if possible, until the pericardium is open.[10, 11, 53, 71, 80]

In a series of 459 patients with cardiac wounds, 43% of the patients who had pericardiocentesis as a definitive treatment died, whereas only 16% of those operated on died.[10] Pericardiocentesis is no longer an accepted definitive treatment for pericardial tamponade.[10, 26, 37, 80, 87] Small pericardial and myocardial wounds (e.g., from ice picks) might be treated successfully with pericardiocentesis, but delayed hemorrhage may occur hours or more later.[71, 83, 84] The mortality in patients treated with pericardiocentesis is usually secondary to recurrent tamponade.[83]

Emergency department subxyphoid pericardial window may relieve a tamponade so efficiently that it may allow the patient to exsanguinate before transfer to the operating room is possible. However, if pericardiocentesis is unsuccessful, the diagnosis of tamponade is still suspected; if the patient still has a discernible pulse, a pericardial window should be created.[31, 53, 83, 100] If blood pressure and pulse are no longer present, an emergency thoracotomy should be performed.[53] The definitive therapy of cardiac tamponade requires pericardial exploration and control of the source of bleeding.

Late Sequelae of Tamponade

Pericardial hemorrhage is probably more common following blunt injury than is appreciated because of the number of cases of pericardial defects and pericarditis discovered months to years later.[10, 53, 54] A small pericardial hemorrhage that is hemodynamically insignificant may produce con-

strictive pericarditis.[63, 75] Such a small hemopericardium may be undetected initially or may even develop a few weeks after injury, possibly secondary to venous bleeding. Patients with significant blunt chest trauma should probably be followed with weekly chest roentgenogram and echocardiogram for at least 3 weeks.[53]

Hemopericardium may also be followed by acute pericarditis or postpericardiotomy syndrome.[53, 74] Although this syndrome is probably multifactorial, it is believed to occur secondary to an inflammatory response caused by blood in the pericardium.[53, 83]

With severe blunt thoracic injuries, the diaphragmatic or pleuropericardium may be disrupted. Although this is usually associated with other cardiac injuries, it may not be recognized acutely. Visceral herniation from the abdomen into the pericardium may occur. The heart may herniate into the pleura and may be associated with ECG position changes and cardiomegaly by chest radiograph. This disruption may be asymptomatic and is sometimes associated with sudden death. Both injuries should be repaired when recognized.[53, 54, 109]

CASE

A 17-year-old white male was kicked by a horse near the xiphoid process. Seen at a community hospital, he was noted to have a hemoglobin of 5 grams. Despite resuscitative efforts he deteriorated, and on arrival the patient was in profound shock. His abdomen was distended, and because of the low hemoglobin, emergency midline celiotomy was performed. Marked gastric distention was present, but no other abnormality was identified in the abdomen. The pericardium, however, was tense. The diaphragmatic surface of the pericardium was incised, releasing a large amount of blood. The patient improved rapidly. The wound was extended as a sternotomy to proceed with definitive treatment. Except for a mild myocardial contusion, no other injury could be identified. The bleeding probably originated from a small lacerated pericardial vessel. Tamponade of this nature is unusual. Definitive surgical therapy must follow release of tamponade.

Pneumopericardium

Pneumopericardium is usually seen in the presence of pneumothorax or pneumomediastinum.[10] Air from alveolar or bronchial rupture is thought to track along the pulmonary vessels with that of tamponade. Chest radiograph is diagnostic. The only clinical differentiation that might be helpful is bruit de moulin. These splashing heart sounds were described by Bricheteau, and air and fluid must both be present in the pericardium to induce this auscultory phenomenon.[35] Air tamponade is a rare and sometimes fatal complication of blunt chest trauma.[26]

Hemothorax

Any collection of blood in the pleural cavity constitutes a hemothorax. In one series of great vessel injuries, hemothorax was discernible in 35% of cases.[28] Massive hemothorax in children is more likely to result from penetrating injuries than from blunt injuries, but ruptured pulmonary parenchyma, heart, or great vessels may occur with blunt injury.[37, 53, 74] More frequently in children, a fractured rib lacerates the lung, internal mammary artery, or intercostal artery.[4, 74] Rarely, a fractured rib may also cause great vessel laceration.[38] Overall, significant hemothorax in children is usually secondary to intercostal artery laceration, and bleeding is self-limited.[26, 74] In only 15 to 25% of patients is the source of hemorrhage from the heart, lungs, pericardium, or great vessels, but the mortality from massive hemothorax is 50 to 75%.[53, 59]

Children do not tolerate hemothorax or hemopneumothorax because of mediastinal mobility.[101] Large amounts of blood may compress the ipsilateral lung, the mediastinum, and ultimately the contralateral lung, resulting in severe respiratory distress.[37, 50, 74] Thirty to 40% of a patient's blood volume can quickly collect in the pleural space.[19] Hemorrhage from systemic vessels is more likely to be life threatening than is bleeding from pulmonary vessels.[18, 50, 59] Blood that has been in the pleural cavity may not clot because it has clotted once and subsequently lysed, but this result is not consistent.[74, 110]

When hemothorax is present, a proportionately large chest tube should be placed, utilizing aseptic technique, to remove blood from the pleural cavity, re-expand the lung, and assess blood loss.[37, 50, 53, 58, 74, 100, 110] Inadvertent lung injury from chest tube placement occurs in up to 25% of children, so this procedure should be performed carefully by an experienced surgeon.[26]

In a series of 51 children with crushing chest injuries, two patients required thoracotomy for ongoing bleeding, one had lacerated intercostal vessels, and the other a subclavian artery injury.[58] In another series of 68 children with both blunt and penetrating injuries, 14 patients had hemopneumothorax.[65] No patients had sustained rib fractures, 21 patients required chest tube placement, and four patients underwent thoracotomy for bleeding; one patient had a negative thoracotomy, one patient had intercostal artery bleeding, one patient had a right upper lobectomy for persistent air leak, and one patient had a gunshot wound to the subclavian artery and vein. Thoracotomy should be performed for exsanguinating or persistent bleeding, uncontrolled shock, and suspected mediastinal injury.[38, 50, 53, 65, 74, 100]

Children with obvious rib fractures should be observed carefully because delayed hemothorax or pneumothorax may occur up to 48 hours after the injury.[65]

Cardiac Concussion

Cardiac concussion may follow blunt chest injury and is a "physiologic" abnormality. Grossly, no contusion or coronary artery thrombosis is identifiable, and histology shows no evidence of cell death.[77, 94] The patient may have a variety of arrhythmias, including immediate refractory ventricular fibrillation.[77, 98, 105, 109] Windsor reported a 17-year-old male who was hit in the chest with a cricket ball and developed ventricular fibrillation that was not reversible.[109] In addition, low cardiac output may be present without arrhythmias. Concussion arrhythmias may be associated

with complete recovery or with death by cardiogenic shock.[33, 53]

Animal studies have documented that sudden death with blunt chest injury can occur from intractable *apnea* without initial arrhythmias, pump failure, or gross cardiac lesion.[103]

Supportive care including antiarrhythmic agents, pressors, pacemaker, or intra-aortic balloon pump should be utilized as indicated.[53]

Echocardiography should be part of the evaluation of suspected cardiac concussion. Coronary angiography may be necessary to rule out coronary laceration or thrombosis in the patient with unclear clinical presentation.[94]

Cardiac Contusion

Cardiac contusion is an increasingly recognized entity but still a frequently missed diagnosis.[53, 65, 74, 109] Motor vehicle and motorcycle accidents account for most heart and great vessel injuries in children.[74] This injury is more common in adolescents than in young children and most commonly follows steering wheel injury, as in the adult.[37, 53, 59] It is believed that 15% of fatal chest injuries in all ages are secondary to contusion, with subendocardial hemorrhage in 90% and moderate chest trauma in 50%.[54] Series analyzing only pediatric trauma report the incidence of myocardial contusion to occur in from 0.4 to 30.0% of blunt chest injuries.[17, 33, 47, 49] Seemingly trivial injuries can produce cardiac contusion in children.[33] Myocardial contusion may occur as a result of being kicked by an animal or hit with a fist, club, or ball.[53] Also, the forward-facing infant car seat with a supporting bar across the front has been associated with myocardial contusion.[33] Falls from great heights, upper abdominal trauma, and blast injuries have also been reported to produce myocardial contusion with considerable frequency.[53]

Pathology

The contusion may vary from a small, superficial ecchymosis to extensive transmural and septal hemorrhage.[53, 98, 109] Coronary artery injury secondary to contusion is rare.[94] The transition from normal to injured tissue is abrupt.[53, 94] Myocardial contusion may be complicated by the same factors as a myocardial infarction, and differentiation at a later date between contusion and infarction may be difficult.[53, 54]

Pathophysiology

Arrhythmias may occur because of local hypoxia, reentry patterns from electrical gradients in the transition zone, direct conduction system injury, or activation by myocardial stretching and hemorrhage.[30, 53, 60, 74] The presence of arrhythmias and conduction abnormalities correlate to some degree with the severity of injury.[60]

Late sequelae of myocardial contusion consist of pericarditis, cardiac rupture, ventricular septal defect, aneurysm, calcification, and emboli.[53, 54, 94, 98, 104, 109] Some degree of pericarditis after blunt cardiac injury almost always occurs and may become chronic or constrictive.[60]

Cardiac output is depressed by 30 to 50% in myocardial contusion; hence, the response to stress is somewhat blunted.[33, 53, 59, 94, 98, 109] Small amounts of alcohol in the blood may enhance the effect of contusion by decreasing ventricular arrhythmias.[53]

Diagnosis

Pain analogous to angina is present in approximately 70% of patients.[53, 54, 59, 60, 109] Tachycardia is the most common sign.[53, 59] The ECG is an important screening tool and is abnormal in up to 56% of cases when subtle conduction delays and tachycardia are included as abnormalities.[74, 98] The ECG changes may not appear for 72 hours and usually consist of ST-T wave changes consistent with pericarditis and infarction.

Enzyme changes may or may not be present or may be delayed.[53, 59, 60, 78, 94, 105, 109] Autopsy studies have confirmed significant contusion in the presence of normal enzymes.[98] Tellez and colleagues reported the diagnosis of contusion by enzyme in 7.7%, by ECG in 20%, and by echocardiography in 34%. Enzyme elevations do not correlate with the severity of the injury.[98] Generally, no patients with normal enzyme levels and normal ECGs had clinically significant cardiac contusions.[94] False elevations of enzymes can be seen in crush injuries, tachyarrhythmias, muscle disease, gas gangrene, Reye syndrome, idiopathic myoglobulinemia, Rocky Mountain spotted fever, and tongue trauma.[94, 98]

Myocardial scintiscans may be helpful in the diagnosis of myocardial contusion. If they produce positive results, they can be a good assessment of severity of injury.[94] Echocardiography allows estimation of the ejection fraction and wall motion, identification of intracardiac anatomy, and easy repetition for follow up. An ejection fraction of less than 50% is compatible with significant contusion and was seen in 34% of children in one study.[98]

Therapeutic Measures

Patients with blunt chest trauma should be monitored carefully because of the risk of significant arrhythmias.[53, 94, 98] Prophylactic lidocaine, however, is unnecessary and may or may not be useful in patients needing urgent surgical intervention.[53, 94] Necessary operations should not be postponed because of myocardial contusion.[94]

Nitroglycerin is of no value in the therapy of myocardial contusion.[53, 54, 60] Anticoagulation medication is contraindicated because of potential hemorrhagic extension.[53, 105] Appropriate therapy for arrhythmias is necessary and indicated.[53, 98] The therapy for myocardial contusion should be the same as for myocardial infarction.[37, 59, 60, 74, 87]

Patients with myocardial contusion should be followed closely for late myocardial dysfunction.[65] What Burchell said in 1954 is still true: "always, with a heart contusion, arise both doubt and much confusion."[109]

Death may occur immediately or years later as a result of blunt cardiac injury. Late deaths are usually secondary to delayed rupture of the ventricular septum, ventricular aneurysm, or ventricular pseudoaneurysm.[53]

CASE

A 9-year-old white boy fell off a tractor on an incline in heavy snow. The rear tire ran over his chest. He was taken to the local medical facility and subsequently was transferred to a regional hospital intensive care unit, where he was given bolus doses of lidocaine for frequent premature ventricular contractions, and a lidocaine drip was started after a six-beat run of ventricular tachycardia. He was then transferred to our facility.

Creatine phosphokinase levels were elevated at 1260 and 1660 with MB fractions of 8.25% and 5.1%. Serum glutamic-oxaloacetic transaminase (SGOT) and lactate dehydrogenase levels were also elevated. The chest radiograph (Fig. 18–1) revealed a pulmonary contusion, a widened mediastinum, and an apical fluid cap on the left. The ECG showed lateral wall injury with ST elevation and Q waves in V5 and V6 as well as reciprocal ST depression in V2 (Fig. 18–2). The echocardiogram showed dyskinesis of the inferior ventricular segment. An aortogram was performed because of mediastinal widening on the chest radiograph. The aorta and coronary arteries were normal.

The patient was treated as though he had a myocardial infarction. He was discharged 14 days after the injury and has done well.

Chamber Disruption

Mechanism of Injury

Animal studies have demonstrated that cardiac rupture is not caused by displacement only but by a combination of

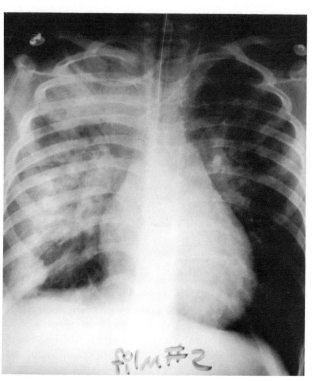

FIGURE 18–1

Cardiac contusion. The pulmonary contusion and widened mediastinum are evidence of significant injury. The vascular congestion seen correlates with decreased myocardial function, as documented by an echocardiogram.

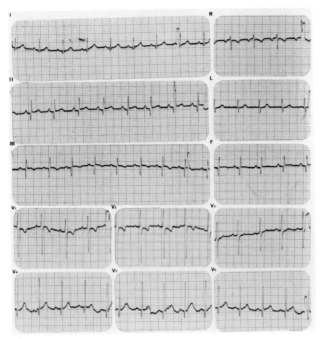

FIGURE 18–2

The subtle changes resulting from cardiac contusion. The electrocardiogram shows q waves in V5 and V6. The ST elevation in V5 and V6 and the reciprocal ST depression in V2 are consistent with lateral wall injury.

velocity and compression. Impacts of this nature may increase aortic blood pressure to levels of 400 to 800 mm Hg. Anterior cardiac compression displaces tissue and blood to create rapid lateral acceleration and potential chamber rupture.[103] Six mechanisms of lethal cardiac disruption injuries have been described.

1. Direct anterior chest wall blow during maximum filling of the heart[31] (e.g., a 20-year-old man who died of left ventricular rupture during a football game[77]).
2. Indirect extremity or abdominal crush, or both, that increases blood pressure and causes cardiac rupture without chest trauma.[31]
3. Compression of the heart between the sternum and the vertebral bodies, especially likely in children.[31, 103]
4. Acceleration-deceleration injury in which the atria tear at venous insertion sites. Twenty percent of patients with such injuries also have aortic rupture.[31]
5. Blast injury causing septal or ventricular rupture.[31]
6. Sternum or rib fracture with penetration of the heart by bone.[31]

Chamber rupture is commonly encountered at autopsy[31, 47, 59, 75, 109] and is responsible for death in 10 to 17% of motor vehicle accident victims. A significant number of these victims also have great vessel disruption. Ventricular rupture occurs twice as often as atrial rupture and is almost always immediately fatal.[75] The ventricle is most vulnerable to rupture at the thinner apical area, and both atria and ventricles are most susceptible to rupture when the chamber is maximally distended and the valves are closed.[31, 53] Chamber rupture reported in clinical series suggests that

atrial rupture is more common than ventricular, probably because the longer survival of live patients with atrial rupture accounts for the disparity between clinical and autopsy series.[31, 33, 36, 87] Patients with atrial rupture frequently survive *long* enough to reach treatment because an atrial tear may seal before tamponade.[31, 53, 87]

Less force is necessary to cause myocardial rupture in children because of the pliability of the thorax. This was unfortunately demonstrated in the report of a 4-year-old boy who sustained atrial rupture and tamponade from overzealous cardiopulmonary resuscitation administered by his father.[79]

Diagnosis

The diagnosis of cardiac rupture should be suspected when hypotension or hypovolemia seems out of proportion to the injury or is unresponsive to treatment. There may also be ongoing acidosis after apparently adequate resuscitation.[31, 53] Upper body cyanosis often occurs with cardiac rupture. The exact mechanism for this is not known but may be analogous to traumatic asphyxia.[53]

Treatment of Chamber Rupture

Successful therapy for a ruptured cardiac chamber requires prompt diagnosis and operation. Only patients who come to operation for definitive repair within the first 2 hours after injury survive.[87] Blunt or penetrating injuries may destroy cardiovascular anatomy so extensively that cardiopulmonary bypass is necessary to facilitate repair.[74, 83] Heparinization required for bypass utilization is extremely hazardous in these traumatized patients, and anticoagulation in the presence of a contused lung may be fatal.[33, 87, 109] Intracranial hemorrhage is also a risk, as these patients often have associated head injuries. Fortunately, bypass is rarely needed.[31, 59, 74, 100]

If uncontrolled hemorrhage is encountered, caval occlusion or induced cardiac fibrillation may be necessary. Fibrillation the heart and associated brain ischemia is tolerated for 4 to 10 minutes in the adult patient who has not been in shock.[53, 83, 87] Suture repair usually takes 2 to 3 minutes.[53]

Atrial lacerations may be repaired with a pursestring suture, but pledgets may be needed. Ventricular laceration should be closed with mattress sutures. If a large defect is present, Teflon strip pledgets should be incorporated into the mattress closure. A second continuous suture should be utilized for reinforcement. A prosthetic patch can be used if the defect cannot be closed by direct suture.[53] Care must be taken, however, to avoid inclusion of a main coronary artery if at all possible.

Coronary Artery Injury

Coronary artery injury occurred in 10 out of 546 (2%) blunt cardiac injuries reported by Parmley and colleagues, and all were fatal.[75] The eight patients with associated heart and aortic rupture died immediately, and the other two died of tamponade.[75] Some have survived blunt coronary artery injury, however, and an ECG pattern of myocardial ische- mia or infarction may be seen secondary to thrombosis or disruption.[53] Coronary angiography may be needed to de- fine the abnormality.[87] Although some success has been reported with coronary artery ligation, bypass grafting of the injured artery is preferred.[53] Morbidity is more signifi- cant with more proximal or with left anterior descending coronary artery lesions.[87] All patients with coronary artery injuries should be treated with the same precaution and observation as a patient with myocardial infarction. Seque- lae such as aneurysm may develop.[53]

Valve Injury

Sudden compression of the heart against closed valves can cause laceration or detachment of cusps. The valve injury is usually an extension of a subendocardial laceration and can be associated with severe myocardial disruption.[109] Less than 5% of blunt cardiac injuries are accompanied by valve laceration, and these cases are usually missed.[53, 83] Preexist- ing valvular disease increases the risk of injury.[60]

Untreated valve injury is followed by heart failure, pul- monary edema, and death, except possibly in tricuspid valve injury with regurgitation.[5, 53, 60, 109] Early operation is necessary, but if the patient is tolerating the lesion well, surgical intervention may be delayed for 6 to 8 weeks.[53, 59, 60] Windsor and Shanahan described successful surgical treatment of an isolated mitral valve injury with partial anterior leaflet detachment and ruptured chordae in a 7- year-old boy.[109] However, results of repair of the trauma- tized valve are poor, and valve replacement is usually nec- essary.[60]

The aortic and mitral valves are the most frequently injured valves.[36, 53, 54, 60] Aortic valve injury occurs most commonly as an isolated event and is associated with the worst prognosis.[5, 54, 109] Physical examination is variable: even the murmur can be difficult to appreciate because of low cardiac output.

Pulmonic and tricuspid valve injuries are rare.[54, 60] Pres- entation of tricuspid valve injuries may be delayed owing to lack of symptoms except when there is papillary muscle rupture, which is usually fulminating.[109] Acute tricuspid valve insufficiency is not tolerated as well as chronic leak- age; valve replacement is usually necessary.[53] Any trauma- tized valve may develop late stenosis.[54] Also, any intracar- diac or valvular injury may become a locus of bacterial endocarditis.[54, 70]

Traumatic Ventricular Septal Defect

Mechanism of Injury

Acute septal rupture occurs when the heart is compressed between the sternum and the spine.[5, 53, 88] Peak vulnerability occurs when the ventricles are full and the valves closed.[53, 60, 88] Multiple traumatic ventricular septal defects (VSDs) may occur.[88] The most common location for traumatic sep- tal defect is at the apex.[60, 90] When traumatic VSD occurs acutely, it is usually associated with multiple cardiac inju-

ries or other thoracic injuries.[34, 90, 109] If the defect is large, immediate death may ensue.[88, 90] If the conduction system is involved, arrhythmias will be present.[53, 88] Isolated trau- matic VSD may occur with no external evidence of injury.[55, 88]

Delayed septal defect occurs after contusion of the ven- tricular septum with subsequent liquefaction necrosis.[34, 53, 88] This is one of many important reasons why children with documented contusion and those with seemingly benign chest injury should be followed for at least 2 months after injury.

Diagnosis

Twenty percent of patients with traumatic VSD have no symptoms, but 80% demonstrate symptoms of cardiac fail- ure such as dyspnea and palpitations.[53] Symptoms depend on the size of the defect and the shunt. A systolic thrill at the left sternal border associated with a harsh holosystolic murmur may be present, but low cardiac output may mask physical findings.[5, 34, 53, 60, 72, 88, 90] Diaphoresis, tachycardia, and other stigmas of congestive heart failure appear as decompensation occurs.[5, 88, 90]

The ECG may reveal biventricular hypertrophy, right axis deviation, right bundle branch block, and other con- duction delays or arrhythmias.[5, 53] Echocardiography should be part of the diagnostic evaluation. The chest radiograph may show cardiomegaly and increased pulmonary vascular- ity due to the left to right shunt.[88] This may be difficult to distinguish from a mild pulmonary contusion.

Cardiac catheterization is necessary to establish the di- agnosis. Oxygen saturation increases at the level of the defect, and the degree of pulmonary hypertension and shunting can be evaluated.[16, 53, 60, 88, 90]

Therapy for Traumatic Ventricular Septal Defect

Management of traumatic VSD in the pediatric population has been set forth by several investigators.[5, 25, 34, 53, 60, 81, 88, 90] The patient who is not severely decompensated or who responds favorably to medical management should undergo surgical repair if the defect is still documented 2 to 6 months after the injury. This healing period not only allows some traumatic VSDs to close spontaneously, but also al- lows tissue organization in the area of the injury and makes the repair much safer and simpler.[32, 34, 53, 88] Improved suc- cess with delayed VSD repair is probably also influenced by elimination of the associated injuries as a factor in sur- vival.[53] Instances of apparent successful nonoperative man- agement alone have been reported, but this approach cannot be recommended because of the mortality rate of approxi- mately 50% in patients so managed.[5, 60, 88, 90]

During the observation period between diagnosis and surgical intervention, the patient must be monitored closely for signs of pulmonary hypertension, congestive heat fail- ure, or both. The presence of pulmonary hypertension or worsening heart failure, despite adequate decongestive measures, mandates urgent repair before irreversible changes take place.[5, 53, 90]

Patients who develop severe congestive heart failure, pulmonary hypertension, or both immediately following injury must undergo an emergency operation.[5, 15, 23, 53, 90, 102] These hemodynamically unstable patients have a higher operative mortality rate than those who have delayed, elective VSD repair.[67] The morbidity and mortality rates for surgical repair in delayed posttraumatic VSD are quite low but depend on the degree of disruption of cardiac anatomy and the severity of associated injuries. Some degree of residual shunt postoperatively is not uncommon, and septal aneurysm has also been reported.[88, 90] Small residual shunts following repair often close spontaneously.[56]

Acute VSD repair may require a left ventriculotomy in the presence of left ventricular transmural necrosis and should be accomplished in a manner analogous to repair of a VSD in association with myocardial infarction.[21, 53, 86] Otherwise, a right ventriculotomy with primary closure or a prosthetic patch and pledgets should be utilized as indicated.[53]

CASE

A 6-year-old white boy was playing under a tree that his father was trimming when a limb, 10 to 12 inches in diameter, fell from a height of 10 feet, striking him on the left chest, head, and abdomen. After mouth-to-mouth resuscitation by the father, the apneic child resumed respirations. Arriving at the emergency department approximately 1 hour after injury, he was combative and hypotensive, with a systolic blood pressure of 50 to 60 mm Hg, a pulse of 120 beats per minute, and a respiratory rate of 40 per minute with retractions. Physical examination revealed swelling and tenderness over the left parietal region, tenderness over the left clavicle, crackling rales bilaterally, and a harsh 3/6 holosystolic murmur at the lower left sternal border. No marks appeared on the chest. Arterial blood gases revealed a pH of 7.16, a PCO_2 of 58, and a PO_2 of 15 mm Hg. Following intubation, a repeat PAO_2 measurement rose to 90. Peritoneal lavage revealed no evidence of intra-abdominal injury; hemoglobin was 11.6, and a computed tomography scan of the head revealed a left parietal skull fracture. He was also found on chest radiograph to have a left pulmonary contusion.

On his arrival in the intensive care unit, blood pressure was 72/54, pulse 158, and respirations 26, and he was cyanotic. He developed bilateral pulmonary consolidation and pleural effusions (Fig. 18–3). Hemodynamic deterioration prompted a pericardial tap, and 10 ml of fluid was withdrawn with no improvement. Blood gases also deteriorated, with a pH of 7.25, a PCO_2 of 40, and a PO_2 of 69. The patient suffered cardiac arrest during echocardiography and died. Autopsy revealed a 4.8 cm disruption of the interventricular septum near the apex of the heart.

Posttraumatic Cardiac Aneurysm and Pseudoaneurysm

Mechanism of Injury

A *pseudoaneurysm* is a pulsating hematoma that communicates with the ventricular cavity.[44, 73] The walls are formed by pericardium or other extracardiac tissue.[53, 73] By definition, the injury is tamponaded by pericardium, which prevents exsanguination.[44] *Ventricular aneurysm* is a process of fibrosis and dilation following injury and muscle

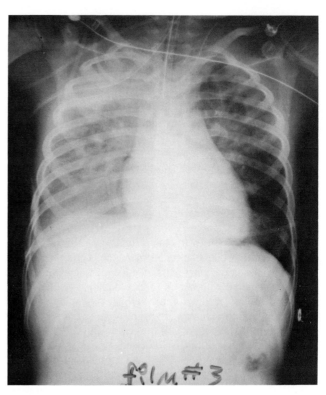

FIGURE 18–3
Traumatic ventricular septal defect. Pulmonary contusion, right pulmonary consolidation-effusion, and vascular congestion are appreciated on this radiograph.

necrosis.[44, 61] Paradoxical systolic motion develops in both true and false aneurysms.[78]

The incidence of development of aneurysm and pseudoaneurysm after cardiac injury is unknown, but these injuries have been reported in children.[34, 44, 73, 78] Posttraumatic aneurysm is thought to occur more frequently than pseudoaneurysm.[44] The number of hours or days necessary for aneurysmal development after injury is unknown.[34] Most of the time, pseudoaneurysm or aneurysm evolves from liquefaction necrosis following blunt trauma.[44, 53, 73, 78] Penetrating injuries may form pseudoaneurysm at the site of the defect. Coronary artery injury increases the risk of aneurysm formation due to infarction.

Diagnosis

The diagnosis should be suspected in children with a history of blunt or penetrating chest trauma.[73] This is usually a delayed manifestation and is another reason why follow up is important, specifically in the patient who has had a hemothorax.[44] Frequently, a systolic murmur is present, and although the ECG may be normal, many patients have conduction delays, blocks, arrhythmias, or changes consistent with an aneurysm.[34, 44, 48, 61, 73, 78] Calcification or globular extension of the left ventricular wall may be appreciated by chest radiograph.[44, 48, 53, 61, 73, 78]

Echocardiography is useful to visualize the paradoxical wall motion of ventricular wall aneurysm.[14] Cardiac catheterization is the preferred diagnostic procedure because it allows visualization of the dyskinesis as well as associated defects and also differentiates aneurysm from pseudoaneurysm that communicates by a narrow neck (usually a centimeter or less) with the ventricular cavity.[34, 44, 48]

The patient may be asymptomatic and the physical examination may be normal if left ventricular dysfunction is minor.[44, 73] At the other end of the spectrum, congestive heart failure and peripheral emboli may occur.[53, 73] Laminated ventricular thrombus has been documented and is probably the source of emboli.[44] In one series of untreated left ventricular aneurysms, nine patients (four of whom were children) died from rupture.[73] The incidence of thromboembolism approaches 50% and is a cause of death in nearly 20% of the cases.[61] Sudden death from arrhythmias or rupture may occur.[53, 73, 75]

Surgical repair should not be performed immediately if the patient is tolerating the defect so that postinjury tissue organization can occur.[34] Immediate operation is necessary in the presence of emboli or heart failure.[61] Elective resection should be performed when ventricular aneurysm or pseudoaneurysm is identified because of the lethal nature of this entity.[44, 48, 53, 61, 73, 78]

PENETRATING CARDIAC INJURIES

Mechanism of Injury and Etiology

Penetrating cardiac injuries are rare in children but appear to be increasing in frequency.[16, 18, 33, 37, 45, 49, 59, 64, 68, 72, 74, 83, 84, 91, 92, 108] The true incidence of penetrating cardiac trauma is unknown.[83] In 1900, needles were the most common wounding agent in cardiac injuries. Knives and guns are now more common.[76] Death from a penetrating wound of the heart is most commonly caused by hemorrhage, which produces tamponade.[70, 76, 83] Rarely, coronary artery injury may be the cause of death.[70, 108] Overall, penetrating ventricular injury appears more common and more lethal than blunt injury.[92, 100, 108]

Knife and ice pick wounds are more likely to produce tamponade than exsanguinating hemorrhage and thus have a better prognosis than gunshot wounds.[10, 19, 59, 108] Patients who die from these smaller wounds usually succumb to tamponade.[74] Although the ventricular chambers may seal more efficiently than the atrial chambers, this potential benefit is probably offset by the higher pressure, which allows enough blood loss to produce tamponade.[45, 108] Fifty to 80% of patients with penetrating cardiac injuries develop tamponade.[63]

Only 19% of all patients with penetrating heart wounds reach a hospital alive—11% of patients with gunshot wounds and 39% of patients with stab wounds.[59, 63, 83, 100] When multiple gunshot wounds exist, the cardiac injury is the main prognostic factor, but mortality rates rise with associated organ injuries.[83, 84] Age has not been identified as a prognostic factor, but mortality appears to be *higher* in the pediatric population sustaining penetrating cardiac injuries.[108]

Two to 3% of all penetrating wounds of the thorax involve the heart.[76] Although a penetrating wound almost anywhere in the chest may injure the heart, the presence of a wound near the area of the mediastinum should strongly raise suspicion of cardiac or great vessel injury, even though the wound may appear to be deceptively benign.[33, 71, 108] If the wound overlies the cardiac silhouette, the chance of cardiac penetration is 60%.[80] In addition, any penetration of the base of the neck or the upper abdomen is potentially associated with cardiac or great vessel injury.[71] A penetrating injury of the thoracic wall or diaphragm, especially if accompanied by hemothorax or pneumothorax compromises an already tenuous patient.[19] During active expiration, the diaphragm may rise to the fourth rib anteriorly, so thoracic wounds at or caudal to this level may also involve abdominal organs.[19]

Patients with penetrating cardiac injuries may appear stable, and the entrance wound may seem deceptively small for the degree of injury.[19, 30, 45] When potential cardiac injury exists, the patient should be monitored continuously and transported outside critical care areas minimally, as several deaths from cardiac wounds have occurred while patients were undergoing radiographic evaluation.[45]

As with blunt cardiac injury, pericardiocentesis may be a temporizing measure before thoracotomy in those patients presenting with cardiac tamponade.[14, 16, 33, 59, 68, 75, 108] The ability of the pericardium to prevent exsanguination is a critical survival factor. Moreno and associates reported survival in 36% of emergency department thoracotomies and 100% of operating room thoracotomies with tamponade following penetrating cardiac injury. Of the patients *without* tamponade, 63% who had operations and *none* who had emergency department thoracotomies survived.[68] Also, time is of the essence.[76, 83, 108] A series of 200 patients with penetrating cardiac injuries revealed a mortality rate of 10% in patients operated on within 30 minutes of arrival and 26% in the remainder.[108] The mortality rate in patients with gunshot wounds of the heart who were not operated on is 100%.[84]

Close-range shotgun wounds do extensive direct damage. High-velocity gunshot wounds are associated with extensive contusion even though the penetrating wound may be small. Overall, knife wounds produce much less injury.[16, 19] If a weapon or a large penetrating foreign body is embedded in the patient, it should not be removed before operative exposure is provided.[30, 71]

If penetrating cardiac injuries have associated coronary artery laceration, the mortality rate is even higher.[63, 83, 108] In a series of more than 500 penetrating cardiac injuries reported from Parkland Hospital in Dallas, 4.4% had coronary artery involvement. Myocardial or pericardial injury may be present, and lethal arrhythmias may occur.[16, 64, 76, 108]

Operative Therapy

Although bypass may be needed and should certainly be available to repair cardiac penetrations, most frequently the surgeon's finger can control bleeding while suturing is performed.[20, 83, 87, 100] If the hole is large, two mattress sutures may be placed and held with countertraction to facilitate visualization. Once mattress sutures have been placed, a continuous reinforcing suture layer is recommended by some.[83] If the laceration is adjacent to but does not involve a coronary artery, the wound is best managed by using a horizontal mattress suture that passes under the coronary artery.[83, 100] Partial occlusion clamps may be helpful in atrial and great vessel injuries.[80, 83, 100] Inflow occlusion of the cavae may be utilized for 60 to 90 seconds if necessary to gain exposure.[83, 100]

Induced fibrillation should be employed only if absolutely necessary. It may be useful in patients who have not been in shock or had evidence of cerebral ischemia preoperatively.[83, 100] Patients with cardiac injuries have extreme myocardial stress, and warm fibrillation alone incurs further ischemic damage.

Penetrating valve injuries are usually rapidly fatal and are believed to have a worse prognosis than blunt valve injuries.[70, 76] If valve injury is suspected, some believe cardiac catheterization should be carried out and, if confirmed, an emergency operation should be performed. Time may make this unnecessary.

Sequelae of Penetrating Cardiac Injury

Late complications of penetrating cardiac injury include recurrent pericarditis, VSD, ventricular aneurysm, or ventricular pseudoaneurysm. Reaction from a retained foreign body may also produce late cardiac dysfunction.[83] Delayed VSD may be associated with penetrating cardiac lesions.[16, 70, 72] Instances have been reported in which a traumatic VSD clotted and sealed shortly after its creation.[72, 89]

CASE

An 11-year-old boy was shot in the left anterior chest with an air gun. On arrival at the emergency department approximately 1 hour after the injury, systolic blood pressure was 60 mm Hg, pulse was 120 beats per minute, and respirations were 20. He was conscious but agitated. His neck veins were distended, his heart sounds were muffled, and his CVP was 39 mm HG. When the systolic blood pressure dropped to 40 mm Hg and the pulse rate to 100, pericardiocentesis was performed, yielding 70 ml of non-clotting blood. His blood pressure rose to 90, and his pulse increased to 120.

The entry wound was about 3 cm superior and medial to the left nipple. Chest roentgenogram showed a pellet that was possibly within the heart. A median sternotomy was performed, and clotted blood was evacuated from the pericardial sac. The systolic blood pressure immediately improved to 110 mm Hg. A right ventricular outflow tract injury was present. The pellet could not be located, and attempts to retrieve it were abandoned. The right ventricular defect was closed with two 3-0 Prolene sutures with pledgets. A postoperative chest radiograph revealed the pellet's position to be unchanged.

GREAT VESSEL INJURIES

Blunt Aortic Injury

Incidence and Etiology

In the general population, 10 to 15% of victims of motor vehicle accidents die from aortic rupture.[52, 82, 99] The incidence approaches 30% in patients ejected from a crashed vehicle.[52, 82] The incidence of blunt aortic rupture rises sharply beginning at age 17 and peaks at about age 20.[66] The reported incidence of this injury is lower in children.[13, 37, 51–53, 66, 77, 82, 85, 87, 99] One series estimated the incidence of aortic disruption in children to be one in 1000 serious injuries.[37] Other reported causes of aortic rupture include airplane crashes, airplane accidents, falls from heights, compression of the chest, direct blows to the chest, pedestrian-vehicle accidents, and cardiopulmonary resuscitation.[83, 85]

Whatever the cause, the mechanism of injury involves horizontal or vertical deceleration of the arch away from the fixed descending aorta, crushing injury, or marked compression.[13, 52, 99, 109] If there is associated cardiac injury, 52% of patients will have disruption of the ascending aorta within the pericardium and will rapidly succumb to tamponade.[10, 36, 52] Approximately 7% of aortic disruptions are associated with heart or other great vessel injuries.[47] Usually the disruption occurs at the isthmus, just distal to the left subclavian artery; most aortic disruptions at other locations are rapidly fatal.[13, 27, 36, 37, 47, 52, 77, 82, 99] Disruption occurs at multiple sites in 15 to 20% of patients.[27, 51, 99] Those who survive may develop a pseudoaneurysm.[109]

Studies of aortic tensile strength have shown that it takes 600 to 2500 mm Hg to rupture a normal aorta.[27] Sixty percent of the aortic tensile strength is maintained by the adventitia, which limits the hemorrhage and may explain why as many as 40% of patients who have complete aortic transection survive.[13, 27, 52, 82, 99]

Aortic disruptions outside the pericardium may produce no discernible signs or symptoms. In a series of 275 patients who had aortic injuries, 33% had no external evidence of chest trauma.[27] Also, the patient may be unable to relate symptoms owing to other frequently present associated injuries.[27, 52, 82, 83, 85, 99] Thirty percent have dyspnea secondary to tracheobronchial compression, and 30% have back pain as the symptom of aortic injury.[51, 52, 85, 99] Systolic murmur, dysphagia, hoarseness, and superior vena caval obstruction have all been reported.[27, 99] The physiologic picture of coarctation may be present with reduced femoral pulses and upper extremity hypertension.[13, 27, 51, 52, 85, 87] Paraplegia may result from interrupted spinal cord circulation.[85, 109] Anuria secondary to loss of renal circulation may also occur.[109]

Although 85% of patients exsanguinate immediately with aortic rupture, approximately 15% survive the initial injury because bleeding is controlled by adventitia, pleura, and surrounding tissue.[13, 36, 37, 51, 52, 83, 85, 109] Thirty percent of the patients who arrive at a hospital alive will exsanguinate in 24 hours without treatment.[87] Forty-five percent of those surviving this period will exsanguinate within 3 weeks without treatment.[51, 85, 87] Thus, if untreated or unrecognized, aortic injury is 95% fatal.

If exsanguination does not occur initially, a pseudoaneurysm will form in approximately 2 months, and in the 2 to 5% of patients who develop aortic pseudoaneurysm, rupture may be delayed for years.[13, 27, 66, 83, 87] Delayed rupture has been reported in seven children. One child, 4 years old at the time of injury, died with aortic rupture 15 years later.

The chest roentgenogram is an important diagnostic

study in these patients. Portable films of the supine chest produce some mediastinal magnification and are thus more difficult to interpret than the upright chest roentgenogram done at the standard tube to cassette distance, but mediastinal widening is seen in almost all cases of aortic disruption.[83] A mediastinal hematoma causes loss of sharpness of the aortic knob, inferior displacement of the left bronchus, and displacement of the trachea and esophagus to the right.[27, 37, 51, 52, 99] Left pleural effusion with an apical cap may also be present.[37, 51, 52, 99] The presence of first or second rib fractures denotes violent impact and is often associated with great vessel injury.[37]

Aortic rupture can occur without appreciable mediastinal widening, and mediastinal widening may be present without great vessel injury.[27, 51] An example is that of torn intercostal veins.[99] Development of a mediastinal hematoma may be delayed, so that the injury can be detected only by repeated roentgen examinations.[27, 82]

Aortography should be performed in patients with a suspected aortic disruption, specifically in those with a wide mediastinum.[27, 51, 66, 82, 83, 85, 87] The angiogram also helps to diagnose other associated great vessel injuries and to identify multiple disruptions.[27] Negative angiography in the presence of aortic disruption has been reported.[82]

Magnetic resonance imaging (MRI) has no current role in the treatment of acute aortic injuries. The equipment and personnel are not readily available. The procedure takes a considerable amount of time, and the typically unstable patient is inaccessible to critical care monitoring during the examination. It has, however, been valuable in demonstrating the presence of the traumatically induced aortic pseudoaneurysm days or weeks later, particularly in visualizing the area of the ligamentum arteriosum, where injury usually occurs. In this setting, both the defect and any related vessels are defined.[106] Intimal tears can also be identified with MRI.[24]

Operative Therapy

When the diagnosis has been established, emergency thoracotomy should be performed.[52, 83] Before opening the thorax, the femoral artery and vein should be exposed in case bypass is necessary.[83] Some investigators recommend routine utilization of bypass or of a shunt.[52, 81, 85] Aortic clamping for longer than 20 minutes without distal circulatory support increases the risk of distal thrombosis, renal failure, cerebral hypertension, and paraplegia.[82, 83] Paraplegia may occur despite the utilization of bypass as a result of injury to the anterior spinal artery. If at all possible, blood-saving techniques should be utilized at the time of operation.[83]

Sternotomy is the preferred exposure for ascending aortic injuries and lateral thoracotomy for descending injuries.[83] Thoracoabdominal incisions should not be utilized when celiotomy is also necessary because of the risk of graft contamination from abdominal visceral wounds.[82]

Before opening the hematoma, proximal and distal control of the aorta should be achieved.[83] Proximal control may need to be established within the pericardium. Injury to the recurrent laryngeal nerve, which often lies within the hematoma coursing around the ligamentum arteriosum, should be avoided if possible.[52, 83]

A prosthetic graft is usually required because the retracted ends may be farther than 6 cm apart, making reunion impossible.[13, 52, 83, 87, 99] Long-term results from homografts utilized for this procedure are not known, but early degeneration is a concern.[83, 85] At least one case of graft infection following repair of aortic disruption has been reported. Repair of this injury may be an indication to use a homograft.[85] The surgical mortality in patients with aortic disruption ranges from 18 to 30%.[82, 85]

Uncontrollable hemorrhage and coagulopathy may occur intraoperatively.[52, 82, 99] Respiratory problems, including aspiration, are relatively common postoperatively.[52, 82, 99] Postpericardiotomy syndrome and congestive heart failure may also develop.[85]

CASE

A 16-year-old white adolescent was an unrestrained passenger in a high-speed motor vehicle accident. Ejected approximately 90 feet from the vehicle, he was taken to an outlying hospital, where evaluation by six specialists over a period of 8 hours was accomplished. The chest roentgenogram, taken approximately 30 minutes after the accident, was suggestive of aortic injury, but the problem was not recognized until the sixth consultant, a surgeon, saw him. He was transferred immediately with a diagnosis of "possible aortic disruption."

On arrival, pulmonary artery and arterial monitoring catheters were in place. Central venous, right ventricular and diastolic, and pulmonary artery diastolic pressures were equal, ECG voltage was low, and blood pressure was marginal. The chest radiograph was repeated, and the results were unchanged (Fig. 18–4). Emergency echocardiogram excluded the presence of tamponade.

Within 20 minutes of arrival, the patient was in the angiography suite, but while arterial access was being accomplished, he suffered cardiac arrest, and fluoroscopy showed the left hemithorax to be filling rapidly. All resuscitative efforts were futile, and the patient died of aortic rupture. Myocardial fractions of creatine phosphokinase and lactate dehydrogenase were significantly elevated, indicating that he probably also had severe myocardial contusion.

Penetrating Aortic Injury

Incidence and Etiology

Only 20% of patients with penetrating aortic injuries survive the initial insult.[27, 76] Most patients who sustain penetrating injury of the intrapericardial aorta succumb to sudden tamponade, and such aortic injuries outside the pericardium are usually accompanied by rapid exsanguination.[27, 76] However, an aortic laceration may develop a thrombus temporarily so that exsanguination occurs a few days later.

Pseudoaneurysm may also develop following penetrating aortic injury.[76] Small wounds, such as from an ice pick, allow the patient the best chance of survival; survival after aortic injury caused by a high velocity missile is rare.[83] When the aortic injury is caused by a gunshot, the heart is frequently injured as well.[82, 100]

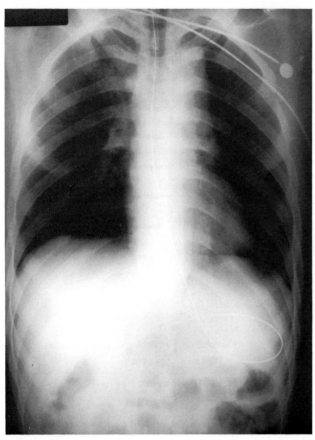

FIGURE 18–4

Aortic disruption. The most striking findings are loss of the aortic knob and widening of the superior mediastinum.

Operative Therapy

Prompt operation is indicated as soon as the diagnosis is suspected.[76] There is little time to perform diagnostic maneuvers. The survival rate is much higher when rapid, definitive therapy is instituted, preferably in the operating room.[82] The surgical approach is much the same as that for blunt injuries, and partial occlusion clamps frequently are quite helpful in controlling hemorrhage in such instances.[96]

Aortic Arch Branch Vessel Injuries

Anatomy, Incidence, and Etiology

The anatomy of the aortic branches in the thorax varies in up to 30% of patients.[83] This fact, in conjunction with the difficulty in controlling hemorrhage from them, makes their management extremely challenging.[8] The overall mortality rate is reported to approach 30%, but because these injuries are frequently fatal before treatment begins they are probably more common than the literature reflects.[7, 8, 18, 28] Innominate, carotid, and subclavian injuries usually are associated with upper extremity or rib fractures, with bone fragments being primarily responsible for the vascular injury.[12, 97, 109] A second great vessel injury is present in 10% of patients, and 30% have associated thoracic aortic injuries.[12, 28, 47, 53, 82]

Intimal disruption with dissection and occlusion may occur after blunt trauma or high-velocity gunshot wounds. The adventitia is intact, and little or no hemorrhage occurs. Bony fractures may not be present. Arteriosclerotic vascular disease is not a prerequisite for this injury; the youngest reported case was that of a 3-year-old boy.[40]

Because these traumatized patients typically present in a low-flow state, the subtle changes of intimal injury may be difficult to detect.[40] Intimal flat formation has occurred in the innominate and subclavian arteries with no abnormality in extremity perfusion.[12, 40] Distal injuries seem to be more symptomatic. When the diagnosis is suspected, arteriography should be performed to evaluate the nature of the occlusion and to rule out arterial spasm.[40]

Operative Therapy

At operation, contused arteries should be explored because the outer arterial layers may appear to be nearly normal, even though clot and disruption are present within. Proximal and distal Fogarty catheter thrombectomy typically yields a large amount of thrombus.[40] If possible, resection and primary anastomosis should be performed. Frequently, adequate mobilization is not possible, in which case the intima should be débrided and fixed to the vessel to prevent further dissection.[40]

An intraoperative arteriogram should be performed because additional thrombectomy is frequently needed. Total body heparinization should be used during but not after the operative procedure because of the degree of soft tissue injury these patients usually have.[40]

Innominate Vessel Injuries

Innominate artery or vein injuries are rare but have been reported more frequently than those to the carotid or subclavian vessels.[1, 7, 8, 12, 27, 28, 82, 91] Innominate artery injury usually occurs in young people who have a pliable thorax. On impact, the vessel is crushed between the sternum and spine. Displacement of the heart into the left chest may also cause shearing at the origin of the innominate.[7]

This injury is usually not recognized at the time of initial trauma.[7] Only 50% of patients have diminished pulse or blood pressure in the extremities, and of the patients who present more than 15 days after injury, only about 20% have pulse or blood pressure change.[12, 53] Signs of distal ischemia are rare.[53] A systolic murmur may be present, and some patients complain of dysphagia.[12, 53, 109]

Mediastinal, axillary, or supraclavicular hematoma or persistent bleeding from a chest tube may be the most consistent finding on physical examination. Brachial plexus deficits or neurologic findings of carotid occlusion warrant assumption of great vessel injury.[7, 8, 12, 109] If the patient is stable, arteriography of the aorta and its major branches should be performed immediately.[8, 12, 53]

Operative Therapy

Sternotomy is the incision that provides the best opportunity of proximal control.[7, 8, 12] If there is associated carotid artery injury, an extension of the incision can be carried obliquely into the neck.[7, 53] Otherwise, a right supraclavicular incision should be extended from the sternotomy.[8, 12] If possible, musculoskeletal flaps should not be used owing to the morbidity of rib fractures and subclavian and innominate vein injuries.[8] Femoro-femoral bypass should be available in patients with associated aortic or other great vessel injuries.[8]

Innominate vein injuries are best repaired, but ligation is acceptable if the vessel is severely injured or if division is necessary to expose an intimal injury.[8]

Frequently, the physician must operate on a hypovolemic, unstable patient without knowing the exact location of the injury.[8] If intrathoracic bleeding is so severe that blood pressure cannot be maintained, anterolateral thoracotomy should be performed on the side of the injury and large packs placed into the apex for compression. Pressure should also be maintained at the supraclavicular space on the side of the injury while the patient's blood volume is restored.[8] Sternotomy and supraclavicular incisions should then be carried out.[8, 12] The subclavian artery should be clamped and pressure held on the innominate artery while an aortic-carotid shunt is established.[8, 12, 53]

Subclavian Vessel Injuries

Incidence, Anatomy, and Mechanism of Injury

The subclavian vessels are usually injured in their proximal portion, and injuries to them are frequently associated with other great vessel injuries.[53, 109] The mechanism of injury is more frequently penetrating than blunt.[1]

Diagnosis should be suspected if there is a large or expanding hematoma, usually in the mediastinum.[1] This may present as a pulsatile mass at the base of the neck, which may have a bruit, and the ipsilateral radial pulse may be absent secondary to thrombosis.[1, 53] Subclavian "steal" has also been described to occur acutely.[12, 53] If possible, angiography should be performed to demonstrate the location of the injury as well as any potentially coexisting great vessel injuries.[1] Anatomically, this is a difficult area to expose, especially when hematoma obscures landmarks.[97]

Operative Therapy

Subclavian artery ligation is no longer recommended as a definitive form of therapy. Although the acute effects are variable, long-term effects in children include retarded longitudinal bone growth, decreased muscle mass, and weakness in the affected arm of most patients.[20]

Exposure of the innominate and subclavian vessels on the right is best done by sternotomy with right supraclavicular extension.[8, 12, 53] On the left side, posterolateral thoracotomy through the fourth intercostal space should be performed, because sternotomy does not yield adequate exposure.[8] Exposure of the distal subclavian vessels may require division of the sternocleidomastoid, scalenus anterior, and strap muscles or removal of the first rib.[8, 12, 53, 97]

Subclavian vein injuries are usually associated with massive blood loss into the pleural space.[1, 97, 109] Major venous injuries should be repaired when possible, but collateral circulation permits ligation if necessary.[1, 28]

Carotid Artery Injury

Incidence, Anatomy, and Mechanism of Injury

Patients who present with carotid artery injury may vary from an asymptomatic patient (30%) with an innocuous-appearing wound to those who present in shock. Much of the variation is explained by the ability of the local tissues to contain hemorrhage and the extensive collateral cerebral circulation.[28]

Carotid artery injuries are usually not isolated.[12] When signs and symptoms are present, hemorrhage, pulse deficit, bruit, expanding hematoma, or neurologic changes may be seen.[1, 28] Thirty-five percent have lateralizing neurologic abnormalities.[28] Under such circumstances, exploration of the wound should be carried out if the platysma is penetrated or the mediastinum is widened.[28] Patients with cervical spine injuries are at risk for carotid contusion and thrombosis.[77] If the patient is stable, an aortogram may be helpful, but evaluation and treatment must be expedient and without delay.

Operative Therapy

Both proximal and distal control should be established.[28] Distal carotid artery injury is usually manageable via a neck incision.[3] Proximal carotid artery injury is well exposed by sternotomy with an oblique neck extension to whatever side is necessary.[12, 28] Before repair, compression should be utilized to control bleeding while the patient is being resuscitated.[28]

It is not possible to predict which patients will develop cerebral injury during carotid occlusion, although the risk probably increases linearly with age.[3] An electroencephalogram should be utilized intraoperatively if possible.[7] A carotid shunt should be available and may decrease cerebral injury, although selective shunting based on electroencephalographic monitoring may be utilized.[3, 12, 37] Grafts are needed in a significant percentage of patients.[1, 3, 12]

HEART AND GREAT VESSEL PERFORATIONS FROM FOREIGN BODY

Incidence and Mechanism of Injury

Young children who are mobile enough to gain access to sharp objects may ingest them, and this history is often difficult to obtain. Presentation is usually nonspecific, consisting of fussiness, low-grade fever, and vomiting. Heart and great vessel perforation from foreign body ingestion is rare.[2, 6, 30, 42, 62] The most common mechanism of perforation is from the esophagus into the aorta, but the heart may be involved.[6, 42] Intravascular foreign body perforation into the esophagus has also been reported.[30]

Operative Therapy

A single bleeding episode usually precedes exsanguination and may occur 2 hours to 10 days after the injury.[2, 6, 42] Hematemesis in association with a foreign body seen on the chest roentgenogram should arouse suspicion of major vessel penetration. Early operation with closure, drainage, and broad spectrum antibiotics is recommended.[42] To date, this injury has been uniformly fatal in children, with the diagnosis being made only at postmortem examination.

Cardiovascular Foreign Bodies

Patients who sustain penetrating injuries are at risk for residual foreign body and secondary injury from them. Bullets or pellets constitute the most common foreign bodies. Ten percent of patients with penetrating cardiac injury have a foreign body remaining in the heart. Migration into the right heart and pulmonary vessels may occur, but more commonly the missile penetrates the heart or great vessels and migrates from there.[22, 29, 30, 41, 46, 69, 72, 74, 76, 83, 89, 95, 96]

If patients are able to provide a good history, they usually describe a rapid onset of extremity pain, numbness, or weakness occurring after a gunshot injury.[29, 46, 96] Frequently, however, they are unable to communicate because of the trauma, and the subtle changes of paresis and vascular insufficiency may go unrecognized. Embolic foreign body should be suspected when there is an entrance wound with no exit wound.[29, 46, 83] Roentgenogram of the area of bullet entry confirms whether the missile remains or may have embolized.[29, 46] Late recognition usually results in ischemia and amputation.[29, 46, 69]

Most missile foreign body emboli go to the lower extremity, three times more common on the left than on the right.[29, 83, 96] This is believed to be secondary to the less acute angle of the left common iliac artery as it branches from the aorta.[29] Vessel occlusion is typically at the femoral level.[83, 95]

Extremity missile embolus should be removed when discovered because of the risk of limb loss.[69, 72, 89, 95] The decision to remove a cardiac or great vessel missile is not simple, as they may be very difficult to locate and remove. Pericarditis, bronchial erosion via the pulmonary artery, pulmonary infarction, sudden death, esophageal erosion, angina, and coronary arterial-venous fistula have all been reported to occur from cardiac foreign bodies.[22, 30, 41, 76, 83] In addition, 30% of missiles are accompanied by other foreign bodies such as clothing, and cultures of missile tracts yield bacteria in 67% of cases.[76] Hence, infection is a serious threat.[22, 76]

Surgical removal of a foreign body may itself incur significant damage.[76] The entrance wounds must be closed because of the risk of hemorrhage, late rupture, and aneurysm.[107] A missile capable of embolization or local penetration should probably be removed to avoid vascular occlusion and prevent erosion into a vital structure.[22, 41, 76, 83]

EMERGENCY DEPARTMENT THORACOTOMY FOR HEART AND GREAT VESSEL INJURIES IN CHILDREN

Emergency department thoracotomy is rarely necessary in children.[37] Although emergency department thoracotomy has improved survival for patients with some types of lesions, the survival rate is much higher if the patient is stable enough to be transported to the operating room for thoracotomy.[68, 82] A stable status should not reassure the physician, as abrupt deterioration may occur.[71, 80, 83]

Emergency department thoracotomy is indicated in traumatized children in the following settings:

1. When the patient has an abrupt loss of vital signs.[26, 82]
2. When closed-chest resuscitation has been unsuccessful for 5 minutes.[26, 68]
3. When the patient has sustained cardiac arrest associated with a probable penetrating great vessel or heart injury or when there has been blunt chest injury.[26, 37]
4. When there is profound shock and massive chest tube blood loss.[26]
5. When there is uncontrolled blood loss in the abdomen, open thoracotomy with descending aortic compression should be performed to increase cerebral perfusion temporarily and to decrease hemorrhage from the injury.[26, 37]

Left anterolateral thoracotomy should be performed unless a right-sided penetrating injury of the subclavian region appears to be present. Exsanguination from subclavian vessel injury responds best to anterolateral thoracotomy on the side of the injury with apical packing.[8, 97] After thoracotomy, any tamponade should be relieved, and a finger should be placed in the perforation or compression held on the great vessel injury while volume resuscitation proceeds.[64] Definitive repair should then be accomplished.

References

1. Bar-Ziu J, Eger M, Feuchtwanger M, et al: Angiography in diagnosis of subclavian vessel injury. Clin Radiol 23:471–473, 1972.
2. Barrie HJ, Townrow V: Perforation of the aorta by a foreign body in the esophagus. J Laryngol Otol 61:38–42, 1946.
3. Beall AC Jr, Shirkey AL, DeBakey ME: Penetrating wounds of the carotid arteries. J Trauma 3:276–287, 1963.
4. Bellinger SB: Penetrating chest injuries in children. Ann Thorac Surg 14:635–644, 1972.
5. Berman RW, Rook GD, Bronsther B, et al: Traumatic nonpenetrating VSD: Recovery under conservative management. J Pediatr Surg 1:275–283, 1966.
6. Bokat R, Fife J, Galen R: Foreign body ingestion with perforation of one of the great vessels of the mediastinum. J Maine Med Assoc 64:129–130, 1973.
7. Bosher LH, Freed TA: The surgical treatment of traumatic rupture or avulsion of the innominate artery. J Thorac Cardiovasc Surg 54:732–739, 1967.
8. Brawley RK, Murray GF, Crisler C, et al: Management of wounds of the innominate, subclavian and axillary blood vessels. Surg Gynecol Obstet 13:1130–1140, 1970.
9. Burrington JD: Childhood trauma. In: Holder TM, Ashcraft KW (eds): Pediatric Surgery. Philadelphia, WB Saunders, 1980, pp 138–161.
10. Callaham M: Pericardiocentesis in traumatic and nontraumatic cardiac tamponade. Ann Emerg Med 13:924–945, 1984.

11. Casson WR: Delayed cardiac tamponade. Anesthesia 40:48–50, 1985.
12. Castagna J, Nelson RJ: Blunt injuries to branches of the aortic arch. J Thorac Cardiovasc Surg 69:521–532, 1975.
13. Chalant C-H, Ponlot R, Tremouroux J, et al: Surgical treatment of post-traumatic aneurysms of the thoracic aorta. J Cardiovasc Surg 12:108–112, 1971.
14. Choo MH, Chia BL, Chia KC, et al: Penetrating cardiac injury evaluated by two-dimensional echocardiography. Am Heart J 108:417–420, 1984.
15. Cleland WP, Ellman P, Goodwin J, et al: Repair of ventricular septal defect following indirect trauma. Br J Dis Chest 55:17–22, 1961.
16. Cleveland RJ, Benfield JR, Nemhauser GM, et al: Management of penetrating wounds of the heart. Arch Surg 97:517–520, 1968.
17. Colombani PM, Buck JR, Dudgeon DL, et al: One year experience in a regional pediatric trauma center. J Pediatr Surg 20:8–13, 1985.
18. Conn JH, Hardy JD, Fain WR, et al: Thoracic trauma: Analysis of 1022 cases. J Trauma 3:22–40, 1963.
19. Creech O, Pearce CW: Stab and gunshot wounds of the chest. Am J Surg 105: 469–483, 1963.
20. Currarino G, Engle MA: The effects of ligation of the subclavian artery on the bones and soft tissues of the arms. J Pediatr 67:808–811, 1965.
21. Daggett WM: Surgical technique for early repair of posterior ventricular septal rupture. J Thorac Cardiovasc Surg 84:306–312, 1982.
22. Decker HR: Foreign bodies in the heart and pericardium—Should they be removed. J Thorac Surg 9:62–79, 1939.
23. Deforges G, Abelmann WH: Interventricular septal defect due to blunt trauma. Report of a case repaired surgically under total cardio-pulmonary bypass. N Engl J Med 268:128–131, 1963.
24. Dinsmore RE, Wedeen VJ, Miller SW, et al: MRI of dissection of the aorta: Recognition of the intimal tear and differential flow velocities. AJR 146:1286–1288, 1986.
25. Dunseth W, Ferguson TB: Acquired cardiac defect due to thoracic trauma. J Trauma 5:142–149, 1965.
26. Eichelberger MR, Randolph JG: Thoracic trauma in children. Surg Clin North Am 61:1181–1197, 1981.
27. Fishbone G, Robbins DI, Osborn DJ, et al: Trauma to the thoracic aorta and great vessels. Radiol Clin North Am 11:543–554, 1973.
28. Flint LM, Snyder WH, Perry MO, et al: Management of major vascular injuries in the base of the neck. Arch Surg 106:407–413, 1973.
29. Garzon A, Gliedman ML: Peripheral embolization of a bullet following perforation of the thoracic aorta. Ann Surg 160:901–904, 1964.
30. Gerbode F: Surgical treatment of emergencies of the heart and vessels in the thorax. JAMA 154:898–901, 1954.
31. Getz BS, Davies E, Steinberg SM, et al: Blunt cardiac trauma resulting in right atrial rupture. JAMA 255:761–763, 1986.
32. Glancy DL, Roberts WC: Complete spontaneous closure of VSD: Necropsy study 5 subjects. Am J Med 43:846–953, 1967.
33. Golladay ES, Donahoo JS, Haller JA: Special problems of cardiac injuries in infants and children. J Trauma 19:526–531, 1979.
34. Green L, Oakley CM, Davies DM, et al: Successful repair of left ventricular aneurysm and VSD after indirect injury. Lancet 2:984–986, 1965.
35. Gupta K: Cardiac air tamponade following closed chest injury. J R Coll Surg 31:120–121, 1986.
36. Hallen A, Hansson HE, Norlund S: Thoracic injuries. Scand J Thorac Cardiovasc Surg 8:34–35, 1974.
37. Haller JA Jr: Thoracic injuries. In: Welch KJ, Randolph JG, Ravitch MM, et al (eds): Pediatric Surgery. Chicago, Year Book Medical Publishers, 1986.
38. Haller JA, Shermeta DW: Major thoracic trauma in children. Pediatr Clin North Am 22:341–347, 1975.
39. Haller JA, Shermeta DW: Acute thoracic injuries in children. Pediatr Ann 5:71–79, 1976.
40. Hare RR, Gaspar MR: The intimal flap. Arch Surg 102:552–555, 1971.
41. Harken DE, Williams AC: Foreign bodies in and in relation to the thoracic blood vessels and heart. Am J Surg 72:80–90, 1946.
42. Henry WJ, Miscall L: Aortic-esophageal fistula. J Thorac Cardiovasc Surg 39:258–262, 1960.
43. Hood RM: Trauma to the chest. In: Sabiston DC Jr, Spencer FC (eds): Gibbon's Surgery of the Chest. 4th ed. Philadelphia, WB Saunders, 1983, p 291.
44. Jamshidi A, Berry RW: Left ventricular pseudoaneurysm secondary to cardiac stab wound. Am J Cardiol 16:601–604, 1965.
45. Jones EW, Helmsworth J: Penetrating wounds of the heart—Thirty years' experience. Arch Surg 96:671–682, 1968.
46. Keeley JL: A bullet embolus to the left femoral artery following a thoracic gunshot wounds. J Thorac Surg 21:608–620, 1951.
47. Kemmerer WT, Eckert WC, Gathright JB, et al: Patterns of thoracic injuries in fatal traffic accidents. J Trauma 1:595–599, 1961.
48. Killen DA, Gobbel WG, France R, et al: Post-traumatic aneurysm of the left ventricle. Circulation 39:101–108, 1969.
49. Kilman JW, Charnock E: Thoracic trauma in infancy and childhood. J Trauma 9:863–873, 1969.
50. King DR: Trauma in infancy and childhood: Initial evaluation and management. Pediatr Clin North Am 32:1299–1310, 1985.
51. Kirsh MM, Crane JD, Kahn DR, et al: Roentgenographic evaluation of traumatic rupture of the aorta. Surg Gynecol Obstet 131:900–904, 1970.
52. Kirsh MM, Kahn DR, Crane JD: Repair of acute traumatic rupture of the aorta without extracorporeal circulation. Ann Thorac Surg 10:227–236, 1970.
53. Kirsh MM, Sloan H: Blunt Chest Trauma: General Principles of Management. Boston, Little, Brown & Co, 1977, pp 75, 143–210.
54. Kissane RE: Traumatic heart disease: Nonpenetrating injuries. Circulation 6:421–425, 1952.
55. Knapp JF, Sharma V, Wasserman G, et al: Ventricular septal defect following blunt chest trauma in childhood: A case report. Pediatr Emerg Care 2:242–243, 1986.
56. Krajcer Z, Cooley DA, Leachman RD: Ventricular septal defect following blunt trauma: Spontaneous closure of residual defect after surgical repair. Cathet Cardiovasc Diagn 3:409–415, 1977.
57. Lasky II, Nahum AM, Siegel AW: Cardiac injuries incurred by drivers in automobile accidents. J Forensic Sci 14:13–33, 1969.
58. Levy JL: Management of crushing chest injuries in children. South Med J 65:1040–1044, 1972.
59. Lewis FR, Krupski WC, Trunkey DD: Management of the injured patient. In: Way LW (ed): Current Surgical Diagnosis and Treatment. Los Altos, Calif, Lange, 1985, pp 193–196.
60. Liedtke AJ, DeMuth WE: Nonpenetrating cardiac injuries: A collective review. Am Heart J 86:687–697, 1973.
61. Lyons C, Perkins R: Resection of a left ventricular aneurysm secondary to cardiac stab wound. Ann Surg 147:256–260, 1958.
62. McDaniel JR, Krepper PA: Esophagopericardial fistula. J Thorac Surg 34:173–176, 1957.
63. Maynard AL, Brooks HA, Froix CJL: Penetrating wounds of the heart. Arch Surg 90:680–686, 1965.
64. Melick DW: Traumatic laceration of right ventricle. Arizona Med 31:98–100, 1974.
65. Meller JL, Little AG, Shermeta DW: Thoracic trauma in children. Pediatrics 74:813–819, 1984.
66. Meyer JA, Neville JF, Hansen WG: Traumatic rupture of the aorta in a child. JAMA 208:527–529, 1969.
67. Moraes R, Victor E, Arruda M, et al: Ventricular septal defect following nonpenetrating trauma. Angiology 24:222–229, 1973.
68. Moreno C, Moore EE, Majure JA, et al: Pericardial tamponade: A critical determinant for survival following penetrating cardiac wounds. J Trauma 26:821–825, 1986.
69. Movin R, Russell J, Valle AR: A migratory arterial foreign body. Am J Surg 91:118–120, 1956.
70. Mulder DG: Stab wound of the heart. Ann Surg 160:287–291, 1964.
71. Naclerio EA: Penetrating wounds of the heart. Dis Chest 46:1–22, 1964.
72. Neerken AJ, Clement FL: Air rifle wound of the heart with embolization. JAMA 189:133–134, 1964.
73. O'Reilly RJ, Kazenelson G, Spellberg RD: Traumatic pseudoaneurysm of the left ventricle. Am Dis Child 120:252–254, 1970.
74. Othersen HB: Cardiothoracic Injuries. In: Touloukian RH (ed): Pediatric Trauma. New York, John Wiley & Sons, 1978, pp 305–368.
75. Parmley LF, Manion WC, Mattingly TW: Nonpenetrating traumatic injury of the heart. Circulation 18:371–396, 1958.
76. Parmley LF, Mattingly TW, Manion WC: Penetrating wounds of the heart and aorta. Circulation 17:953–973, 1958.
77. Petty C: Soft tissue injuries: An overview. J Trauma 10:201–219, 1970.
78. Pupello DF, Daily PO, Stinson EB, et al: Successful repair of left ventricular aneurysm due to trauma. JAMA 211:826–827, 1970.

79. Reardon MJ, Gross DM, Vallone AM, et al: Atrial rupture in a child from cardiac massage by his parent: Ann Thorac Surg 43:557–558, 1987.

80. Reece IJ, Davidson KG: Emergency surgery for stab wounds to the heart. Ann R Coll Surg 65:304–307, 1983.

81. Rees A, Symons J, Joseph M, et al: VSD in a battered child. BMJ 1:20–21, 1975.

82. Reul GJ, Rubio PA, Beall AC Jr: The surgical management of acute injury to the thoracic aorta. J Thorac Cardiovasc Surg 67:272–281, 1974.

83. Rich NM, Spencer FC: Vascular Trauma. Philadelphia, WB Saunders, 1978, pp 384–440.

84. Ricks RK, Howell JF, Beall AC Jr, et al: Gunshot wounds of the heart: A review of 31 cases. Surgery 57:787–790, 1965.

85. Rittenhouse EA, Dillard DH, Winterscheid LC, et al: Traumatic rupture of the thoracic aorta. Ann Surg 170:87–100, 1969.

86. Robicsek F: Repair of posterior postinfarction septal defects. Surg Rounds, November 1985, pp 24–28.

87. Roe BB: Cardiac trauma including injury of great vessels. Surg Clin North Am 52:573–583, 1972.

88. Rosenthal A, Parisi LF, Nados AS: Isolateral interventricular septal defect due to nonpenetrating trauma. N Engl J Med 283:338–341, 1970.

89. Saltzstein EC, Freeark RJ: Bullet embolism to the right axillary artery following gunshot wound of the heart. Ann Surg 158:65–69, 1963.

90. Scheinman JI, Kelminson LL, Vogel JHK, et al: Early repair of VSD due to nonpenetrating trauma. J Pediatr 74:406–412, 1969.

91. Schramel R, Kellum H, Creech O Jr: Analysis of factors affecting survival with chest injuries. J Trauma 1:600–607, 1961.

92. Sinclair MC, Moore TC: Major surgery for abdominal and thoracic trauma in childhood and adolescence. J Pediatr Surg 9:155–162, 1974.

93. Smyth BT: Chest trauma in children. J Pediatr Surg 14:41–47, 1979.

94. Snow N, Richardson JD, Flint LM Jr: Myocardial contusion; implications for patients with multiple traumatic injuries. Surgery 92:744–750, 1982.

95. Spencer FC, Kennedy JH: War wounds of the heart. J Thorac Surg 33:361–370, 1957.

96. Stanford W, Crosby VG, Pike JP, et al: Gunshot wounds of the thoracic aorta with peripheral embolization of the missile. Ann Surg 165:139–141, 1967.

97. Steenburg RW, Ravitch MM: Cervico-thoracic approach for subclavian vessel injury from compound fracture of the clavicle. Ann Surg 157:839–846, 1963.

98. Tellez DW, Hardin WD Jr, Takahashi M, et al: Blunt cardiac injury in children. J Pediatr Surg 22:1123–1128, 1987.

99. Thomford NR, Pace WG, Meckstroth CV: Traumatic rupture of the thoracic aortas. Am Surg 35:244–249, 1969.

100. Trinkle JK, Marcos J, Grover FL, et al: Management of the wounded heart. Ann Thorac Surg 17:230–236, 1974.

101. Trunkey DD: Advanced Trauma Life Support Course: Student Manual. 2nd ed. Chicago, American College of Surgeons, 1984, p 169.

102. Turney SZ, Mathai J, Singleton R, et al: Traumatic ventricular septal defect. Surgical repair in 2 patients. Ann Thorac Surg 13:36–43, 1972.

103. Viano DC, Lau V-K: Role of impact velocity and chest compression in thoracic injury. Aviat Space Environ Med 54:16–21, 1983.

104. Vincenti W, Bukhanov K, Semelhago L, et al: Increased susceptibility of fibrillating hearts to irreversible ischemia: A comparison of adult versus neonatal hearts. Surgical Forum. Chicago, American College of Surgeons, pp 199–202.

105. Watson JH, Bartholomal WM: Cardiac injury due to nonpenetrating chest trauma. Ann Int Med 52:871–880, 1960.

106. White RD, Dooms GC, Higgins CB: Advances in imaging thoracic aortic disease. Invest Radiol 21:761–778, 1986.

107. Williams DJ: Embolization of a bullet to the posterior tibial artery following a gunshot wound of the thorax. J Trauma 4:258–261, 1964.

108. Wilson RF, Bassett JS: Penetrating wounds of the pericardium or its contents. JAMA 195:513–518, 1966.

109. Windsor HM, Shanahan MX: The crushed chest. Med J Austr 18:877–882, 1970.

110. Haller JA, Talbert JL, Shermeta DW: Trauma and the child. In: Zuidema GD, Rutherford RB, Ballinger WF (eds): Management of Trauma. 3rd ed. Philadelphia, WB Saunders, 1979, pp 731–753.

Denis R. King
William E. Wise, Jr.

Vascular Injuries

Although the basic principles for management of vascular trauma in infancy and childhood follow the guidelines established for adult patients, the differences between adult and pediatric patients who have vascular injury are considerable and involve incidence, etiology, anatomic distribution, diagnostic evaluation, therapeutic intervention, and eventual outcome. The special problems of vascular injuries in childhood have been reviewed by Stanford, Shaker, Whitehouse, and Villavicencio and their colleagues,[81, 83, 88, 90] all of whose clinical reports focused on the unique diagnostic and therapeutic considerations of children.

In children, vascular elasticity and abundant collateral blood flow frequently mask underlying vascular injuries, delaying diagnosis and repair. The small caliber of pediatric blood vessels requires meticulous attention to operative technique if prolonged patency is to be achieved. The potential for subsequent abnormalities in growth and development demands both prompt evaluation and long-term follow-up in any child experiencing either accidental or iatrogenic vascular trauma. This chapter presents information on a wide variety of pediatric vascular injuries, with a discussion of both iatrogenic and traumatic lesions.

IATROGENIC INJURIES

During the first 2 years of life, the overwhelming majority of vascular injuries are iatrogenic in nature.[39, 81] Invasive monitoring is required frequently in tiny premature infants with severe cardiopulmonary disease, and management of these critically ill neonates often necessitates placement of umbilical arterial catheters for pressure measurement, blood gas sampling, or infusion of therapeutic agents. In addition, arterial access is often required for diagnostic cardiac catheterization in children with complex congenital heart disease. The polycythemia and hyperviscosity that accompany cyanotic heart disease predispose patients with this disease to arterial and venous thrombosis[28, 41] following arterial catheterization. Complications of umbilical artery catheter (UAC) placement and diagnostic cardiac catheterization represent the bulk of vascular "trauma" in children younger than 2 years of age.

Umbilical Artery Catheters

Umbilical artery catheters have been utilized clinically for more than 25 years and currently remain the standard method for monitoring the adequacy of cardiopulmonary function, including the necessity for continuous blood pressure monitoring and frequent blood gas sampling.[30] About half of all neonates admitted to intensive care nurseries undergo placement of umbilical artery lines, and it has been estimated that 2% of all newborn infants at large obstetric referral centers require arterial access.[10] More than 250,000 umbilical artery catheters were sold during 1983. Unfortunately, umbilical artery catheterization is associated with considerable morbidity and occasionally is the source of infant mortality. In 1970 Wigger and associates reported a catheter-related mortality rate of 11.6% in 43 neonatal patients who underwent umbilical artery catheterization.[91]

Marsh and co-workers subsequently reviewed 165 neonates with UACs and found that 15 deaths (9.1%) were directly attributable to catheter complications.[46] Although recent reports present a more optimistic outlook, catheter-related mortality rates of 2 or 3% are not considered unusual.[11]

Complications of umbilical artery catheterization include. (1) thrombosis, (2) sepsis, (3) hemorrhage, and (4) hypertension.[24, 35, 51, 60, 64, 77, 80, 84] Less frequent but equally serious sequelae include emboli with visceral or extremity infarction, aneurysm formation in the thoracic and abdominal aorta, injury to the urinary bladder, and other less common problems.[5, 14, 19, 34, 36, 45, 60, 67] The principles of catheter care that have been learned painfully during the past 2 decades must not be ignored if complications are to be kept to a minimum.

Chidi and colleagues described the natural history of the vascular injury associated with umbilical artery catheterization in a rabbit model.[12] Within 24 hours of insertion, the catheter routinely produced substantial aortic endothelial injury with loss of large segments of the intimal lining of the aorta (Fig. 19–1). Once the nonthrombogenic surface of the vessel was damaged, platelets and cellular elements of the blood had an opportunity to react with the newly exposed underlying tissue, triggering a cascade of cellular and biochemical activities that resulted in thrombus formation (Fig. 19–2). When the protective layer of the endothelial cells was lost, the arterial wall became permeable, allowing contact between the low-density lipoproteins that were products of platelet aggregation and the medial smooth muscle cells. This stimulated smooth muscle cell proliferation, producing intimal thickening, a phenomenon similar to the progression observed in atherosclerotic plaque formation. In the experimental model of Chidi and associates, the extent of vascular damage and the intensity of the arterial injury were directly related to the duration of catheter placement.[12] When the catheter was removed, the intima typically regenerated, and healing ensued with gradual resolution of much of the intramural inflammatory process.

The clinical correlate of the ultrastructural changes observed in this rabbit model is thrombosis. Wigger reported a 12.5% incidence of catheter-related thrombosis which produced a visceral infarction rate of 75%[91] (Fig. 19–3). Neal performed aortography in 19 asymptomatic infants with indwelling umbilical artery catheters, and thrombus formation was demonstrated in 18.[60] In addition, in seven of 12 autopsies (58%) had evidence of arterial thrombosis at postmortem. These data were confirmed by Mokrohisky and colleagues, who studied 23 asymptomatic infants by contrast injection before removal of their umbilical artery catheters.[54] Thrombus formation was documented in 21. This report was of particular significance because it was a prospective randomized study comparing the incidence of complications in infants with high and low aortic catheter placement. Although no catheter-related deaths were reported, the overall UAC complication rate was 59%, and catheter removal was required in 36% of the patients. A significantly higher complication rate was observed in infants with low aortic catheter placement. This observation has been confirmed in two subsequent studies. There was a significant difference between high and low catheter position with reference to the incidence of arterial thrombosis

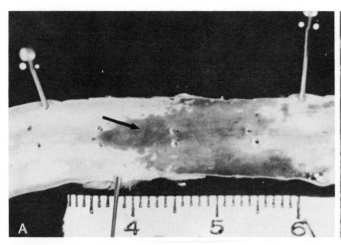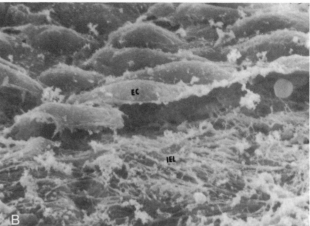

FIGURE 19–1

A, An area of endothelial injury caused by an umbilical artery catheter is apparent in this rabbit aorta (*arrow*). *B,* This electron micrograph shows the junction between the intact endothelial cells (EC) and the denuded surface of the aorta with the internal elastic lamina (IEL) exposed.

in the study by Wesstrom and co-workers, and Harris and Litte observed an increase in the incidence of blanching and cyanosis of the lower extremities in infants whose UACs were positioned in the lumbar area.[29, 89] On the basis of these papers, thoracic positioning of umbilical artery catheters is usually recommended.

Some researchers have suggested adding heparin to the catheter infusate to reduce the incidence of thrombosis. Bosque and Weaver reported a decreased incidence of catheter clotting in infants who received a continuous heparin infusion (1 unit/ml).[7] Heparin at this dose did not prolong the prothrombin time or partial thromboplastin time and did not increase the risk of intracranial hemorrhage. Horgan and colleagues studied ill infants who required UAC placement and found no difference in the incidence of aortic thrombosis between those infants who received heparinized infusions and those who did not.[31] In this study the addition of heparin decreased the risk of catheter malfunction, how-

ever, and lowered the incidence of UAC-associated hypertension. The risk of intra-aortic thrombus formation as defined by ultrasound was 31% in the study by Horgan and associates. Although the majority of the thrombotic lesions were sleevelike fibrin sheaths at the catheter tip, bulky intraluminal thrombi were observed in 10 patients (Fig. 19–4). Jackson and colleagues studied a heparin-bonded polyurethane UAC and concluded that endothelial trauma was primarily related to catheter size and stiffness and that these appeared to be more important factors in thrombus formation than the use of thromboresistant catheters.[32]

Krueger and co-workers reported seven infants who developed complete aortic thrombosis as a result of umbilical artery catheterization.[37] The seven patients were estimated to represent 0.13% of all neonates who required umbilical artery catheterization. Placement-related features (sepsis, hypoxia, and low cardiac output) and catheter characteristics (size and duration of catheterization) were implicated

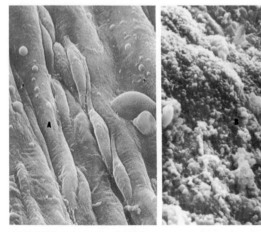

FIGURE 19–2

The intact endothelial surface (*A*) is nonthrombogenic. Once the endothelial cells are damaged (*B*), platelet deposition occurs and thrombus formation is initiated.

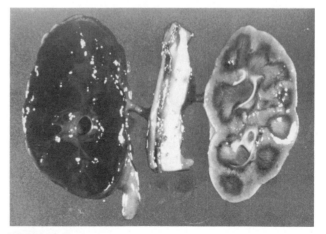

FIGURE 19–3

Thrombus has formed about the umbilical artery catheter. It has obstructed the renal artery completely, leading to an infarction of the right kidney.

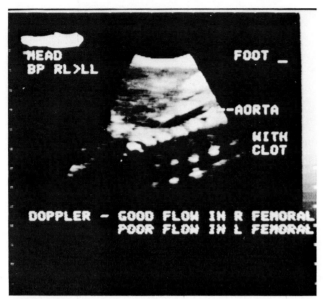

FIGURE 19–4
A thrombus is apparent within the lumen of the distal aorta in this ultrasound study.

as important factors predisposing to thrombosis. The clinical presentation of aortic occlusion was frequently heralded by the onset of congestive heart failure, hypertension, extremity ischemia, or hematuria. Diagnostic evaluation of the extent of thrombosis was established utilizing ultrasound and radionuclide scans, and surgical management yielded a successful outcome in six of the seven infants treated by transabdominal aortic thrombectomy.

The optimal management of complete aortic thrombosis remains a controversial issue, however. Other investigators have described the use of heparin or fibrinolytic agents, or both, with equally good results.[42, 78] In Horgan and colleagues' report, supportive care alone provided spontaneous resolution of the aortic thrombus in 11 patients.[31] Our own experience confirms the latter observation. Direct operative intervention is usually not required and would not be recommended unless uncontrolled metabolic acidosis or progressive tissue ischemia demanded immediate resolution of the low-flow state.

Infection is another common problem in infants who require umbilical artery catheterization. Bacterial colonization has been reported in up to 57% of UACs but catheter-related bacteremia is much less frequent (about 5%).[35, 65] As with all central vascular access devices, the quality of catheter care is a major determinant of the risk of infection. Prophylactic antibiotics are not indicated because they do not decrease the incidence of infection. *Staphylococcus epidermidis* is a common pathogen in UAC-associated sepsis, and this dictates the use of vancomycin as part of the initial antimicrobial protocol whenever catheter sepsis is suspected.

A related problem is the development of aneurysms in the aorta and iliac vessels. Although the natural history of this lesion is not well defined, Drucker and co-workers have implicated a combination of intravascular trauma at the catheter tip and bacterial infection of the vessel wall in the formation of neonatal aortic aneurysms.[15] These lesions are usually asymptomatic but should be suspected in any infant with an umbilical artery catheter who develops systemic sepsis. Occasionally hypertension, localized arterial insufficiency, or a pulsatile abdominal mass is observed. An ultrasound examination is usually sufficient for diagnostic screening of infants in the neonatal nursery, but aortography should be performed for precise delineation of the vascular anatomy before surgical reconstruction is considered.[34] Resection and reconstruction of vascular continuity are recommended because spontaneous rupture with exsanguination may occur.[67]

Other less frequent complications of umbilical artery catheterization include buttock ischemia, paraplegia, renal and mesenteric emboli, vessel penetration with exsanguination, and bladder perforation with the development of uroascites. The majority of these problems can be avoided by careful attention to appropriate techniques of catheter position (thoracic versus lumbar remains controversial); all authorities agree that placement of the catheter tip adjacent to the ostia of the visceral arteries should be avoided. Correct catheter position can be estimated using the distance between shoulder and umbilicus as described by Dunn, but the exact level of placement within the aorta must be confirmed utilizing a portable radiograph.[16] The UACs should always be end-hole catheters and should be continuously infused with a heparin-containing solution to maintain patency. All external connections should be taped securely, and stopcocks should be capped and cleansed with povidone-iodine (Betadine) before use. Umbilical artery catheters should be removed when distal ischemia is observed, when embolic phenomena are suspected, when the pressure tracing becomes dampened, when blood withdrawal becomes difficult, or when continuous pressure monitoring and frequent blood gas analyses are no longer necessary.

Peripheral Arterial Access

Many other vessels have been utilized for continuous blood pressure monitoring in critically ill or injured pediatric patients, including the radial, dorsalis pedis, posterior tibial, ulnar, axillary, and femoral arteries. It should be emphasized that the superficial temporal artery should never be used because of the risk of central nervous system damage. The radial artery is considered the safest peripheral arterial access site, and a vast clinical experience has been accumulated with an acceptably low incidence of significant complications.[53] Although thrombosis of the radial artery is relatively common, the risk of hand ischemia is low because the blood supply of the superficial palmar arch is usually derived from the ulnar artery (88%).[56]

A number of principles must be followed if complications are to be avoided, however.

1. The nondominant hand should be utilized for initial arterial access.
2. Before attempting arterial access, the collateral circulation of the hand should be evaluated by performing an Allen test. Although delayed reperfusion is not an absolute contraindication to ipsilateral radial artery catheterization,

in such instances the use of an alternative access site is recommended.

3. Percutaneous insertion of the catheter is preferred.

4. The shortest possible length of intravascular catheter should be used to prevent occlusion of proximal collateral vessels.

5. The catheter should be fixed to the skin and the wrist immobilized to minimize intimal damage from catheter motion.

6. A continuous infusion of heparinized fluid should be administered.

7. High-pressure bolus injections should be avoided to prevent retrograde central embolic phenomena.[40]

Although the risk-benefit ratio of peripheral arterial access is quite acceptable, Cartwright and Schreiner[11] and Mayer and colleagues[47] have reported children who required amputation of the hand and forearm following percutaneous radial artery catheterization. As with any invasive angioaccess procedure, definite indications for arterial monitoring should be established, and the cannula should be removed at the first indication of catheter malfunction. The incidence of significant complications following radial artery catheterization is low, but some clinical evidence of hand ischemia can be anticipated in 0.2 to 0.5% of patients.[4, 92]

Arterial Access—Diagnostic

Arteriography is a valuable diagnostic tool that is used with increasing frequency in the pediatric age group. Our ability to cannulate the vascular system and to directly image complex cardiac anomalies, vascular malformations, and solid organ tumors has greatly facilitated the diagnosis and management of a wide variety of clinical problems in childhood. The thromboembolic complications of diagnostic angiography have been well documented, however, and are known to occur with much greater frequency in children. In a report of 3500 adults who underwent cardiac catheterization, only 15 patients (0.4%) required surgical intervention for the correction of arterial injuries.[43] In pediatric patients, thromboembolic problems have been identified in up to 37% of cases.[55]

In 1968, Bassett and associates reported an alarming incidence of limb length inequality following cardiac catheterization.[3] Twenty-four of 28 randomly selected children who had previously undergone diagnostic left ventricular catheterization had evidence of limb length shortening and diminished distal circulation in the extremity utilized for arterial catheter introduction. Surprisingly, none of the children had a history of noticeable ischemic sequelae in the extremity immediately following cardiac catheterization, and all but one were asymptomatic at the time of reevaluation. Mortensson performed follow-up angiography of previously catheterized femoral arteries in 44 children to evaluate the incidence and anatomic extent of late thrombotic complications.[55] Complete occlusion of the external iliac artery was observed in six patients (12%), significant arterial narrowing was noted in three cases (6%), and small mural abnormalities were apparent in four children (8%).

The vascular anatomy was normal in the remaining patients (74%). Age was noted to be a primary predisposing factor in the development of vascular occlusion. Arterial injury was much more common (24%) in the children who were younger than 8 years of age at the time of cardiac catheterization. Only one older child developed arterial thrombosis (6%). Four of the reported patients had measurable leg length discrepancies at the time of follow-up.

Mansfield and co-workers evaluated the management of 29 children who developed the clinical appearance of acute arterial insufficiency following diagnostic angiography.[44] In all of the patients in whom distal pulses were absent for 8 hours after catheterization, arterial thrombosis was found to be complete at the time of exploration. Even though overt tissue ischemia was rarely observed, the researchers recommended early re-exploration and thrombectomy to avoid future problems with growth and development of the extremity. Wigger and colleagues postulated that these ischemic complications occurred as a result of thrombus formation on the surface of the catheter that was stripped off as the catheter was removed from the vessel.[91] Freed and associates initiated a prospective double-blind study of 161 children who required diagnostic arterial access to evaluate the efficacy of heparin in preventing this complication.[21] None of the 84 children older than 8 years of age developed thrombotic problems. Of the 40 younger children who received a single bolus dose of heparin (1 mg/kg) during cardiac catheterization, only three patients (8%) developed a pulseless extremity and none required surgical intervention for limb salvage. By contrast, 15 of the 37 children in the placebo group developed complete loss of pulses, and embolectomy was required on seven occasions (19%). The researchers concluded that heparinization was effective in preventing thrombosis associated with percutaneous arterial access procedures and recommended the routine use of heparin during diagnostic angiography.

Franken and colleagues emphasized the role of vascular spasm in the pathophysiology of the arterial thrombosis associated with angiography.[20] Arterial spasm was observed in 62% of the 100 children studied and was quantified as severe (complete loss of distal pulses) in 28%. Return of pedal pulses was delayed for more than 1 hour in 20 patients, but pulses were palpable by 6 hours in all but two children, both of whom developed complete arterial thrombosis. On the basis of radiographic evidence, Franken and associates concluded that the primary factor that produced severe vascular spasm was the relatively large catheter-to-artery size required for angiography in pediatric patients. It was suggested that the development of thin-walled catheters with increased flow rates would result in a substantial decrease in the incidence of thrombotic complications.

With continued improvement in technique and equipment, this problem has become less frequent. In 1979, Rubenson and co-workers evaluated the incidence of acute and chronic thromboembolic complications in a group of 253 children who underwent diagnostic angiography utilizing a percutaneous "catheter-over-wire" arterial access technique.[76] Only six patients (2.4%) developed evidence of acute vascular insufficiency, and at the time of arterial exploration obstructing thrombotic masses were observed at the arterial puncture site in five children. The remaining

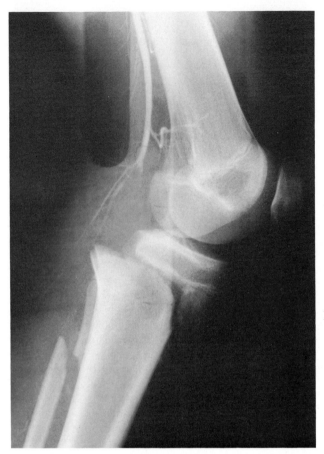

FIGURE 19–5

This femoral arteriogram was obtained in a 15-year-old boy who sustained a fracture dislocation of the proximal tibia and fibula. Complete obstruction of the popliteal artery is apparent, and very little collateral blood flow is observed.

patient developed a distal embolus that responded to heparin administration. In the remote follow-up period, Rubenson and colleagues noted no evidence of impaired limb growth, but three patients had significantly decreased arterial pulsations as measured by oscillography.

Adar and colleagues reviewed the outcome of 180 children who required left ventricular catheterization and reported a 12.6% incidence of postcatheterization ischemia.[1] In 11 patients (5.5%), surgical intervention was needed for management of either thrombosis (8) or traumatic laceration of the vessel (3). Late follow-up of 95 children demonstrated no evidence of leg length discrepancy or functional disability, however.

Because of potential problems with growth disturbance and functional disability, we recommend that the thromboembolic complications associated with diagnostic angiography be managed aggressively.[52] If arterial spasm is the problem, it should resolve spontaneously within 3 to 4 hours. If extremity ischemia as evaluated by absent pulses or decreased oscillography persists beyond 4 hours, exploration of the arterial access site should be performed. Fogarty catheter thrombectomy with meticulous repair of the arteriotomy site provides relief of acute ischemic symptoms in the vast majority of patients. Remote postoperative fol-

low up of all children who require diagnostic arterial access is recommended, and particular attention should be focused on the potential for abnormalities of limb growth and exercise intolerance in the affected extremity.

VASCULAR TRAUMA

In contrast to the overwhelming predominance of iatrogenic injuries in patients younger than 2 years of age, vascular trauma in older children and adolescents is usually not iatrogenic in origin.[81, 83, 88, 90] Increased mobility unaccompanied by improved judgment, access to vehicles for transportation, and availability of weapons predispose children to a wide variety of blunt and penetrating injuries that may damage the vascular system. Vascular involvement should be suspected in all patients with penetrating injuries that are in proximity to vessels and in all blunt trauma victims with crush injuries, displaced long bone fractures, and fractures or dislocations involving joints (Fig.19–5). A high index of suspicion is necessary if prompt diagnosis and timely therapeutic intervention are to be achieved. Most investigators emphasize that vascular repair should be accomplished within 6 hours of the injury if an optimal outcome is to be expected.

Since April 1985, the National Pediatric Trauma Registry has been accumulating data from 38 pediatric trauma centers.[38] During the first 2 years of registry activity, 5267 trauma patients have required admission at the participating hospitals and 60 children (1.1%) have been documented to have major vascular injuries (Table 19–1). The majority of the patients were male, and 80% were older than 5 years of age. Penetrating injuries were more frequent than blunt impact trauma. Surgical management was required for 33 of the 60 patients (55%). The mortality rate for the children who sustained vascular trauma was increased almost tenfold (23% vs. 2.8%) compared with that of all of the children in the registry population. This suggests that severe associated injuries are common in children sustaining major vascular trauma.

Penetrating Trauma

Although the mechanism of injury in most pediatric trauma victims is blunt impact, this is not the cause of the majority

Table 19–1

Data from the National Pediatric Trauma Registry on Patients with Vascular Trauma

Total patients	5267	
Patients with vascular injury	60	1.1%
Male to female ratio	43:17	
Age Distribution		
1—5 years	12	20%
6–10 years	21	35%
11–15 years	20	33%
16–20 years	7	12%
Mechanism of Injury		
Penetrating	35	58%
Blunt	23	38%
Operating management required	33	55%
Mortality	14	23%

of vascular injuries. At the Columbus Children's Hospital, 92 children with 98 arterial injuries have been treated during the past 14 years.[18] The cause of these injuries included broken glass (47), motor vehicle accidents (16), knife wounds (7), gunshots (6), crush injuries (5), lawn mower accidents (4), and miscellaneous (7). The upper extremity was involved most frequently, accounting for more than 60% of the injuries observed. Lower extremity trauma was noted in 28% of the children, visceral vessels accounted for 6%, and vascular injuries in the neck were least common (4%). A number of important clinical observations were apparent on review of our patient population.

1. Associated nerve injuries were common (40%).
2. Orthopedic injuries were observed in 22%.
3. Delay in diagnosis (longer than 6 hours) was frequent (24%).
4. Poor functional results with chronic ischemia or amputation were uncommon (6%).
5. Four of the six children who had an unsatisfactory outcome had a delay in diagnosis.
6. All of the poor results occurred in patients with injuries adjacent to the knee or elbow.

Table 19–2 presents data from five clinical reports on vascular trauma in 243 pediatric patients.[18, 48, 59, 72, 81] More than three fourths of the reported injuries were the result of penetrating trauma (78%). Broken glass was the source of injury in 85 children; 46 sustained gunshot wounds, and stabbing accounted for 10 injuries, whereas motor vehicle incidents accounted for 61 injuries, or 25%, of the cases. In this collated series the male-to-female ratio was 3:1; upper extremity damage was observed in 132 patients (50%); the lower extremity was involved in 80 (31%); visceral vessels were injured in 26 children (10%); and neck injuries were least common (7%). Associated neural and orthopedic trauma was noted in the majority of the patients. Delay in

diagnosis was common (15%) and appeared to substantively increase the risk of a poor outcome. Amputation was infrequently required (3.7%). Fifteen children died, yielding an overall mortality rate of 6%.

Injuries to major vessels in the neck represent a very small percentage of the vascular trauma in childhood. Of the 243 patients listed in Table 19–2, only 19 arterial injuries occurred in the neck. Despite this low incidence, the mortality from penetrating neck trauma in children has been reported to be as high as 20%. Ordog and associates attribute the increased mortality rate in children to anatomic considerations: a high concentration of vital structures in a very small cross-sectional area and little subcutaneous fat and muscular tissue to protect these structures.[62]

Injuries to the neck vessels are almost always the result of penetrating trauma. The available literature is divided on selective versus mandatory exploration of neck wounds that penetrate the platysma. To facilitate the decision-making process following penetrating neck injury, the neck has been divided into anatomic zones.[69] Zone I includes the structures between the cricoid cartilage and the clavicle. Zone II is the area between the cricoid cartilage and the angle of the mandible. Zone III includes injuries above the angle of the mandible. The vast majority of traumatic events affect the structures in zone II.[2, 6, 50] Diagnostic and therapeutic controversies center on (1) the need for arteriography and (2) selective versus mandatory exploration of penetrating injuries. Narrod and Moore recommend preoperative angiography in all patients with a zone I injury, with multiple wounds in zone II, or with injuries in zone III that are thought to involve the carotid arteries.[58] Patients with active hemorrhage, expanding hematomas, or pulse deficits and children with esophageal or tracheal injuries as demonstrated by dysphagia, crepitus, or radiographic evidence of extraluminal air should also undergo mandatory neck exploration.[69] Very little data exist on the accuracy of

Table 19–2
The Etiology and Anatomic Distribution of Pediatric Vascular Trauma

Author	Year	Male/ Female	Penetrating/ Blunt	Etiology				
				MVA	Glass	GSW	Knife	Other
Shaker	1976	— —	22/8	8	9	9	2	2
Meagher	1979	26/13	28/11	9	5	22	1	2
Richardson	1981	19/6	14/11	11	5	9	—	—
Navarre	1982	51/8	— —	17	19	—	—	24
Evans	1988	66/26	71/21	16	47	6	7	16
TOTALS		162/53	135/51	61	85	46	10	44
PERCENT		75/25	73/27	25	35	19	4	18

Author	Year	Patients/ Injuries	Delay in Diagnosis	Location					Outcome	
				Arm	Leg	Visceral	Neck	Other	Death	Amputation
Shaker	1976	28/30	1	14	6	3	2	5	3	2
Meagher	1979	39/—	—	14	9	11	5	—	7	1
Richardson	1981	25/33	2	7	15	4	7	—	2	0
Navarre	1982	59/60	10	34	23	2	1	—	0	4
Evans	1988	92/100	23	63	27	6	4	—	3	2
TOTALS		243/262	36	132	80	26	19	5	15	9
PERCENT			15	50	31	10	7	2	6	3.7

MVA, Motor vehicle accident; GSW, gunshot wound.

panendoscopy and contrast radiographs in the pediatric age group, but these techniques have been helpful in adults.[61, 73]

Blunt Trauma

Arterial injuries that occur as a result of blunt trauma are unusual in children, and they represent a particularly insidious clinical problem.[13, 22] Patients who sustain major blunt impact trauma frequently have life-threatening multiple organ system injuries that require immediate attention and that may initially distract the physician and delay recognition of a vascular lesion. Because blunt impact trauma is a relatively unusual cause of arterial injury, a high index of suspicion must be maintained if early diagnosis is to be achieved (Fig. 19–6). The clinical appearance of the extremity in a patient with a significant blunt vascular injury may not include the classical signs of arterial insufficiency (pain, pallor, pulselessness, paresthesias, paralysis). Associated peripheral or central nervous system damage may make an assessment of sensory and motor deficits difficult, if not impossible. Absent or diminished pulses distal to the area of injury are the single most reliable physical finding, but palpable pulses have been documented in up to 20% of pediatric patients with arterial injuries. Arteriography should be utilized whenever vascular injury is suspected.

Long bone fractures and dislocations are responsible for the vast majority of blunt arterial trauma. Arterial injuries have been documented to occur in up to 3% of patients with long bone fractures who require hospital admission.[27] The orthopedic injuries that are well known to be associated with extremity ischemia are fractures of the mid and distal portion of the femur, dislocations of the elbow and knee, tibial plateau injuries, and midshaft fractures of the humerus. The lower extremity injuries are usually sustained in motor vehicle accidents, and substantial associated soft tissue trauma occurs as a result of falls.

The anatomic distribution of the arterial injuries associated with blunt impact trauma in 278 adults and children is presented in Table 19–3.[27, 49, 63, 68, 85] Lower extremity trauma predominated, representing 70% of the total. Almost one half of all of the lower extremity injuries involved the popliteal vessels; 28% were observed in the femoral artery; and vessels distal to the knee were affected in 25% of the patients. In the upper extremity, brachial artery injuries were most common (55%). Axillary artery trauma was observed in 20% of the patients, and in 25% the radial or ulnar vessels, or both, were occluded.

The spectrum of potential anatomic abnormalities associated with blunt trauma includes (1) contusion with vascular spasm, (2) intimal tear, (3) complete or partial arterial disruption, (4) formation of a pseudoaneurysm, (5) creation of an arteriovenous fistula, and (6) arterial entrapment. The most common anatomic finding encountered at surgery is an intimal tear with thrombosis, and this was observed in 75% of the patients reported by Meek and Robbs.[49] A number of important points should be considered in the surgical management of patients with blunt arterial injuries.

1. Expeditious diagnosis and immediate repair are necessary if an optimal outcome is to be expected.

2. Preoperative evaluation should include a detailed evaluation of neurologic function because of the high incidence of associated disabling nerve injuries.

3. If definitive vascular repair must be delayed because of associated life-threatening injuries, temporary placement of an intravascular shunt should be considered.

4. Fasciotomy should be utilized liberally, particularly in patients with lower extremity trauma.

5. If a fasciotomy is not performed, compartment pressures should be monitored.

6. Major venous injuries should be repaired simultaneously.

7. Circumferential casts should not be applied to an extremity with a suspected vascular injury.

8. External fixation may provide the best method of immobilizing open fractures.

Despite early diagnosis and aggressive surgical management, the outcome for patients with blunt impact vascular trauma is far from ideal. Ransom and co-workers reported that major amputations were required in 13 of 58 patients (22%).[68] The amputation rate was 18% in patients with upper extremity injuries and was somewhat higher in those with lower extremity trauma (25%). Sturm and colleagues have reported similar results in a group of 29 patients with blunt impact arterial injuries (17% amputations).[85] The majority of the amputations were required because of injuries to vessels about the knee and elbow.

The overall results of management of patients with blunt impact vascular damage compares very unfavorably with the 3 to 5% amputation rate routinely reported in patients with penetrating civilian arterial trauma. Even when preservation of the extremity is achieved, functional integrity may be lost because of associated nerve injuries. The inci-

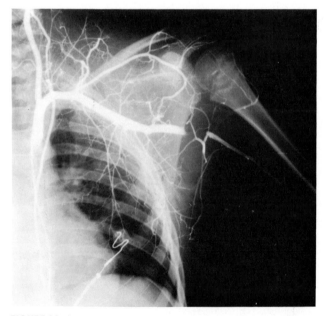

FIGURE 19–6

Thrombosis of the axillary artery is evident in this 8-year-old boy, who sustained a hyperextension injury of the shoulder in a snowmobile accident. The left upper extremity was viable but pulseless on physical examination.

Table 19-3
Anatomic Distribution of Arterial Injuries in Patients with Blunt Impact Injuries

Author/ Year	Sturn 1980	Ransom 1981	Meek 1984	Guercio 1984	Palazzo 1986
Patients	29	58	100	64	27
Upper Extremity 91 cases—30%					
Axillary	4	9	1	3	1
Brachial	7	12	17	8	6
Radial/Ulnar	5	3	0	6	9
Lower Extremity 211 cases—70%					
Femoral	7	10	26	11	4
Popliteal	5	14	57	17	10
Distal	5	21	0	15	9

dence of disabling neurologic damage is highest in patients with upper extremity trauma and is most commonly observed in those individuals with axillary or brachial artery injuries.

Because of the complex nature of these lesions, a team approach to the initial evaluation and management of these patients should be recommended. Primary amputation rather than vascular reconstruction may be appropriate if extensive soft tissue damage or major neurologic deficits are apparent. The need for prolonged and intensive physiotherapy in the postoperative period should be anticipated.

Compartment Syndromes

Vascular compromise as a result of either blunt or penetrating injury may produce hemorrhage and edema in the injured extremity, which can progress to the development of a compartment syndrome. Failure to promptly recognize and treat increased compartment pressures may result in sensory and motor deficits, contractures, and loss of function in the affected extremity. The diagnosis of a compartment syndrome should be considered in any patient with either blunt or penetrating trauma who develops increasing localized pain and swelling in the area of injury with pain on passive motion of the affected muscle group. In the lower extremity, a sensory deficit in the web space between the great and second toes is a valuable early sign of increased compartment pressure. Arterial pulses may be intact initially and are diminished only when compartment pressures approach systemic blood pressures.

If a compartment syndrome is suspected, immediate action must be taken either to evaluate the intracompartmental pressure directly or to perform an emergency fasciotomy. Compartment pressures can be measured by insertion of a Wick catheter into the muscle.[57] Pressures greater than 30 mm Hg are considered elevated in the normotensive patient, and fasciotomy is required. Absolute indications for a fasciotomy at the time of initial revascularization include (1) an arterial injury with concomitant venous compromise, (2) an arterial injury with severe soft tissue trauma, and (3) progressive postoperative edema resulting in vascular insufficiency. A prolonged delay between injury and revascularization (longer than 10–12 hours) is a relative indication for decompression.

Ernst and Kaufer have proposed a fibulectomy as the best method of four-compartment fascial decompression in the lower extremity.[17] Richardson and associates noted that four of 29 children suffering arterial injuries required fasciotomy and recommended four-compartment decompression through the bed of the fibula.[72]

Pelvic Fractures

In adults fractures of the pelvis are associated with an inordinately high mortality rate (10–15%), which is usually the result of exsanguinating extraperitoneal hemorrhage.[33, 75] In the pediatric patient the pelvis is far less rigid than its adult counterpart and is subject to deformation without fracture. Identification of disruption of the pelvic ring in children, therefore, is indicative of severe trauma, and the possibility of injury to the pelvic viscera and vessels must be considered. Torode and Zieg reported 40 children with unstable pelvic fractures (type IV); laparotomy was required in 40% of the patients, and a mortality rate of 12% was observed.[87]

In Table 19–4 data from four clinical reports on pelvic fractures in childhood are presented.[9, 66, 70, 71] Overall, the incidence of associated visceral injuries was 16.0%, and the risk of significant vascular trauma was 4.7%. Thirteen of the 276 children died (4.7%). Clearly, pelvic fractures are significant injuries that deserve careful evaluation and management. On initial assessment, extensive soft tissue trauma, disruption of the sacroiliac joint, absence of a femoral pulse, or loss of sciatic nerve function are all indicators of severe pelvic trauma and should suggest potential major vascular damage. Shock secondary to significant blood loss is common in such patients, and blood transfusion is frequently required to maintain the circulating blood volume and hemodynamic stability. In Quinby's report, four of the five children with exsanguinating hemorrhage associated with pelvic fractures required an operation for control of vascular injuries.[66] Lacerations and avulsions of the iliac, gluteal, and lumbar arteries were observed. Estimated blood loss ranged from 3500 to 8000 ml, and four of the five children died.

At present, an initial trial of external counterpressure utilizing medical anti-shock trousers (MAST) is advised for

Table 19–4
The Mortality Rate and Incidence of Visceral and Vascular Trauma in Children with Pelvic Fractures

Author	Year	Patients	Vascular Injury	Visceral Injury	Death
Quinby	1966	20	5	12	5
Reed	1976	84	—	16	2
Bryan	1979	52	4	8	4
Reichard	1980	120	4	8	2
TOTALS		276	13	44	13
PERCENT			4.7	16	4.7

any child with a pelvic hemorrhage. Failure of transfusion and MAST to maintain circulatory stability indicates the necessity for urgent diagnostic and therapeutic intervention.

If the hemorrhage persists and the hemodynamic status remains unstable, an aortogram should be obtained to evaluate the retroperitoneal and pelvic vasculature. Angiographic occlusion of arterial vessels disrupted by pelvic trauma has provided good clinical results. Brown and colleagues reported on a 13-year old boy with a false aneurysm of the superior gluteal artery that was obliterated with Gelfoam.[8] Sundaram and associates also reported the successful use of embolization for control of a bleeding gluteal artery,[86] and Reichard and co-workers have suggested the use of radiopaque silicone balloons for management of ongoing pelvic hemorrhage.[71] Other researchers have utilized direct operative repair of the involved vessels or ligation of the hypogastric arteries, but current reports appear to favor early angiographic evaluation and embolotherapy over direct surgical intervention.[93]

The Role of Arteriography

The incidence of pediatric vascular injuries appears to be increasing, particularly in the major metropolitan areas where use of weapons is common among children and adolescents. The need for an accurate evaluation of the presence and extent of injury in patients with suspected vascular trauma is obvious. Although the issue of emergency angiography has been widely debated in the literature on adults, little data exist that would help to define the precise role of arteriography in the pediatric trauma victim. The published reviews on repair of pediatric vascular injuries have reported infrequent use of angiography, and no specific guidelines have been developed for its use in the emergency setting. Preoperative angiography has been employed with varying degrees of apparent benefit. Meagher states that arteriography is "seldom indicated," whereas Richardson describes it as "valuable" in selected situations.[48, 72]

Because the complication rate following diagnostic angiography in young children is relatively high, the indiscriminate use of arteriography should be discouraged. In patients with penetrating injuries and such obvious signs of significant vascular trauma as brisk arterial bleeding, pulse deficits, or expanding hematomas, arteriography may not be helpful, and clinical management should include immediate operative exploration.[23, 25] The remaining patients with penetrating injuries "in proximity" to major vessels have been managed by various investigators with mandatory exploration, selective operation based on clinical findings, or arteriography.[26, 74, 79, 82] Geuder and colleagues compared routine exploration with arteriography for "proximity" injuries and demonstrated a reduction in the negative exploration rate from 84.0% to 2.4%.[23] Exploration for proximity of injury would have resulted in an 83% negative exploration rate in the study by Gorman and associates compared with a 1.3% false negative arteriographic result.[26] The low incidence of vascular injuries associated with penetrating trauma in proximity to major vessels has led some researchers to question the need for angiography in this situation. Gomez and co-workers obtained normal arteriograms in 55 of 72 patients with penetrating injuries when proximity was the only indication for contrast study.[25] The investigators felt that angiography was not indicated for penetrating injuries that are "in proximity" to major vascular structures. Our current indications for angiography in pediatric vascular trauma include the following:

1. Any penetrating neck wound in zone I or II or multiple injuries in zone II
2. Pelvic fractures with ongoing massive blood loss
3. Failure of peripheral pulses to reappear after closed reduction of long bone fractures
4. Injuries resulting from multiple wounds (i.e., shotgun blast injuries)
5. Severe crush injuries with extensive soft tissue damage
6. Fractures or dislocations about the elbow and the knee

Using these criteria, we have been satisfied that the majority of diagnostic angiographic studies obtained are definitely indicated and that very few injuries are overlooked on initial evaluation.

References

1. Adar R, Rubinstein N, Blieden L: Immediate complications and late sequelae of arterial catheterization in children with congenital heart disease. Pediatr Cardiol 4:25–28, 1983.
2. Ayuyao AM, Kaledzi YL, Parsa MH, et al: Penetrating neck wounds: Mandatory versus selective exploration. Ann Surg 202:563–567, 1985.
3. Bassett FH III, Lincoln CR, King TD, et al: Inequality in the size of the lower extremity following cardiac catheterization. South Med J 61:1013–1017, 1968.
4. Bedford RF, Wollman H: Complications of percutaneous radial-artery

cannulation: An objective prospective study in man. Anesthesiology 38:228–236, 1973.

5. Bergqvist D, Bergentz SE, Hermansson G, et al: Late ischaemic sequelae after umbilical artery catheterization. Br J Surg 74:628–629, 1987.

6. Bishara RA, Pasch AR, Douglas DD, et al: The necessity of mandatory exploration of penetrating zone II neck injuries. Surgery 100:655–660, 1986.

7. Bosque E, Weaver L: Continuous versus intermittent heparin infusion of umbilical artery catheters in the newborn infant. J Pediatr 108:141–143, 1986.

8. Brown JJ, Green FL, McMillin RD: Vascular injuries associated with pelvic fractures. Am Surg 50:150–154, 1984.

9. Bryan WJ, Tullos HS: Pediatric pelvic fractures: Review of 52 patients. J Trauma 19:799–805, 1979.

10. Caeton AJ, Goetzman BW: Risky business: Umbilical artery catheterization. Am J Dis Child 139:120–121, 1985.

11. Cartwright GW, Schreiner RL: Major complications secondary to percutaneous radial artery catheterization in the neonate. Pediatrics 65:139–141, 1980.

12. Chidi CC, King DR, Boles ET Jr: An ultrastructural study of the intimal injury induced by an indwelling umbilical artery catheter. J Pediatr Surg 18:109–115, 1983.

13. Cole WG: Arterial injuries associated with fractures of the lower limbs in childhood. Injury 12:460–463, 1980–81.

14. Dmochowski RR, Crandell SS, Corriere JN Jr: Bladder injury and uroascites from umbilical artery catheterization. Pediatrics 77:421–422, 1986.

15. Drucker DEM, Greenfield LJ, Ehrlich F, et al: Aorto-iliac aneurysms following umbilical artery catheterization. J Pediatr Surg 21:725–730, 1986.

16. Dunn PM: Localization of the umbilical catheter by postmortem measurement. Arch Dis Child 41:69–75, 1966.

17. Ernst CB, Kaufer J: Fibulectomy-fasciotomy: An important adjunct in the management of lower extremity arterial trauma. J Trauma 11:465–380, 1971.

18. Evans WE, King DR, Hayes JP: Arterial trauma in children: Diagnosis and management. Ann Vasc Surg 2(3):268–270, 1988.

19. Fok TF, Ha MH, Leung KW, et al: Sciatic nerve palsy complicating umbilical artery catheterization. Eur J Pediatr 145:308–309, 1986.

20. Franken EA Jr, Girod D, Sequeira FW, et al: Femoral artery spasm in children: Catheter size is the principal cause. AJR 138:295–298, 1982.

21. Freed MD, Keane JF, Rosenthal A: The use of heparinization to prevent arterial thrombosis after percutaneous cardiac catheterization in children. Circulation 50:565–569, 1974.

22. Friedman RJ, Jupiter JB: Vascular injuries and closed extremity fractures in children. Clin Orthop 188:112–119, 1984.

23. Geuder JW, Hobson RW II, Padbert FT Jr, et al: The role of contrast arteriography in suspected arterial injuries of the extremities. Am Surg 51:89–93, 1985.

24. Goetzman BW, Stadalnik RC, Bogren HE, et al: Thrombotic complications of umbilical artery catheters: A clinical and radiographic study. Pediatrics 56:374–379, 1975.

25. Gomez GA, Kreis DJ Jr, Ratner L, et al: Suspected vascular trauma of the extremities: The role of arteriography in proximity injuries. J Trauma 26:1005–1008, 1986.

26. Gorman RB, Feliciano DV, Bitondo CG, et al: Emergency center arteriography in the evaluation of suspected peripheral vascular injuries. Arch Surg 119:568–572, 1984.

27. Guercio N, Orsini G: Fractures of the limbs complicated by ischaemia due to lesions of the major vessels. Ital J Orthop Traumatol 10:163–185, 1984.

28. Gross RE: Arterial embolism and thrombosis in infancy. Am J Dis Child 70:61–73, 1945.

29. Harris MS, Litte GA: Umbilical artery catheters: High, low, or no. J Perinatal Med 6:15, 1978.

30. Hodson WA, Troug WE: Peripheral arterial catheterization. In: Avery GB (ed): Neonatology. 3rd ed. Philadelphia, JB Lippincott, 1983, pp 469–474.

31. Horgan MJ, Bartoletti A, Polansky S, et al: Effect of heparin infusates in umbilical arterial catheters on frequency of thrombotic complications. J Pediatr 111:774–778, 1987.

32. Jackson JC, Troug WE, Watchko JF, et al: Efficacy of thrombo-resistant umbilical artery catheters in reducing aortic thrombosis and related complications. J Pediatr 110:102–105, 1987.

33. Kam J, Jackson H, Ben-Menachem Y: Vascular injuries in blunt pelvic trauma. Radiol Clin North Am 19:171–186, 1981.

34. Katz ME, Perlman JM, Tack ED, et al: Neonatal umbilical artery pseudoaneurysm: Sonographic evaluation (case report). AJR 147:322–324, 1986.

35. Kraus AN, Albert RF, Kannan MM: Contamination of umbilical vessel in the newborn infant. J Pediatr 77:963, 1970.

36. Krishnamoorthy KS, Fernandez RJ, Rodres ID, et al: Paraplegia associated with umbilical artery catheterization in the newborn. Pediatrics 58:443–445, 1976.

37. Krueger TC, Neblett WW, O'Neill JA, et al: Management of aortic thrombosis secondary to umbilical artery catheters in neonates. J Pediatr Surg 20:328–332, 1985.

38. LaScala C, National Pediatric Trauma Registry. Personal communication, August 1987.

39. Leblanc J, Wood AE, O'Shea MA, et al: Peripheral arterial trauma in children. J Cardiovasc Surg 26:325–331, 1985.

40. Lowenstein E, Little JW III, Lo HH: Prevention of cerebral embolization from flushing radial-artery cannulas. N Engl J Med 285:1414–1415, 1971.

41. McFaul RC, Keane JF, Nowicki ER, et al: Aortic thrombosis in the neonate. J Thorac Cariovasc Surg 81:334–337, 1981.

42. Mackereth MRN, Lennihan R Jr: Gangrene of the extremity in infants and children. Angiology 23:688–698, 1972.

43. McMillan I, Maurie JA: Vascular injury following cardiac catheterization. Br J Surg 71:832–835, 1984.

44. Mansfield PB, Gazzaniga AB, Litwin SB: Management of arterial injuries related to cardiac catheterization in children and young adults. Circulation 62:501–507, 1970.

45. Mares AJ, Siplovich L: Obliterated umbilical artery abscess simulating a strangulated umbilical hernia: A late complication of neonatal umbilical artery catheterization. Isr J Med Sci 20:1197–1198, 1984.

46. Marsh JL, King W, Barrett C, et al: Serious complications after umbilical artery catheterization for neonatal monitoring. Arch Surg 110:1203–1208, 1975.

47. Mayer T, Matlak ME, Thompson JA: Necrosis of the forearm following radial artery catheterization in a patient with Reye's Syndrome. Pediatrics 65:141–143, 1980.

48. Meagher DP Jr, Defore WW, Mattox KL, et al: Vascular trauma in infants and children. J Trauma 19:532–536, 1979.

49. Meek AC, Robbs JV: Vascular injury with associated bone and joint trauma. Br J Surg 71:341–344, 1984.

50. Meyer JP, Barrett JA, Schuler JJ, et al: Mandatory vs selective exploration for penetrating neck trauma: A prospective assessment. Arch Surg 122:592–597, 1987.

51. Miller D, Kirkpatrick BV, Kodroff M, et al: Pelvic exsanguination following umbilical artery catheterization in neonates. J Pediatr Surg 14:264–269, 1979.

52. Mills JL, Wiedeman JE, Robison JG, et al: Minimizing mortality and morbidity from iatrogenic arterial injuries: The need for early recognition and prompt repair. J Vasc Surg 4:22–27, 1986.

53. Miyasaka K, Edmonds JF, Conn AW: Complications of radial artery lines in the paediatric patient. Can Anaesth Soc J 23:9–14, 1976.

54. Mokrohisky ST, Levine RL, Blumhagen JD, et al: Low positioning of umbilical-artery catheters increases associated complications in newborn infants. N Engl J Med 229:561–564, 1978.

55. Mortensson W: Angiography of the femoral artery following percutaneous catheterization in infants and children. Acta Radiologica Diag 17:581–593, 1976.

56. Mozersky DJ, Buckley CJ, Hagood CO Jr, et al: Ultrasonic evaluation of the palmar circulation. Am J Surg 126:810–812, 1973.

57. Mubarah JJ: The Wick catheter technique for measurement of intramuscular pressure: A new research and clinical tool. J Bone Joint Surg 58:1016, 1976.

58. Narrod JA, Moore EE: Selective management of penetrating neck injuries: A prospective study. Arch Surg 119:574–578, 1984.

59. Navarre JR, Cardillo PJ, Gorman JF, et al: Vascular trauma in children and adolescents. Am J Surg 143:229–231, 1982.

60. Neal WA, Reynolds JW, Jarvis CW, et al: Umbilical artery catheterization: Demonstration of arterial thrombosis by aortography. Pediatrics 50:6–13, 1972.

61. Noyes LD, McSwain NE Jr, Markowitz IP: Panendoscopy with arteriography versus mandatory exploration of penetrating wound of the neck. Ann Surg 204:21–31, 1986.

62. Ordog GJ, Prakash A, Wasserberger J, et al: Pediatric gunshot wounds. J Trauma 27:1272–1278, 1987.

63. Palazzo JC, Ristow AVB, Cury JM, et al: Traumatic vascular lesions associated with fractures and dislocations. J Cardiovasc Surg 27:688–696, 1986.
64. Plumber LB, Kaplan GW, Mandoza SA: Hypertension in infants: A complication of umbilical arterial catheterization. J Pediatr 89:802, 1976.
65. Powers WF, Tooley WH: Contamination of umbilical vessel catheters: Encouraging information. Pediatrics 49:470, 1972.
66. Quinby WC Jr: Fractures of the pelvis and associated injuries in children. J Pediatr Surg 1:353–364, 1966.
67. Rabin E, Vye MW, Farrell EE: Umbilical artery catheterization complicated by multiple mycotic aortic aneurysms. Arch Pathol Lab Med 110:442–444, 1986.
68. Ransom KJ, Shatney CH, Soderstrom CA, et al: Management of arterial injuries in blunt trauma of the extremity. Surg Gynecol Obstet 153:241–246, 1981.
69. Rao PM, Bhatti KJ, Ivatury RR, et al: Selective management of penetrating neck wounds. Contemp Surg 23:41–47, 1983.
70. Reed MH: Pelvic fractures in children. J Can Assoc Radiol 27:255–261, 1976.
71. Reichard SA, Helikson MA, Shorter N: Pelvic fractures in children—Review of 120 patients with a new look at general management. J Pediatr Surg 15:727–734, 1980.
72. Richardson JD, Fallat M, Nagaraj HS, et al: Arterial injuries in children. Arch Surg 116:685–690, 1981.
73. Roon AJ, Christensen N: Evaluation and treatment of penetrating cervical injuries. J Trauma 19:391–397, 1979.
74. Rose SC, Moore EE: Emergency trauma angiography: Accuracy, safety, and pitfalls. AJR 148:1243–1246, 1987.
75. Rothenberger DA, Fischer RP, Perry JF Jr: Major vascular injuries secondary to pelvic fractures: An unsolved clinical problem. Am J Surg 136:660–662, 1978.
76. Rubenson A, Jacobsson B, Sorensen S-E: Treatment and sequelae of angiographic complications in children. J Pediatr Surg 14:154–157, 1982.
77. Sasidharan P: Umbilical artery rupture: A major complication of catheterization. Indiana Med 78:34–35, 1985.
78. Schmidt B, Wais U, Furste HO, et al: Arterial occlusion in a preterm infant: Successful non-surgical treatment with urokinase and low-dose heparin. Helv Paediat Acta 37:483–488, 1982.
79. Sclafani SJA, Cooper R, Shafton GW, et al: Arterial trauma: Diagnostic and therapeutic angiography. Radiology 161:165–172, 1986.
80. Seibert JJ, Taylor BJ, Williamson SL, et al: Sonographic detection of neonatal umbilical-artery thrombosis: Clinical correlation. AJR 148:965–968, 1987.
81. Shaker IJ, White JJ, Signer RD, et al: Special problems of vascular injuries in children. J Trauma 16:863–867, 1976.
82. Sirinek KR, Gaskill HV, Dittman WI, et al: Exclusion angiography for patients with possible vascular injuries of the extremities—A better use of trauma center resources. Surgery 94:598–603, 1983.
83. Stanford JR, Evans WE, Morse TS: Pediatric arterial injuries. Angiology 27:1–7, 1976.
84. Stringel G, Mercer S, Richler M, et al: Catheterization of the umbilical artery in neonates: Surgical implications. Can J Surg 28:143–145, 1985.
85. Sturm JT, Bodily KC, Rothenberger DA, et al: Arterial injuries of the extremities following blunt trauma. J Trauma 20:933–936, 1980.
86. Sundaram M, Patel B, Wolverson MK, et al: Superior gluteal artery haemorrhage following pelvic fractures controlled by embolization. Clin Radiol 32:187–190, 1981.
87. Torode I, Zieg D: Pelvic fractures in children. J Pediatr Orthop 5:76–84, 1985.
88. Villavicencio JL, Gonzalez-Cerna JL, Velasco P: Acute vascular problems of children. Curr Probl Surg 22:1–85, 1985.
89. Wesstrom G, Finnstrom O, Stemport G: Umbilical artery catheterization in newborns. Acta Paediatr 68:575–581, 1979.
90. Whitehouse WM, Coran AG, Stanley JC, et al: Pediatric vascular trauma. Arch Surg 111:1269–1275, 1976.
91. Wigger HJ, Bransilver BR, Blanc WA: Thromboses due to catheterization in infants and children. J Pediatr 76:1–11, 1970.
92. Wilkins RG: Radial artery cannulation and ischaemic damage: A review. Anaesthesia 40:896–899, 1985.
93. Yellin AE, Lundell CJ, Finck EJ: Diagnosis and control of posttraumatic pelvic hemorrhage: Transcatheter angiographic embolization techniques. Arch Surg 118:1378–1383, 1983.

Frank P. Lynch III

CHAPTER TWENTY

Liver Injuries

MECHANISM OF INJURY

ANATOMY

DIAGNOSIS

RESUSCITATION

PATTERNS OF INJURY

GRADING SYSTEMS

OPERATIVE APPROACH

Table 20-1
Hepatic Injury

Series	Child Struck		Passenger	Misc*	GSW	Bicycle	Stab	ATV
No. of patients	42	21	7	5	2	2	1	4
Age (years)	5.63	5.2	5.3	4.6	8.0	7.0	2.0	8.8
Male	28	15	3	2	1	2	1	3
Female	14	6	4	3	1	0	0	1
Trauma score	12.29	11.1	12.0	12.2	15.0	16.0	16.0	14.0
ISS	32	38	35	24	22	17	4	27
Ps	77	0.65	0.81	0.75	0.96	0.99	0.99	0.98
Survivors	36	17	6	4	2	2	1	4
Nonsurvivors	6	4	1	1	0	0	0	0
Observed survival	0.86	0.71	0.86	0.80	1.0	1.0	1.0	1.0

*Includes falls, crutches, and the like.
GSW, Gunshot wound; ATV, all-terrain vehicle; ISS, injury severity score; Ps, P score (probability of survival).

The importance of trauma in childhood cannot be overemphasized. It is the leading cause of mortality and morbidity in young people. Although head injury is the leading cause of death, abdominal trauma still plays a significant role. Touloukian and Welch, in separate reviews, reported that blunt injury accounts for more than 90% of all injury in childhood.[59, 63] In San Diego, where all injured children are brought directly to Children's Hospital, the liver is the most commonly injured intra-abdominal organ, and 90% of all hepatic injury in this group is caused by blunt forces.

Hepatic injury accounts for a significant number of all deaths due to trauma and for nearly all of the deaths related to abdominal trauma.[40] Recognition and treatment of hepatic injury, then, is of paramount importance to the surgeon managing the injured child.

Children are usually innocent victims, happening to be in the wrong place at the wrong time, and the incidence of childhood trauma seems to be increasing. The number of patients admitted to Children's Hospital in San Diego has increased by a threefold number of patients each year of the 4-year trauma system operation. Part of the increase is accounted for by an increasing population and the rest by an increase in automobile density. In 599 patients discharged between March 1986 and March 1987, 28% of the patients admitted were pedestrians struck by automobiles, an additional 12% were struck while riding bicycles, and 18% were passengers in automobiles. Of all our pediatric trauma, 58% of the cases involved the automobile. Persons struck by automobiles versus persons who were not were more likely to die: 15 deaths out of 167 patients, a mortality of 9.0%. Cyclists so injured also have a high risk of death: 7 of 79 admissions, or 8.9%. If the child is a passenger and is injured, the chance of death is only 4%. The other usual mechanisms of injury are less lethal. Falls, for example, have a mortality rate among patients in our institution of 2.7%.

In children, trauma is usually an unplanned event. In most families in which children are highly valued members, the event is devastating, even more so if the child is permanently disabled or dies. The loss to society of a child who dies or, perhaps more significantly, is disabled is enormous. Dealing with disability places a special burden on those managing the injured child. Such health care professionals must be expert in all areas of pediatric trauma and must ensure that their institutions are responsive to the special needs and requirements of children.

MECHANISM OF INJURY

The usual pediatric trauma victim is approximately 6 years of age and is male two thirds of the time. Sixty percent of these patients have isolated closed-head injuries. Approximately 20% have an abdominal injury, and the majority of these have multiple associated injuries, often some that include the head. These statistics are the same for the child with hepatic injury.

In a 3½-year period, 42 hepatic injuries were treated at Children's Hospital in San Diego (Table 20-1). Three of the children had penetrating injuries; two were gunshot wounds, and one was a miscellaneous missile wound, leaving 39 blunt injuries. The blunt injuries included 21 pedestrians and two bicyclists struck by motor vehicles and seven passengers in automobiles. The remaining patients had miscellaneous mechanisms of injury; however, the automobile was the vector in 76% of these hepatic injuries.

The severity of hepatic trauma depends on the mechanism of injury. In this series of 42 patients, there were six deaths—a mortality rate of 14%. Four of the six deaths occurred in the 21 pedestrians, a mortality rate of 19%. Only one of the seven automobile passengers was killed, and the final death was caused by a falling wall.

Current measures of severity commonly in use include the trauma score, the injury severity score (ISS), and the probability of survival derived mathematically from the first two. A low trauma score indicates severe metabolic derangement. A high ISS indicates the presence of multiple severe injuries. The probability of survival is self-explanatory: a low probability indicates a high chance of death. Children struck by automobiles are admitted with greater physiologic derangement, that is, a lower trauma score and a greater number of more severe injuries and therefore a high ISS. They are expected to have a lower probability of survival. Passengers in automobiles have less physiologic derangement and less severe injuries. Those with miscellaneous mechanisms of injury are even less severely injured.

The ISS reflects in numeric fashion the presence and severity of associated injuries. It has been amply documented in the literature that mortality from hepatic injury depends on the number of associated injuries.[11, 14, 24, 36, 56] Clearly, in children the nature and extent of injury and mortality is determined by the mechanism of injury; hence, the child struck by a motor vehicle should arouse the greatest suspicion of serious injury.

ANATOMY

To understand the nature and pattern of hepatic injury in children, a brief discussion of anatomy is in order. The surgical anatomy of the liver has been of great interest in the last 30 years, and a number of descriptions are available in the literature.[2, 4–6, 21, 30, 33]

The liver occupies the majority of the right upper quadrant of the abdomen and is divided into two lobes, right and left. Reflections of the parietal peritoneum serve as ligaments that fix the liver to the abdominal wall and diaphragm. The right lobe of the liver is securely fixed to the abdominal wall and diaphragm by the coronary ligament, and the large area between the anterior and posterior layers of the coronary ligament is referred to as the bare area. The left lobe is fixed somewhat less securely to the diaphragm by the triangular ligament, which has a much smaller bare area that communicates with that on the right. The coronary and triangular ligaments join to form the falciform ligament, which attaches to the anterior abdominal wall and continues from the diaphragm to the umbilicus. In its margin runs the usually obliterated umbilical vein, the ligamentum teres.

Although the falciform ligament would seem to divide the liver into right and left lobes, the true anatomic lobar division runs on a line connecting the gallbladder fossa and the lateral border of the vena cava. The falciform ligament marks the division between the medial and lateral segments of the left lobe. The right lobe of the liver is divided into an anterior and posterior segment. This is of some importance because in children it is the posterior segment that is most commonly injured.[39, 55] The liver has been further divided into eight functional segments, but from the standpoint of the trauma surgeon these are not important. The important divisions are the left lobe medial and lateral segments and the right lobe anterior and posterior segments.

The liver has two afferent and one efferent set of vessels. The afferent vessels are the hepatic artery and portal vein. The hepatic artery supplies approximately 30% of the blood and 50% of the oxygen and has several common anomalies. The left hepatic artery can arise from the left gastric artery. In this instance, it is to be found in the gastrohepatic ligament. The right hepatic artery may arise from the superior mesenteric artery. These anomalies are important if hepatic artery ligation is used for control of hemorrhage.

The common hepatic artery usually arises from the celiac axis, lies medial to the common duct in the hepatoduodenal ligament, and divides to the left of the lobar fissure, giving a long right hepatic artery and a relatively short left hepatic artery. The right hepatic artery enters the liver behind the right hepatic duct and when it enters the liver it divides into an anterior and posterior branch. It is this posterior branch of the right hepatic artery that is commonly injured in children. The left hepatic artery is rather short and divides almost immediately into its terminal branches.

The portal vein is formed by the confluence of the inferior mesenteric, splenic, and superior mesenteric veins. It enters the liver via the hepatoduodenal ligament. Just before entering the liver, it divides into a right and a left branch. The right portal vein is particularly short. It is located deep in the porta hepatis and is easily injured during dissection. Controlling the right portal vein is difficult in an elective controlled lobectomy, a difficulty magnified manyfold in the patient with hepatic injury and torrential blood loss. The dissection of the porta hepatis and its difficulties, particularly the portal vein, probably accounts for the poor results in right hepatic resection for trauma.

The anatomy of the extrahepatic biliary system is well known to all trauma surgeons. The right and left hepatic ducts join to form the common hepatic duct. The common hepatic duct is joined by the cystic duct on its right side to form the common bile duct. The common bile duct passes behind the duodenum to the ampulla of Vater, where it terminates. The intrahepatic ducts follow closely the anatomy of the hepatic artery.

The efferent drainage is of great interest to the trauma surgeon for it is from these vessels and the vena cava that torrential blood loss commonly occurs. Injury to these vessels is lethal in 50 to 100% of patients.[31, 44, 52, 53, 60]

The liver is drained by three hepatic veins: right, left, and middle. The right hepatic vein drains both the anterior and posterior segments of the right lobe, and it is commonly injured in children. The left hepatic vein drains the lateral segment of the left lobe. The middle hepatic vein drains a portion of the anterior segment of the right lobe and the medial segment of the left. The left and middle hepatic veins usually join the vena cava as a single trunk. The entrance of the right hepatic vein and the confluence of the middle and left into the vena cava occur just below the diaphragm and may be obscured by the parenchyma of the liver. It is usually not possible to gain proximal control of the hepatic veins without splitting the liver parenchyma. Various shunt systems have been used to control bleeding from the confluence of the hepatic veins and inferior vena cava. Difficulty in obtaining control of these vessels contributes significantly to the lethal nature of injuries in this area.

DIAGNOSIS

Hepatic injury must be suspected in any childhood injury that involves high-energy transfer. The child struck by a rapidly moving vehicle is the chief example. Passengers in high-energy crashes—especially unbelted passengers—are also at risk. Crush injuries can result in hepatic trauma, although falls seldom do. The chest wall, ribs, and abdominal musculature are reasonably resilient in children and may not reflect the magnitude of intra-abdominal injury. Tire marks, abrasions, and puncture wounds may offer clues to the diagnosis. A description of the event such as "the tire passed over the child" is also helpful. Paramedics are often the only adults accompanying the child, and the history must be a part of their report.

The pattern of injury and the number of associated injuries are determined by the mechanism of injury. Children struck by motor vehicles are much more likely to have multiple injuries, including central nervous system and chest injuries.

Intra-abdominal hemorrhage with resultant hypovolemia is the most common physiologic consequence of hepatic injury. The physiologic state of the patient depends on the severity of the anatomic injury and the amount of bleeding that has occurred. The amount of bleeding depends on the injury and the time elapsed from the time of the injury. Children may present as alert, talkative, and communicative or scared and crying or silent. Oftentimes they are unconscious, either from central nervous system injury or from hypovolemia. If the child is able to communicate, he or she may or may not complain of abdominal pain, but most will demonstrate abdominal tenderness and approximately half will have evidence of peritoneal irritation. Both abdominal tenderness and peritoneal irritation may be the result of acute gastric dilation. Although abdominal distention can be present if there has been a great deal of bleeding, the most common cause in children is swallowed air, causing acute gastric dilation. Placement of a nasogastric tube should be routine in the resuscitation area.

Hypovolemia is commonly present but may not be apparent. The San Diego paramedics have become uncommonly proficient in intravenous access, and more than half of our patients arrive with appropriate lines in place. Intravenous fluids and short transport times may mask significant blood loss. Moreover, children are remarkably able to compensate for hypovolemia. The earliest sign of hypovolemia in children is tachycardia. Children compensate in this fashion until they can no longer increase cardiac output by increasing rate. At this point they may go into profound shock, the so-called stairstep phenomenon. Children with vena caval injuries have come to the emergency department with stable vital signs. The most useful diagnostic tool is a suspicious nature and a willingness to utilize the ancillary diagnostic equipment available.

RESUSCITATION

When the seriously injured child is brought to the emergency department, a very rapid assessment of the child's condition is made following the Advanced Trauma Life Support guidelines. In a child (perhaps more than in an adult) a secure airway is of paramount importance. If an airway is inadequate or not secure, the patient is intubated immediately. An associated head injury occasions hyperventilation. The awake, communicative patient can be questioned regarding the nature and extent of injuries as the lungs are evaluated and vital signs are taken. At this point the child requiring multiple painful procedures and computed tomography (CT) is anesthetized electively after the cervical spine has been cleared.

Decreased compliance in the intubated patient means a plugged tube, a tube not in the trachea, or a hemopneumothorax. This situation must be remedied appropriately and immediately. With the airway secured and ventilation ensured, restoration of circulation is then paramount. Multiple upper extremity lines, large in diameter and short in length, are necessary. In our hands, the subclavian route has proved to be very useful, but peripheral antecubital lines are preferred. An arterial catheter, usually in the right radial artery; a Foley catheter, and a nasogastric tube are all placed. Routine screening radiographs are obtained next, including chest, abdomen, and pelvis films as well as any indicated long bone roentgenograms.

When the child has been stabilized and blood is available, CT is considered. The benefits of a CT scan are several; most important, both quantitative and qualitative evaluations of the injuries are obtained. A CT scan has proved extremely useful in evaluating solid abdominal viscera injuries, and studies have documented its accuracy in both adults and children.[3, 16, 17, 27, 29, 32, 34, 46, 48, 57, 58] In our hands, CT is the imaging study of greatest usefulness and sensitivity. The usefulness of a CT scan depends in large measure on the speed and safety with which the service can be delivered. In the modern trauma center, CT should be available almost instantaneously—24 hours a day. The trauma patient must take precedence over the routine elective case despite being disruptive of schedules. The situation in the radiology department clinically becomes then similar to that in the operating suite, with continuous monitoring and nursing care.

Patient safety is maintained by providing the speed and the equipment and personnel to ensure that the level of care taken to obtain the CT scan is the same as the patient was receiving in the resuscitation area and will receive in the operating suite. The CT suite must therefore be equipped much like an operating room with the ability to monitor the child in a similar fashion. An oxygen saturation monitor; a Doppler blood pressure monitor; an electrocardiogram monitor; and arterial, venous, and intracranial pressure monitors must all be available.

Computed tomography in injured children commonly requires anesthesia, and in our institution indications for early intubation include severe head injury for hyperventilation and maintenance of optimal oxygenation, extreme pain, uncontrolled fear, or inability to cooperate. Hence, the anesthesia equipment in the CT scan area should be of the same quality and design as that in the operating suite.

Protocols need to address the personnel available in the CT scan area. The staff should include everyone necessary to respond to any change in the patient's condition. Certainly this should include the surgeon, anesthesiologist, and any resident staff required. It is very useful to have a trauma nurse follow the patient from the emergency department through evaluation to the operating room or intensive care unit. It is unacceptable to abandon the patient in the radiology department to a nurse or radiology technician.

PATTERNS OF INJURY

In most settings, hepatic injury in children is the result of blunt trauma, and examination of hepatic injuries by CT scan has enabled a better definition of the injuries that usually occur. Hardy examined 50 adult victims of fatal blunt trauma and documented the frequency of injury to the right lobe of the liver, particularly the posterior superior portion.[23] Two studies based on CT scan analysis confirmed the frequency of right hepatic injury in children.[55, 61] The study by Stalker and colleagues is particularly helpful.[55] Of all patient injuries, 83% were to the right lobe; 65% of these were to the posterior segment, 21% to the anterior segment, and 15% to the dome. Twenty-three percent of all patients had injury to the left lobe, 15% to the medial segment, and 10% to the lateral segment.

The experience from Children's Hospital in San Diego is similar. Of 42 patients with hepatic injury, 39 were the result of blunt trauma. Of these 39 patients, 32 had CT scans (Table 20–2). The other seven patients were admitted directly to the operating room or died in the emergency department. Four of these seven arrived with cardiopulmonary resuscitation in progress, but the three remaining patients were potentially salvageable. All of these seven patients had hepatic transections, four had inferior vena cava lacerations, and one patient had a burst injury involving both lobes. Of the three children who had the potential to survive, all had inferior vena cava lacerations, and one survived.

Thirty-two patients had abdominal CT scans. In these 32 patients, two had bilobar injuries. The resulting distribution of injuries was (1) right lobe: 28 patients, with 15 or 46% in the posterior segment; (2) eight (or 28%) in the anterior segment; and (3) five (or 15%) in the dome. Six patients had injuries of the left lobe, and four of these were in the medial segment including the two with bilobar injuries. It is interesting to note that all of the patients requiring surgery had injuries of the posterior segment or dome.

GRADING SYSTEMS

Over the last 15 years, the surgical literature has exploded with articles extolling or condemning the nonoperative therapy of abdominal trauma. In an attempt to define the approach or practice of nonoperative therapy more precisely, efforts have been made to determine the severity of injury and its likelihood of life-threatening hemorrhage. These judgments can be made on clinical grounds, for example, how much blood is replaced to maintain isovolemia; however, if anatomic criteria are used as proposed by some,

Table 20–2
Pattern of Injury

	Patients	Percent
Right Lobe		
Anterior segment	8	28
Posterior segment	15	46
Dome	5	15
TOTAL	28	87
Left Lobe		
Medial segment	4	12
Lateral segment	2	5
TOTAL	6	17

NOTE: Two patients had bilobar injuries.

imaging is required. The two studies most rapidly available are ultrasound and CT. The information derived from the CT scan is much more amenable to the grading of injury severity than that from ultrasound. Buntain and Gould have suggested a CT scan grading system for splenic trauma, relating the severity of injury to the need for surgical intervention.[8]

In hepatic trauma, currently available grading systems are based on direct observation. In general, the more severe the trauma the greater the likelihood of death.[7, 10, 15, 42, 45] These systems are obviously of no help if operative exploration is not undertaken. The operative grading system can be used as a guide to construct a CT scan grading system that can be used to predict outcome and necessity of operative intervention (Table 20–3).

In general, class I and class II injuries are minor, superficial injuries that do not by themselves require operative therapy. Injuries that fall into class III may require surgery; however, many, if not most, deep lacerations located peripherally can be monitored carefully without surgical intervention. Those involving the posterior segment of the right lobe or the dome, however, probably should be explored. Similarly, complex, that is, stellate lacerations may be followed and monitored carefully. Others, confirmed at Children's Hospital in San Diego, have shown that intrahepatic hematoma does not require operative intervention unless a coagulopathy is present.[1, 19, 35]

Class IV injuries that involve extensive tissue destruction all need exploration, however. Many patients with these injuries have hepatic vein or vena caval injuries. The CT scan is beneficial here if the patient is stable, so that time can be given to the proper planning of an operative approach and the proper marshaling of resources. There is no CT counterpart for class V injuries. These severe injuries usually require prompt exploration because of hemodynamic instability, and CT is not undertaken. Injury to the vena cava or hepatic veins or both must be suspected in all class IV injuries.

OPERATIVE APPROACH

Blood loss is the cause of death in the vast majority of patients who die from liver injury. "Unquestionably death from hemorrhage is the patient's greatest hazard and the surgeon's greatest challenge."[62] Hemostasis is the most immediate priority. Lucas reported a series of blunt and penetrating hepatic trauma in which 51% of injuries had stopped bleeding by the time of surgery. He further stated that the incidence of rebleeding is nil.[37] In children, Stone and Ansley reported that 137 of 203 hepatic injuries in children, (67%) had stopped bleeding by the time surgery was performed.[56]

It appears that a significant number of isolated hepatic injuries can be treated safely without immediate laparotomy. Of 42 patients treated in our institution for hepatic injury, 13 (30%) required celiotomy. Two of these patients were explored for penetrating trauma. The incidence of celiotomy in the blunt trauma group was 28%. One associated injury required surgery, an associated splenic laceration that bled secondarily following open reconstruction of

Table 20–3
Hepatic Injury Grading

	Surgical Grade	Computed Tomography Grade
I	Capsular avulsion and parenchyma <1 cm deep.	Subcapsular hematoma.
II	Parenchyma fracture 1–3 cm deep. Subcapsular hematoma ≤10 cm and peripheral penetrating wound.	Simple laceration 1–3 cm small, 1–3 cm hepatic contusion.
III	Parenchyma fracture >3 cm deep. Subcapsular hematoma ≥10 cm and central penetrating wound.	Simple or complex lacerations >3 cm deep. Peripheral in location. Large intrahepatic hematoma.
IV	Lobar tissue damage and massive central hematoma.	Hepatic transection. Extensive laceration, stellate dome, or posterior segment right lobe.
V	Injury to hepatic view or retrohepatic vena cava.	Not applicable.

a complicated pelvic injury. Alternatively, patients who required surgery often had extensive and complex injuries, and 30% of patients taken to the operating suite with hepatic injuries died from hepatic vein–vena cava or head injuries. Of the 11 patients operated on secondary to blunt trauma, five had hepatic transections, and four of these had injury to the hepatic vein–vena cava junction. In this group one survived. Three additional patients had extensive injuries to the posterior segment of the right lobe. The remaining three patients had incidental hepatic injuries and were operated on for other reasons. The only patients who died of hepatic injury had extensive vena caval injuries as well. Two of these cases were particularly troubling because the patients were responsive on admission and therefore were potentially salvageable.

The pattern of injury and its extent mandates adequate exposure and rapid mobilization. On occasion, if injury to the vena cava is suspected, sternotomy before laparotomy with control of the vena cava in the pericardium and the aorta and placement of a right atrial pursestring suture may prove life saving. Otherwise, a midline incision long enough to allow adequate exposure is required, which if necessary can be lengthened cephalad to include a median sternotomy.

The liver must be adequately mobilized. Usually this requires transection of the falciform ligament to the hepatic veins. Because injury to the right lobe is most common in children, the coronary ligament must also be taken down. This procedure allows the entire liver to be rotated to the patient's left, exposing the posterior segment of the right lobe and the dome. If further exposure is needed, it is best obtained by sternotomy and transection of the central tendon of the diaphragm to the inferior vena cava, allowing access to the hepatic veins and vena cava.

Recent series in the literature have emphasized several points.[11, 14, 18, 43, 47, 49, 56] First, most hepatic injury can be handled by employing simple techniques. Direct suture ligation of individual bleeding vessels is preferable to mass ligation. Formal resection has a high mortality rate, 59 to 83% and has subsequently fallen into disfavor and been replaced by nonanatomic resection.[14, 49] This technique, termed *resectional débridement*, has been described by Pachter and associates as having several consecutive steps[50]:

1. Temporary hemostasis with compression
2. Occlusion of the portal triad

3. Resection of devitalized liver to achieve exposure
4. Ligation and repair of lacerated vessels and bile ducts

Mortality from employment of this approach has been reported as low as 4.5%.[49]

Hepatic artery ligation, as popularized by Mays, has also been abandoned in favor of direct suture ligation of bleeding vessels.[14, 18, 38, 41, 49, 50] The vast majority of injuries can be treated by nonanatomic resection and direct control of bleeding vessels. It is generally accepted that resection should include all nonviable tissue. In penetrating trauma it may be necessary to open into areas of viable liver to achieve hemostasis. It is not often necessary to invade viable tissue in coping with blunt trauma injuries, but if it is necessary to control arterial hemorrhage there should be little hesitation.

Temporary hepatic inflow occlusion was first described by Pringle in 1905.[51] The Pringle maneuver is usually accomplished by placing a vascular clamp across the portal triad. Complications resulting from use of the maneuver have been rare but include delayed bile duct stricture. Occlusion times have been increased from 15 minutes to 1 hour.[49, 50] This technique has proved invaluable in the immediate control of torrential hepatic hemorrhage. It is important to keep in mind that bleeding from hepatic veins is unaffected by inflow occlusion.

If torrential bleeding occurs after attempting the Pringle maneuver, hepatic vein or vena caval injury must be suspected. Hepatic vein injury is also suggested by injuries to the dome of the liver or transections, either between the anterior and posterior segments of the right lobe or between the right and left lobes. If the patient has evidence of injury to the right side of the abdomen and arrives severely volume deficient, it is important to assume major venous injury. In this situation children can exsanguinate in minutes after releasing the tamponade by opening the abdomen; "air embolus" has been implicated as the cause of death in these patients, but Walt has demonstrated that death is due to exsanguination.[62] Because death in these children is so rapid, opening the sternum for control of the inferior vena cava and aorta may prove life saving. Circulation to the lower half of the body can thus be controlled while the hepatic injury is assessed. Occasionally it is possible to repair or ligate the right hepatic vein, but frequently the vena cava has extensive injuries as well. If the injury to the vena cava is simple, a partially occluding clamp may control the injury and complete occlusion of the vena cava and aorta may be released. While the vena cava is repaired, bleeding from the liver is controlled by occlusion of the porta hepatis.

When injury to the hepatic veins and inferior vena cava are complex and require some time for repair, vascular isolation of the liver is required. Several methods of hepatic exclusion have been reported, but only two seem applicable to children. Heany and colleagues in 1966 described a technique of hepatic isolation by occluding the aorta below the superior mesenteric artery and the inferior vena cava above the renal veins and below the liver.[25] A Pringle maneuver is also necessary to control bleeding from the hepatic artery.

The second method was popularized by Schrock and coworkers.[54] It involves placement of an intracaval shunt through the right atrium into the inferior vena cava. The vena cava is occluded at the diaphragm and above the renal veins by Rumel tourniquets. A Pringle maneuver completes isolation of the liver and intrahepatic vena cava. Yellin and colleagues have discussed the relative merits of the two techniques.[64] Vascular isolation by clamps is quicker and requires less skill to perform. However, the shunt protects the kidneys and is less likely to produce arrest from reduced venous return. The ability of the shunt to maintain venous return has been disputed by Caln and associates.[9]

Experience at Children's Hospital in San Diego indicates that patients with isolated liver injuries should survive. The same can be said of patients with hepatic vein injuries that do not involve the vena cava. To save children with juxtahepatic vein–vena cava injuries, certain procedures can be instituted if one suspects either vena caval or hepatic vein injury. (This approach is considered very aggressive because these children exsanguinate in minutes, and the technique of compressing the liver against the body wall has not proved to be effective in controlling torrential hemorrhage in this age group, probably because of the extensive hepatic parenchymal injuries that these children sustain.) The following steps are recommended:

1. Restore blood volume. This may be accomplished with or without medical antishock trousers. Operation is not begun until the central venous pressure is 20 mm Hg and acidosis has been at least partially corrected. These children are resuscitated in the operating suite while the cell saver and rapid infusion warmer are prepared and packed red cells, platelets, and fresh-frozen plasma in adequate volumes are readied.

2. With a relatively stable patient, a sternotomy is performed, a Rumel tourniquet is placed about the inferior vena cava within the pericardium, and an atrial appendage pursestring suture is placed.

3. With control of the inferior vena cava and potential control of the aorta at the diaphragm, celiotomy is accomplished and the liver quickly palpated.

4. If bleeding cannot be controlled by pressure, both the inferior vena cava and aorta are occluded. This allows inspection of the injury in a relatively bloodless field, and blood is evacuated into the cell saver for reinfusion.

5. The liver is fully mobilized by incising the falciform ligament, the coronary ligament, and the central tendon of the diaphragm.

6. Injury to the vena cava can be inspected directly.

7. Placement of a shunt depends on the time required for vena caval repair.

8. Segmental resection with control of the hepatic artery and portal vein is accomplished after vena caval circulation is restored.

Evidence indicates that warm ischemic times up to 1 hour are well tolerated by the normothermic patient.[26]

In treating juxtahepatic venous injuries, time is of the essence. Once the abdominal tamponade has been released, there is very little time for thought or contemplation. If children with these injuries are to be saved, planning and preparation must be accomplished in advance of patient arrival. The trauma team must be experienced and technically proficient. A thorough familiarity with hepatic anatomy should be a part of team training. A step-by-step plan familiar to all needs to be in place. The planning should include obtaining all equipment including cell savers, rapid infusion warmers, sternal saw, and caval cannulae of various sizes. The equipment should be packaged to be readily available. A liver modular cart is appropriate. All of the necessary equipment can be moved into the operating suite at one time, before the start of surgery. This will save the circulating nurse from running for needed equipment. Two circulators may be necessary in these cases.

It may not be possible to train all surgeons on the trauma team to care for these seriously injured patients. Pachter and associates have noted that a senior surgeon was present on each of the major liver cases.[50] It should be restated that this series has the lowest mortality rate reported.

Hepatic injury in children is the most significant cause of mortality, following head injury. It is certainly the most challenging problem that the trauma surgeon interested in children faces. The number of such patients who require surgery is approximately 30%. The nonsurgical treatment of hepatic injury has been amply discussed in the literature.[12, 13, 20, 22, 28, 48] The experience at Children's Hospital in San Diego is consistent with that of previously published studies. The problem of missed intra-abdominal injuries, although always a concern, has not proved to be significant. Utilization of nonoperative treatment depends on a clear and rapid definition of the injury, which is most readily accomplished by rapid resuscitation and immediate torso CT. Based on the anatomic location, extent of injury, and physiologic status of the patient, a decision for or against immediate surgery can be made. In general, patients who require operative intervention require very aggressive surgical therapy, with an extended midline incision and splitting of the diaphragm required on many. Most patients with isolated hepatic injuries should be expected to survive with proper planning and expeditious surgery where indicated. The major unsolved problem at present is the treatment of juxtahepatic vena caval injuries.

References

1. Athey GN, Rahan SU: Hepatic haematoma following blunt injury: Non-operative management. Injury 13(4):302–306, 1982.
2. Balasegaram M: Hepatic surgery: Present and future. Ann R Coll Surg Engl 47(3):139–158, 1970.

3. Berger PE, Kuhn JP: CT of blunt abdominal trauma in childhood. AJR 136(1):105–110, 1981.

4. Bismuth H: Surgical anatomy and anatomical surgery of the liver. World J Surg 6(1):329, 1982.

5. Bismuth H: Surgical anatomy of the liver: Recent Results in Cancer Research 100:197–284, 1986.

6. Bismuth H, Houssin D, Castainy D: Major and minor segmentectomies ''réglées'' in liver surgery. World J Surg 6(1):10–24, 1982.

7. Bootman S, Oliver G, Oster-Granile ML, et al: The treatment of 179 blunt trauma-induced liver injuries in a statewide trauma center. Am Surg 50(11):603–608, 1984.

8. Buntain WL, Gould HR: Splenic trauma in children and techniques of splenic salvage. World J Surg 9(3):398–409, 1985.

9. Caln DG, Crighton J, Schom N: Successful management of hepatic vein injury from blunt trauma in childhood. Am J Surg 140:858–864, 1980.

10. Calne RY: Injuries to the liver. Br J Hosp Med 36(3):166–173, 1986.

11. Carmona RH, Lim RC, Clark CC: Morbidity and mortality in hepatic trauma, a 5 year study. Am J Surg 144(1):88–94, 1982.

12. Cheatham JE, Smith IE, Tunnell WP, et al: Non-operative management of subcapsular hematomas of the liver. Am J Surg 140:852–857, 1980.

13. Cywes S, Rode H, Miller AJ: Blunt liver trauma in children: Non-operative management. J Pediatr Surg 20(1):14–18, 1985.

14. DeSore WW Jr, Mattox KL, Mordon GL, et al: Management of 1590 consecutive cases of liver trauma. Arch Surg 3:493–497, 1976.

15. Elerding SC, Aragon GE, Moore EE: Fatal hepatic hemorrhage after trauma. Am J Surg 138:883–888, 1979.

16. Federle MP, Goldberg HI, Kaiser JA, et al: Evaluation of abdominal trauma by computed tomography. Radiology 135:637–644, 1981.

17. Federle MP, Jeffery RB: Hemoperitoneum studied by configured tomography. Radiology 148(1):187–192, 1983.

18. Feliciano DB, Mattox KL, Jordan GL, et al: Management of 1000 consecutive cases of hepatic trauma. Ann Surg 204(4):438–445, 1986.

19. Geis WP, Schulz KA, Giacchino JL, et al: The fate of unruptured intrahepatic hematomas. Surgery 90(4):689–697, 1981.

20. Giacomantonio M, Filler RM, Rich RH: Blunt hepatic trauma in children: Experience with operative and non-operative management. J Pediatr Surg 19(5):519–522, 1984.

21. Goelford PW: Anatomy of the liver. Radiol Clin North Am 18(2):187–193, 1980.

22. Grisoni ER, Baucher MW, Ferron J, et al: Nonoperative management of liver injuries following blunt abdominal trauma in children. J Pediatr Surg 19(5):515–518, 1984.

23. Hardy KJ: Patterns of liver injury after fatal blunt trauma. Surg Gynecol Obstet 134:39–43, 1972.

24. Hasselgren PO, Almersjo O, Gustavsson B, et al: Trauma to the liver during a ten year period. Acta Chir Scand 147(6):387–393, 1981.

25. Heany JP, Stanton WK, Halbert DS, et al: Improved technique for vascular isolation of the liver: Experimental study and case report. Ann Surg 163(2):237–241, 1966.

26. Huguet C, Nordlinger B, Bloch P, et al: Tolerance of the hema liver to prolonged harmothermic ischemia, a biologic study of 20 patients submitted to extensive hepatectomy. Arch Surg 113:1448–1451, 1978.

27. Karp MP, Cooney DR, Berger PE, et al: The role of computed tomography in the evaluation of blunt abdominal trauma in children. J Pediatr Surg 16(3):316–232, 1981.

28. Karp MP, Cooney DR, Pros GA, et al: The nonoperative management of pediatric hepatic trauma. J Pediatr Surg 18(4):512–518, 1983.

29. Kaufman RA, Tomkin R: Upper abdominal trauma in children: Imaging evaluation. AJR 142(3):449–459, 1984.

30. Kennedy PH, Madding GF: Surgical anatomy of the liver. Surg Clin North Am 157(2):233–243, 1977.

31. Kudsk KA, Sheldon GF, Lin RC: Atrio-caval shunting (ACS) after trauma. J Trauma 22(2):81–85, 1982.

32. Kuhn JP, Berger PE: Computed tomography in the evaluation of blunt abdominal trauma in children. Radiol Clin North Am 19(3):503–513, 1981.

33. Kune GH: The anatomical basis of liver surgery. Aust N Z J Surg 39(2):117–125, 1969.

34. Kurtna RS: Radiology of blunt abdominal trauma. Surg Clin North Am 57(1), 1977.

35. Lanketch W, Rubin BE: Non-operative management of intra-hepatic hemorrhage and hematoma following blunt trauma. Surg Gynecol Obstet 148:507–511, 1979.

36. Levin H, Gover P, Nance FC: Surgical restraint in the management of hepatic injury: A review of the charity hospital experience. J Trauma 18(6):399–404, 1978.

37. Lucas CE: Liver injury, a modern day surgical challenge. S Afr J Surg 14(4):163–174, 1976.

38. Lucas DE, Ledgerwood AM: Prospective evaluation of thermostatic techniques for liver injuries. J Trauma 16(6):442–450, 1976.

39. Lynch FP: Unpublished data.

40. Lynch FP, Kitchen L, Wotherspoon L: Unpublished data.

41. Mays ET, Conti S, Fallah Zadeh H, et al: Hepatic artery ligation. Surgery 86(4):536–543, 1979.

42. Micas CE, Ledgerwood AM: Factors influencing morbidity and mortality after liver injury. Am Surg 44(7):406–412, 1978.

43. Miller DR, Bernstein JM: Hepatic trauma, a review of 56 consecutively treated patients. Arch Surg 115(2):175–178, 1980.

44. Misra B, Wagner R, Boneval H: Injuries of hepatic veins and retro-hepatic vena cava. Am Surg 49(19):55–60, 1983.

45. Moore EE: Critical decisions in the management of hepatic trauma. Am J Surg 148:712–716, 1984.

46. Moore KL, Federle MP: Computed tomography in hepatic trauma. AJR 141(2):309–314, 1983.

47. Nevin A, Crover P, Nance F: Surgical restraint in the management of hepatic injury: A review of charity hospital experience. J Trauma 18(6):399–404, 1978.

48. Oldham KT, Guice KS, Ryckman F, et al: Blunt liver injury in childhood: Evaluation of therapy and current perspective. Surgery 100(3):542–549, 1986.

49. Pachter HL, Spencer FC: Recent concepts in the treatment of hepatic trauma. Ann Surg 190(4):423–429, 1979.

50. Pachter LH, Spencer FC, Hofstetler SR, et al: Experience with the finger fracture technique to achieve intra-hepatic hemostasis in 75 patients with severe injuries of the liver. Ann Surg 197(6):771–778, 1981.

51. Pringle JH: Notes on the arrest of hepatic hemorrhage due to trauma. Ann Surg 48:541–548, 1908.

52. Rovito PF: Atrial caval shunting in blunt hepatic vascular injury. Ann Surg 205(3):318–321, 1987.

53. Schrock T, Blaisdell WF, Mathewson C: Management of blunt trauma to the liver and hepatic veins. Arch Surg 96(5):698–704, 1968.

54. Schrock T, Blaisdell FW, Mathewson C Jr: Management of blunt trauma to the liver and hepatic veins. Arch Surg 96(5):698–704, 1968.

55. Stalker HP, Kaufman RH, Towkin R: Patterns of liver injury in childhood: CT analysis. Am J Radiol 147(6):1199–2005, 1986.

56. Stone HH, Ansley JD: Management of liver trauma in children. J Pediatr Surg 12(1):3–10, 1977.

57. Toombs BD, Lester RG, Ben-Menachem Y, et al: Computed tomography in blunt trauma. Radiol Clin North Am 19(1):17–35, 1981.

58. Toombs BD, Sandler CM, Rauschkolb EN, et al: Assessment of hepatic injuries with computed tomography. J Comput Assist Tomogr 6(1):72–75, 1982.

59. Touloukian RJ: Abdominal Injuries in Pediatric Trauma. New York, Wiley Medical Publishing, 1978.

60. Turpin I, State D, Schwartz A: Injuries to the inferior vena cava and their management. Am J Surg 134:25–32, 1977.

61. Vock P, Kehrer B, Tschaeppeler H: Blunt liver trauma in children: The role of computed tomography in diagnosis and treatment. J Pediatr Surg 21(5):413–418, 1986.

62. Walt A: The mythology of hepatic trauma—Or Babel revisited. Am J Surg 135:12–18, 1978.

63. Welch KJ: Abdominal Injuries in Pediatric Surgery. 3rd ed. Chicago, Year Book Medical Publishers, 1979.

64. Yellin AE, Chaffee CG, Donovan AJ: Vascular isolation in treatment of juxtahepatic venous injuries. Arch Surg 102:566–573, 1971.

William L. Buntain

Spleen Injuries

Since the observation by Aristotle centuries ago that congenitally asplenic patients led apparently normal lives, there has been disagreement over his conclusion that the spleen was not essential to life.[134, 177] The landmark study in 1952 by King and Shumacher that reported fatal sepsis in children following removal of their spleens generated considerable interest in reassessing the management of splenic injuries. Over the next 25 years, as the importance of splenic function and immune competency has clarified, emphasis has shifted from removal to preservation of the spleen following injury.[99] It is now recognized that the risk of bacterial sepsis increases after splenectomy performed at any age and for any reason. Few would now disagree that every effort should be made to save the injured spleen if it can be done without increased risk to the patient.

As this evolving therapeutic change has occurred, precise guidelines to define the criteria that enter into the decision of how to manage splenic injuries have proved to be controversial. Although these guidelines were meant to be based on experienced surgical judgment in a setting in which close clinical and laboratory observation is possible, individual preference and bias based on inadequate or insufficient information have unfortunately influenced management decisions.[18, 133] Although conflicting opinions still exist, more definitive guidelines for management are being developed as published experience accumulates.

HISTORICAL PERSPECTIVES

The spleen has been of interest for much of recorded history. Rosner found references to the spleen in ancient Jewish writings, citing Judah Halevi (1086–1145) in the book of Kuzari and Maimonides (1135–1204) who attributed to the spleen the functions of "promoting cheerfulness and laughter" and "cleansing both the blood and the spirit from unclean and obscuring matter."[167]

The earliest reported splenectomies were by Fioravanti in 1541 and by Zaccairelli in 1549.[4] The scholarly influence of Aristotle, Wren, and Morgagni prompted more reports over the next few hundred years, all under the premise that the spleen was not essential to life. A brief interlude in this philosophy occurred in Germany in the midnineteenth century, however, when sepsis, imperfect technique, and suspect indications all contributed to a mortality rate from splenectomy of 90%. Simon, the most influential surgical authority of the time, opposed the operation, and it was temporarily abandoned. However, as Simon's influence waned, splenectomy was again advocated and popularized by Kuchenmeister in 1866, Nussbaum and Edler in 1877, and Moyer in 1878.[4] Except for the brief cautionary challenge of Morris and Bullock in 1919, splenectomy remained the procedure of choice for the injured spleen for the next 60 years; resistance to surgical repair of the spleen following injury as well as the myth of the impossibility of suturing the spleen continued.[11, 163]

In fact, parts of the injured spleen have been preserved through the ages by either cautery or massive ligation.[131] In 1902, Berger, as cited by Ross in 1908, collected 360 cases of traumatized spleens.[9, 168] Pointing out that the mortality

rate was 92% in 220 nonoperative cases, he reported that splenectomy in 67 cases had a mortality rate of *only* 57%. He also reported six patients who were explored and underwent tamponade of their injured spleens with five recoveries, and he added two more patients who had splenorrhaphies for splenic trauma with one recovery—the first known case of successful splenorrhaphy. In 1914, Barnes quoted Brogsitter's work from 1909 in which he (Brogsitter) reported 47 traumatic injuries to the spleen, of which six were treated with tamponade successfully, one with tamponade and splenorrhaphy successfully, and one with splenorrhaphy alone successfully.[4] Barnes added six more cases, including one successful splenorrhaphy, and finished his dissertation with a plea to "preserve the spleen if it is possible."

In 1930 Dretzka reported 27 cases, 17 of which were operated on. Of these 17, seven were treated with tamponade, seven with tamponade plus splenorrhaphy, and three with splenorrhaphy alone. Of the 17 who were operated on, seven died, but all of those managed with splenorrhaphy alone survived.[49] In 1932, Mazel added another splenic injury successfully managed with splenorrhaphy and cautiously suggested that "the individual case must be decided upon by the surgeon at the time of the operation."[117] By 1945, however, he had reported another case successfully managed with splenorrhaphy and stated that the spleen "should be preserved whenever possible."[118]

The classic study in 1919 of Morris and Bullock demonstrating the susceptibility of splenectomized rats to overwhelming infection was refuted clinically by several small retrospective clinical reports.[131, 134] However, in 1952 King and Shumacher reported overwhelming sepsis in five infants undergoing splenectomy for congenital hemolytic anemia, and similar reports in 1958 and 1962 confirmed a 5 to 8% incidence of life-threatening infection in children under the age of 1 who had undergone splenectomy for disease or trauma.[86, 91, 99]

Information gained from the study of postsplenectomy infections is difficult to interpret unless it can be compared with the frequency of similar infections in various control situations.[22] Evaluating illness from organisms similar to those primarily involved in postsplenectomy infections, the infection rate for the Thousand Family Survey for the Newcastle-upon-Tyne study in England was 0.7%, and the same rate of bacterial meningitis in the borough of Brooklyn for 1955 to 1965 was 0.2%.[46, 122] From these studies it was determined that in children with intact spleens, the mortality rate due to these similar infections is 0.3% in the first year of life, 0.07% between 1 and 7 years, and 0.02% between 7 and 14 years.[46]

In 1972, Eraklis and Filler directed a multicenter survey by the American Academy of Pediatrics to determine the incidence of postsplenectomy complications.[58] Of 342 children who underwent splenectomy for trauma, three, or 0.88%, died from overwhelming sepsis. In 1973, Singer collected cases of 2796 patients following splenectomy; 921 splenectomies had been done for trauma or incidental to other procedures, and there were six deaths, or a 0.65% mortality rate. In the total series of 2796 cases, sepsis occurred in 119, or 4.25%, and 71—60% of the ones infected and 2.52% of the total—died. Singer concluded that regardless of the reason for splenectomy, the mortality rate from overwhelming sepsis varies from 50 to more than 200 times more than that of the incidence in the population at large.[189]

While these problems with asplenia were evolving, Michels and Nguyen and colleagues demonstrated anatomically the segmental end-arterial system of the spleen, observing that blunt fractures along the avascular intersegmental planes provided an anatomic basis for operative salvage.[121, 141] In addition, the development of topical hemostatic agents that further aided controlled segmental resection and favorable results of splenic salvage in children with splenorrhaphy led to even more aggressive efforts at splenic preservation.[9, 29–35] Such salvage efforts are now considered "standard of care."

INCIDENCE

The exact incidence of splenic trauma is unknown.[135] The only controlled general population study addressing the issue of sepsis following splenectomy for any reason based the incidence rate on the United States population of 1980 and projected more than 40,000 splenectomies per year.[176] Twenty-five percent of these splenectomies were for trauma, and no attention was given to splenorrhaphies or those treated by nonoperative observation. Excluding primary splenic disease or hematologic malignancies, 46% were "incidental" at the time of abdominal surgery. Exactly how many of these incidental splenectomies represent iatrogenic injury is unknown, but injury to the spleen is much more common than one might think if operative injury is included.[105] These patients correspond closely to those with splenic trauma in their susceptibility to infection, and the mortality rate, although seemingly low, is still at least 86 times greater than that of the population at large.

The pervasive belief in the expendability of the spleen and the likelihood of recurrent hemorrhage if attempts are made to stop the bleeding led to an almost universal dictum in dealing with such trauma: remove the injured spleen to ensure no further problems.[157] Peck and Jackson reported that 23% of 95 patients requiring splenectomy in their series did so because of iatrogenic injury, that the incidence of splenic injury in all abdominal operations was 0.5%, in gastric resections 2.7%, and in vagotomies 3.7%.[153] Four of 22 patients died 1 to 30 days after surgery (18%). These investigators discussed the possible legal consequences of inadvertent removal of the spleen, emphasizing that the mortality in any major operation is increased when splenectomy is added. They also noted that details of surgical trauma to the spleen are often vague in operative reports. Indeed, the older literature is replete with reports associating iatrogenic splenic injury with other abdominal operations; however, these have noticeably decreased since the importance of an intact spleen to immune function has been better elucidated.

Demographically, a peak incidence of splenic injury is noted in the second and third decades of life with males predominating, while a secondary small peak is observed in women older than 70.[135] Mortality appears to parallel age.

PHYSIOLOGY AND IMMUNE FUNCTION

Total circulation of the spleen is estimated at between 150 to 250 ml per minute, representing 5% of the total cardiac output.[135] Intimately related to its architectural anatomy is the ability of the spleen to remove blood-borne particulate matter and abnormal red blood cells. However, the historical concept of the spleen functioning only as a filter is somewhat obsolete. Data now demonstrate unequivocally that the regulatory functions exerted by the spleen and its immunologic role are extensive.[99, 109, 185] The spleen represents 25% of the total lymphoid body mass or reticuloendothelial system and has a direct impact on distinct populations of lymphocytes, that is, the T and B cells.[2, 70, 76, 198, 215] Impaired capacity for clearance of blood-borne particles; decreased phagocytic activity directed against encapsulated bacteria; decreased antibody response to specific antigens; and decreased opsonization of bacteria, together with an absence of circulating tuftsin, other decreased antibody responses, and decreased properdin, have all been demonstrated in the asplenic state.[12, 24, 27, 31, 47, 64, 70, 76, 88, 106, 138, 218]

Clearly, an asplenic patient can survive severe infection because the liver is capable of assuming the reticuloendothelial function of the spleen.[179] Despite having fixed tissue macrophages, however, the liver cannot provide the optimal environment for clearance of intravascular antigen, and this deficiency is the apparent basis for the infectious complications associated with the asplenic state.

Of particular importance clinically has been the recognition of the phenomenon of overwhelming postsplenectomy sepsis.[10, 41, 42, 52, 59, 61, 73, 185, 189] This type of overwhelming infection is characterized clinically by early systemic symptoms of fever, chills, nausea, vomiting, and malaise, and it often follows an upper respiratory infection. It may progress rapidly to fulminant sepsis with associated disseminated intravascular coagulation, adrenal insufficiency, coma, hypotension, and death within hours of onset. Early recognition and aggressive treatment are mandatory. The classic findings at postmortem include bilateral adrenal hemorrhage, positive blood culture, and an occult or subclinical focus of infection.[179]

Healthy individuals splenectomized for trauma appear to be at slightly less risk than those splenectomized for hematologic reasons, and younger children seem to fare worse than older children and adults.[85] The severity of the sepsis, however, appears to be worse in the older patients.[22] Regardless of the reason for splenectomy, the mortality rate for overwhelming postsplenectomy sepsis varies from 40 to 70%, with infection occurring an estimated 50 to 200 times more than in the normal population.[18, 73, 131, 176, 189] The majority of serious infections following splenectomy occur within 24 months, with almost 50% occurring within 12 months, but there is no specific time period beyond which an asplenic person can be considered to be safe.[18, 85]

In addition to overwhelming postsplenectomy sepsis, an increased susceptibility to almost any type of infection appears to be evident following splenectomy.[22, 85, 109, 178] Of considerable concern is the unexpectedly high incidence of viral illness in asplenic individuals, indicating that overwhelming postsplenectomy sepsis is not confined to encapsulated bacteria.[18, 109, 178] Early postoperative septic morbidity and mortality in splenectomized trauma patients is also believed to be greater than in a comparable group of non-splenectomized trauma patients or similar patients with splenorrhaphy.[80, 178] Long-term follow up of 740 American servicemen splenectomized during World War II revealed a statistically significant excess mortality from pneumonia and ischemic heart disease.[165]

Recognition of overwhelming postsplenectomy sepsis aroused interest in the immune function of the spleen. In septic postsplenectomy patients, large numbers of bacteria are found in peripheral blood smears, indicating at least 1 million organisms per mm. Causative microorganisms are typically encapsulated and include *Streptococcus pneumoniae,* 50%; *Meningococcus,* 12%; *Escherichia coli,* 11%; *Haemophilus influenzae,* 8%; staphylococci, 8%; and other streptococci, 7%. The remarkable virulence of the pneumococcus is related to its rapid multiplication and its encapsulated state, which resists opsonization and therefore phagocytosis.

The spleen reaches its maximum weight at puberty, and it is perfused with 200 ml of blood per minute in the adult. Blood passes first through the central arteries of the germinal centers, bringing particulate matter in contact with lymphocytes for antigen processing. More than 90% is then forced through the cords of Billroth. Phagocytosis occurs during this percolation process by fixed macrophages. This unique anatomy increases contact time, thus decreasing opsonic requirements. This is the major reason that encapsulated organisms require greater opsonization for hepatic clearance and that patients with chronic liver disease are more prone to postsplenic infections.[131]

The spleen's other major role is that of an immunologic factory, producing immunoglobulin (Ig), properdin, and tuftsin.[24, 25, 30, 82, 106, 138, 197, 220] As the first antibody formed in response to an antigen, the primary role of IgM is the initiation of other immune mechanisms. Compared with IgG, IgM has a shorter half-life and a lower serum concentration. Its large size limits it to the intravascular space but enhances its ability to activate complement and agglutinate bacteria. IgG is produced later, remains longer, and is free to exude into the interstitial space. The body has immunologic memory with respect to IgG production, and on second exposure to an antigen, there is a more rapid, higher, and sustained IgG response. Of particular significance is the fact that this immunologic imprinting does not occur in children younger than 2 years of age.

Complement activation is also vital to host defense. It increases vascular permeability and promotes chemotaxis, phagocytosis, and intracellular killing. Complement is activated in the classic sense by antibody-antigen interaction or via the alternative pathway in which properdin is a crucial mediator.[24]

Tuftsin is a substance made predominantly by the spleen.[24, 30] This tetrapeptide binds the leukokinen, which coats circulating neutrophils, inducing a nonspecific enhancement of phagocytosis. Low IgM, properdin, and tuftsin levels characterize the asplenic state and contribute to the increased susceptibility to overwhelming postsplenectomy sepsis. In addition, the spleen affects the helper-to-suppressor T-cell ratio and modulates distant monocyte function.[48, 51, 76, 103, 187, 197] The spleen may also protect against the induction of cancer and is important in immune surveillance.[90]

Asplenia leads to an impairment in the initial response to blood-borne particulate antigen, resulting in a variety of immunologic defects, a deficiency of phagocytosis-promoting peptides—tuftsin—of up to 50%, a significant and constant decrease in IgM in all cases, and a decreased level of properdin.[28, 30, 31, 81, 101, 154, 163, 170, 175, 191]

The spleen appears to be somewhat selective in its role as a defense mechanism, being more important when the site of bacterial invasion is via the blood stream.[54, 189] Splenectomized individuals form antibodies to subcutaneous antigens quite normally and respond well to soluble intravenous antigens. However, when particulate antigen is injected intravenously for the first time, the asplenic individual forms little or no antibody, particularly the young infant.[28, 111, 190]

ANATOMY

The spleen is a purple, wedge-shaped organ that lies in the uppermost portion of the left upper quadrant of the abdomen. It is the most friable of the abdominal viscera, making it the most frequently injured abdominal visceral organ in blunt torso trauma. The lateral surface of the spleen is in contact with the diaphragm, its medial surface is in contact with the kidney, stomach, and pancreas, the latter extending just below the entrance of the splenic vessels into the splenic hilum.

The spleen develops from multiple anlagen in the dorsal mesogastrium at the 6 to 8 mm embryonic stage, when the stomach has begun its rotation. The multiple anlagen develop close to the pancreas to form the mature organ. Incomplete fusion of these parts may result in a lobulated spleen, or failure of fusion may lead to formation of one or more accessory spleens. The development of the spleen in proximity to the pancreas in the dorsal mesogastrium explains its location in relation to the pancreas when rotation of the viscera is complete. It also explains its ease of mobilization by division of its lateral peritoneal attachments during surgery.[157]

The spleen becomes morphologically mature during the first year of life and reaches its maximum weight of 100 to 150 gm at puberty; thereafter it decreases in weight by 25 to 30% in a normal adult. The spleen is encapsulated by an external serous coat derived from the peritoneum and an internal fibroelastic coat, which is invaginated at the hilum and carried inward with the splenic artery and its branches. In the child there is more functional smooth muscle and elastic in the parenchyma, and the capsule is relatively thicker compared with that of the adult.

The peritoneum of the anterior and posterior walls of the stomach is reflected onto the spleen as the gastrosplenic ligaments that carry the short gastric vessels from the splenic artery to the stomach.[5] Below this, the gastrosplenic ligament contains the gastroepiploic vessels and is continuous with the greater omentum through the splenocolic (lienocolic) ligament. The peritoneum is reflected off the spleen superiorly, laterally, and inferiorly to form the splenophrenic, splenorenal, and splenocolic ligaments, respectively.

The spleen receives its blood supply from the splenic artery, which divides into an arcade of between six and 36 branches before entering the splenic parenchyma, usually at right angles.[120] Gupta and colleagues and others demonstrated segmental anatomy, with the artery dividing into dorsal and ventral primary branches to dorsal and ventral segments of the spleen, with no communications visualized between the branches of the two main divisions.[37, 45] This arterial division and segmental distribution is extremely important to the trauma surgeon, for it is this feature that allows partial splenic resection. As blood enters the parenchyma through these segmental arteries, the branches traverse the trabeculae of the capsule, further branching into central arteries that give off follicular arterioles at right angles. These arterioles enter focal areas of lymphoid tissue (the white pulp) located in the splenic parenchyma (the red pulp).

MECHANISMS OF INJURY

Splenic injuries include capsular tears, parenchymal lacerations, bursting or macerating disruptions, hilar disruptions, and subcapsular hematomas.

Blunt Injuries

Following blunt mechanisms of abdominal or torso trauma, the spleen is consistently reported as the most common abdominal organ to be injured.[177] If all trauma victims with nonpenetrating injuries to the spleen are included (that is, those who are dead on arrival or who expire in the emergency department), mortality rates range from 18 to 25%.[65, 177, 185, 203, 224] This alarmingly high death rate reflects the magnitude of multisystem injury and, in particular, associated injuries to the head and chest. Until the advent of diagnostic peritoneal lavage (DPL) and computed tomography (CT), part of this high mortality rate was also attributed to difficulties and delays in diagnosis and operative intervention.[135]

Moore and co-workers have described clearly the pathophysiology of blunt deceleration splenic trauma:

In the typical blunt deceleration injury, the mobility of the stomach and transverse colon is transferred to the relatively fixed spleen via the gastrolienal ligaments and splenic flexure, producing capsular avulsion or tears in the polar and short gastric vessels. With severe deceleration, the spleen may be totally avulsed from the retroperitoneum and its hilar vessels. Blunt compression injury transverse to the axis of the spleen usually fractures the organ according to the segmental arterial anatomy. In most cases only the parenchyma is injured, producing predominantly venous bleeding, however, deeper lacerations may involve the trabecular arteries. With greater energy transfer, the blunt injury does not parallel segmental anatomy, and stellate fractures occur, with extensive arterial and venous disruption.[128]

The mechanism of injury most often responsible for blunt trauma continues to be motorized vehicles. Such high-speed, energy-dissipating events also account for the high incidence of associated extra-abdominal injuries, reportedly occurring in up to 80 to 85% of cases.[65, 136, 203, 224] Associated intra-abdominal injuries have been reported in 30 to 61% of blunt splenic trauma cases and remain the strongest argument for those supporting abdominal exploration in cases of blunt splenic injury.[108, 123, 136, 178, 203] Ten to 33% of these associated injuries require operation themselves; hence, careful evaluation and selection of patients for nonoperative management following blunt trauma to the spleen are important.[18, 135]

Isolated blunt splenic injury occurs in less than 25% of cases and usually involves less disruptive forces, such as direct blows to the left upper quadrant of the abdomen following minor falls or contact sports.[135] With access to appropriate emergency care systems, the mortality rate secondary to isolated splenic injury should ideally be less than 1%.

The type of hospital and population served determines the cause and type of injuries seen and managed. A community hospital with limited emergency facilities generally manages cases of less severe trauma, and patients may not be seen rapidly after injury. Splenic injuries under these low–energy transmission circumstances are more likely to be isolated and less severe, and significant systemic manifestations are less striking.[113] Trauma centers treat victims of major blunt and penetrating trauma regularly. Such patients are seen early following the event, and splenic injury is usually more severe and is associated with other abdominal visceral and extra-abdominal injuries. These combinations of injuries may be immediately life threatening, and specific circumstances determine approaches to management.[157] Recommendations applicable to a stable, healthy 14 year old with an apparently minor splenic tear following a sports injury are considerably different from those for the same-aged patient who is unconscious and hypotensive with multiple system injuries following a high-speed motorcycle accident.

Penetrating Injuries

The incidence of penetrating splenic injury in reported series of operative abdominal trauma approximates less than 10%, reflecting the volume of intraperitoneal space occupied by the spleen as compared with that of other intra-abdominal organs.[135, 177] The mortality rate for penetrating splenic injury varies with the mechanism of injury, ranging from 0 to 1% with stab wounds to 10% with gunshot wounds.[65, 108, 177] Noteworthy with regard to penetrating splenic injuries is the reported 90% incidence of associated injuries, the majority of which require surgical intervention, thereby justifying the consensus that penetrating injuries to the spleen demand operative intervention.[65, 108, 203]

Delayed Rupture of the Spleen

In 1932, McIndoe described a patient with delayed manifestations of hemorrhage from traumatic injury to the spleen and collected 45 similar cases from the literature.[112] Pointing out that the latency period of time between injury and hemorrhage may vary from days to weeks, he operatively classified the injuries to the spleen in terms of their severity and reported the incidence to be 35%, varying from 5 to 40%.[94, 223]

Delayed rupture of the spleen remained an accepted diagnosis in the spectrum of splenic injuries until better diagnostic methods such as arteriography, radionuclide scanning, and DPL became available.[157] Once these modalities became acceptable, if the strict criteria of McIndoe were followed for diagnosing delayed hemorrhage from spleen injuries, the true incidence would be 0.3%, confirming that delayed rupture is usually only delayed diagnosis.

Occult Rupture of the Spleen

The trauma may be trivial and the initial signs and symptoms so mild that major rupture of the spleen may go completely undiagnosed, and hence untreated, early after injury. This has been termed *occult rupture of the spleen.* However, as with delayed rupture, this diagnosis should be extremely rare with the advent of more aggressive diagnostic maneuvers, primarily CT.

INJURY CLASSIFICATION

Precise criteria to ensure the safety, timing, and method of splenic salvage have been difficult to develop and thus remain controversial. Current debate revolves around whether the most acceptable means to accomplish splenic salvage is by nonoperative or operative means, and if the latter, when to surgically intervene.

It is important to emphasize and be mindful that the objective of splenic injury management is *to salvage sufficient splenic tissue to preserve immune competence.* Too often this objective has been influenced by personal preference or bias, and if management decisions are based on inadequate or insufficient information, unfortunate outcome can result. Because splenic salvage is really the objective, a classification that determines the severity of splenic injury as well as the presence of associated injuries with recommendations for prompt intervention when appropriate would seem to contribute significantly to management of the injured spleen. However, the gold standard of care for splenic injuries in children at this time seems to be "the management of splenic trauma without operating."[152] Indeed, so emphatically has this concept been propagated that many physicians responsible for caring for these injured children do not study them for early determination of severity of injury or for possible associated injuries, and CT classification of injury severity is not only not recognized or practiced but also not addressed.[152, 212]

Despite the declaration that "what we are trying to accomplish with nonoperative splenic management is to preserve the spleen as much as preserve the patient, rather than just to avoid a laparotomy,"[69] *the objective of salvaging sufficient splenic tissue to maintain immune protection has often seemingly been replaced by efforts to avoid operation.* The management of splenic injuries by nonoperative means

is a commendable objective and is certainly acceptable, indeed preferable, if based on sufficient diagnostic information and subsequent surgical judgment with regard to patient safety, *but not at all costs.* Further, it is my opinion that the ability to manage a child with a proven "shattered" spleen without intervening surgically does not substantiate its wisdom and is not necessarily in the best interest of the patient. Indeed, although occasionally successful, it more closely represents the probable limits to which we can subject injured children.

Because it is well accepted that *severity of injury* and *delay in diagnosis and intervention* can adversely influence outcome, a classification of the splenic injury in terms of severity and presence or absence of associated injuries that is based on early postresuscitative and reproducible diagnostic findings is important. It allows a more predictable therapeutic approach, helps to avoid potential late complications or sequelae by identifying early on which injuries can be safely observed and which require operative intervention, and improves the ability to standardize and compare results.[67]

Initial attempts to classify splenic injuries were based on operative findings.[112] Later, arteriographic findings were used and clearly demonstrated that severity of injury could be classified and was related to outcome, clinically and prognostically.[14, 67, 77] However, invasive angiography is cumbersome and is not recommended for routine evaluation, particularly in small children.[18]

Oakes and Charters described and diagrammed the location, extent, and nature of splenic injuries, defining them as "minor" or "major."[143, 144] All injuries, however, were classified at celiotomy, obviating the ability to preoperatively assess the injury to determine the direction of management should the patient be a candidate for nonoperative care. Traub and Perry also surgically categorized the extent and nature of such injuries and clearly showed that both morbidity and mortality increased with severity of injury.[203]

In 1981, Shackford and associates developed a much more detailed classification based on operative findings.[180] Grading splenic injury in terms of severity from grade I through grade V, they suggested that splenic salvage should be achieved in more than 90% of grade I and II injuries, 60 to 65% of grade III injuries, and 5 to 10% of grade IV injuries. Splenectomy was recommended for grade V injuries. Using this system, experience has suggested that ultimate success depends on the surgeon's experience, ingenuity, and persistence.[65, 180] This classification system, further refined, later proved very comparable to findings based on CT and was subsequently adopted by the American Association for the Surgery of Trauma's Organ Injury Scaling Committee as its definitive mechanism for consistently classifying and standardizing splenic injuries to enable improved comparison of results and care.[128]

In 1983 and 1984, Barrett and colleagues and Buntain independently described workable and remarkably similar classifications for splenic injuries based on CT, identifying and grading the injuries qualitatively as well as quantitatively.[6, 16] This enabled identification of the severity of injury and often, but not always, the presence of associated injuries *early in the postresuscitative and preoperative phase of management.* Physicians could be provided with essential information that was comparable to operative findings, which helped the managing physician decide between an operative and a nonoperative approach to care. In 1985 we added to this classification ''subtype'' injuries to account for associated injuries that may also be present in an attempt to improve predefinitive management recognition of severity and extent of injuries sustained[18] (Table 21–1). ''A'' represents ''isolated'' splenic injuries without other associated intra-abdominal or extra-abdominal injuries; ''B'' represents splenic injuries with associated intra-abdominal injuries: ''B_1'' for those involving a solid viscus and ''B_2'' for those involving a hollow viscus. ''E'' represents splenic injuries with associated extra-abdominal injuries. It is important to note that *hemodynamically unstable patients are not candidates for CT* and this type of classification of their injuries; instead, operative intervention is indicated for these patients as per usual accepted criteria.

We later confirmed the usefulness of this classification and reported on our experience with 46 patients, 10 children, and 36 adults.[20] All of these patients were evaluated additionally with regard to injury severity by using the Trauma Score (TS), the Pediatric Trauma Score (PTS), and the Injury Severity Score (ISS), and these scores were compared with the classification system described previously in an attempt to correlate our system of grading spleen injuries with other better-known indices of injury severity, particularly the ISS.[3, 26, 201] Although the correlation coefficient between our classification and both the TS and the PTS implied a weak relationship, that between our classification and the ISS (the generally accepted gold standard for such comparisons) was indeed positive and significant (p = 0.0204). In addition, the overall ''accuracy'' of this classification was 97%; the specificity, using operative findings as the gold standard, was 100%; and the sensitivity (i.e., the number of positives that were correct) was 93%.

Table 21–1
Classification of Splenic Injury

Grade	Description
I	Localized capsular disruption or subcapsular hematoma, without significant parenchymal injury
II	Single or multiple capsular or parenchymal disruptions, transverse or longitudinal, that do not extend into the hilum or involve major vessels; intraparenchymal hematoma may or may not coexist
III	Deep fractures, single or multiple, transverse or longitudinal, extending into the hilar area and involving major segmental blood vessels
IV	Completely shattered or fragmented spleen or spleen separated from its normal blood supply at the pedicle

Subclass	Description
A	Without other associated intra-abdominal injuries
B	With associated intra-abdominal injuries; B_1 = solid viscus B_2 = hollow viscus
E	With associated extra-abdominal injuries

Adapted from Buntain WL, Gould HR: Splenic trauma in children and techniques of splenic salvage. World J Surg 9:398–409, 1985.

We also demonstrated that patients who were operated on for splenic injury had a 38% higher ISS (25 vs. 18) and a 13% higher hospital bill. Similarly, patients with grade III injuries had a 47% higher ISS (28 vs. 19), a 23% higher hospital bill ($22,400 vs. $18,200), and a 13% longer hospital stay (18 vs. 16 days) than patients with grade II injuries. Also patients with splenectomies had an 89% higher ISS (35 vs. 18, p = 0.0036) than patients with splenorrhaphies, remained in the hospital 27% longer, and had a 35% higher hospital bill. Patients with isolated splenic injuries or subclass A had an average ISS of 15, an average hospital stay of 10 days, and an average hospital bill of $9800. If the patient had an associated intra-abdominal and extra-abdominal injury along with the spleen injury, they also had a statistically significant higher ISS (27 vs. 15 or 80%, p = 0.0290), a 100% longer hospital stay (20 days vs. 10, p = 0.0198), and a 170% higher hospital bill ($24,900 vs. $9800, p = 0.0084). In this time of dramatically changing remuneration for health care delivery, both physician and institutional, these figures would seem important in determining what remuneration will be. In essence, all splenic injuries are not the same and cannot be treated the same, and the expected results are intimately related to the severity of injury and the presence of associated injuries.

In January 1988 at the Eastern Association for the Surgery of Trauma meeting, we presented our experience with 30 children utilizing this classification, the pediatric experience coming from a busy level I trauma center where mechanism of injury, as suggested by Perry, is more severe and is often associated with other abdominal visceral and extra-abdominal trauma.[19, 157] In previously unpublished data, hemodynamically unstable patients were not candidates for torso CT, but all 30 children in this study presented with or soon achieved hemodynamic stability with resuscitation. Spleen injuries were classified according to severity by CT and, provided no associated injuries necessitated surgical intervention, children with grade I (five patients) or uncomplicated and usually isolated grade II injuries (13 patients) were directly admitted to the critical care unit for observation and monitoring. Children with grade III (eight patients) or grade IV injuries (one patient) and those with grade I or II injuries accompanied by what appeared to be other significant intra-abdominal injuries (four patients) were taken directly to the operating room for celiotomy, and splenic salvage was accomplished whenever possible.

Seventeen children (57%), four with grade I and 13 with grade II injuries, had their injuries managed nonoperatively. Thirteen patients underwent operative intervention (43%), four for associated intra-abdominal injuries with less severe splenic damage (one grade I injury and three grade II injuries) and nine for major splenic injury (grade III and IV). Twelve of those operated on (92%) had successful splenic salvage. Hence, including the 17 children with splenic injuries who were successfully managed nonoperatively and did not require surgery, the overall splenic salvage rate was 29 of 30, or 97%.

There were three deaths, all secondary to associated severe head injuries. In only one instance was the splenic injury considered to have possibly contributed to the death of the patient. This 7-year-old patient with a grade IV injury

Table 21-2

Operated versus Nonoperated Injury Severity, Morbidity, and Cost (30 Children)

	Mean PTS	Mean ISS	Mean Hospital Cost	Mean Hospital Stay
Nonoperated (17)	8	19	$16,200	16 days
Operated (13)	6	29	$33,000	21 days
Difference	33%	53%	104%	31%

PTS, Pediatric Trauma Score; ISS, Injury Severity Score.

Table 21-4

Associated Injuries: Injury Severity, Morbidity, and Cost (30 Children)

Subclass (No.)	Mean PTS	Mean ISS	Mean Hospital Cost	Mean Hospital Stay (Days)
A (5)	10	13	$ 9400	6
BE (7)	8	23	$25,900	24
E (18)	6	26	$26,500	19

PTS, Pediatric Trauma Score; ISS, Injury Severity Score.

was the only splenectomy in the group, the splenectomy having been done because of the severity of the splenic injury and the necessity to obtain prompt hemodynamic control. A 2-year-old physically abused child and a 16-year-old child ejected from a motor vehicle suffered massive head injuries and at autopsy or organ harvesting were found to have minor or grade I splenic injuries that almost certainly could have been managed nonoperatively.

Blunt trauma was responsible for all injuries. There were 21 (70%) motor vehicle accident victims, including 15 passengers (eight unrestrained), five pedestrians struck by vehicles, and one bicycle rider also struck by a vehicle. In addition, five patients were injured riding motorcycles, two were injured while riding bicycles, one was injured in a fall, and another was physically abused. Importantly, only five of the 30 (or 17%) had isolated splenic injuries: subclass A. Eighteen, or 60%, had associated extra-abdominal injuries. Seven children (23%) had associated intra-abdominal injuries: subclass B. Injuries to another solid viscus, subclass B_1, occurred in five with two significant liver injuries and four significant renal injuries. All were managed nonoperatively. Two associated injuries to hollow viscera—subclass B_2—however, required additional procedures, an intestinal disruption and a torn iliac artery. Hence, two of the seven patients (29%) with associated injuries needed an operative procedure in their own right. Among this subclass B, there were also 16 associated extra-abdominal injuries—subclass BE—in the seven patients.

Our data also allowed us to look at injury severity, morbidity, and cost as these related to operation versus nonoperation cases (Table 21-2), injury grade (Table 21-3), and associated injuries (Table 21-4). Of the patients managed with operative intervention versus those managed nonoperatively (see Table 21-2), those who underwent surgical

intervention had more serious injuries as indicated by a 33% more serious PTS, a 53% more serious ISS, and a 31% longer hospital stay. As expected, patients who had operations had larger hospital bills, more than twice those of patients who were managed nonoperatively.

In evaluating injury grade with regard to severity, morbidity, and cost (see Table 21-3), as the injury grade worsened, the severity as indicated by the PTS and ISS became progressively worse, as did the hospital charges. Although the number of patients was not large, one of the primary reasons to stratify these injuries is to allow for the collection of appropriate numbers with which to perform adequate statistical comparisons, such as with a multi-institutional or cooperative study.

Table 21-4 illustrates this importance for it is clearly seen that associated injuries were very influential in terms of injury severity, morbidity, and cost. If there were no associated injuries (e.g., an isolated splenic injury or subclass A), the injury severity was distinctly less, indicated by a higher PTS, a lower ISS, and a shorter and considerably less expensive hospital stay. We had no patients with associated intra-abdominal injuries only, but if the child had a spleen injury and another associated injury within the abdomen as well as an associated extra-abdominal injury (as happened in each instance when more than one intra-abdominal injury was encountered), the severity of injury worsened by 25% with regard to the PTS and by 77% with regard to the ISS, and the hospital stay reflected this, increasing by 300%. Of course, the cost increased significantly also, by 176% from $9400 to $25,900. In addition, if the splenic injury was associated *only* with an extra-abdominal injury (subclass E), the severity of injury worsened even more, with the PTS decreasing from 10 to 6, or 40%; the ISS increasing from 13 to 26, or 100%; and the hospital stay increasing from 6 to 19 days, or by 216%. This was primarily due to the associated head and orthopedic injuries.

In evaluating the severity of splenic injury and the presence or absence of associated injuries (Table 21-5), only

Table 21-3

Injury Grade: Injury Severity, Morbidity, and Cost (30 Children)

Grade (No.)	Mean PTS	Mean ISS	Mean Hospital Cost	Mean Hospital Stay (Days)
I (5)	8	20	$22,300	19
II (16)	8	21	$18,900	17
III (8)	7	25	$35,200	22
IV (1)*	0	59	$ 9300	1

*Expired 24 hr after the injury from severe closed-head injury.
PTS, Pediatric Trauma Score; ISS, Injury Severity Score.

Table 21-5

Injury Grade versus Associated Injuries (30 Children)

Grade I	3 of 5 or 60%
Grade II	15 of 16 or 94%
	11 extra-abdominal (69%)
	4 intra-abdominal (25%)
Grade III	6 of 8 or 75%
Grade IV	1 of 1 or 100%

two of the grade I injuries had isolated splenic injuries and 3, or 60%, had associated extra-abdominal injuries. However, as the grade of injury to the spleen increased in severity, so did the number of associated injuries. Fifteen of the 16 grade II injuries had an associated injury, 11 (69%) extra-abdominal and four (25%) intra-abdominal. Hence, a child with a grade II injury had a 69% chance of having a significant associated extra-abdominal injury and a 25% chance of an associated intra-abdominal injury. Similarly, for grade III injuries, six of eight (75%) had associated injuries, three intra-abdominal and three extra-abdominal. Thus, a child with a grade III injury had a 38% chance of having an intra-abdominal injury and a similar incidence for an extra-abdominal injury. Our solitary grade IV injury had a severe head injury that eventually caused his death. I believe that the relatively low incidence of grade IV injuries illustrates the fact that patients with these injuries most often present with hemodynamic instability and thus go directly to the operating room without CT evaluation.

Using this approach to classifying splenic injuries and intervening surgically for the more serious ones, we successfully salvaged 29 of 30 spleens, a splenic salvage rate of 97%. We were able to salvage 12 of 13 injured spleens that were operated on, an operative salvage rate of 92%. I have personally managed 42 consecutive splenic injuries since first beginning this approach, with an overall salvage rate of 98% (41 of 42) and an operative salvage rate of 94% (17 of 18).

Stratifying patients in this manner improves the ability to standardize and compare the experiences of other investigators. Indeed, Elmore and colleagues, in a review of 143 consecutive adult patients with splenic injuries, included CT scoring of these patients "for academic purposes. We wanted other investigators to be able to compare their results with ours. We also documented with CT scores that these were not trivial splenic injuries but rather significant injuries to the spleen."[55]

Malangoni and associates also addressed this, noting that comparison of reports of splenic injuries in adults, particularly those dealing with nonoperative management, are difficult to interpret because the extent of splenic injury has often not been stratified or analyzed carefully.[115] Because a major goal of nonoperative management of splenic injuries is to select patients with injuries that are likely to have a high probability of success with nonoperative care, the ability of torso CT not only to determine the pattern and degree of splenic injury but to allow an estimate of free blood in the abdomen (hence blood loss) and to identify potential associated injuries is important. As Malangoni and associates stated:

The increased use of CT to evaluate blunt abdominal trauma has led to recognition of splenic injury in some patients who may not have had their injuries diagnosed previously because of minimal findings on physical examination alone. Most of these are minor, but the augmentation of reports of splenic trauma with patients who may have minor injuries accentuates the need for a classification system for injury to the spleen so that series can be compared with appropriate consideration given to the impact of degree of splenic injury on the success of management.[115]

They compared CT evaluation of injury with operative assessment and eventual management and found that operations increased in frequency, in both adults and children, as the injury score worsened.

Cogbill and co-workers, using the Organ Injury Scale for splenic trauma outlined by the American Association for the Surgery of Trauma, demonstrated that nonoperative management of splenic injuries is most successful in patients with less severe injury by severity grading.[29] They looked at 112 patients with splenic injuries that were intentionally managed by observation, 40 of whom (36%) were younger than 16 years old. Diagnosis was established by CT in 89%: 28 grade I injuries, 51 grade II injuries, 31 grade III injuries, two grade IV injuries, and no grade V injuries. They concluded that patients with grade I, II, or III splenic injuries are candidates for nonoperative management if there is no hemodynamic instability after initial resuscitation, no serious associated intra-abdominal organ injury, and no extra-abdominal condition that precludes assessment of the abdomen. This has been confirmed by others.[126, 211]

Failure of nonoperative management was defined as clinical or laboratory evidence of ongoing hemorrhage requiring celiotomy for control or any evidence of a missed or delayed diagnosis of serious associated abdominal injury.[29] All injuries were blunt. The children had a 93% overall nonoperative salvage rate, 39 of 40, and the one who required an operation also had a successful splenic salvage procedure. Thus, there was a 100% overall success of salvage rate in the children marked for nonoperative management based on CT classification of injury severity. When they stratified these patients by severity of splenic injury, none of 28 grade I injuries, four of the 51 (8%) grade II injuries, six of the 31 (19%) grade III injuries, and two of the two (100%) grade IV injuries failed nonoperative management because of persistent hemorrhage. Hence, as the injury severity increased, so did the failure rate for nonoperative management.

It has also been our belief that following a policy of early operative intervention after appropriate identification of the severity of injury ensures that the injured organ is more amenable to surgical repair, easier to work with, less friable, and more responsive to manipulation. Perhaps related to the ability to improve splenic salvage if operative intervention is instituted earlier is the "volume change" in splenic size following trauma as reported by Goodman and Aprahamian.[78] They pointed out that after blunt abdominal trauma the spleen often increases in volume on serial CT scans. They looked at 44 hemodynamically stable patients ranging in age from 5 to 78 years, and 25, or 57%, had greater than a 10% enlargement, the average being 56%, on follow-up CT. Although this increasing organ volume did not correlate with clinical deterioration, it did correlate with hemoperitoneum as determined by CT; the number of units of blood transfused; and two clinical indexes of systemic trauma, the Glasgow Coma Score (GCS) and the Revised Trauma Score (RTS). The average splenic volume increase was 25.6%, but 19 patients (43% of their series) had less than a 10% increase in splenic volume and 25 patients (57% of their series) had greater than a 10% increase, with an average enlargement of 56%. Notably, three spleens more than doubled in size.

In healthy adult volunteers, the average splenic volume is 219 ± 75 cm³.[83] No such standards for splenic volume exist in children. In Goodman and Aprahamian's study, the initial splenic volume was slightly below this and follow-up splenic volume slightly above it. They believe that the initial less than normal splenic size with eventual return to normal size is not a sign of deteriorating splenic status but appears to be due to the systemic effect of trauma, a physiologic contraction and perhaps spontaneous transfusion, rather than to the local abdominal injury, because the GCS, the RTS, and the ISS all correlated significantly with changing splenic size. They point out that splenic contraction in response to exercise, hemorrhage, or administration of epinephrine is well documented in dogs, providing a source of autotransfusion in response to stress.[83, 208] In humans, the visceral circulation is known to contract in response to adrenergic stimulation such as stress, thus decreasing blood flow to the spleen.[172] It is likely that in these acutely injured patients, the spleen contracted under heavy adrenergic stimulation. With time, volume replacement, and equilibration, the spleen returned to normal size, seen physiologically on the CT scan as progressive splenic enlargement, *peaking in size at 6 days after the injury.*

It is plausible that as the spleen returns to normal size, or larger, as part of the physiologic response to injury and resuscitation, increasing parenchymal and extrasinusoidal edema or hemorrhage would provide a more difficult organ to work with in terms of splenic salvage procedures because of the increased risk of adversely aggravating ongoing bleeding and disrupting temporarily ceased bleeding, particularly with regard to mobilization for repair and holding sutures. In terms of the amount of intra-abdominal bleeding, the amount of blood transfused, the GCS, and the RTS, it is conceivable that the grade I and II injuries therefore have less volume change and hence are more conducive to nonoperative management. At the same time, the more severe grade III, IV, and V injuries would be more likely to have greater volume changes and so be more difficult to work with and less tolerant of splenic salvage attempts.

Addressing the criticism that splenic salvage techniques are less likely to be successful in patients who fail observation, Cogbill and colleagues concentrated on patients with minor injuries, those who had the lower ISSs and the ones in whom splenic enlargement from autotransfusion would be the least.[29] In these, one would expect operative salvage rates to be high, and, in fact, seven of the 12 patients who required surgical intervention and who were operated on within 5 days of injury had their spleens salvaged. However, the successful salvage at 9 days had a mesh splenorrhaphy and the one salvaged at 10 days a hemisplenectomy, results that could reflect the increasing inability of the spleen to be manipulated or sutured as the number of days following the injury increases. Their conclusion was similar to others, namely, that improvement in the success of nonoperative management can result from using the CT scan to select patients according to the degree of splenic injury.[29, 115, 159, 164]

Scatamacchia and associates looked at how scoring affected treatment rather than how accurately it correlated with the degree of splenic injury.[173] Using their own splenic injury severity scoring system, they graded their patients in terms of severity of injury. In an initial group in whom nonoperative management was attempted, they found that there was a significantly higher splenic trauma score for patients who subsequently required abdominal exploration than for those who were successfully managed nonoperatively. Using this finding as a baseline, in a second very similar group of patients, the managing surgeon determined the advisability of operative intervention based on their "splenic trauma score" when they were first seen. The incidence of splenic salvage was increased significantly from 21 to 67%, *thereby increasing the overall splenic salvage rate for the group.* The researchers concluded that delaying surgery for 24 hours after the injury "practically excluded the chances for successful splenic salvage." They pointed out that the nonoperative management of splenic trauma works, but without a mechanism to identify candidates for a trial of nonoperative management, significant complications can occur and the chance of operative splenic salvage is decreased. Among their high-risk patients (as determined by stratifying the injury severity) operated on because of splenic injury, successful splenorrhaphy was accomplished in 67% in the second group of their study compared with 21% in the first, with similar patients in terms of injury severity scores and *with no increase in the overall operative rate in the two groups.*

Admitting that their scoring system may indeed prompt occasional unnecessary operations, Scatamacchia and associates concluded that an early operation in a high-risk patient is not necessarily a bad strategy because of the demonstrated difficulty in salvaging the spleen when operative intervention is delayed more than 24 hours.[173] They further reported that their results using a splenic injury CT grading system in the clinical decision-making process confirm that patients with lower scores can more often be treated safely without operation than those with more severe injuries; thus, patients with higher scores are more likely to need surgery. Importantly, in this study, use of their splenic trauma score did not increase the operation rate but did prompt earlier surgical intervention and nullified the number requiring surgery after an initial trial of nonoperative management, which increased the rate of splenic salvage significantly.

Nonetheless, the gold standard of care for splenic injuries in children continues to be nonoperative management, and indeed a considerable body of evidence has accumulated supporting and confirming that the injured spleen is capable of satisfactory healing either spontaneously or following surgical repair. The most commonly affected organ in blunt abdominal trauma despite its relatively well-protected anatomic location, the spleen is frequently damaged in association with other injuries as evidenced by postmortem findings in cases in which the fatal lesion involved a head injury.[124, 148, 181, 206, 214] Bleeding of the spleen in such cases had stopped, seemingly controlled by clotted blood. Had these patients survived, surgical intervention most likely would never have occurred.[49]

Foster and Prey wondered about the recovery of such injured spleens, questioning if they ever recovered spontaneously.[72] He quoted Turnbull of London as saying that he "never had seen at necropsy a spleen containing the scar of an old injury," and McCartney of the University of Minnesota reviewed 25,000 autopsies without finding evidence of healed splenic injuries. However, Barnes disclosed a report by Lukis in Lancet in 1909, stating that there were two such specimens in the St. Bartholomew's Hospital Museum, confirming that this occurs.[18]

The Toronto group has contributed immensely and importantly to our understanding of spleen injuries. In 1940, Wansborough, Chief of General Surgery at The Hospital for Sick Children in Toronto, observed a healed spleen several months following an apparent abdominal injury, and he postulated very appropriately that splenic injury was probably not an absolute indication for splenectomy. Over the ensuing years the Toronto group developed its current practice of "conservative management for splenic injury" and documented that approach in several publications, culminating in the 1989 report of their latest 75 cases over a 5-year period.[44, 52, 53, 66, 152, 182, 183, 206, 217] Reported in the *Journal of Pediatric Surgery,* patients varied in age from 1 day to 18 years, with a mean age of 9.6 years. All injuries were the result of blunt trauma, and diagnosis was by emergency celiotomy, spleen scan (radioisotope), ultrasound, and CT.[152] Operative intervention was based on clinical parameters only, and documented splenic injury was not an indication for surgery. Immediate surgery was performed on patients for "massive hemorrhage," defined as more than 40 ml per kg estimated blood loss; "patients who could be stabilized with fluid resuscitation were admitted and treated without surgery," initially to the intensive care unit, but later only those who required close monitoring were admitted to the intensive care unit. The rest were admitted to a regular surgical floor. In patients who required surgery, preference was given to splenorrhaphy or partial splenectomy. Total splenectomy was performed only when the spleen was irreparable or when other abdominal injuries precluded attempts at splenic salvage.

The motor vehicle was the responsible mechanism of injury in 48% of the patients, and 45 of the 75, or 60%, had "isolated" splenic injuries. In our series alluded to previously, only 17% had isolated splenic injuries and the motor vehicle was responsible for the injuries in 70%, implying a more severe transfer of energy with the mechanism of injury in our series. Sixty-five of the 75 patients were successfully managed nonoperatively (87%), but, as Malangoni and colleagues pointed out, "patients in their study were not stratified according to the degree of splenic injury."[115] Indeed, the 45 isolated spleen injuries most likely represented grade I or II injuries, perhaps some grade III injuries, implying less energy transfer with trauma, and the type of injury most would appropriately manage nonoperatively.

Of additional importance was the disclosure that of 10 patients who were operated on, three underwent total splenectomy, four had splenorrhaphies, one had a partial splenectomy, and two required no operative manipulation, an overall splenectomy rate of 4% for the series and 30% for the patients who had operations. Hence, in this review of 75 patients with splenic injuries, salvage of the spleen and thus presumed immunity overall was 95% and the operative salvage rate was 70%. Three other very reliable and reputable centers reported 173 total patients (in the three series) who were also managed by clinical observation without

regular CT and with operative intervention for clinical deterioration only and reported 37 patients who had operations with 22 splenectomies, or complete loss of splenic tissue surgically in 59% of operated cases.[162, 171, 217] These four series combined, then, represent an overall operative intervention rate of 19% in 248 injured children, an overall operative splenic salvage rate of 53%, and an overall total management salvage rate of 90%.

Lally and associates confirmed this, reviewing their experience for the decade 1965 to 1975 in the management of splenic injuries, when the primary mode of management was splenectomy, and compared it with their experience for the decade 1976 to 1985, when the primary mode of management was observation or splenorrhaphy if possible, splenectomy if necessary.[100] All the patients in the first decade had splenectomies; however, in the second decade reviewed, 44 of 70 patients (63%) were successfully managed nonoperatively. Of the 26 patients who had operations, an operative intervention rate of 37%, 10 still underwent splenectomy, for an overall splenic salvage rate for the second decade—the decade of modern splenic trauma management—of 85%. Once again, stratification of splenic injuries in terms of severity was not done; hence, it is difficult to interpret these results.

It is also difficult to interpret O'Neill's figures.[147] Commenting on Malangoni and associates' study, he reported 123 patients from the Children's Hospital of Philadelphia who were all evaluated with double contrast CT following splenic injury. Seventy percent, or 86 patients, were managed nonoperatively, and 30%, or 37 patients, underwent operation, with only three splenectomies. This implies an operative salvage rate of 92% and an overall splenic salvage rate of 98%, but exact figures and mechanisms of injury were not available and stratification of injuries was not done. Many of the patients had injured spleens that were not suspected, and these may well have been "isolated" injuries. If so, it is not surprising that most did very well.

What do these results mean? They suggest that in these centers, the gold standard of care for children with spleen injuries is primarily observation; operative intervention is reserved for clinical deterioration. However, they also suggest that reports supportive of a nonoperative approach that does not stratify splenic injuries in terms of their severity treat all splenic injuries as equal when obviously they are not. Insufficient information is being utilized in this approach to management, information that can and does improve splenic salvage.

How does one tell which injuries are potentially severe and perhaps accompanied by a significant associated intra-abdominal injury that may require operative intervention if it is not investigated? Blunt trauma to the abdomen results in injuries to the intraperitoneal as well as the retroperitoneal viscera, and most researchers believe that early diagnosis is imperative to obtain maximal results with minimal morbidity.[34, 63] The detection of intra-abdominal injury by physical examination alone continues to be a diagnostic enigma in the multiply injured, particularly in young uncooperative injured children, and delay in diagnosis and treatment can increase morbidity and mortality substantially.[65] Unstable patients are usually diagnosed rapidly, and management is initiated with minimal diagnostic procedures required. However, even the less severe presentations are diagnosed correctly by physical examination alone in only 42 to 87% of cases.[1, 57, 63, 145, 158] Therefore, physical examination, which is essential, of course, for all injuries regardless of severity, can be difficult and its results misleading in at least 13 to 58% of situations, particularly in the uncooperative child; in the presence of neurologic injury; or when lower rib fractures, abdominal wall contusions or abrasions, pelvic fractures, or drug or alcohol influence are contributing factors.

In addition, despite the low incidence of associated injuries (40%) in the study by Pearl and co-workers, the argument that "associated injuries to major organs are uncommon" is not supportable; in fact, the opposite is true, and isolated splenic injury in blunt trauma is uncommon. In a previous paper that reviewed eight separate series totaling 1048 cases, isolated splenic injuries occurred only 14% of the time and in our series alluded to above only 17% of the time.[17, 18, 26, 158, 196, 200, 201, 203, 205] In this group of 1048 patients, 55% had associated intra-abdominal injuries, and in reports that addressed the issue in children, 33% of these concomitant intra-abdominal injuries required operative management by themselves, including renal and hepatic lacerations, diaphragmatic injuries, mesenteric rents, vascular injuries, and intestinal injuries.[18, 200, 201, 203] Gross contamination of the abdomen from gastrointestinal injuries occurred in 31% of the associated injuries, and, although not common, failure to recognize intestinal injury with contamination occurs more frequently than is generally appreciated.[201] Symptoms may be few and diagnosis greatly delayed. Patients may even continue to eat initially because adjacent bowel and omentum can temporarily occlude the injury.[213, 214] In one series, five of seven children with jejunal injuries had their operations delayed from 24 hours to 4 days because of this delay in diagnosis.[214] Delayed recognition of splenic injury is, in fact, one of the most common causes of preventable death following blunt trauma.[131]

The real misfortune, however, is that regardless of which approach is correct or more appropriate, results cannot be compared adequately until the injuries are stratified consistently. Polk, in discussing Villalba's study, emphasized the need to standardize data:

> What we need are some data similar to [those] for the treatment of certain kinds of very favorable cancers. We need a huge number of patients treated in a standard way and followed up for a very long time. That is the only way to tell whether no treatment, aggressive treatment, or conservative treatment works.[160]

A combined or multicenter cooperative study, standardized with stratification of injuries for proper comparison, would seem the best approach to this. For example, the high incidence of apparently "isolated" splenic injuries from the Toronto series (compared with ours) and the higher incidence of motor vehicles being the mechanism of injury in a significantly larger number of our cases suggests a greater energy transfer causing the trauma in our patients and hence the higher ISS scores in our operated versus unoperated cases. It seems likely that our unoperated cases were very similar to the unoperated cases from the Toronto series, but our operated cases may have presented us with a

group of more seriously injured children, and our overall salvage results were related to a more favorable injured organ to deal with because we did not wait for clinical deterioration.

Many splenic injury grading systems have been proposed to help unify reporting among practitioners and to evaluate the results of treatment.[179] Recognizing this, the Organ Injury Scaling Committee of the American Association for the Surgery of Trauma in 1989 proposed a Splenic Injury Scale that combined previous scales with ICD-9 codes and abbreviated injury scores[128] (Fig. 21–1). Based on careful accurate assessment at autopsy, celiotomy, or by radiologic

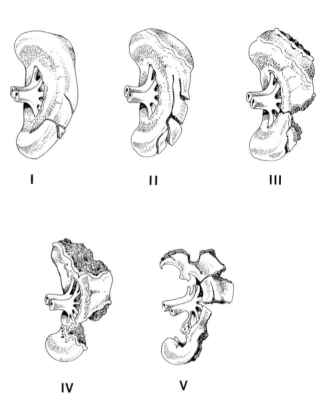

FIGURE 21–1

Classification of splenic injuries as recommended by the Organ Scaling Committee of the American Association for the Surgery of Trauma. Class I splenic injuries can manifest as a hematoma (subcapsular, nonexpanding, and <10% of the surface area), a laceration (capsular tear, nonbleeding, <1 cm parenchymal depth), or both. Class II injuries can manifest as a hematoma (subcapsular, nonexpanding, 10–50% surface area; intraparenchymal, nonexpanding, <2 cm in diameter), a laceration (capsular tear, mild active bleeding, 1–3 cm parenchymal depth, which does not involve a major trabecular vessel), or both. Class III injuries can manifest as a hematoma (subcapsular, >50% surface area or expanding; ruptured subcapsular hematoma with active bleeding; intraparenchymal hematoma (<2 cm or expanding)), a laceration (>3 cm parenchymal depth or involving trabecular vessels), or both. Class IV injuries manifest as a hematoma (ruptured intraparenchymal with active bleeding), a laceration (involving segmental or hilar vessels producing major devascularization—>25% of the spleen), or both. Class V injuries represent the severely lacerated spleen, disrupted, with extensive vascular compromise, and the completely shattered spleen with a devascularizing hilar vascular injury. (Adapted from Shackford SR, Molin MR: Management of splenic injuries. Surg Clin North Am 70: 604–608, 1990.)

study, this classification is important because it represents a compilation of all previous classifications and standardizes splenic injury scaling to one very workable mechanism with regard to management as well as outcome. Grade I splenic injuries can manifest themselves as a hematoma (subcapsular, nonexpanding, and <10% of the surface area), a laceration (capsular tear, nonbleeding, <1 cm parenchymal depth), or both. Grade II injuries also manifest themselves as a hematoma (subcapsular, nonexpanding, 10–50% of the surface area; intraparenchymal, nonexpanding, <2 cm in diameter), a laceration (capsular tear, active bleeding, 1–3 cm parenchymal depth that does not involve a trabecular vessel), or both. Grade III injuries also can manifest as a hematoma (subcapsular, >50% surface area or expanding; ruptured subcapsular hematoma with active bleeding; intraparenchymal hematoma, <2 cm or expanding), a laceration (>3 cm parenchymal depth or involving trabecular vessels), or both. Grade IV injuries also can manifest as a hematoma (ruptured intraparenchymal with active bleeding), a laceration (involving segmental or hilar vessels producing major devascularization—>25% of the spleen), or both. Grade V injuries represent spleens that are severely lacerated, disrupted, with extensive vascular compromise, or completely shattered with a devascularizing hilar injury.

I believe this is an acceptable and a workable classification for the early postresuscitative *and* preoperative phases of management. Using these criteria, we would expect all grade I and II injuries and most likely some grade III injuries to be manageable nonoperatively and most grade III injuries and all grade IV and V injuries to require operative intervention for the best opportunity for splenic salvage. Universal adoption of this standardized classification is recommended to help clarify our future understanding of splenic trauma. Once comparison becomes possible with general use, disagreement in terms of management will most likely center on the grade III injuries, and more specific criteria for operative intervention should be then attainable as documented standardized experience is achieved.

DIAGNOSIS

Before the advent of the more specific radiographic imaging modalities and DPL, diagnosis of splenic injury was largely based on clinical findings. Splenic injury can often be assumed to be present based on the results of the history, with critical details of the traumatic event often revealing the type of force suffered (deceleration or compressive). It should be remembered, however, that an accurate appraisal of the actual status of the spleen and hence some ability to predict outcome requires a more precise diagnostic assessment.

Clinical Presentation

Physical examination in the assessment of splenic injuries has an accuracy of 65%.[161] The signs and symptoms suggestive of splenic injury are those associated with intra-abdominal bleeding from any cause and vary according to the severity and degree of hemorrhage and possible associated injuries. They are due to the irritating effect of intraperitoneal blood, the acute blood volume loss, or the adjacent chest and abdominal wall tenderness.

Generalized abdominal pain and nausea are common. Pain localized to the left upper quadrant is reported in approximately 30% of both adults and children.[135] The reported incidence of pain at the tip of the left shoulder—Kehr's sign—varies from 15 to 75%, is secondary to irritation of the diaphragm, and can be enhanced by placing the patient in the Trendelenburg position. Tachycardia, hypotension, or both may be present. Palpation of the abdomen usually reveals tenderness and muscle spasm. Signs of peritoneal irritation secondary to hemoperitoneum are not uncommon. Occasionally, a tender mass or fullness can be appreciated in the left upper quadrant at the costal margin with an area of fixed dullness that can be outlined by percussion—Ballance's sign.

Although the diagnosis of isolated splenic trauma may be relatively easy in the cooperative patient, usually it is not, particularly when there may be multiple injuries; when the child is obtunded, unconscious, or uncooperative; or when there are other factors of importance such as drug involvement. In such cases, symptoms and abdominal findings are not reliable criteria for diagnosis of splenic injury, especially when other injuries are potential or present.[157]

Laboratory Findings

Laboratory findings after acute injuries are frequently not helpful. The hematocrit and hemoglobin values are often normal, even in the presence of arterial hypotension, unless sufficient time (18 to 24 hours) has elapsed following the injury to allow for transcapillary refill to occur.[157] Rapid modern transport of the injured patient to emergency facilities does not usually allow such time, and even leukocytosis, assumed by many to be a reliable sign of splenic rupture, in Perry's series was only elevated over 10,000/cu mm in 50% of the patients.[155] A base deficit of 3 mEq per liter or less obtained from an arterial blood sample suggests significant hemorrhage in healthy trauma patients and has been a useful indicator of ongoing intra-abdominal hemorrhage.[35]

Recognition of the usually inaccurate results utilizing conventional methods and the modern philosophy of aggressively identifying any and all organ injuries as soon as possible to optimize a trauma victim's care prompted the aggressive search for other diagnostic methods to find intra-abdominal injuries. Among these was DPL.

Diagnostic Peritoneal Lavage

The introduction of DPL by Root and colleagues in 1965 provided a rapid, inexpensive, accurate, and relatively safe diagnostic adjunct, which when performed properly has a reported 91% sensitivity, a 99% specificity, and a 97% accuracy.[156, 166] Although it remains an integral part of the evaluation of the seriously injured, it does not necessarily mandate celiotomy.[20, 131]

Diagnostic peritoneal lavage is widely accepted in the evaluation of patients with potential abdominal injuries, and despite the development of other more specific modalities it is still the most reliable method for diagnosis of abdominal visceral injury in the hemodynamically unstable patient.[157] When nonoperative management has been used for presumed isolated splenic injury, DPL may also be useful when associated intra-abdominal injury is suspected.

Diagnostic peritoneal lavage demonstrates free blood or intestinal content in the peritoneal cavity, but it is invasive, is not organ specific, may result in false positive findings in pelvic or retroperitoneal injuries, has a high false negative rate with disruptive injuries to the urinary bladder and the diaphragm, and results in a nontherapeutic celiotomy in 6 to 25% of patients.[63, 65, 74, 157] In addition, blood in the peritoneal cavity is no longer necessarily an indication for celiotomy, particularly in the pediatric age group.

Conventional Radiography

The chest radiograph may be abnormal in up to 50% of patients with splenic injury, but none of the changes is specific.[128] The supine radiograph of the abdomen may be helpful, the most common finding being free blood within the abdomen. However, at least 800 ml of intraperitoneal blood must be present to be evident on plain abdominal radiographs.[131] Findings that may support the diagnosis of splenic injury are the medial displacement of the left colon, making the "flank stripe sign" less obvious; the gravitation upward along each side of the bladder of blood accumulated in the pelvis, the so-called dog ear sign; the obliteration of the angle of the lower edge of the liver as blood accumulates along the right lateral side wall between it and the liver, the so-called hepatic angle sign; and, with extensive hemoperitoneum, the floating of the small bowel toward the center of the abdomen with the appearance of ground glass. Also, the injured spleen may displace the gastric bubble medially; indent the splenic flexure; or, with bleeding into the gastrosplenic ligament, cause "scalloping" along the gastric border as the bleeding indents the greater curvature while the stretched short gastric vessels resist. Other suggestive findings include coexisting rib or transverse process fractures in the area of concern and the suggestion of a soft tissue mass in the left upper quadrant.

Radioisotope Scan

Radioisotope scan has enjoyed extensive application in the investigation of splenic injury, the first report for a subcapsular hematoma being in 1967.[216] An added benefit of this study is that the liver is visualized along with the spleen, and coexisting liver injuries may also be identified. Witek and associates reported finding eight splenic injuries in 21 patients with abdominal trauma, and in only one of the eight were the classical physical findings evident.[221] They also found only one case in the literature in which a ruptured spleen was discovered at surgery following a scan that revealed no defect; however, false positive results reportedly occur in 3% of cases secondary to fetal lobulations.[131] Now outmoded, these scans are used primarily to follow the progress of healing of splenic injury when nonoperative management has been utilized.[89, 146] Their major disadvantages in the evaluation of acute abdominal trauma, however, include the time required for obtaining nuclear scanning, its qualitative limitation in assessing severity of injury as well as other intra-abdominal injuries with the possible exception of the liver, its inability to quantify intraperitoneal hemorrhage, and its inability to evaluate the retroperitoneum.[135] However, the overall sensitivity of technetium splenic scanning for acute injury is 98%.[140, 146] Direct comparisons of scintigraphy and CT for hepatosplenic trauma have found the former modality superior with respect to sensitivity, but scintigraphy is less specific with regard to the previously mentioned disadvantages.[131] These scans are useful during healing, however, and are also indirect measures of residual splenic function.

Ultrasonography

Ultrasonography, which is popular in Europe, should be mentioned as an additional noninvasive diagnostic modality that may be useful in the assessment of splenic trauma.[135] A positive feature is its bedside application. Free intraperitoneal blood and splenic capsular disruption can be identified readily, but limitations again include a lack of specificity and a decreased sensitivity when compared with those of the other diagnostic modalities, especially CT. In a controlled study comparing ultrasonography to CT for abdominal trauma in children, ultrasound had an unacceptable false negative rate of 50%.[97] In addition, Spencer and Gupta pointed out that ultrasonography is technically difficult with chest wall trauma and is not as sensitive as radionuclide study. Also intrasplenic changes are difficult to interpret in the presence of perisplenic, intraperitoneal, or pleural fluid.[194]

Angiography

In 1957, Norell described the first case of splenic injury identified by abdominal aortography.[142] Since then, because angiography is organ specific and has demonstrated a high degree of accuracy in the diagnosis and delineation of splenic injury with excellent correlation with operative and autopsy specimens, angiography has become to some investigators the gold standard against which all other modalities were compared.[20, 149] In fact, Sclafani, in discussion of Buntain and co-workers, suggested that angiography is the best means of identifying CT-diagnosed splenic injuries that are actively bleeding and thus candidates for operative intervention or therapeutic selective embolization.[20]

However, most centers do not advocate routine angiography, particularly for children, unless the patient requires angiography for other suspected conditions such as traumatic injury to the thoracic aorta, diagnostic and therapeutic embolization of pelvic fracture bleeding, or peripheral vascular trauma.[135] Hence, in the acutely injured, arteriography has largely been replaced by diagnostic methods that are less invasive and less time consuming.

Computed Tomography

Most major trauma centers use CT as the primary diagnostic modality in the evaluation of torso injuries. Contrast-enhanced CT, both intravenous and oral and sometimes colonic, offers potential advantages over all other diagnostic tests previously used and is our diagnostic method of choice.[184] The major advantage is that CT can simultaneously evaluate intra-abdominal and retroperitoneal structures, and, in combination with clinical observation and DPL, *CT has enabled the identification and usually the classification of solid viscus injury both qualitatively (i.e., which organ is involved) and quantitatively (i.e., to what degree the organ is involved).* The application of CT scanning also reduces the number of ancillary tests required for diagnosis, provides more accurate information regarding the extent and severity of injury, and results in more appropriate decisions regarding the need for exploration versus nonoperative management of the specific injuries. CT provides also a rapid, clear, and understandable presentation of findings in the third dimension, and the sensitivity and specificity are above 96%.[18, 93, 96, 114, 155, 184] The paracolic gutters, the subhepatic space, and the cul-de-sac can be examined for intraperitoneal blood, which can be quantified. Intravenous contrast for vascular and renal assessment as well as contrast opacification of the first portion of the small intestine is also important, and colonic contrast with CT in flank or posterior penetrating injuries is sometimes helpful.

Because delayed hemorrhage may occur with even minor splenic injuries seen at the initial study, there is some rationale for repeating CT scans at regular intervals early in the clinical course—the so-called delayed second look scans.[92]

It should be noted, however, that CT does have limitations, primarily in the evaluation of pancreatic injuries. Combination with DPL is most likely the appropriate mechanism to diagnose these injuries. Some have also questioned the ability of CT to demonstrate hollow viscus injuries, particularly in the gut.[116] My experience with CT and hollow viscus injury is very encouraging in that we now have 12 consecutive cases in children in which intestinal injury was suggested by CT. The diagnosis was based on the finding of significant intraperitoneal fluid in the presence of no solid organ injury in nine cases; of significant intraperitoneal fluid with minor grade II splenic injuries in two cases, both of which had the intestinal injury confirmed by DPL; and of significant intraperitoneal fluid along with a grade IV splenic injury (American Association for the Surgery of Trauma's Organ Injury Scale) in one case. This last patient, a 15-year-old unrestrained boy ejected from a pickup truck as it rolled over, underwent celiotomy for an extensively disrupted spleen with successful vicryl mesh splenorrhaphy and for an unsuspected solitary jejunal disruption that was discovered and repaired.

A technically adequate and normal CT virtually excludes a clinically significant traumatic spleen lesion. With the ability to detect the less severe injuries, the CT-based classification thereby helps determine which patients can be safely managed nonoperatively and which require operative intervention.[20]

MANAGEMENT

Four factors have most influenced change in the management of splenic injury from prompt splenectomy in all cases to splenic salvage when possible: (1) recognition of the risk of overwhelming postsplenectomy sepsis, (2) identification and understanding of the anatomic basis for splenic repair, (3) increasing experience with techniques of operative splenic salvage, and (4) advances in organ-specific imaging technology.[179]

Initial Evaluation, Resuscitation, and Stabilization

Initial maneuvers in the evaluation, resuscitation and stabilization of the acutely injured patient with suspected splenic trauma follow the general steps taken for all the acutely injured (see Chapter 10). Specific management of the child with a possible splenic injury is determined by hemodynamic status; age; interval from time of injury; associated injuries; and, of importance but to a lesser extent in the child, the mechanism of injury and the possible presence of associated abnormalities or disease processes. In children these are usually congenital, such as sickle cell disease.

The ultimate manner in which any patient with a splenic injury is managed is dictated by the patient's needs. Clearly, urgent celiotomy is indicated for the acutely injured child who is hemodynamically unstable and has a possible splenic injury. Diagnostic peritoneal lavage is often helpful in confirming or eliminating the potential for intra-abdominal injury in such patients, particularly when other injuries with potentially significant blood loss such as pelvic or long bone fractures may be present. Usually, however, the majority of children are hemodynamically stable on arrival or shortly thereafter with appropriate fluid resuscitation. Management of these patients should progress through the completion of stabilization along with appropriate definitive evaluation to determine, as accurately as possible, the presence of the injury; the severity of the injury; the presence or absence of associated injuries, including the identification of all potentially lethal or life-threatening injuries; and the appropriate management, nonoperative or operative, depending on the previously mentioned findings. *The objective of care is the salvage of sufficient splenic tissue to preserve normal or near normal immunity* (Fig. 21–2).

Nonoperative Management

The long-believed myth that the spleen was not necessary for normal survival, the technical ease of splenectomy, the persistent natural aversion of many surgeons to suturing the spleen, and the protracted belief that nonoperative management of spleen injuries carries considerable morbidity and mortality have significantly contributed to the unfortunate tendency toward operative intervention and splenectomy for splenic injury even today. However, an accumulation of knowledge that the spleen is not expendable, a natural inclination to avoid an operation if less invasive management

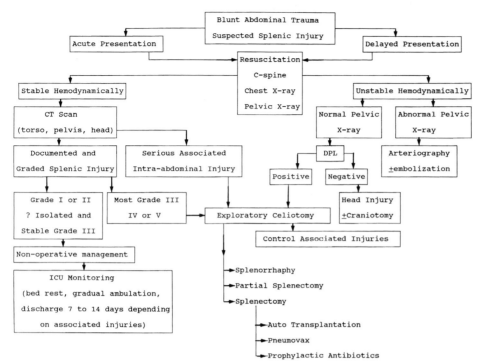

FIGURE 21–2

Algorithm of management for blunt abdominal trauma and suspected splenic injury. C-spine, Cervical spine; CT, computed tomography; ICU, intensive care unit; DPL, diagnostic peritoneal lavage.

sufficed, and a recognition that the injured spleen in certain instances stops bleeding and heals following injury led to the nonoperative approach to managing the injured spleen. The approach has been promulgated primarily by pediatric surgeons, initially at The Hospital for Sick Children in Toronto, and is now accepted as the gold standard for children almost universally.

In 1971, Douglas and Simpson reported on 32 children with suspected splenic injury, of whom 25 survived without operative intervention. Patients were managed with transfusions and required support otherwise, and all 25 left the hospital after an average of 16 days without apparent significant complications. Cautiously, because existing knowledge was meager and this was a radical change from accepted means of treating these injuries, they recommended this type of management be restricted to selected children and that they be observed under optimal circumstances.[44] They even cited some of the problems with this approach: the potential for missing associated injuries, the lack of confirmation of the potential for septic complications in older children, and the possibility of delayed consequences.

A 1976 editorial from the same institution by Shandling addressed the impaired initial response to blood-borne antigens and the lack of antibody formation after splenectomy and questioned why a stable patient with a splenic injury should undergo celiotomy with probable removal of one fourth of the lymphatic mass of the body.[181] He also cautioned that this management be selectively limited to children observed under optimal conditions.

A report from Australia a year later confirmed these observations, reporting on 39 children with splenic injuries, 25 of whom were initially managed without operation; one eventually required operative intervention and splenectomy.[95] Commenting on the spleen's ability to heal without operative intervention, they also recommended close obser-

vation and the availability of appropriate facilities for immediate operative intervention.

Since then many large series of children with splenic injuries managed nonoperatively have been reported.[8, 39, 53, 66, 89, 98, 192, 193, 217, 222] The majority of these children, "if chosen carefully," have not required operative intervention; complications have been few, delayed bleeding has been very rare, and mortality rates have been negligible.[157] However, all investigators have recommended that the child's condition be stable initially or stable after fluid or blood transfusion and closely monitored, preferably in an intensive care unit, and that adequate blood and an operating room must be readily available. Operative intervention is recommended if there is evidence of acute or delayed hemorrhage or if transfusion requirements exceed 40 ml per kg or one half the child's estimated total blood volume.[89, 157, 217]

Muehrcke and colleagues evaluated 24 children with splenic injury to attempt to determine which of them could be managed nonoperatively.[137] Six underwent operation, but 18 were managed nonoperatively, and these latter children were younger; had fewer associated injuries; required fewer blood transfusions; and suffered injury secondary to falls, sports, or altercations. Those requiring surgery were older, had multiple injuries, lost more blood, and were injured in motor vehicle accidents. They recommended that ISS, amount of blood required, age, and mechanism of injury encountered be used to help select patients who can be safely managed nonoperatively.

The criteria for utilization of nonoperative management of splenic injuries in adults is much less clear cut; however, clearly nonoperative management is a rational policy in selected patients. Elmore and associates reviewed 143 consecutive adult patients and, confirming Muehrcke and colleagues' findings, divided them into categories based on the

ISS: "isolated" splenic trauma with an ISS of less than or equal to 20, and polytrauma with an ISS of more than 20.[55] They confirmed that the nonoperative group's injuries were primarily due to falls, sporting injuries, and assaults, whereas the mechanism of injury in the operative group was primarily motor vehicle related (p = 0.005). Associated intra-abdominal injuries requiring surgery occurred in 22% of those who underwent immediate operation, and blood transfusions were significantly less in the nonoperative group. They concluded that if CT is used to detect and classify injuries, nonoperative management is also safe and effective in properly selected adult patients.

An important and prudent note of caution was stated by Grabowski, in a discussion of Elmore and associates, who addressed the issue of nonoperative management in the community hospital.[55] He pointed out several important caveats: If the physician is not in the hospital with the patient, as perhaps the physician should be for the first 24 to 48 hours, he or she must live only a few minutes away from the hospital; the monitoring personnel must be experienced and dedicated trauma or critical care nurses with the same degree of sophistication as more senior surgical residents; and the surgeon must have a ready, quality CT scanner, blood bank, and operating room on call at all times.

A frequent criticism promulgated by opponents of nonoperative management has been that splenic salvage is not successful in patients who fail observation.[9] In a multicenter experience sponsored by the Western Trauma Association, in which nonoperative trauma alone was successful in 60 (83%) of 72 adults, seven of the 12 failures, or 58%, were managed with splenic preservation techniques.[29] This well-controlled study followed precise criteria for nonoperative management, selecting patients carefully, and limiting nonoperative management to grade I and II injuries. In fact, splenic salvage would be expected in most of these injuries if operative intervention were initiated at the onset of care, at least in more than 90%, as suggested by Shackford and colleagues.[180]

The potential for missing a seriously associated abdominal injury is a legitimate concern and has been discussed previously. Traub and Perry noted serious concomitant intra-abdominal injuries in 37% of patients with blunt splenic trauma.[203] Fisher and co-workers documented gastrointestinal disruption after blunt abdominal trauma in 26.5% of adults compared with 6.5% in children.[68]

The risk to benefit issue with respect to blood transfusions in patients managed nonoperatively has also been addressed. Luna and Dellinger advocate a threshold limit of two units of blood, based on the known calculated risk of transmitting infectious diseases.[110] Because many patients treated nonoperatively require blood transfusion for replacement of losses, they questioned whether nonoperative management of splenic injuries is a safe therapeutic option and they studied splenic salvage with nonoperative and operative treatment, the incidence of overwhelming postsplenectomy sepsis and posttraumatic hepatitis, and related mortality in survivors of splenic injury. They estimated the amounts of blood transfused for operative and nonoperative therapy and calculated that the posttransfusion death rate per unit of blood from posttransfusion hepatitis is 0.14%. This frequency had previously been reported to vary from 7 to 50%, with chronic active hepatitis developing in 20 to 50% of those infected and 5 to 10% of these die from hepatitis-related complications.[110] Luna and Dellinger compared the risks of mortality from overwhelming postsplenectomy sepsis with the risks of dying from transfusion-related complications occurring during attempts at splenic salvage. Developing a "conditional probability model" and using available clinical data, they reviewed the world's literature and suggested several important observations:

1. The quoted incidence of 1 to 2% for overwhelming postsplenectomy sepsis in trauma patients may be a ten- to twentyfold overestimation;
2. The increased number of units of blood transfused during nonoperative therapy of splenic injury may lead to an increased probability of mortality when compared to early celiotomy because
   A. Early celiotomy with control of hemorrhage may decrease or eliminate the need for transfusion, and
   B. Splenorrhaphy is far more likely to be successful when performed soon after the injury rather than after a period of failed observation.

They concluded that the conditional probability of eventual death in a child treated initially nonoperatively was 0.17% compared with 0.06% for initial operative treatment. They suggested that this concern with potential transmission of the human immunodeficiency virus as well as hepatitis antigen by blood transfusion may make prompt operation to repair the injured spleen a preferable option to nonoperative management with its possible greater blood replacement requirements. However, this concern has proved to be unfounded because injuries of greater severity, those that usually prompt a decision for surgical intervention early, have been demonstrated to have even greater transfusion requirements.

Perry summarizes the nonoperative management of the injured spleen by noting that it clearly appears to be an option in the child. Patients with splenic injuries that appear to be isolated and unassociated with other intra-abdominal visceral trauma or with extra-abdominal injuries appear to be the best candidates.[157] Further, Perry states that circumstances most likely to produce such an injury are sports accidents, minor falls, or other trauma in which the forces applied to the body are of medium severity and more localized. Patients with major deceleration injuries with multiple injuries and hemodynamic instability are less liable to be candidates for nonoperative management.

Our approach is to follow the recommendations best stated by Shackford, who summarized the indications for embarking on a course of nonoperative management[179]:

The success of nonoperative [management] does not make it a routine practice in all children with abdominal trauma. Candidates for nonoperative management must have suffered blunt trauma, have an isolated splenic injury, be sufficiently alert to comply with repeated physical examination, and be hemodynamically stable. When nonoperative management is contemplated, diagnosis of splenic injury is usually established by CT and an assessment of the severity of injury is made. The child is hospitalized in the intensive care unit (ICU) and managed by a pediatric surgeon. Serial physical examinations of the abdomen are complemented with CT scans repeated on the third and seventh hospital days.

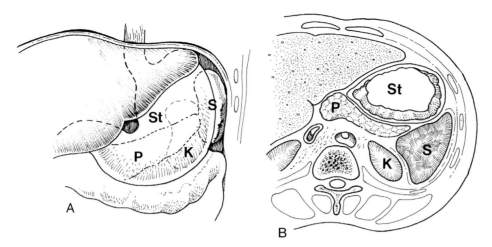

FIGURE 21-3

Surface (A) and cross-sectional (B) anatomy of the spleen in the posterolateral left upper quadrant of the abdomen, bounded superiorly by the lateral segment of the left lobe of the liver, the stomach (St), and the diaphragm; laterally and posteriorly by the diaphragm and the chest wall; inferiorly by the splenic flexure (S) and kidney (K); medially by the pancreas (P) and colon; and anteriorly by the stomach.

Vital signs and hematocrit are followed carefully, and the child is transfused to maintain hemodynamic stability and a hematocrit greater than 20 to 25%. If the child should become hemodynamically unstable or if the transfusion requirement exceeds an explicitly stated predetermined limit, nonoperative management is aborted and the child taken expeditiously to surgery.

Guidelines on ICU stay, duration of hospitalization, frequency of repeat CT scanning, and duration and frequency of outpatient management vary. We hospitalize the child in the ICU until the need for transfusion is abated, during which time the child remains prepared for surgery with consent signed, NPO, and intensive monitoring. The child is transferred to the ward setting and remains prepared for surgery for an additional 24 to 48 hours. A CT scan is obtained at discharge and at the first follow-up visit. Another scan is obtained at 3 months. If the injury is more severe, we are more conservative, prolonging the hospitalization and restricting activity. We realize that others have advocated prolonged ICU stays, hospitalizations, and restricted activities (for up to 3 months), but our experience does not justify this amount of conservatism. Moreover, we doubt that compliance with activity restriction is maintained well in this age group.

Operative Management

Surgical Approach and Mobilization of the Spleen with Injury Assessment

The surgical approach to splenic injuries, like the surgical approach to the spleen for elective problems, is straightforward and simple and can be accomplished expeditiously provided the operator has a thorough understanding of the anatomy and location of the spleen (Fig. 21-3A and B). With the patient in the supine position on the operating table, the spleen lies in the posterior-lateral area of the left upper quadrant, bounded superiorly by the lateral segment of the left lobe of the liver, the stomach, and the diaphragm; laterally by the diaphragm and rib cage–costal margin; inferiorly by the splenic flexure and the kidney; medially by the pancreas and the colon; posteriorly by the posterior chest wall; and anteriorly by the stomach.

Exploration of the abdomen for blunt trauma is usually done through a midline incision (Fig. 21-4) because appropriate operative surgical management of trauma requires the entire abdomen, its contained viscera, and the retroperitoneum, to be carefully assessed. The incision starts just below the xiphoid and extends down to the umbilicus. This incision can be made quickly, is associated with minimal blood loss, and can be extended cephalad or caudad rapidly if necessary to manage associated injuries.

Before making the incision, an appropriately sized nasogastric sump tube (size adjusted for age) is placed in the stomach. On opening the peritoneum, free intraperitoneal nonclotting blood is almost always encountered and is evacuated. However, excess time is not immediately taken to do this, attention being directed promptly to the left upper quadrant. In the hypotensive patient, the first maneuver should be to palpate the suprarenal aorta at the diaphragmatic hiatus to ascertain systemic perfusion pressure.[131] This information is shared with anesthesia, and if

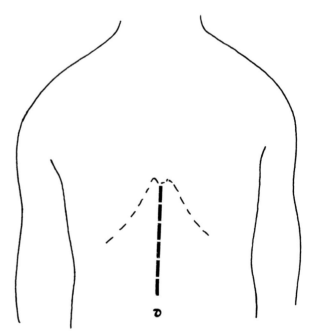

FIGURE 21-4

A midline incision allows access to the spleen and the remainder of the abdomen for evaluation of possible associated injuries.

ongoing intraperitoneal hemorrhage from the liver and spleen is identified, these areas are packed. If circulatory insufficiency exists and the spleen is believed to be contributing significantly, splenectomy is performed.

An essential feature in successfully performing a splenic salvage procedure is complete gentle mobilization of the spleen up onto the operative field, exactly as if one were going to do a splenectomy.[18] The spleen is secured deep in the left upper quadrant by generally avascular ligamentous tissue and peritoneum. With an assistant retracting the left side of the upper abdominal incision laterally and somewhat superiorly, the intragastric sump tube is manipulated to lie along the greater curvature. Grasping the sump through the stomach at the greater curvature with the right hand, it and the stomach are gently lifted anteriorly and to the patient's right or toward the operator, exposing the gastrosplenic ligament and closely attached spleen deep in the left upper quadrant. As the stomach comes up and out of the abdomen the spleen moves up and out of its bed as well. Nonclotting and partially clotted blood is gently aspirated clear, after which possible ongoing splenic bleeding is assessed. If a totally shattered spleen or one avulsed from its vascular pedicle is found, the surgeon may have no other alternative but splenectomy. If indeed this is the finding, we temporarily compress the splenic artery where it crosses the vertebral column with a sponge stick followed by prompt mobilization and then finger control of bleeding at the hilum or application of a noncrushing vascular hilar clamp. Usually, however, lesser degrees of hemorrhage are present.

The left hand then replaces the right and maintains stomach and sump traction, hence exposure (Fig. 21–5). The right hand then slides down over the spleen cupping the

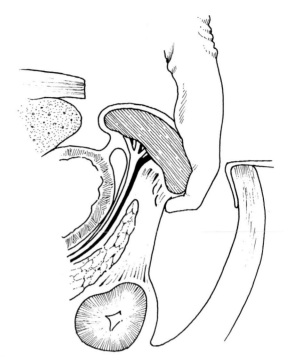

FIGURE 21–6

The right hand then slides down over the spleen with the fingers slightly spread, gently palpating the extent of injury, "gathering" and carefully lifting the organ anteromedially, exposing and tensing up the retrosplenic and peritoneal attachments.

organ with the tips of the fingers posteriorly, gently feeling the injury and gaining some insight as to its extent. Spreading the fingers to gently "gather" the entire organ, including the injured areas, it is lifted anteriorly and medially toward the pancreatic head, exposing the retrosplenic and suprasplenic area and the lienorenal and phrenicolienal ligaments (Fig. 21–6). Using forceps in the left hand, a damp lap sponge is placed over the right hand and then the left hand replaces the right and gently adds further traction so as to stretch the ligamentous attachments (Fig. 21–7). The entire posterior area of the left upper quadrant is now exposed and is irrigated and aspirated clear, no attempt to formally examine the extent of injury to the spleen having been made thus far.

The lienorenal ligament, now stretched, is opened with scissors and, working in a caudad to cephalad direction, sharply incised by working the deep blade just under the ligament and "push cutting" (Fig. 21–8). Elevation of the ligament by an assistant is helpful but is not absolutely necessary. As the right hand cuts, the left hand holding and retracting the spleen gently continues to lift the spleen and tail of the pancreas anteromedially. Care is taken to avoid injury to the more deeply positioned left kidney and adrenal gland. Cephalad dissection stops just after the lienorenal ligament incision is completed and the phrenicolienal ligament is freed at the top of the greater curve of the stomach. The incision must be carried up this far because the superior pole of the spleen is often intimately attached to the stomach at this point and excessive traction may avulse the short gastric vessels and result in troublesome bleeding.

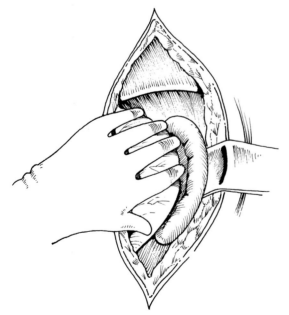

FIGURE 21–5

Splenic exposure is accomplished by applying medial and anterior traction on the nasogastric tube within the stomach at the greater curvature, pulling gently with the right hand, and then placing the left hand over the stomach, exposing the spleen.

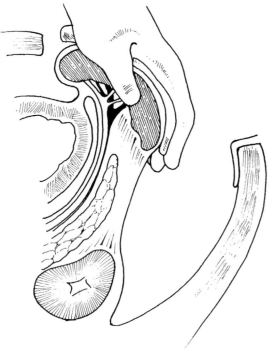

FIGURE 21-7

With a damp sponge placed over the right hand, the left hand replaces the right, further tenting the peritoneal attachments and exposing the entire area for irrigation and packing.

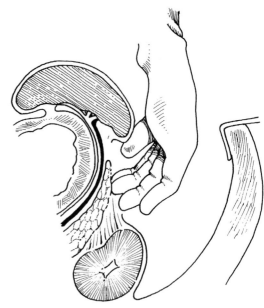

FIGURE 21-9

Completion of the incision of these peritoneal attachments further releases the spleen and tail of the pancreas, and the fingers, first of the supporting left hand and then of the right hand, assist this maneuver by gently and bluntly working into the retropancreatic space.

On completion of the release of these ligaments, the spleen freely retracts even more anteromedially and the right hand is placed over the left so that the fingers of the right hand can bluntly develop a plane between the underside of the pancreatic tail and the kidney (Fig. 21-9). As

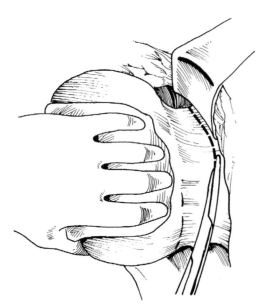

FIGURE 21-8

The peritoneal attachments, now exposed and under tension, are incised with scissors, in a cephalad direction up to the diaphragmatic crus, ''push-cutting'' as the left hand gently lifts and maintains traction.

this plane develops, the spleen and pancreatic tail are gently brought anteriorly out of the abdomen and placed on the anterior abdominal wall. This mobilization can be done rapidly. Once completed, one or two damp lap sponges are packed into the left upper quadrant to help support the elevated structures as well as to tamponade small vessel oozing from incised raw surfaces in the splenic fossa.

The spleen can now be thoroughly and gently examined and the extent of injury determined in a less hurried fashion. Ongoing bleeding is controlled, but it is often minimal. Although most recommend gentle removal of existing clot, I do not because removal is almost certain to result in the resumption of bleeding, which can be dangerous and can threaten organ salvage. If bleeding has ceased or is very minimal, it seems inappropriate to allow it to start again. In fact, it is our belief that some of the apparent inability to accomplish splenorrhaphy is because the surgeon removes this clot unnecessarily, and significant and possibly uncontrollable bleeding results. Large clots on the surface must be removed; however, the clot between the edges of the disruption is left undisturbed. If bleeding does become troublesome, finger pressure on the vessels in the hilus or the noncrushing hilar clamp is a very helpful maneuver to enable isolation of the bleeding area and appropriate control. Unless complete disruption of the spleen from its blood supply has occurred, a splenic salvage procedure rather than splenectomy is clearly indicated whenever it can be performed safely. Once the severity or grade of the injury and whether to undertake splenorrhaphy or partial splenic resection are determined, major clots are removed, actively bleeding vessels ligated or controlled with mattress sutures, and loose and devitalized tissue removed.

Operative Techniques of Splenic Salvage

Once the injury has been evaluated and operative salvage is an option, there are basically seven mechanisms to repair or salvage the spleen, alone or in combination.[18, 22, 132, 143]

1. Application of omentum or a topical hemostatic agent, with or without simple capsular sutures
2. Direct repair of the splenic parenchyma and capsule with simple or mattress sutures, with or without pledgets or omentum
3. Suture ligation of individual splenic vessels
4. Ligation of segmental vessels in the hilum or the splenic artery, or both, with or without ligation of selective short gastric vessels also
5. Partial splenectomy
6. Capsular, parenchymal, and vessel compression with application of an absorbable net (Vicryl or Dexon)
7. Large entire organ through-and-through absorbable mattress sutures, perpendicular to the plane of injury

Appropriately accomplished by knowledgeable surgeons, these procedures should be completed in essentially the same time it takes to do a splenectomy, management of any associated intra- and extra-abdominal injuries being the major determinant of the length of surgery.[204]

It seems reasonable to assume that all grade I and most grade II injuries can be managed nonoperatively, provided information regarding potential associated intra-abdominal injuries is complete and they are minor or absent. Careful monitoring in an appropriate critical care unit with advanced technologic backup is important. However, if these injuries are encountered in the course of emergency celiotomy in the face of hemodynamic instability or while performing celiotomy for other important associated injuries, topical hemostasis, direct pressure, or simple capsular sutures may be used if further management is necessary.

Our current preference is fibrin glue for the simple avulsion-type injuries and the same with or without simple capsular sutures for the superficial or shallow grade II injuries. Fibrin glue is a useful adjunct in the management of trauma to all the abdominal solid viscera.[84] It is formed by mixing a source of concentrated fibrinogen with thrombin and has been found to be hemostatic in mild to moderate splenic trauma.[13, 174] Intraparenchymal injection and direct application to the raw surface of an avulsion injury are the mechanisms of choice for application. The fibrin glue is allowed to seep into the injury, sealing it, and compression of the injected parenchyma until the glue polymerizes is useful to maximize local adherence as well as to eliminate the theoretic danger of embolism to the lungs.

For superficial injuries, electrocautery may be effective when applied as an arc current, avoiding deep parenchymal penetration with the cautery tip, which may stir up or initiate more serious hemorrhage. Electrocautery has been of little use to us, however, except for partial splenic resections when we use it to transect the devascularized tissue. The Argon Beam Coagulator (Bard Electro Medical Systems, Englewood, Colo.) has reportedly been highly effective.[131]

In my opinion, most of the patients with grade III injuries (American Association for the Surgery of Trauma, Organ Injury Scaling) and all of those with grade IV and V injuries should be resuscitated, stabilized if possible, and then surgically explored and should have their splenic injuries repaired when possible and clinically feasible. Active bleeding from deeper parenchymal disruptions requires suturing, controlled with direct suture transfixion of responsible vessels.[131] More diffuse bleeding, particularly if arterial, requires horizontal mattress sutures that incorporate bleeding vessels. We use 3–0 or 4–0 PDS sutures with Teflon, Gelfoam, or omental bolsters when necessary.

Extensive splenic disruption with devascularized segments usually requires segmental resection. This can be done safely because of the segmental vascular arrangement of the secondary divisions of the splenic artery. Segmental resection of the spleen preferably follows anatomic principles used for other solid organ resections. In reality, this is often very difficult because of hematoma and edema in the hilar area secondary to the injury. If the segmental vessel can indeed be isolated and surgically occluded, vascular demarcation should result. However, much of the segment intended for resection is already devascularized, and reliance on this demarcation to aid resection is unwise.

Some recommend the finger fracture technique used for liver resections to be used on the spleen in these circumstances; we suspect undesirable, indeed perhaps uncontrollable, bleeding and perhaps splenectomy would result from this unnecessary maneuver. Our approach is to identify the devascularized segment to be resected and if the hilus is not swollen and edematous with associated hematoma we will identify and ligate if possible the appropriate segmental vessels and resect the devascularized segment as described above. This is done using electrocautery and a row of horizontal mattress sutures placed over teflon pledgets across the spleen perpendicular to the hilus and just inside the remaining well vascularized portion of the spleen (Fig. 21–10A and B). Each mattress suture is tied with placement, completely traversing the spleen before removal of the devascularized portion. If however, as is often the situation in our experience, there is associated swelling and hematoma at the hilus such that a surgical approach to this area may threaten splenic salvage, the same row of horizontal mattress sutures is placed along the segmental plane of resection and the same result is accomplished. If any residual bleeding results, it is usually controlled with an overlapping or interlocking mattress suture at the particular site.

It has been postulated that preservation of immunity requires an as yet undetermined mass of splenic tissue, estimated by some to be approximately a third of the spleen that is originally present.[123] When performing partial resection, residual splenic volume should be considered. A substantial immunologic advantage exists if sufficient splenic tissue remains, but this may not offer sufficient protection from encapsulated bacteria if residual splenic arterial blood flow is reduced in the process. Horton and colleagues evaluated experimentally the rate of pneumococcal clearance by the spleen to define the relationship between splenic blood flow and amount of splenic tissue to bacterial clearance from the blood.[87] Comparing splenic blood flow in normal spleens, spleens with ligated splenic arteries, splenic autotransplants, hemisplenectomies, and splenectomies, they demonstrated, as expected, that autotransplanted splenic tis-

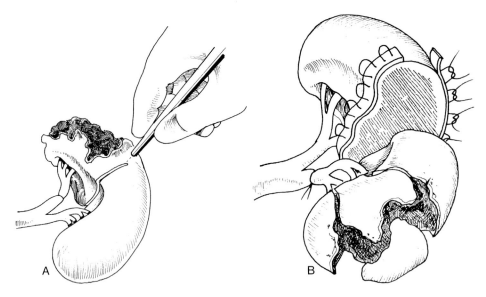

FIGURE 21–10

Partial splenectomy, with ligation of the segmental vessels to the injured area and transection of the subsequently devascularized area with electrocautery (A) or with multiple horizontal mattress sutures, with or without pledgets (B).

sue had the greatest reduction in blood flow (21% of control) and the smallest amount of splenic tissue (46% of control). Those with splenic artery ligation had splenic weights slightly greater than the control animals but had only half the blood flow. The hemisplenectomized animals had splenic weights that were 73% of controls and had 79% as much splenic blood flow as the controls. Because 50% of the spleen was removed, this was less of a reduction than expected because residual splenic tissue hypertrophied during the 3-month recovery period. In evaluating pneumococcal bacterial clearance, it occurred most rapidly with intact spleens, as expected, being complete at 2 hours. Hemisplenectomized animals had clearance rates an hour longer than the controls, and no clearance occurred with the splenectomized animals. *Animals with the ligated splenic arteries and those with autotransplanted splenic tissue failed to clear the blood of pneumococcal organisms.*

Immunologically, the absence of the spleen impairs the initial response to blood-borne particulate antigen or bacteria. Splenectomized individuals form antibodies to subcutaneous antigens quite normally, but when a particulate antigen is given intravenously, asplenic individuals form few or no antibodies.[170] Preserving even small amounts of splenic tissue results in normal immunologic responses, but the question is whether these smaller remnants will respond normally to protect against blood-borne bacteria. Singer pointed out that a 4 year old with a 15-gm splenic implant 2 years after splenectomy died from overwhelming postsplenectomy sepsis; hence, splenic remnants, whether implants, accessory spleens, or splenosis, may not be effective filters against blood-borne infection.[189] Horton and associates believed this was because of inadequate arterial blood flow to the implants and postulated that perhaps another site of autotransplant or longer periods before evaluation may be required to gain this extra blood supply and so offer better protection.[87] Their study demonstrated that an intact splenic artery was important in the removal of encapsulated organisms from the peripheral blood despite normal or greater than normal splenic weights. This finding is impor-

tant because one of the techniques for operative splenic salvage for trauma is ligation of the splenic artery. If arterial supply is maintained, small volumes of splenic tissue may afford protection, as compensatory hypertrophy does occur, at least experimentally.

Splenic artery ligation, either alone or in combination with topical hemostatic agents or suture techniques, or both, has been used. A major concern of this in the past was the creation of a completely devascularized spleen if the short gastric vessels are injured at the initial trauma or are compromised with mobilization of the spleen. If the spleen can receive adequate blood supply from the remaining or residual short gastric vessels, splenic size increases; however, clearance of encapsulated organisms will not be normal and the presumed protection of an otherwise intact spleen is greatly jeopardized.

When operative intervention for splenic injury is deemed necessary, the spleen can be and frequently is repaired using the previously discussed techniques. As surgeons have gained experience with these techniques, greater numbers of spleens have been salvaged.[65]

In 1979 I discussed two new techniques for splenorrhaphy.[22] Using principles previously reported for repairing liver injuries, large through-and-through absorbable mattress sutures perpendicular to the plane of injury are passed through a spinal needle (Fig. 21–11). Once protruding through the capsule above and below the injury, the metal needle is touched with the electrocautery to discourage local bleeding around the needle. Absorbable suture—usually 3–0 or 4–0 PDS—is threaded through the needle, and the needle is withdrawn. Several such sutures are placed to secure the injury anatomically, and then the sutures are tied at each end, firmly securing the injured area to its near normal anatomy. Concern regarding the potential creation of ischemic areas after securing these large horizontal mattress sutures in a plane perpendicular to the segmental blood supply of the spleen has been unfounded, and postoperative spleen scans 6 months after repair have been normal. Indications to use this technique are infrequent, but

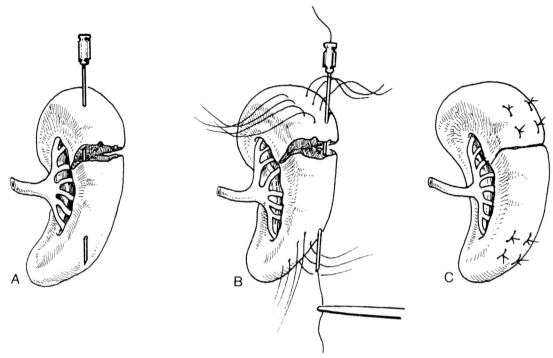

FIGURE 21–11

The Lynn technique of splenorrhaphy, using large through-and-through absorbable mattress sutures passed through a transinjury spinal needle (A and B) and tied (C). (Adapted from Buntain WL, Lynn HB: Splenorrhaphy: Changing concepts for the traumatized spleen. Surgery 86:748–760, 1979.)

when we have found splenic parenchyma fractured segmentally into large viable pieces, this technique has worked well.

Reluctance to suture repair splenic injuries continues to be prevalent, and despite the very significant implications of surgical removal of the spleen, splenectomy continues to be done unnecessarily. Various negative inclinations to do splenorrhaphy consist of an apparently time-honored aversion to suturing the spleen; a fear of delayed splenic rupture, traumatic splenic cyst, or abdominal splenosis; or a belief that the time taken for splenorrhaphy is too long. These complications have been reported very rarely and have not occurred in my experience.

However, in an effort to obviate these objections early in the course of the splenorrhaphy movement, we developed and used successfully an absorbable suture ladder (Vicryl or Dexon) that was easily and quickly constructed at the operating table and shortly thereafter began using woven Dexon or Vicryl mesh.[18, 22] Variations of this *parenchymal compression* technique have been reported by others.[38, 102, 131] The mesh is very user friendly, and our technique is relatively simple, accomplishes the same hemostatic and repair principles as the ''ladder,'' is very effective, and can be accomplished quickly, avoiding suturing the spleen yet accomplishing the same results. This has become our preferred method of splenorrhaphy in almost all situations (Fig. 21–12A, B, C, D, and E).

Once the spleen has been mobilized adequately, including the upper pole where occasionally unusually adherent short gastric vessels may hinder manipulation, the extent of injury is assessed. If arterial bleeding is brisk, it is con-

trolled directly with suture ligature. Venous or arterial oozing is not addressed immediately but is managed by the technique described here. With bleeding thus controlled, the mesh, in its semistretched state, is easily and expeditiously trimmed to a strip the length of which is equal to the circumference of the spleen at its outer edge. The width is measured in the nonstretched state and is equal to 1.5 times the thickness of the spleen (see Fig. 21–12A). Top (nonhilar) and bottom (hilar) pursestring sutures are then placed by folding the strip *along its length* like an accordion and 3–0 or 4–0 PDS on a Keith needle passed through the folded mesh at its top and bottom (see Fig. 21–12B). It helps to tag each of the four ends once the needles are removed to prevent inadvertent dislodgment during manipulation. The material is then opened to its previously unstretched length, and starting posteriorly so the spleen lies with the mesh stabilized between it and the abdominal wall, the mesh is wrapped around the spleen just overlapping the hilar side as well as the nonhilar side—like attaching a chain for snow driving around a tire (see Fig. 21–12C). The mesh is then stretched gently lengthwise along the circumference to make it snug, the overlapping ends are trimmed to approximate, and two sutures to secure this are placed— 3–0 or 4–0 PDS ''stick ties.'' Both pursestring sutures are now snugged up gently, and then first the hilar side suture is tied with a nonslipping knot so as to overlap the spleen's edge by 1.5 to 2.0 cm—enough so that it does not slip off when the nonhilar compressing side is tied and just enough to ''bend'' the contour of the spleen *very slightly* in a concave manner toward the hilus (see Fig. 21–12D and E). The nonhilar side pursestring is then tied, gathering the

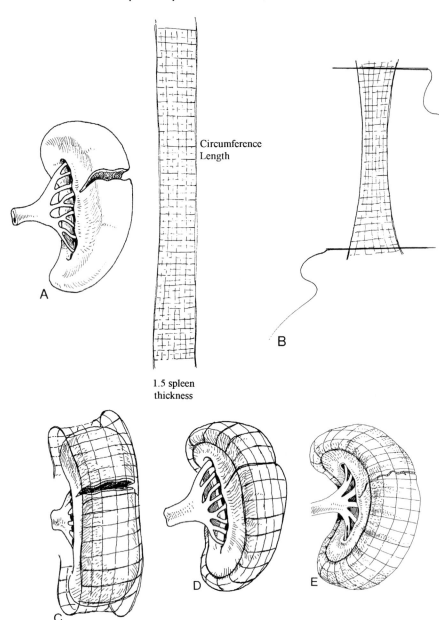

Circumference
Length

1.5 spleen
thickness

FIGURE 21–12

The "parenchymal compression" technique of splenic repair, using Vicryl or Dexon mesh. In its semi-stretched state, the mesh is trimmed to a strip the length of which is equal to the circumference of the spleen at its outer edge; the width, in the non-stretched state, is equal to 1.5 times the thickness of the spleen (A). Folding the mesh accordion-like lengthwise, end-to-end, Keith needles with absorbable suture are passed through the top and bottom (B). These are the purse strings. The mesh is then spread open and placed under the spleen between it and the abdominal wall and is then wrapped around the injured organ, stretching it to make the ends meet (C). These are secured with two or three stick ties. The slightly overlapping hilar side (1.0–1.5 cm) purse string is then tied snugly so as not to slip off when the nonhilar side is tied, just bending the organ in a concave manner toward the hilus (D). The nonhilar side is then snugged down, drawing the spleen together hemostatically, compressing the parenchyma toward the center of the organ (E).

spleen together toward its natural normal contour *until the capsule starts to wrinkle.* The stretch component of the mesh pulls the spleen together, hemostatically compressing the parenchyma toward the center of the organ (see Fig. 21–12E and F). In our experience mild oozing, arterial or venous, ceases. The entire procedure takes 5 to 10 minutes, and on completion the spleen is returned to its normal position in the left upper quadrant provided any previous peritoneal or ligamentous oozing is dry.

Splenectomy

Regardless of the ability to utilize these techniques for splenorrhaphy or partial splenic resection, some patients will always have such substantial injuries that splenectomy will be mandatory, such as separation of the spleen from its blood supply or total maceration of splenic parenchyma.

With all the enthusiasm over splenorrhaphy, the practicing surgeon may feel compelled to pursue repair at all costs, because failure may seem to imply technical shortcomings. A realistic approach in achieving what is best for any given patient recognizes that not all spleens can be repaired, nor should they be, especially if one is going to leave behind nothing more than a mass of devitalized splenic tissue.

The technical aspects of splenectomy are well known; mobilization of the spleen for splenic salvage procedures is identical for performing splenectomy. Mobilization should be done quickly, and in the presence of ongoing bleeding finger pressure or a noncrushing clamp across the hilus should control hemorrhage to allow precise maneuvers to remove the spleen. Following this, we usually begin at the posterior aspect of the mobilized and reflected hilar area, with the spleen, hilus, and tail of the pancreas folded over on the right side of the abdominal incision. In this position,

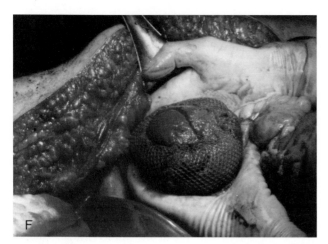

FIGURE 21–12 *Continued*
The capsule starts to wrinkle *(F)*.

the splenic artery and vein are much more accessible as they usually run along the posterior superior edge of the body and tail of the pancreas, and approaching them from that side helps to avoid potential injury to the pancreas. Identifying and isolating the hilar vessels, first the splenic artery if possible and then the splenic vein, the vessels are individually ligated and transected (Fig. 21–13*A* and *B*). We usually doubly ligate the nonresected side. The short gastric vessels are then easily rotated into view and individually ligated and transected. As is our routine with elective splenectomies, we usually suture ligate the stomach side of the highest short gastric vessels to avoid postoperative lig-

ature slip and bleeding from these vessels. We do not drain the splenic bed for splenectomy or splenorrhaphy.

Splenic Autotransplantation

Despite aggressive splenic salvage efforts, splenectomy may still be required, and an important consideration in any trauma patient undergoing this procedure is autotransplantation. Although somewhat controversial, routine reimplantation of a portion of the spleen should be considered in all patients who have had splenectomies for trauma. Experimental studies have confirmed the viability of reimplanted revascularized splenic tissue that is apparently capable of phagocytizing pneumococcal organisms and contributing to a higher level of antibody formation following pneumococcal vaccination.[32, 33, 64, 195] Although several sites for reimplantation have been suggested, the most popular technique is the one recommended by the Denver group[123, 131] (Fig. 21–14). The removed splenic tissue is sectioned into five fragments measuring approximately 40 mm × 40 mm × 3 mm, and these are enclosed in a greater omental pouch, secured with sutures and marked with radiopaque surgical clips. The omental pouch separates the splenic fragments from the small intestine, theoretically averting the risk of splenosis-induced adhesions, and attempts to take advantage of the portal venous drainage.[107, 169]

Several clinical reports corroborate the viability of these implants and indicate that the procedure is safe and effective.[130, 151, 202] After a period of apparent necrosis, implants regenerate, and in animal models growth is progressive over 2 years.[199, 210] Mizrahi and co-workers, definitively stating that "autotransplantation of irreparably damaged

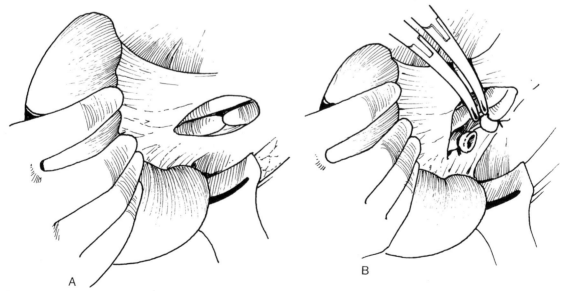

FIGURE 21–13
With the completely mobilized spleen gently reflected medially, the posterior aspect of the hilar area with the splenic vessels coursing along the posterior superior border of the pancreas is easily approached. The vessels, first the artery and then the vein, are individually isolated and ligated *(A)* and then divided *(B)*. Ligation and division of the individual short gastric vessels can be accomplished before or after major vessel control.

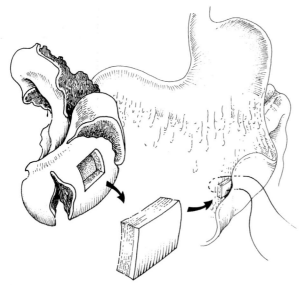

FIGURE 21–14
Removed splenic tissue is sectioned into four or five fragments approximately 40 × 40 × 3 or 4 mm, secured in an omental pouch, and marked with radiopaque surgical clips. (Adapted from Moore FA, Moore EE, Abernathy CM: Injuries to the spleen. In: Moore EE, Mattox KL, Feliciano DV (eds): Trauma. 2nd ed. East Norwalk, Conn, Appleton & Lange, 1991, pp 465–483.)

spleens in humans preserved splenic functions,'' reported 10 patients with splenectomy and autotransplantation of roughly 50 gm of splenic tissue.[125] Postoperative studies of splenic function revealed disappearance of Howell-Jolly bodies from peripheral blood, and levels of IgM that were initially significantly depressed returned to normal. In addition, technetium Tc 99m sulfur colloid scans were normal 10 weeks after surgery. Pointing out the usual splenic deficiencies after splenectomy, such as ''failure of antibody response to particulate antigen,'' all patients received pneumococcal polysaccharide vaccine subcutaneously, 0.5 ml, following surgery. No mention was made of the importance of blood flow in contributing to patient immunity.

Greco and Alvarez, reporting that if 80% of the spleen is removed the remnant will hypertrophy and protect the host against subsequent bacteremia, supported the contention that hilar vessels may not be essential for function if identifiable blood vessels remain in continuity with the splenic remnant.[79] In animals, this revascularized hypertrophied splenic tissue appears to phagocytize pneumococci from the blood stream and to contribute to higher levels of pneumococcal antibody following immunization.[33, 64] Their data are subject to further interpretation, however, because although greater survival with transplanted tissue over the splenectomized rats occurred at 24 hours, at 72 hours there was no difference statistically.

However, although animal studies are compelling, supporting clinical data continue to be less than definitive. The Denver group, using the technique described earlier, since 1978 confirmed uniform implant viability by technetium scanning at 6 months with normalization of IgM levels and platelet numbers.[123] They also reported a case with docu-

mented growth of intraperitoneal splenic implants at 7 years, and the patient survived an episode of pneumococcal sepsis with oral penicillin, suggesting graft function.[60] Patel and colleagues confirmed these findings and documented the disappearance of Howell-Jolly bodies and the return of normal complement levels at 4 weeks.[151]

What quantity of the reimplanted splenic tissue is necessary for complete protection against overwhelming postsplenectomy sepsis? Van Wyck and associates found experimentally that the splenic mass correlates directly with production of antibody to particulate intravenous antigen, and possession of greater than one third of the normal splenic mass showed a clear-cut protective edge over asplenia.[207] To confer protection, however, the critical splenic mass has to receive a critical volume of blood flow.[87] When part of the spleen left was in situ while reimplantation of the remnant occurred, only 1.5% of total splenic blood flow participated in the replanted particles.[209] Moore agreed with the concept of autotransplantation and of transplanting splenic tissue in a place to utilize the portal circulation.[127] However, he also pointed out that support for objective evidence of immunologic–host-defense benefit is not definitive yet. Hence, the suggestion that a critical mass of spleen that is more than 30% of the normal is required to ensure immune function remains controversial.[36, 150, 207] Although numerous animal studies have strongly suggested immunologic benefit, indeed this may be related to the mechanism of inoculation challenge, that is, subcutaneous versus intravenous. The importance of pneumococcal vaccine given subcutaneously then has become obvious. Additional work is required to answer this problem definitively.

POSTINJURY MANAGEMENT

Early Postoperative Complications

Following splenic repair, by whatever technique, the remainder of the operation and immediate postoperative care proceeds in a normal manner, and morbidity depends primarily on the presence or absence of associated injuries. Acute gastric dilation is prevented by nasogastric suction for 48 hours. Recurrent bleeding, pancreatitis, and intraabdominal abscesses have not occurred in our experience. Postsplenectomy thrombocytosis has not been a problem or required therapeutic intervention; we reserve prophylactic anticoagulation for platelet counts well in excess of 1 million.

If the spleen injury was an isolated event with no other injuries, 48 hours in a critical care unit followed by 5 to 7 days of routine postoperative care usually is all that is required, and the patient is then followed on an outpatient basis for at least 6 weeks. After this time, a gradual return to normal activity is accomplished.

Dulchavsky and associates, in a very elegant and widely referred to experimental study using dogs and pigs, demonstrated that repaired spleens had a higher wound-breaking strength than normal or unrepaired spleens at 3 weeks after the injury, but at 6 weeks after the injury, the wound-breaking strength for all three types of spleens was the same.[50] This report prompted many trauma surgeons to release their patients to full activity after 6 weeks of convalescence. However, we routinely obtain CT scans at discharge or 14 days after the injury on most of our patients, again at 1 month, and then at monthly intervals until resolution has occurred. Grade I and II injuries are invariably healed by 6 weeks; however, the grade III and more severe injuries take progressively longer, sometimes up to 3 months. Our policy is to allow the resumption of restricted activities at 6 weeks, but when healing is not complete, strenuous physical activity, including contact sports, is to be avoided until healing is complete as visualized by CT scan, particularly for those who were managed nonoperatively.

Alternatives to Splenic Salvage

Regardless of the ability to successfully utilize splenic salvage procedures for splenic injuries, there will always be patients with such substantial injuries that splenectomy will be mandatory. Prophylaxis against overwhelming postsplenectomy sepsis in these patients is the surgeon's responsibility.[186] Autotransplantation of splenic remnants at the operating table followed by postoperative prophylactic antipneumococcal vaccine and antibiotic prophylaxis are important viable adjuncts in such situations.

Pneumovax

Even though only slightly more than 50% of all cases of overwhelming postsplenectomy sepsis are attributed to pneumococcal organisms—primarily *Streptococcus pneumoniae*—there is general agreement that pneumococcal vaccine (Pneumovax) should be administered to all splenectomized patients.[104] The currently available vaccines contain 23 serotypes, which account for 90% of the pneumococcal infections.[119] The antibody response to *subcutaneous* vaccination of an otherwise normal asplenic patient is nearly equal to that of controls, but the duration of elevated titre is unknown.[75, 197]

The question of timing of the vaccination is controversial. Ideally, it is preferable to give the vaccine preoperatively, but this is usually not possible in the trauma patient. Some recommend immediate vaccination, experience implying that the antibody response is the same whether vaccination is immediate or delayed.[7, 23] However, others have demonstrated altered B-cell function with suppression of antibody response following major trauma.[62] This may be particularly relevant as injury severity increases.[131]

The need for revaccination is also unclear. Reports of severe Arthus reactions with the newer 23-valent vaccine have tempered enthusiasm for a booster injection.[131] Hence, at present revaccination is not recommended for adults; however, after 5 years or more, pending long-term data, some recommend revaccination for children.[21]

Prophylactic Penicillin

It is clear that pneumococcal sepsis occurs despite vaccination, and therefore long-term oral penicillin or erythromycin prophylaxis has been recommended, especially for children younger than 2 years of age. Unfortunately, the documented compliance rate with antibiotic prophylaxis programs is less than 50%.[15, 40, 43] In addition, sepsis can occur from organisms that are not sensitive to the antibiotic being used, and resistant strains of organisms may evolve during therapy. However, it is recommended that continuous antibiotic prophylaxis should be given to all children, particularly those under the age of 2 years, until they are old enough to understand the significance of the problem and can complain or bring attention to the signs and symptoms of impending infection. After that, antibiotics are given only therapeutically but *early and for even trivial problems*.[16]

The patient and the family must be properly educated concerning the risks of overwhelming postsplenectomy sepsis, and we recommend a MedicAlert bracelet be worn to alert health care providers of the presence of a splenectomized patient and the potential for overwhelming postsplenectomy sepsis.

Of interest, an unexpectedly high incidence of viral illness in splenectomized individuals has also been suggested in both children and adults.[71, 178] Most complain of an increased number of viral infections of the upper respiratory tract and a greater severity and duration of illness when compared with their experience before splenectomy. This suggests that the cause of overwhelming postsplenectomy sepsis may not be confined to encapsulated bacteria.[178]

Asplenic Registry

It is recommended that every institution—indeed perhaps every surgeon—that has cared for trauma victims maintain an asplenic registry.[135] Splenectomized patients should be informed about the potential long-term complications of splenectomy such as ischemic heart disease, carotid occlusive disease, cirrhosis, and, of course, increased susceptibility to infection including overwhelming postsplenectomy sepsis. Such a registry would allow splenectomized patients to be updated regarding recent developments and reminded of the importance of seeking medical attention for what may seem like even a minor viral illness.

Accessory Spleens and Splenosis

Accessory spleens occur presumably as a result of failure of fusion of elements of the splenic anlagen in early embryonic development.[56] They are found in 10 to 44% of normal persons, and the locations in which they are found is fairly constant.[157] Similar to true spleens including the configuration of the blood supply, accessory spleens show evidence of function as some of the disease processes that affect the true spleen also can affect accessory spleens. This is evidenced by the fact that with some hematologic disorders, failure to remove accessory spleens at the time of splenectomy may result in recurrence of that disorder.

This physiologic ability to functionally resemble normal spleens has raised the question of whether accessory spleens left behind at the time of splenectomy for trauma can protect the host from overwhelming postsplenectomy sepsis. Evidence that accessory spleens do protect against overwhelming postsplenectomy sepsis is currently not available; however, there is some limited evidence that protection is not conferred by accessory spleens.[139] The critical factor here is probably the critical mass of functioning splenic tissue that must be present to preserve immunity.

Splenosis following traumatic splenic disruption does not appear to provide protection from immune consequences such as overwhelming postsplenectomy sepsis. The presence of normal levels of circulating red blood cells that are pitted or have inclusions may indicate residual splenic tissue, but this is not indicative of sufficient immune function and thus protection for the host.

SUMMARY

The spleen is not an expendable organ, and splenectomy creates an iatrogenic disease. The asplenic state is associated with loss of much of the spleen's ability to protect the host from certain infections, primarily those caused by encapsulated bacteria. The risk of developing overwhelming postsplenectomy sepsis is not great for the asplenic trauma victim, but is probably 50 to 100 times greater than that of the population who have intact spleens. However, when overwhelming postsplenectomy sepsis does occur, the mortality for affected subjects is 50 to 70%. Given these circumstances, splenectomy and creation of the asplenic state should be avoided if at all possible. Following traumatic injury to the spleen, the managing surgeon must assume the responsibility for splenic salvage by whatever means appropriate for each individual patient as well as for making sure that certain alternate methods of immune protection are entertained and utilized. Decisions in this regard are helped considerably by knowing the severity of injury to the spleen and the presence or absence of associated injuries.

References

1. Ahmad A, Polk WC: Blunt abdominal trauma: A study of the relation between diagnosis and outcome. South Med J 66:1127–1131, 1973.
2. Amsbaugh DF, Prescott B, Baker PJ: Effect of splenectomy on the expression of regulatory T cell activity. J Immunol 121:1483–1485, 1978.
3. Baker SP, O'Neill B, Haddon W Jr, et al: The injury severity score: A method for describing patients with multiple injuries and evaluating emergency care. J Trauma 14:187–196, 1974.
4. Barnes AF: Subcutaneous traumatic rupture of the normal spleen. Ann Surg 59:597–609, 1914.
5. Baronofsky ID, Walton W, Noble JF: Occult injury to the pancreas following splenectomy. Surgery 29:852–857, 1951.
6. Barrett J, Sheaff C, Abuabara S, et al: Splenic preservation in adults after blunt and penetrating trauma. Am J Surg 145:313–317, 1983.
7. Barringer M, Meredith W, Sterchi M, et al: Effect of anesthesia and splenectomy on antibody response to pneumococcal polysaccharide immunization. Am Surg 48:628–633, 1982.
8. Beasley SW, Auldist AW: Management of splenic trauma in childhood. Aust N Z J Surg 55:199–202, 1985.
9. Berger E: The injuries to the spleen and their surgical treatment [in German]. Arch Klin Chir 68:865–871, 1902.
10. Bisno AL, Freeman JC: The syndrome of asplenia, pneumococcal sepsis and disseminated intravascular coagulation. Ann Inter Med 72:389–393, 1970.
11. Bodon GR, Verzosa ES: Incidental splenic injury: Is splenectomy always necessary? Am J Surg 113:303–304, 1967.
12. Bogart D, Biggar WD, Good RA: Impaired intravascular clearance of pneumococcus type-3 following splenectomy. J Reticuloendothel Soc 11:77–87, 1972.
13. Brands W, Menniken C, Beck M: Preservation of the ruptured spleen with highly concentrated human fibrinogen: Experimental and clinical results. World J Surg 6:366–368, 1982.
14. Brindle MJ: Arteriography and minor splenic injury. Clin Radiol 23:174–180, 1972.
15. Buchannan GR, Siegel JD, Smith SJ, et al: Oral penicillin prophylaxis in children with impaired splenic function: Study of compliance. Pediatrics 70:926–930, 1982.
16. Buntain WL: Splenic trauma. In: Cameron JL (ed): Current Surgical Therapy, 1984–1985. New York, Decker/Mosby, 1984, pp 501–505.
17. Buntain WL: Splenic trauma. In: Hurst J (ed): Current Problems in Trauma/Critical Care. Chicago, Year Book Medical Publishers, 1987, pp 78–89.
18. Buntain WL, Gould HR: Splenic trauma in children and techniques of splenic salvage. World J Surg 9:398–409, 1985.
19. Buntain WL, Gould HR: Enhancement of splenic salvage in children following injury by computed tomography classification of injury severity. Presented at the second annual meeting of the Eastern Association for the Surgery of Trauma, Longboat Key, Florida, January 1988. Previously unpublished data.
20. Buntain WL, Gould HR, Maull KI: Predictability of splenic salvage by computed tomography. J Trauma 28:24–34, 1988.
21. Buntain WL, Lynch FP, Ramenofsky ML: Management of the acutely injured child. In: Maull KI (ed): Advances in Trauma, Volume 2. Chicago, Year Book Medical Publishers, 1987, pp 43–86.
22. Buntain WL, Lynn HB: Splenorrhaphy: Changing concepts for the traumatized spleen. Surgery 86:748–760, 1979.
23. Caplan ES, Boltansky H, Snyder MJ, et al: Response of traumatized splenectomized patients to immediate vaccination with polyvalent pneumococcal vaccine. J Trauma 23:801–805, 1983.
24. Carlisle HN, Soslaw S: Properdin levels in splenectomized persons. Proc Soc Exp Biol Med 102:150–154, 1959.
25. Chaimoff C, Douer D, Pick IA, et al: Serum immunoglobulin changes after accidental splenectomy in adults. Am J Surg 136:332–333, 1978.
26. Champion HR, Sacco WJ: Management of injury severity and its practical application. Trauma Q 1:25–36, 1984.
27. Chu DZJ, Nichioka K, El-Hagin T, et al: Effects of tuftsin on postsplenectomy sepsis. Surgery 97:701–706, 1985.
28. Claret I, Morales L, Montoner A: Immunological studies in the postsplenectomy syndrome. J Pediatr Surg 10:59–64, 1975.
29. Cogbill TH, Moore EE, Jurkovich GJ, et al: Nonoperative management of blunt splenic trauma: A multicenter experience. J Trauma 29:1312–1317, 1989.
30. Constantopoulos A, Najjar VA, Smith JW: Tuftsin deficiency: A new syndrome with defective phagocytosis. J Pediatr 80:564–572, 1972.
31. Constantopoulos A, Najjar VA, Wish JB, et al: Defective phagocytosis due to tuftsin deficiency in splenectomized subjects. Am J Dis Child 125:663–665, 1973.
32. Cooney DR, Dearth JC, Swanson SE, et al: Relative merits of partial splenectomy, splenic reimplantation, and immunization in preventing postsplenectomy infection. Surgery 86:561–569, 1979.
33. Cooney DR, Swanson SE, Dearth JC, et al: Heterotopic splenic autotransplantation in prevention of overwhelming postsplenectomy infection. J Pediatr Surg 14:336–342, 1979.
34. Cox EF: Blunt abdominal trauma: A 5-year analysis of 870 patients requiring celiotomy. Ann Surg 199:467–474, 1985.
35. Davis JW, Shackford SR, Mackersie RC, et al: Base deficit as a guide to volume resuscitation. J Trauma 28:1464–1467, 1988.
36. Dawes LG, Malangoni MA, Spiegel CA, et al: Response to immunization after partial and total splenectomy. J Surg Res 39:53–58, 1985.
37. Dawson DL, Molina ME, Scott-Conner CEH: Venous segmentation of the human spleen. A corrosion cast study. Am Surg 52:253–256, 1986.
38. Delany HM, Porreca F, Mitsudo S, et al: Splenic capping: An experimental study of a new technique for splenorrhaphy using woven polyglycolic acid mesh. Ann Surg 196:187–193, 1982.
39. Delius RE, Frankel W, Coran AG: A comparison between operative and nonoperative management of blunt injuries to the liver and spleen in adult and pediatric patients. Surgery 106:788–793, 1989.

40. DePalma A, Buraschi G, Canpani G, et al: Compliance with oral penicillin prophylaxis in splenectomized phalocemic patients. Hematologica 70:221–226, 1985.
41. Diamond LK: Splenectomy in childhood and the hazard of overwhelming infection. Pediatrics 43:886–889, 1969.
42. Dickerman JD: Traumatic asplenia in adults: A defined hazard? Arch Surg 116:361–363, 1981.
43. Dorgna-Pignatti C, DeStefano R, Barone F, et al: Penicillin compliance in splenectomized phalocemics. Eur J Pediatr 142:83–85, 1984.
44. Douglas GJ, Simpson JS: The conservative management of splenic trauma. J Pediatr Surg 6:565–570, 1971.
45. Douglass BE, Baggenstoss AH, Hollinshead WH: The anatomy of the portal vein and its tributaries. Surg Gynecol Obstet 91:562–576, 1950.
46. Dover CC, Korns RF, Schuman LM: Infectious Diseases. Cambridge, Harvard University Press, 1968, p 134.
47. Downey EC, Catanzaro A, Ninnemann JC, et al: Long-term depressed immunocompetence of patients splenectomized for trauma. Surg Forum 29:41–44, 1980.
48. Downey EC, Shackford SR, Fridlund PH, et al: Long-term depressed immune function in patients splenectomized for trauma. J Trauma 27:661–663, 1987.
49. Dretzka L: Rupture of the spleen. Surg Gynecol Obstet 51:258–261, 1930.
50. Dulchavsky SA, Ledgerwood AM, Lucas CE, et al: Wound healing of the injured spleen with and without splenorrhaphy. J Trauma 27:1155–1160, 1987.
51. Durig M, Landmann RMA, Harder F: Lymphocyte subsets in human peripheral blood after splenectomy and autotransplantation of splenic tissue. J Lab Clin Med 104:110–115, 1984.
52. Ein SH, Shandling B, Simpson JS, et al: The morbidity and mortality of splenectomy in childhood. Ann Surg 185:307–310, 1977.
53. Ein SH, Shandling B, Simpson JS, et al: Nonoperative management of the traumatized spleen in children: How and why. J Pediatr Surg 13:117–119, 1978.
54. Ellis EF, Smith RT: The role of the spleen in immunity with special reference to the post-splenectomy problems in infants. Pediatrics 37:111–119, 1966.
55. Elmore JR, Clark DE, Isler RJ, et al: Selective nonoperative management of blunt splenic trauma in adults. Arch Surg 124:581–586, 1989.
56. Emmett JM, Dreyfuss ML: Accessory spleens in the scrotum. Ann Surg 117:754–759, 1943.
57. Engrav LH, Benjamin CI, Strate RG, et al: Diagnostic peritoneal lavage in blunt abdominal trauma. J Trauma 15:854–859, 1975.
58. Eraklis AJ, Filler RM: Splenectomy in childhood: A review of 1413 cases. J Pediatr Surg 4:382–388, 1972.
59. Eraklis AJ, Kevy SV, Diamond LK: Hazard of overwhelming infections after splenectomy in childhood. N Engl J Med 276:1225–1229, 1967.
60. Erdoes L, Moore FA, Moore EE, et al: Fivefold enlargement of implants in a splenic autotransplant recipient. Surgery 113:462–465, 1993.
61. Erikson WD, Burgert EO, Lynn HB: The hazard of infection following splenectomy in children. Am J Dis Child 116:1–12, 1968.
62. Ertel W, Faist E, Nestle C, et al: Dynamics of immunoglobulin synthesis after major trauma. Arch Surg 124:1437–1441, 1989.
63. Fabian TC, Mangiante EC, White TJ, et al: A prospective study of 91 patients undergoing both computed tomography and peritoneal lavage following blunt abdominal trauma. J Trauma 26:602–608, 1986.
64. Fasching MD, Cooner DR: Reimmunization and splenic autotransplantation: A long-term study of immunologic response and survival following pneumococcal challenge. J Surg Res 28:449–458, 1980.
65. Feliciano DV, Bitondo CG, Mattox KL, et al: A four year experience with splenectomy versus splenorrhaphy. Ann Surg 201:568–575, 1985.
66. Filler RM: Experience with the management of splenic injuries. Aust N Z J Surg 54:443–445, 1984.
67. Fisher RG, Foucar K, Estrada R, et al: Splenic rupture in blunt trauma. Correlation of angiographic and pathological records. Radiol Clin North Am 19:141–165, 1981.
68. Fisher RP, Miller-Crotchett P, Reed RL: Gastrointestinal disruption: The hazard of nonoperative management with blunt abdominal injury. J Trauma 28:1445–1449, 1988.
69. Flancbaum L, in discussion of Delius[39].
70. Ford WL, Smith ME: Lymphocyte recirculation between the spleen and the blood. In: Role of the Spleen in the Immunology of Parasitic Diseases. Basel, Schwabe, 1979, pp 29–41.
71. Forward AD, Ashmore PG: Infection following splenectomy in infants and children. Can J Surg 3:229–332, 1960.
72. Foster JM, Prey D: Rupture of the spleen. Am J Surg 47:487–493, 1948.
73. Francke EL, Neu HC: Postsplenectomy infection. Surg Clin North Am 61:135–155, 1981.
74. Freeman T, Fischer RP: The inadequacy of peritoneal lavage in diagnosing acute diaphragmatic rupture. J Trauma 16:538–542, 1976.
75. Giebink GS, Foker JE, Kim Y, et al: Serum antibody and opsonic response to vaccination with pneumococcal capsular polysaccharide in normal and splenectomized children. J Infect Dis 141:404–412, 1980.
76. Gill PG, Deyoung NJ, Kiroff GK, et al: Monocyte antibody-dependent cellular cytotoxicity in splenectomized subjects. J Immunol 132:1244–1248, 1984.
77. Gold RE, Redman HC: Splenic trauma: Assessment of problems in diagnosis. Am J Radiol 116:413–418, 1972.
78. Goodman LR, Aprahamian C: Changes in splenic size after abdominal trauma. Radiology 176:629–632, 1990.
79. Greco RS, Alvarez FE: Protection against pneumococcal bacteremia by partial splenectomy. Surg Gynecol Obstet 152:67–69, 1981.
80. Green JB, Shackford SR, Sise MJ, et al: Late septic complications in adults following splenectomy for trauma: A prospective analysis of 144 patients. J Trauma 26:999–1004, 1986.
81. Grosfeld JL, Ranochak JE: Are hemisplenectomy and/or primary splenic repair feasible? J Pediatr Surg 11:419–424, 1976.
82. Gross P: Zur kindlichen traumatischen milzuptur. Beitr Klin Chir 208:396–401, 1965.
83. Guyton A: Textbook of Medical Physiology. 7th ed. Philadelphia, WB Saunders, 1986, p 343.
84. Hauser CJ: Hemostasis of solid viscus trauma by intraparenchymal injection of fibrin glue. Arch Surg 124:291–293, 1989.
85. Holschneider AM, Kreiz-Klimeck H, Strasser B, et al: Complications of splenectomy in childhood. Z Kinderchir 35:130–139, 1982.
86. Horan M, Colebatch JH: Relation between splenectomy and subsequent infection: A clinical study. Arch Dis Child 37:398–412, 1962.
87. Horton J, Ogden ME, Williams S, et al: The importance of splenic blood flow in clearing pneumococcal organisms. Ann Surg 195:172–176, 1982.
88. Hosea SW, Brown EJ, Hamburger MI, et al: Opsonic requirements for intracellular clearance after splenectomy. N Engl J Med 304:245–250, 1981.
89. Howman-Giles R, Gilday DL, Venugopal S, et al: Splenic trauma—Nonoperative management and long-term follow-up by scintiscan. J Pediatr Surg 13:121–126, 1978.
90. Hull CC, Galloway P, Gordon NC, et al: Splenectomy and the induction of murine colon cancer. Arch Surg 123:462–464, 1988.
91. Huntley CC: Infection following splenectomy in infants and children. A review of the experience at Duke Hospital in infants and children during a twenty-two year period (1933–1954). Am J Dis Child 95:477–480, 1958.
92. Jeffery RB: CT diagnosis of blunt hepatic and splenic injuries: A look to the future. Radiology 171:17–18, 1989.
93. Jeffery RB, Laing FC, Federle MP, et al: Computed tomography of splenic trauma. Radiology 141:729–732, 1981.
94. Johnson N: Traumatic rupture of the spleen. A review of eighty-five cases. Aust N Z J Surg 24:112–124, 1954.
95. Joseph TP, Wyllie GG, Savage JP: The nonoperative management of splenic trauma. Aust N Z J Surg 47:179–182, 1977.
96. Karp MP, Cooney DR, Berger PE, et al: The role of computed tomography in the evaluation of blunt abdominal trauma in children. J Pediatr Surg 16:316–323, 1981.
97. Kaufmann RA, Towbin R, Babcock DS, et al: Upper abdominal trauma in children: Imaging evaluation. AJR 142:449–460, 1984.
98. King DR, Lobe TE, Haase GM, et al: Selective management of the injured spleen. Surgery 90:677–682, 1981.
99. King H, Shumacher HB Jr: Splenic studies. I. Susceptibility to infection after splenectomy performed in infancy. Ann Surg 136:239–242, 1952.
100. Lally KP, Rosario V, Mahour GH, et al: Evolution in the manage-

ment of splenic injury in children. Surg Gynecol Obstet 170:245–248, 1990.

101. LaMura J, Chung-Fat S, San Felippo JA: Splenorrhaphy for the treatment of splenic rupture in infants and children. Surgery 81:497–501, 1977.

102. Lange D, Zaert PH, Merlotti GJ, et al: The use of absorbable mesh in splenic trauma. J Trauma 28:269–274, 1988.

103. Lau HT, Hardy MA, Altman RP: Decreased pulmonary alveolar macrophage bacterial activity in splenectomized rats. J Surg Res 34:568–571, 1983.

104. Lennard ES: Pneumococcal vaccine: A surgeon's overview (editorial). Am J Surg 137:283–284, 1979.

105. Lieberman RC, Welch CS: A study of 248 instances of traumatic rupture of the spleen. Surg Gynecol Obstet 127:961–965, 1968.

106. Likhite VV: Opsonin and leukophilic gamma-globulin in chronically splenectomized rats with and without heterotropic autotransplanted splenic tissue. Nature 253:742–744, 1975.

107. Livingston CD, Levine BA, Sirinek KR: Site of splenic autotransplantation of the spleen following pneumococcal pneumonia. Surg Gynecol Obstet 156:761–766, 1983.

108. Livingston CD, Sirinek KR, Levine BA, et al: Traumatic splenic injury: Its management in a patient population with a high incidence of associated injury. Arch Surg 117:670–674, 1982.

109. Llende M, Santiago-Delpin EA, Lavergne J: Immunological consequences of splenectomy: A review. J Surg Res 40:85–94, 1986.

110. Luna GK, Dellinger EP: Nonoperative observation therapy for splenic injuries: A safe therapeutic option? Am J Surg 153:462–468, 1987.

111. Lynch MJ: Mechanisms and defects of the phagocytic systems of defense against infection. In: Perspectives in Pediatric Pathology. Chicago, Year Book Medical Publishers, 1973, pp 33–115.

112. McIndoe AH: Delayed hemorrhage following traumatic rupture of the spleen. Br J Surg 20:249–268, 1932.

113. Mackersie RC, Tiwary AD, Shackford SR, et al: Intra-abdominal injury following blunt trauma: Identifying the high risk patient using objective risk factors. Arch Surg 124:809–813, 1989.

114. Mahboubi S: Abdominal trauma in children: Role of computed tomography. Pediatr Emerg Care 1:37–39, 1985.

115. Malangoni MA, Cue JI, Fallat ME, et al: Evaluation of splenic injury by computed tomography and its impact on treatment. Ann Surg 211:592–599, 1990.

116. Marx JA, Moore EE, Jorden RC, et al: Limitations of computed tomography in the evaluation of acute abdominal trauma: A prospective comparison with diagnostic peritoneal lavage. J Trauma 25:933–945, 1985.

117. Mazel MS: Traumatic rupture of the spleen. Ill Med J 62:170–173, 1932.

118. Mazel MS: Traumatic rupture of the spleen. J Pediatr 26:82–88, 1945.

119. Medical Letter 27:701, November 1985.

120. Michels NA: The variational anatomy of the spleen and splenic artery. Am J Anat 70:21–72, 1942.

121. Michels NA (ed): Blood Supply and Anatomy of the Upper Abdominal Organs. Philadelphia, JB Lippincott, 1955, p 210.

122. Miller FJW: Childhood morbidity and mortality in Newcastle-upon-Tyne: Further report on the Thousand Family Study. N Engl J Med 275:683–690, 1966.

123. Millikan JS, Moore EE, Moore GE, et al: Alternative to splenectomy in adults after trauma. Am J Surg 144:711–716, 1982.

124. Mishalany H: Repair of the ruptured spleen. J Pediatr Surg 9:175–178, 1974.

125. Mizrahi S, Bickel A, Haj M, et al: Posttraumatic autotransplantation of spleen tissue. Arch Surg 124:863–865, 1989.

126. Molin MR, Shackford SR: The management of splenic trauma in a trauma system. Arch Surg 125:840–843, 1990.

127. Moore EE: In invited commentary of Mizrahi[124].

128. Moore EE, Shackford SR, Pachter HL, et al: Organ injury scaling: Spleen, liver, and kidney. J Trauma 29:1664–1666, 1989.

129. Moore FA, Moore EE, Moore GE, et al: Risk of splenic salvage following trauma: Analysis of 200 adults. Am J Surg 148:800–805, 1984.

130. Moore FA, Moore EE, Abernathy CM: Injuries to the spleen. In: Moore EE, Mattox KL, Feliciano DV (eds): Trauma. 2nd ed. East Norwalk, Conn, Appleton & Lange, 1991, pp 465–483.

131. Morgenstern L: The surgical inviolability of the spleen: Historical evolution of a concept. Proceedings of the XXXII Congress of History of Medicine. London, Sept 2–9, 1972, p 62.

132. Morgenstern L, Shapiro S: Techniques of splenic conservation. Arch Surg 114:449–454, 1979.

133. Morgenstern L, Uyeda RY: Nonoperative management of injuries to the spleen in adults. Surg Gynecol Obstet 157:513–518, 1983.

134. Morris DH, Bullock FD: The importance of the spleen in resistance to infections. Ann Surg 70:513–518, 1919.

135. Mucha P Jr, Buntain WL: Spleen Injuries. In: Kreis DJ Jr, Gomez GA (eds): Trauma Management. Boston, Little, Brown, 1989, pp 194–260.

136. Mucha P Jr, Daly RC, Franell MB: Selective management of blunt splenic trauma. J Trauma 26:970–979, 1986.

137. Muehrcke DD, Kim SH, McCabe CJ: Pediatric splenic trauma: Preceeding the success of nonoperative therapy. Am J Emerg Med 5:109–112, 1987.

138. Najjar VA, Nishioka K: Tuftsin: A physiological phagocytosis-stimulating peptide. Nature 228:672–673, 1970.

139. Navarro C, Kondlapoodi P: Failure of accessory spleens to prevent infection following splenectomy. Arch Intern Med 145:369–370, 1985.

140. Nebesar RA, Rabinov KR, Potsaid MS: Radionuclide imaging of the spleen in suspected splenic injury. Radiology 110:609–614, 1974.

141. Nguyen HH, Person H, Hong R, et al: Anatomical approach to vascular segmentation of the spleen (lien) based on controlled experimental partial splenectomies. Anat Clin 4:265–281, 1982.

142. Norell HG: Traumatic rupture of the spleen diagnosed by abdominal aortography. Acta Radiol 48:449–452, 1957.

143. Oakes DD: Splenic trauma. Curr Prob Surg 17:342–401, 1981.

144. Oakes DD, Charters AC: Changing concepts in the management of splenic trauma. Surg Gynecol Obstet 153:181–185, 1981.

145. Olsen WR, Redman HC, Hildreth DH: Quantitative peritoneal lavage in blunt abdominal trauma. Arch Surg 104:536–543, 1971.

146. O'Mara RE, Hall RC, Dombroski DL: Scintiscanning in the diagnosis of rupture of the spleen. Surg Gynecol Obstet 131:1077–1084, 1970.

147. O'Neill J: In discussion of Malangoni[114].

148. Orland JC, Moore TC: Splenectomy for trauma in childhood. Surg Gynecol Obstet 134:94–96, 1972.

149. Panetta T, Scalfani SJ, Goldstein AS, et al: Percutaneous transcatheter embolization for massive bleeding from pelvic fractures. J Trauma 25:1021–1029, 1985.

150. Patel JM, Williams JS, Hinshaw JR: Effect of splenectomy, hemisplenectomy, splenic artery ligation and splenic tissue reimplantation on antibody response to T-dependent antigen. J Trauma in press.

151. Patel JM, Williams JS, Shmigel B: Preservation of splenic function by autotransplantation of traumatized spleen in man. Surgery 90:683–688, 1981.

152. Pearl RH, Wesson DE, Spence LJ, et al: Splenic injury: A 5-year update with improved results and changing criteria for conservative management. J Pediatr Surg 24:121–124, 1989.

153. Peck DA, Jackson FC: Splenectomy after surgical trauma. Arch Surg 89:54–65, 1964.

154. Pedersen B, Videback A: On the late effects of removal of a normal spleen. Acta Chir Scand 131:89–98, 1966.

155. Peitzman AB, Makaroun MJ, Slasky S, et al: Prospective of computed tomography in the initial management of blunt abdominal trauma. J Trauma 26:585–592, 1986.

156. Perry JF: Current status of peritoneal lavage for blunt abdominal trauma. In: Najarian JS, Delaney JP (eds): Trauma and Critical Care Surgery. Chicago, Year Book Medical Publishers, 1986, pp 41–45.

157. Perry JF: Injuries of the spleen. Curr Prob Surg 25:757–832, 1988.

158. Perry JF, Strate RG: Diagnostic peritoneal lavage in blunt abdominal trauma: Indicators and results. Surgery 71:898–901, 1972.

159. Pickhardt B, Moore EE, Moore FA, et al: Operative splenic salvage in adults: A decade perspective. J Trauma 29:1386–1391, 1989.

160. Polk HC: In discussion of Villalba[211].

161. Powell DC, Bivins BA, Bell RM: Diagnostic peritoneal lavage. Surg Gynecol Obstet 155:257–262, 1982.

162. Randolph JG: In discussion of Feliciano[65].

163. Ratner MH, Garrow E, Valda V, Shashikumar VL, et al: Surgical repair of the injured spleen. J Pediatr Surg 12:1019–1026, 1977.

164. Resciniti A, Fink MP, Raptopoulos V, et al: Nonoperative treatment of adult splenic trauma: Development of a computed tomography scoring system that detects appropriate candidates for expectant management. J Trauma 28:828–831, 1988.

165. Robinette CD: Splenectomy and subsequent mortality in veterans of the 1935–1945 war. Lancet 2:127, 1977.

166. Root HD, Hauser CW, McKinley CR, et al: Diagnostic peritoneal lavage. Surgery 57:633–637, 1965.

167. Rosner F: The spleen in the Talmud and other early Jewish writings. Bull Hist Med 46:82–85, 1972.

168. Ross GG: Subcutaneous rupture of the spleen. Ann Surg 48:66–71, 1908.

169. Roth H, Waldherr R: Problems in spleen autotransplantation: Comparative study of types of implantation in animal experiments. In: Warnig P (ed): Progress in Pediatric Surgery. Vol. 18. Berlin and Heidelberg, Springer Verlag, 1985, p 182.

170. Rowley DA: The formation of circulating antibody in the splenectomized human being following intravenous injection of heterologous erythrocytes. J Immunol 65:515–521, 1950.

171. Rychman FC, Noseworthy J: Multisystem trauma. Surg Clin North Am 65:1287–1302, 1985.

172. Sandler P, Kronenberg MW, Forman MB, et al: Dynamic fluctuations in blood and spleen radioactivity: Splenic contraction and relation to clinical radionuclide volume calculations. J Am Coll Cardiol 3:1205–1211, 1981.

173. Scatamacchia SA, Raptopoulos V, Fink MP, et al: Splenic trauma in adults: Impact of CT grading on management. Radiology 171:725–729, 1989.

174. Scheele J, Gentche HH, Matteson G: Splenic repair by fibrin tissue adhesive and collagen fleece. Surgery 95:6–13, 1984.

175. Schumacher MJ: Serum immunoglobulin and transferrin levels after childhood splenectomy. Arch Dis Child 45:114–117, 1970.

176. Schwartz PE, Storioff S, Mucha P Jr, et al: Postsplenectomy sepsis and mortality in adults. JAMA 248:2279–2283, 1982.

177. Schwartz SI: Spleen. In: Schwartz SI (ed): Principles of Surgery. New York, McGraw-Hill, 1974, p 1281.

178. Sekikawa T, Shatney CH: Septic sequelae after splenectomy for trauma in adults. Am J Surg 145:667–673, 1983.

179. Shackford SR, Molin MR: Management of splenic injuries. Surg Clin North Am 70:595–620, 1990.

180. Shackford SR, Sise MJ, Virgilio RW, et al: Evaluation of splenorrhaphy: A grading system for splenic trauma. J Trauma 21:538–542, 1981.

181. Shandling B: Splenectomy for trauma. A second look. Arch Surg 111:1325–1326, 1976.

182. Shandling B: Conservative management of the ruptured spleen. S Afr Med J 57:655–658, 1980.

183. Shandling B: Nonoperative management of splenic trauma. Contemp Surg 29:50–53, 1986.

184. Sherck JP, Oakes DD: Computed tomography in the management of thoracic, abdominal, and pelvic trauma. J Surg Infect 4:505–512, 1985.

185. Sherman R: Perspectives in management of trauma to the spleen: 1979 Presidential Address. American Association for the Surgery of Trauma. J Trauma 20:1–13, 1980.

186. Sherman R: Rationale and methods of splenic preservation following trauma. Surg Clin North Am 61:127–134, 1981.

187. Sieber G, Breyer HG, Herrman F, et al: Abnormalities of B-cell activation and immunoregulation in splenectomized patients. Immunology 169:263–271, 1985.

188. Silverstein ME, Chvapil M: Experimental and clinical experiences with collagen fleece as a hemostasis agent. J Trauma 21:388–393, 1981.

189. Singer DB: Postsplenectomy sepsis. In: Rosenburg AD, Bolande RP (eds): Perspectives in Pediatric Pathology. Vol. 1. Chicago, Year Book Medical Publishers, 1973, pp 285–311.

190. Sodeman WA, Sodeman WA Jr.: Pathologic Physiology: Mechanisms of Disease. 4th ed. Philadelphia, WB Saunders, 1967.

191. Solheim K: A plea for a conservative approach in the treatment of splenic injuries. Curr Surg 35:373–379, 1978.

192. Solheim K: Nonoperative management of splenic rupture. Acta Chir Scand 145:55–58, 1979.

193. Solheim K, Hoivil B: Changing trends in the diagnosis and management of rupture of the spleen. Injury 16:221–226, 1985.

194. Spencer RP, Gupta SM: Radionuclide studies of the spleen in trauma and iatrogenic disorders. Semin Nucl Med 15:305–316, 1985.

195. Steely WM, Satava RM, Brigham RA, et al: Splenic autotransplantation: Determination of the optimal amount required for maximal survival. J Surg Res 45:327–332, 1988.

196. Strate RG, Perry JF, Quattlebaum FW: Pediatric blunt trauma. Minn Med 65:15–18, 1982.

197. Sullivan JL, Ochs HD, Schiffman G, et al: Immune response following splenectomy. Lancet 1:178–181, 1978.

198. Sy MS: Splenic requirement for the generation of suppressor T-cells. J Immunol 119:2095–2099, 1977.

199. Tavassoli M, Ratzan RJ, Crosby WH: Studies on regeneration of heterotopic splenic autotransplants. Blood 41:701–709, 1973.

200. Tepas JJ, Mollitt DL, Talbert JL, et al: The pediatric trauma score as a predictor of injury severity in the injured child. J Pediatr Surg 22:14–18, 1987.

201. Tepas JJ, Wears R, Alexander RH, et al: An improved scoring system for assessment of the injured child. J Trauma 25:720–724, 1985.

202. Traub AC, Giebink GS, Smith C, et al: Splenic reticuloendothelial function after splenectomy, spleen repair and spleen autotransplantation. N Engl J Med 317:1559–1564, 1987.

203. Traub AC, Perry JF: Injuries associated with splenic trauma. J Trauma 21:840–847, 1981.

204. Traub AC, Perry JF: Splenic preservation following splenic trauma. J Trauma 22:496–501, 1982.

205. Trunkey D, Federle MP: Computed tomography in perspective (editorial). J Trauma 26:660–661, 1986.

206. Upadhyaya P, Simpson JS: Splenic trauma in children. Surg Gynecol Obstet 126:781–790, 1968.

207. Van Wyck DB, White MH, Witte CL, et al: Critical splenic mass for survival from experimental pneumococcemia. J Surg Res 28:14–17, 1980.

208. Vatner SF, Higgins CB, Millam RW, et al: Role of the spleen in the peripheral vascular response to severe exercise in untethered dogs. Cardiovasc Res 8:276–282, 1974.

209. Vega A, Howell C, Krasna I, et al: Splenic autotransplantation: Optimal function factors. J Pediatr Surg 16:898–904, 1981.

210. Velcek FT, Kugaczewski JT, Jongco B, et al: Function of the reimplanted spleen in dogs. J Trauma 22:502–506, 1982.

211. Villalba MR, Howells GA, Lucas RJ, et al: Nonoperative management of the adult ruptured spleen. Arch Surg 125:836–839, 1990.

212. Vinograd I, Filler RM: Splenic trauma. In: Schiller M (ed): Pediatric Surgery of the Liver, Pancreas and Spleen. Philadelphia, WB Saunders, 1991, pp 247–262.

213. Vock P, Kehrer B, Tschaeppeler A: Blunt liver trauma in children: The role of computed tomography in diagnosis and treatment. J Pediatr Surg 21:413–418, 1986.

214. Welch KJ: Abdominal injuries. In: Ravitch MM, Welch KJ, Benson CD (eds): Pediatric Surgery. Chicago, Year Book Medical Publishers, 1979, pp 125–140.

215. Wells WL, Battisto JR: Splenic regulation of humoral and cellular immunological responses in other domains. In: Role of the Spleen in the Immunology of Parasitic Diseases. Basel, Schwabe, 1979, pp 59–84.

216. Wener L, Boyle CD: Splenic scintiscanning in the preoperative diagnosis of subcapsular hematoma. N Engl J Med 277:35–37, 1967.

217. Wesson DE, Filler RM, Ein SH, et al: Ruptured spleen: When to operate? J Pediatr Surg 16:324–326, 1981.

218. Whitaker AN: Effect of previous splenectomy on the course of pneumococcal bacteremia in mice. J Pathol Bacteriol 95:357–376, 1968.

219. Whitesell FB Jr: A clinical and surgical anatomic study of rupture of the spleen due to blunt trauma. Surg Gynecol Obstet 110:750–754, 1960.

220. Winkelstein JA, Lambert GH: Pneumococcal serum opsonizing activity in splenectomized children. Pediatrics 87:430–433, 1975.

221. Witek JT, Spencer RP, Pearson HA, et al: Diagnostic spleen scans in occult splenic injury. J Trauma 14:197–199, 1974.

222. Wolf Y, Vinograd I, Katz S, et al: Nonoperative management of traumatized spleen in children: The role of open abdominal tap. Z Kinderchir 42:23–25, 1987.

223. Zabinski EJ, Harkins HN: Delayed splenic rupture: A clinical syndrome following trauma. Arch Surg 46:186–213, 1943.

224. Zucker K, Browns K, Rossman D, et al: Nonoperative management of splenic trauma: Conservative or radical treatment? Arch Surg 119:400–404, 1984.

CHAPTER TWENTY-TWO

Richard R. Ricketts

Duodenal and Biliary Tract Injuries

Duodenal and biliary tract injuries are rare in children, and their diagnoses and treatment is often delayed for several reasons:

1. The majority of trauma to children is blunt trauma.
2. Blunt trauma in children is often managed nonoperatively unless the patient exhibits peritoneal irritation or hemodynamic instability.
3. Duodenal and biliary tract injuries frequently do not cause peritonitis initially.
4. The duodenum and biliary tract are often not evaluated adequately during an acute celiotomy for trauma.

These delays in diagnosis and management often result in a higher complication rate and a potentially higher mortality rate. This chapter discusses trauma to these two areas separately.

DUODENAL INJURIES

Anatomy and Function

The duodenum is classically divided into four portions (Fig. 22–1). The first portion, or superior duodenum, consists almost entirely of the duodenal "bulb" and extends from the pylorus to the neck of the gallbladder at the level of the first lumbar vertebra. It is the most mobile portion of the duodenum and is completely covered by serosa. The second portion, or descending duodenum, extends along the right side of the vertebral column from the body of the first lumbar vertebra to that of the fourth. It has close relationships with the transverse colon and liver above; the right kidney, renal vessels, and inferior vena cava behind; and the head of the pancreas and the common bile duct medially. The common bile duct enters its medial wall obliquely at the ampulla of Vater. Its anterior surface is covered by serosa, but its posterior portion is not. The third portion, or transverse duodenum, extends from the right side of the body of the fourth lumbar vertebra over the spinal column and great vessel to the left side of the aorta. It is crossed anteriorly by the superior mesenteric vein artery and is partially covered by mesentery that loosely forms a serosal coat; it has no serosal covering posteriorly but rather rests directly on the inferior vena cava, aorta, and crus of the diaphragm. The fourth portion, or ascending duodenum, extends from the left side of the aorta to the upper border of the second lumber vertebra where it turns anteriorly at the ligament of Treitz to become the jejunum. It is partially covered by serosa.[29]

The duodenum receives gastric, biliary, and pancreatic secretions and transports these to the jejunum. The volume of fluid that passes through the duodenum daily is impressive when one considers that the average adult secretes about 1 to 2 liters of saliva, 2500 ml of gastric juice, 750 ml of bile, and more than 1000 ml of pancreatic juice per day.[67] In addition to water and electrolytes, these secretions contain bile acids and salts, proteases, lipases, and amylase, all of which can be irritating and destructive to surrounding tissues should they escape from the confines of the duodenum.[15, 22, 26, 69]

These anatomic and functional characteristics of the duodenum are important when considering injury to the organ. Although its deep retroperitoneal location provides protection from frequent injury, its relationship with the spine also makes it vulnerable to injury from localized and at times seemingly insignificant traumatic forces.[39, 40] In such instances, it may be the only organ injured. However, major trauma in which the duodenum is injured is frequently accompanied by injury to other organs closely associated with it, namely, the liver, colon, pancreas, biliary tract, and great vessels (see Associated Injuries). Hence, because of the volume and nature of the duodenal contents, leakage of these following traumatic disruption of the bowel wall results in significant retroperitoneal tissue injury and often sepsis, particularly if the diagnosis is delayed.[15, 22, 26, 69]

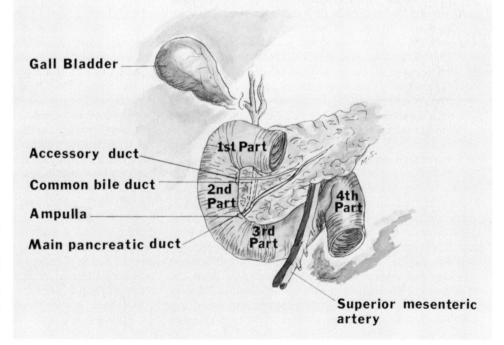

FIGURE 22–1

Anatomy of the duodenum showing its intimate relationship with the pancreas, distal common bile duct, and mesenteric vessels. (Adapted from Adkins RB, Keyser JE: Recent experiences with duodenal trauma. Am Surg 51:121–131, 1985.)

Gall Bladder

Accessory duct

Common bile duct

Ampulla

Main pancreatic duct

1st Part

2nd Part

3rd Part

4th Part

Superior mesenteric artery

These factors, plus the lack of a serosal coat in the retroperitoneal portion of the duodenum, can render repair of the duodenal wall tenuous and with a propensity for leakage and fistula formation.[22, 52, 80] This has resulted in an array of surgical techniques designed to decompress, defunctionalize, and drain repairs of such injuries (see Treatment).

Incidence

Duodenal injuries at all ages are rare, occurring in from 3 to 5% of patients sustaining abdominal trauma.[1, 26, 43] In children, the incidence is about 2%.[58] Although penetrating injuries account for the majority of instances in adults from urban settings, blunt trauma is responsible for the vast majority of cases in children or for all ages in rural settings.[1, 11, 22, 26, 41, 43, 50, 52, 58, 69, 74, 79, 80, 83]

Duodenal injuries account for 25% of all small bowel injuries from blunt or penetrating sources. However, because of the relatively fixed position of the duodenum and its relationship to the vertebral column, it accounts for 50% of the small bowel injuries following blunt trauma.[13] Blunt duodenal trauma is most commonly caused by motor vehicle accidents, falls, or altercations.[10, 11, 15, 22, 43, 46, 76, 80] In addition, children frequently suffer blunt duodenal trauma from bicycle accidents and child abuse.[43, 58, 67, 86]

Mechanisms of Injury

Several mechanisms of injury have been proposed to explain blunt duodenal disruption. Direct compression of the duodenum against the vertebrae, a sudden increase in intraluminal pressure, a shearing force between the fixed portions of the duodenum and the nonfixed stomach or jejunum, mural ischemia, and infarction have all been incriminated.[10, 34, 85] Direct compression against the vertebral column can adequately account for injuries to the third and fourth portion of the duodenum; however, compression does not explain injuries to the second portion, which are much more common (see Location of Duodenal Injuries).[62, 85] Because the pylorus is closed approximately one third of the time, this and the acute angulation formed by the ligament of Treitz at the duodenojejunal junction could theoretically create a closed duodenal loop.[10, 62] Traumatic forces thus applied to this closed loop could cause an acute rise in intraduodenal pressure, resulting in disruption.

A similar mechanism could also create shearing forces in the duodenal wall rupturing intramural vessels and leading to hematoma formation. Such a hematoma has the potential to produce infarction of the wall with delayed rupture.[10] Such shearing forces between fixed portions of the duodenum and its surrounding structures have been studied experimentally and have correlated with duodenal injuries seen clinically.[18, 19] Sudden upward movement of the liver and diaphragm from abrupt abdominal wall compression can also theoretically exert traction on the hepatoduodenal ligament and common bile duct and potentially injure the duodenum distal to the ampulla of Vater, another common site for injury.[62] In addition, a sudden deceleration can allow the mobile stomach and first portion of the duodenum to move forward abruptly, resulting in a shearing force on the fixed second and third portions of the duodenum, with a resultant tear. A similar mechanism can explain injuries at the duodenojejunal junction.

Associated Injuries

Duodenal injury is nearly always associated with injuries to adjacent viscera. One clear exception of this is the isolated duodenal hematoma (see Intramural Duodenal Hematoma). Penetrating injuries to the duodenum have an associated intra-abdominal organ injury rate of 93 to 100%, whereas 69 to 83% of patients with blunt duodenal trauma have associated injuries.[15, 33, 46, 58, 69, 74] The most common organs sustaining concomitant injury are the liver, colon, stomach, small bowel, and pancreas. Major vascular injuries to the inferior vena cava, aorta, mesenteric or renal vessels, or portal vein occur in about 30 to 35% of these patients.[1, 43, 69, 74] Overall, patients with duodenal injuries have an average of 2.7 associated intra-abdominal organ injuries; those with penetrating injury have a slightly higher rate than those with blunt injury.[1, 11, 26, 41, 43, 74] Similar statistics apply to children; one study reported an average of 2.25 associated injuries per patient.[58]

Diagnosis

Most duodenal injuries are diagnosed during emergency abdominal exploration for exsanguinating hemorrhage or peritonitis. In fact, when performing a celiotomy under these circumstances, it is mandatory to assess the status of the duodenum through careful mobilization, visual inspection, and palpation. As many as 10 to 30% of duodenal injuries are overlooked at the time of initial celiotomy.[34, 76] Unless identified, the complications subsequently manifest are serious and associated with significant mortality.[1, 10, 15, 82, 83]

At celiotomy, evidence indicating a possible duodenal injury includes bile staining of the retroperitoneum, periduodenal or pancreatic hematoma, crepitance or "bubbles" in the retroperitoneum, free intraperitoneal bile or gas, saponification of the retroperitoneal tissues, or proximity of a missile tract.[26, 43, 73] Any of these findings mandates full exposure and inspection of the duodenum.

The duodenum can be exposed in its entirety by dividing the gastrohepatic ligament to free the first portion; performing an extensive Kocher maneuver from the foramen of Winslow to the superior mesenteric vessels to free the second portion; mobilizing the right colon and small bowel mesentery medially as described by Cattell and Braasch to free the third portion; and dividing the ligament of Treitz to free the fourth portion.[8, 15, 22, 26, 43, 82] The anteriomedial surface of the duodenum can be inspected through the lesser sac by taking down the gastrocolic omentum. A policy of routine duodenal exploration despite absent intraoperative signs is recommended by some so that occult retroperitoneal injuries are not missed.[1, 22]

Duodenal injuries, particularly from blunt trauma, that are not associated with concomitant injuries that cause hemorrhage or peritonitis are even more subtle and difficult to diagnose preoperatively. This often leads to a delay in treatment, which increases morbidity and mortality significantly (see Treatment; Results).[11, 26, 45, 46, 69, 78, 82] The most common symptom and sign of such a duodenal injury is mild epigastric pain and tenderness that persists or increases in severity during several hours' observation.[43, 46, 82] Accompanying this pain may be back or flank pain or radiation of pain down into the testes.[82] The abdominal pain and tenderness may be maximal in the right lower quadrant after several hours because of seepage of duodenal contents along the right colic gutter; this may lead to a preoperative diagnosis of appendicitis, especially in children.[58]

Laboratory values are nonspecific and of little help.[76] The white blood cell count is elevated in approximately 40% of patients, and the serum amylase is elevated in 50 to 70% of patients.[15, 43, 69, 82] Peritoneal lavage is not useful because of a reported 60 to 75% false negative rate.[43, 76]

Several nonspecific radiographic findings may be present, including intraperitoneal gas, obliteration of the right psoas shadow, scoliosis to the right, and generalized ileus. More specific radiographic findings of duodenal disruption include retroperitoneal gas around the right kidney and right crus of the diaphragm, bubbles of gas in the transverse mesocolon mimicking feces in the colon, and extravasation of water-soluble contrast given with the patient lying right-side down.[11, 15, 43, 45, 69, 78] One or more of these specific radiographic signs is found in 33 to 50% of patients evaluated within 6 hours from injury and in virtually all patients studied within 24 hours.[46, 78] Computed tomography is more definitive, superseding plain radiographs in diagnostic accuracy by identifying retroperitoneal gas bubbles or fluid and duodenal hematomas, as well as disruptions, earlier when done in conjunction with gastrointestinal contrast.[27, 51]

Still, however, the diagnosis of duodenal injuries requires a high index of suspicion. The duodenum should be inspected in all patients undergoing abdominal exploration for blunt or penetrating trauma, especially if there are periduodenal findings indicating a possible injury. In patients who appear not to require immediate exploration, repeated physical examination, judicious use of serial radiographs, and abdominal computed tomography should be done to expedite the diagnosis and treatment to avoid the increased morbidity and mortality that accompanies delayed diagnosis and intervention.

Location of Duodenal Injuries

Overall, approximately 15% of single duodenal injuries occur in the first portion, 40% in the second portion, 25% in the third portion, and 20% in the fourth portion of the duodenum.[11, 22, 36, 41, 69, 74] Approximately 20% of patients have multiple duodenal injuries. Penetrating injuries tend to be more evenly distributed along the course of the duodenum (Fig. 22–2). Overall mortality is directly related to the portion of the duodenum that is injured, being lowest in the first and fourth portions (4–8%) and highest in the second and third portions (20%).[74] The reasons for this are many but almost certainly relate to the lack of a serosal

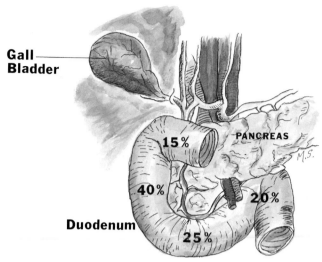

FIGURE 22–2

Location of injuries in blunt duodenal trauma. (Adapted with permission from Fabian TC, Mangiante EC, Millis M: Duodenal rupture due to blunt trauma: A problem in diagnosis. South Med J 77:1078–1082, 1984.)

covering over a major part of the second and third portions of the duodenum (see Anatomy and Function).

Classification of Duodenal Injuries

The commonly accepted classification system for duodenal injuries was proposed by Lucas and Ledgerwood in 1975.[45, 46] Class I injuries are duodenal hematomas, contusions, or incomplete disruptions (serosal tears) without pancreatic injury. Class II injuries are complete duodenal disruptions without pancreatic injury. A class III injury is any duodenal injury with an associated minor pancreatic injury such as a contusion, hematoma, or laceration but without a main pancreatic ductal injury. Class IV injuries are severe combined injuries of the duodenum and pancreas (Table 22–1). Class III injuries have been further subclassified into class IIIA, when the combined pancreatic or duodenal injury consists of a hematoma or a contusion only, and Class IIIB, when a perforation, laceration, or transection of either the duodenum or pancreas is associated with a hematoma or a contusion of the other.[1]

Other factors critical to determining the severity of duodenal injury are often tabulated to have a basis for comparison of different treatment methods (see Treatment; Re-

Table 22–1
Classification of Duodenal Injuries

Class I	Minor duodenal injury
	Normal pancreas
Class II	Major duodenal injury
	Normal pancreas
Class III	Minor or major duodenal injury
	Minor pancreatic injury
Class IV	Major duodenal injury
	Major pancreatic injury

sults). These include the extent of the duodenal wall circumference that is injured (<20%, 20–70%, or >70% of the circumference); the portion of the duodenum that is injured (see Location of Duodenal Injuries); the time interval between injury and operative repair; the mechanism of injury (blunt vs. penetrating); and the presence of associated injuries with particular reference to major vascular, hepatobiliary, and pancreatic injuries.[1, 11, 22, 43, 45, 46, 69, 74] The possible effects these factors have on choosing one surgical method over another and on the results of management are discussed later in this chapter (see Treatment; Results).

Treatment

Although a multitude of complex operative procedures have been described to treat duodenal injuries, the vast majority can be managed with meticulous primary closure of the wound, with or without drainage.[1, 22, 26, 43, 69, 76, 83] More extensive procedures designed to "defunctionalize," decompress, or "exclude" the duodenum during healing of the repair are indicated in certain instances, as is discussed. It is useful to consider the various treatment alternatives relative to the class of duodenal injury involved. It should be noted that this classification system does not take into account other important variables such as the associated visceral injuries, other than pancreatic; the time between injury and treatment; the mechanism of injury; or the portion of the duodenum that is injured, any one of which may influence the type of procedure indicated.

Because duodenal trauma is rare in children, most of the information on treating patients has derived from experiences in treating adults. With few exceptions, the principles utilized in treating adults with duodenal trauma can be applied to children effectively. In fact, the two largest series of duodenal trauma in children report results superior to those of adult series that utilized the same methods.[58, 73]

Class I Injuries

Class I duodenal injuries (hematoma, contusion, serosal tear) are usually managed without operative intervention. Serosal tears can be sutured, and drainage is neither required nor indicated. If a hematoma is found at celiotomy, it should be gently unroofed or evacuated to ensure that the underlying duodenal wall is intact; drainage may or may not be employed.[1, 45, 46, 79, 87] Duodenal hematomas diagnosed preoperatively represent a unique injury in children and are discussed separately.

Intramural Duodenal Hematoma. An intramural duodenal hematoma is a collection of blood in the subserosal layer of the duodenal wall in most instances.[39] In some, the hematoma may be located in the submucosal layer or within the muscular layer itself.[12, 24, 39] Sometimes distention, discoloration, and edema are significant, sufficient to make viability of the duodenal wall questionable.[24] Full-thickness duodenal disruptions have apparently resulted in 4.0 to 37.5% of patients.[39, 86]

The hematoma usually affects the second or third portion of the duodenum (Fig. 22–3). It quite frequently affects both of these portions and may extend proximally or dis-

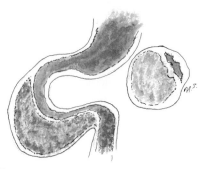

FIGURE 22–3
Intramural duodenal hematoma along the second, third, and fourth portion of the duodenum. (From Freeark RJ, Corley RD, Norcross WJ, et al: Intramural hematoma of the duodenum. Arch Surg 92:463–475, 1965. Copyright 1965, American Medical Association.)

tally to involve the first or fourth portion in 15% and 40% of patients, respectively.[12, 39]

Blunt trauma, most commonly from a narrow object such as a handle bar, a steering wheel, an edge of a chair, or a fist, is the usual etiologic event. In many cases the trauma is so trivial as to be forgotten.[12, 23, 24, 28, 39, 60, 61, 81, 86] Other etiologic factors include anticoagulant therapy, blood dyscrasias (hemophilia), Henoch-Schönlein purpura, clotting disorders, and pancreatic disease.[12, 39, 60, 61, 77] Additional factors that may be of etiologic importance include the rich submucosal vascular plexus in the duodenum, the tangential insertion of the duodenal mesentery, the varying tensile strength of the layers of the duodenal wall, and the lack of a completely circumferential serosal layer capable of tamponading active intramural hemorrhage.[12, 39] These factors, combined with shearing forces applied to the duodenum, can result in intramural hemorrhage and hematoma formation.[23, 39, 60] Often there is a significant delay (up to 12 days; average of 4 days) between the traumatic event and the appearance of obstructive symptoms.[12, 23, 24, 86] This may be the result of a slowly enlarging mass secondary to the hyperosmotic effect of a liquefying hematoma, analogous to that of a chronic subdural hematoma.[23, 39, 61]

The incidence of duodenal hematoma is unknown because many may resolve spontaneously without medical attention. In Stone and Fabian's large series of patients (adults and children) with duodenal trauma (blunt and penetrating), only 19 of 321, or 6%, had duodenal hematomas.[74] In considering patients treated for blunt duodenal trauma only, 10 to 35% have duodenal hematomas; the remainder have more severe injuries.[1, 11, 43, 73] The incidence of duodenal hematoma is higher in males than in females and is also higher in children than in adults; approximately 50% of the patients are younger than 14 years old, and two thirds are younger than 20 years old.[24, 38, 39]

Associated visceral injuries are uncommon but can occur. Biliary and pancreatic injuries occur in approximately 15% and 25% of patients, respectively.[39] Jaundice occurs in about 8% and may be related to compression of the common bile duct by the hematoma or to hemolysis or to both.[5, 12, 39, 60] Hyperamylasemia occurs in 15 to 35% and results from direct pancreatic trauma or ampullary obstruction by the hematoma, or both.[12, 24, 38, 39, 86] Other duodenal or prox-

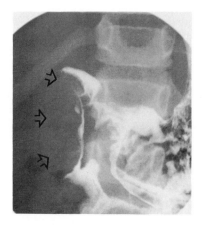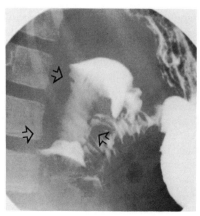

FIGURE 22–4

Anteroposterior and lateral views demonstrating an intramural hematoma *(arrows)* with near total duodenal obstruction on an upper gastrointestinal series.

imal jejunal injuries such as serosal lacerations or full thickness disruptions occur in up to 35% of the patients with duodenal hematomas.[39, 86] The high percentage of injuries in the last-mentioned category points to the importance of careful and repeated physical examination and diagnostic evaluation when a nonoperative approach is chosen.

Diagnosis is based on the characteristic history, physical examination, and radiographic findings. The classical history is that of a child who sustains direct blunt trauma to the epigastrium that may seem trivial and for which medical attention is not sought. Several days later bilious vomiting ensues.[12, 23, 39, 61] Symptoms of upper gastrointestinal tract obstruction are present in 95% of the patients.[12] A much less common presentation is that of an acute abdominal emergency following blunt trauma.[23, 39, 61] In the latter presentation, serious associated injuries should be suspected. Abdominal pain is invariably present, being in the right upper quadrant when the first, second, or third portion of the duodenum is involved and in the left upper quadrant when the fourth portion or proximal jejunum is involved.[12, 39, 60] Pain may also be referred to the back, flank, or testes.[39, 60]

Specific physical findings include epigastric abdominal tenderness and a mass that is palpable in approximately 40% of the patients.[39] The remainder of the abdomen is soft and scaphoid owing to the high-grade proximal obstruction that is present. The presence of diffuse abdominal tenderness should alert one to the possibility of associated visceral injuries.[23, 86]

The diagnosis is confirmed by the typical upper gastrointestinal series finding of an intramural mass with a "coiled spring" mucosal pattern overlying it, as described by Felson and Levin in 1954 (Fig. 22–4).[17] The coiled spring pattern represents an intramural extramucosal mass with crowding of the circular folds adjacent to the mass.[39, 57] Another mucosal pattern seen on the upper gastrointestinal series is the "picket fence" sign, which represents disappearance of the circular folds of the duodenum with mucosal pinching and spiculation perpendicular to the lumen. This is caused by more diffuse infiltration of the wall of the duodenum by blood.[12, 57] Ultrasound is also useful in demonstrating the size of the hematoma and in observing its gradual resolution without exposing the patient to repeated irradiation. Computed tomography (Fig. 22–5) and now magnetic resonance imaging with its characteristic "ring"

sign on T1-weighted images are also useful for establishing the diagnosis and for following patients who are treated nonoperatively.[31, 51, 57]

Management of patients found to have a duodenal hematoma during exploration for an acute abdominal emergency is straightforward: the hematoma should be evacuated, and any other associated injuries should be managed appropriately. To evacuate the hematoma, a short longitudinal incision is made along the lateral aspect of the duodenum over the surface of the hematoma. The hematoma, which is usually subserosal but may be submucosal, is carefully evacuated with irrigation and a blunt sponge forceps. Care must be taken not to injure the underlying and intact mucosa; if there is a question concerning mucosal integrity, dilute methylene blue can be instilled via the nasogastric tube and milked through the duodenum into the jejunum, observing for leaks.

The hematoma may extend to the fourth portion of the duodenum and into the proximal jejunum; in such instances, a second, transverse incision should be made just distal to the ligament of Treitz to be certain that all of the clot is evacuated.[61] Specific bleeding vessels, if identified, should be ligated. The seromuscular layer at the distal inci-

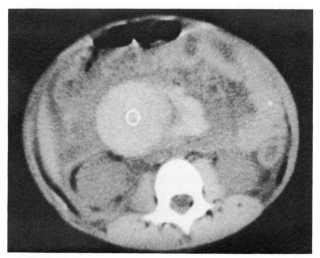

FIGURE 22–5

A computed tomography scan of an intramural duodenal hematoma (note the cursor).

sion can be closed with interrupted sutures; the proximal incision over the duodenum is left open or only partially closed to allow for continued drainage.[73] Whether to leave a drain in place, either in the cavity previously occupied by the hematoma or along the side of the duodenum, is controversial.[12, 39, 61, 73] The current trend is to drain any associated injuries but not to drain the duodenal injury itself.

Management of duodenal hematomas diagnosed before surgical intervention is more controversial: some investigators favor a nonoperative approach, whereas others advocate surgical drainage.[12, 23, 24, 39, 61, 77, 86] The nonoperative approach consists of nasogastric suction, intravenous fluid and nutrition administration, and serial radiographic examination until the obstruction is relieved and oral alimentation can be instituted. Nonoperative therapy is indicated only when the surgeon can confidently exclude a full thickness perforation or significant associated injuries; such therapy may require 2 to 38 days of nasogastric suction (average 13 days) and 5 to 53 days of hospitalization (average 18 days) to be successful.[77] Nonoperative therapy has most often been successful in young children with partial obstruction; older patients or those with near total obstruction more often require surgical intervention.[23]

The advantages of nonoperative therapy are the avoidance of general anesthesia and operative and postoperative (short-term and long-term) complications. It is perhaps less costly, although perhaps not when one considers the prolonged hospitalization time and the long-term need for total parenteral nutrition that is required. These advantages must be balanced against the possibility of delaying the diagnosis of a duodenal disruption or associated visceral injury, the possibility of fibrous organization of the clot with persistent obstruction, and the possible septic hazards of prolonged total parenteral nutrition.[12, 86]

Operative intervention allows one to exclude or manage associated injuries, relieve the obstruction quickly, and lower hospitalization time (and cost?) and the need for parenteral nutrition. The operation is generally not associated with significant morbidity or mortality. These advantages must be weighed against the small risk of general anesthesia and the potential long-term postoperative complications that can occur following any celiotomy.

Considering the previously mentioned factors, the current management of a child with duodenal hematoma in whom full thickness disruption or associated visceral injuries can be reliably excluded by physical examination and laboratory or radiographic evaluation is a trial nonoperative therapy period of 5 to 10 days. If there is no evidence for partial resolution of the obstruction in 5 days or complete resolution with resumption of oral intake in 10 days, operative intervention with evacuation of the hematoma without drainage should be done.[12, 24, 61, 86] This approach should result in the least morbidity and mortality and at the same time lessen the time and cost of hospitalization.

Class II Injuries

Full thickness disruption of the duodenum without associated pancreatic injury, especially that resulting from penetrating trauma, can usually be managed by meticulous débridement of devitalized tissue and two-layer transverse

closure in the vast majority of cases.[1, 26, 36, 43, 46, 69, 76] Class II injuries resulting from blunt trauma may devitalize a large portion of the duodenal wall and therefore may require a more complex procedure.[43] In extensive longitudinal injuries, the closure may narrow the duodenal lumen; in such cases consideration of a gastrojejunostomy added to the repair should be made.[45, 46]

The use of drains, either simple or sump, is controversial. Those favoring use of a drain believe that if an anastomotic leak occurs, a controlled duodenal fistula will result, thus sparing the patient widespread intraperitoneal contamination.[1, 22] Others believe that drains themselves may be responsible for fistula formation.[15, 73, 74] Another technique used in class II injuries to ''protect'' a tenuous suture line is to place a jejunal serosal patch over the repair (Fig. 22–6).[87] However, McInnis and colleagues could find no significant difference in the outcome of patients treated by primary closure with or without the addition of a jejunal patch.[50]

It is clear that all class II injuries are not the same. If a secure two-layer closure with good blood supply and without tension can be achieved, one should not feel compelled to drain the suture line or to protect it with a serosal patch. If, on the other hand, the diagnosis was delayed and the

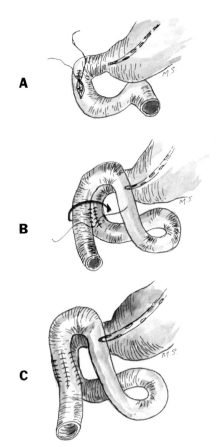

FIGURE 22–6

A technique for covering a duodenal repair with a ''serosal patch.'' (From McInnis WD, Aust JB, Cruz AB, et al: Traumatic injuries of the duodenum: A comparison of 1° closure and the jejunal patch. J Trauma 15:847–853, 1975.)

tissues are edematous and friable, or if some tension is noted on the suture line, or if any other factors raise concern about the integrity of the injury, some type of protective measures should be taken, in the form of either internal or external drainage, as discussed under class III injuries.

Class III Injuries

Major duodenal injuries with minor pancreatic injuries that do not involve the main pancreatic duct generally can be managed by direct repair of the duodenal wound with the addition of internal or external drainage of the repair and drainage of the pancreatic injury.[1, 45, 46, 74, 83] Severe class III injuries are effectively managed by repair plus pyloric exclusion and gastrojejunostomy or by duodenal "diverticularization."[4, 41, 43, 45, 46, 52, 80] These last-mentioned methods are more commonly used in class IV injuries that are not severe enough to warrant pancreaticoduodenectomy.

Stone and Fabian reported the successful use of a three-tube technique in managing complex duodenal wounds or those associated with pancreatic injury.[74] This technique utilizes a tube gastrostomy to decompress the stomach, a retrograde tube jejunostomy to decompress the duodenum, and an antegrade feeding jejunostomy for enteral nutrition (Fig. 22–7).[33, 74] Utilizing this technique, the postinjury incidence of duodenal fistula formation was reduced markedly.[74] Most agree that internal decompression is superior to external drainage in decreasing the rate of fistula formation. In addition, the mortality resulting from fistulas is lower in repairs in which decompression is used than in repairs performed without the use of decompression.[11, 22, 33, 74] Others have found that morbidity may actually be increased with the use of tubes for decompression and argue against their routine use; in situations in which decompression is indicated, they favor pyloric exclusion and gastrojejunostomy.[35, 36, 69]

Pyloric exclusion was first described in 1977.[80] This technique involves repair of the duodenal injury, an antral gastric incision through which the pylorus is closed with either absorbable or nonabsorbable sutures (or staples), and construction of a loop side-to-side gastrojejunostomy (Fig. 22–8).[80] Follow-up studies have shown that the pylorus reopens in 94% of patients after 3 weeks regardless of the method of closure and that marginal ulceration occurs infrequently (less than 10%).[52, 58, 80] Pyloric exclusion is indicated when

the operation has been delayed for more than 24 hours after injury, when more than 75% of the circumference of the duodenal wall is involved, when the blood supply is compromised, or when there are severe regional injuries to the head of the pancreas or distal common bile duct.[41] This procedure has lowered the incidence of fistula formation and has decreased the complications resulting from duodenal leakage.[4, 52, 80] Fistulas that do form are "end" duodenal fistulas rather than "lateral" fistulas, are less difficult to manage, and have a high rate of spontaneous closure.[4, 48, 52]

Duodenal "diverticularization," first described in 1968, consists of repair of the duodenal injury, gastric antrectomy with end-to-side gastrojejunostomy, tube duodenostomy, and extensive drainage. Truncal vagotomy and biliary tract drainage may be advisable in some instances (Fig. 22–9).[3, 4] This technique was developed to treat extensive duodenal wounds or duodenal wounds combined with severe pancreatic injuries.[4] It reduced the morbidity (especially from duodenal fistulas) and mortality from such injuries reported up until that time.[4] Currently the use of this procedure is limited because the same protective and physiologic effect can be achieved with the simpler pyloric exclusion procedure and because if the latter procedure is not advisable, a pancreaticoduodenectomy should be performed.[1, 36, 45]

Class IV Injuries

Extensive combined injuries of the duodenum and pancreas require more complex procedures for a successful outcome. When tissue destruction is not so extensive that repair is impossible, pyloric exclusion or duodenal diverticularization is the procedure of choice.[4, 43, 45, 46, 52, 54, 80] When tissue destruction is massive, however, and especially when the terminal bile duct is injured, pancreaticoduodenectomy (Whipple procedure) is indicated.[1, 15, 36, 55, 80, 83, 89] The latter procedure is required in less than 1% of patients undergoing celiotomy for trauma and in a minority (3–15%) of patients who have class III or IV duodenal injuries.[22, 36, 55, 69, 80] Pancreaticoduodenectomy should be regarded as a "débridement" procedure when no other alternative forms of treatment are available. It is used for injuries that are nonreconstructible, for those with proven injury to the terminal common bile duct, or for those with devascularization of the duodenum and head of the pancreas.[4, 55, 82] A summary

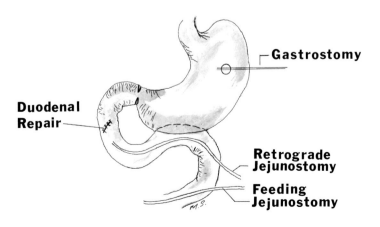

FIGURE 22–7

Gastrostomy and retrograde jejunostomy to decompress the duodenal repair with an additional feeding jejunostomy. (From Hasson JE, Stern D, Moss GS: Penetrating duodenal trauma. J Trauma 24:471–474, 1984.)

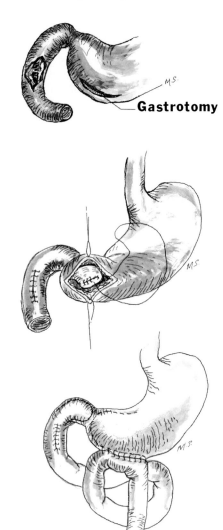

Gastrotomy

FIGURE 22–8

Technique of "pyloric exclusion": A 1-degree repair of a duodenal wound, closure of the pylorus through an antral gastrotomy, gastrojejunostomy. (From Vaughn GD III, Frazier OH, Graham DY, et al: The use of pyloric exclusion in the management of severe duodenal injuries. Am J Surg 134:785–790, 1977.)

of the methods used to treat duodenal injuries is shown in Table 22–2.

Results

The major complication resulting from repair of a duodenal injury is a duodenal fistula, which occurs in 1 to 30% of patients and accounts for a 4 to 50% mortality rate.[4, 11, 22, 33, 36, 48, 52, 69, 74, 80, 83] As a result of this, procedures have been designed to lower the incidence of this complication. External drainage does not lower the rate of fistula formation and may actually increase it.[15, 73, 74] Internal decompression, as advocated by Stone and Fabian, has resulted in a markedly lower fistula formation rate; only one in 237 of their patients developed a duodenal leak.[74] Others using this technique have found that fistula formation after decompression

can be reduced to 0 to 2.3% versus 11.8 to 30% when decompression is not used.[22, 33] In addition, the mortality rate resulting from a duodenal leak is decreased from 42% to 14% when decompression is employed.[33] At variance with these reports is an analysis of a series of 100 patients that compared repair plus "ostomies" (of all types) versus repair without ostomies; 27% of those with ostomies developed a duodenal fistula, whereas only 1.6% of those having primary repair did so.[36]

The rate of fistula formation following repair of complex duodenal injuries utilizing the pyloric exclusion procedure is from 2 to 5%.[52, 80] Fistula formation following the more complex duodenal diverticularization procedure is 14%.[4] However, if a fistula forms following the employment of either of these techniques, it is an end fistula rather than a lateral fistula, is less difficult to manage, nearly always closes spontaneously, and has a lower mortality rate (14% vs. 40%) when compared with that of a lateral fistula.[4, 48, 52, 80] In one series of lateral duodenal fistulas, only four of 14 closed spontaneously, seven of 10 were successfully closed at the first reoperation, but three recurred; of these, two were treated successfully with another operation, and one patient died (7% of the total).[48]

The mortality rate for duodenal trauma ranges from 10 to 40%.[4, 11, 13, 15, 22, 26, 33, 35, 41, 43, 46, 52, 69, 74, 80, 83, 87] Interestingly, the lowest mortality, 10 to 14%, has been reported in the two series dealing with duodenal and pancreatic trauma in children.[58, 73] The vast majority of the deaths are attributable to associated visceral and vascular injuries.[1, 22, 26, 33, 35, 36, 41, 69, 74, 80] If these are excluded, deaths directly attributable to the duodenal wound occur in 0 to 6% of patients.[1, 26, 36, 41, 52, 69, 74, 80] However, of late deaths among those who survive the initial surgery, 50% are related to the duodenal injury itself or to complications relating to its repair.[43, 74] These deaths result from suture line leaks with abscess or fistula formation, sepsis, and subsequent multisystem failure.[15, 35, 43, 80, 83, 87]

Blunt duodenal trauma has a higher mortality rate than that of penetrating trauma (12.5 to 30% vs. 7.5 to 20%) in

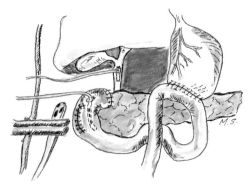

FIGURE 22–9

Technique of duodenal "diverticularization": A 1-degree repair of the duodenal wound, an antrectomy with a Billroth II gastrojejunostomy, tube drainage of the duodenum, drainage of the duodenal repair and pancreas; a vagotomy and T-tube drainage of the common bile duct in some cases. (From Berne CJ, Donovan AJ, White EJ, et al: Duodenal "diverticularization" for duodenal and pancreatic injury. Am J Surg 127:503–507, 1974.)

Table 22–2
Treatment of Duodenal Injuries

	Class I	Class II	Class III	Class IV
Duodenal repair	Serosa only	2 layer	2 layer	2 layer
External drainage	No	No	Yes	Yes
Tube decompression	No	No	Yes	Yes
Pyloric exclusion	No	No	Yes	Yes
Diverticularization	No	No	No	Yes
Whipple procedure	No	No	No	Yes*/No†

*With distal common bile duct injury.
†Without distal common bile duct injury.

all series.[11, 15, 43, 69, 74, 80] Patients treated after 24 hours has elapsed from the time of the injury have a higher mortality rate than patients treated within 24 hours (40% vs. 11%).[46] Patients who have extensive injuries that are treated with repair only have a higher mortality rate than those having repair plus decompression (30% vs. 15%).[11] Patients with combined duodenal and pancreatic injuries (classes III, IV) have a higher mortality rate than those with duodenal injuries alone (classes I, II). Patients with class I and II injuries have a 0 to 20% mortality rate, whereas those with class III and IV injuries have a 20 to 100% mortality rate (Table 22–3).[43, 83, 87] The highest mortality rates (30 to 100%; 40% average) are in patients who require a Whipple procedure for combined pancreatic and duodenal trauma, the one exception being a report of 10 patients, all of whom survived.[36, 55, 87, 89]

BILIARY TRACT INJURIES

The overall incidence of trauma to the extrahepatic biliary tract is approximately 2 to 5%.[59] In most cases the gallbladder in involved (74%), followed in frequency by the common bile duct and the porta hepatis (26%).[37] Injury to the extrahepatic biliary system is most often secondary to penetrating trauma, although in children blunt trauma predominates.[37, 56, 59] Because trauma to each of these parts of the extrahepatic biliary system has different presentations, managements, and outcomes, each is discussed separately.

Gallbladder

Gallbladder injuries occur in approximately 2% (range 0.5 to 8.6%) of patients who sustain penetrating and blunt ab-

Table 22–3
Overall Mortality from Duodenal Trauma

Blunt trauma	12.5–30%
Penetrating trauma	7.5–20%
Repair after 24 hours	40%
Repair before 24 hours	11%
Class III, IV	20–100%
Class I, II	0–20%
Repair alone	30%
Repair plus decompression	15%

dominal trauma.[56, 66] Of these, 90% are from penetrating trauma, and 10% are from blunt trauma.[37, 56] Almost all blunt traumatic injuries to normal gallbladders occur in children.[66]

Gallbladder injuries resulting from penetrating trauma nearly always have associated visceral injuries and therefore should be recognized at the time of initial celiotomy. Treatment is cholecystectomy, with uniformly good results. Morbidity and mortality rates are related to the associated visceral or vascular injuries rather than to the gallbladder injury per se.[37, 56, 59]

Gallbladder injuries are classified into four categories: *lacerations or disruptions,* which are the most common; *avulsions,* which are the next most common; and *contusions,* probably more common than reported, because all patients with blunt trauma are not routinely explored surgically.[30, 56, 70, 72] A fourth category, *traumatic cholecystitis,* may result from bleeding into the gallbladder with subsequent obstruction of the cystic duct, infection, and the clinical manifestations of cholecystitis accompanied by jaundice, melena, and hematemesis.[56]

Three factors predisposing the gallbladder to injury from blunt trauma have been proposed: (1) a thin-walled, normal gallbladder is more prone to rupture than a thick-walled, diseased one, hence the relatively high incidence in children; (2) the degree of filling at the time of trauma; and (3) alcohol ingestion, which by increasing the flow and production of bile and by increasing the tone of the sphincter of Oddi effectively increases the pressure within the biliary tree.[30, 59, 70] Shearing forces between the fluid-filled gallbladder and the solid parenchyma of the liver produce rapid deceleration forces and result in avulsions or disruptions, whereas contusions result from direct trauma.[59, 70]

Because most patients with gallbladder injuries resulting from blunt trauma have associated visceral injuries (50–93%; 2.5 associated injuries per patient), the majority of gallbladder injuries should be noted at the time of celiotomy.[56, 70, 84] Any noticeable tissue bile staining requires a thorough exploration of the biliary tree, including the gallbladder.

Isolated injuries to the gallbladder resulting from blunt trauma are usually subtle and difficult to diagnose. The reason for this is that sterile bile within the peritoneal cavity, choleperitoneum ("bile peritonitis"), is relatively innocuous initially. It does not have the same irritating and catastrophic effects as infected bile released within the peritoneal cavity. However, the bile salts and bile acid do initiate a chemical peritonitis resulting in an effusion, with the development of ascites, nausea and vomiting, low-grade fever, abdominal pain, and hypovolemia. Eventually jaundice, dark urine, and in some cases acholic stools become evident.[20, 56, 66, 70, 84] This process may take from 1 day to 6 weeks (average 36 hours) depending on whether the leaking bile becomes encysted.[20, 30, 56, 66]

Although peritoneal lavage may be diagnostic when bile is free within the peritoneal cavity, the high incidence of "pseudocyst" formation results in a high rate of false negative lavages, making this test useless in most cases.[70, 84] When diagnosis is delayed beyond 3 days because of pseudocyst formation, a mass may become palpable in the right upper quadrant. Plain abdominal radiographs may reveal a soft tissue mass displacing the hepatic flexure of the colon downward and medially and causing elevation of the right hemidiaphragm.[18, 72] Ultrasonic examination may show an encapsulated fluid collection with septa; aspiration of this fluid using ultrasonic guidance is diagnostic if bile is found.[72] This in combination with a rising serum direct bilirubin level confirms the diagnosis of gallbladder rupture.[18] Another diagnostic test for gallbladder rupture and other injuries to the biliary tract is the Technetium-labeled iminodiacetic acid scan.[44, 75]

Cholecystectomy is the standard treatment of choice for nearly all gallbladder injuries.[30, 37, 59, 66, 70, 84] Cholangiography is indicated if injury to other portions of the biliary tract is suspected.[84] Drainage is unnecessary for isolated injuries but may be indicated if associated injuries are present.[70] Tube cholecystostomy has been used in children and adults in the past in attempts to preserve the gallbladder; currently this procedure should be reserved for patients who are desperately ill or hemodynamically unstable or in whom obscured anatomy makes cholecystectomy a hazardous procedure.[37, 56, 66, 70, 71] Cholecystorrhaphy, reported in children with small lacerations, should probably be avoided because of the potential risk of calculus formation along the scar.[14, 59, 66, 84] Minor contusions of the gallbladder may be managed expectantly because no delayed ruptures have been reported.[59, 70] However, with moderate or severe contusions, cholecystectomy should be performed, if feasible, to prevent the possible development of a calculous gangrenous cholecystitis in the postoperative period in a severely traumatized patient.[70]

Morbidity and mortality in patients with gallbladder injuries are directly related to associated visceral injuries.[37, 59] The overall mortality rate is less than 5%, with no reported deaths following isolated injury of the gallbladder.[59, 84]

Extrahepatic Bile Ducts

Trauma to the extrahepatic bile ducts accounts for only 0.5% of patients undergoing celiotomy for acute trauma.[59] Penetrating wounds predominate, but a small number of cases, particularly in children, are caused by blunt trauma.[2, 7, 16, 32, 37, 42, 47, 59, 63, 88] Patients with penetrating wounds to the biliary tract virtually always have associated visceral injury.[16, 37, 59] The bile duct injury should be discovered at the initial celiotomy for acute trauma, although 3% are missed.[37] To avoid this, careful exploration of the biliary tract is required when free intraperitoneal bile is noted or when bile staining or a hematoma of the hepatoduodenal ligament is seen. Operative cholangiography through the gallbladder is indicated if dissection does not reveal the injury.[16, 37, 59]

Injuries of the extrahepatic bile duct resulting from blunt trauma are rare. The force required to injure these ducts by blunt trauma is considerable, and therefore nearly all patients have severe associated visceral injury; isolated bile duct injury from blunt trauma is exceedingly rare.[6, 53, 59, 63]

The mechanisms by which blunt trauma causes injury to the extrahepatic bile ducts have been studied experimentally. It has been postulated that three factors are necessary: (1) a short cystic duct to allow for rapid emptying of the gallbladder; (2) a force applied adjacent to the gallbladder to empty it rapidly; and (3) a simultaneous shearing force to the common duct.[21] Observations of injury to the common bile duct after the gallbladder has been removed previously indicate that the shearing force is the main etiologic factor.[59, 63] Nearly 55% of blunt injuries to the extrahepatic bile duct occur in the distal common bile duct, mainly at the superior border of the pancreas where the common bile duct becomes intrapancreatic. Nearly 25% occur at the bifurcation where the ducts become intrahepatic. The common bile duct is relatively fixed at these points, explaining why a lateral or upward shearing force causes the duct to be stretched and torn at these locations.[5, 6, 37, 53, 59, 63, 90] Another possible etiologic factor in cases in which the diagnosis is delayed for several weeks may be ischemia of the common bile duct secondary to injury to its axial blood supply.[25, 47, 90] It is interesting to note that the hepatic artery and portal vein are almost never injured in association with blunt trauma to the common bile duct. The reason cited for this is that the elasticity and mobility of the hepatic artery, in comparison with the relatively fixed position of the common bile duct, protect the artery from injury. The portal vein, being in a valveless system, can rapidly dissipate applied pressure proximally or distally, whereas the common bile duct is limited in doing so by the narrow cystic duct at one end and sphincter of Oddi at the other end.[7, 59, 63]

Patients sustaining blunt injury to the extrahepatic bile duct have two distinct clinical presentations. The first, and most common, is an acute presentation because of injury to other viscera. In these patients celiotomy is carried out within 24 hours after the traumatic event, and injury to the bile duct should be discovered at that time.[2, 6, 53, 63, 68] However, a large review found that injuries were not discovered at the initial operation in 12.1% of patients.[53] Failure to diagnose and treat the injury at the initial operation increases morbidity and mortality.[32, 47, 63]

The second clinical presentation is slower in onset because of an isolated bile duct injury or because the bile duct injury is associated with less serious visceral injuries not requiring urgent celiotomy. The presentation is similar to that described for blunt gallbladder injuries: initial abdominal pain followed by a symptom-free interval varying from several days to several weeks (average 15 days).[42] Progressive abdominal pain, distention, nausea and vomiting, and fever associated with direct hyperbilirubinemia then develops.[2, 5, 37, 47, 53, 63, 88] Acholic stools are present with complete ductal transection, but the stools may be normal with partial transection.[47] In patients having this clinical presentation, abdominal paracentesis is the most important diagnostic procedure.[53, 63]

Treatment of injuries to the extrahepatic bile ducts is determined by the extent of injury. Primary suture of the duct with absorbable sutures is indicated for simple partial lacerations when a tension-free repair can be accomplished.[6, 16, 37, 59, 68] A T-tube or stent should probably be placed if the duct is of adequate size or if associated duodenal or pancreatic injuries are present; otherwise repair and external drainage alone should suffice, particularly in children in whom the duct is small.[2, 6, 37, 88]

Extensive partial lacerations and complete transections or avulsion of the common bile duct should be treated by biliary-enteric anastomosis rather than by primary repair over a stent.[6, 16, 37, 59, 68] End-to-end anastomosis in these circumstances leads to a 55% stricture rate as opposed to the 3.6% stricture rate in those managed by biliary-enteric anastomoses.[37] Roux-en-Y choledochojejunostomy is the preferred procedure, although choledochoduodenostomy and cholecystojejunostomy have also been used effectively.[7, 59, 63] It is not necessary to ligate or drain the distal common bile duct, which usually remains buried in the head of the pancreas, because no complications have resulted from leaving it undisturbed.[16, 53]

Complications from repair of extrahepatic bile duct injuries are frequent. One large review found a biliary fistula rate of 23%, a stricture rate of 16%, and a need for reoperation for a biliary complication in 25% of patients.[37] Many of these biliary complications are avoidable by adhering to the principles stated previously. Mortality from injuries to the extrahepatic bile ducts ranges from 20 to 33% and is almost always from associated visceral or vascular injuries.[7, 16, 42, 59] Approximately 80% of the deaths occurred during surgery or in the immediate postoperative period.[42]

Porta Hepatis

Injuries to the porta hepatis are usually the result of penetrating trauma and always have major associated visceral or vascular injuries, averaging 3.6 organs injured per patient.[68] The most common associated injuries are to the liver (62%), pancreas (29%), and aorta or inferior vena cava (24%).[6, 68] In one large review, 23% of the patients had injuries to two of the three structures in the porta, whereas no patient had injuries to all three (portal vein, hepatic artery, and bile duct).[68]

These patients generally present in hypovolemic shock and require immediate resuscitation followed by celiotomy. The first priority is to control hemorrhage from the aorta or inferior vena cava; a Pringle maneuver or packing is useful for controlling hemorrhage from the portal vein and hepatic artery while other life-threatening injuries are managed. After that, extensive anatomic delineation of the porta hepatis and paraduodenal area is required.[6, 68]

Extrahepatic bile duct injuries are treated as previously described: partial, clean lacerations can be primarily closed if no undue tension results. Complete laceration or those involving more than 50% of the circumference of the duct and complete transections or avulsions are best treated by a biliary-enteric anastomoses.[6, 68]

Hepatic artery injuries are best and most expeditiously managed by ligation. If the portal vein is also injured, at least one of these structures, preferably the vein, should be repaired.[6, 68] Fortunately, the combination of hepatic artery and portal vein injury occurs in only 13% of these patients.[68]

Portal vein injuries should be repaired if possible, either by lateral suture, end-to-end anastomosis, or vascular or vein bypass grafts.[6] In desperate situations, the portal vein can be ligated. It is not necessary to perform an emergency portasystemic shunt, as this is too time consuming and will undoubtedly cause severe encephalopathy.[6] Isolated reports reveal long-term survival after acute portal vein ligation in 60 to 80% of patients.[6, 57, 68] These patients develop splanchnic hypervolemia and peripheral hypovolemia and thus must be monitored very closely to maintain normal circulating volume. This may require an overtransfusion of blood equal to the patient's normal blood volume.[6]

Injuries to the porta hepatis are highly lethal, with an overall mortality rate of 35%.[68] Most of these result from the associated vascular injuries. Biliary tract trauma associated with portal vein injury has a 50 to 75% mortality rate, a 40 to 60% mortality rate with associated inferior vena caval injuries, and a 60 to 80% mortality rate with associated hepatic arterial injuries.[68]

Intrahepatic Bile Ducts

Intrahepatic bile duct injuries occur as a consequence of blunt or penetrating trauma to the liver. In addition to management of the parenchymous and vascular injuries of the liver, attention must be directed to management of the intrahepatic bile duct injury. This is usually accomplished by placing multiple drains around the injured liver to allow for the controlled escape of bile until the ductal injury seals.[9]

If a major intrahepatic bile duct injury is suspected, and if the condition of the patient allows it, an intraoperative cholangiogram should be performed to direct the management.[9, 49] Major ductal lesions that are accessible through liver fractures should be sutured. Bile "lakes" within the liver should be drained. Complete disruption of the right or left hepatic duct within the liver substance should be repaired over stents or via a Kasai-type Roux-en-Y portojejunostomy.[9, 32, 49, 90] Strictures that develop late are associated with dilated intrahepatic ducts; these can be managed more easily and successfully by secondary hepatic-enteric drainage procedures performed electively than in the acute traumatic setting.[9]

Hemobilia

Hemobilia—gastrointestinal hemorrhage secondary to bleeding within the biliary tract—results from trauma in more than half of the cases.[5, 64, 65] Of these, one third are from iatrogenic trauma, and two thirds are from accidental trauma (67% of the total).[65]

The bleeding may be occult or massive and can lead to

death in 25% of patients. Massive hemobilia results from arterial bleeding. In half of the reported cases, the bleeding originates from within the liver and in one quarter each from the gallbladder or extrahepatic ducts.[64] Hemobilia associated with trauma is nearly always from the liver, with only 5% originating from the extrahepatic biliary tract.[5]

The classic triad of symptoms is biliary colic, jaundice, and gastrointestinal bleeding. These symptoms occur intermittently and may last for years without any hope for spontaneous cure.[5, 64] Diagnosis is confirmed by arteriography, which not only shows the source of bleeding but also delineates the type and exact location of the lesion.[64]

Treatment is either hepatic resection for peripheral and well-localized lesions or hepatic artery ligation or embolization for centrally located lesions.[64]

SUMMARY

Duodenal and biliary tract injuries are rare, especially in children. However, they must always be considered when caring for a child suffering from blunt trauma because of the devastating consequences that result from delayed diagnosis and treatment. In this era of conservative nonsurgical management of the blunt trauma victim, the potential for missing an injury to the duodenum or biliary tract is increased. The surgeon should not be lulled into a false sense of security that there are no intra-abdominal injuries because the abdominal computed tomography scan does not reveal them; if the patient has clinical signs and symptoms, an exploration should be undertaken in spite of this. Only in this way will subtle injuries to the duodenum and biliary tract be discovered early when their repair uniformly leads to a favorable outcome.

References

1. Adkins RB, Keyser JE: Recent experiences with duodenal trauma. Am Surg 51:121–131, 1985.
2. Ahmed S: Bile duct injuries from non-penetrating abdominal trauma in childhood. Aust N Z J Surg 46:209–212, 1976.
3. Berne CJ, Donovan AJ, Hagen WE: Combined duodenal pancreatic trauma. Arch Surg 96:712–722, 1968.
4. Berne CJ, Donovan AJ, White EJ, et al: Duodenal "diverticularization" for duodenal and pancreatic injury. Am J Surg 127:503–507, 1974.
5. Burt TB, Nelson JA: Extrahepatic biliary duct trauma. West J Med 134:283–289, 1981.
6. Busuttil DW, Kitahama A, Cerise E, et al: Management of blunt and penetrating injuries to the porta hepatis. Ann Surg 191:641–648, 1980.
7. Carmichael DH: Avulsion of the common bile duct by blunt trauma. South Med J 73:166–168, 1980.
8. Cattell RB, Braasch JW: A technique for the exposure of the third and fourth portions of the duodenum. Surg Gynecol Obstet 111:378–379, 1960.
9. Charters AC, Bardin J: Intrahepatic bile duct rupture following blunt abdominal trauma. Arch Surg 113:873–876, 1978.
10. Cocke WM, Meyer K: Retroperitoneal duodenal rupture—Proposed mechanism, review of literature, and report of a case. Am J Surg 108:834–839, 1964.
11. Corley RD, Norcross WJ, Shoemaker WC: Traumatic injuries to the duodenum. Ann Surg 181:92–98, 1975.
12. Debroede GJ, Tirol FT, Lo Russo VA, et al: Intramural hematoma of the duodenum and jejunum. Am J Surg 112:947–954, 1966.
13. Donohue JH, Crass RA, Trunkey DD: The management of duodenal and other small intestinal trauma. World J Surg 9:904–913, 1985.
14. Evans JP: Traumatic rupture of the gallbladder in a three-year-old boy. J Pediatr Surg 11:1033–1034, 1976.
15. Fabian TC, Mangiante EC, Millis M: Duodenal rupture due to blunt trauma: A problem in diagnosis. South Med J 77:1078–1082, 1984.
16. Feliciano DV, Bitondo CG, Burch JM, et al: Management of traumatic injuries to the extrahepatic biliary ducts. Am J Surg 150:705–709, 1985.
17. Felson B, Levin EJ: Intramural hematoma of the duodenum. A diagnostic roentgen sign. Radiology 63:823–831, 1954.
18. Fielding JWL, Stachan CJL: Jaundice as a sign of delayed gallbladder perforation following blunt abdominal trauma. Injury 7:66–67, 1975.
19. Fish JC, Johnson GL: Rupture of duodenum following blunt trauma: Report of a case with avulsion of the papilla of Vater. Ann Surg 162:917–932, 1965.
20. Fletcher WS: Nonpenetrating trauma to the gallbladder and extrahepatic bile ducts. Surg Clin North Am 52:711–717, 1972.
21. Fletcher WS, Mahnke DE, Dunphy JE: Complete division of the common bile duct due to blunt trauma. J Trauma 1:87–95, 1961.
22. Flint LM, McCoy M, Richardson JD, et al: Duodenal injury. Analysis of common misconceptions in diagnosis and treatment. Ann Surg 191:697–702, 1980.
23. Freeark RJ, Corley RD, Norcross WJ, et al: Intramural hematoma of the duodenum. Arch Surg 92:463–475, 1965.
24. Fullen WD, Selle JG, Whitely DH, et al: Intramural duodenal hematoma. Ann Surg 179:549–556, 1974.
25. Gately JF, Thomas EJ: Post-traumatic ischemic necrosis of the common bile duct. Can J Surg 28:32–33, 1985.
26. Ghuman SS, Pathak VB, McGovern PJ Jr, et al: Management and complications of duodenal injuries. Am Surg 48:109–113, 1982.
27. Glaser GM, Buy JN, Moss AA, et al: CT detection of duodenal perforation. Am J Roentgenol 137:333–336, 1981.
28. Gornall P, Ahmed S, Jolleys A, et al: Intra-abdominal injuries in the battered baby syndrome. Arch Dis Child 47:211–214, 1972.
29. Gray H: Gray's Anatomy. 5th ed. New York, Bounty Books, 1977, p 912.
30. Greenwald G: Perforation of the gallbladder following blunt abdominal trauma. Ann Emerg Med 16:452–454, 1987.
31. Hahn PF, Stark DD, Vici LG, et al: Duodenal hematoma: The ring sign in MR imaging. Radiology 159:379–382, 1986.
32. Hartman SW, Greaney EM: Traumatic injuries to the biliary tract in children. Am J Surg 108:150–156, 1964.
33. Hasson JE, Stern D, Moss GS: Penetrating duodenal trauma. J Trauma 24:471–474, 1984.
34. Hawkins ML, Mullen JT: Duodenal perforation from blunt abdominal trauma. J Trauma 14:290–292, 1974.
35. Ivatury RR, Gaudino J, Ascer E, et al: Treatment of penetrating duodenal injuries: Primary repair vs. repair with decompressive enterostomy/serosal patch. J Trauma 25:337–341, 1985.
36. Ivatury RR, Nallathambi M, Gaudino J, et al: Penetrating duodenal injuries. Analysis of 100 consecutive cases. Ann Surg 202:153–158, 1985.
37. Ivatury RR, Rohman M, Nallathambi M, et al: The morbidity of injuries of the extra-hepatic biliary system. J Trauma 25:967–973, 1985.
38. Janson KL, Stockinger F: Duodenal hematoma. Critical analysis of recent treatment of techniques. Am J Surg 129:304–308, 1975.
39. Jones WR, Hardin WJ, Davis JT, et al: Intramural hematoma of the duodenum: A review of the literature and case report. Ann Surg 173:534–544, 1971.
40. Judd DR, Taybi H, King H: Intramural hematoma of the small bowel. Arch Surg 89:527–535, 1964.
41. Kashuk JL, Moore EE, Cogbill TH: Management of intermediate severity duodenal injury. Surgery 92:758–764, 1982.
42. Khodadadi J, Mihich M, Finally R, et al: Avulsion of the common bile duct after blunt abdominal injury: A review of the literature. Injury 14:447–450, 1983.
43. Levison MA, Petersen SE, Sheldon GF, et al: Duodenal trauma: Experience of a trauma center. J Trauma 24:475–480, 1984.
44. Lineaweaver W, Robertson J, Rumley T: PIPIDA scan diagnosis of traumatic rupture of the gallbladder. Injury 16:238–240, 1985.
45. Lucas CE: Diagnosis and treatment of pancreatic and duodenal injury. Surg Clin North Am 57:49–65, 1977.
46. Lucas CE, Ledgerwood AM: Factors influencing outcome after blunt duodenal injury. J Trauma 15:839–846, 1975.

47. Maier WP, Lightfoot WP, Rosemond GP: Extrahepatic biliary ductal injury in closed trauma. Am J Surg 116:103–108, 1968.

48. Malangoni MA, Madura JA, Jesseph JE: Management of lateral duodenal fistulas: A study of fourteen cases. Surgery 90:645–651, 1981.

49. McFadden PM, Tanner G, Kitahama A: Traumatic hepatic duct injury. New approach to surgical management. Am J Surg 139:268–271, 1980.

50. McInnis WD, Aust JB, Cruz AB, et al: Traumatic injuries of the duodenum: A comparison of 1° closure and the jejunal patch. J Trauma 15:847–853, 1975.

51. Martin B, Mulopulos GP, Butler HE: MR imaging of intramural duodenal hematoma. J Comput Assist Tomogr 10:1042–1043, 1986.

52. Martin TD, Feliciano DV, Mattos KL, et al: Severe duodenal injuries. Arch Surg 118:631–635, 1983.

53. Michelassi F, Ranson JHC: Bile duct disruption by blunt trauma. J Trauma 25:454–457, 1985.

54. Moore JB, Moore EE: Changing trends in the management of combined pancreatoduodenal injuries. World J Surg 8:791–797, 1984.

55. Oreskovich MR, Carrico CJ: Pancreaticoduodenectomy for trauma: A viable option? Am J Surg 147:618–623, 1984.

56. Penn I: Injuries of the gall-bladder. Br J Surg 49:636–641, 1962.

57. Petersen SR, Sheldon GF, Lim RC Jr: Management of portal vein injuries. J Trauma 19:616–620, 1979.

58. Pokorny WJ, Brandt ML, Harberg FJ: Major duodenal injuries in children: Diagnosis, operative management, and outcome. J Pediatr Surg 21:613–616, 1986.

59. Posner MC, Moore EE: Extrahepatic biliary tract injury: Operative management plan. J Trauma 25:833–837, 1985.

60. Prathikanti V, Bhuti I: Intramural hematoma of the duodenum. South Med J 69:490–492, 1976.

61. Raffensperger GJ: Swenson's Pediatric Surgery. 4th ed. New York, Appleton-Century-Crofts, 1980, p 248.

62. Resnicoff SA, Morton JH, Bloch AL: Retroperitoneal rupture of the duodenum due to blunt trauma. Surg Gynecol Obstet 125:77–81, 1967.

63. Rydell WB: Complete transection of the common bile duct to blunt abdominal trauma. Arch Surg 100:724–728, 1970.

64. Sandblom P: Hemobilia. Surg Clin North Am 53:1191–1201, 1973.

65. Sandblom P, Saegesser F, Mirkovitch V: Hepatic hemobilia: Hemorrhage from the intrahepatic biliary tract, a review. World J Surg 8:41–50, 1984.

66. Schechter DC: Solitary wounding of the gallbladder from blunt abdominal trauma. N Y State Med J 69:2895–2901, 1969.

67. Schwartz SI: Principles of Surgery. New York, Blakiston, 1969, p 56.

68. Sheldon GF, Lim RC, Yee ES, et al: Management of injuries to the porta hepatis. Ann Surg 202:539–545, 1985.

69. Snyder WH, Weiglet JA, Watkins WL, et al: The surgical management of duodenal trauma. Arch Surg 115:422–429, 1980.

70. Soderstorm CA, Maekawa K, DuPriest RW Jr, et al: Gallbladder injuries resulting from blunt abdominal trauma. Ann Surg 193:60–66, 1981.

71. Songsanand P, Groff DB: Treatment of gallbladder rupture in an infant. Ann Surg 38:335–337, 1972.

72. Spigos DG, Tan WS, Larson G, et al: Diagnosis of traumatic rupture of the gallbladder. Am J Surg 141:731–735, 1981.

73. Stone HH: Pancreatic and duodenal trauma in children. J Pediatr Surg 7:670–675, 1972.

74. Stone HH, Fabian TC: Management of duodenal wounds. J Trauma 19:334–339, 1979.

75. Sty JR, Starshak RJ, Hubbard AM: Radionuclide hepatobiliary imaging in the detection of traumatic biliary tract disease in children. Pediatr Radiol 12:115–118, 1982.

76. Talbot WA, Shuck JM: Retroperitoneal duodenal injury due to blunt abdominal trauma. Am J Surg 130:659–666, 1975.

77. Touloukian RJ: Protocol for the nonoperative treatment of obstructing intramural duodenal hematoma during childhood. Am J Surg 145:330–334, 1983.

78. Toxopeus MD, Lucas CE, Krabbenhoft KL: Roentgenographic diagnosis in blunt retroperitoneal duodenal rupture. AJR 115:281–288, 1972.

79. Vargish R, Urdaneta LF, Cram AE, et al: Duodenal trauma in the rural setting. Am Surg 49:211–213, 1983.

80. Vaughn GD III, Frazier OH, Graham DY, et al: The use of pyloric exclusion in the management of severe duodenal injuries. Am J Surg 134:785–790, 1977.

81. Vellacott KD: Intramural haematoma of the duodenum. Br J Surg 67:36–38, 1980.

82. Ward GP, Fabian TC, Mangiante EC: Blunt duodenal disruption. J Tenn Med Assoc 78:224–226, 1985.

83. Whalen GF, Robbs JV, Baker LW: Injuries of the pancreas and duodenum—Results of a conservative approach. S Afr J Surg 25:15–18, 1987.

84. Weiner I, Watson LC, Wolma FJ: Perforation of the gallbladder due to blunt abdominal trauma. Arch Surg 117:805–807, 1982.

85. Williams Rd, Sargent FT: The mechanism of intestinal injury in trauma. J Trauma 3:288–294, 1963.

86. Wooley MM, Mahour GH, Sloan T: Duodenal hematoma in infancy and childhood. Changing etiology and changing treatment. Am J Surg 136:8–14, 1978.

87. Wynn M, Hill DM, Miller DR, et al: Management of pancreatic and duodenal trauma. Am J Surg 150:327–332, 1985.

88. Yadav K, Pathak IC: Biliary peritonitis following blunt abdominal trauma in children. Am J Gastroenterol 72:444–447, 1979.

89. Yellin AE, Rosoff L Sr: Pancreatoduodenectomy for combined pancreatoduodenal injuries. Arch Surg 110:1177–1183, 1975.

90. Zollinger RM, Keller RT, Hubay CA: Traumatic rupture of the right and left hepatic ducts. J Trauma 12:563–569, 1972.

Pancreatic Injuries

Injuries to the pancreas have increased during the past three and a half decades. In 1950 the incidence of pancreatic injury was only 2% in patients sustaining abdominal trauma, and the low percentage was attributed to the relatively protected position of the pancreas in the retroperitoneum.[34] This percentage has increased, however, to nearly 12% and reflects the increased incidence of violent injuries, including gunshot wounds and stab wounds, and of severe blunt injuries resulting from motor vehicle accidents. Although children are not frequently involved in these types of injuries, pancreatic injuries occur in 4% of children who require operative intervention for blunt abdominal trauma.[80]

ANATOMY AND MECHANISM OF INJURY

In young children with flat diaphragms and high costal margins the pancreas lies in a relatively unprotected position across the spine (Fig. 23–1). The poorly developed abdominal musculature and thin abdominal wall in children also contribute to pancreatic injuries that result from what in the adult would be an insignificant blow or trauma. However, in children the operative dissection and repair of the pancreas is facilitated by the well-defined anatomic structure, the lack of fat, and the ease of mobilization of the spleen and tail of the pancreas into the operative field, allowing a clear but tedious dissection of the pancreatic vessels and the splenic artery. This allows both the resection of the distal pancreas with preservation of the spleen and, conversely, mobilization, repair, or resection of the spleen without injury to the pancreas.

The pancreas shares its blood supply with the duodenum through the superior and inferior gastroduodenal arteries, and the tail and body of the pancreas are supplied by branches from the splenic artery. Therefore, it should be remembered that resection of or injuries to these adjacent structures may compromise the blood supply to the pancreas. During childhood and infancy, the collateral blood supply of the duodenum is excellent so that the head of the

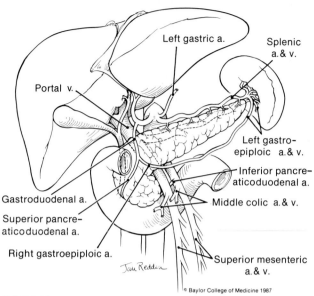

FIGURE 23–2

The proximity of major vessels accounts for the frequent life-threatening associated injuries with pancreatic injuries. a, artery; v, vein.

pancreas, including the gastroduodenal arteries, may often be resected without sacrificing the duodenum.

Because of the relatively protected location of the pancreas in the retroperitoneum of the more mature patient, injuries to the pancreas occur in only 5% of patients who incur blunt abdominal injuries. An unfortunate corollary, however, is that patients who do have pancreatic injuries following blunt trauma usually have sustained severe injuries.[2] The mortality rate for these patients is approximately 20%, and associated injuries are common, occurring in 90% of such patients.[68, 70]

The close proximity of numerous major vascular structures as well as the duodenum accounts for the frequent life-threatening injuries that are associated with pancreatic injuries (Fig. 23–2). The location of pancreatic injury in blunt abdominal trauma depends on the relationship between the impact forces and the spine. When impact forces are concentrated to the right of the spine, the head of the pancreas is crushed and the duodenum may also be crushed and torn. The liver may be displaced superiorly, leading to liver laceration and avulsion of the common bile duct and gastroduodenal artery. The colon is thrust downward, thus lacerating the right and midcolic vessels and omentum. When the impact forces are midline, transection of the neck and body of the pancreas occurs. This is frequently seen as an isolated injury. If the impact forces occur to the left of the spine, distal pancreatic injuries occur, usually with associated splenic injuries. Steering wheel trauma to the abdomen typically results in a crushed head of the pancreas with tears of the second portion of the duodenum and is frequently a lethal injury.[82, 84]

In contrast to blunt trauma, penetrating wounds are common and account for the majority of the pancreatic injuries in adults. This simply reflects the types of injuries that patients in urban centers sustain. At the large urban trauma

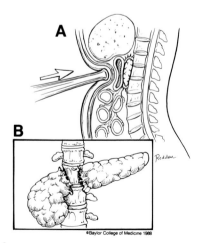

FIGURE 23–1

Blunt trauma to the epigastrium (A) may result in a compression fracture of the pancreas across the vertebral column (B).

centers in Houston, Atlanta, and Los Angeles nearly 80% of the injuries to the pancreas and duodenum are the result of violent penetrating wounds, including knife and gunshot wounds.[34, 65, 71] Of the remaining 20%, the vast majority (between 60 and 80%) are the result of motor vehicle accidents. This is in contradistinction to the pediatric age group patients who typically have injuries as the result of blunt trauma that are mainly from falls, bicycle accidents, and auto-pedestrian accidents. The force of impact in these cases is frequently less, resulting in fewer associated injuries.

Penetrating injuries are almost always associated with other significant visceral and vascular injuries. Nearly 50% of patients with penetrating injuries have liver and gastric injuries, and one third may have an injury to a major vessel. By contrast, when the pancreas is injured by blunt trauma, the liver, the spleen, and the duodenum are each injured in 15 to 18% of patients.[44, 74, 77]

DIAGNOSIS AND DELAYED DIAGNOSIS

When first examined, the majority of patients with pancreatic injuries exhibit signs of intraperitoneal injury, indicating the need for early exploration. However, many of these patients, particularly those whose injuries are caused by less forceful impact, may have a delay of 4 to 12 hours before the onset of symptoms.[7, 65, 79, 83] It is not uncommon for a patient with a contused or even transsected pancreas as the result of a bicycle or other childhood accident to be discharged from the emergency center within hours or even days with peritoneal signs or sometimes weeks later with a pancreatic pseudocyst.

Abdominal Radiographs

The early radiographic findings of pancreatic injury vary depending on the site and extent of the injury and the amount of hemorrhage. The initial examination may disclose only free intra-abdominal fluid, which indicates intraperitoneal hemorrhage.[23] An oral contrast medium, given to rule out gastric and duodenal injuries, may also be helpful in showing displacement of the duodenum and edema of the pancreas.[25] In the acute stage, edema of the pancreas with duodenal atony is usually present with or without organ displacement. In patients in whom there is a question of pancreatic injury, serial radiographs may show further displacement of the duodenum and stomach by an expanding pancreatic or retroperitoneal hematoma or fluid within the lesser sac.

Peritoneal Aspiration and Lavage

Retroperitoneal pancreatic injuries are among the small group of lesions associated with false negative results from peritoneal aspiration and lavage, normally a highly sensitive clinical diagnostic test. The accuracy of open diagnostic peritoneal lavage in detecting intra-abdominal injury in children following blunt trauma is 95 to 100%.[19, 21, 63] However, the reported experience with peritoneal lavage in children with pancreatic injuries has been small. Powell and colleagues reported three patients with pancreatic injuries.[63] Two had strongly positive lavage findings, but one had equivocal findings, which resulted in a significant delay in operative intervention. Other investigators who used peritoneal lavage in children with blunt trauma report that no significant retroperitoneal injuries were missed because all the children had concomitant intraperitoneal injuries that were responsible for a positive peritoneal lavage.[19, 21] An elevated amylase level in the lavage fluid is an indication of either pancreatic injury or disruption of intestinal continuity with leakage of amylase into the free peritoneum.

Amylase Determinations

Complete blood count, urinalysis, blood urea nitrogen (BUN), creatinine, and blood sugars are all routinely drawn in patients who sustain abdominal trauma. In addition, a serum amylase should be obtained specifically for those who sustain pancreatic injuries. The serum amylase is seldom of value in establishing the presence of a pancreatic injury due to penetrating trauma and is elevated in only approximately 10% of these patients. Similarly, in blunt trauma, the serum amylase drawn immediately following the injury is elevated in only approximately 60% of these patients.

Elman and associates were the first, in 1929, to associate an elevated serum amylase with pancreatitis and pancreatic injury.[24] Fourteen years later Naffziger and McCorkle described eight patients with pancreatic trauma and hyperamylasemia and commented that an elevated serum amylase is good evidence that the pancreas has been damaged.[56] It is also recognized that the source of the elevated serum amylase may be of extrapancreatic origin, including the following: salivary glands, liver, striated muscle, fallopian tubes, and adipose tissue. Hyperamylasemia has also been associated with a number of diseases, as well as with the user of narcotics, alcohol, steroids, and drugs that alter carbohydrate metabolism.

Although it is generally agreed that serum amylase determinations should be made in patients with blunt abdominal trauma, a single elevated amylase level in a recently injured patient with no evidence of intra-abdominal injury is of questionable significance. Olsen reviewed 179 patients who had sustained blunt abdominal trauma and who had a serum amylase drawn within 30 minutes of admission.[58] Of the total 179 patients, 36 had an elevated serum amylase level, but only four patients overall had a pancreatic injury; of these four, one had a normal amylase reading, and one had only a slightly elevated amylase level. Hence, in Olsen's series, only 8% of patients with an elevated serum amylase level immediately after trauma had a pancreatic injury. In addition, the level of hyperamylasemia did not correlate with pancreatic injury. Of the five patients with a markedly elevated amylase level, only one had a pancreatic injury.

Moretz and co-workers in 1975 corroborated Olsen's findings that in blunt trauma there is a poor correlation between elevated serum amylase levels and pancreatic injury. They concluded that decisions regarding the advisability of laparotomy in patients with suspected pancreatic injury should be based on factors other than the serum amylase level.[55]

Organ-specific isoamylases renewed surgical interest in the serum amylase as a means of identifying patients with pancreatic injuries. Greenlee and colleagues did find a statistically significant difference in the elevations of the pancreatic and salivary fractions of serum amylase between patients sustaining head and facial trauma and patients sustaining abdominal trauma.[36] Unfortunately, when Bouwman and associates measured the serum pancreatic and nonpancreatic isoamylases on admission of a large number of patients with blunt abdominal trauma injuries and compared the admission sera with the findings at laparotomy, they found no improvement of pancreatic isoamylase over the serum amylase in evaluating patients with blunt abdominal trauma.[9] They concluded with earlier researchers that regulation of serum amylase is multifactorial and variable. However, if the diagnosis is delayed, the serum amylase typically becomes elevated, and persistent elevation of the serum amylase is a strong indication of pancreatic injury.[13]

Ultrasonography

Occasionally a hematoma surrounding the pancreas may be detected by ultrasonography and is suggestive of pancreatic injury. Particularly in late cases, posttraumatic pancreatic pseudocysts and abscesses may also be seen and the progression or resolution of these may be satisfactorily followed by ultrasound.[32]

Computed Tomography

In many trauma centers, including our own, computed tomography (CT) is an accepted diagnostic tool in the evaluation of the child with blunt abdominal trauma. Its role in evaluating splenic, hepatic, and renal injuries has been demonstrated clearly.[5, 46] With the addition of oral contrast medium, it has been helpful in diagnosing gastric and duodenal injuries, particularly retroperitoneal duodenal injuries.

Because the CT examination requires 30 to 45 minutes to perform, patients must be hemodynamically stable. Unstable patients who require rapid blood transfusion or who have increasing peritoneal irritation should undergo immediate operative intervention. However, it is our policy to obtain a CT scan on all children with major blunt truncal injury who are hemodynamically stable and who do not have increasing peritoneal signs. Following this policy and observing patients with known and stable splenic and hepatic injuries, we have dramatically decreased the number of children who undergo negative celiotomy.

When initially used to evaluate abdominal trauma, the CT scans were believed helpful in identifying pancreatic injuries, particularly those with a hematoma of the pancreas and duodenum. More recent experience has shown an unacceptably high number of false negative and false positive results in patients with pancreatic injuries who underwent

CT scans for evaluation of blunt abdominal trauma within a few hours of the injury.[41, 67] Jeffrey and associates found the diagnosis of pancreatic injury by CT scan performed soon after the injury to be difficult in selected patients.[41] They attributed the diagnostic errors to the following: (1) Lacerations or fractures of the pancreas may produce little change in density and therefore may not be detectable by CT; (2) There may be minimal separations of the lacerated parenchymal fragments. These areas of injury may be difficult to distinguish from motions or streak artifacts on scans; and (3) Patients who are scanned immediately after trauma may demonstrate little evidence of posttraumatic pancreatitis. The radiologist must give careful attention to scanning techniques and keep in mind that unexplained thickening of the left anterior renal fascia might suggest a possible pancreatic injury (Fig. 23–3).

Other Studies

Abdominal angiography is now infrequently used due to the development of computerized axial tomography.

Endoscopic retrograde cholangiopancreatography (ERCP) is of little help in acutely injured patients in that it is quite time consuming. However, in evaluating complications developing from missed ductal injuries such as fistulas and pseudocysts, ERCP may be of considerable help.[10, 32, 33]

MANAGEMENT OF PANCREATIC INJURIES

Operative Management and Intraoperative Evaluation

The approach to managing a child with a suspected pancreatic injury is the same as that for any child with an

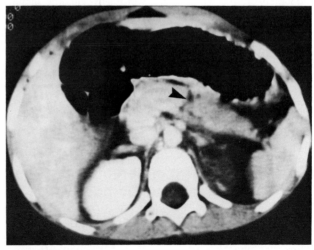

FIGURE 23–3

A computed tomography scan of the abdomen of a 6-year-old girl taken 24 hours after a horse had fallen on her shows her pancreas to be transected (*arrow*).

abdominal injury. Preoperative management is determined most often by management of associated injuries rather than by management of the pancreatic injury itself. Similarly, at celiotomy, after a thorough evaluation of the entire abdominal contents, the first priority is control of hemorrhage, the second priority is control of contamination of the peritoneal cavity by gastrointestinal perforations, and the third priority is treatment of the pancreatic injury. In the presence of other serious life-threatening injuries, the pancreas may be the last organ to be treated and, depending on circumstances, may be treated by simple drainage of the pancreatic wound.[42, 44]

Operative management of pancreatic injury must include the following[35, 70]:

1. Careful definition of the injury
2. Control of hemorrhage
3. Control of pancreatic secretions
4. Conservation of pancreatic function

Careful operative exposure of the pancreas is necessary to establish the presence of a pancreatic injury. This is accomplished by opening the lesser sac through the gastrocolic omentum to examine the anterior surface of the pancreas. A Kocher maneuver provides exposure of the head of the pancreas, posteriorly as well as anteriorly. In children the pancreas is usually quite mobile, with little surrounding adipose tissue, which allows precise palpation and inspection. However, if there is still a question of pancreatic injury, the peritoneum along the inferior border of the pancreas may be incised to allow further mobilization and inspection of the posterior surface. Peripancreatic hematomas that occur after trauma must be explored thoroughly because underlying pancreatic injury is common.[28]

Berni and co-workers have advocated the use of intraoperative pancreatography in patients suspected of having injuries to the ductal system.[8] This technique is difficult in a small child; hence, we prefer to rely on careful examination of the pancreas and take into account the type of injury to determine the presence of a ductal injury.

It seems clear that important determinants of the selection of operative repair and the ultimate outcome include the following: ductal injury; site of ductal injury; and presence of associated injuries, particularly duodenal. Classifications of the extent of injury include the following: glandular injury, including ductal injury; site of injury, that is, proximal injury to the head or neck versus injury to the tail of the gland; and associated duodenal injury.[51, 64] All of these factors have been incorporated into a grading system that is well accepted and utilized in most major trauma centers (Table 23–1).

Grade I: Contusion or Hematoma (Minimal Parenchymal Damage)

Nonoperative Management (Fig. 23–4). A simple pancreatic contusion within an intact capsule that results from blunt abdominal trauma may be treated nonoperatively in most cases. This has been commonly referred to as *traumatic pancreatitis*. As with the nonoperative management of any intra-abdominal injury, the surgeon must continue to

Table 23–1
Classification of Pancreatic Injury

Grade I	Contusion or hematoma (minimal parenchymal damage).
Grade II	Capsular or parenchymal disruption without major ductal injury.
Grade IIIa	Capsular or parenchymal disruption with ductal involvement distal to the superior mesenteric vessels. The duodenum is intact.
Grade IIIb	Capsular or parenchymal disruption with ductal involvement to the right of the superior mesenteric vessels. The duodenum is intact.
Grade IV	Combined extensive pancreatic and duodenal crush injuries.

evaluate the child for the presence of associated injuries and delayed complications of the pancreatic injury.[35, 39] Death from an overlooked duodenal rupture has been reported in a patient with a known pancreatic contusion that was treated nonoperatively. Many children with pancreatic pseudocysts have been initially treated nonoperatively for pancreatic contusion or incidental abdominal trauma.

Operative Management. After a thorough examination confirming that there is just a simple contusion, simple drainage is the only treatment necessary.

Grade II: Capsular or Parenchymal Disruption without Major Ductal Injury

As with grade I injuries, adequate drainage is the cornerstone of treatment (Fig. 23–5). Larger lacerations should be carefully approximated with monofilament polyglycolic acid or nonabsorbable suture. Catgut is not acceptable because it dissolves rapidly in the presence of pancreatic enzymes. Severe parenchymal disruption of the distal tail may be simply excised and the proximal surface closed with figure-of-eight or mattress sutures to control bleeding.[78, 84] Care must be taken not to injure the splenic vessels.

Grade III: Capsular or Parenchymal Disruption with Ductal Involvement

Grade IIIa: Involvement Distal to the Superior Mesenteric Vessels

In grade IIIa injuries the duodenum is intact (Fig. 23–6). The most serious pancreatic wounds include those with

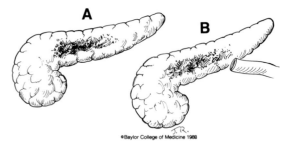

©Baylor College of Medicine 1988

FIGURE 23–4

Grade I pancreatic injury. *A*, Contusion-hematoma with minimal parenchymal damage. *B*, Operative management consists of drainage after thorough exploration.

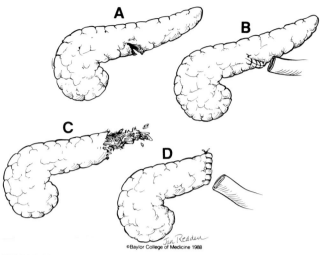

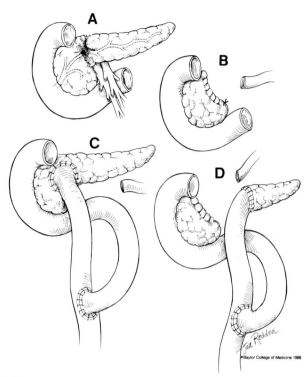

FIGURE 23–5

Grade II pancreatic injury. *A,* Capsular-parenchymal disruption without major ductal injury. *B,* Careful approximation and drainage. *C and D,* Simple excision and closure with drainage.

transection of the major pancreatic duct and those in which a portion of the gland is devitalized. The selection of operative repair depends on the location of the pancreatic injury and associated visceral injuries, particularly splenic and duodenal injuries. As discussed in the introduction, blunt injuries of the neck and midportion of the pancreas may occur without duodenal or splenic injuries, whereas more distal injuries to the tail of the pancreas are more likely to be associated with splenic injuries.

Distal pancreatic ductal injuries, particularly when devitalized tissue is present, should be managed by distal pancreatectomy with preservation of the splenic vessels and

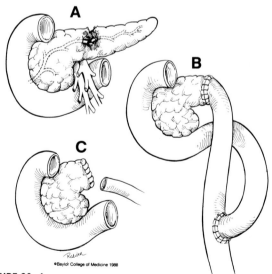

FIGURE 23–6

Grade IIIa pancreatic injury. *A,* Capsular-parenchymal disruption with ductal involvement distal to the superior mesenteric vessels. The duodenum is intact. *B,* Distal pancreatectomy with anastomosis of the transected pancreas to a Roux-en-Y of jejunum. *C,* Distal pancreatectomy with closure and drainage.

FIGURE 23–7

Grade IIIb pancreatic injury. *A,* Capsular-parenchymal disruption with ductal involvement to the right of the superior mesenteric vessels. The duodenum is intact. *B,* Distal pancreatectomy with closure and drainage. *C,* Anastomosis of the transected pancreas and duct to a Roux-en-Y loop of jejunum and drainage. *D,* Closure of the proximal transected end of pancreas and anastomosis of the distal transected end to a Roux-en-Y loop of jejunum.

splenic salvage if possible.[64, 78, 79] If the splenic vessels are injured or if the spleen itself is injured and is not reparable, or if the patient's associated injuries and general poor condition warrant expedient management, rapid ligation of the splenic vessels and removal of the spleen as part of the resection are indicated.[84]

In children distal pancreatectomy with preservation of the spleen is technically simpler than in adults and, when possible, is preferred. Splenic repair is also technically simpler in children because the capsule is less brittle than in adults.

Grade IIIb: Involvement to the Right of the Superior Mesenteric Vessels

As in grade IIIa injuries, the duodenum is intact in grade IIIb injuries (Fig. 23–7). Injuries to the head of the pancreas are almost twice as lethal as injuries to the body or tail. This increased mortality is due to a higher frequency of associated duodenal and vascular injuries with proximal pancreatic injuries.

The distal devitalized gland should be resected and the spleen preserved if possible, as is done with grade IIIa injuries. When total transection occurs through the neck or head of the pancreas without a devitalization of the distal gland, an effort should be made to conserve pancreatic tissue. Experimental animals will grow normally after pancreatectomies in which 75 to 90% of the pancreas is removed.[18, 38] Although pancreatic endocrine insufficiency is rare following resection of distal pancreatic fragments to the left of the superior mesenteric vessels, a literature review in 1982 found six patients out of 348 who had undergone distal pancreatectomy who developed insulin deficiency.[42, 57, 64] Conservation of tissue seems warranted.

The simplest and most common reconstructive procedure for transection injuries has been anastomosis of the transected pancreas to a Roux-en-Y loop of jejunum.[17] The Roux-en-Y loop may be anastomosed to both the proximal and distal pancreatic ends, or, more commonly, the proximal transected end is closed and the Roux-en-Y loop is anastomosed to the distal transected end of the pancreas.[30, 43, 50] Pancreatogastrostomy has been reported, which is anastomosis of the transected pancreas into the posterior wall of the stomach, as one would do for a pancreatic pseudocyst.[73]

When performing closure of the proximal end of the transected gland, the pancreatic duct is identified and the suture ligated. The end of the pancreas is closed with a series of figure-of-eight or mattress nonabsorbable monofilament sutures that are tied only tightly enough to approximate the gland and to provide homeostasis. This can be reinforced with a pedicle of omentum. The use of the autostapler to transect and close the gland has also been advocated.[1, 25]

Although the majority of patients with pancreatic injuries do not develop a fistula and consequently do not theoretically require drainage, the development of complications of a poorly or undrained pancreatic injury can be life threatening. For this reason all pancreatic wounds requiring operative intervention should be drained.[44] If parenchymal or capsular disruption is significant, sump drains, in addition to Penrose drains, should be used.[2]

Injuries to the head of the gland present the most difficult problem when there is a ductal injury. In some series, up to 5% of patients require pancreaticoduodenectomy and rarely a total pancreatectomy.[12, 13, 37] If possible an anastomosis to an onlay Roux-en-Y loop of jejunum creating an internal fistula conserves pancreas and decreases the risk of fistula formation.[10] Intraoperative pancreatography may be helpful in defining the injury in cases of suspected proximal ductal injury.[8] While successful primary repairs of disrupted pancreatic duct have been reported, reanastomosis of a transected duct is time consuming, technically difficult, and almost always unsuccessful.[52, 69]

Grade IV: Combined Extensive Pancreatic and Duodenal Crush Injuries

The principles for treatment of pancreatic injuries with associated duodenal injury remain the same as those for grade IIIb injuries: control of hemorrhage, drainage of pancreatic secretions, and conservation of pancreatic tissue (Fig. 23–8). Unfortunately, pancreatic injuries associated with duodenal injuries have a high rate of complication, particularly fistula formation. The procedures to divert the duodenal flow away from the repair are discussed in Chapter 22.

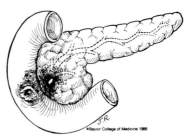

FIGURE 23–8

Grade IV pancreatic injury. Combined, extensive pancreatic-duodenal crush injuries.

COMPLICATIONS OF PANCREATIC INJURIES

Complications as a direct result of the pancreatic injury occur in one third of patients with pancreatic trauma.

Fistula

The formation of a fistula is the most common postoperative complication of pancreatic injury.[81] Most fistulas are minor, close readily, and are rarely a cause of death.[81] Persistent or large-volume fistulas occur when the major pancreatic duct is injured, particularly when the injury occurs to the head or neck regions. Nearly all injuries with capsular or parenchymal disruption have some drainage of pancreatic secretions for a few days. For this reason a fistula should be considered to exist only if the drainage persists for longer than a few days or if it starts draining 3 to 4 days postoperatively. Jones and Shires considered only fistulas that drained more than 1 month to be major.[43]

Jordan classified pancreatic fistulas in adults as minor (draining less than 200 ml per day), moderate (200 to 700 ml per day), and major (more than 700 ml per day).[44] Minor fistulas usually close within a few days. Pure pancreatic fistulas usually have an amylase concentration of 50,000 units. However, values of 5000 to 10,000 units may also indicate a pancreatic fistula in which the pancreatic fluid has been diluted by fluid from the surrounding tissue or lymphatics. Those with a relatively low amylase concentration are more likely to close rapidly.

The vast majority of fistulas that develop in children close spontaneously within 1 week of operation. Occasionally a fistula persists, and attention must be given to management of the fistula, which includes (1) adequate drainage, usually with a sump drain; (2) skin care with stomal bags and sump drains to clear secretions from the skin; (3) sinogram to confirm that adequate drainage exists; (4) metabolic and nutritional support for the patient; and, rarely, (5) operative intervention. However, when operative intervention is necessary, the Roux-en-Y loop of jejunum should be anastomosed to the pancreas itself. Placing the anastomosis of the Roux-en-Y loop directly to the fistula tract is not recommended owing to a high complication rate. Nutritional support with total parenteral nutrition of the patient while allowing spontaneous closure of the traumatic pancreatic fistula is helpful.[15, 20, 31]

Abscess

True pancreatic abscess is the result of either inadequate débridement of devitalized tissue or failure to drain an accumulation of peripancreatic fluid effectively. Occasionally a pancreatic abscess develops as a complication of the inflammatory pancreatitis following the injury rather than as a result of the original injury. The diagnosis is confirmed by an ultrasound or a CT scan, and management consists of drainage and broad-spectrum antibiotic therapy.

Pancreatic Pseudocyst

Cysts of the pancreas include congenital cysts, parasitic cysts, neoplastic cysts, fibrocystic disease, and pseudocysts resulting from pancreatic inflammation. Pseudocyst of the pancreas is cystic structure located primarily in the lesser sac of the peritoneum but may extend into the transverse mesocolon, the pericolic gutter, the mediastinum, or, rarely, within the pancreas itself.[29] The wall consists of the adjacent viscera and is lined by granulation and fibrous tissue and is devoid of epithelium. Although its lumen may or may not communicate with a pancreatic duct, at some point most pseudocysts connect with pancreatic glandular tissue or the ductal system.[54]

The occurrence of pancreatic pseudocysts in children is low but has been reported in 12 to 30% of children sustaining pancreatic injuries.[35, 59, 67] Only 75 cases had been reported as late as 1975.[14] The majority of these patients sustained blunt trauma, and either their acute injuries were treated nonoperatively or the pancreatic injury was not appreciated until the child presented with a pancreatic pseudocyst. Because the number of missed pancreatic injuries is not known, the true incidence of pseudocyst formation following pancreatic trauma cannot be calculated and the previously stated percentage may be high.

However, the majority of children who present with a pancreatic pseudocyst have a history of blunt trauma to the epigastrium, frequently from a bicycle handlebar; the injury is often considered inconsequential with or without a short period of hospitalization.[27] The patient typically presents 1 week to several months later with abdominal pain, fever, and vomiting.[16] The history of trauma may have been forgotten and must be sought specifically. Other diagnoses such as peptic ulcer, appendicitis, and tumor are considered.[14] An abdominal mass is present in about two thirds of these patients. Persistent hyperamylasemia is nearly always present. The diagnosis is confirmed by upper gastrointestinal series and ultrasonography or CT scan.

The etiology, pathophysiology, management, and prognosis of pseudocysts in childhood are different from that seen in adults. Nevertheless, many of the rules described for the treatment of adults with pseudocysts are too commonly applied to children. To properly manage children with pancreatic injuries and pseudocyst formation, one must understand the difference in the pathophysiology of this disorder in children from that in adults. In adults nearly 75% of pancreatic pseudocysts are due to alcoholic or biliary pancreatitis, and 3 to 15% are primary neoplastic cysts or are secondary to a proximal primary carcinoma.[6, 45, 75] Trauma is a predisposing factor in only 10 to 24% of adult patients with pseudocysts. In contrast, trauma is responsible for the majority of pancreatic pseudocysts seen in children.[14, 49, 59, 62] A significant number of children, 32% in one series, have no etiology of their underlying pancreatitis.[14] In these patients mumps, hereditary pancreatitis, biliary tract disease, hyperlipidemia, hypercalcemia, and therapy with steroids and L-asparaginase should be excluded. In younger children without a history of trauma, innocuous injuries may be responsible and child abuse should be suspected.[54, 60]

Because the etiology of pseudocyst in adults is a chronic or progressive inflammatory process or tumor, recurrent pseudocysts and chronic fistula formation following external drainage are common—11 to 34% and 23 to 31%,

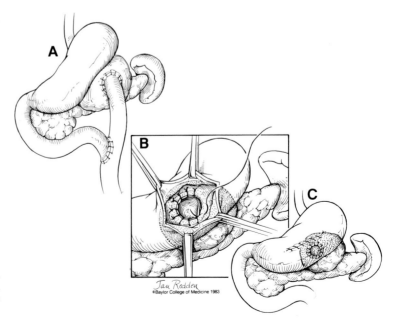

FIGURE 23–9

Internal drainage of a pancreatic pseudocyst. *A,* A cystojejunostomy using a Roux-en-Y technique. *B and C,* Cystogastrostomy with drainage of the pseudocyst directly into the stomach.

respectively.[76] In contrast, following external drainage of pancreatic pseudocysts in children, recurrence is rare, and when fistulas occur they usually close spontaneously within a few weeks.[59, 61] The proximal ductal obstructions due to trauma usually resolve.

As in adults, children undergoing internal drainage of a mature pseudocyst have fewer complications and leave the hospital sooner than those undergoing external drainage.[61, 72] Unfortunately, internal drainage is frequently impossible in children owing to the thin, poorly formed wall of the pseudocyst.[26] Because patients usually undergo external drainage in the acute phase of pseudocyst development, the higher complication rate may be the result of the phase of pancreatic injury rather than the type of drainage utilized.[61]

Spontaneous resolution of pancreatic pseudocysts that have been followed by ultrasound studies have been reported.[11, 16, 32] Patients with these pseudocysts must be followed closely because untreated pancreatic pseudocysts may develop serious complications.[22, 53, 67] Becker and Pratt reported 42% of their patients with pseudocysts developed complications, including the following: infection, perforation, hemorrhage, jaundice, and intestinal obstruction.[6] In our experience, nearly all children with pancreatic pseudocysts present with one or more of the triad of symptoms of pain, vomiting, and fever.[61] Anorexia is also a common symptom. For these reasons, operative delay is unwarranted in children with large or symptomatic pancreatic pseudocysts.

When a cyst with a mature, well-formed wall is found, internal drainage is the operation of choice.[16, 61] Numerous methods of internal drainage have been described (Fig. 23–9).[40, 47] Depending on the location and relationship of the pseudocyst to adjacent organs, the pseudocyst can be drained directly into the stomach or the duodenum. If these options are not possible, a cystojejunostomy using a Roux-en-Y technique can be done. Complications, including recurrence of the pseudocyst, are low.

If the cyst wall is thin and poorly formed or if the

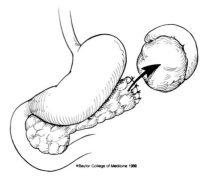

FIGURE 23–11

Excision of a pseudocyst that involves only the tail of the pancreas.

patient's condition indicates a short operative procedure, external drainage is done (Fig. 23–10).[48] Drainage should include the placement of a large sump drain in addition to Penrose drains that are brought out through a separate adequate incision in a dependent position in the flank.[61] Pseudocysts involving only the tail of the pancreas may be resected with the spleen if necessary (Fig. 23–11).

MORTALITY OF PANCREATIC INJURY

The mortality rate for adults sustaining pancreatic trauma is 10 to 27%.[25, 43, 44, 65, 68] However, the mortality rate for children is lower, 8 to 10%.[30, 35, 70] Mortality is directly related to the major vessels injured, not to the number of organs injured and not to the pancreatic injury itself.[3, 42, 66] Mortality in recent experience has been related to hemorrhage in the perioperative period or to severe neurologic damage; earlier series reported multiorgan system failure and sepsis to be major factors in mortality.[25] Patients with associated colon injuries also have a high mortality rate and a higher incidence of intra-abdominal abscess and fistula formation.[65] Injuries to the head of the pancreas are nearly twice as lethal as injuries to the body and tail.[2, 4] This is due to a higher frequency of associated duodenal and vascular injuries with proximal pancreatic injuries. Similarly, blunt trauma due to steering wheel injuries has a particularly high mortality rate, but again, this injury has a high incidence of associated vascular and duodenal injuries.[57]

References

1. Andersen D, Bolman R, Moylan J: Management of penetrating pancreatic injuries: Subtotal pancreatectomy using the auto suture stapler. J Trauma 20:347–349, 1980.
2. Anderson C, Connors J, Mejia D, et al: Drainage methods in the treatment of pancreatic injuries. Surg Gynecol Obstet 138:587–590, 1974.
3. Babb J, Harmon H: Diagnosis and management of pancreatic trauma. Ann Surg 42:390–394, 1976.
4. Bake RJ, Dipple WF, Freeark RJ, et al: The surgical significance of trauma to the pancreas. Arch Surg 86:1038–1043, 1963.
5. Beaver B, Colombani PM, Fal A, et al: The efficacy of computed tomography in evaluating abdominal injuries in children with major head trauma. J Pediatr Surg 22:1117–1122, 1987.

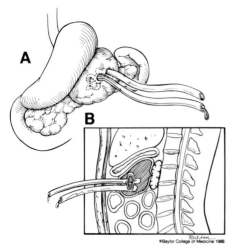

FIGURE 23–10

External drainage of a pseudocyst using a large mushroom catheter and Penrose drains.

6. Becker W, Pratt H: Pseudocysts of the pancreas. Surg Gynecol Obstet 127:744–747, 1968.

7. Berger J, Sauvage P, Levy M, et al: Pancreatic trauma in childhood. Ann Chir Infant 13:602–605, 1982.

8. Berni G, Bandyk D, Oreskovich M, et al: Role of intraoperative pancreatography in patients with injury to the pancreas. Am J Surg 143:602–605, 1982.

9. Bouwman D, Weaver D, Walt A: Serum amylase and its isoenzymes: A clarification of their implications in trauma. J Trauma 24:573–578, 1984.

10. Bozymski E, Orlando R, Holt J: Traumatic disruption of the pancreatic duct demonstrated by endoscopic retrograde pancreatography. J Trauma 21:244–245, 1981.

11. Bradley E, Clements L: Spontaneous resolution of pancreatic pseudocysts: Implications for timing of operative intervention. Am J Surg 129:23–28, 1975.

12. Cameron A, Southcott R, Blake J, et al: Successful Whipple's operation for pancreatic injury. Injury 16:233–234, 1985.

13. Cogbill T, Moor E, Kashuk J: Changing trends in the management of pancreatic trauma. Arch Surg 117:722–728, 1982.

14. Cooney D, Grosfeld J: Operative management of pancreatic pseudocysts in infants and children: A review of 75 cases. Ann Surg 182(5):590–596, 1975.

15. Cummins G, Grace A, Beardmore H: Supportive use of total peripheral parenteral alimentation in children with severe pancreatic injuries. J Pediatr Surg 11:961–965, 1976.

16. Dahman B, Stephens C: Pseudocysts of the pancreas after blunt abdominal trauma in children. J Pediatr Surg 16:17–21, 1981.

17. Dawson A, Webster C, Howe H, et al: Rupture of the head of the pancreas by blunt trauma. S Afr Med 67:560–562, 1985.

18. Dragstedt LR: Some physiological problems in surgery of the pancreas. Ann Surg 118:576–593, 1943.

19. Drew R, Perry J, Fischer R: The expediency of peritoneal lavage for blunt trauma in children. Surg Gynecol Obstet 145:885–888, 1977.

20. Dudrick S, Wilmore D, Steiger E, et al: Spontaneous closure of traumatic pancreatoduodenal fistulas with total intravenous nutrition. J Trauma 10:542–553, 1970.

21. DuPriest R, Rodriguez A, Shatney C: Peritoneal lavage in children and adolescents with blunt abdominal trauma. Am Surg 48:460–462, 1982.

22. Eisebaum S, Grant RN, Cohen A: Hemorrhagic pseudocyst and pancreatitis in a ten-year-old boy. Am Surg 36:387, 1970.

23. Ekengren K, Soderlund S: Radiological findings in traumatic lesions of the pancreas in childhood. Ann Radiol (Paris) 9:279–284, 1929.

24. Elman R, Arneson N, Graham EV: Value of blood amylase estimations in the diagnosis of pancreatic disease. Arch Surg 19:943, 1929.

25. Fitzgibbons T, Yellin A, Maruyama M, et al: Management of the transected pancreas following distal pancreatectomy. Surg Gynecol Obstet 154:225–231, 1982.

26. Fonkalsrud E, Henney R, Riemenschneider T, et al: Management of pancreatitis in infants and children. Am J Surg 116:198–203, 1968.

27. Fraser G: "Handlebar" injury of the pancreas: Report of a case complicated by pseudocyst formation with spontaneous internal rupture. J Pediatr Surg 4:216–219, 1969.

28. Freeark R, Kane J, Folk F, et al: Traumatic disruption of the head of the pancreas. Arch Surg 91:5–18, 1965

29. Galligan J, Williams H: Pancreatic pseudocysts in childhood. Am J Dis Child 112:479–482, 1966.

30. Gillesby W: Traumatic injuries of the pancreas and the management of traumatic pancreatic pseudocysts. Ill Med J 128:429–433, 1965.

31. Goodgame J, Fischer J: Parenteral nutrition in the treatment of acute pancreatitis: Effect on complications and mortality. Ann Surg 186:651–658, 1977.

32. Gorenstein A, O'Halpin D, Wesson D, et al: Blunt injury to the pancreas in children: Selective management with ultrasound. J Pediatr Surg 22:1110–1116, 1987.

33. Gougeon F, Legros G, Archaqmbault A, et al: Pancreatic trauma: A new diagnostic approach. Am J Surg 132:400–402, 1976.

34. Graham J, Mattox K, Jordan GL, et al: Traumatic injuries of the pancreas. Am J Surg 136:744–748, 1978.

35. Graham J, Pokorny W, Mattox K, et al: Surgical management of acute pancreatic injuries in children. J Pediatr Surg 13:693–697, 1978.

36. Greenlee T, Murphy K, Ram M: Amylase isoenzymes in the evaluation of trauma patients. Am Surg 50:637–640, 1984.

37. Halgrimson C, Trimble C, Gale S, et al: Pancreaticoduodenectomy for traumatic lesions. Am J Surg 118:877–882, 1969.

38. Hallman GL, Jordan GL: Subtotal pancreatectomy and growth of young mice. JAMA 191:167–168, 1965.

39. Henarejos A, Cohen D, Moossa A: Management of pancreatic trauma. Ann R Col Surg Engl 65:297–300, 1983.

40. Hillson R, Taube R: Surgical management of pancreatic pseudocysts. Am Surg 41:492–496, 1975.

41. Jeffrey R, Federle M, Crass R: Computed tomography of pancreatic trauma. Radiology 147:491–494, 1983.

42. Jones R: Mangement of pancreatic trauma. Ann Surg 187:555–564, 1978.

43. Jones R, Shires G: The management of pancreatic injuries. Arch Surg 90:502, 1965.

44. Jordan G: Injury to the pancreas and duodenum. In: Mattox KL, Moore EE, Feliciano DV (eds): Trauma. East Norwalk, Conn, Appleton & Lange, 1988, pp 473–494.

45. Jordan G, Howard J: Pancreatic pseudocysts. Am J Gastroenterol 45:444–453, 1966.

46. Karp M, Cooney D, Berger P, et al: The role of computed tomography in the evaluation of blunt abdominal trauma in children. J Pediatr Surg 16:316–323, 1981.

47. Koch A, Rehbein F: Special surgical precautions in traumatic pancreatic cysts in children. Ann Chir Infant 13:401–404, 1972.

48. Kummer M, Bettex M: External drainage of pseudocysts of the pancreas. Ann Chir Infant 13:417–418, 1972.

49. Leistyna J, Macaulay J: Traumatic pancreatitis in childhood. Am J Dis Child 107:644–648, 1964.

50. Letton D, Wilson J: Traumatic severance of pancreas treated by Roux-en-Y anastomosis. Surg Gynecol Obstet 109:473–478, 1959.

51. Levine R, Glauser F, Berk J: Enhancement of the amylase-creatinine clearance ratio in disorders other than acute pancreatitis. N Engl J Med 292:329–332, 1975.

52. Martin L, Henderson B, Welsh N: Disruption of the head of the pancreas caused by blunt trauma in children: A report of two cases treated with primary repair of the pancreatic duct. Surgery 63:697–700, 1968.

53. Moazzenzadah A, Fernandez L, Zamora B: Intraperitoneal rupture of pancreatic pseudocyst: Report of a case and review of the literature. Am Surg 42:589–592, 1976.

54. Moossa A: Pancreatic pseudocysts in children. J R Coll Surg Edinb 19:149–158, 1974.

55. Moretz J, Campbell D, Parker D, et al: Significance of serum amylase level in evaluating pancreatic trauma. Am J Surg 130:739–741, 1975.

56. Naffziger HC, McCorkle HJ: The recognition and management of acute trauma to the pancreas: With particular reference to the use of the serum amylase test. Ann Surg 118:594, 1943.

57. Northrup W, Simmons R: Pancreatic trauma: A review. Surgery 71:27–43, 1972.

58. Olsen W: The serum amylase in blunt abdominal trauma. J Trauma 13:200–204, 1973.

59. Othersen H, Moore F, Boles E: Traumatic pancreatitis and pseudocyst in childhood. J Trauma 8:535–545, 1968.

60. Pena S, Medovy H: Child abuse and traumatic pseudocyst of the pancreas. J Pediatr 83:1026–1028, 1973.

61. Pokorny W, Raffensperger J, Harberg F: Pancreatic pseudocysts in children. Surg Gynecol Obstet 151:182–184, 1980.

62. Pollard P, Chavrier Y: Pseudocyst of the pancreas in a child aged 13 years. Ann Chir Infant 13:395–398, 1972.

63. Powell R, Smith D, Zarins C, et al: Peritoneal lavage in children with blunt abdominal trauma. J Pediatr Surg 11:973–977, 1976.

64. Robey E, Mullen J, Schwab C: Blunt transection of the pancreas treated by distal pancreatectomy, splenic salvage and hyperalimentation. Ann Surg 196:695–699, 1982.

65. Sims E, Mandal A, Schlater T, et al: Factors affecting outcome in pancreatic trauma. J Trauma 24:125–128, 1984.

66. Smego DR, Richardson JD, Flint LM: Determinants of outcome in pancreatic trauma. J Trauma 5:771–776, 1985.

67. Smith S, Nakayama D, Gantt N: Pancreatic injuries in childhood due to blunt trauma. J Pediatr Surg 7:610–614, 1988.

68. Steele M, Sheldon G, Blaisdell F: Pancreatic injuries. Arch Surg 106:544–549, 1973.

69. Stone H: Pancreatic and duodenal trauma in children. J Pediatr Surg 7:670–675, 1972.

70. Stone H, Fabian T, Satiani B, et al: Experiences in the management of pediatric trauma. J Trauma 21:257–262, 1981.
71. Stone HH, Stowers KB, Shippey SH: Injuries to the pancreas. Arch Surg 85:525–530, 1962.
72. Stone H, Whitehurst J: Pseudocysts of the pancreas in children. Am J Surg 114:448–453, 1967.
73. Strauch G: The use of pancreatogastrostomy after blunt traumatic pancreatic transection: A complete and efficient operation. Ann Surg 176:16–18, 1972.
74. Thompson RJ, Hinshaw DB: Pancreatic trauma: Review of 87 cases. Ann Surg 163:153–159, 1966.
75. Van Heerden J, ReMine W: Pseudocysts of the pancreas. Arch Surg 110:500–505, 1975.
76. Warren W, Marsh W, Sandusky W: An appraisal of surgical procedures for pancreatic pseudocyst. Ann Surg 147:903, 1958.
77. Waters RL, Gaspard DJ, Germann TD: Traumatic pancreatitis. Am J Surg 3:364, 1966.
78. Weitzman J, Rothschild P: The surgical management of traumatic rupture of the pancreas due to blunt trauma. Surg Clin North Am 48:1347–1353, 1968.
79. Weitzman J, Swenson O: Traumatic rupture of the pancreas in a toddler. Surgery 57: 309–312, 1965.
80. Welch K: Abdominal trauma: Pancreatic-duodenal injury. In: Welch K (ed): Pediatric Surgery. Chicago, Year Book Medical Publishers, 1986, pp 168–174.
81. Werschky L, Jordan G: Surgical management of traumatic injuries to the pancreas. Am J Surg 116:768–772, 1968.
82. Wilson R, Tagett J, Pucelik J, et al: Pancreatic trauma. J Trauma 7:643–651, 1967.
83. Woolley M, Joergenson E: Transection of the pancreas by blunt trauma. Calif Med 92:210–211, 1960.
84. Yellin A, Vecchione T, Donovan A: Distal pancreatectomy for pancreatic trauma. Am J Surg 124:135–142, 1972.

Neil J. Sherman

CHAPTER TWENTY-FOUR

Traumatic Injuries to the Stomach and Small Bowel

MECHANISM OF INJURY

DIAGNOSIS

MANAGEMENT

DISCUSSION

Injuries to the stomach and small intestine have plagued humankind since the invention of the spear, and hollow viscus injuries have contributed significantly to mortality rates in wartime since prehistoric times. Aristotle was among the first to recognize bowel injury from blunt trauma and described rupture of the intestine in a deer without penetration of the skin.[60] The successful repair of a small intestinal injury was first reported in 1720 by Sacherus, and Ramdorh successfully repaired a completely transected bowel in 1730.[42] Most experience and knowledge has been acquired during the last 50 years; the advent of mass transportation and an increasingly mobile population have contributed to the increase in the number of these injuries, and advances in technology have contributed to the successful management and treatment of them.

Although not frequently reported, isolated injuries to the stomach or small bowel in the pediatric population are most commonly due to blunt trauma. In a combined large series of cases of blunt abdominal trauma, injury occurred to the stomach in 0 to 1.7% and to the small bowel in 2.1 to 9.8%.[1, 2, 14, 16, 21–23, 28, 30, 32, 36, 39, 41, 43, 46, 47, 49, 56, 58, 59] Predictably, infants and small children sustain these isolated injuries less frequently than the school-aged child, and although the mechanism by which such injuries occur differs at various ages, vehicular accidents predominate in all series at all ages (Fig. 24–1). Boys are more often involved than girls, indicating behavioral differences. A large variety of blunt forces strike the child's abdomen regularly, whether in or on a moving vehicle or a playground or at home; however, the relative position and lack of fixation of both the stomach and small bowel provide some inherent protection.

Penetrating injuries occur randomly throughout the abdomen, however, and, predictably, the extensive area occupied by the stomach and small bowel means that these organs are at great risk for injury. The likelihood of any penetrating wound affecting the stomach or intestine is high.

Associated intra-abdominal injuries include most often the liver, spleen, and duodenum.[58] Damage to these organs may produce dramatic symptoms and prompt early surgical intervention only to have injuries to the stomach and small intestine discovered concurrently. In children, extra-abdominal injuries, usually involving the head or extremities, attract initial attention and may take precedence over the potentially serious but less obvious intra-abdominal problem.

In addition to early rupture, significant blunt injury may be manifest later by a variety of symptoms. Perigastric adhesions that produce gastric outlet obstruction, delayed rupture, and traumatic ulceration with upper gastrointestinal bleeding have been reported.[10, 31, 52] In addition, small intestinal strictures can result following blunt abdominal trauma, as a later manifestation.[6, 8, 34, 45]

Less common causes of rupture of the stomach and small intestine have been reported from sports activities, seat belts, child abuse, cardiopulmonary resuscitation, electrical shock, carrying out the Heimlich maneuver, and ingesting syrup of ipecac.[12, 17–19, 25, 29, 38, 52, 57, 62, 64]

This chapter focuses on injury to the stomach and small bowel, whether isolated or in combination with other injuries, and delineates its diagnosis and management. Experience with such injuries, classified as blunt or closed as opposed to penetrating, has been multiplied greatly in modern times with the ready availability of the bicycle and the automobile.

MECHANISM OF INJURY

The child's abdomen sustains innumerable episodes of blunt trauma, most of which are mild and inconsequential. One is often surprised by the lack of significant injury in contact sports, for example. With this knowledge, a high degree of suspicion and diagnostic inquiry is required to identify episodes that cause injury to an intra-abdominal organ.

Several important factors predispose the abdominal contents to damage regardless of the organ or direction of the force encountered. When the stomach and the upper small bowel contain a recent meal the likelihood of damage is far greater.[11, 57] In fact, an empty stomach is so well protected by its location and lack of fixation that blunt injuries to it are very unusual. However, when the history suggests a major force has been applied, injuries to the intra-abdominal viscera must be expected. Significant trauma does occur through the relaxed abdominal wall in a child, even if the blow is such that it may hardly be remembered or is presumed to be insignificant.

The infrequency of isolated stomach and small bowel injuries is understandable because these structures have few points of fixation and usually slide away from an offending force. Those few points of attachment, such as the pylorod-

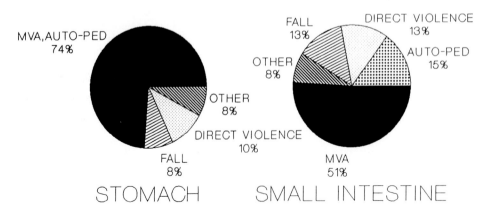

FIGURE 24–1

Summary of modes of injury. MVA, Motor vehicle accident. PED, pedestrian.

Table 24–1

Incidence of Stomach and Small Intestinal Rupture in Series of Blunt Abdominal Trauma

	Stomach	Small Intestine	Number of Cases
Courcy[16]	0.4%	2.1%	1412
Levy*[30]	0.04%	4.1%	49
Sinclair*[56]	0	3%	99
Rodkey[49]	1.7%	7.9%	177
Morton[39]	1.7%	5.0%	120
Tank*[59]	1.2%	9.8%	82

*Indicates pediatric series.

uodenal junction, the ligament of Treitz, and the cecum, are in fact the most injured sites. In addition, congenital bands or adhesions from prior surgical procedures likewise can create fixed areas and therefore make those sites more prone to injury. The incidence of stomach and small bowel injuries from blunt trauma, both isolated and combined with other organs, is shown in Table 24–1. Understandably, the diagnosis requires a very high index of suspicion, because stomach and small bowel ruptures occur so rarely. The stomach was ruptured in approximately 1% and the small bowel in 2 to 10% in reported series. These were often discovered at the time of laparotomy for concurrent injuries. Depending on the child's age and activity at the time of the accident, the vehicle of injury may be a skateboard, a bicycle, a scooter, a sled, or an automobile. Sports injuries are far less common, and injury from child abuse is generally limited to the smaller child.

Rupture of a hollow viscus secondary to blunt force occurs when the intraluminal pressure exceeds the resistance of the wall. Such a blowout follows the principles of Laplace's law, wherein the transmural pressure (P) is directly proportional to the ratio between the tension (T) and the radius (R) of the curve. The formula $P = K (T/R)$ describes this principle mathematically, in which K is the geometric shape and predicts that a rise in intraluminal pressure leads to rupture at the point of the greatest radius.[63]

In experimental animals, rupture occurs first in the seromuscular layer, followed by rents in the mucosa and submucosa.[55] This is characteristic of both the stomach and the small bowel. One would predict that the greater curvature of the stomach would be the most frequent site of perforation, but this is only true in infants and children.[15, 33, 63] In adults the lesser curvature more frequently perforates, the theory being that there are fewer mucosal folds, less elasticity, and lack of a peritoneal surface in that area. Also, the anterior wall is ruptured much more frequently than the posterior one.[24] This is believed to result from a shearing force, enhanced by a full stomach, and by the sudden forward motion from the relatively unfixed greater curvature.

Penetrating injuries in children are less common than blunt injuries; however, the management of these injuries does not differ substantially from that in adults, and celiotomy is routinely advised. Studies of the wound tract, either by using a probe or a catheter and subsequent contrast, are difficult in the uncooperative, constantly moving child. This technique may be appropriate for the older child

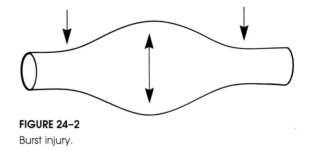

FIGURE 24–2

Burst injury.

or teenager depending on the frequency with which such injuries are managed at a particular institution and the expertise of the surgeon.

Figures 24–2, 24–3, and 24–4 illustrate diagrammatically the three mechanisms by which any hollow viscus sustains damage.[13] It seems only logical that most instances of blunt force are not purely of one type or another but a mixture of all three. Although analysis of the injury might favor a specific mechanism, this compartmentalization is artificial when discussing a particular patient.

When exposed to a comparable force, the child is more susceptible than the adult to internal injury from blunt trauma because of anatomic differences, especially the prepubertal child. These include a more prominent abdomen with wider flaring costal margins that may not protect the intra-abdominal contents as well, a less-developed abdominal musculature, and a narrower anteroposterior diameter. Hence, the abdomen of a small child is less prepared to resist an oncoming force, and the relaxed abdominal wall provides almost no protection.[53]

Most small bowel injuries occur as a direct crush or shearing because even after a meal little or no bulk is contained within it. Blunt trauma from the left side tends more often to produce injuries to the stomach than trauma from the right because of the relative protection afforded by the liver from forces directed from that side.

The physiology of delayed rupture involves a partial thickness injury, which in time becomes a full thickness injury and clinically apparent. These late injuries rarely perforate but can gradually produce stenosis in unpredictable scattered sites in the small bowel.[34] Mesenteric rents can also cause strictures.[8] Shearing injuries from seat belts can

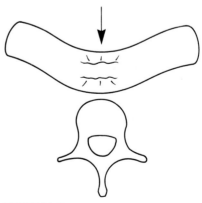

FIGURE 24–3

Crush injury.

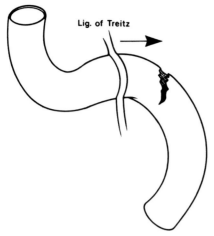

FIGURE 24–4
Shear injury.

produce either immediate or delayed damage and are usually, but not always, confined to the older child and adult.[45] Smaller children sustain such injuries from seat belts less frequently, presumably because the relationship between the size of the child and the efficacy of the seat belt is much more favorable than in the larger, heavier adult.

DIAGNOSIS

The history of the mechanism of injury may suggest the presence of an intra-abdominal injury even though other injuries are more obvious; when life threatening, the other injuries make the abdominal trauma of secondary importance. Confirmation of head injuries, which may produce altered levels of consciousness, and stabilization of the cardiorespiratory system take precedence over investigation of the abdomen. These associated injuries tend to make the diagnosis of an intra-abdominal injury even more difficult. The use of an algorithm (Fig. 24–5) provides an overview as to the suggested management of the child with a possible injury to the stomach or small bowel. Tables 24–2 and 24–3 summarize the diagnostic studies most valuable in diagnosing stomach and small intestinal injuries and show how these findings influence morbidity and mortality, illustrating and emphasizing how the patient's sensorium affects the physician's ability to diagnose and isolate a blunt injury to the stomach or intestine.

During this process the other organ systems involved may point to or mask additional problems, for example, when an abdomen is expanding from a hemoperitoneum from an injured liver or spleen. Only in patients who require prompt surgical intervention will a bowel injury be diagnosed early. It is exactly because so many pediatric patients who have sustained blunt abdominal trauma are treated nonoperatively that the diagnosis of stomach and small bowel injuries is delayed in this age group.

History and Physical Examination. The history of a direct blow or assault to the abdomen is helpful. A witness to the blow or the child's symptoms can direct the physician's attention early in the investigative process. The physical examination should specifically assess for the presence or absence of peritoneal irritation. Tenderness must be pres-

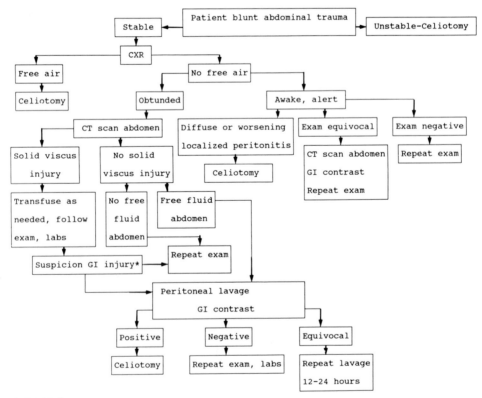

FIGURE 24–5
Evaluation algorithm for gastrointestinal injuries in blunt abdominal trauma. CXR, Chest radiograph; CT, computed tomography; GI, gastrointestinal.

Table 24–2
Stomach Injuries Due to Blunt Trauma

	No.	Tap/ Lavage	Exam	Evidence of Sepsis	Free Air	Associated Injuries	Infectious Complication	Mortality
		Diagnosis					**Outcome**	
Courcy[16]	6	5	0	1	0	5	2	0
Siemans[54]	6	1	2	0	3	3	3	2
Vassy*[61]	4	2	0	0	2	3	3	0
Asch*[3]	2	0	0	0	2	1	2	0
Yajko[63]	2	0	0	0	2	1	2	1
Brunsting[7]	6	3	2	1	0	5	2	3
Hunt[26]	67				40	46	35	20

*Indicates pediatric series.

ent for an injury to be likely, providing the child is alert and cooperative. Significant injury is usually accompanied by decreased bowel sounds, abdominal distention, and peritoneal irritation. If marked tenderness or distention is present, a nasogastric tube should be inserted because acute gastric dilation following injury is usually present and makes abdominal evaluation difficult. Initial resuscitative efforts always include routine blood studies, but no specific laboratory values point to an injury to the stomach or small bowel.

Radiographs. Chest and abdominal radiographs to search for pneumoperitoneum are done early, and a left lateral decubitus film may reveal even small amounts of free air. However, less than 20% of instances of traumatic perforation of the small intestine demonstrate free air, although 50 to 60% of stomach perforations reveal free air on radiographic examination. Although this finding is an absolute indication for celiotomy, its absence does not give complete reassurance that a traumatic disruption has not taken place.

Computed Tomography. After the initial evaluation and stabilization, a computed tomography (CT) scan is often the first specific study obtained, usually because the head needs to be studied and if the abdomen can be scanned at the same time it is more efficient and convenient. The CT scan

has definite value in assessing injuries to solid organs but is of limited help in uncovering injuries to the stomach and small bowel. Free fluid in the abdomen in the absence of an injury to a solid organ should alert the physician that the fluid could be secondary to damage to a hollow viscus. This finding alone would not prompt surgical intervention, but in the child with an altered sensorium, it should prompt further studies.[9] Ideally, this would include a water-soluble contrast study of the stomach and proximal small bowel. Traditionally, the use of barium has been avoided, diatrizoate meglumine (Gastrografin or Hypaque) being preferred instead in cases of possible gastrointestinal disruption. Recently iopamidol has been preferred because it has isotonic characteristics with fewer side effects.[4]

Diagnostic Peritoneal Lavage. The use of diagnostic peritoneal lavage (DPL) is well documented in the literature, although it has fallen into some disfavor for use in the pediatric population because of the frequent nonoperative management of children with blunt abdominal trauma. Hence, the presence or absence of blood in the peritoneal cavity as detected by DPL is, in some hands, less important in clinical decision making in this age group.

It is this combination of avoiding DPL and nonoperative treatment of blunt trauma that leads to delays in the diagnosis of injury to the stomach and small bowel. When

Table 24–3
Small Intestinal Injuries Due to Blunt Trauma

	No.	Tap or Lavage	GI Series	Exam	CT Scan	Sepsis	Free Air	Associated Injuries	Infectious Complication	Mortality
		Diagnosis							**Outcome**	
Cerise[13]	20	4	0	20	0	0	4	10	1	2
Schenk[51]	13	7	0	6	0	0	2	10	4	2
Kakos*†‡[27]	26	0	8	24	0	0	7	7	1	2
Maull[37]	20	4	0	15	0	0	1	16	2	2
Phillips[44]	12	10	0	12	0	0	0	6	1	1
Rouse[50]	4	1	1	1	0	0	1	0	1	1
Hunt[26]	22	14	0	0	0	0	2	13	3	5
Reilley*†[48]	14	1	13	0	0	0	3	7	0	0
Dickinson*[20]	5	1	0	4	0	0	1	1	1	0

*Indicates pediatric series.
†Includes duodenal trauma.
‡Includes intramural hematoma.
GI, Gastrointestinal; CT, computed tomography.

explorations were formerly done for a positive tap or lavage, the entire gastrointestinal tract could be examined carefully. Perhaps more liberal use of DPL should be considered but with a specific purpose. This would include a search not only for blood, but also for cells, amylase, bacteria, and food debris, the last two being diagnostic for a bowel injury. Also, DPL is indicated in the child with a diminished sensorium when the usual clinical parameters are absent or unreliable.[9]

It has been suggested that at the time of DPL an analysis of the fluid for alkaline phosphatase might assist in the diagnosis of a bowel injury within 1 hour following the accident.[35] This thinking is because alkaline phosphatase is present in the intestinal mucosa and hepatobiliary secretions. When the amylase in the fluid is high, it is nonspecific. The cell count may take as long as 3 hours or more to become elevated in the peritoneal fluid. When lavage fluid is associated with a stomach perforation, it may have a characteristic reddish-brown color due to the mixture of acid and hemoglobin.[40]

For children in whom DPL is done, the laboratory parameters are shown in Table 24–4. Each extreme of the spectrum has valid diagnostic accuracy, but the wide range of values in the center limits its usefulness. For example, a white blood cell count of more than 500 cells per ml is believed to be positive, less than 100 cells per ml is negative, and from 100 to 500 cells per ml indeterminate.

The combination of an abdominal CT scan and a gastrointestinal contrast study is an important technique in searching for injury to a hollow viscus. It is less accurate than a formal contrast study but does have the advantage of immediate availability and interpretation by the attending physician on an emergency basis.

In my experience and that of others, the indications that eventually lead to surgical exploration are the traditional findings of an intra-abdominal insult. Characteristically, in isolated stomach and small bowel injuries a 6- to 12-hour delay ensues before sufficient peritoneal irritation develops to change the clinical picture. Progressive distention, tenderness, and guarding are reliable criteria, especially if not present initially.

Delays in diagnosis and surgical repair predictably increase the morbidity, which is often manifested by an increased incidence of infection (see Tables 24–2 and 24–3). Earlier intervention decreases the incidence of postoperative infections, and therefore repeated examination and

evaluation are most valuable in establishing an earlier diagnosis. When surgical exploration is deferred until fever or other late signs of injury to a hollow viscus appear, the morbidity rises accordingly.[5] Incomplete injuries may be impossible to differentiate early and might require intervention a few days after the trauma. The clinical differentiation among a partial bowel tear, an intramural hematoma, a mesenteric rent, an intramesenteric hemorrhage, or a bowel contusion, depends on the child's clinical course during the first few days. To maintain a high degree of accuracy, some of the previously recommended studies must be repeated and trended to elicit important changes that may have adverse effects.

MANAGEMENT

Preoperative Preparation. The preoperative management of a child with a penetrating injury of the stomach or small bowel does not differ substantially from that of any injured patient. The vital signs should be stabilized when necessary, and, when possible, appropriate vascular access should be established for infusion and monitoring. A nasogastric tube should be inserted to prevent gastric dilation that commonly accompanies blunt abdominal trauma, and broad spectrum antibiotics should be administered as early as possible to achieve satisfactory blood levels intraoperatively.

Operative Intervention. Surgical exploration is recommended through a midline incision to allow both an expeditious and a flexible exposure. If bowel disruption has been documented preoperatively by a pneumoperitoneum, it is imperative that this site be identified. Although this procedure seems straightforward and routine, experience has shown that small perforations that occur high up and posteriorly on the stomach may be difficult to locate, especially in the presence of significant contamination and associated retroperitoneal edema or hematomas. Intraluminal installation of a dilute solution of methylene blue may be helpful in finding small holes.

Localized full thickness areas of injury should be débrided conservatively and closed using primarily a single- or double-layered technique. Both the stomach and the small bowel have an excellent blood supply and are quite forgiving in even seriously contused areas that are disrupted. Occasionally, a limited resection may be required if the injured area has many confluent perforations or is devascularized. Primary anastomotic repair is invariably possible. Postoperative gastric decompression is essential, but the use of a gastrostomy is discouraged. Complications from the gastrostomy itself can occur, and it is rarely necessary to perform even in the severely traumatized stomach.

In unusual cases in which a bowel injury is suspected but never confirmed at surgery, it is reasonable to obtain a contrast study before discharge or at an early follow-up visit. This might uncover cases that develop late strictures. With the exception of adhesive small bowel obstruction in future years, there is little to suggest any long-term sequelae for most instances of blunt trauma to the stomach and small bowel.

Table 24–4
Peritoneal Lavage Findings Associated with Intestinal and Stomach Injuries

WBC >500/mm³
Alkaline phosphatase >31 U/L
Food particles
Bacteria or Gram stain
Equivocal Findings
WBC >100/mm³, <500/mm³
Amylase >200 U/dl
Bile

WBC, White blood count.

DISCUSSION

Isolated injuries to the stomach and small bowel represent less than 2% of all cases of blunt abdominal trauma requiring hospital admission. The ratio of penetrating to blunt injuries depends on how heavily weighted the series is with teenagers in large urban hospitals.

A thorough review of the literature pertaining to stomach and small bowel injuries, both isolated and in combination with other injuries, is documented in Tables 24–2 and 24–3. My own experience from a large metropolitan children's hospital is shown in Table 24–5. The increasing trend toward nonoperative treatment of most intra-abdominal injuries in children has resulted in delays in the diagnosis of a disruptured hollow viscus. The acceptability of this is questionable, as the literature has shown conclusively an increased morbidity and mortality with delay in diagnosis of such injuries.

For children who require exploratory surgery for other injuries, stomach and small bowel injuries will be detected. Obviously patients presenting with free air need urgent celiotomy. However, in the large group of patients treated expectantly, even though blood is present in the peritoneal cavity producing peritoneal irritation, the diagnosis of bowel perforation is more difficult, particularly in children with associated head injuries. The value of repeated physical examinations cannot be overstated, but *aggressive* radiographic investigation is recommended when the patient demonstrates borderline findings, especially when a decision is made *not* to operate.

On rare occasions, rupture of a hollow viscus can result in subcutaneous emphysema in the absence of pneumoperitoneum. Unless there is an obvious explanation, the gastro-esophageal junction and upper gastrointestinal tract should be investigated carefully. I am unaware of instances of pneumoperitoneum from the dissection of mediastinal air secondary to trauma. During cardiopulmonary resuscitation, the stomach has occasionally been injured or ruptured, but this occurs less often in small children because of the technique of closed cardiac massage. At least one adult has sustained a gastric rupture from performance of the Heimlich maneuver.

References

1. All RB, Curry GJ: Abdominal trauma: A study of 297 consecutive cases. Am J Surg 93:398, 1957.
2. Arcari FA: Blunt trauma in infants and children. J Mich Med Soc 61:335, 1962.
3. Asch MJ, Coran AG, Johnston PW: Gastric perforation secondary to blunt trauma in children. J Trauma 15:187–189, 1975.
4. Bell KE, McKinstry CS, Mills JOM: Iopamidol in diagnosis of suspected upper gastro-intestinal perforation. Clin Radiol 38:165–168, 1987.
5. Bose SM, Kumar A, Chaudhary A, et al: Factors affecting mortality in small intestinal perforation. Indian J Gastroenterol 5:261–263, 1986.
6. Braun P, Dion Y: Intestinal stenosis following seat belt injury. J Pediatr Surg 8:549, 1973.
7. Brunsting LA, Morton JH: Gastric rupture from blunt abdominal trauma. J Trauma 27:887–891, 1987.
8. Bryner UM, Longerbeam JK, Reeves CD: Post traumatic ischemic stenosis of the small bowel. Arch Surg 115:1039–1041, 1980.
9. Buntain WL, Stevens S, Gould HR: Early diagnosis of intestinal injury with computed tomography and diagnostic peritoneal lavage (abstract). Presented at the Kiwanis Second National Meeting on Pediatric Trauma, Boston, September 1987.
10. Burke AM, Harley HAJ: Traumatic gastric ulceration. Aust N Z J Surg 53:379–380, 1983.
11. Bussey HJ, McGehee RN, Tyson KRT: Isolated gastric rupture due to blunt trauma. J Trauma 15:190–191, 1975.
12. Case MES, Nanduri R: Laceration of the stomach by blunt trauma in a child: A case of child abuse. J Forensic Sci 28:496–450, 1983.
13. Cerise EJ, Scully JH: Blunt trauma to the small intestine. J Trauma 10:46–50, 1970.
14. Clarke R: Closed abdominal injuries. Lancet 2:877, 1954.
15. Cole DA, Burcher SK: Accidental pneumatic rupture of the esophagus and stomach. Lancet 1:24, 1961.
16. Courcy CA, Soderstrom C, Brotman S: Gastric rupture from blunt trauma: A plea for minimal diagnosis. Am Surg 50:424–427, 1984.
17. Cowan M, Bardole J, Dlesk A: Perforated stomach following the Heimlich maneuver. Am J Emerg Med 5:121–133, 1987.
18. Custer JR, Polley TZ, Moler F: Gastric perforation following cardiopulmonary resuscitation in a child: Report of a case and review of the literature. Pediatr Emerg Care 3:24–27, 1987.
19. Dajee H, MacDonald AC: Gastric rupture due to seat belt injury. Br J Surg 69:436–437, 1982.
20. Dickinson SJ, Shaw A, Santulli TV: Rupture of the gastrointestinal tract in children by blunt trauma. Surg Gynecol Obstet 130:655, 1970.
21. Donohue JH, Crass RA, Trunkey DD: The management of duodenal and other small intestinal trauma. World J Surg 9:904–913, 1985.
22. Fitzgerald JB, Crawford ES, DeBakey ME: Surgical considerations of non-penetrating abdominal injuries: An analysis of 200 cases. Am J Surg 100:22, 1960.
23. Fock G: Closed abdominal injuries in children. Ann Paediatr Fenn 12:167, 1966.
24. Frankel P: Untersuchungen zur Entstehung der sogenannten Magenrupture. Schr Klin Med 89:113, 1906. Cited by Yajko et al. J Trauma 15:177–183, 1975.
25. Halpern P, Sorkine P, Leykin Y, et al: Rupture of the stomach in a diving accident with attempted resuscitation. Br J Anaesth 58:1059–1061, 1986.

Table 24–5
Children's Hospital of Los Angeles Experience 1971–1986: Small Intestinal Injuries

Penetrating	12
Gunshot wound	4
Stab	8
Associated injuries	5 (41%)
Mortality	1 (8%)
Blunt	13
Mechanism of Injury	
Fall	6 (46%)
Motor vehicle accident	3 (23%)
Automobile/pedestrian	3 (23%)
Direct violence	1 (7%)
Injury–Diagnosis Interval	
0–12 hr	6 (46%)
12–24 hr	6 (46%)
1–3 days	0 (0)
73 days	1 (7%)
Method of Diagnosis	
Examination	8 (61%)
Lavage	1 (7%)
Free air	2 (15%)
Upper gastrointestinal	0 (0)
Celiotomy	2 (15%)
Associated Injuries	6 (16%)
Mortality	2 (15%) (unrelated to injury)

26. Hunt KE, Garrison RN, Fry DE: Perforating injuries of the gastrointestinal tract following blunt abdominal trauma. Am Surg 46:100–104, 1980.
27. Kakos GS, Grosfeld JL, Morse TS: Small bowel injuries in children after blunt abdominal trauma. Ann Surg 174:238–241, 1971.
28. Kanfer C, Wulfing D: Darmverlet Zungen bei Kindern als folge stumpter bauch traumen. Z Kinder Chir 6:55, 1969.
29. Knight KM, Doucet HJ: Gastric rupture and death caused by ipecac syrup. South Med J 80:786–787, 1987.
30. Levy JL, Linder LH: Major abdominal trauma in children. Am J Surg 120:55–58, 1954.
31. Lloyd RG: Delayed rupture of stomach after blunt abdominal trauma. BMJ 285(6336):196, 1982.
32. Luccioni L, Mammucari R: In temaditraumichiusi dell'addome; considerazioi anatomo-cliniche e terapeutiche chirurigiche su alcune osservazioi di lesioi gastriche da scoppio. J Ann Ital Chir 45:226, 1969.
33. McCormick WF: Rupture of the stomach in children; review of the literature and report of seven cases. Am Arch Pathol 67:416, 1959.
34. Marks CG: Small bowel strictures after blunt abdominal trauma. Br J Surg 69:236–238, 1982.
35. Marx JA, Bar-Or D, Moore EE, et al: Utility of lavage alkaline phosphatase in detection of isolated small intestinal injury. Ann Emerg Med 14:10–14, 1985.
36. Mathieson AJM: Closed abdominal injury. BMJ 2:749–756, 1962.
37. Maull KI, Reath DB: Impact of early recognition on outcome in nonpenetrating wounds of the small bowel. South Med J 77:1075–1077, 1984.
38. Miller EF, Peterson D, Miller J: Abdominal visceral perforation secondary to electrical injury: Case report and review of the literature. Burns 12:505–507, 1985.
39. Morton JH, Hinshaw HR, Morton JJ: Blunt trauma to the abdomen. Ann Surg 145:699, 1957.
40. Munafo WW: In discussion of: Branstirg LA, Morton JH: Gastric rupture from blunt abdominal trauma. J Trauma 27:891, 1987.
41. Nadkarni KM, Shetty SD, Kagzi RS, et al: Small bowel perforations. Arch Surg 116:53–57, 1981.
42. Newing A: Rupture of the small bowel in association with procedentia. Med J Aust 2:901–902, 1955.
43. Orloff MJ, Charters AC: Injuries of the small intestine and mesentery and retroperitoneal hematoma. Surg Clin North Am 52:729, 1972.
44. Phillips TF, Brotman S, Cleveland S, et al: Perforating injuries of the small bowel from blunt abdominal trauma. Ann Emerg Med 12:75–79, 1983.
45. Pohl MJ, Cook WJ: Small bowel stenosis after seat belt injury. Med J Aust 2:156, 1980.
46. Portius GV, Kilbourne BC, Paul EG: Nonpenetrating abdominal trauma. Arch Surg 72:800, 1956.
47. Rajagopalan AE, Pickleman J: Free perforation of the small intestine. Ann Surg 43:229–233, 1977.
48. Reilley A, Marks M, Nance F, et al: Small bowel trauma in children and adolescents. Am Surg 51:132–135, 1985.
49. Rodkey GV: The management of abdominal injuries. Surg Clin North Am 46:627, 1966.
50. Rouse T, Collin J, Daar A: Isolated injury to the intestine from blunt abdominal injury. Injury 16:131–133, 1984.
51. Schenk WG, Lonchyna V, Myolan JA: Perforation of the jejunum from blunt abdominal trauma. J Trauma 23:54–56, 1983.
52. Sclafani SJA: Post-traumatic gastric stenosis due to perigastric adhesions. Radiology 54:14, 1985.
53. Semel L, Frittelli G: Gastric rupture from blunt abdominal trauma. N Y State J Med 81:938–939, 1981.
54. Siemens RA, Fulton RL: Gastric rupture as a result of blunt trauma. Am Surg 43:229–233, 1977.
55. Silbergleit A, Berkus EM: Neonatal gastric rupture. Minn Med 49:65, 1966.
56. Sinclair MD, Morre TC: Major surgery for abdominal and thoracic trauma in children and adolescents. J Pediatr Surg 9:155–162, 1974.
57. Speakman M, Reece-Smith H: Gastric and pancreatic rupture due to a sports injury. Br J Surg 70:190, 1983.
58. Swartzbauch S, Curtin JE: Rupture of stomach, spleen, and left hemidiaphragm. Am J Dis Child 87:616–620, 1954.
59. Tank ES, Eraklis AJ, Gross RE: Blunt abdominal trauma in infancy and childhood. J Trauma 8:439, 1968.
60. Vance BM: Traumatic lesions of the intestine caused by non-penetrating blunt force. Arch Surg 7:197–212, 1923 (quotes Aristotle, cited by Morgagni, Epistola 54:141–142, 1761).
61. Vassy LE, Klecker RL, Koch E, et al: Traumatic gastric perforation in children from blunt trauma. J Trauma 15:184–186, 1975.
62. Wangensteen OH: Intestinal Obstruction. Springfield, Ill, Charles C Thomas, 1955, p 35.
63. Yajko RD, Seydel F, Trimble C: Rupture of the stomach from blunt abdominal trauma. J Trauma 15:177–183, 1975.
64. Yand JY, Tsai YC, Noordhoff MS: Electrical burn with visceral injury. Burns 11:207–212, 1985.

Michael W. L. Gauderer
Thomas A. Stellato

Colonic and Rectal Injuries

The management of injuries to the colon and rectum is one of the most challenging and controversial areas of torso trauma. The "large bowel," which traverses all quadrants of the abdomen as well as the pelvis, can frequently be disrupted by penetrating or blunt force. Because the colon contains particulate matter and abundant bacterial flora, spillage of colonic contents can lead to serious local and systemic septic complications, adversely affecting the outcome of patients with other intra-abdominal or extra-abdominal injuries. Few clinical situations require more acumen in judgment and surgical experience.[112] Because most trauma to children is blunt, colonic injuries are relatively uncommon. In contradistinction to the rarity of colonic injury in children, obvious or occult anorectal injuries are regularly encountered in major pediatric centers.

Most guidelines for the management of colorectal injuries in infants and children are based on the adult experience. However, the surgeon caring for a child with colorectal injuries must exhibit a certain flexibility in adapting time-honored measures to the pediatric patient.

EVOLUTION OF MANAGEMENT

Improvement in the management and outcome of adult patients with injuries to the colon and rectum directly reflects the experience of military surgeons during some of the major conflicts of the nineteenth and twentieth centuries. Nearly 4000 abdominal wounds were recorded during the American Civil War. Both the lethality of these wounds and the inadequacy of surgical intervention are illustrated by an overall mortality rate of 90%. All soldiers who underwent surgery for these injuries died.[49]

During World War I, the practice of nonoperative management of military abdominal wounds was abandoned. Most colorectal injuries were treated by primary closure, with mortality rates as high as 60%.[61] For extraperitoneal colonic injuries (i.e., injuries to the ascending or descending colon and rectum), exteriorization through colostomy was occasionally employed, although the mortality rate was even higher with this procedure.[111]

Suture closure without proximal diversion was also the generally accepted approach to civilian colon injuries until the early years of World War II. A switch to exteriorization of the injured colon or primary closure with proximal decompression by colostomy resulted in a reduction of mortality to approximately 30%.[24, 53, 83, 86] During these years, rectal injury was managed by repair when possible, with presacral drainage and proximal sigmoid colostomy. An additional 15% decrease in mortality rates occurred during the Korean conflict; this decrease has been attributed to improved resuscitation techniques, improved prehospital transport, and continued application of exteriorization or diverting colostomy.[16]

The Vietnam War provided the most recent opportunity to review a large series of colon and rectal injuries sustained during combat. Refinements in techniques and continued improvement in resuscitation, evacuation, and selectivity in surgical management depending on anatomic location of the injury resulted in a mortality rate of less than 12% in patients with colorectal injuries.[45, 60] Right colon injuries in the absence of multiple intra-abdominal visceral injuries were treated by resection and anastomosis. Primary anastomosis was not attempted in the transverse, left, or sigmoid colon. Injuries of the rectum were routinely treated by primary repair, diverting colostomy, extraperitoneal presacral drainage, and irrigation of the distal segment of colon.

These guidelines have also been applied to the civilian population. However, because the nature of the injuries sustained by civilians is often not as severe as those sustained by combat patients, a more selective approach favoring primary suture repair has been generally advocated. Since the early 1950s, ample evidence has accumulated supporting the safety and efficacy of simple closure in the majority of civilian colonic wounds.[8, 13, 17, 41, 44, 54, 63, 87, 96, 99, 104, 114]

Another option for treating colonic wounds is exteriorized primary repair.[25, 58, 70, 79] In this technique, the injured colon is repaired and secured above the approximated fascia. The affected colonic segment is returned to the abdominal cavity 5 to 10 days after proper healing has taken place. If the repair breaks down prior to reoperation, the segment functions as a colostomy.

Although controversy about ideal management persists, it is clear that each of the previously described approaches has a place in the treatment of colorectal injury. The surgeon should choose a procedure based on the specific findings and conditions in each individual patient.

MECHANISMS OF INJURY AND INCIDENCE

Injuries to the colon and rectum can be isolated or can coexist. For the purpose of clarity, injuries to the colon and the rectum are considered separately in this section.

Colon

In children, injuries can result from intraluminal trauma, blunt or crushing external trauma, perforating trauma that includes the abdominal wall, perforating trauma that does not include the abdominal wall, and suction trauma.

Intraluminal Trauma

Thermometers. The distance between the anus and the rectosigmoid junction is approximately 3 cm in the newborn. When thermometers are inserted too far into the anus, perforation of the upper rectum or lower sigmoid can result.[33, 51] Typically, this injury occurs in healthy newborns. Illness develops rapidly, frequently on the first day of life, with abdominal distention and evidence of peritonitis. Pneumoperitoneum and shock are common, and the site of perforation is often difficult to identify.[93] Although the number of publications on this subject is substantial,[33, 51, 98] the incidence of this mishap is unknown. With proper instruction of parents and health care personnel in the correct technique of thermometer insertion, the incidence of this injury should be low. Any use of rectal thermometers in children has been challenged by some; however, when used rectally, thermometers should never be inserted forcefully and should not be advanced beyond 3 cm.

Endoscopy, Diagnostic or Therapeutic. Perforation of the gastrointestinal tract is a well-recognized complication of endoscopy in both adults and children.[20, 42, 59] The rate of perforation during diagnostic colonoscopy varies from 0.14 to 0.65%.[42] As would be expected, the incidence of perforation increases during therapeutic endoscopy, and the rate of perforation is higher in the diseased colon. In addition, injury to organs other than the colon during colonoscopy has also been reported.[42, 105]

Perforation should be recognized either at the time of occurrence by the endoscopist, or shortly thereafter when signs of peritoneal irritation become apparent. Because colonoscopy will be performed using general anesthesia in most infants and children, recognition of perforation may be delayed.

A rare complication is intraluminal explosion during endoscopy. This occurs when electrocautery is used in an incompletely prepared colon or in a colon in which mannitol has been used for mechanical preparation.[6, 29, 66]

Contrast Enema, Diagnostic or Therapeutic. Although uncommon, perforation of the colon during attempted reduction of ileocolic intussusception in children is a well-recognized complication with a reported incidence of about 0.7%.[7, 29] Bowel perforation can also occur from enema tips or as a result of nontherapeutic studies.[66, 77, 90]

Air Insufflation. High-pressure air insufflation by applying the tip of an air hose to the buttocks is usually the consequence of a prank. It can lead to immediate and sometimes extensive tearing of the colon.[3] The incidence of this condition is unknown. Excessive air pressure can also be a complication of colonoscopy.[59] Air insufflation has been used therapeutically for the reduction of ileocolic intussusception.

Impalement. Impalement can produce some of the most serious colorectal injuries with an attendant excessive morbidity.[34, 103] These lesions are often associated with perineal and urogenital trauma. Each injury requires careful evaluation of structures adjacent to the rectum as well as other intra-abdominal organs. In children, these injuries can be the consequence of play. There is often a delay in diagnosis of the unsuspected lesion.

Foreign Bodies. Occasionally, swallowed pins or other sharp objects perforate the colonic wall. Most commonly, such perforations result in a localized abscess rather than diffuse peritonitis.[23, 43, 67]

Blunt, Crushing, or Decelerating Trauma

External Blow. Forces applied to the abdomen either accidentally (e.g., motor vehicle, bicycle handlebars, furniture edges, tree stumps) or purposely (e.g., child abuse) can also lead to bowel disruptions.[5, 21, 26, 28, 52, 57, 68, 97, 110, 113] There is, as in most other colonic injuries, a male preponderance for this type of injury. In a series of 870 patients with blunt abdominal trauma, Cox encountered 11 colonic injuries (1.3%).[21] The reported incidence of bowel disruption (duodenum, small bowel, and colon) following blunt trauma in children is between 1 and 9%.[5, 28, 57] These lesions can be deceiving, because external signs of trauma are unfortunately frequently absent.

Welch, in a series of 89 children with gastrointestinal injuries, found that 65 were the result of blunt trauma and 24 were caused by penetrating trauma.[113] Of these 89 injuries, nine involved the colon (four blunt, five penetrating). Of the four children who had blunt trauma, three were associated with a pelvic crush. Avulsions or ruptures of the gastrointestinal tract occur in areas adjacent to fixed points, such as the ligament of Treitz, the ileocecal angle, or the sigmoidorectal angle.[28, 57, 113] The cecum is particularly prone to both avulsion and disruption. In patients with intestinal injury secondary to blunt abdominal trauma, the incidence of associated intra-abdominal injuries is high. Nonperforating damage to the bowel wall may lead to constrictive lesions of the colon.[2]

Crushing. Crushing injuries are usually secondary to pelvic compression and have a high incidence of associated trauma. Welch encountered three cases of crushing injury among nine colonic injuries in children.[113]

Seat Belt Compression. When small children are restrained with adult lap seat belts, the belt often rests above the bony pelvis. With acute deceleration, there is compression of intra-abdominal organs, including compression of the colon against the spine.[52, 73] The signs and symptoms of compression injury may include one or all of the following: bruises over both lower quadrants, early or late peritoneal signs, or pneumoperitoneum. Because this injury is uncommon, its incidence in children is unknown.

Blast Injury. Propagation of an intense shock wave can lead to colonic disruption.[36]

Perforating Trauma That Includes the Abdominal Wall

Stabbing. In children, particularly young children, stabbing is not nearly as common as it is in adolescents or adults. In a series of 75 children 16 years of age or younger with stab wounds, Barlow and colleagues encountered 20 abdominal and eight flank wounds.[10, 113] Of these, only one involved the colon.

Gunshot. The increased incidence of gunshot wounds in children has paralleled, among other factors, the greater availability of guns. Barlow and associates reviewed the records of 108 children 16 years of age or younger who sustained firearm wounds during a 10-year period.[9] In these 108 children, there were 15 gastrointestinal injuries, of which four were colonic. None of the children with colonic injuries died; however, a fecal fistula developed in one child. Slim and colleagues reviewed 44 children from Lebanon with perforating injuries secondary to shrapnel and high-velocity bullets.[99] This important report represents the first study limited to this type of injury in the pediatric age group.

Perforating Trauma That Does Not Include the Abdominal Wall

Intraoperative Mishaps. The incidence of this iatrogenic lesion is difficult to determine and depends on the difficulty of the operation (e.g., dense adhesions) and the experience of the surgeon.

Perforation by Intraperitoneal Foreign Bodies. Fisher and associates have described a case in which the colon was penetrated by the tip of a ventriculoperitoneal shunt.[31] The outcome in this case was fatal.

Suction Trauma

In a series by Cain and colleagues, severe transanal suction injuries were sustained by five children when they sat on uncovered swimming pool drain sites.[18] This occurrence led to rectosigmoid perforation and intestinal evisceration. With surgical intervention, salvage of these children was possible, but short-gut syndrome occurred.

Rectum

In the pediatric age group, a wide variety of causes can lead to perianal and anorectal injury.

Injuries Related to the Stool or Foreign Material in the Stool

Hard Stool. Anal fissure due to hard stool is well known and a common occurrence in children.[15]

Swallowed Foreign Bodies. Injury caused by swallowed foreign bodies is similar to the mechanism of colonic injury previously discussed.[43] Our experience includes two children in whom swallowed pins became lodged in the anorectum. In both cases, the manifestation was severe anal pain.

Injuries from Foreign Bodies Introduced through the Anus

Multiple Foreign Bodies. An incredible variety of objects have been introduced into the rectum.[11, 91] The incidence of this problem in children is very small compared with that in the adult population. In this age group, child abuse should be suspected.[15] Trauma by thermometers and enema nozzles has been discussed previously.[33, 51, 56, 66, 98]

Endoscopy. In addition to the well-recognized potential complication of perforation, which has been discussed previously, forceful insertion of flexible or rigid endoscopes may result in anal or rectal injuries.[20, 42, 59]

Impalement Injuries

Impalement injuries have been discussed previously.

External Perforating Injuries

Stab and Gunshot Wounds. Because of the location of the rectum, these injuries are rare in children.[15, 99] However, penetrating wounds of the buttock can be associated with extensive pelvic and intra-abdominal damage.[73]

Sexually Related Injuries

Child Abuse. Nonaccidental trauma is associated with both significant physical and emotional morbidity. Several features of child abuse must be stressed: The victims range from infants and toddlers to adolescents,[15] and although it is commonly believed most victims are girls, a report by Hobbs and Wynne suggests that an equal frequency of injury from abuse occurs in girls and boys.[50] Such trauma is associated with a high rate of serious anal and perianal injuries in assaulted boys.[30, 50] Other signs of child abuse, such as emotional deprivation, failure to thrive, developmental delay, and behavioral disturbances, are often present.[50] The exact incidence of this problem is unknown.

Rape. Underreporting of this injury in children may be even more problematic than in the adult rape victim. Serious rectovaginal tears can occur.[88]

Injuries Associated with Pelvic Fractures

Rectal Disruption. With severe crush injuries, the rectum can be severed. Damage to the blood supply from these injuries can lead to ischemic necrosis, resulting in perforation or subsequent stricture.[68, 89]

Perforation by Bony Spiculae. Sharp bony fragments can perforate both the rectum and the urogenital tract.

Perineal Injuries

Straddle Injuries. These lesions are seen with regularity in pediatric centers, but they rarely produce significant rectal injury. However, rectovaginal tears and serious urogenital lesions can occur.[15]

Avulsions. Avulsion injuries may arise from a variety of insults (e.g., crushing, farm machinery). Serious perineal trauma can lead to tissue loss involving the rectum and its sphincter mechanism.

Burns. Whether they occur accidentally or are intentionally sustained, as in child abuse, these lesions can lead to scarring and eventual anal stenosis.

Miscellaneous Rectal Injuries

Self-Inflicted Rectal Trauma. Local injury leading to bleeding was reported by Srinivasan and colleagues in a 9-year-old child with emotional problems.[101]

Iatrogenic Injury. Iatrogenic injury is a well-recognized risk in a variety of rectal and perineal procedures as well as endoscopy.[43]

Parturition. Spontaneous as well as instrument-aided delivery can lead to injury of the anorectal sphincter mechanism in young mothers.[43]

DIAGNOSIS

The diagnosis of colorectal injuries can be difficult. A thorough history is very helpful, but, as with many trauma victims, a history may be unavailable. Unless the injury is obvious (e.g., gunshot wound), the surgeon must have a high index of suspicion, particularly if the perforation has occurred in an extraperitoneal segment of the colon.

Physical Examination

After adequate resuscitation and general evaluation, the child's abdomen, back, and perineum are examined. Gastric decompression with a nasogastric tube should precede abdominal evaluation. Distention, discoloration, and bruising are noted. Abdominal palpation must be gentle. Peritoneal irritation, ranging from mild to severe, is the single most important finding. It must be remembered, however, that in the very early stages of intra-abdominal colonic perforation or somewhat later in retroperitoneal perforation, symptoms may be minimal or absent. Peritoneal irritation may be nearly impossible to determine in the very severely injured child. Bowel sounds are usually present initially; however, their absence after several hours is strongly suggestive of peritoneal irritation.

The site of any abdominal wall wound is carefully evaluated topographically and recorded. Probing of the wound or injection of contrast into the wound is avoided. A rectal examination is essential; however, it must be undertaken with extreme care, particularly in the very young patient or in those in whom a crushing injury to the pelvis or sexual abuse is suspected. We prefer to perform this examination with the child in a supine position.

Blood in the rectum, severe pain, the presence of foreign material, or bony spiculae can give important clues to the presence of a significant rectal injury. However, the absence of blood does not exclude the presence of trauma. The position of the prostate is determined. Whenever possible, the sphincter tone is evaluated. Anoscopy can occasionally be performed in the emergency department, but any further endoscopy should be done in the operating room with the patient under general anesthesia.[103]

Imaging Techniques

Plain abdominal roentgenograms are routinely obtained and should include the pelvis. These are useful in the diagnosis of fluid collections, foreign bodies, bony fractures, and, occasionally, free air. The optimal radiograph to identify pneumoperitoneum is the upright chest radiograph. However, in the multiply injured child, especially when unstable, obtaining such a film may not be possible. In this situation, an abdominal roentgenogram with the patient in the lateral decubitus position or a cross-table lateral film is employed. Computed tomography, ultrasonography, isotope scanning, and nuclear magnetic resonance, which may be extremely helpful in the diagnosis of injuries to solid intra-abdominal viscera, are also believed by many to be useful in the initial diagnosis of colorectal trauma and may be invaluable in demonstrating complications such as abscesses, especially in the postoperative patient.[80]

Contrast enemas may be employed in selected instances. Specifically, this technique is more useful in a stable patient without peritoneal signs or in a child who presents late in the course of the injury. In these patients, water-soluble contrast material is used and administered with great care.

Other Diagnostic Methods

A complete blood count and amylase determination is routinely obtained. A urinalysis is essential in the evaluation of any trauma patient but is particularly important in assessing colorectal injury. If the child is unable to void spontaneously, a urethral catheter is gently inserted. The possibility of urethral injury or any difficulty in advancing the catheter mandates a urethrogram.

Occasionally, peritoneal lavage can provide evidence of bowel disruption when the effluent is examined for bile and white blood cells. When the amount of either of these is increased, a Gram stain of the fluid is helpful.

MANAGEMENT

General Guidelines

When colorectal trauma is identified or strongly suspected, the child should be resuscitated expeditiously, stabilized with blood pressure and urine output reestablished, and then taken directly to the operating room if necessary. With penetrating trauma secondary to a gunshot wound, celiotomy is mandatory. A selective approach, however, can be applied to penetrating trauma resulting from stab wounds. Celiotomy is mandatory in the presence of peritonitis, evisceration, or leaking of bile, intestinal contents, or urine. In the absence of obvious signs of intraperitoneal injury, the hemodynamically stable patient is admitted for careful observation, which includes serial abdominal examination in addition to the plain radiographs previously described. If signs of peritoneal irritation, hemodynamic instability, or free air on abdominal radiographs develop, operative intervention is indicated. Thus, physical examination is the cornerstone of management of the patient with a stab wound to the abdomen.

Rectal injuries are managed by diversion, débridement, and drainage. Perineal and anal lesions are managed selectively, depending on the severity of the injury and the absence or presence of associated injuries. Minor perineal or anal injuries (i.e., no major tissue loss, minimal contamination, and no associated injuries) may be managed by débridement and primary repair without proximal diversion. Major perineal or anal injury, especially when associated with rectal injury or pelvic fractures, generally requires débridement, repair, and proximal diversion.

Because sepsis is an ever-present threat in colorectal injuries, antibiotic coverage should be instituted early in the course of the injury. The selected antibiotics should cover aerobic and anaerobic organisms and are given intravenously prior to celiotomy. If no perforation is identified, antibiotics can be discontinued; however, with established contamination, the antibiotics are continued for at least 5 to 7 days.

Although advocated by some, the efficacy of adding antibiotics to irrigating solutions has not been definitively established.[80, 81] Copious amounts of warm saline to irrigate any area of suspected contamination are usually sufficient to dilute and wash away debris and bacteria.

Surgery for Colonic Injury

Access

The child is positioned to allow maximal abdominal and, if necessary, perineal exposure. Surgical drapes are placed in a manner that allows access to all areas of the abdominal cavity. In older children, a midline incision is used. For infants and toddlers, a transverse abdominal incision may be equally appropriate.[40] At celiotomy, major hemorrhage requires immediate attention. Any obvious bowel perforation site is packed with moist gauze to avoid further contamination. The abdominal cavity is then systematically explored after blood, fecal material, or other fluids are evacuated. Extensive lavage is employed in an attempt to remove all debris and minimize bacterial contamination. The colon is then carefully examined from the ileocecal area to the pelvic peritoneal reflection. Mobilization of the colon to reach retroperitoneal areas is used selectively, and simultaneous colonoscopy can be useful in special instances. If the site of injury is not identified or a suspected second site remains elusive, colonic air insufflation with a colonoscope or rectal tube is a helpful adjunct. In this technique, the abdominal cavity is filled with saline, and a search for bubbling is made. After the location and extent of any colonic injury is determined, the mesenteric blood supply is evaluated.

Because different types of injury and associated factors such as age and general condition of the child, interval between injury and repair, number and severity of associated injuries, and degree of soiling necessitate different approaches, no standard method for treatment of colonic trauma is possible. The surgeon must weigh all possible options and then choose the approach that best suits the patient.

Options for Surgical Management and Techniques

Primary Repair without Colostomy. Increasing evidence supports the management of favorable colonic wounds by primary repair (Fig. 25–1A).[4, 12–14, 27, 32, 35, 38, 48, 49, 55, 63, 64, 71, 82, 92, 102] However, considerable controversy as to what constitutes a favorable wound exists. Most investigators agree that punctures, clean stab wounds, and low-velocity missile wounds can be primarily closed. Stone and Fabian have outlined seven contraindications to primary closure in adults.[104]

1. Shock preoperatively
2. An interval of 8 hours or more between injury and repair
3. Gross fecal contamination of the peritoneal cavity
4. Presence of hemoperitoneum greater than 1 liter
5. Two or more concomitant organ injuries in the abdomen
6. Colon wound so destructive that it requires resection
7. Extensive loss of abdominal wall

These guidelines are useful for the adult population but may not be indicated for the injured child. Some believe that the first five items are not absolute contraindications;

for example, it may be that delay is of major importance only if there is frank peritonitis, and there is also a preference among surgeons to primarily repair right colonic injuries only.[80, 94] However, the safety of primary closure of selected left colonic wounds has also been demonstrated, suggesting that despite known anatomic and physiologic differences, trauma to the right and left colon can be managed similarly.[41, 72, 80, 99, 107] Primary closure offers distinct advantages: absence of a stoma and its complications, elimination of stomal care and closure, and decreased length of hospitalization.[99] It seems feasible that primary closure should be employed whenever it is deemed safe by the operating surgeon.

Technique. The colonic wound is isolated using moist gauze or other appropriate wound protection. Simple punctures are closed with interrupted synthetic absorbable sutures. Lacerations and low-velocity bullet wounds require limited débridement followed by suture repair. A catheter may be inserted through the colonic wound to aspirate excess fluid and air. Single-or double-layer closure using synthetic absorbable suture material is employed; we prefer to use single-layer closure. Whenever possible, a transverse closure is used to minimize luminal narrowing. Serosal lacerations with intact mucosa can either be left alone or reinforced with Lembert-type sutures. The latter choice is more appropriate when the underlying subserosa has been attenuated because of colonic distention or injury. Although staples can be employed in older children, they may not be applicable in younger patients because of the small size of the colon. The suture line can be covered by an omental patch, although the efficacy of this maneuver is unproven.

Primary Repair with Proximal Colostomy. A proximal colostomy (Fig. 25–1B) is employed to protect the repair of a complex left colonic wound. It can also be used in the case of a mesenteric or subserosal hematoma of the distal colon; however, in this particular setting, resection of the affected areas with either primary anastomosis and proximal colostomy or exteriorization of the injury is preferable. For extensive right colonic wounds, resection of the damaged segment, closure of the distal bowel, and proximal end colostomy or ileostomy are recommended.

Technique. Primary repair is performed as outlined previously. For left-sided colonic repairs, a transverse loop colostomy is constructed without mobilizing the colon. A small window is made in the avascular portion of the mesocolon, and a Penrose drain placed through the window and encircling the bowel allows the colon to be exteriorized through a counterincision. The exteriorized bowel is then secured without tension to the peritoneum and posterior fascia with interrupted synthetic absorbable sutures, and the Penrose drain is replaced with a short plastic rod. Twenty-four hours later, the stoma is opened at the bedside with a disposable battery-operated cautery unit. Suturing of the mucosa is not necessary. Because complications related to stomas in children are common, great care in their construction is essential.[74]

Limited Resection with Exteriorization or Wide Resection with Proximal Enterostoma. These procedures are the most expeditious options for management of colonic injuries deemed unsuitable for primary closure or resection and anastomosis. The procedure of choice when there is

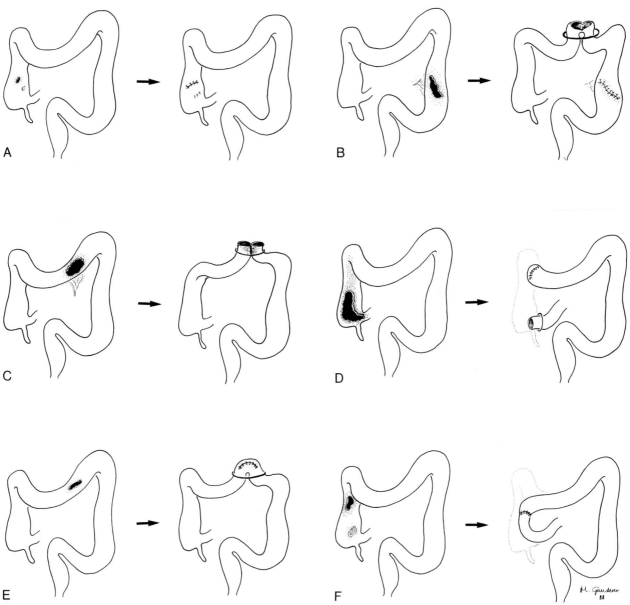

FIGURE 25–1

Schematic representation of the options for surgical management of colonic injuries. *A*, Primary repair without colostomy. Through-and-through colonic perforation managed by minimal débridement and transverse closure of both sites. *B*, Primary repair with proximal colostomy. A more extensive perforation of the colon managed by débridement and closure and protected by a loop colostomy proximal to the injury. *C*, Limited resection with exteriorization. Excision of the perforated segment with double-barrel exteriorization. If the perforation is smaller and the back wall of the colon is healthy, a loop colostomy can be used. The end colostomy and the mucous fistula may also be brought out separately. *D*, Wide resection with proximal enterostoma. Extensive destruction managed by resection of the cecum and ascending colon, ileostomy, and oversewing of the distal colon. *E*, Exteriorization of primary repair. The edges of the laceration are débrided and a primary closure performed. The closed segment is then exteriorized and allowed to heal before being returned to the abdominal cavity. *F*, Resection and primary anastomosis. An extensive double perforation is managed by resection of the affected segment followed by end-to-end ileocolostomy.

damage to a short segment of colon in the presence of extensive peritonitis or many other intra-abdominal lesions is limited resection of that segment with exteriorization (Fig. 25–1*C*). With extensive injuries to the right colon, wide resection with proximal ileostomy is recommended

(Fig. 25–1*D*).[39] All segments of the colon except the low sigmoid can be mobilized and exteriorized.

Although colostomies are intended to minimize the occurrence of intra-abdominal septic complications, in practice, this is not always accomplished. Several reports suggest that the incidence of intra-abdominal infection can be higher in patients with stomas than in those treated by primary closure or resection and anastomosis.[17, 80, 94, 107] Nance compiled eight major series in which selective management of colonic injury with and without colostomy was compared.[13, 14, 55, 64, 80, 94, 102, 104] The percentage of patients, primarily adults, treated with colostomy in any one institution ranged from 19 to 75%. Overall, the mortality rate for patients treated with colostomy was higher than that for patients treated without colostomy. All of the series except one were retrospective.[104] It is possible, however, that colostomies were employed in the more seriously ill or injured patients.[80]

Despite these shortcomings, colostomy is still one of the mainstays of the treatment of children with serious colonic injury. An enterostoma is preferred when primary colonic repair or resection with primary anastomosis is not judged to be safe.

Technique. After adequate mobilization of the injured colon segment to be exteriorized, a suitable site for the stoma is chosen on the abdominal wall. Stomas should generally not be brought through the incision. A separate incision is made over the rectus muscle, away from the celiotomy incision, bony prominences, and natural folds, allowing comfortable placement and handling of an appliance. The damaged colon is temporarily closed with either sutures or a stapler to avoid contamination of the subcutaneous tissues during exteriorization. In smaller children, the peritoneum and the fascia are carefully sutured circumferentially to the exteriorized colon using interrupted stitches; failure to do so can lead to parastomal hernias and prolapse. A loop colostomy is usually adequate for fecal diversion.[43] A small rod or rubber catheter holds the colon above the skin maintaining the spur. Tension must be avoided. A double-barreled colostomy or a divided colostomy can also be employed.

Exteriorization of Primary Repair. In this two-staged repair (Fig. 25–1*E*), an attempt is made to combine the advantages of primary wound closure with the safety of exteriorization. The injured segment is closed and exteriorized above the skin level, similar to a loop colostomy. The segment is protected with moist gauze, and if healing occurs properly, the patient is reoperated on after 5 to 10 days, at which time the exteriorized colon is mobilized and returned to the abdominal cavity, and the abdominal wall is closed. If healing fails to occur in the exteriorized loop, the loop is transformed into a colostomy. This method has some advocates, but a less than optimal success rate has led others to abandon it.[1, 17, 25, 32, 58, 76, 78, 80, 92] This technique does offer an attractive alternative for the child with multiple intra-abdominal injuries in whom resection and primary anastomosis seems unsafe; however, there is currently no reported experience with this repair in the pediatric age group.

Technique. If exteriorization of primary repair is employed, the guidelines are the same as those for a colostomy. Tension and venous stasis must be avoided.[58]

Resection and Primary Anastomosis. This approach (Fig. 25–1*F*) is most frequently applied to injuries of the right colon that are not amenable to primary repair.[4, 19, 39, 45, 85] However, evidence is increasing that, in other selected patients, resection and primary anastomosis are also applicable to the other colonic segments.[63, 82, 107] Slim and colleagues demonstrated that, in children, primary anastomosis without colostomy following resection for penetrating trauma is equally effective on both sides of the colon.[99] Resection and primary anastomosis have been advocated by some researchers as superior to ileostomy, even in the presence of peritonitis.[32, 39] However, any primary anastomosis following colonic resection must be approached cautiously. An example of colonic perforation in young children occurred during attempted hydrostatic reduction of ileocolic intussusception.[29, 66] The usual procedure for this mishap is right colectomy and ileocolostomy, but the technique chosen depends on the site and extent of disruption.

The contraindications outlined in the section on primary repair must be carefully observed.[104] If there is sufficient doubt as to whether anastomosis is contraindicated, exteriorization is advisable.

Technique. We prefer single-layer end-to-end anastomosis using interrupted synthetic absorbable sutures for colonic as well as small bowel anastomoses.

Surgery for Anorectal Injury

Access

The child with suspected rectal injury is positioned in the lithotomy position in such a way that the legs can be moved down and access to the abdomen gained. Suspending the legs of a small child by means of a frame that can be tilted down is very useful if an abdominoperineal approach is anticipated. Gentle digital palpation precedes endoscopy. A nasal speculum is helpful in small children. Rectoscopy and sigmoidoscopy follow endoscopy. We prefer the rigid, open scopes, because they allow for better simultaneous evacuation of stool and blood as well as irrigation. In girls, vaginoscopy precedes rectosigmoidoscopy, and in some severe perineal injuries, cystoscopy may be indicated. If sexual abuse is suspected, appropriate sampling is necessary. When there is minimal or no identifiable injury, the child is returned to the ward and observed.

Options for Surgical Management and Techniques

Local Repair Only. This approach is indicated only if the injury is at the level of the anus, superficial to the sphincter mechanism, or limited to the rectal mucosa.[47] If there is doubt about the extent or depth of the lesion, proximal diversion is indicated.

Technique. The affected area is cleaned and débrided. A few fine absorbable sutures may be used in the deep layer. The skin is loosely approximated, but the portion close to the anus is left open.

Repair, Proximal Diversion, and Drainage. This approach is the mainstay of management in major anorectal injuries.[47, 60, 65, 80, 89, 108] When primary repair is not possible, management consists of débridement, proximal diversion, and perineal drainage. In addition to colostomy, presacral drainage, rectal repair, and evacuation of intestinal contents by irrigation of the distal segment are recommended, especially if primary repair cannot be achieved.[60, 95] These maneuvers are believed to prevent ongoing contamination of the perirectal space. When properly constructed, a sigmoid loop colostomy provides excellent diversion of the fecal stream.[7, 43] We prefer this approach, because this stoma is faster to construct and easier to take down than a divided colostomy or an end sigmoidostomy and Hartmann closure. After any perineal and anorectal repair, the site must be periodically inspected for early signs of infection. If signs of infection are noted, prompt reexploration is indicated.

Technique. If the wound is mainly perineal, it is extensively irrigated and cautiously débrided. Excessive débridement is avoided, because this can inadvertently result in sphincter dysfunction. Viable muscle tissue is reapproximated with synthetic absorbable sutures, suction catheters are placed in areas of potential fluid accumulation, and mucosa and skin are loosely approximated. If there is any concern about the viability of tissue or tension on the edges, the mucosa, the skin, or both are left open.

Drains

Drainage of intraperitoneal colonic repair or anastomoses usually is not indicated and may in fact be detrimental.[62, 69, 100, 116] It is inappropriate to rely on drains to salvage a nonviable or questionably viable intestinal segment. In such instances, exteriorization or a protective colostomy should be employed.[80]

Drainage of rectal injuries, however, is essential. We prefer soft, silicone rubber drains placed in the retrorectal space and connected to a closed, constant suction system. The drains can be brought out either through the perineum just anterior to the coccyx, through the abdominal wall without opening the perineum in select cases, or through both sites.

Wound Closure

Midline incisions are closed with either nonabsorbable monofilament or synthetic absorbable sutures using age-appropriate sizes. We prefer interrupted sutures, although a continuous running suture technique can also be employed. Transverse incisions are closed in layers using the same suture materials for each layer. Retention sutures are not used in children. Irrigation of each layer prior to closure is advisable. Unless there is massive contamination, we approximate the skin without tension using interrupted monofilament sutures. Skin sutures may be removed between postoperative days 4 and 6, at which time adhesive strips are applied.

Colostomy Closure

Reestablishment of large bowel continuity can be performed between 4 to 6 weeks after the initial operation; however, we prefer to wait 6 to 8 weeks, which allows an additional 2 weeks for nutritional repletion, lessening of the inflammatory response, and decrease of edema. Colostomy closures at 6 to 8 weeks or longer after the initial procedure seem to have a lower complication rate.[23, 84] We believe it to be a misconception that colostomy construction and closure are simple procedures. Both are associated with considerable morbidity and occasional mortality in both adults and children.[37, 74, 84, 106, 115] To achieve low morbidity with colostomy closure after colon injury, the patient must be carefully prepared and the procedure meticulously performed.[17, 22] In preparation for closure, the child should have a barium enema to demonstrate adequate patency of the distal bowel. If the colostomy was established for rectosigmoid trauma, endoscopy should precede colostomy closure. We prefer antegrade, whole-bowel irrigation with an oral lavage solution, as well as distal segment irrigation with saline. Intravenous antibiotics are given prior to the operation and continued for at least 24 to 48 hours postoperatively.

The colostomy is fully taken down, and a formal end-to-end approximation if performed. We prefer single-layer anastomoses using synthetic absorbable suture material. The abdominal wall is closed in the previously described manner.

PITFALLS IN MANAGEMENT

Because of the variety of etiologic factors in colonic and rectal injuries in children, the difficulties associated with obtaining a history and doing a thorough examination, and the complexity of some of these injuries, opportunities for pitfalls in management abound. The lesion can be missed altogether; this is often the case with anorectal injuries, particularly impalements and sexually related trauma. Children often play in areas that are off-limits, and they have a tendency to conceal mishaps incurred in these situations. Young children are often not aware of what really happened to them. Victims of sexual abuse are usually afraid to relate their traumatic experience to others.

Failure to identify a colonic injury with the resultant continual fecal soiling can lead to disastrous consequences. Lack of recognition of associated injuries in other organs is a substantial cause of morbidity and mortality. The presence of blood, bile, pancreatic juice, urine, or barium compound the consequences of fecal soilage. Any bowel wall damage that interferes with blood supply, as well as partial thickness damage or hematomas, can lead to delayed rupture or fecal fistula.

Although pneumoperitoneum, as a rule, mandates celiotomy, in rare settings free air in the peritoneal cavity of a child on high-pressure respiratory support may be secondary to mediastinal air dissection.[109]

COMPLICATIONS

Colonic and rectal injuries have a high potential for both intra-abdominal and extra-abdominal morbidity and mortality. The complication rate is directly proportional to the number of serious associated injuries and does not seem to be influenced by the method of colon management.[12, 41, 60, 63, 75, 82, 85, 99, 104, 107, 108, 117] Moore and colleagues and other researchers have correlated the number and severity of organs injured with the morbidity and outcome using a penetrating abdominal trauma index.[41, 75, 79] Flint and associates developed a grading system for evaluating patients with colon injuries based on the degree of contamination, the number of associated injuries, the presence or absence of shock, and the time between injury and operation.[32]

The predominant complications are of septic origin, including intra-abdominal or intrapelvic abscess formation, wound infection, wound dehiscence, fecal fistulas, urinary tract fistulas, pelvic osteomyelitis, and adhesive bowel obstruction.[9, 12, 32, 41, 60, 75, 80, 82, 99, 104] Extra-abdominal septic complications such as systemic sepsis, pneumonia, and meningitis can also occur.[60]

Although the mortality associated with well-managed colonic and rectal injuries is relatively low, the morbidity of these lesions is considerable. The incidence of intra-abdominal abscess formation is estimated to be from 5 to 15% in adults.[32, 41, 80, 104] In the pediatric age group, however, because there is a great variety of etiologic agents and management modalities as well as the possibility of associated injuries, exact figures regarding morbidity are currently not available. Because sepsis is one of the gravest complications, any patient whose postoperative course is accompanied by fever, leukocytosis, prolonged ileus, or other signs of sepsis should be aggressively investigated for the presence of intra-abdominal abscesses. Ultrasonography is noninvasive and allows frequent examinations, often at the bedside, without radiation. When an abscess is identified, prompt drainage should be performed. For a well-localized single abscess, ultrasonographically or CT-guided percutaneous drainage can be attempted.[46] Multiple intra-abdominal abscesses require open drainage.

The incidence of wound infection is difficult to determine, because multiple factors, including the type of celiotomy closure, play a role. In our experience using mostly primary closures, infections have occurred in 5 to 10% of pediatric patients. Incisions managed by primary closure must be carefully monitored to allow early recognition and management of cellulitis, fascitis, synergistic infections, and abscess formation. The incidence of wound infection is reportedly higher in patients with stomas.[41]

The occurrence of fecal and urinary fistulas is uncommon, as is pelvic osteomyelitis.[9, 41, 60] The incidence of adhesive bowel obstruction, a complication with potential long-lasting morbidity, is enhanced by intra-abdominal infection or the presence of foreign material.[77]

Complications related to colostomy placement include poor site choice, stomal necrosis, wound separation, abscess formation, retraction, stricture, and prolapse.[74] The need for meticulous technique in the construction of a pediatric colostomy has been discussed previously. Failure to recognize or appropriately treat sphincter damage can lead to serious consequences and interfere with the child's future sociability.

The importance of preventing or recognizing and managing the psychological complications of anorectal injuries must be emphasized. The older child or adolescent with a colostomy will need not only help with stomal care, but also reassurance.

CASE STUDIES

CASE 1 (Fig. 25–2)

A 6-year-old boy fell from a porch, landing on a freshly pruned hedge. On the following day, he developed fever and abdominal pain followed by vomiting. Initially admitted to a local hospital, he was subsequently referred to the Children's Hospital 36 hours after the accident. A small perineal laceration from a twig was noted. Upon insertion of a urethral catheter, bloody urine was obtained. Upright radiographic films of the abdomen revealed free air evident below the right hemidiaphragm (two arrows) and air present in the urinary bladder (three arrows). This finding was not appreciated at the initial radiographic evaluation.

The operative findings were rectosigmoid perforation, bladder laceration, and tears in the ileum and jejunum. The patient underwent bladder closure and drainage, repair of ileal and jejunal tears, limited rectosigmoid débridement, pelvic drainage, and sigmoid loop colostomy. The patient recovered well and underwent colostomy closure 2 months after the initial operation.

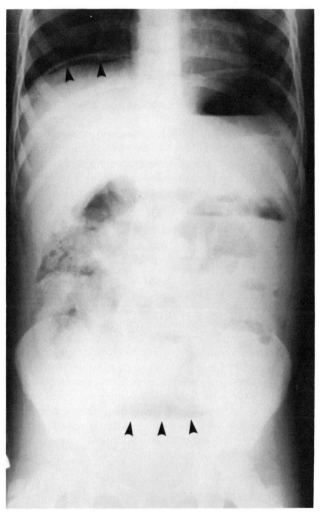

FIGURE 25–2

Radiograph of a 6-year-old boy with an impalement injury that caused trauma to the bladder, ileum, jejunum, and colon. Upright films show free air below the right hemidiaphragm (*two arrows*) and air in the urinary bladder (*three arrows*).

Comment

Severe impalement injuries through the anorectum may present with few external signs. A high index of suspicion, a thorough physical examination, and careful interpretation of radiographic films are essential. These injuries carry a high morbidity and can be lethal.

CASE 2 (Fig. 25–3)

A 2½-month-old premature boy presented with lower gastrointestinal bleeding following colonoscopy. After transfer to our institution, rapid resuscitation and celiotomy were performed. The suspected sigmoid perforation was identified. Because of the child's prematurity and the prolonged interval between injury and celiotomy, the surgeon chose exteriorization of the affected area as a sigmoid loop colostomy. Reestablishment of bowel continuity was performed 6 months after the initial operation. The patient recovered well.

Comment

Because of the small size of the colon, endoscopic examination in small children requires great skill and judgment. If a perforation is immediately recognized, primary closure is a possible option, provided that the colon has been mechanically cleansed and the affected bowel segment is otherwise healthy.

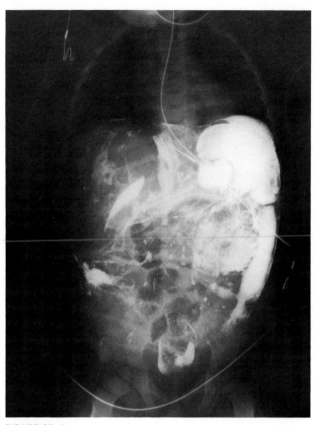

FIGURE 25–4
Radiograph of a 9-month-old boy with a perforated colon with air and scattered contrast free in the peritoneal cavity.

CASE 3 (Fig. 25–4)

A 9-month-old boy presented with a 3-day history of abdominal pain, bilious vomiting, and rectal bleeding. The diagnosis of ileocolic intussusception was made and confirmed radiologically. Hydrostatic reduction was attempted, resulting in partial reduction, but the procedure also caused cecal perforation. At operation, the intraperitoneal barium was evacuated, the ileocecal reduction was completed, and the cecum was resected. Because of the extravasation of barium and the ischemic appearance of the reduced intussusceptum, the surgeon exteriorized the ileum and the ascending colon. Bowel continuity was reestablished 2 months after the initial operation, and the child recovered well.

Comment

Bowel perforation is a well-recognized complication of attempted hydrostatic reduction of ileocolic intussusception. Reduction is more difficult in the patient with a long history of intussusception and in the younger child. In such situations, attempts at reduction should be made with extreme care. Although in this case, the operating surgeon chose diversion, in most children resection with primary ileocolic anastomosis is possible.

CASE 4 (Fig. 25–5)

A 4-week-old girl presented with Hirschsprung disease. A barium enema done 4 days following full thickness rectal biopsy clearly demonstrates extravasation of contrast material into the

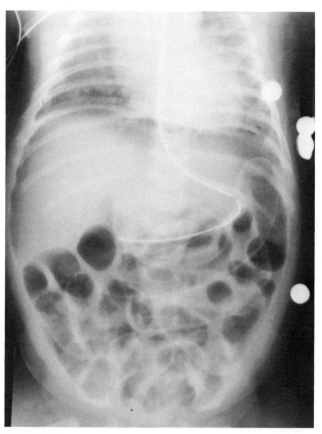

FIGURE 25–3
Radiograph showing sigmoid perforation in a 2½-month-old child with extensive free intraperitoneal air.

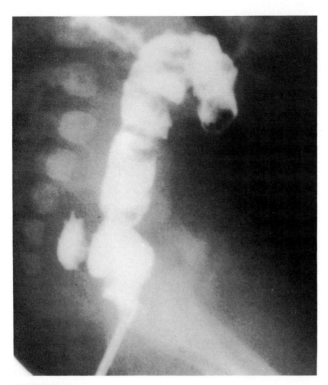

FIGURE 25–5
Radiograph of a 4-week-old infant with Hirschsprung disease showing extravasation of contrast material into the perirectal space.

perirectal space. A sigmoid diverting colostomy was constructed immediately above the transition zone in bowel with normal ganglion cells. Subsequently, the patient underwent a pull-through operation and recovered.

Comment

Deep, full thickness biopsies are not necessary in this condition. The barium enema, performed too soon after the biopsy, should have preceded it. This avoidable complication can lead to pelvic sepsis and will create difficulties at the time of the eventual definitive pull-through procedure.

CASE 5 (Fig. 25–6)

A 5-year-old girl fell onto the telescoping antenna of a television set placed on the floor while playing with siblings. The patient was wearing pants, and there was no blood on the antenna, the garment, or the rectum. Because of pain, the patient was admitted to the pediatric service for evaluation. Although her temperature rose to 39.4°C and the white blood cell count increased to 32,600/mm³ with a shift to the left, it was thought that no rectal injury occurred and she was discharged.

Two weeks after discharge, the child was readmitted to the pediatric surgical service, still febrile with a large, tender, right gluteal mass (see Fig. 25–6). The diagnosis of perirectal abscess was made, and 100 ml of purulent material was evacuated. No site of perforation could be identified at endoscopy. The patient became afebrile and recovered rapidly.

Comment

Although rectal trauma as well as child abuse were suspected during the first admission, endoscopy was not performed. Follow up was inadequate, and the child returned quite ill with a large abscess. Any suspected anorectal injury mandates careful evaluation. The absence of external signs should not deter from performing endoscopic examination, particularly in a symptomatic child. Close follow up is essential.

CASE 6 (Figs. 25–7, 25–8)

A 17-month-old boy was run over by a riding lawn mower operated by a sibling. The vehicle backed over the child, who was trapped under the raised cutting deck. The findings included severe perineal laceration with transection of right gluteal muscles, transection of the right sciatic nerve, and a comminuted fracture of the right hip joint and ischial tuberosity. The lower rectum was lacerated and part of the sphincter mechanism avulsed.

The rectal exam (see Fig. 25–7) preceded the endoscopic evaluation. The patient underwent extensive lavage and conservative débridement followed by repair of the lower rectum and its musculature, primary repair of the sciatic nerve, repair of the gluteal muscle, and drainage. The repair was protected by a sigmoid loop

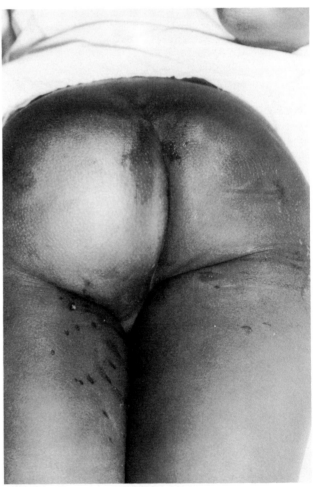

FIGURE 25–6
A 5-year-old girl with a large right gluteal mass, which was the result of an infection sustained after she fell on a television antenna while playing.

colostomy, and the patient was placed in a half-body spica cast. Three months after the initial operation, the diverting colostomy was closed.

The follow-up photograph (see Fig. 25–8), 6 months after stomal closure, shows good anatomic appearance. The child had normal gait and sphincter control 3 years following the injury.

Comment

This severe lawn mower injury was associated with extensive soiling and some devitalized tissue. Thorough irrigation and limited débridement allowed primary anatomical reconstruction. Local suction catheter drainage and the diverting colostomy were essential in the prevention of septic complications.

SUMMARY

Although colorectal trauma is not common in children, failure to recognize or properly treat this injury can lead to substantial morbidity and mortality. A wide variety of etiologic agents can produce colonic or rectal injury. Some of the mechanisms are specific for the pediatric age group (e.g., colonic perforation through barium enema in attempts to reduce ileocolic intussusceptions, colorectal perforations by thermometers in infants, damage to sphincter mechanisms through sexual abuse). If the need for surgical intervention is not immediately apparent, the most useful diagnostic approach after a thorough initial exam is frequent, careful reexaminations.

The majority of simple colonic perforations can be treated by primary repair. After the edges of the wound are conservatively trimmed, a transverse closure is done. Right colonic injuries, which are not amenable to primary closure, are usually managed by resection and primary anastomosis. This technique is not so readily applicable to the left colon. In very sick children, particularly those with associated intra-abdominal injury, or in those with extensive colonic damage or soilage, exteriorization by means of colostomy is the preferred management.

The key for successful management of anorectal injuries

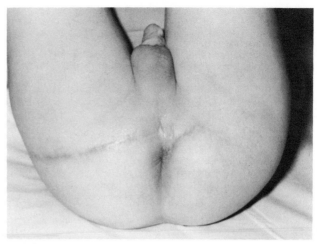

FIGURE 25–8
Follow-up photograph of the boy shown in Figure 25–7 taken 6 months after the injury.

and severe perineal trauma involving the rectum or its sphincter mechanism is cautious débridement, closure if possible, generous drainage, and proximal diversion, usually by using a sigmoid loop colostomy.

When treating colorectal trauma in the young patient, a few differences between children and adults must be stressed:

1. The history is more difficult to obtain.
2. Physical examination can be confusing.
3. The pelvis of very young children is small and fairly flat. Consequently, most intrapelvic organs occupy an intra-abdominal position.
4. The colon is thinner and therefore easier to perforate.
5. The omentum in very young children is not fully developed and therefore does not reach all colonic segments.
6. Congenital or acquired anatomic abnormalities (i.e., malrotation, scoliosis) will displace the colon.
7. The child needs additional nutritional support, because growth must be taken into account.

The management of colorectal injury in children can be challenging, and poor treatment can lead to serious long-lasting physical and psychological disability. Properly treated children, however, will reward the surgeon with prompt healing and recovery.

References

1. Adkins RB, Zirkle PK, Waterhouse G: Penetrating colon trauma. J Trauma 24:491–499, 1984.
2. Altner PC: Constrictive lesions of the colon due to blunt trauma to the abdomen. Surg Gynecol Obstet 118:1257–1262, 1964.
3. Andrews EW: Pneumatic rupture of the intestine, or a new type of industrial accident. Surg Gynecol Obstet 12:63–72, 1911.
4. Arango A, Baxter CR, Shires T: Surgical management of traumatic injuries of the right colon. Arch Surg 114:703–706, 1979.
5. Arcari FA: Blunt abdominal trauma in infants and children. J Mich Med Soc 61:335–336, 1962.
6. Armstrong EA, Dunbar JS, Gravvis ER, et al: Intussusception com-

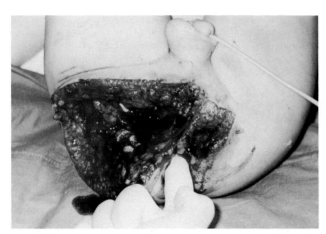

FIGURE 25–7
Rectal examination of a 17-month-old boy who was run over by a lawn mower and trapped under the raised cutting deck shows extensive gluteal and perineal destruction.

plicated by distal perforation of the colon. Radiology 136:77–81, 1980.

7. Armstrong RG, Schmitt HJ Jr, Patterson LT: Combat wounds of the extraperitoneal rectum. Surgery 74:570–574, 1973.
8. Axelrod AJ, Hanley PH: Treatment of perforating wounds of the colon and rectum: A reevaluation. South Med J 60:811–814, 1967.
9. Barlow B, Niemirska M, Gandhi RP: Ten years' experience with pediatric gunshot wounds. J Pediatr Surg 17:927–932, 1982.
10. Barlow B, Niemirska M, Gandhi RP: Stab wounds in children. J Pediatr Surg 18:926–929, 1983.
11. Barone JE, Sohn N, Nealon TF Jr: Perforations and foreign bodies of the rectum: Report of 28 cases. Ann Surg 184:601–603, 1976.
12. Bartizal JF, Boyd DR, Folk FA, et al: A critical review of management of 392 colonic and rectal injuries. Dis Colon Rectum 17:313–318, 1974.
13. Beall AC, Bricker DL, Alessi FJ, et al: Surgical considerations in the management of civilian colon injuries. Ann Surg 173:971–978, 1971.
14. Biggs TM, Beall AC, Gordon WB, et al: Surgical management of civilian colon injuries. J Trauma 3:484–492, 1963.
15. Black CT, Pokorny WJ, McGill CW, et al: Anorectal trauma in children. J Pediatr Surg 17:501–504, 1982.
16. Bowers WF: Surgical treatment in abdominal trauma: Comparison of results in war and peace. Mil Med 118:9–22, 1956.
17. Burch JM, Brock JC, Gewirtzman L, et al: The injured colon. Ann Surg 203:701–711, 1986.
18. Cain WS, Howell CG, Ziegler MM, et al: Rectosigmoid perforation and intestinal evisceration from transanal suction. J Pediatr Surg 18:10–13, 1983.
19. Chilimindris C, Boyd DR, Carlson LE, et al: A critical review of the management of right colon injuries. J Trauma 11:651–660, 1970.
20. Classen JN, Martin RE, Sabagal J: Iatrogenic lesions of the colon and rectum. South Med J 68:1417–1428, 1975.
21. Cox EF: Blunt abdominal trauma. A 5-year analysis of 870 patients requiring celiotomy. Ann Surg 199:467–474, 1984.
22. Crass RA, Salbi F, Trunkey DD: Colostomy closure after colon injury: A low morbidity procedure. J Trauma 27:1237–1239, 1987.
23. Crass RA, Tranbaugh RF, Kudsk KA, et al: Colorectal foreign bodies and perforation. Ann Surg 141:85–88, 1981.
24. Cutler EC: Military surgery—United States Army. European theatre of operations, 1944–1945. Surg Gynecol Obstet 82:261–274, 1946.
25. Dang CV, Peter ET, Parks SN, et al: Trauma of the colon: Early drop-back of exteriorized repair. Arch Surg 117:652–656, 1982.
26. Dauterive AH, Flancbaum L, Cox EF: Blunt intestinal trauma: A modern day review. Ann Surg 201:198–203, 1985.
27. Demetriades D, Rabinowitx B, Sofianos C, et al: The management of penetrating injuries of the back. A prospective study of 230 patients. Ann Surg 207:72–74, 1988.
28. Dickinson SJ, Shaw A, Santulli TV: Rupture of the gastrointestinal tract in children by blunt abdominal trauma. Surg Gynecol Obstet 130:655–657, 1970.
29. Ein SH, Mercer S, Humphry A, et al: Colon perforation during attempted barium enema reduction of intussusception. J Pediatr Surg 16:313–315, 1981.
30. Ellerstein NS, Canaven JW: Sexual abuse of boys. Am J Dis Child 134:255–257, 1980.
31. Fisher G, Goebel H, Latta E: Penetration of the colon by a ventriculo-peritoneal drain resulting in an intra-cerebral abscess. Zentralbl Neurochir 44:155–160, 1983.
32. Flint LM, Vitale GC, Richardson JD, et al: The injured colon: Relationship of management to complications. Ann Surg 193:619–623, 1981.
33. Fonkalsrud EW, Clatworthy HW Jr: Accidental perforation of the colon and rectum in newborn infants. N Engl J Med 272:1097–1100, 1965.
34. Fox PF: Impalement injuries of the perineum. Am J Surg 82:511–516, 1951.
35. Freeark RJ: The injured colon (editorial). J Trauma 17:563–564, 1977.
36. Frykberg ER, Tepas JJ III: Terrorist bombings: Lessons learned from Belfast to Beirut. Ann Surg 208:569–576, 1988.
37. Garber HI, Morris DM, Eisenstat TE, et al: Factors influencing the morbidity of colostomy closure. Dis Colon Rectum 25:464–470, 1982.
38. Garfinkle SE, Cohen SG, Matolo NM, et al: Civilian colon injuries. Arch Surg 109:402–404, 1974.
39. Garrison RN, Shively EH, Baker C, et al: Evaluation of management of the emergency right hemicolectomy. J Trauma 19:734–739, 1979.
40. Gauderer MWL: A rationale for the routine use of transverse abdominal incisions in infants and children. J Pediatr Surg 16:583–586, 1981.
41. George SM Jr., Fabian TC, Mangiante EC: Colon trauma: Further support for primary repair. Am J Surg 156:16–20, 1988.
42. Ghazi A, Grossman M: Complications of colonoscopy and polypectomy. Surg Clin North Am 62:889–896, 1982.
43. Goligher J: Injuries of the rectum and colon. In: Goligher J (ed): Surgery of the Anus, Rectum and Colon. London, Bailliere Tindall, 1984, pp 1119–1136.
44. Grablowsky OM, Gage JO, Ray JE, et al: Traumatic colonic and rectal injuries. Dis Colon Rectum 16:296–299, 1973.
45. Granchow MI, Lavenson GS Jr, McNamara J: Surgical management of traumatic injuries of the colon and rectum. Arch Surg 100:515–520, 1970.
46. Haaga JR, Weinstein AJ: CT guided percutaneous aspiration and drainage of abscesses. Am J Roentgenol 135:1187–1194, 1980.
47. Haas PA, Fox RA Jr.: Civilian injuries of the rectum and anus. Dis Colon Rectum 22:17–23, 1979.
48. Haygood FD, Polk HC: Gunshot wounds of the colon. A review of 100 consecutive patients, with emphasis on complications and their causes. Am J Surg 131:213–218, 1976.
49. Haynes CD, Gunn CH, Martin JD: Colon injuries. Arch Surg 96:944–948, 1968.
50. Hobbs CJ, Wynne JM: Buggery in childhood—A common syndrome of child abuse. Lancet 2:792–796, 1986.
51. Horwitz MA, Bennett JV: Nursery outbreak of peritonitis with pneumoperitoneum probably caused by thermometer-induced rectal perforation. Am J Epidemiol 104:632–644, 1876.
52. Howell HS, Bartizal JF, Freeark RJ: Blunt trauma involving the colon and rectum. J Trauma 16:624–632, 1976.
53. Imes PR: War surgery of the abdomen. Surg Gynecol Obstet 81:608–616, 1945.
54. Isaacson JE Jr, Buck RL, Kahle HR: Changing concepts of treatment of traumatic injuries of the colon. Dis Colon Rectum 4:168–172, 1961.
55. Josen AS, Ferrer JM Jr, Forde KA, et al: Primary closure of civilian colorectal wounds. Ann Surg 176:782–786, 1972.
56. Kassner EG, McAlister WH, Siegel MJ: Complications of diagnostic radiology. In: Kassner EG (ed): Iatrogenic Disorders of the Fetus, Infant and Child. Vol. 1. New York, Springer Verlag, 1985, pp 1–37.
57. Kaufer C, Wulfing D: Darmverletzungen bei Kinder als Folge stumpfer Bauchtraumen. Z Kinderchir 6:55–66, 1968.
58. Kirkpatrick JR, Rajpal SC: The injured colon: Therapeutic considerations. Am J Surg 129:187–191, 1975.
59. Kozarek R, Earnest D, Silverstein M, et al: Air-pressure induced colon injury during diagnostic colonoscopy. Gastroenterology 78:7–14, 1980.
60. Lavenson GS Jr, Cohen A: Management of rectal injuries. Am J Surg 122:226–230, 1971.
61. Lee BL: Wounds of the colon in the medical department of the United States Army in the World War. Vol. 11. Washington DC, Government Printing Office, 1927, pp 460–461.
62. Lennox MS: Prophylactic drainage of colonic anastomoses. Br J Surg 71:10–11, 1984.
63. LoCicero J III, Tajima T, Drapanas T: A half-century of concepts. J Trauma 15:575–579, 1975.
64. Lucas CE, Ledgerwood AM: Management of the injured colon. Curr Surg 43:190–193, 1986.
65. Lung JA, Turk RP, Miller RE, et al: Wounds of the rectum. Ann Surg 172:985–990, 1970.
66. McAllister WH, Siegel MJ: Complications of diagnostic radiology. In: Kassner EG (ed): Iatrogenic Disorders of the Fetus, Infant and Child. Vol. 1. New York, Springer Verlag, 1985, pp 1–37.
67. McCanse D, Kirchin A, Hinshaw JR: Gastrointestinal foreign bodies. Am J Surg 142:335–337, 1981.
68. McKenzie AD, Bell GA: Non-penetrating injuries of the colon and rectum. Surg Clin North Am 53:735–746, 1972.
69. Marc CW, La Tendresse C, Sako Y: The detrimental effect of drains on colonic anastomoses: An experimental study. Dis Colon Rectum 13:17–25, 1974.
70. Mason JM: Surgery of the colon in the forward battle area. Surgery 18:534–541, 1945.

71. Matolo NM, Cohen SE, Wolfman EF Jr.: Experimental evaluation of primary repair of colonic injuries. Arch Surg 111:78–80, 1976.

72. Matolo NM, Wolfman ER Jr: Primary repair of colonic injuries: A clinical evaluation. J Trauma 17:554–556, 1977.

73. Maull KI, Snoddy JW, Haynes BW Jr: Penetrating wounds of the buttock. Surg Gynecol Obstet 149:855–857, 1979.

74. Mollit DL, Malangoni MA, Ballantine TVN, et al: Colostomy complications in children. Arch Surg 115:455–458, 1980.

75. Moore EE, Dunn EL, Moore JB, et al: Penetrating abdominal trauma index. J Trauma 21:439–445, 1981.

76. Mulherin JL, Sawyers JL: Evaluation of three methods for managing penetrating colon injuries. J Trauma 15:580–587, 1975.

77. Nahrwold DL, Isch JH, Benner BA, et al: Barium peritonitis. Surgery 70:778–781, 1971.

78. Nallathambi MN, Ivatury RR, Rohman M, et al: Penetrating colon injuries: Exteriorized repair versus loop colostomy. J Trauma 27:876–882, 1987.

79. Nallathambi MN, Ivatury RR, Shah PM, et al: Aggressive definitive management of penetrating colon injuries: 136 cases with 3.7 percent mortality. J Trauma 24:500–505, 1984.

80. Nance FC: Injuries to the colon and rectum. In: Mattox KL, Moore EE, Feliciano DV (eds): Trauma. Norwalk, Connecticut, Appleton and Lange, 1988, pp 495–504.

81. Noon GP, Beall AC, Jordon GL, et al: Clinical evaluation of peritoneal irrigation with antibiotic solution. Surgery 62:73–78, 1967.

82. Obeid FN, Sorensen V, Gilford V, et al: Management of colonic trauma: Six-year experience at Henry Ford Hospital. Henry Ford Hosp Med J 31:17–20, 1983.

83. Ogilvie WH: Abdominal wounds in the western desert. Surg Gynecol Obstet 78:225–238, 1944.

84. Parks SE, Hastings PR: Complication of colostomy closure. Am J Surg 149:672–675, 1985.

85. Parks TG: Surgical management of injuries of the large intestine. Br J Surg 68:725–728, 1981.

86. Poer OH: Evaluation of colostomy for present day surgery. Review of 4,939 cases of injury of the colon and rectum. Arch Surg 61:1058–1065, 1950.

87. Pontius RG, Creech O Jr, Debakey ME: Management of large bowel injuries in civilian practice. Ann Surg 146:291–295, 1957.

88. Rabkin JG: The epidemiology of forcible rape. Am J Orthopsychiatry 49:634–647, 1979.

89. Robertson HD, Ray JE, Ferrari BT, et al: Management of rectal trauma. Surg Gynecol Obstet 154:161–164, 1982.

90. Santulli TV: Perforations of the rectum or colon in infancy due to enema. Pediatrics 23:972–976, 1951.

91. Schofield PF: Foreign bodies in the rectum: A review. J R Soc Med 73:510–513, 1980.

92. Schrock TR, Christensen N: Management of perforating injuries of the colon. Surg Gynecol Obstet 135:65–68, 1972.

93. Segnitz RH: Accidental transanal perforation of the rectum. Am J Dis Child 93:255–258, 1957.

94. Shannon FL, Moore EE: Primary repair of the colon: When is it a safe alternative? Surgery 98:851–860, 1985.

95. Shannon FL, Moore EE, Moore FA, et al: Value of distal colon washout in civilian rectal trauma—Reducing cut bacterial translocation. J Trauma 38:989–994, 1988.

96. Shorr RM, Gottlieb MM, Webb K, et al: Selective management of abdominal stab wounds. Importance of the physical examination. Arch Surg 123:1141–1145, 1988.

97. Shuck JM, Lowe RJ: Intestinal disruption due to blunt abdominal trauma. Am J Surg 136:668–673, 1978.

98. Siebner M: Instrumentelle Verletzungen des Mastdarms, insbesondere durch Fieber-thermometer. Chirurg 3:208–215, 1931.

99. Slim MS, Makaroun M, Shamma AR: Primary repair of colorectal injuries in childhood. J Pediatr Surg 16:1008–1011, 1981.

100. Smith SRG, Connolly JC, Crove PW, et al: The effect of surgical drainage materials in colonic healing. Br J Surg 69:153–155, 1982.

101. Srinivasan K, Babu RK, Machado T, et al: Self-injurious bleeding per rectum. Indian J Pediatr 52:679–681, 1985.

102. Steele M, Blaisdell W: Treatment of colon injuries. J Trauma 17:557–562, 1977.

103. Sterioff S Jr., Izant RJ Jr., Persky L: Perineal injuries in children. J Trauma 9:56–61, 1969.

104. Stone HH, Fabian TC: Management of penetrating colon trauma: Randomization between primary closure and exteriorization. Ann Surg 190:430–436, 1979.

105. Telmos A, Mittal V: Splenic rupture following colonoscopy. JAMA 237:2718, 1977.

106. Thal ER, Yeary EC: Morbidity of colostomy closure following colon trauma. J Trauma 20:287–291, 1980.

107. Thompson JS, Moore EE, Moore JB: Comparison of penetrating injuries of the right and left colon. Ann Surg 193:414–418, 1981.

108. Trunkey D, Hays RJ, Shires GT: Management of rectal trauma. J Trauma 13:411–415, 1973.

109. Udassin R, Zamir O, Nissan S: Pneumoperitoneum in the ventilated infant. Diagnostic and therapeutic paracentesis in selected patients. Pediatr Surg Int 4:260–262, 1988.

110. Vance BM: Traumatic lesions of the intestine caused by non-penetrating blunt force. Arch Surg 7:197–212, 1923.

111. Wallace C: A study of 1200 cases of gunshot wounds of the abdomen. Br J Surg 4:679–733, 1917.

112. Walt AJ: Abdomen. In: Walt AJ (ed): Early Care of the Injured Patient. Committee on Trauma, American College of Surgeons. 3rd ed. Philadelphia, WB Saunders, 1982, pp 142–159.

113. Welch KJ: Abdominal Injuries. In: Randolph JG, Ravitch MM, Welch KJ, et al (eds): The Injured Child. Chicago, Year Book Medical Publishers, 1979, pp 155–213.

114. Woodhall JP, Ochsner A: The management of perforating injuries of the colon and rectum in civilian practice. Surgery 29:305–320, 1951.

115. Yajko RD, Norton LW, Bloemendal L, et al: Morbidity of colostomy closure. Am J Surg 132:304–306, 1976.

116. Yates JL: An experimental study of the local effect of peritoneal drainage. Surg Gynecol Obstet 1:473–480, 1905.

117. Yaw PB, Smith RN, Glover JL: Eight years experience with civilian injuries of the colon. Surg Gynecol Obstet 145:203–205, 1977.

CHAPTER TWENTY-SIX

Hernan M. Reyes

Retroperitoneal and Pelvic Injuries

The retroperitoneal space is that part of the body located between the sac-like peritoneum and the posterior parietal wall of the abdominal cavity extending from the twelfth vertebrae and the twelfth rib superiorly to the base of the sacrum and iliac crest inferiorly. For practical purposes, the retroperitoneal space can be defined as the space beneath the peritoneum that extends from the diaphragm to the pelvis and includes both flanks. Bleeding and extravasation of intestinal, fecal, and urinary contents into this space may result from penetrating or blunt injuries to the lower chest, abdomen, or pelvis.

ZONES OF INJURY

The various organ system injuries in the retroperitoneal space have variegated severity, incidence, and prognosis. Furthermore, diagnostic evaluations and complex management considerations vary depending on the anatomic location of the organ system, so much so that overall clinical concepts have been developed along the lines of dividing the retroperitoneal space into three anatomic zones (Fig. 26–1).[10, 19] Zone 1 represents the centromedial area of the retroperitoneal space. Zone 2 includes the areas of the flank. Zone 3 represents the entire pelvis. The various organ systems that can be injured in zone 1 consist of the pancreas and the posterior wall of the transverse colon and mesocolon. Zone 2 includes both kidneys, the adrenal glands, the ureters, and the posterior walls of the descending and ascending colon. Zone 3 includes the iliac vessels, rectum, and lower genitourinary tract.

RETROPERITONEAL HEMATOMA

Hemorrhage is the most common complication of an injury to the retroperitoneal organ system.[7, 13, 21] In the adult patient, retroperitoneal hematoma occurs secondary to blunt forces in two thirds of patients; penetrating injuries account for the other one third. Uncontrolled hemorrhage is responsible for the high incidence of early deaths in the adult population (18–31%).[7, 18] This incidence is especially high when hemorrhage occurs in the pelvis or the zone 3 region. Late death in these patients is usually the result of sepsis and respiratory failure.

Hemorrhage into the retroperitoneal space in the pediatric patient is infrequent except in the region of the pelvis (i.e., zone 3), where it occurs in nearly half of children with a fracture of the pelvic bones.[12, 15, 16] Nearly all of these patients were involved in motor vehicle accidents—two thirds as pedestrians.

Hemorrhage into zone I in all age groups is frequently due to penetrating injuries of major blood vessels.[2, 9] Bleeding can be expected to occur from blunt or penetrating pancreatic or duodenal injuries as well, although the bleeding is usually of lesser severity. A typical example of zone I injury from blunt abdominal trauma in the pediatric patient is the development of a pancreatic pseudocyst from ductal disruption or an intramural duodenal hematoma, both of which may resolve spontaneously or require operative intervention to resolve the complication.

Hemorrhage into zone II is almost invariably secondary to renal parenchymal disruption from either blunt or penetrating injuries.[9]

PELVIC HEMATOMA

Retroperitoneal hematoma occurring in the pelvis is a common complication of pelvic bone fracture in the pediatric patient, occurring in about half of these patients.[4, 11, 12, 14–16] Half of these children bleed sufficiently to require crystalloid resuscitation and blood transfusion; the mean blood loss is approximately 20% of the estimated blood volume. Although pelvic hemorrhage is common, only 3% of these patients bleed massively enough that their injuries are life threatening.[12, 15, 16] Uncontrolled hemorrhage from pelvic fractures in the pediatric population accounts for only 1.4 to 5% of all trauma deaths.[12, 15] In another report on the impact of pelvic fracture on mortality, there were no deaths from the resulting pelvic hemorrhage.[11] In most pediatric trauma series, the majority of deaths have been caused by associated closed head injuries.[12, 14–16]

The less severe retroperitoneal bleeding observed in children with pelvic fractures may be explained by a host of factors. The pelvic fractures produced may be less comminuted and nondisplaced; this appears to be a reflection of the immature bony structure with increased cartilaginous content in this age group.[12] This makes the pelvic bony

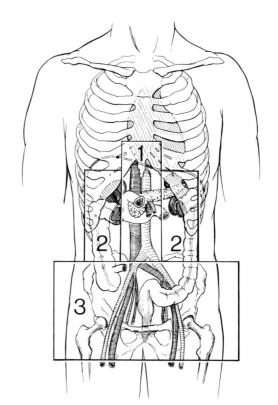

FIGURE 26–1

Retroperitoneal zones of injury. (Reprinted with permission from Kudsk KA, Sheldon GF: Retroperitoneal hematoma. In: Blaisdell FW, Trunkey DD (eds): Abdominal Trauma. New York, Thieme-Stratton, 1982, pp 279–293.)

structures more elastic, thereby reducing the chances of major disruption of the rich arterial venous network in the pelvis. Although other investigators refute this concept, the less severe nature of the resultant pelvic hemorrhage can only be assumed to be related to the distinct structure of the child's pelvic bones and, to some degree, is a reflection of a more competent tamponade effect provided by an intact peritoneum.

The posttraumatic pelvic hemorrhage almost invariably results from multiple lacerations of the pelvic arteries and veins. In the pelvis, there is a rich network of interconnecting blood vessels (Fig. 26–2). The high pressure gradient maintained in the injured vessel promotes continued bleeding and prevents clotting. Furthermore, the venous collaterals represent connections between the valveless portal circulation and the systemic pelvic veins, thus allowing hepatofugal venous flow and resultant excessive pelvic bleeding.

Diagnosis of a Pelvic Hematoma

Any patient with a fracture of the pelvic bones should be considered to have a retroperitoneal hematoma.[3, 4] The diagnosis can be readily confirmed with an intravenous pyelogram, voiding cystourethrogram, or double-contrast infusion CT scan of the abdomen and pelvis. These studies are invariably obtained to evaluate intra-abdominal and retroperitoneal injuries to the viscus. Close to one half of these patients are hypotensive upon admission and require crystalloid resuscitation and blood transfusion.[4, 11–13, 19]

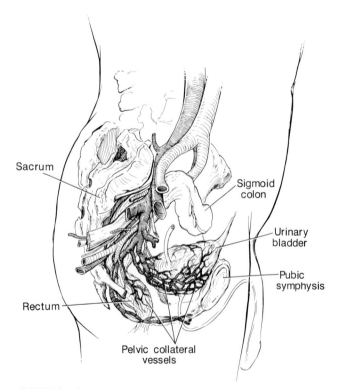

FIGURE 26–2

Relationship of pelvic structures to the network of collateral vessels.

In some patients, peritoneal lavage may be necessary to help identify the presence of associated intra-abdominal injuries, and certain precautions should be exercised when performing this procedure and interpreting the results.[1] The peritoneal lavage should be performed at a site above the umbilicus to avoid the retroperitoneal hematoma. The lavage fluid aspirated should contain greater than 50,000 red blood cells per cubic millimeter, greater than 500 white blood cells per cubic millimeter, food, foreign particles, bile, and bacteria, and it should be amylase-rich to indicate injury. Unless the retroperitoneal hematoma has ruptured into the peritoneal cavity or has been inadvertently entered during the surgical procedure, the presence of any of the above findings indicates an associated injury to a major solid or hollow viscus in the peritoneal cavity.

As a general rule, whenever the patient is stable, even following resuscitation with crystalloid or blood transfusion, a double-contrast CT scan of the abdomen is important in evaluating the entire spectrum of injuries, whether intra-abdominal or retroperitoneal. We do not routinely perform peritoneal lavage or peritoneal tap in a stable patient.

Local Associated Injuries

Although one half of the patients with retroperitoneal hematoma will manifest gross or microscopic hematuria on admission, bladder rupture occurs in only 2 to 6% of patients. Furthermore, the urethra is less frequently injured, with an incidence of 0 to 2%. If the urethra is injured, the prostatomembranous segment appears to be the most vulnerable. Although infrequent, the rectum (1.7 to 3%), vagina (3.5 to 5%), and perineum (2%) were likewise observed to be injured following pelvic fractures in children.[12]

Associated Intra-abdominal and Retroperitoneal Organ Injury

Associated injuries to the kidneys, spleen, and liver are less frequent in children than in adults, occurring in from 5 to 10% of patients.[12, 15, 16] In a series of 120 patients with pelvic fractures, Reichard and colleagues reported that although liver laceration was observed in five patients, only one required operative treatment because of uncontrolled bleeding.[16] Nevertheless, every attempt should be made to evaluate these organs by an infusion CT scan of the abdomen, provided the patient is stable.[3, 4, 8] If the patient remains unstable despite replacement of greater than 50% of the estimated blood volume, peritoneal lavage should immediately be performed.[19] Negative or equivocal lavage findings require that the patient immediately be taken to the x-ray department for a transfemoral arteriography to evaluate the site and determine the source of pelvic hemorrhage.[5, 6]

Associated System Injuries

Craniocerebral injuries are frequently encountered in children with pelvic fractures.[12] The literature gives an incidence of 22 to 32.5%; this figure is supported by our own experience.[12] This association with craniocerebral injuries is not unusual, considering the strong force necessary to produce a pelvic fracture. In a recent report of 57 patients with pelvic fractures, the only cause of death was due to closed head injury.[16] Lung contusions and pneumothorax were also observed in some patients with retroperitoneal hematoma, although this was not a major cause of increased morbidity or mortality (Fig. 26–3).

Management of Pelvic Hematoma

Retroperitoneal bleeding caused by pelvic fracture is best treated nonoperatively. Celiotomy to control pelvic hematoma should be universally avoided. Most investigators agree that a retroperitoneal hematoma should be left undisturbed when found at the time of celiotomy unless it is pulsatile and expanding. Evidence of uncontrolled hemorrhage, as indicated clinically by multiple transfusions and continued instability of the patient, is an indication for immediate arteriography using the femoral approach on the least traumatized side.[5, 6, 11, 12] An attempt should be made to delineate and localize the pelvic arterial laceration. If identified, the lesion should be treated by embolization using a variety of embolic agents, such as gelatin sponge, stainless-steel coils, autologous clot, detachable balloons, polyvinyl alcohol, and silicone microspheres. The reported

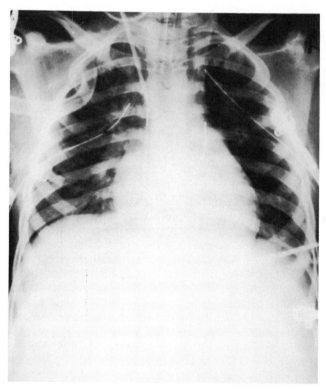

FIGURE 26–3

Chest radiograph of a child with multiple injuries (including a retroperitoneal hematoma from a pelvic fracture) indicating the need for critical care monitoring and management of associated respiratory injury and complications.

success rate of controlling hemorrhage with treatment by embolic agents is approximately 90 to 95% (Fig. 26–4).

Intraoperative control of pelvic arteriovenous bleeding by direct suture or hypogastric arterial ligation has been uniformly unsuccessful in providing effective hemostasis. Packing of the retroperitoneal space with gauze pads should be resorted to only when, in the course of a celiotomy for associated intra-abdominal organ injury, an open pelvic hematoma with bleeding into the peritoneal area is discovered and remains uncontrolled despite measures for local hemostasis. In the event that bleeding persists despite packing of the pelvis, percutaneous selective arteriography using the femoral approach and therapeutic embolization of the source of bleeding should be attempted.[5, 6, 12] A recent alternative procedure to control pelvic hemorrhage is the technique of operative hypogastric artery embolization with proximal ligature control; countertraction; and injection of a slurry of autologous clot, microfibrillar collagen, topical thrombin, and calcium chloride as described by Saueracker and associates.[17] This is a logical approach to an expanding and pulsatile pelvic hematoma found at celiotomy in a hemodynamically unstable patient.

It must be understood that arteriography and embolization also may be associated with serious complications.[5, 6, 16] A large volume of dye in a hypovolemic patient may increase the renal toxicity of the contrast agent. Embolization may precipitate distal tissue ischemia or infarction. Distal embolization or migration of embolic agents through arteriovenous fistulas into the pulmonary circulation may occur with life-threatening complications. These potential serious complications of pelvic embolization are, however, far outweighed by the alternative for life-threatening hemorrhage, hemipelvectomy, or exsanguinating hemorrhage.

The major limiting factor for successful embolization treatment is the size of the femoral artery. With current techniques, inability to insert a 5-Fr polyethylene catheter into the femoral artery precludes a successful embolization procedure.[12]

DIAGNOSIS AND MANAGEMENT OF OTHER RETROPERITONEAL HEMATOMAS

Centromedial hematomas secondary to penetrating injuries are best explored after initially establishing proximal and distal control of the aorta or vena cava above or below the diaphragm using a combined thoracoabdominal incision. This incision provides excellent access to both the thoracic and abdominal cavity for evaluation and treatment of associated injuries.

Pulsatile centromedial hematoma secondary to blunt trauma found at laparotomy, especially when the hematoma extends cephalad beyond the aortic hiatus, should not be explored until an angiogram is obtained to define the nature and the extent of the aortic disruption. Life-threatening injuries to the viscus should be promptly recognized and managed. If there is a reason to suspect aortic disruption preoperatively by virtue of the radiologic studies, a history of a direct thoracic steering-wheel injury, or a high-speed

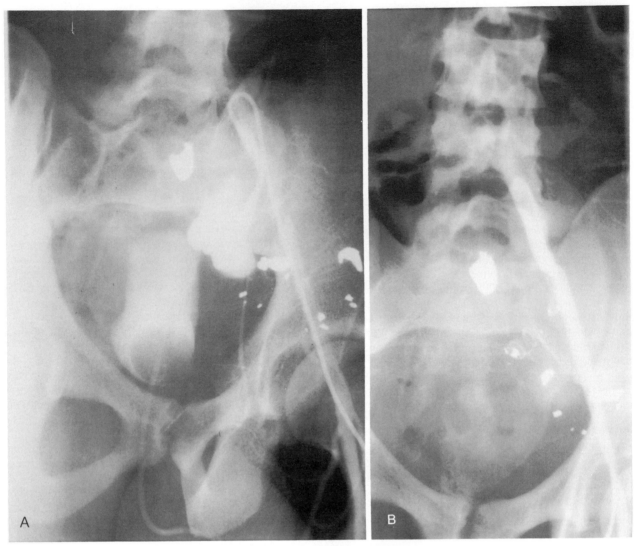

FIGURE 26–4

A, Pseudoaneurysm of the left hypogastric artery secondary to a gunshot wound of the pelvis in a male adolescent. *B,* Pseudoaneurysm successfully managed by embolization utilizing a femoral approach.

vehicle injury with chest contusion in a patient who is otherwise stable, angiographic evaluation is initially performed before other diagnostic CT scans or surgical intervention is undertaken (Fig. 26–5).

MANAGEMENT OF EXTRARENAL UROLOGIC COMPLICATIONS

Whenever a urologic injury is suspected in a patient with pelvic fracture, even in the absence of any obvious findings of urinary extravasation or hematuria, an appropriate-sized Foley catheter should be carefully inserted through the external meatus into the urinary bladder and a cystourethrogram obtained. On the other hand, whenever gross or microscopic hematuria is present and there is evidence of swelling and bogginess in the anterior rectal wall within the vicinity of the prostate gland on rectal examination, insertion of a urethral catheter should be cautiously avoided. An

injured urethra may be converted into a more serious problem if a false passage is created by forceful insertion of a urethral catheter. It is our practice and our recommendation to perform an antegrade urethrogram initially. If the urethra is found to be normal and the dye has not adequately outlined the urinary bladder, a catheter can then be inserted to the urinary bladder for a prompt cystogram examination. A double-contrast CT scan of the abdomen and pelvis should simultaneously be obtained.

Posterior bladder wall injury with retroperitoneal urinary extravasation is best treated by primary repair through a midline cystotomy. Care must be exercised during the dissection to avoid an associated pelvic hematoma. A suprapubic cystostomy tube is routinely inserted. The bladder neck and each ureteral orifice must be inspected for signs of injury. Intravenous injection of methylene blue or careful cannulation of the ureteral orifice may be necessary.

The presence of an anterior bladder wall rupture identified by a cystogram is an indication for immediate celi-

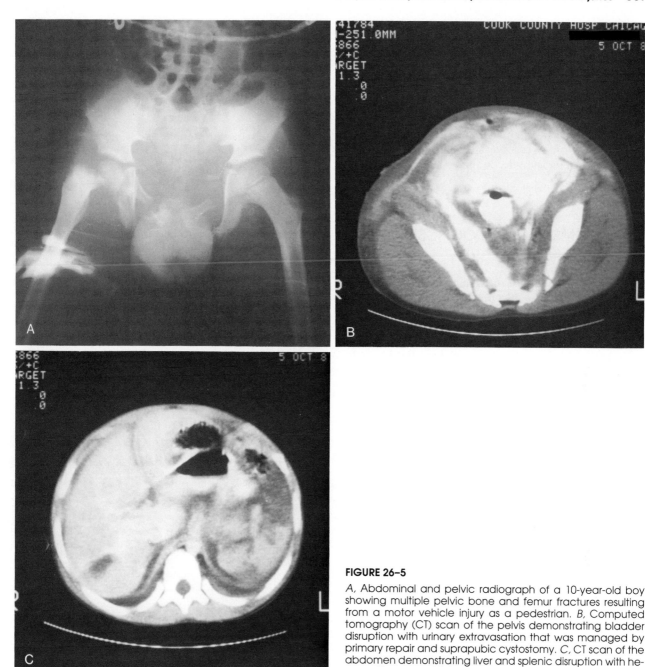

FIGURE 26–5

A, Abdominal and pelvic radiograph of a 10-year-old boy showing multiple pelvic bone and femur fractures resulting from a motor vehicle injury as a pedestrian. *B*, Computed tomography (CT) scan of the pelvis demonstrating bladder disruption with urinary extravasation that was managed by primary repair and suprapubic cystostomy. *C*, CT scan of the abdomen demonstrating liver and splenic disruption with hemoperitoneum, which was managed nonoperatively.

otomy. The bladder rupture should be repaired after appropriate inspection, and suprapubic cystostomy for urinary drainage should be established. The retroperitoneal hematoma must not under any circumstances be entered into unless it is pulsatile and expanding. If this finding exists or if the patient remains unstable postoperatively because of uncontrolled pelvic hemorrhage, percutaneous arteriogram with selective embolization of the arterial bleeder should be promptly performed. Alternatively, intraoperative hypogastric embolization as previously described may be an option.

Urethral injury should be treated with a suprapubic cystostomy. The diagnosis is established by a finding of urinary extravasation into the perineum and scrotal sac as well as the suprapubic region of the anterior abdominal wall.

The absence of urine, the presence of blood at the urethral meatus, and findings on rectal examination as previously described further suggest the presence of a urethral injury. Diagnosis is confirmed using an antegrade urethrogram. No attempt should be made to insert a catheter into the urethra and splint the injury. Primary repair is best avoided to gain a better functional result.

Rectal laceration, although a rare complication of pelvic fractures, should be recognized and treated promptly. Rectal bleeding or the presence of blood on rectal examination should be immediately investigated.[20] The diagnosis is best confirmed by endoscopic examination. Any penetrating injury to the rectal wall is preferentially treated with a complete diverting colostomy (i.e., end colostomy with a mucous fistula) and perineal drainage. The distal rectum should be irrigated with copious amounts of normal saline to reduce fecal contamination of the pelvis. The patient should receive broad-spectrum antibiotics to reduce the incidence of abscess formation in the pelvis. Active hemorrhage through the anorectal canal originating from a communicating pelvic hematoma should be initially treated by gauze packing the entire length of the anorectum. Failure to achieve control of bleeding is an indication for percutaneous arteriogram and selective embolization of the bleeding arterial vessel or for intraoperative hypogastric artery embolization.

MANAGEMENT AND PROGNOSIS OF PELVIC FRACTURES

Unlike in adults, the type of fracture in the pelvis in children does not seem to influence the severity of retroperitoneal hematoma that subsequently develops. Likewise, there is no increase in mortality associated with the type of pelvic fracture. Three fourths of these patients are usually treated by bed rest, and less than 10% of patients need open reduction and internal fixation.[12-14] A smaller percentage are treated by external fixation, traction, or immobilization using a hip spica cast.

References

1. Alyono D, Morrow CE, Perry JF: Reappraisal of diagnostic peritoneal lavage criteria for operation in penetrating and blunt trauma. Surgery 11:751–757, 1982.
2. Barlow B, Niemirska M, Gandhi R: Ten years' experience with pediatric gunshot wounds. J Pediatr Surg 17(12):927–932, 1982.
3. Bryan WJ, Tullos HS: Pediatric pelvic fractures—Review of 52 patients. J Trauma 19:799–805, 1979.
4. Buckley SL, Burkus JK: Computerized axial tomography of pelvic ring fractures. J Trauma 27:496–502, 1987.
5. Flint LM, Brown A, Richardson JD, et al: Definitive control of bleeding from severe pelvic fractures. Ann Surg 189:709–716, 1979.
6. Gerlock AJ: Hemorrhage following pelvic fracture controlled by embolization: Case report. J Trauma 15:740–742, 1975.
7. Grieco JG, Perry JF: Retroperitoneal hematoma following trauma: Its clinical importance. J Trauma 20:733–736, 1980.
8. Hauser CJ, Huprich JE, Posco P: Triple-contrast computed tomography in the evaluation of penetrating posterior abdominal injuries. Arch Surg 122:1112–1115, 1987.
9. Henao F, Jiminez H, Tawil M: Penetrating wounds of the back and flank: Analysis of 77 cases. South Med J 80:21–25, 1987.
10. Kudsk KA, Sheldon GF: Retroperitoneal hematoma. In: Blaisdell FW, Trunkey DD (eds): Abdominal Trauma. New York, Thieme Stratton, 1982, pp 279–293.
11. Musemeche CA, Fischer RP, Cotler HB, et al: Selective management of pediatric pelvic fractures: A conservative approach. J Pediatr Surg 22:538–540, 1987.
12. Quinby WC Jr: Fractures of the pelvis and associated injuries in children. J Pediatr Surg 1:353–364, 1966.
13. Quinby WC Jr: Pelvic fractures with hemorrhage. N Engl J Med 283(12):668–669, 1971.
14. Rang M: Children's fractures. Philadelphia, JB Lippincott, 1974.
15. Reed MH: Pelvic fractures in children. J Can Assoc Radiol 27:255–261, 1976.
16. Reichard SA, Helikson MA, Shorter N, et al: Pelvic fractures in children—Review of 120 patients with a new look at general management. J Pediatr Surg 15:727–734, 1970.
17. Saueracker AJ, McCroskey BL, Moore EE, et al: Intraoperative hypogastric artery embolization for life-threatening pelvic hemorrhage: A preliminary report. J Trauma 27:1127–1129, 1987.
18. Selivanov V, Chi HS, Alverdy JC: Mortality in retroperitoneal hematoma. J Trauma 24:1022–1027, 1984.
19. Trunkey DD, Chapman MW, Lim RC, et al: Management of pelvic fractures in blunt trauma injury. J Trauma 14:912–923, 1974.
20. Weil PH: Injuries of the retroperitoneal portions of the colon and rectum. Dis Colon Rectum 26:19–21, 1983.
21. Yellin AE, Lundell CJ, Finck EJ: Diagnosis and control of posttraumatic pelvic hemorrhage. Arch Surg 118:1378–1383, 1983.

Thom E. Lobe
Dennis C. Gore
Leonard E. Swischuk

Urinary Tract Injuries

Although injury to the genitourinary tract is common in trauma in infancy and childhood, second only to closed-head injuries, death from these injuries is rare. When death occurs, it is usually because of associated injuries.[13] Fifty percent of children with documented urinary tract injuries have injuries to other organs as well.[12] Renal damage from trauma in this age group is four times more frequent than liver or hollow viscus injury and 10 times more common than damage to the pancreas, lung, or bladder. In children, the ureter and urethra are injured 100 times less frequently than the kidney.

Classification of urinary tract injuries according to severity is somewhat arbitrary and subject to the opinions of the researcher (Table 27–1). Injuries that require immediate intervention (e.g., an intimal tear of the renal artery) may be only a relatively mild injury of that structure but can jeopardize the viability of the kidney and are usually classified as severe injuries. In general, injuries that can be managed by simple observation or by catheter drainage alone are considered minimal-to-moderate injuries, whereas injuries that require major operative reconstruction are considered severe.

DIAGNOSTIC CONSIDERATIONS

Secondary Survey Considerations

The diagnosis of genitourinary trauma begins with the secondary survey, during which most well-trained physicians routinely insert a Foley catheter. Blood at the urethral meatus, blood in the scrotum, or an abnormally positioned or abnormally mobile prostate should signal to the resuscitation team that a urethral injury is highly likely and that a retrograde urethrogram is indicated. When blood is absent, a urinary catheter is usually placed. We believe that in small boys younger than 5 years of age, the passage of a urinary catheter by an inexperienced or a hurried practitioner may predispose the child to the development of urethral strictures later in life.[57] Accordingly, our preference is to avoid routine urethral catheter placement in all boys younger than 5 years of age unless their condition specifically warrants it.

In the absence of gross blood at the meatus or grossly traumatized genitalia, hematuria is the classic indicator of genitourinary trauma. The question, ''How much, if any, blood in the urine is necessary before the physician should suspect urinary tract injury?'' always must be addressed. Sklar and colleagues assessed the contribution of the introduction of a Foley catheter into the bladder to the magnitude of hematuria in otherwise healthy individuals and observed that all of the study subjects had fewer than four red cells per 400-power field.[65] They concluded that male subjects exhibited more red blood cells per 400-power field than female subjects and that more than three red blood cells per 400-power field could not be attributed to catheter placement. Guice and colleagues, after reviewing the records of 156 trauma victims, suggested that microscopic hematuria alone is a poor predictor of significant genitourinary tract injury.[27] Griffen and associates have documented major renal trauma in the absence of hematuria,[26] and in some series, as many as 24% of patients with renal trauma documented by intravenous pyelogram and approximately 50% of patients who have vascular pedicle injuries have no associated hematuria.[9, 11]

Overt signs of renal trauma are subtle and usually result from retroperitoneal hemorrhage or extravasation of urine. Flank tenderness or ecchymosis suggests the possibility of retroperitoneal hemorrhage. Owing to the confined space and high likelihood of tamponade within an intact Gerota fascia, the amount of blood lost from an isolated renal injury is unlikely to precipitate shock. Evidence of urinary extravasation is usually delayed and may be associated with the development of flank tenderness or an indistinct mass. Sepsis with fever and paralytic ileus occurring as late as 7 to 10 days after an accident may be the only sign of extravasated urine. In our view, any child who has sustained a major impact or has multiple injuries at opposite ends of the body (e.g., closed-head injury and femur fracture) warrants evaluation of the urinary tract by appropriate diagnostic imaging.

Computed Tomography

In the past, the physician usually relied for diagnosis on the intravenous pyelogram. Although this study may have diagnostic merit in minor injuries with questionable clinical findings, when serious injury is suspected computed tomography with contrast enhancement is indicated. It is generally considered that computed tomography is the best primary imaging modality in the assessment of blunt abdominal trauma in general, and urinary tract trauma in particular.[2, 5, 30, 33]

Ultrasonography is also often used as a screening test in patients with blunt abdominal trauma. Although ultrasonography readily can detect the presence of abnormal fluid

Table 27–1
Classification of Urinary Tract Injuries by Severity

Severity	Renal	Ureter	Bladder	Urethral
Minimal	Contusion	Contusion	Contusion	Contusion
Moderate	Cortical laceration Calyceal tear Rupture	Small tear	Extraperitoneal rupture Intraperitoneal rupture	Anterior disruption Posterior disruption (partial)
Severe	Vascular injury Pelviureteral disruption	Disruption	Combined rupture Vesicourethral disruption Vesicovaginal disruption	Posterior disruption (complete)

collections in the abdomen and can suggest renal injury, it provides no information regarding function of the kidney or whether blood supply to the kidney is intact. Magnetic resonance imaging does not yet have a large role in examining patients with abdominal trauma, and it seems doubtful that it will replace computed tomography.

With computed tomography, the physician can assess the following: (1) whether the kidney is intact; (2) the presence of intrarenal hematomas; (3) various fractures and tears through the kidney; and (4) the extent of perirenal blood and urine collection (Fig. 27–1). Because contrast material is excreted into the bladder, enhanced computed tomography also provides adequate information regarding the condition of the bladder and surrounding soft tissue. Information is also derived regarding renal function and residual functioning renal tissue.

Retrograde Cystourethrography

With the advent of these diagnostic techniques, there has been a decrease in the need for formal retrograde cystourethrography in many of these patients. In this regard, however, when lower urinary tract trauma is suspected, or if gross hematuria persists in the presence of a normal computed tomography scan of the urinary tract, retrograde cystourethrography is indicated. In such patients, it is most important that the physician first exclude a urethral injury, and this is accomplished by performing a retrograde urethrogram. When the urethra is deemed normal and no leaks are present, the physician can advance the catheter into the bladder and perform the cystogram. If a bladder tear is present, there will be extravasation of contrast material into the soft tissues of the pelvis or into the peritoneal cavity (Fig. 27–2).

Arteriography

When vascular pedicle injury is suspected, either clinically or on computed tomographic studies that show the presence of a normally contoured kidney that is not functioning (i.e., contrast is not being delivered to and excreted by the kidney), the physician should proceed immediately to arteriography. Nuclear scintigraphy can provide similar data as arteriography, but eventually, an arteriogram will have to be performed; therefore, an arteriogram probably is best performed initially. Arteriography usually shows the commonest problem: occlusion of the renal artery (Fig. 27–3). Occasionally, lesser degrees of trauma with intimal tears can also be detected by arteriography.

Ultrasonography

Because most renal injuries can be treated conservatively, the patient requires follow up with some imaging modality. For the most part, such follow up is directed at detecting complications and determining the rate or extent of healing. Complications include problems such as subcapsular hematomas, abscesses, urinomas, and eventually, stenoses of the urinary tract. Most of these complications are best detected using ultrasonography (Fig. 27–4); if assessment of renal function is required, nuclear scintigraphy is probably the most efficient diagnostic modality. Nuclear scintigraphy also can be used to detect obstructive lesions such as post-traumatic strictures, although retrograde pyelography is usually required in these cases.

Special Considerations

Ureteral lesions are difficult to detect in their initial stages with any imaging modality. Later, extravasation of urine or the development of urinary tract obstruction can be detected with ultrasound, and scintigraphy can be used to determine residual renal function. Retrograde pyelography may also be required in some instances. It also should be noted that occult hydronephrotic kidneys are more prone to injury than normal kidneys. Minor trauma of these dilated structures may lead to nothing more than hematuria and vague abdominal pain. In such cases, ultrasonography is worthwhile, because it can define clearly the hydronephrotic kidney, which is most often due to ureteropelvic junction obstruction (Fig. 27–5).

Intraoperative imaging of the genitourinary tract may occasionally be required, as indicated in the following discussion. Generally, doses of contrast material are the same as those used for a regular intravenous pyelogram. These doses differ depending on the contrast material used, but adult doses must be scaled down in young children and infants. Because trauma patients receive intravenous fluids at the time of study, there should be a prompt diuresis, and adequate studies are not difficult to obtain.

With genitourinary trauma in the neonate as opposed to the older infant and child, often the first imaging modality used is ultrasonography. Ultrasound is very useful in neonatal patients in general, and because injuries such as renal lacerations and caliceal tears are not the major injury, most often the physician requires little else than the ultrasound study for upper urinary tract evaluation. However, if a bladder injury is suspected, retrograde cystourethrography as in the older child is required.

KIDNEY TRAUMA

The greater vulnerability to damage from blunt trauma of kidneys of young patients compared with those of adults has been ascribed to several factors: the kidneys' greater proportional size within the torso and the greater magnitude of fetal renal lobulation; the kidneys' lack of equivalent structural support with diminished perinephric fat and a less-well-developed Gerota fascia; the fact that the ribs in infants and children are not fully ossified, allowing for greater flexibility of the lower ribcage and likelihood of impact against the kidney; and the higher incidence of abnormally enlarged kidney due to congenital anomalies, hydronephrosis, or renal tumors.[23, 66] Enlarged kidneys are more likely to be damaged and may constitute as much as 20% of documented renal trauma during childhood; as

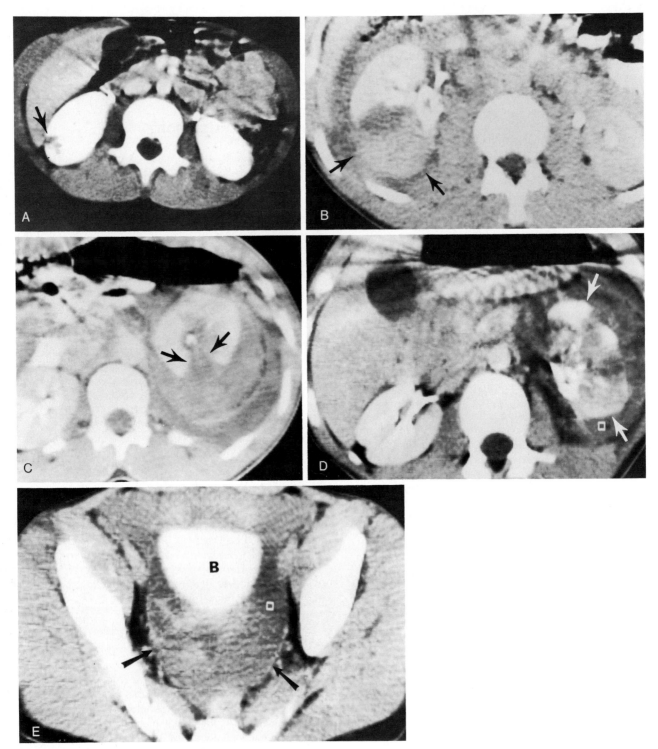

FIGURE 27-1

Computed tomography (CT) findings of renal trauma. *A*, Note the small intraparenchymal hematoma *(arrow)*. *B*, CT scan of another patient with a large hematoma and associated area of contusion that are still confined by the renal capsule *(arrows)*. The radiolucent halo around the kidney indicates associated bleeding into the pararenal space. *C*, Note the laceration in the left kidney *(arrows)*. The kidney is displaced forward by a large subcapsular hematoma. The crescentic area of radiolucency represents compressed fat in the perirenal space. The surrounding gray area beyond the fat stripe represents blood in the posterior pararenal space. *D*, Note the completely fractured kidney with numerous residual fragments *(arrows)*. Also note that subcapsular blood surrounds the kidney. *E*, Blood in the cul-de-sac *(arrows)* surrounds the urinary bladder (B), which has been displaced forward. Same patient as in *D*.

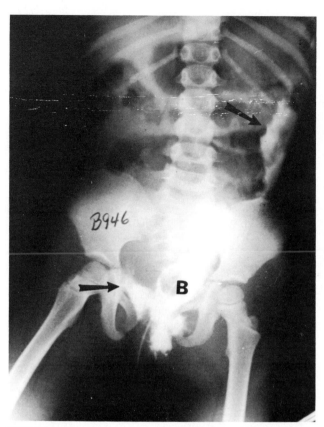

FIGURE 27–2

Bladder tear. Note in this patient that contrast material has extravasated into the perineal soft tissues (lower arrow) and into the peritoneal cavity (upper arrow). A Foley bulb is in the bladder (B).

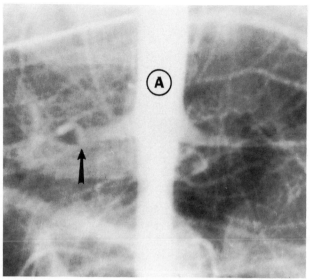

FIGURE 27–3

Renal artery injury. On this aortogram note the aorta (A) and the abrupt obstruction due to laceration (arrow) of the right renal artery. The left renal artery, just opposite, is normal.

Eleven percent of renal injuries from blunt trauma are bilateral.[29]

Management

Renal trauma rarely requires immediate operative exploration except for those few cases in which the patient is at risk of near exsanguination because of an open wound or

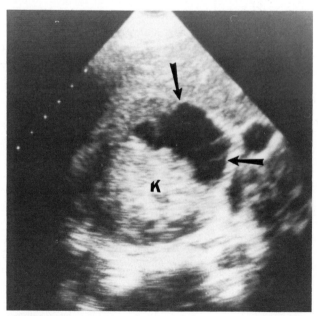

FIGURE 27–4

Subcapsular hematoma. Ultrasound clearly demonstrates a sonolucent subcapsular hematoma (arrows) 1 week after the initial injury. The kidney (K) is somewhat compressed.

many as 10% of renal anomalies are first diagnosed during the evaluation of blunt abdominal trauma.[7, 38, 75]

Incidence

The overall ratio of blunt to penetrating trauma in childhood is 4:1, with an increased incidence of penetrating trauma occurring in urban settings and during adolescence. Stabbings and gunshots are the most common causes of penetrating injuries. Iatrogenic renal damage is rare and is usually a complication of such frequently performed procedures as amniocentesis, liver biopsy, or percutaneous nephrostomy.

Mechanism of Injury

Blunt renal trauma is most often due to the rapid deceleration that occurs in falls and in motor vehicle accidents. Because the kidney is relatively fixed by the vascular pedicle, rapid deceleration may disrupt arterial flow by causing an intimal tear or vascular spasm, may sever the ureteropelvic junction, or may completely avulse the entire renal pedicle.[69] Direct injury may also occur to the renal parenchyma from the impact against the lower ribs or vertebrae.

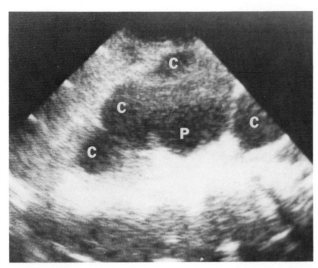

FIGURE 27–5

Occult obstruction of the ureteropelvic junction. Note the marked hydronephrosis with a large dilated renal pelvis (P) and numerous dilated calices (C). This child sustained minor abdominal trauma and presented with abdominal pain and hematuria.

an avulsion injury of the vascular pedicle. After the hemorrhage is controlled, renal exploration should proceed only after diagnostic evaluation of the contralateral kidney, the integrity and function of which may have an impact on immediate operative decisions. When preoperative studies have not been performed because of the urgency of operation, an intraoperative intravenous pyelogram can and should be performed.

Frequently, a perirenal hematoma is discovered during abdominal exploration for other visceral injuries. An intraoperative intravenous pyelogram should be obtained if preoperative studies have not documented renal integrity and function. With evidence of adequate renal perfusion and a nonexpanding hematoma, no exploration of the retroperitoneum is required, regardless of the size of the hematoma.[45] Operative evaluation is recommended, however, when there is evidence of urinary extravasation or an absence of renal perfusion, indicating a possible renal pedicle injury. Emergency correction of a vascular injury is imperative for any chance of preserving the kidney.[42, 45] Although it is well established that the allowable warm ischemic time is only a few hours at best, it is impossible to tell when renal perfusion stopped in relation to the time of the accident, and collateral blood flow to the capsule or a portion of the kidney may be sufficient to allow more time for successful repair than would ordinarily be expected. Good return of renal function in apparently devascularized kidneys has been reported to occur when vascularization is accomplished as long as 24 hours after the time of injury. Thus, even though the chance of salvage of the kidney with prolonged warm ischemia may be slight, our preference is to attempt to repair any renovascular damage within 24 hours of the injury unless the renal parenchyma is also damaged beyond repair.

Penetrating trauma mandates a thorough radiologic evaluation of the kidneys. The need for operative exploration of flank stab wounds without evidence of intra-abdominal injury is dependent on the severity of the hemorrhage or urinary extravasation. The extent and trajectory of gunshot injuries are unpredictable, and complete evaluation is most safely accomplished with compulsory exploration.

Cass evaluated 219 children who sustained blunt renal injuries.[12] He noted that all of the children with renal laceration, rupture, or pedicle injury had associated injuries, and more than three fourths of these patients required celiotomy for an intra-abdominal injury. His review suggested that up to 70% of conservatively managed blunt renal injuries will require a second operation for the renal injury during the child's recovery from the initial surgery for associated injuries, and he estimated that the incidence of renal loss with this approach is between 5 and 40% and the significant complication and renal surgery rate is between 32 and 80%. He advocated immediate operative intervention in patients with severe injuries, quoting a nephrectomy rate of 11% for renal lacerations, 100% for ruptures, and 33% for pedicle injuries in the 16 patients so managed.

In contrast, Kuzamarov and colleagues, in their assessment of 240 children who suffered from blunt renal trauma, concluded that the conservative approach is satisfactory, resulting in a 12% nephrectomy rate and only a few complications that were easily managed with simple, temporary drainage.[34]

Classification of Injury

Woodward and Smith emphasized the value of classifying renal injuries when considering the indications for operative intervention of blunt renal trauma.[74] They used the following classification:

Type 1: Renal contusion
Type 2: Cortical laceration
Type 3: Caliceal tear
Type 4: Complete tear or rupture
Type 5: Vascular pedicle injury
Type 6: Ureteropelvic disruption

these researchers advised conservative (i.e., nonoperative) management for injuries of types 1 through 3 and found that only 4% of their patients in this category required operation. However, they performed operations on 89% of their patients who were classified as having injuries of types 4 through 6. When operation was indicated, these researchers used a transperitoneal approach, isolating and controlling the renal vessels before opening the Gerota fascia. They also cooled the kidney locally with crushed ice to control hemorrhage and facilitate the repair of parenchymal and pelvic tears.

Before incising the Gerota fascia, proximal control of the renal vessels is recommended. Lacerations of renal parenchyma or calyces should be closed with absorbable sutures.[71] Omentum can be used to bolster the repair and may provide improved hemostasis.[54] Dependent drainage of the retroperitoneum is recommended to prevent collections of blood and urine that would otherwise delay healing.

Duckett and Pfister recommend the use of ureterocalicostomy for renal salvage in cases of severe pelvic disease.[19]

This technique can be used in selected patients with severe renal pelvic trauma.

Vascular injuries usually can be repaired with a primary excision of the injured segment and end-to-end anastomosis.[9] The normal appearance of the vessel does not preclude an intimal injury. When renal perfusion appears to be compromised, it cannot be safely assumed that arterial spasm is at fault. Arteriography is essential to clarify the nature of the vascular injury, and if necessary, this technique should be performed at the time of celiotomy.

Venous repair is especially important for the right renal vein, the simple ligation of which is associated with a high incidence of renal loss due to inadequate collateral circulation. When necessary, ligation of the left renal vein or segmental renal veins bilaterally may allow sufficient venous drainage for renal salvage.[68]

Complications

The complications that commonly occur with renal injuries of childhood include clot obstruction, which rarely produces symptoms; acute or persistent hemorrhage, which may indicate the need for surgery; posttraumatic polar hydronephrosis, which requires repair in approximately one half of the cases; hypertension, which requires close follow up and evaluation for the need for therapy; and loss of renal parenchyma.[1]

There is a small incidence of urinary fistulas following extensive renal trauma. These fistulas are frequently related to foreign material within the wound. The vast majority of these fistulas (>85%) close spontaneously within 3 to 4 weeks. Radionuclide imaging of the proximal renal unit and retrograde pyelography may be required to exclude a distal urinary obstruction as a predisposing factor to fistulas. Operative exploration is indicated for persistent urinary fistulas (i.e., those lasting >6 weeks) or when there is evidence of urinary tract obstruction.

Trauma may also result in a renal arteriovenous fistula. Simple ligation of the arteriovenous fistula is ineffective, and nephrectomy may be required.[15]

URETERAL TRAUMA

Ureteral disruption caused by blunt trauma is rare, and its diagnosis is usually delayed because of the lack of early symptoms. Careful evaluation of posttraumatic flank masses or of perinephric fluid collections detected using diagnostic imaging is indicated. Ureteral injuries in the patient with multiple injuries have been known to form fistulas to other injured sites, such as the perineum.[70] Despite their typically delayed recognition, most ureteral injuries can be managed successfully, although their early recognition and repair is more desirable.[4, 11, 59, 68]

Mechanism of Injury

Although penetrating or iatrogenic injuries may occur anywhere along the course of the ureters, blunt injuries most often occur at the renal pelvis or below the bony pelvic brim.[21, 71] Children appear to be particularly susceptible to ureteral avulsion in acute acceleration or deceleration trauma, which for some unexplained reason occurs more often on the right side.[50] These injuries may be bilateral and are thought to occur with sudden hyperextension and ureteral stretching followed by a snap against the bony prominence, causing disruption at or near the ureteropelvic junction.[36] The ureter also has been known to become injured by entrapment or by penetration or laceration by bony spicules in cases of pelvic trauma in children.[47]

The only sign of a ureteral injury may be leakage of urine from a wound, oliguria, or an enlarging flank mass. Hematuria is absent in 30% of patients with documented ureteral damage.[54] The manifestations of sepsis, peritonitis, progressive oliguria and azotemia, a tender flank, or a urinary fistula, all of which may result from ureteral damage, are often delayed for several days.[21, 35]

Upper ureteral injuries are the most commonly missed, and their delayed recognition usually is associated with a higher nephrectomy rate (32%) than that in injuries detected and corrected immediately.[40]

Early detection and repair of ureteral injury appears to lower the morbidity associated with the injury. Mendez and McGinty reported that four of nine patients with delayed diagnosis required nephrectomies, whereas only three of 33 patients whose injuries were recognized early lost their kidneys.[43]

When ureteral injury is suspected on clinical grounds and confirmed by ultrasonography or computed tomography, retrograde pyelography may be useful to locate precisely the site of the defect.[10, 61]

Management

The management of ureteral injuries is operative. Primary anastomosis is preferred for lesions that are detected early and noncontaminated. The basic surgical tenets of tensionless anastomoses using absorbable sutures after adequate débridement cannot be overemphasized.[21, 54] We prefer to use magnifying optical loupes to assure a more precise anastomosis. Ureteral damage within infected wounds or in the unstable, critically injured patient may be more appropriately managed with urinary diversion and antibiotics and the postponing of definitive repair. Urine can be diverted using a cutaneous ureterostomy by simply exteriorizing the ureter proximal to the defect or by placement of a nephrostomy tube with stenting across the damaged segment of ureter.

Several techniques are available to obtain urinary tract continuity when a primary ureteroureterostomy or pyeloplasty are not possible. For lesions along the proximal ureter, autotransplantation of the kidney into a pelvic location, although technically challenging, has been demonstrated to be safe and effective.[21, 25] The interposition of a segment of bowel may facilitate midureteral repair and obviates the risks of vesicoureteral reflux.[37] For distal ureteral lesions at or below the pelvic brim, a ureteroneocystostomy or a transureteroureterostomy combined with a Boari flap (i.e., tubularization of bladder wall to form the distal ureter attachment) or a psoas bladder hitch to provide extra length, if necessary, aids in establishing a tensionless anastomosis.[21, 25]

Many researchers advise a spatulated ureteral anastomosis in hopes of decreasing the incidence of ureteral stricture.[21, 53] Other experts stress the importance of prolonged drainage of the wound to remove any surrounding urine, which may impede healing and reepithelization.[54]

Stenting ureteral anastomosis is controversial. Stents provide an adequate ureteral lumen for internal urine drainage, which minimizes subsequent extravasation; however, stents are foreign bodies, which may increase the incidence of infection and prolong convalescence.[21, 53] An internal stent should be removed before discontinuing external drainage if both are used.[53] We prefer to use the double-J Silastic stent when stenting is required. This device usually stays in place well, provides good drainage, causes minimal tissue reaction, and is easy to remove cystoscopically.

Penetrating injuries to the ureter in childhood are rare but usually can be treated with stented ureteroureterostomy after débridement of devitalized tissue in conjunction with a primary anastomosis or the interposition of a segment of bowel in the more severe cases, in which a primary anastomosis is likely to create too much tension.[55]

Complications

Long-term complications of ureteral repair include urinary fistulas, chronic infections, and strictures.[70] Strictures may result either from fibrosis of the ureter intrinsically or from diffuse retroperitoneal fibrosis from previously existing stagnant, extravasated urine.[35]

BLADDER TRAUMA

In the adult, the urinary bladder lies primarily within the protection of the bony pelvis. The bladder of the infant and child is largely an abdominal organ, thus predisposing it to an increased risk of trauma.

Mechanism of Injury

Bladder injuries can be placed into four classes in order of decreasing frequency: (1) contusion, (2) extraperitoneal rupture, (3) intraperitoneal rupture, and (4) combined extraperitoneal and intraperitoneal rupture. Injury can occur from blunt or penetrating trauma or result from iatrogenic causes. Rarely, the bladder is subject to spontaneous rupture.

Vesical contusion resulting from direct impact is probably the most common of bladder injuries, occurring in approximately one third of cases.[58] This condition may go unrecognized and rarely is of any consequence. The bladder wall remains intact, although all layers may show evidence of hemorrhage, swelling, or histologic disruption. This type of injury may be associated with nonpenetrating pelvic fracture or may be iatrogenic, resulting from endoscopy, retraction of the bladder at the time of operation, or the Credé

maneuver. Self-inflicted injuries from foreign bodies placed in the urethra may occasionally have an impact on the inner bladder wall. Additionally, active teenagers who jog may occasionally present with hematuria from bladder contusion.[6]

The diagnosis of bladder contusion is usually one of exclusion based on the presence of hematuria without evidence of diagnostic imaging to suggest renal injury and without extravesical extravasation of contrast. Confirmation is unnecessary but usually can be made by endoscopy, at which time mucosal hemorrhage or disruption is seen.

Bladder rupture from blunt trauma nearly always occurs because of a sudden increase in intravesical pressure. Extraperitoneal vesical rupture is most often associated with a pelvic fracture (98%) but also may result from penetrating injury.[14] The diagnosis is usually made when diagnostic imaging demonstrates extravasation of contrast material. The lacerations are usually on the anterolateral surface of the bladder near the bladder neck and are usually caused by penetrating bony fragments of the disrupted pubic rami. Occasionally, acetabular blowout fractures send fragments toward the bladder, and displaced femoral head penetration of the bladder has been reported.[62]

Intraperitoneal vesical rupture also occurs with the transmission of force through fluid under pressure and typically affects the dome of the bladder. Recognition of this lesion may be delayed because the symptoms mimic those of commonly associated abdominal visceral injury (e.g., spleen, kidney, liver), and these lesions are usually treated nonoperatively.[8] Penetrating injuries from sharp objects or projectiles can also occur. Neonatal bladders have been ruptured during attempts at performing the Credé maneuver or umbilical artery catheterization.[18, 64]

Management

When surgery for associated injuries is unnecessary, catheter drainage alone, using a Foley catheter or percutaneous suprapubic cystostomy, is adequate therapy and rarely results in persistent leakage or complications after the wound has been proved healed.[14] Although many researchers urge formal repair of extraperitoneal bladder lacerations when operative exploration for other injuries in undertaken, placement of a suprapubic drainage catheter usually proves adequate. The magnitude of the bladder injury cannot be judged by the extent to which radiopaque contrast leaks from the bladder. Accordingly, the degree of injury cannot be assessed without operative exploration. Such assessment is unnecessary, however, because essentially all of these lesions heal with adequate catheter drainage.

Penetrating injuries probably should be managed by surgical débridement of the missile tract or of devitalized tissue, closure of the defect, and catheter drainage (generally for 10 days), particularly when a missile or bony spicule remains lodged in the bladder wall. There have been only rare reports of successful treatment by catheter drainage of these injuries, most of which were caused by iatrogenic trauma. We have used catheter drainage alone to treat one such injury in a child whose urinary reservoir (colon) we perforated at the time of stone removal.

Three fourths of intraperitoneal bladder injuries are associated with pelvic fractures. Most patients appear more acutely ill than those with other types of bladder injuries, but they have pain that is difficult to distinguish from the pain of the associated pelvic fracture. Occasionally, these patients also have associated bladder spasm to a degree that makes voiding difficult despite an intact urethra. The essential features of management of this type of injury include pelvic exploration, during which the surgeon should examine the sigmoid colon and rectum for associated injuries; débridement of devitalized tissues; multilayer closure with absorbable sutures; perivesical drainage; and urinary diversion with a suprapubic catheter for 7 to 10 days. If injury to the trigone is suspected, careful examination of this area to exclude distal ureteral injury should be performed. This examination may include the passage of ureteral stents or the intravenous administration of indigo carmine, awaiting its appearance in the urine to document the extent of injury. Ureteral injuries should be repaired immediately if discovered.

Nearly all patients with combined extraperitoneal and intraperitoneal vesical disruption have an associated pelvic fracture. The major difficulty in treating patients with these combined injuries is the identification of all of the injured sites. The abdominal domicile of the bladder in children makes it particularly susceptible to vesicourethral or vesicovaginal injuries. Retrograde urethrograms or carefully performed endoscopy can aid in the diagnosis of suspected combined lesions. Immediate repair under direct vision, using a suprapubic urinary catheter for diversion, is advised to maximize the potential for retaining urinary continence and to minimize the potential for vesicovaginal fistulas in girls.[44] Short-term urethral stenting in patients with vesicourethral injury should be considered to facilitate proper alignment of these structures.

Unfortunately, iatrogenic injuries to the bladder are common. Abdominal paracentesis should not be performed in trauma victims without proper urinary tract drainage to empty the bladder beforehand. These injuries are usually recognized immediately or are discovered when the instilled paracentesis fluid runs out the urethra. Drainage by a Foley catheter for 7 to 10 days is usually sufficient to treat these injuries. Occasionally, the novice or the experienced surgeon may injure the infant bladder at the time of herniorrhaphy. Tragedy only occurs when the injury goes unrecognized. When the rent in the bladder is small, we prefer to use a multilayer closure with nonabsorbable sutures and to place a suprapubic catheter for drainage. Rarely, a near total cystectomy is performed inadvertently, if the bladder is mistaken for the hernia sac. Careful attention to the anatomic layers helps avoid making this mistake. The surgeon should be suspicious if a particularly thick ''hernia sac'' (i.e., the bladder) is discovered on the asymptomatic side of a bilateral exploration. Immediate reconstruction, with ureteral reimplantation into an enteric conduit if one or both ureters are involved, should be performed.[60] In these cases, when the surgeon is liable to be distracted by the significance of the error, he or she should not forget to attend to the hernia sac on the affected side, which was most likely missed when the bladder was selected instead.

Spontaneous bladder rupture has been reported in a fetus, and vesical prolapse can occur in patients with epispadias or with preliminary closure of an exstrophy. Fetal bladder rupture is indicated by urinary ascites in the newborn. The prolapsed bladder should be reduced expeditiously to avoid gangrene. With heavy sedation, reduction of the prolapse can be performed without general anesthesia.

URETHRAL TRAUMA

Mechanism of Injury

Traumatic injuries to the prostatomembranous portion of the urethra are the most common type of urethral injury, occurring in slightly more than one half of the cases. In children, these injuries usually are associated with pelvic fractures from motor vehicle accidents, or they may occur with straddle injuries. Urethral injuries from break dancing have been reported also.[22] Injury to this structure may be partial or complete. Blood at the tip of the meatus should alert the examiner to the strong probability of a urethral disruption. The physician should refrain from passing a urethral catheter until a retrograde urethrogram has allowed visualization of the entire urethra. Although rectal examination to assess the position and degree of fixation of the prostate is often recommended, the findings may be difficult to interpret in the small child whose prostate is not well developed or in the child with a large hematoma from pelvic fracture, which is the most common cause of posterior urethral injuries.

Management

The management of urethral injuries remains a subject of controversy. Glassberg and colleagues suggest that the outcome in patients with a partial tear of the proximal urethra is best with initial suprapubic drainage alone.[24] The largest review of this subject, evaluating the results and complications in 576 patients, adults and children, concludes that the procedure of choice is initial operative suprapubic cystostomy alone, delaying urethroplasty until later.[72] These researchers cite the apparently lower overall incidence of impotence (11.6% compared with 44% in the immediate repair group) and of incontinence (1.7% compared with 20% in the immediate repair group) as their primary argument. They recommend immediate reapproximation be performed only in specific instances of rectal injury, extremely large pelvic hematoma with a high-riding bladder, and concomitant bladder neck injury. Their review suggests that urethral strictures occur in all patients treated with delayed repair but in only 69% of those treated by immediate repair. Patil also recommends initial suprapubic drainage with delayed urethroplasty based on his experience with some long-term follow up in 30 children.[51] This approach has resulted in no apparent impotence; only one case of urinary incontinence, which occurred after the delayed repair; and no apparent strictures. In contrast to these data, Patterson and colleagues treated 10 children with primary realignment in their series, which also included 19 adults.[52] They described a stricture rate of 38%, an incontinence rate of 3%, and an impotence rate of 15%.

Several different types of urethroplasty have been advocated. Kramer and associates report successful reconstruction using the transpubic approach in 12 children.[32] As described previously, Patil also reports excellent results with this approach.[51] He believes the important operative technical points to be adequate support of the thighs to prevent their sudden displacement during excision of the pubis; no mobilization of the prostate; extensive mobilization of the distal urethra to the glans penis,, swinging the mobilized urethra anterior to the strictured site; opening the prostatic urethra close to the stricture, creating a 24- to 26-Fr–caliber stoma; anchoring of the prostatic urethral mucosa to the prostatic capsule to prevent anastomotic stricture; and anchoring of the mobilized penile urethra to the corpora to prevent anastomotic tension. Harshman and associates report similarly successful urethral stricture repair using excision and reanastomosis for short strictures,[28] and Devine and colleagues report success with full thickness patch grafts for longer strictures.[17] Barbagli and associates report 31 children who required urethroplasty for traumatic injuries.[3] Twenty of these patients were managed by transpubic urethroplasty, with 13 cases of absence of erectile function, two cases of incontinence, and two cases of restricture. They stress the importance of using omentoplasty in conjunction with this repair. Nine of their patients underwent a perineal urethroplasty with 5 cases of absence of erectile function, 1 case of incontinence, and 1 case of restricture.

Marshall and colleagues and McCoy and associates report the successful endoscopic management of urethral injuries.[39, 41] This technique involves placement of a flexible nephroscope through the suprapubic tract to the end of the proximal urethra and passing a rigid endoscope through the distal urethra. Under C-arm fluoroscopic control, a small, hollow needle is passed into the apex of the prostatic urethra through the scar. A Rosen wire is then passed through a straight-needle trocar, and urethral continuity is restored with balloon dilation. A 22-Fr catheter is then passed over the wire into the bladder and is left in place for at least 4 weeks. Additional endoscopic resection accompanied by triamcinolone injection is performed as indicated, and the catheter is removed 2 to 4 weeks later.

Traumatic injury to the anterior or distal urethra is much less common in boys because of the mobile nature of this structure. Injuries in this portion of the urethra are much more likely to be iatrogenic. These strictures have been reported to occur in nearly 5% of children in whom urinary catheters were placed for cardiac surgery and after 8 to 25% of cases of posterior valve ablation.[35, 57] Accidents in which the bulbous urethra is crushed against the bony symphysis also may result in stricture. Many of these lesions can be dealt with successfully by temporary suprapubic urinary diversion alone, by either catheter or vesicostomy.[56] Noe reports an 80% success rate using visual urethrotomy with intralesional steroid injections and suggests that this treatment is preferable to dilation.[48] We prefer using the KTP/532 Laser (Laserscope, Santa Clara, Calif.) to electrocautery for the endoscopic treatment of these lesions.

Injury to the urethra in girls is rare. The most severe injuries occur in association with pelvic fractures, and these nearly always involve the vagina.[73] Contusion or minor lacerations may result from foreign bodies or self-inflicted trauma and are best treated conservatively. Blunt trauma from straddle injuries or suction injuries from swimming pool drains may result in contusion and hematoma of the periurethral tissues. Direct visualization under anesthesia or heavy sedation, with endoscopy as indicated, is mandatory to rule out more serious injuries.

Uniform treatment of severe urethral disruption in girls has not been established and depends to a great extent on the exact nature of the lesion and the experience of the surgeon. Suprapubic drainage is indicated and may be all that is required in the occasional lesion that does not involve the vagina. Vaginal, transpubic, and retropubic approaches have all been used successfully, with incontinence being the major complication in high lesions.[46]

NEONATAL URINARY TRACT TRAUMA

Genitourinary injuries may occur in utero, or during delivery. Amniocentesis is often performed and has been known to injure the kidney.[16] Although massive hemoperitoneum usually occurs from visceral injury, one case has been reported after suprapubic bladder aspiration.[31]

We have seen one case of a neonate with a massive intracapsular renal hematoma from trauma that caused infarction of the kidney. This patient presented with hematuria in the first 24 hours of life, and a nephrectomy was required to control the hypertension that later occurred.

CHILD ABUSE

Hematuria in cases of suspected child abuse should make the physician suspicious of urinary tract injury. Occasionally, a battered child presents with oliguria and pigmented urine that is positive for blood but without red blood cells on microscopic examination of the urine. These children should be assessed for rhabdomyolysis and myoglobinuria, which may be associated with their trauma.[63]

PELVIC FRACTURES

As previously mentioned, most lower urinary tract injuries are seen in association with pelvic fractures. There appears to be no particular correlation between the extent of pelvic injury and the degree of hematuria. Microscopic hematuria is rarely associated with significant urinary tract injury (1 of 77 cases), but gross hematuria always indicates that there is an associated urinary tract injury.[20, 49] Urologic injury in these cases occurs primarily with anterior arch fractures.

References

1. Ahmed S, Morris LL: Renal parenchymal injuries secondary to blunt abdominal trauma in childhood: A 10 year review. Br J Urol 54:470–477, 1982.

2. Amparo EG, Hayden CK Jr, Schwartz MZ, et al: Computerized tomography and ultrasonography in evaluating blunt abdominal trauma in children. In: Brooks BF (ed): The Injured Child. Austin, Texas, University Park Press, 1985, pp 61–70.

3. Barbagli G, Stomaci N, Rose AD, et al: Posterior urethroplasty in children. Pediatr Urol 13:110–115, 1987.

4. Beamud-Gomez A, Martinez-Verduch M, Estronell-Moragues F, et al: Rupture of the ureteropelvic junction by nonpenetrating trauma. J Pediatr Surg 21:702–705, 1986.

5. Berger PE, Kauhn JP: CT of blunt abdominal trauma in childhood. AJR Am J Roentgenol 136:105–110, 1981.

6. Blacklock N: Bladder trauma in the long distance runner: 10,000 metres haematuria. Br J Urol 49:129–132, 1977.

7. Brower P, Paul J, Brosman SA: Urinary tract abnormalities presenting as a result of blunt abdominal trauma. J Trauma 18:719–722, 1978.

8. Brown D, Magill HL, Black TL: Delayed presentation of traumatic intraperitoneal bladder rupture. Pediatr Radiol 16:252–253, 1986.

9. Carlton CE Jr: Injuries of the kidney and ureter. In: Harrison JH, Gittes R, Perlmutter A, et al (eds): Campbell's Urology. 4th ed. Philadelphia, WB Saunders, 1978, pp 891–905.

10. Cass AS: Immediate radiological evaluation and early surgical management of genitourinary injuries from external trauma. J Urol 122:772–774, 1979.

11. Cass AS: Blunt renal pelvic and ureteral injury in multiple-injured patients. Urology 22:268–270, 1983.

12. Cass AS: Blunt renal trauma in children. J Trauma 23:123–127, 1983.

13. Cass AS, Luxenberg M, Gleich P, et al: Deaths from urologic injury due to external trauma. J Trauma 27:319–321, 1987.

14. Corriere JN, Sandler CM: Management of the ruptured bladder: Seven years of experience with 111 cases. J Trauma 26:830–833, 1986.

15. Cosgrove MD, Mendez R, Morrow JW: Branch artery ligation for renal arteriovenous fistula. J Urol 110:632–638, 1973.

16. Cromie WJ, Bates RD, Duckett JW: Penetrating renal trauma in the neonate. J Urol 119:259–260, 1978.

17. Devine PC, Fallon B, Devine CJ Jr: Free full thickness skin graft urethroplasty. J Urol 116:444–446, 1976.

18. Dmochowskin RR, Crandell SC, Corriere JN: Bladder injury and uroascites from umbilical artery catheterization. Pediatrics 77:421–442, 1986.

19. Duckett JW, Pfister RR: Ureterocalicostomy for renal salvage. J Urol 128:98–101, 1982.

20. Fallon B, Wendt JC, Hawtrey CE: Urological injury and assessment in patients with fractured pelvis. J Urol 131:712–714, 1984.

21. Garrett RA: Pediatric urethral and perineal injuries. Pediatr Clin North Am 22:401–406, 1975.

22. Gearhart JP, Lowe FC: Genitourinary injuries secondary to break dancing in children and adolescents. Pediatrics 77:922–924, 1986.

23. Giyanani VL, Gerlock AJ Jr, Grozinger KT, et al: Trauma of occult hydronephrotic kidney. Urology 25:8–12, 1979.

24. Glassberg KI, Tolete-Velcek F, Ashley R, et al: Tears of prostato-membranous urethra in children. Urology 13:500–504, 1979.

25. Godec CJ: Genitourinary trauma. Urol Radiol 7:185–191, 1985.

26. Griffen WO, Belin RP, Ernst CB, et al: Intravenous pyelography in abdominal trauma. J Trauma 18:387–391, 1978.

27. Guice K, Oldham K, Eide B, et al: Hematuria after blunt trauma: When is pyelography useful? J Trauma 23:305–311, 1983.

28. Harshman MW, Cromie WJ, Wein AJ, et al: Urethral stricture disease in children. J Urol 126:650–654, 1981.

29. Javadpour N, Guinan P, Bush IM: Renal trauma in children. Surg Gynecol Obstet 136:237–240, 1973.

30. Kaufman RA, Towbin R, Babcok DS, et al: Upper abdominal trauma in children: Imaging evaluation. AJR 142:449–460, 1984.

31. Kimmelstiel FM, Holgersen LO, Dudell GG: Massive hemoperitoneum following suprapubic bladder aspiration. J Pediatr Surg 21:911–912, 1986.

32. Kramer SA, Furlow WI, Barrett DM, et al: Transpubic urethroplasty in children. J Urol 126:767–769, 1981.

33. Kuh JP, Berger PE: Computed tomography in the evaluation of blunt abdominal trauma in children. Radiol Clin North Am 19:503–512, 1981.

34. Kuzmarov IW, Morehouse DD, Gibson S: Blunt renal trauma in the pediatric population: A retrospective study. J Urol 126:648–649, 1981.

35. Livne PM, Gonzales FT: Genitourinary trauma in children. Urol Clin North Am 12:53–65, 1985.

36. Lowe P, Hardy BR: Isolated bilateral blunt renal trauma with pelvi-ureteric disruption. Urology 19:420–422, 1982.

37. Lytton B, Schiff M: Interposition of an ileal segment for repair of ureteral injuries. J Urol 125:739–741, 1981.

38. Malek RS: Genitourinary trauma. In: Kelalis PP, King LR, (eds): Clinical Pediatric Urology. Philadelphia, WB Saunders, 1976, pp 1029–1064.

39. McCoy GB, Barry JM, Lieberman SF, et al: Treatment of obliterated membranous and bulbous urethras by direct vision internal urethrotomy. J Trauma, 27:883–886, 1987.

40. McGinty DM, Mendez R: Traumatic ureteral injuries with delayed recognition. Urology 10:115–117, 1977.

41. Marshall FF, Chang R, Gearhart JP: Endoscopic reconstruction of traumatic membranous urethral transection. J Urol 138:306–309, 1987.

42. Mendez R: Renal trauma. J Urol 118:698–703, 1977.

43. Mendez R, McGinty DM: The management of delayed recognized ureteral injuries. J Urol 119:192–193, 1978.

44. Merchant WC III, Gibbons MD, Gonzales ET: Trauma to the bladder neck, trigone and vagina in children. J Urol 131:747–750, 1984.

45. Mitchell JP: Trauma to the urinary tract. BMJ 2:567–573, 1971.

46. Netto NR Jr, Ikari O, Zuppo VP: Traumatic rupture of female urethra. Urology 22:601–603, 1983.

47. Noakes JE, Wese FX, Churchill BM: Ureteral entrapment injury in blunt pelvic trauma: A case report. J Urol 127:764–765, 1982.

48. Noe HN: Complications and management of childhood urethral stricture disease. Urol Clin North Am 10:531–536, 1983.

49. Palmer JK, Benson GS, Corriere JN Jr: Diagnosis and initial management of urological injuries associated with 200 consecutive pelvic fractures. J Urol 130:712–714, 1983.

50. Palmer JM, Drago JR: Ureteral avulsion from non-penetrating trauma. J Urol 125:108–111, 1981.

51. Patil UB: Long-term results of transpubic prostatomembranous urethroplasty in children. J Urol 136:186–187, 1986.

52. Patterson DE, Barrett DM, Myers RP, et al: Primary realignment of posterior urethral injuries. J Urol 129:513–516, 1983.

53. Persky L, Hoch WH: Genitourinary tract trauma (monograph). Curr Probl Surg September:1–64, 1972.

54. Peters PC, Bright TC III: Management of trauma to the urinary tract. Adv Surg 10:197–224, 1976.

55. Peterson NE, Pitts JC III: Penetrating injuries of the ureter. J Urol 126:587–590, 1981.

56. Pontes JE, Pierce JM: Anterior urethral injuries: Four years of experience at the Detroit General Hospital. J Urol 120:563–564, 1978.

57. Prabhu S, Cochran W, Raine PAM, et al: Postcatheterization urethral strictures following cardiac surgery in children. J Pediatr Surg 20:69–71, 1985.

58. Prather GC: Injuries of the bladder. In: Campbell MF, Harrison JH (ed): Urology. 3rd ed. Vol. 1. Philadelphia, WB Saunders, 1970, pp 852–865.

59. Reda EF, Lebowitz RL: Traumatic ureteropelvic disruption in the child. Pediatr Radiol 16:164–166, 1986.

60. Redman JF, Jacks DW, O'Donnell PD: Cystectomy: A catastrophic complication of herniorrhaphy. J Urol 133:97–98, 1985.

61. Richter MW, Lytton B, Grnja V: Radiology of genitourinary trauma. Radiol Clin North Am 11:593–631, 1973.

62. Riehle RA: Trauma to the lower urinary tract and genitals. In: Kendall AR, Karafin L, Stein BS (eds): Goldsmith: Practice of Surgery. Vol. 2. Thomastown, Conn, Practice of Surgery Ltd, 1987, pp 1–25.

63. Rosenberg HK, Gefter WB, Lebowitz RL, et al: Prolonged dense nephrograms in battered children. Urology 21:325–330, 1983.

64. Roth DR, Krueger RP, Barraza M: Bladder disruption in the premature male neonate. J Urol 137:500–501, 1987.

65. Sklar DP, Diven B, Jones J: Incidence and magnitude of catheter-induced hematuria. Am J Emerg Med 4:14–16, 1986.

66. Smith MJV, Seidel RJ, Bonacarti AF: Accident trauma to the kidneys in children. J Urol 96:845–847, 1986.

67. Snyder JM III, Caldamone AA: Genitourinary injuries. In: Welch KJ, Randolph JG, Ravitch MM, et al (eds): Pediatric Surgery. 4th ed. Chicago, Year Book Medical Publishers, 1986, pp 174–185.

68. Stampfel G, Joost J: Die Ureterruptur nach stumpfem Bauchtrauma. Fortschr Rontgenstr 141:570–573, 1984.

69. Tank ES: Upper urinary tract injuries. Dial Pediatr Urol 3:1, 1980.

70. Wallijn E, DeSy W, Fonteyene E: Blunt ureteral trauma with perineal urine fistulization: Review of the literature. J Urol 114:942–945, 1975.

71. Waterhouse K, Gross M: Trauma to the genitourinary tract: A 5 year experience with 251 cases. J Urol 101:241–246, 1969.

72. Webster GD, Mathes GL, Selli C: Prostatomembranous urethral injuries: A review of the literature and a rational approach to their management. J Urol 130:898–902, 1983.

73. Williams DI: Rupture of the female urethra in childhood. Eur Urol 1:129–130, 1975.

74. Woodward A, Smith ED: Closed renal trauma in children. Aust N Z J Surg 52:66–70, 1982.

75. Young JD: Trauma to the kidney and ureter. In: Kendall AR, Karafin L, Stein BS (eds): Goldsmith: Practice of Surgery. Vol. 2. Thomastown, Conn, Practice of Surgery Ltd, 1987, pp 1–40.

Sterling H. Blocker
John F. Redman

CHAPTER TWENTY-EIGHT

Genital and Perineal Injuries

VULVAR INJURIES
  Straddle Injuries
  Vaginal Injuries
  Rape and Sexual Abuse
  Water Skiing Injury

ANAL (ANORECTAL) INJURY
  Straddle Injury
  Sexual Abuse

PENILE INJURIES
  Crush Injury
  Strangulation Injury
  Circumcision
  Bites
  Flexion of Erect Penis
  Vacuum Cleaner Injury
  Avulsion (Power Takeoff) Injuries
  Burns

  Gunshot Wounds
  Blade Injuries
  Child Abuse

SCROTAL INJURIES
  Blunt Trauma
  Avulsion (Power Takeoff) Injuries
  Impalement
  Burns
  Gunshot Injury
  Animal Bites
  Birth Trauma

TESTICULAR INJURIES
  Forcible Direct Compression (Blunt Trauma)
  Avulsion
  Penetrating Trauma
  Burns

Injuries of the perineum and genitalia of children include injuries to the anus, vulva, vagina, penis, scrotum, and testes. Injuries to these areas are usually minor but can be severe and associated with significant physical morbidity and emotional trauma. The mechanisms of injury are diverse. Unfortunately, an increasingly common mechanism is nonaccidental: child abuse. Hence, the need for heightened suspicion; careful elicitation of history; and diligent, meticulous physical examination on the part of the examining physician is repeatedly emphasized in this chapter.

VULVAR INJURIES

The vulvar area in little girls, is most commonly injured by ''straddle'' mechanisms (with or without penetration), such as kicks or direct blows, falls, sudden forced stretching of the perineum, sexual abuse (including rape), and motor vehicle accidents. Less commonly, injuries have been reported from human bites and water skiing and even as a result of breech delivery[15, 31] (Fig. 28–1). All children with vulvar injuries should be approached with a high index of suspicion that sexual abuse could be involved. Generally, a history of prompt referral, a clear description of the accident, and appropriate physical findings consistent with the described mechanisms will clarify the issue. However, if there are inconsistencies in the history, then careful inquiry into the social environment of the child should be initiated.[55]

Straddle Injuries

With straddle injuries, the soft tissues of the vulva are compressed between the straddle object and the symphysis pubis and pubic rami.[55, 59] If the straddle object is blunt and no penetration occurs, the anatomic areas at greatest risk are the perineum, labia, clitoris, and urethra (Fig. 28–2). The two most common resulting injuries are hematoma formation and linear lacerations.

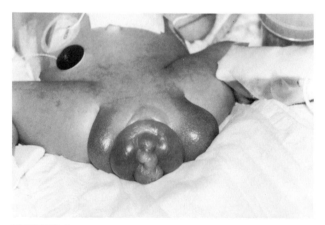

FIGURE 28–1

Vulvar hematoma secondary to breech delivery in a female infant with ambiguous genitalia.

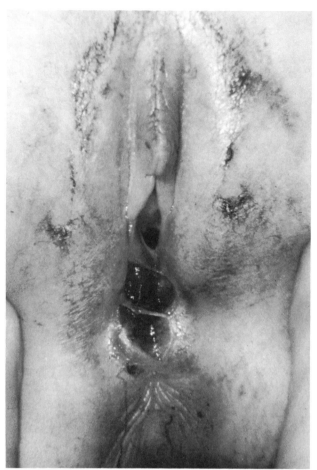

FIGURE 28–2

Straddle injury. Blunt superficial tears into posterior fourchette and labia. Also superficial tear into anus.

If the child is cooperative and permits an examination in which it can be determined that the introitus is not involved and that no blood and discharge are emanating from the introitus, then appropriate local treatment can be initiated. However, if the child will not permit good visualization of the external genitalia, as is quite often the case, or if there is a suggestion of a vaginal injury, then the child should be examined under anesthesia.[57]

Vulvar hematomas generally require no specific treatment, although a large hematoma that is increasing in size should be considered for incision, drainage, and, if possible, ligation of the offending vessel or vessels.[34] Lacerations may or may not be closed, depending on size and elapsed time before diagnosis (Fig. 28–3). Closure is accomplished with fine, simple absorbable sutures, and broad spectrum antimicrobial coverage, both systemic and topical, should be employed and tetanus prophylaxis ensured. Sitz baths can help reduce contamination from perineal secretion and reduce the need for analgesics. Physical therapy devices such as rubber or inflatable rings can aid in comfort with sitting and prevent early disruption of repaired lacerations, especially in older children. The discussion of management of vulvar injuries associated with rape and other sexual abuse is found in the section on vaginal injuries.

Vaginal Injuries

The vagina may be injured by falls astride a projection that may be penetrating (impalement), motor vehicle accidents, rape, and even water skiing.[15] In any instance in which vulvar or perineal trauma has occurred in a female child, the introitus should be examined for any slight degree of trauma, and blood or discharge from that area should be sought. If there is vaginal introital involvement or introital blood, a concomitant vaginal injury must be ruled out, a process that probably does not require examination under general anesthesia. Sometimes patients with vaginal injuries present with only a modicum of introital physical findings. As described under vulvar injuries, any injury to the vagina should be suspected as having occurred as the result of sexual abuse, and careful attention should be given to the history of injury, the apparent emotional status of the child, and the physical findings themselves.

Rape and Sexual Abuse

If penetration does not occur, the most common physical findings are those of vulvar trauma, including bruising and

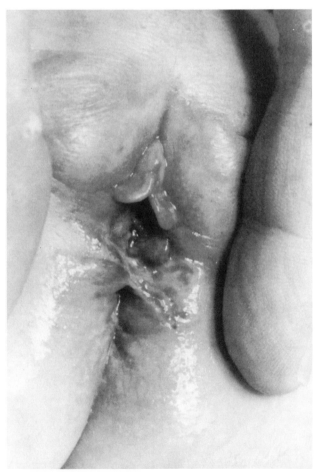

FIGURE 28-3

Chronic secondary laceration in a 3-month-old-girl that was inflicted by a psychotic parent using a "hairbrush."

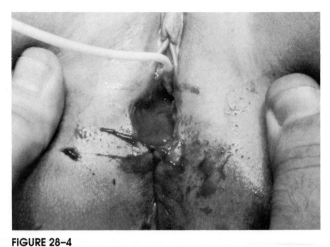

FIGURE 28-4

Second-degree posterior vaginal laceration in a 5-year-old girl that extended through the perineum into the anal sphincter.

lacerations.[16, 59] At times, severe trauma occurs, including vaginal laceration, tears into the anal sphincter and rectum, and even penetration into the peritoneal cavity (Fig. 28-4).

A most complete and valuable forensic examination protocol for the evaluation of a sexually abused child is that of Enos and colleagues.[16] Their guidelines are important reading for physicians given the responsibility of ascertaining the occurrence of sexual abuse. As these investigators indicated, professionals, functioning from a medical rather than a forensic perspective, must be mindful that "the forensic aspects of care are often not considered, or may be poorly handled, for lack of proper guidelines. It has to be appreciated that sexual child abuse is a determination made by the courts and not by medical diagnoses."[16] If sexual abuse is suspected in childhood genital trauma, care should be taken initially in structuring the history taking and physical examination so that the proper evidence is obtained and legally documented. It is therefore very important for professionals called to manage victims of child abuse to be knowledgeable of the legal requirements for data collection and documentation extant in their area.

In brief, the history should be obtained in a gentle, sympathetic manner using language that fits the age and educational level of the child.[16] The physical examination should begin with the least invasive procedures first and include a general body examination. Any trauma, no matter how minimal it may seem, should be documented and even photographed.[41] Swabs should be obtained systematically during the perineal and anal examination and should be carefully labeled and stored. The vulvar and vaginal examination, which in most cases should be undertaken under general anesthesia, may not disclose injury in one third of children known to have been abused sexually. A greater percentage appear to be uninjured if the suspected abuse occurred more than a week before the examination.[36] Subtle findings of abuse may become more apparent to the examiner if he or she uses a colposcope or is aided by the addition of dye, such as 1% toluidine blue.[25, 58]

Young children who have undergone penile penetration of the vagina usually sustain posterior midline lacerations

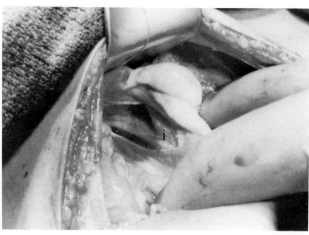

FIGURE 28–5

Perforation through the broad ligament in an 8-year-old rape victim. Note the exposed iliac artery (i).

that extend into the perineal body.[59] First-degree injuries are defined as those in which the muscle is intact; second-degree injuries are those in which the muscle is torn; and third-degree injuries are those that extend into the rectum.[59] With full penile penetration, tears may extend to the posterior lateral wall of the vagina (Fig. 28–5), at times to the lateral fornix or fornices, with the most extreme injury being that of intraperitoneal penetration with massive retroperitoneal hemorrhage (Fig. 28–6).

Management of such vaginal injuries begins with a careful examination under anesthesia utilizing endoscopy of the vagina when applicable. Distal lacerations may be closed primarily if they are less than 24 hours old. If there is concern regarding soiling, the skin and mucosa may be left open. In instances of anal sphincter damage, when a complete primary closure is not prudent, an attempt should be made primarily to retrieve the sphincter, which may be retracted, and to secure the muscle with sutures. The major difficulty in managing trauma to the vagina itself is brisk bleeding, which, if staunched initially, may again manifest itself abundantly with the onset of preparation for surgery. Ingenuity, good retraction, and illumination are requisites to ligating bleeding vessels and effecting closure of the vaginal wall. The deeper vaginal injuries should be repaired first; for the most part, these may be accomplished primarily with good healing expected and no introital narrowing. Perforations into the peritoneal cavity mandate celiotomy.

Water Skiing Injury

Severe tearing of the vagina with extension to the fornices has been described following falls while water skiing.[15] The injuries generally occur with outside swings at excessive speeds during which the skier falls with her legs apart. Management is as previously described for other lacerations of the vagina and injuries of the vulva. A preventative measure, other than avoiding high speeds on outside turns while water skiing, is the wearing of a wet suit or cutoff jeans.[15]

ANAL (ANORECTAL) INJURY

The mechanisms of anorectal injury include straddle injuries (with or without penetration), sexual abuse, gunshot wounds, suction from swimming pool drains, and water skiing.

Straddle Injury

A falling child landing forcefully astride a variety of smooth structures, may sustain an injury to the anus, the perineum, and even possibly the rectum.[8] Injuries may consist only of ecchymosis but may also include lacerations extending into the anal sphincter and into the vulva in females. These injuries are usually managed in the operating room with irrigation and primary closure.

A straddle injury in which the child falls onto a vertically oriented object—impalement—can produce extensive rectal injury as well as injury to the bladder, prostate, vagina, and intraperitoneal structures.[8] Impalement injuries require extensive evaluation, including, but not limited to, proctoscopy, vaginoscopy, cystography, and, if necessary, computed tomography. Diverting colostomy may be necessary for proper healing.

Sexual Abuse

Anorectal trauma in children is most frequently caused by child abuse or deviant sexual activity.[8] Black and associates found that one third of children evaluated because of possible rape alleged that they sustained anal trauma.[8] Although male children are sexually abused considerably less than females (7.5%:16.0%, male:female), almost 50% sustain significant anorectal injury.

Examination of the anus, even in a child who is known to have sustained anal abuse, frequently shows no change or changes not unlike those seen in a nonabused child.[20, 28, 35] Children who are able to describe anal assault in detail,

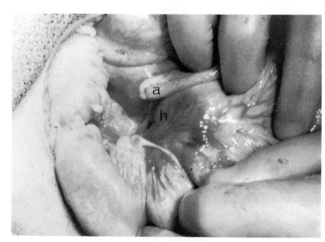

FIGURE 28–6

Large retroperitoneal hematoma (h) beneath the appendix (a) in the same patient as in Figure 28–5.

however, are more likely to have perianal abnormalities.[35] It should be noted and remembered that the anus may appear to be traumatized following chronic constipation or vigorous cleansing or in children with perianal dermatologic conditions. If child abuse is suspected based on the findings of the anal evaluation, however, the matter of sexual abuse should still be pursued.

The majority of anal lacerations may be closed primarily following evaluation of the rectum by palpation and proctoanoscopy to ensure its integrity. Disruption of the sphincter may also be repaired primarily in most instances. If the injury is old or soiled, an attempt should be made to secure the sphincter by sutures to prevent its retraction. Normal healing with good continence can be expected.

PENILE INJURIES

The penis, being a relatively small movable appendage with a centripetal location, is not often injured. However, reported injuries can range from simple bruising and laceration to complete amputation, and the mechanisms of injury include crushing, circumcision, strangulation, bites, flexion

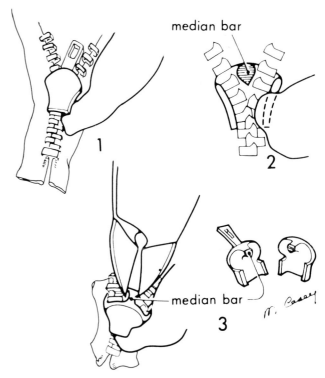

FIGURE 28–8
Technique of disarticulating the zipper by first cutting the median bar with bone- or wire-cutting pliers.

of the erect penis, gunshot wounds, self-inflicted knife wounds, burns, avulsion, vacuum cleaners, and child abuse.

Crush Injury

Crushing-type injuries to the penis have been reported to occur from various mechanisms, including entrapping the prepuce while zippering a pants fly and dropping the toilet seat onto the penis.[19, 42]

Entrapment of the prepuce in young boys by zippers usually occurs with hurried zippering or unzippering of the fly when the penis is not returned to the confines of the underwear or when underwear is not worn (Fig. 28–7). It may also occur in boys who wear night clothing with anterior zippers.[37] It has been suggested that the decreased rate of neonatal circumcision will subject more boys to the risk of this injury.[42] Attempts to free the prepuce by unzippering manipulations cause considerable pain and are generally unsuccessful. The now standardized method of treatment is to employ a bone or wire cutting instrument to cut the median bar of the zipper, which allows its disarticulation through the separation of the anterior and posterior parts[17] (Fig. 28–8). Anesthesia is not required, and healing is usually uneventful with minimal scarring.

Crushing of the glans or prepuce or shaft also occurs in a particular group of small boys who are at the age of potty training and of a size in which the position of the penis, while standing, coincides with the height of the rim of the toilet bowl when the seat is raised. Injury occurs with the dropping of the seat as the penis lies on the anvillike rim of

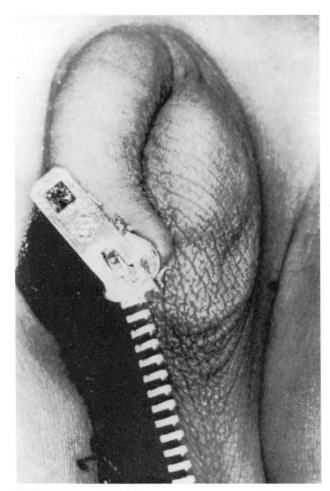

FIGURE 28–7
Prepuce entrapped in zipper.

the toilet bowl. Resulting injuries may include laceration, edema, and ecchymosis, with the potential for anterior urethral stricturing if there is sufficient crushing of the urethra. Although the initial appearance may be dramatic, no specific diagnostic or management measures are required, and healing is usually uneventful. However, as with any non-specific injury to the penis in a child, sexual abuse should be a consideration, and a detailed history of the occurrence of the injury and a thorough physical examination should be completed. Prevention may be facilitated by primary care physicians if they will advise parents with boys undergoing potty training to be certain that adequate clearance is maintained by the spacers between the toilet seat and rim of the bowl.[19]

Strangulation Injury

Penile strangulation may occur when the penis has been placed through a ring, a bottle, or a pipe or has been wrapped with a rubber band, thread, or human hair.[44, 52]

Human hair producing strangulation of the penis has been described for centuries. It is generally thought to occur by accidental wrapping of the shaft, but is also known to occur by deliberate wrapping by parents to control enuresis. As in other instances of penile injury in children, child abuse as a factor should receive consideration. Hair or thread strangulation should be suspected in any boy who presents with the nonspecific complaints of glandular swelling or pain, whether or not discoloration of the glans is present.[47] A careful search is necessary to find the encircling hair or thread. If the hair is not seen but a circumferential depressed area is noted on the penile shaft or glans, an incision in the groove on the lateral aspect of the penis (to avoid injury to the urethra) should be made, incising the hair.[44] The degree of injury is dependent on the length of time that the hair has been in place; therefore, the skin is affected first, with the corpus spongiosum and the urethra being injured next[44] (Fig. 28–9A and B). The neurovascular bundle and corpus cavernosum are the last structures to be injured. A 0 to 3 grading scale has been proposed in which grade "0" indicates skin injury alone; grade 1 indicates partial division of the corpus spongiosum and urethra with fistula formation; grade 2 indicates complete division of the corpus spongiosum and constriction of the corpora cavernosa; and grade 3 indicates gangrene, necrosis, and complete amputation of the glans.[5]

Initial treatment consists of removal of the constriction with local and possibly systemic antimicrobial coverage. Repair is delayed until all signs of induration and erythema have subsided and then consists of closure of the urethrocutaneous fistula and reapproximation of the glans penis, either in one or two stages.[29]

Other constrictive penile band injuries, particularly those involving the shaft of the penis, may require innovation in removing the constricting agent, particularly wide or dense metal bands. Aggressive débridement, skin grafting, and temporary urinary diversion may then be necessary.[52] Wrapping of the shaft distal to the ring with a cord, which is then in turn passed under the ring, may be an effective technique for removal. As the cord is unwrapped proximally the ring is advanced distally. Some rings are so dense and tight that a machinist or even the fire department may need to be enlisted to facilitate removal.[52] If débridement is not accomplished initially, marked chronic penile edema may necessitate skin excision and subsequent grafting. In skin grafting of the penis, contraction of the graft is the primary consideration, and the choice should be, where possible, a full thickness graft. With severe penile skin and urethral injury, urinary diversion by a suprapubic tube is a requisite.[52]

Circumcision

Circumcision as a mechanism of penile injury in children is considered to be one of the most common, particularly if overzealous removal of shaft skin is considered.[12, 39] Generally, the apparently denuded shaft, which may be noted following a neonatal circumcision, may be recovered with the often remaining generous sleeve of the inner leaf of the prepuce. In some instances, vascularized flaps or free full thickness skin grafting may be required.[39] A useful admonition to avoid denuding of the shaft is to withhold circumcision in the neonatal period on boys who do not have a definitive straight shaft protruding from the body. Those with a short or hidden penis should have the circumcision accomplished, if at all, in the operating room at 6 months to 1 year of age, where careful attention to skin measuring may be done.

A devastating injury to the penis with circumcision is that caused by the use of diathermy, particularly in conjunction with a metallic shield such as the Gomco clamp. Severe burns and even sloughing of the entire penis have occurred.[4]

Bites

Animal bites causing genital injury have been infrequently reported, even though 1 to 2 million people are bitten by animals each year in the United States, with dog bites being the most common.[14] Penile injury, including amputation, by dog bites has been described, as well as penile amputation by the bite of a pig.[14, 53] The potential risk of rabies and tetanus should be considered, as well as that of nonspecific bacterial infection. When in doubt regarding the condition of the animal, appropriate antirabies therapy should be given. Tetanus prophylaxis should also be ensured. Management of the penile injury is dependent on the type and degree of injury. Simple lacerations may be cleaned and then closed primarily.[14] Degloving of the shaft should be managed by aggressive débridement and antimicrobial irrigation followed by full thickness or split thickness skin grafting. Child abuse or child neglect should be suspected in any child with a history of animal bites.[14]

Flexion of Erect Penis

Rapid forceful flexion of the erect penis can result in rupture of the corpus cavernosum. In the adolescent such a

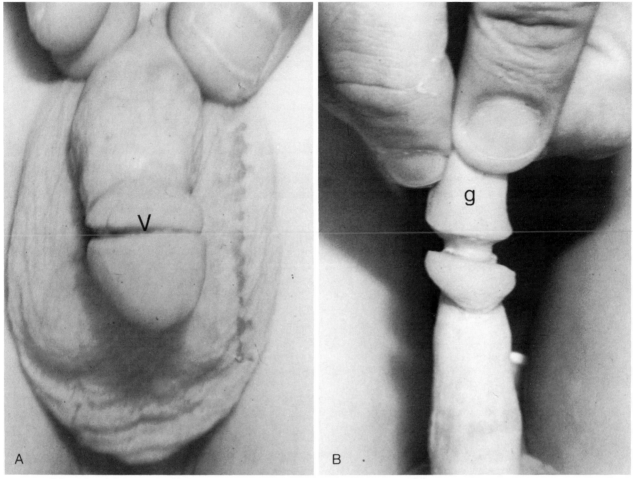

FIGURE 28–9

A, Penile injury (v) resulting from encirclement by a hair. *B*, Note the depth of the injury beneath the glans (g) viewed from above. The patient also had a urethral fistula.

mechanism may occur with intercourse or masturbation. The history is usually specific and includes the hearing by the patient of an audible snapping sound or crack followed by immediate detumescence, abnormal swelling, discoloration, and deformity.[11] The diagnosis may be confirmed by sonography, which should include also examination of the urethra and corpus spongiosum.[18] Management should be immediate surgical exploration. On degloving the penis, the laceration will be revealed and may extend into the corpus spongiosum. Primary closure of the defect should be expected to yield an uneventful convalescence and normal straight erections thereafter.

Vacuum Cleaner Injury

A most unusual and bizarre mechanism of adolescent penile injury occurs with the insertion of the erect penis for the purpose of masturbation into the aperture of the body of an operating vacuum cleaner or electric broom.[6] The fan blades are located 15 cm from the opening, and resultant injuries to the penis range from mild laceration and ecchymosis to degloving injuries and severe lacerations up to and including amputation of the glans. Complete amputation of the glans penis has been reported from the insertion of the penis into a vacuum cleaner hose.[6] Management is dictated by the degree of injury, with most repairs being accomplished primarily.

Avulsion (Power Takeoff) Injuries

Avulsion of the penile or penoscrotal skin may occur when the child's clothing comes in contact with a rapidly rotating wheel or axle or power takeoff. Avulsion may also occur as a deceleration injury, when the genitalia become caught on a stationary object, the most frequent instance being in vehicular accidents.[27, 54] Primary repair may be accomplished. If the skin is still attached, it may be cleaned and reapplied. Completely avulsed skin has seldom been reutilized to effect coverage. When skin grafting is required, skin is most often obtained from the anterior aspect of the thigh utilizing the dermatome. Full thickness grafts are harvested if the skin is hairless, and split thickness grafts are used with hair-bearing skin. Each type of graft has its advantages and disadvantages. A full thickness graft generally does not contract but has the disadvantages of hair growth, difficult take, and requirements for split thickness skin grafting of the donor site.[27] The ideal skin graft is considered to be a relatively thick (0.018″) split thickness graft, which results in only a small degree of contracture and does not require grafting of the donor site. Thin split thickness and meshed split thickness grafts should be avoided. As recommended by McAninich, the graft is applied so that the ventral suture line is on the ventrum of the penis and is approximated with 5-0 chromic catgut suture, with the distal and proximal ends being sutured in similar fashion to the existing epithelium.[27] A portion of the proximal and distal sutures should be left long to tie over a large bolster dressing. Fine mesh impregnated gauze, with all folds removed, is placed over the graft, followed by thin cotton padding soaked in mineral oil, followed by fluff dressing, which is held in place by tying the long suture tags together. An indwelling catheter is placed, and the penis is kept in a vertical position by surrounding it with a plastic housing. The penile dressing and catheter are removed on the fifth day unless signs of infection necessitate an earlier removal. A 90% graft take should be expected. Small areas of skin loss may be appropriately managed by rotational flaps from the scrotum, lower abdomen, or thighs.

Burns

Burns of the penis may occur from fire, electricity, chemicals, or scalding, either as an isolated injury or in association with more extensive bodily burns.[24, 27, 32, 51] Because of the thinness of penile skin, burns are usually full thickness. With flame burns, topical care alone is usually all that is required for second-degree lesions; however, third-degree burns should be managed within the first week of injury by excising devitalized tissue and applying thick split thickness auto skin grafts.[27] Patients with deep burns of the ventrum of the penis should have a suprapubic catheter placed to avoid damage to the urethra. Electrical burns should be managed by conservative débridement as the full extent of injury becomes apparent, with initial conservative treatment and later reassessment. For chemical burns, attention should be given initially to flushing or neutralizing the chemical, with excision of the involved skin in severe cases to prevent deeper injury.[27] For severe penile burns, as for any severe penile injury, attention should also be given to the psychological needs of the patient.[51]

Gunshot Wounds

Penetrating injuries of the penis may occur from gunshot wounds, which include shotguns and other low- and high-velocity projectiles.[33] Retrograde urethrography should be considered because of the possibility of concomitant urethral injury. Management is individualized; however, the majority of patients require surgical intervention, including débridement, either primary or delayed urethroplasty, and primary skin closure where indicated. A circumcising incision at the level of the corona with degloving of the shaft provides good exposure of the penis for exploration of injuries and should be considered for all injuries that penetrate the layers deep to the skin.[33] A primary repair of the urethra should be considered if adequate length exists following débridement. Urinary diversion by either a urethral catheter or a suprapubic cystostomy should be maintained for 7 to 10 days. Wound drainage should be considered. Complications include urethral strictures, fistula formation, or both.

Blade Injuries

Instruments that produce blade injuries to the penises of children and adolescents have included knives, scissors, and razor blades. These injuries may be accidental, self-inflicted, or inflicted as an act of child abuse.[48] Injury may vary from a superficial laceration to an extensive severance of the urethra or a total amputation.[10, 48, 53, 56] In any instance of laceration or cutting of the penis with a blade, psychiatric aberrations should be surmised in adolescents and child abuse suspected in children.

Lacerations, including urethral laceration, should be managed primarily as outlined under gunshot wounds. Amputation of the penis may be managed by primary reanastomosis, if the warm ischemic time is less than 18 hours.[10] Microsurgical skills are required for the vascular anastomoses (at least one artery and two veins). If primary reanastomosis is not a consideration, reconstruction of the partially amputated penis may be accomplished by mobilization of the residual corporal bodies and the corpora spongiosum and urethra to the level of the pubic bones. They either may be buried in the scrotum as a first stage or covered with a free skin or pedicle graft.[53] The advantage of mobilization of the corpora is that erectile and urinary functions are preserved, as well as sensation. Other techniques for phalloplasty include penile construction utilizing skin or myocutaneous flaps, or both, as well as a free vascularized transfer graft.

Child Abuse

Child abuse, which can take many forms including beatings, bruising, lacerations, or even neglect leading to injury, may result in penile trauma.[48] Penile trauma, when recognized, may not suggest child abuse, and only the heightened awareness of the examiner will bring the abuse to light. As stated by Slosberg and co-workers, "Frequently the penile lesion was a vital clue in discovering more serious trauma."[48] In their example, discovery of the penile injury prompted radiologic examination, which disclosed a scapular fracture and, coupled with an investigation of the family dynamics, established the diagnosis of child abuse.

SCROTAL INJURIES

The scrotum, like the penis, a movable, centrally located appendage, is not often injured. Injury may be only a simple laceration or an ecchymosis that can result in total loss of the scrotum. The mechanisms of injury include blunt trauma, avulsion (power takeoff) injuries, impalement, burns, gunshot wounds, animal bites, and birth trauma.

Blunt Trauma

Blunt trauma to the scrotum may occur during sporting events when the participant is kicked or hit in the scrotum or from bicycle straddle or handlebar injuries.[26] Such an injury may produce a laceration but more commonly results in ecchymosis and swelling. All scrota injured by blunt trauma with other than superficial bruising should be evaluated by scrotal ultrasonography to rule out associated testicular injury because a palpatory examination of a painful scrotum is difficult and possibly misleading.[3] The contralateral testicle may be used as the control. If a large hematoma or obvious testicular rupture is present, transscrotal surgical exploration should be undertaken. Testicular torsion as a sequela of blunt scrotal trauma should also be considered.[26]

Avulsion (Power Takeoff) Injuries

Any rapidly rotating device that can catch the clothing can produce injury of the scrotum.[10, 54] These devices include power-driven vehicle chains, washing machines, grain augers, power takeoffs of farm machinery, and fan blades. The resulting injury, other than ecchymosis or laceration, will be partial or complete loss of the scrotal skin and may include also loss of penile skin and trauma to or loss of a testicle. Partial scrotal skin loss may be managed by lavage, débridement, and primary closure owing to the compliance and elasticity of scrotal skin.[27] Not infrequently, an apparently large scrotal skin loss turns out to be less once the scrotal skin is stretched out.

The management of total scrotal skin loss requires considerably more thought and endeavor. After the wound is irrigated and débrided, a primary concern is provision of coverage of the testicles. A time-honored method has been to place the testes in subcutaneous thigh or abdominal pouches with the intent of replacing them in a neoscrotum. Unfortunately, the end result has often been the loss of testicular tissue in the subsequent dissection and transfer process.[7] Also at times, the neoscrotum has been inadequate to replace both testes, and, therefore, one is removed, particularly if its appearance is not optimal.

Two perhaps superior alternatives for primary management exist: initially constructing a scrotum or leaving the testes in situ and uncovered. If scrotal skin cannot be found to cover the testes and immediate skin grafting cannot be accomplished, the best decision is not to bury the testes in the thigh or abdominal pouches but to leave them in situ until time for later skin grafting.[7] If the wound is clean, the testes are sutured together by the remaining tunics to form a solitary mass, which is then covered with a split thickness (0.14–0.018″) meshed skin graft.[27, 54] If a primary closure is not possible because of mitigating factors, free skin grafting may be accomplished at a later stage. Pedicle grafts from the thigh can be utilized but are generally not acceptable as an alternative because the skin of children is not often as loose or as devoid of subcutaneous tissue as that of an adult. A further consideration in delayed repair is the employment of a tissue expander, which may be used to expand both perineal and residual scrotal skin.[40, 50] The results of scrotal reconstruction should be satisfactory, with few postoperative complications.[54]

Impalement

Occasionally impalement on a stationary object has been reported to occur in children with "sledding" type injuries. In these instances, a child was sitting on a sled or a skateboard and ran into or passed over a stationary sharp projection that penetrated the scrotum.[9, 23] The scrotal injury was the most serious of the injuries sustained, but surprisingly minimal damage was done, although abdominal explorations were necessary. The scrotal entrance wounds were drained with through and through drains and left open. We had a case of a 9-year-old boy who became impaled on a 2 inch by 6 inch sharp sapling stump, which entered the left hemiscrotum and penetrated the left groin. The wound was irrigated, explored, and closed primarily without sequelae because no other injury was found.

Burns

Burns to the scrotum may occur from flames, scalding, electrical contact, or chemicals.[1, 30] Scrotal burns generally are not isolated but are associated with extensive burns of the abdomen, thighs, and penis. Management of full thickness burns is conservative with the application of topical antimicrobials and physiologic dressings until a good granulating base has been formed.[30] Débridement should be conservative, with only obviously devitalized tissue removed. A meshed split thickness skin graft may then be applied. With the inherent redundancy of scrotal skin, contraction may be so pronounced that closure of the wound without grafting may be possible.[30] Potential early complications are infections, including suppurative epididymo-orchitis. Late complications are generally contractures that may require release and regrafting. Indwelling catheters can be avoided if the patient is able to void.[38]

Gunshot Injury

Gunshot injury to the scrotum may be caused by either low- or high-velocity projectiles, with the scrotum being the site of entrance and with the course of the projectile involving other bodily structure. Generally, with penetrating wounds of the scrotum, the scrotum should be explored for débridement; removal of foreign material, such as clothing or shotgun wadding; and management of concomitant testicular injury, if present.

Animal Bites

Dog bites of the scrotum with scrotal avulsion and testicular loss have been described in infants.[14] Management is by débridement and delayed meshed split thickness grafting. Attention should be given to antimicrobial coverage and tetanus and rabies prophylaxis. Clean, simple injuries may be managed by primary closure. A sound admonition is that an investigation of the home environment is mandatory when a child is reportedly injured by a domestic animal to search out evidence of deliberate child abuse or neglect.[14]

Birth Trauma

Breech delivery may result in severe contusion of the scrotum and perineum and, in extreme cases, may result in gangrene formation[2, 13] (Fig. 28–10). Traumatic hydroceles and hematoceles have been described. Most such injuries tend to resolve spontaneously without intervention. An important caveat is that scrotal ecchymosis in the newborn may be a sign of intraperitoneal hemorrhage. This sign has been recognized with neonatal sepsis and coagulation disorders and intra-abdominal hemorrhage from birth trauma associated with liver and spleen disruptions.[13]

TESTICULAR INJURIES

Testicular injury may occur in association with scrotal trauma or as an isolated event. Mechanisms of trauma include forcible direct compression (blunt trauma), avulsion, penetrating trauma, and burns.

Forcible Direct Compression (Blunt Trauma)

Forcible direct compression may occur as a result of kicks, straddle injuries, sporting events, falls, and motor vehicle accidents. It is surmised that injury of the testicle, which is most often a rupture of the tunica albuginea, occurs when the testis is trapped between the forceful object and a hard stationary object such as the pubis or ischium.[43] Forcible

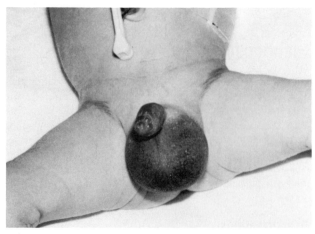

FIGURE 28–10
Hematoma of the penis and scrotum in a newborn resulting from the trauma of a breech delivery.

direct compression has also caused dislocations of the testicle.[46]

Patients with testicular rupture present with no specific sign other than scrotal ecchymosis, pain, and swelling following forceful trauma. This history and these signs should prompt transscrotal exploration because untreated testicular rupture may result in ischemic atrophy, prolonged patient discomfort, and secondary infection.[21] Testicular sonography has been advocated to demonstrate intact testes in instances of scrotal trauma and thus avoid needless surgery.[21] The actual rupture of the tunica albuginea may be linear or stellate with extrusion of seminiferous tubules. However, almost all such injuries may be repaired, although at times, trimming of extruded tubules is required to effect closure of the tunica albuginea, which is accomplished with either absorbable or nonabsorbable suture material. An excellent result should be expected.

Dislocation of the testicle occurs when the mechanism of injury moves the testicle into the subcutaneous tissue along the vector of the force of the trauma.[46] The more common anatomic sites of dislocation include pubic, superficial inguinal, penile, preputial, peritoneal, and crural (superficial to the fascia of the thigh). Initial management should be an attempt to manually accomplish a closed reduction of the testis into the hemiscrotum. If closed reduction is ineffective, an open surgical approach to relocate the testis should be undertaken.

Avulsion

Avulsion of the testis may occur with power takeoff injuries, impalement on stationary objects, or massive trauma such as motor vehicle accidents.[22] In one instance, a child sliding down a flag pole (impalement) lost a testicle, which was later photographed still adhering to the rope-securing cleat at the base of the pole. If the testicle cannot be found or if it is hopelessly traumatized, a search for the remaining spermatic cord should ensue with appropriate ligation. If the testicle is found with an intact pedicle, autotransplantation is an option and may be accomplished by those trained in microsurgical vascular techniques.[45] A concern of parents is whether the loss of a testicle should preclude their child's participation in contact sports. Current opinion is that young athletes and their parents should be counseled regarding risks, equipment for protection, and sport alternatives with the philosophy that active participation in sports rather than exclusion from them is the goal.[45]

Penetrating Trauma

Penetrating injuries of the testicle are usually the result of gunshot or knife trauma.[7] Serious consideration should be given in penetrating injuries of the scrotum to proceed to surgical exploration for the purpose of débridement and repair of testicular rupture.

Burns

Full thickness scrotal burns may involve the testis or testes.[49] Adequate time should be given for clear demarcation before sacrificing scrotal tissue, however; orchiectomy may be required.

References

1. Alghanem AA, McCauley RL, Robson MC, et al: Management of pediatric perineal and genital burns: Twenty-year review. J Burn Care Rehabil 11:308, 1990.
2. Amoury RA, Barth GW, Hall RT, et al: Scrotal ecchymosis: Sign of intraperitoneal hemorrhage in the newborn. South Med J 75:1471, 1982.
3. Anderson KA, McAninich JW, Jeffrey RB, et al: Ultrasonography for the diagnosis and strategy of blunt scrotal trauma. J Urol 130:933, 1983.
4. Azmy A, Boddy SA, Ransley PC: Successful reconstruction following circumcision with diathermy. Br J Urol 57:587, 1985.
5. Bashir AY, El-Barbary M: Hair coil strangulation of the penis. J R Coll Surg Edinb 25:47, 1980.
6. Benson RC Jr: Vacuum cleaner injury to penis: A common urologic problem? Urology 25:41, 1985.
7. Bertini JE Jr, Corriere JN Jr: The etiology and management of genital injuries. J Trauma 28:1278, 1988.
8. Black CT, Pokorny WJ, McGill CW, et al: Ano-rectal trauma in children. J Pediatr Surg 17:501, 1982.
9. Carragher AM, Sulaiman SK, Panesar KJ: Scrotoabdominal impalement injury in a skateboard rider. J Emerg Med 8:419, 1990.
10. Cass AS, Gleich P, Smith C: Male genital injuries from external trauma. Br J Urol 57:467, 1985.
11. Cendron M, Whitmore KE, Carpiniello V, et al: Traumatic rupture of the corpus cavernosum: Evaluation and management. J Urol 144:987, 1990.
12. Conner JP, Hensle TW: Lower tract trauma in children: Causes, presentations, treatment. Contemp Urol 3:35, 1991.
13. Cromie WJ: Genitourinary injuries in the neonate. Perinatal care. Clin Pediatr 18:295, 1979.
14. Donovan JF, Kaplan WE: The therapy of genital trauma by dog bite. J Urol 141:1163, 1989.
15. Edington RF: Vaginal injuries due to water skiing. Can Med Assoc J 119:310, 1978.
16. Enos WF, Conrath TB, Byer JC: Forensic evaluation of the sexually abused child. Pediatrics 78:385, 1986.
17. Flowerdew R, Rishman IJ, Churchill BM: Management of penile zipper injury. J Urol 117:671, 1977.
18. Forman HP, Rosenberg HK, Snyder HM III: Fractured penis: Sonographic aid to diagnosis. Am J Urol 153:1009, 1989.
19. Gorman RL, Oderda GM: Penile trauma: Small slam revisited. Pediatr Emerg Care 5:108, 1989.
20. Hobbs CJ, Wynne JM: Sexual abuse of English boys and girls: The importance of anal examination. Child Abuse Neglect 13:195, 1989.
21. Jeffrey RB, Laing FC, Hricak H, et al: Sonography of testicular trauma. AJR 141:993, 1983.
22. Kalenak A, Gordon SL, Miller S, et al: Power takeoff injuries. J Trauma 18:134, 1978.
23. Knott LH, Barnett WO: Transcorpus impalement: Occurrence in an unusual manner. J Trauma 18:680, 1978.
24. Laitung JKG, Luther PK: Isolated penile burns: A plea for early excision. Br J Plast Surg 41:644, 1988.
25. Lauber AA, Somma ML: Use of toluidine blue for documentation of traumatic intercourse. Obstet Gynecol 60:644, 1982.
26. Livine PM, Gonzales ET Jr: Genitourinary trauma in children. Urol Clin North Am 12:53, 1985.
27. McAninich JW: Management of genital skin loss. Urol Clin North Am 16:387, 1989.
28. McCann J, Voris J, Symon M, et al: Perianal findings in prepubertal children selected for nonabuse: A descriptive study. Child Abuse Neglect 13:179, 1989.
29. McClure WJ, Gradinger GP: Hair strangulation of the glans penis. Plast Reconstr Surg 76:120, 1985.
30. McDougal WS, Peterson HD, Pruitt BA, et al: The thermally injured perineum. J Urol 121:320, 1979.
31. Mathlier AC: Vulvar hematoma secondary to a human bite. J Reproduct Med 32:618, 1987.
32. Mecrow IK: Burn to toddler's penis from an electro-chemical battery. BMJ 297:1315, 1988.
33. Miles BJ, Poffenberger RJ, Farah RN, et al: Management of penile gunshot wounds. Urology 36:318, 1990.
34. Murram D: Genital tract injuries in the prepubertal child. Pediatr Ann 15:616, 1986.
35. Murram D: Anal and perianal abnormalities in prepubertal victims of sexual abuse. Am J Obstet Gynecol 161:258, 1989.
36. Murram D: Child sexual abuse: Relationship between sexual acts and genital findings. Child Abuse Neglect 12:211, 1989.
37. Nolan JF, Stillwell TJ, Sands JP: Acute management of the zipper-entrapped penis. J Emerg Med 8:305, 1990.
38. Peck MD, Boileau MA, Grube BJ, et al: The management of burns to the perineum and genitals. J Burn Care Rehab 11:54, 1990.
39. Radhakrishnan J, Reyes HM: Penoplasty for buried penis secondary to "radical" circumcision. J Pediatr Surg 19:629, 1986.
40. Reid CF, Wright JH Jr: Scrotal reconstruction following an avulsion injury. J Urol 133:681, 1985.
41. Ricci LR: Medical forensic photography of the sexually abused child. Child Abuse Neglect 12:305, 1988.
42. Saraf P, Rabinowitz R: Zipper injury of the foreskin. Am J Dis Child 136:557, 1982.
43. Schuster G: Traumatic rupture of the testicle and a review of the literature. J Urol 127:1194, 1982.
44. Sheinfeld J, Cos LR, Eituak E, et al: Penile tourniquet injury due to a coil of hair. J Urol 133:1042, 1987.
45. Sin-Daw LO, Chung-Sheng L, Pei-Yaun S: Replantation of the testes by microsurgical techniques. Plast Reconstr Surg 76:626, 1985.
46. Singer AT, Das S, Gavrell GJ: Traumatic dislocation of testes. Urology 35:310, 1990.
47. Singh B, Kim H, Wax SH: Strangulation of glans penis by hair. Urology 11:770, 1978.
48. Slosberg EJ, Ludwig S, Duckett J, et al: Penile trauma as a sign of child abuse. Am J Dis Child 132:719, 1978.
49. Smith NJ: Participation of athletes with one testicle (letter). Am J Dis Child 140:90, 1986.
50. Still EF III, Goodman RC: Total reconstruction of a two-compartment scrotum by tissue expansion. Plast Reconstr Surg 85:805, 1990.
51. Stoddard EJ, Chedekel DS, Remensnyder JP: Psychological reactions of a boy to severe electrical burns including the loss of his penis. J Am Acad Child Psych 23:219, 1984.
52. Stoller ML, Lue TF, McAninich JW: Constrictive penile band injury: Anatomical and reconstructive considerations. J Urol 137:70, 1987.
53. Tank Es, Demuth RJ, Rosenberg S: Reconstruction following amputation of the penis in children. J Urol 128:386, 1982.
54. Tripathi FM, Sinha JK, Bhattacharya V, et al: Traumatic avulsion of penile and scrotal skin. Br J Plast Surg 35:302, 1982.
55. West R, Davies A, Fenton T: Accidental vulvar injuries in childhood. BMJ 298:1002, 1989.
56. Westman JC, Zawell DH: Traumatic phallic amputation during infancy. Arch Sex Behav 4:53, 1975.
57. Widholm O: Genital bleeding during childhood. Pediatr Ann 10:16, 1981.
58. Woodling BA, Heger A: The use of the colposcope in the diagnosis of sexual abuse in the pediatric age group. Child Abuse Neglect 10:111, 1986.
59. Wynne JM: Injuries to the genitalia in female children. S Afr Med J 57:47, 1980.

Musculoskeletal Injuries

Because skeletal trauma accounts for approximately 10 to 15% of all childhood injuries,[48] the physician should be familiar with the immature skeleton and how it differs from the mature skeleton. Treatment of many fractures varies markedly depending on the age of the child and whether the injury is isolated or part of a severe multisystem trauma.

Fractures in the immature skeleton are significantly different from those in the mature skeleton. Ligamentous injuries and joint dislocations are less common in children than adults. The periosteum in a child is thicker and more easily elevated from the diaphyseal and metaphyseal bone than in adults; thus, it often plays a role in providing fracture stability and results in a higher number of minimally displaced fractures. This stronger and more biologically active periosteum affects the rate of fracture healing but conversely may impede reduction.

Although the growing child has a greater capacity for remodeling of residual deformity after a fracture, not all deformities remodel completely, particularly those in the older child. The physician should be aware of what type of residual deformity is expected to occur and in what age group remodeling is expected to occur. As a general rule, the younger the child is, or the closer the fracture is to the physis, the greater is the potential for optimal remodeling. Angulation in the plane of motion of the joint has greater potential for remodeling than angulation out of the plane of motion of the joint. Because rotational malalignment does not correct spontaneously, no residual rotational deformity should be accepted. Fractures increase the blood supply to the bone and may stimulate longitudinal growth. Therefore, some degree of overriding of fracture fragments may be satisfactory in younger age groups as long as the overall alignment is acceptable.

PHYSEAL INJURIES

The most important difference in dealing with musculoskeletal injuries in children is the presence of the epiphyseal growth plate or physis. The physis separates the metaphysis of a long bone from the epiphysis and accounts for all longitudinal growth. The radiographic appearance of these secondary centers of ossification varies at different times during skeletal growth and should not be confused with a fracture (Fig. 29–1). The physician who sees pediatric injuries should be familiar with physeal injuries, because the physis is often injured in fractures, and this injury may lead to severe sequelae if there is premature growth arrest resulting in either angular deformity or limb-length discrepancy. These can be very devastating problems in the child with much remaining growth potential.

The age of normal physeal closure varies for different bones and can be used to help determine the amount of remaining growth potential (Fig. 29–2). As a general rule, the majority of growth is completed by 16 years of age in boys and by 14 years of age in girls. A child who has sustained an injury to the physis or a fracture near the physis should be followed up for an appropriate amount of time to make sure premature growth arrest does not occur. Parents should be informed of the possibility of this sequela at the time of any significant injury to this area of the bone.

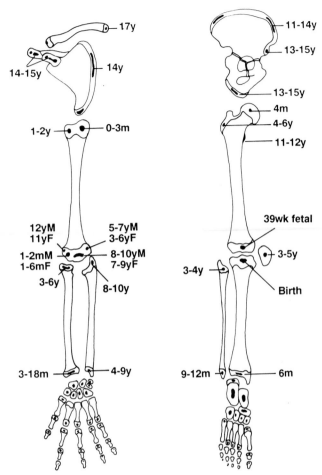

FIGURE 29–1

Schematic representation of the age of onset of secondary ossification centers of the major long bones in the upper lower extremity. M, Male; f, female; m, months; y, years; wk, weeks.

Physeal Fractures

There are several classification systems for growth plate injuries. The most commonly used is the Salter-Harris classification, which was introduced in 1963.[60] This system has important implications regarding intervention as well as prognosis. Originally including five types of injuries, it has now been expanded to six by Rang (Fig. 29–3).[55]

Type I

In the type I injury, the epiphysis is completely separated from the metaphysis. There is no radiographic evidence of a metaphyseal fragment attached to the epiphysis. Type I injury is primarily seen in birth trauma or injuries in the very young child and may be difficult to visualize because of incomplete ossification of the epiphysis. Fortunately, the prognosis for this type of injury is good.

Type II

In type II injury, the most common type of physeal injury, the fracture propagates transversely along the physis and

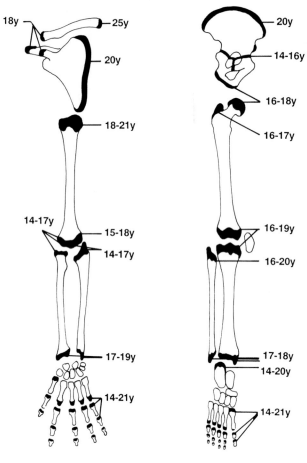

FIGURE 29–2

Schematic representation of the average age (in years) of epiphyseal closure of the bones of the upper and lower extremities.

because incomplete reduction leads to a high incidence of premature growth arrest.

Type IV

Type IV fractures are often referred to as a vertical splitting of the epiphysis. The fracture line crosses the metaphysis, physis, and epiphysis and extends into the joint. In injuries with any significant displacement, the fracture fragment often migrates toward the metaphysis, leading to discontinuity of the physis. If the fracture is allowed to heal in this position, there is not only a step-off in the articular cartilage, but also a premature growth arrest where the fracture

extends into the metaphysis. The metaphyseal fragment is generally on the side opposite the site of fracture initiation and may be either very minute or very large. The periosteum is usually intact on the side of the fragment. It previously was believed that type II injuries rarely cause premature growth arrest, but more current studies suggest that the prognosis may not be as good, particularly in injuries involving the distal femoral physis.[39, 58] Generally, anatomic reductions can be obtained with type II fractures by using closed methods; the intact periosteum on the side of the metaphyseal fragment aids in reduction and stability.

Type III

The type III injury is potentially more serious, because it is intra-articular. The fracture propagates along the physis and extends through the epiphysis into the articular surface. Anatomic reduction is essential, both for realigning the physis and for preventing a step-off in the articular cartilage. Fractures that are initially nondisplaced may displace in the first week or two postinjury; therefore, they need to be followed closely. Most type III injuries require open reduction and internal fixation to obtain the best outcome,

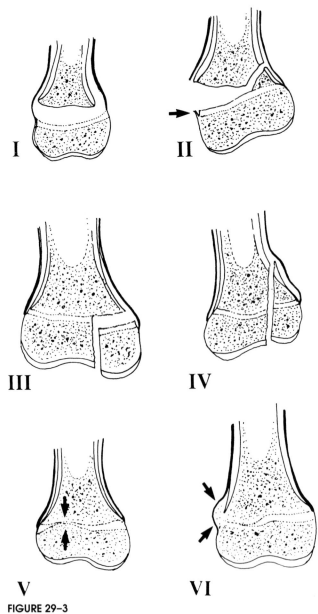

FIGURE 29–3

Schematic representation of the six types of epiphyseal fracture as originally described by Salter and Harris and modified by Rang.

crosses the physis. Most displaced type IV injuries require open reduction and internal fixation for optimal results.

Type V

The type V injury involves physeal crushing and is usually secondary to significant trauma. It is rare, and because there is no fracture, it is virtually impossible to diagnose at the time of injury. When there is significant crushing of the physis, premature growth arrest can occur, resulting in either shortening or angular deformity of the bone. Type V injury is usually diagnosed retrospectively, after the growth plate arrest has been recognized. It can be found in a fracture close to the physis and when no discernible fracture is seen anywhere in the limb. For this reason, it is important to inform the family about the possibility of unrecognized growth plate injury whenever there is significant trauma close to the physis.

Type VI

Not described in the original Salter-Harris classification, the type VI injury does not involve significant damage to the true physis but involves injury to the pericondylar ring and associated periosteum. This could be described as a bruise or soft tissue injury to the periphery of the physis. Because there is no true fracture, preliminary x-rays are often negative, and because this is a peripheral injury, severe angular deformity can develop if premature growth arrest occurs. The type VI injury usually results from a blow to the surface of the extremity, such as from a falling object or in a motor vehicle accident. It can also occur in thermal injuries, such as severe burns to the extremity.

OPEN FRACTURES

Open fractures can occur in children as well as adults, and even though these injuries may heal more quickly in children, initial treatment is the same for both groups. Careful examination of the entire extremity should be performed to rule out any associated injuries. There are three types of open fractures.[24]

Type I

Type I injuries involve a wound less than 1 cm in length. It is usually a clean puncture with very little soft tissue damage.

Type II

The type II injury involves a laceration greater than 1 cm in length with slight or moderate crushing. There is no extensive soft tissue damage or flap.

Type III

Type III injuries are characterized by extensive soft tissue damage, including muscle, skin, and occasionally neurovas-cular structures. There is often a marked amount of contamination. These fractures can be subdivided into type IIIa, in which soft tissue coverage of the bone is adequate; type IIIb, which is associated with extensive loss of soft tissue with periosteal stripping and exposure of the bone with massive contamination; and type IIIc, in which the open fracture is associated with an arterial injury that must be repaired.

Management of open fractures is the same in children as in adults[25] and begins on an emergency basis after initial life-threatening injuries have been addressed. Administration of appropriate antibiotics in the emergency department should be followed by immediate débridement with copious irrigation. Initial antibiotics should include a broad-spectrum cephalosporin accompanied by an aminoglycoside.[8, 20] Penicillin is added to the regimen in farm-related injuries, where there is a high possibility of major clostridial contamination.[8] With more extensive injury, débridement is usually repeated every 24 to 48 hours until the wound is clean. The fracture should then be stabilized, and the wound left open. Closure is obtained with either delayed primary closure, split thickness skin graft, or musculocutaneous flap at a later date.

Débridement of open fractures in the child should include preservation of any possibly viable periosteum, because it has a remarkable ability to regenerate bone in areas where there is segmental bone loss. The fracture should also be stabilized during initial débridement. If there is very little soft tissue injury and the wound is small, stabilization may require only simple plaster immobilization with a window to allow dressing changes and wound inspection. For more significant soft tissue injuries (e.g., types II and III) external fixation provides excellent stabilization in children.[1] External fixation can be applied to any long bone and permits ease of access to the wound. However, when applying an external fixator to the immature skeleton, pin placement must not violate the growth plates. For open fractures involving the growth plate, temporary fixation of the physis with smooth K-wires may also be helpful in addition to the external fixator. Occasionally, the external fixator may have to cross a joint temporarily until soft tissue and bony healing is accomplished.

TREATMENT OF FRACTURES IN PATIENTS WITH MULTIPLE INJURIES

The trend in trauma surgery is for early stabilization of all fractures in patients with polytrauma.[53] This has been shown to be of benefit in adults for decreasing respiratory complications and length of hospital stay. The child with multisystem injuries involving perhaps the head, chest, and abdomen may also have significant long bone fractures, which, though often not life-threatening, may be limb threatening and may produce long-term sequelae if not handled appropriately. Resuscitation of the polytrauma patient takes priority initially, as does the care of life-threatening injuries to the head, chest, and abdomen. If possible, however, early stabilization of long bone fractures makes general care of the patient easier and provides earlier mobilization. Reduction and cast immobilization may be possible for fractures of the upper extremity and distal lower extremity but not for fractures of the femur or multiple fractures in the same limb. In the adolescent, intermedullary fixation of femur fractures has become the method of choice. External fixation is also an excellent means of treating long bone fractures in the polytrauma patient. Spica cast application can be considered but generally is not applicable in the early treatment of these patients, as it may preclude repeat examination of the abdominal cavity and may also partially restrict respiratory function. In general, treatment of fractures in the polytrauma child must be individualized and coordinated with the care of other injuries. Appropriate casting and internal or external fixation may be used in combination, depending on the situation.

NERVE INJURIES

Peripheral nerve injuries remain among the most difficult for the extremity surgeon to manage. Unlike vascular, bony, and even tendinous injuries, the outcome is unpredictable. Because nerves regenerate at a finite rate, significant delay occurs from the time of repair until reinnervation of muscles or sensory end organs. Often, nerve damage in severe crush injuries or complete amputations limits the final outcome.

Peripheral nerve repair is more successful in children than in adults, in part due to the child's superior capability for cerebral cortex reorganization.[42] Studies indicate that the brain of the child has a natural plasticity that is lacking in the adult brain. Children also appear to require less formal sensory reeducation after peripheral nerve repair; their natural curiosity seems to aid this process. Also, hormonal or neurotrophic agents have been demonstrated to play a role in nerve regeneration after repair and may be more effective in children than in adults.[40] In addition, the shorter distances that axons need to regenerate before reaching their end organ may enhance nerve recovery in children.

Generally good results can be obtained by nerve repair in children; therefore, every effort should be made to diagnose nerve injuries and treat them promptly. Unfortunately, diagnosis of these injuries is difficult in the young or uncooperative child. Nerve involvement should be suspected in open injuries that are in proximity to normal anatomic paths of peripheral nerves. In the young child, sensory examination is usually extremely difficult; however, sensory loss can be discerned by lack of sweating in the anatomic distribution of the injured nerve and can be demonstrated by an iodine starch test or a Ninhydrin print test. Possibly the easiest means of establishing sensory loss is the wrinkling test, in which the extremity is immersed in warm water. In skin that is normally innervated, wrinkling occurs; if nerve injury is present, it does not.

Motor examination may also be limited because of noncompliance and pain in the injured child. Thorough knowledge of muscular innervation by peripheral nerves is required to delineate peripheral nerve injury on the basis of absent motor function (Fig. 29–4). Diagnosis of nerve injury can be augmented by electrodiagnostic studies, which show fibrillations and denervation potentials 2 to 4 weeks

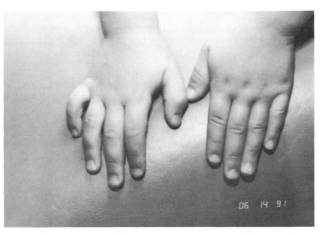

FIGURE 29–4

A 2 year old with complete laceration of the ulnar nerve at the wrist. Subtle clawing of right little and ring fingers is noted secondary to paralysis of the intrinsic muscles of the hand.

after complete nerve injury. If suspicion is high, however, exploration of open wounds is probably warranted rather than waiting for diagnostic changes on electromyelograms.

Nerve injuries are graded I through V, according to anatomic injury, by Sunderland's classification.[69]

1. Grade I nerve injuries consist of a physiologic interruption of conduction with complete axonal continuity. This lesion should be reversible and is consistent with a contusion of the nerve.

2. Grade II nerve injuries are axonal injuries with loss of the axons distal to the injury but with preservation of the endoneurium. Full recovery can be expected.

3. In Grade III nerve injuries, in addition to axonal injury, the endoneurial tube continuity is lost.

4. Grade IV nerve injuries represent total destruction of the internal architecture of the nerve with continuity only of the external epineurium.

5. Grade V nerve injuries consist of complete loss of continuity of the nerve trunk itself. Grades III through V nerve injuries are associated with incomplete recovery.

A somewhat simpler classification was offered by Seddon.[62] In this classification of nerve injury, *neuropraxia* indicates a contusion of the nerve with axonal as well as connective-tissue continuity; *axontomesis* is a disruption of the internal architecture of the nerve with continuity of the epineurium; and *neurotmesis* indicates a completely disrupted nerve trunk.

Open injuries are usually of the Sunderland grade V or the neurotmesis type and require nerve repair to gain optimal neurologic function. Closed injuries, however, can result in nerve injuries of Sunderland grades I through IV, and their management is exceedingly difficult because of the unknown extent of the neural injury. Nerve regeneration of at least 1 mm per day and sometimes more in children can be expected to occur. If recovery of distal muscles is delayed beyond the expected time and the Tinel sign shows a failure to proceed distally, exploration of the nerve is probably warranted. In general, however, closed injuries in children with associated nerve injuries have an excellent prognosis. Delay in exploration is probably warranted unless other considerations such as vascular or bony problems necessitate surgical exploration.

Microsurgical techniques are now standard management for peripheral nerve repairs. These include the use of magnification, usually in the form of the operating microscope, microsurgical instruments, and microsutures. Controversy continues to exist over the preferred type of nerve repair. The impetus toward magnification in microsurgical repair is due to the fact that axonal alignment appears to be critical for nerve recovery. Attempts should be made to align motor fibers proximally to motor fibers distally and sensory fibers to sensory fibers in a similar fashion. In addition, because connective tissue makes up much of the inner contents of a complex mixed nerve, attempts have been made to align individual fascicles of complex nerves and suture the internal connective tissue. Grouped fascicular repairs require alignment of groups of fasciculi in the proximal and distal stumps. Sutures are placed in the internal epineurium surrounding these groups. This type of repair requires definable groups in both the proximal and distal stumps and is particularly applicable in repair of the median and ulnar nerves in the distal forearm, where the motor component is easily distinguished from the rest of the nerve.[14] Identification of motor and sensory fibers, however, is more difficult in proximal portions of these nerves. Histochemical stains, including the enzymes acetylcholinesterase and carbonic anhydrase, have been used to identify specific fibers in nerve stumps. These techniques, however, require a significant amount of time for processing and have not achieved widespread clinical use.

Standard epineural repair with an attempt to align nerve stumps using external and internal topography also achieves excellent clinical results, and clear superiority of grouped fascicular repair to epineural repair has not been shown in clinical studies to date. It is probable that both the grouped fascicular repair and epineural repair are selectively indicated in the repair of peripheral nerve injuries.

In all cases, tension on the site of nerve repair is to be avoided. Small nerve gaps can be overcome by dissection of the stumps and positioning of the extremity. Extreme postural positioning, however, is not recommended. Nerve grafting has been recommended for defects as small as 2.5 cm.[44] Interfascicular nerve grafting as described by Milessi and colleagues has produced excellent results despite the requirement of the axon to pass through two suture lines and through a nonvascularized nerve graft.[45] It is believed that lack of tension on the repair is responsible for these favorable results. In such grafting, attention should be paid to proper microsurgical technique, and significant nerve gaps may be overcome (Fig. 29–5). Suitable donor nerves include the sural for larger nerves and the posterior interosseous at the wrist as well as the medial and lateral antebrachial cutaneous nerves in the forearm for smaller nerves.

When appropriate, nerve repair should be done early but not necessarily immediately. Because of the exacting nature of the repair, it should be performed when adequate equipment and surgeons of necessary expertise are available. Delayed repair of several weeks does not appreciably diminish surgical results. Because there is only one good chance to repair a nerve, all attempts should be made to accomplish the repair under ideal circumstances.

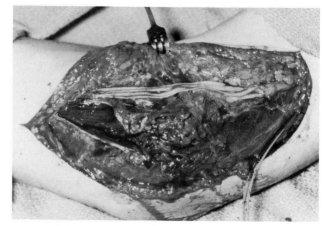

FIGURE 29–5
Cable grafting of the ulnar nerve using multiple sural nerve grafts.

Although the results of nerve repair in children are superior to that in adults, the unpredictability of results should be stressed to the child's parents. Failure to show progressive reinnervation of denervated muscles over a suitable time or failure of the Tinel sign to show improvement are indications for reexploration of the repair. Disruption of the suture line, although unusual, is possible. The formation of a large neuroma incontinuity may necessitate either excision and cable grafting or extensive internal neurolysis. The prognosis after either of these two procedures is much poorer than for a primary repair. In some patients, nerve repair is not possible. In these instances, tendon transfers can be entertained for motor deficits. Fortunately, in children, these transfers are often quite functional. Sensory deficits, however, cannot be entirely compensated for; this emphasizes the importance of performing the ideal nerve repair initially.

REPLANTATION AND MICROSURGERY

Advancements in microsurgical techniques have made possible successful replantation of digits and entire extremities in children as well as adults. Digital plantation in children is somewhat more difficult because of the smaller size of the vessels, resulting in slightly lower viability rates than in adults. However, functional results are often superior in children; this is due to fewer tendon adhesions as well as improved nerve recovery and less joint stiffness.[70] In addition, growth of the replanted part continues to approximately 80% of the predicted normal length.

Although not the case for adult digits, an amputated digit at any level in the child is considered an indication for replantation. Additional importance is placed on replanting thumbs, multiple digits, and proximal amputations through the metacarpals, wrist, or distal forearm.

Sensory reinnervation results in the child who undergoes replantation also tend to exceed those in the adult. Two-point discrimination of less than 10 mm can be expected. Pain does not tend to be a problem, and cosmetic and functional results are superior to any current prosthesis.

Major limb replantation would be expected to provide better results in children than in adults, primarily because of better nerve recovery. Before considering such a replantation, however, systemic factors and the child's overall medical status must be considered. The condition of the amputated extremity also is critical; severe crushing injuries or segmental injuries are contraindications for replantation. In addition, excessive warm ischemia for longer than 6 hours precludes successful replantation, because extensive muscle necrosis due to ischemia could result in renal failure and even death. Consideration should be given to prompt surgical vascular shunting in major limb replantation. The small size of the child's vessels frequently make this difficult, but a small ventricular peritoneal shunt can sometimes be used. It may be necessary to shunt before establishing bony stability; however, venous blood should not be shunted initially due to potential toxins in the amputated part. Although a large blood loss can be expected during these procedures, the use of a cell saver can help minimize it.

Lower extremity replantation is rarely performed in the United States. Indications for leg replantation include clean, sharp amputations in which nerve recovery, as well as good bone growth, can be expected. Children with injuries that would result in severe shortening of the extremity due to growth plate injuries would not be candidates for replantation. Unlike upper extremity prostheses, lower extremity prostheses tend to provide excellent function and can be changed to accommodate growth. Partial amputees requiring revascularization would be ideal candidates for surgical salvage (Fig. 29–6A and B).

Successful replantation requires minimizing warm ischemia time. The severed part should be cooled as soon as possible, kept moist, and placed in a separate container filled with saline or lactated Ringer solution or wrapped in a soaked sponge, which is in turn placed in another con—tainer that is put on ice. To prevent frostbite, the amputated extremity should not be in direct contact with ice. A finger so cooled can be replanted up to 24 hours after the injury; therefore, transportation by heroic measures (e.g., helicop-

ter) often is not required for digit replantation. Because of increased size and muscle mass, larger amputations have significantly less time before revascularization is required due to inadequacy of cooling. Six hours of warm ischemia is considered the maximum allowable time before replantation.

The patient's overall status must be assessed before contemplating replantation. Life-threatening injuries receive top priority. In cases of digital amputations in polytrauma patients, other injuries can be treated initially, and replantation of the digit can take place afterward. However, with major limb replantation, other life-threatening injuries probably preclude replantation of the extremity.

As teenagers join the work force, the incidence of traumatic amputations increases (Fig. 29–7A and B). The indications for replantation in this group are identical to those in adults: (1) amputation of a thumb or multiple digits; (2) amputations at the metacarpal, wrist, or distal forearm level; and (3) amputation of an individual digit distal to the insertion of the flexor digitorum superficialis insertion. Individual digits amputated proximal to the superficialis insertion tend to have considerable stiffness at the proximal interphalangeal joint, which decreases their overall function. More distal amputations leave the patient with a mobile proximal interphalangeal joint and an excellent functional result. The type of amputation is also important in achieving good results. Major crush injuries contraindicate replantation because of poor nerve recovery and tendon function. Segmental injuries are also a contraindication to replantation.

In the more proximal replantations at the midforearm level or higher, results generally are most dependent on eventual nerve recovery. It is critical that nerve repair be done in the most ideal microsurgical fashion, with minimal tension, using nerve grafts when needed. In major limb revascularization with associated disruption, it should be remembered that the final outcome is usually more dependent on the quality of the nerve repair than that of the vascular repair. Many times, vascular repair in a child is not an emergency situation due to excellent collateral circulation. It therefore is important that nerve repair receive

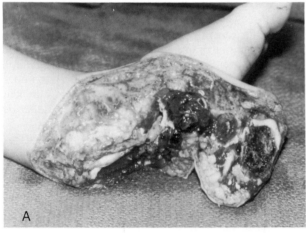 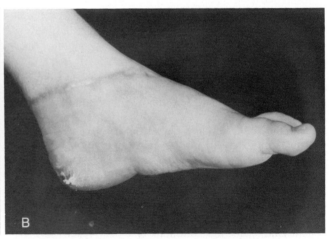

FIGURE 29–6
A, Preoperative photograph of a lawn mower injury that resulted in devascularization of the heel. *B,* Postoperative photograph shows subsequent microvascular reconstruction.

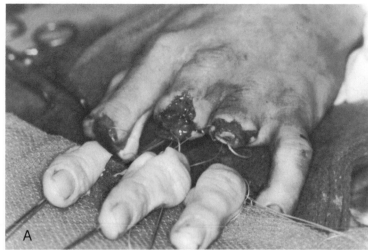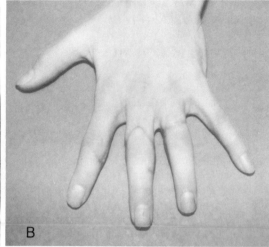

FIGURE 29–7

A, Preoperative photograph of a 16 year old who had three digits amputated by a meat slicer in a delicatessen. *B,* Postoperative photograph shows successful replantation.

priority and be performed by an experienced surgeon with microsurgical expertise, even if a secondary repair is necessary. Care must be taken while performing the vascular repair to avoid injury to adjacent nerves.

TENDON INJURY

Tendon repair or reconstruction is governed by the same principles in children as in adults; however, children are unable to comply with elaborate postoperative rehabilitation protocols for such injuries, particularly of the fingers. Fortunately, children experience less joint stiffness and tendon adhesions after repair, and therefore often can be treated with simpler rehabilitation regimens.

Tendon injuries should be suspected in children with open injuries in the forearm and hand. Diagnosis may be difficult because of refusal to move the extremity or digits secondary to discomfort. Exploration of lacerations in the forearm and hand frequently is required when these injuries occur in proximity to tendons if adequate function cannot be confirmed by physical examination. Adjacent nerves and vessels should also be examined at the time of exploration and repaired if injured.

At the forearm level, lacerations can injure tendons and muscles. Muscle repair is difficult because of the tissue weakness of muscle in holding sutures; however, multiple fine mattress-type sutures and sutures through collagenous structures within the muscle can help approximate the lacerated tissue. The extremity must be splinted for 3 weeks or longer to restrict excessive tension to these repaired structures.

Tendon repair is most difficult in the area of the flexor tendon sheath of the fingers. Between the superficialis insertion and the start of the flexor tendon sheath (i.e., "no man's land"), tendon adhesions and poor results are frequent. It is critical that meticulous surgical technique be used when operating in this area. It is generally accepted that primary repair of these tendons is preferable, if possi-

ble, and if necessary, both the superficialis and the profundus flexor tendons should be repaired. Current recommended techniques include the use of grasping sutures of nonabsorbable material, oversewing with a running suture, and preservation of the flexor tendon pulley system. Controversy exists regarding whether the flexor tendon sheath should be closed, when possible. It is generally believed that preservation of as much of the annular pulley system as possible is the objective. Restoration of the A2 and A4 pulleys over the proximal phalanx and the middle phalanx respectively are the most critical; loss of function in these structures results in bowstringing and decreased range of motion of the digit. The tendons should be handled as little as possible to avoid adhesions, which limit excursion of the tendons.

In the adult, elaborate postoperative regimens have been established to allow for tendon excursion without tension on the repair. In the child, simpler techniques are successful because of a diminished tendency toward scarring. After flexor tendon repair a splint should be applied that flexes the wrist and metacarpophalangeal joints so as to prevent tension upon the repair. The proximal interphalangeal and distal interphalangeal joints should be splinted in near extension to prevent flexion contractures. Passive flexion can be performed by the parents or therapist to allow excursion and prevent tendon adherence. If tendon rupture occurs after repair, prompt exploration and repeat repair should be undertaken.

Lower extremity tendon injuries are less common, and indications for tendon repair in this area are somewhat less clear. Flexor and extensor tendon injuries to toes do not necessarily require repair. It would, however, appear to be prudent to at least repair extensor and flexor tendon injuries to the great toe, and to the lesser toes if it can be easily accomplished. Major tendons that dorsiflex or plantar flex the ankle should always be repaired. In the repair of lower extremity tendons, grasping-type sutures should be used, and the extremity should be immobilized for 3 to 4 weeks.

FRACTURES AND DISLOCATIONS OF THE UPPER EXTREMITY

Shoulder and Humerus

One of the most common fractures in the pediatric age group is that of the clavicle; this type of fracture is usually caused by direct or indirect forces. In the younger age group, injuries tend to be of the low-energy type, but in the older child, more severe injuries are likely. Clavicle fractures are characterized by rapid healing, rare complications, and few nonunions or malunions. Children who have sustained high-energy injuries with fractures of the clavicle should be scrutinized closely for associated neurovascular difficulties. However, despite the proximity of the clavicle to the subclavian artery and brachial plexus, such neurovascular injuries are rare. This relatively low incidence of injury to the underlying nerves and vessels in this age group, despite marked displacement of the clavicular fragments, is probably due to the thick periosteum that envelopes the clavicle.

Clavicular fractures can often occur at the medial border where they are usually Salter-Harris type I or II, and they have an excellent ability to remodel. Surgical treatment is rarely required. True media sternoclavicular dislocations are virtually nonexistent in children.

Injuries to the acromioclavicular joint in children younger than 15 years of age rarely result in true dislocations. Instead, many of these injuries represent a disruption of the periosteum of the distal clavicle with the ligaments remaining intact. Dameron and Rockwood classified six types of acromioclavicular injuries in children.[18] A type I injury is a mild sprain of the acromioclavicular ligaments, consistent with normal radiographic results. A type II injury is a partial disruption of the dorsal periosteal structures with mild instability of the distal clavicle and slight widening of the acromioclavicular joint. In type III injury, the periosteal tube of the distal clavicle is disrupted, and a longitudinal split allows superior displacement of the clavicle. In type IV injury, the distal clavicle is displaced posteriorly and buttonholes into the trapezius muscle. A type V injury is a complete dorsal periosteal split with subcutaneous displacement of the clavicle due to splitting of the deltoid and trapezial attachment. A type VI injury is an inferior dislocation of the distal clavicle. Only injury types IV, V, and VI require open reduction and internal fixation.

Dislocations of the shoulder do occur, particularly in the older child and teenager. Anterior dislocations are associated with exceedingly high rates of redislocation.[30] Immobilization for 3 to 4 weeks after reduction is recommended. Glenohumeral dislocations can be classified as anterior, posterior, or inferior. As in the adult, anterior dislocations are by far the most common, whereas posterior and inferior are exceedingly rare. Most anterior dislocations are due to a fall on the outstretched hand and levering of the humeral head by abduction and external rotation of the arm. Posterior dislocations can occur with extreme trauma, such as motor vehicle accidents and seizures. In the neonate, it is important to rule out epiphyseal separation of the proximal humerus, but due to lack of ossification of the epiphysis, this can be difficult diagnostically and may require a computed tomography scan or arthrogram.

A subset of dislocations include patients who have excessive joint laxity. These individuals may voluntarily dislocate their shoulders, and psychiatric or emotional disturbances without a history of excessive trauma may be present. They tend to respond poorly to surgical procedures to prevent recurrent dislocations, and such individuals may show excessive laxity in other joints and a lack of discomfort in the shoulder.

A child with a traumatic anterior dislocation has a painful, swollen shoulder area and resists movement of the arm. Physical examination should include sensory assessment of the lateral aspect of the upper arm and examination for deltoid function, because axillary nerve injury may be present. With this type of dislocation, the humeral head frequently can be palpated anteriorly. Posterior dislocations can be difficult to diagnose by physical examination alone. Quality radiographs are the standard protocol for diagnosing glenohumeral dislocations. Axillary or lateral views in the plane of the scapula are critical, particularly in patients with posterior dislocations.

Reduction of acute dislocations generally can be obtained with closed manipulation. To avoid injury to the growth plate, gentle reduction is required. Open reduction may be needed in chronic, neglected dislocation, and operative stabilizing procedures are frequently necessary for recurrent involuntary dislocations.

Fractures of the proximal humerus do not tend to involve the physis in the 5- to 12-year-old age group (Fig. 29–8), but in the older adolescent, growth plate involvement is frequent.[17] Rapid growth in the 13- to 16-year-old age group often results in more common fractures of the proximal humerus, primarily due to falls on the outstretched hand. Clinically, pain and swelling are present to a varying extent, but invariably the child avoids any arm movement. Plain radiographs are usually diagnostic. The proximal humerus is responsible for a large portion of the growth of the humerus; therefore, tremendous remodeling capability is present in the young child with such a fracture. In the older child, less remodeling is possible; therefore, manipulation of the fracture is more frequently required. Open reduction and internal fixation is rarely required, primarily in the older individual with an irreducible fracture and in individuals with the rare Salter–Harris type fractures that have intra-articular involvement.

Humeral shaft fractures are quite rare in children. These fractures are often due to twisting injuries producing spiral-type fractures and are frequently the result of child abuse. In older children, direct trauma to the humerus may produce either a short spiral or a true transverse fracture (see Fig. 29–8). Lesser trauma can produce a so-called torus or buckle-type fracture. Examination of a child with a humeral shaft fracture reveals varying degrees of swelling and tenderness, depending on the extent and type of fracture. Radiographs are usually diagnostic. Most patients only require immobilization, although some may require closed reduction. Open reduction and internal fixation is rarely required and is primarily useful in individuals who have sustained multiple trauma, closed-head injuries, vascular injuries, or injuries to the forearm resulting in an unstable elbow.

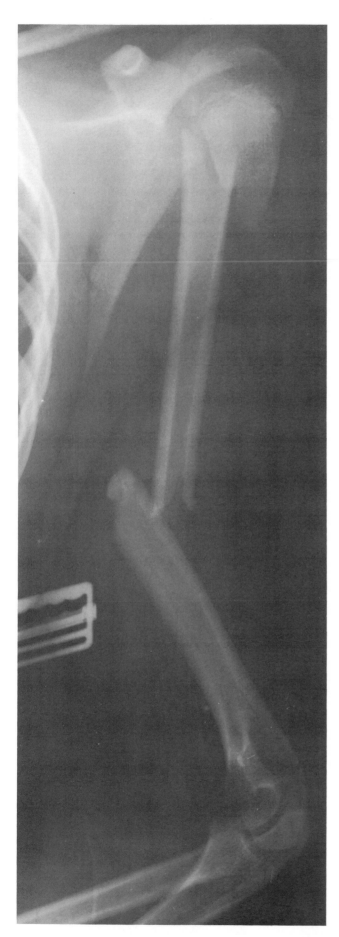

Although humeral shaft fractures are associated with possible radial nerve injury in all age groups, this is less common in children than adults. Fortunately, with closed fractures of the humerus, spontaneous recovery of an injured radial nerve is usual. Exploration of the nerve is rarely required initially, and usually, 12 weeks or more should be allowed for recovery. Indications for immediate exploration of the nerve include loss of its function after manipulation of the fracture, indicating its possible entrapment within the fracture, and major vascular or other open injuries. Radial nerve injuries that fail to show improvement, either by physical examination or electromyelogram, after an adequate amount of time for recovery need exploration and either neurolysis, repair, or grafting.

Elbow

Fractures and dislocations about the pediatric elbow remain challenging diagnostically and therapeutically. Unlike other musculoskeletal injuries, these can have immediate and severe consequences, with the potential for irreversible loss of function. A large portion of the orthopedic literature pertains to treatment of these injuries—specifically, to recognition, possible complications, and initial management, all of which are critically important. Severe injuries usually present with significant swelling, but deformity may or may not be remarkable. Quality radiographs are critical for diagnosis, and often a child needs to be splinted temporarily to achieve good radiographic results. The minimal radiographic examination includes an anteroposterior view of the elbow in as much extension as possible and an anatomic lateral view. Supplementary and comparison views of the opposite elbow are useful and frequently are required.

Examination of an elbow injury begins with the remainder of the extremity, because such fractures frequently are associated with proximal and distal injuries. This is probably because many such injuries are indirect, with force being transmitted from the hand upward, through the arm. Radiographs of other anatomic areas in the extremity may be required, and a thorough physical examination, including a vascular and neurologic assessment, is essential. Doppler examination of the vessels can be performed to augment simple palpation, and it is important to assess and reassess the quality of capillary refill, color, and turgor, because these injuries can be associated with compartment syndromes and Volkmann ischemia of the forearm. Signs and symptoms of compartment syndrome include motor or sensory neurologic deficits, excessive pain, pallor of the extremity, and pain with passive extension of the fingers. A pulse may or may not be palpable. Compartment pressures may be measured if done early after the injury, but measuring should not delay needed fasciotomies if clinically indicated. Arteriograms are rarely required, because direct surgical exploration is the more appropriate. Although a

FIGURE 29–8

Radiograph of an 8-year-old girl who sustained a proximal and midshaft fracture of the humerus in a motor vehicle accident.

neurologic examination is difficult in the injured child, care should be taken to accomplish the best possible evaluation. Motor examination should be done for median, radial, and ulnar nerve function. Additionally, deficits to the anterior and posterior interosseous nerves should be sought. Sensory deficits should also be detected before attempts at closed reduction or operative treatment.

Radiographic diagnosis is complicated by the fact that much of the pediatric elbow is in a nonossified, cartilaginous form. Comparison films of the opposite elbow are sometimes helpful, and a thorough knowledge of the secondary ossification centers is important. At birth, ossification of the humerus extends only to the region of the condyles. Additionally, the ulna shows only partial ossification of the olecranon, and the entire radial head and neck are not ossified.[9] Ossification proceeds at a predictable rate (see Fig. 29–1), with the ossification center of the lateral condyle appearing at approximately 1 to 6 months of age. The proximal radius secondary ossification centers appear around 5 years of age, whereas the medial epicondyle ossification center tends to appear at 5 to 6 years of age, and the trochlear ossification center appears at age 9 years. The olecranon ossifies at about 8 to 10 years of age, and the lateral epicondyle appears near the age of 11 years. Ossification occurs earlier in girls than in boys. The secondary ossification centers can be confused with fractures, and comparison views are often helpful in diagnosis. It should be remembered that fractures can occur through the nonossified cartilage without visualization on radiographic films, and occasionally, an arthrogram of the joint is needed for diagnosis of such fractures.

If plain radiographs of the elbow fail to show a fracture, a joint effusion on the films should be searched for if there is a strong clinical suspicion of injury. Effusion of the elbow can be detected by the appearance of fat pad signs on radiograph. In the elbow, there is an anterior and posterior fat pad in the coronoid fossa and olecranon fossa, respectively. With an effusion, the fat pads displace from the fascia and are visualized on the lateral radiograph as fat density areas (Fig. 29–9). The presence of fat pad signs secondary to an effusion increases the suspicion of an oc-cult fracture (e.g., of the radial head) because of the likelihood of intra-articular bleeding.

Perhaps the most common and certainly the most written about fracture of the pediatric elbow is that of the supracondylar humerus. This type of fracture occurs through the thin bone of the humeral metaphysis proximal to the condyles and usually happens in children younger than 10 years of age because of weakness of the bone in this anatomic area. Supracondylar humerus fractures can be associated with neurological and vascular complications, including Volkmann ischemia. Vascular compromise, in the form of a compartment syndrome in the forearm developing into Volkmann ischemia, is one of the most dreaded complications in orthopedics. In addition to these severe complications, the cosmetic deformity of cubitus varus is a frequent and bothersome sequela to this fracture.

Supracondylar humerus fractures can be separated into extension and flexion types. The extension type is by far the most common and usually involves a fall on the outstretched arm. The humeral condyles are displaced posteriorly, and the anterior soft tissues are at risk of injury by the prominent proximal fracture fragment. The severity of the injury is dependent on the amount of displacement, and the classification system reflects this. A type I injury is a nondisplaced fracture with an intact anterior periosteum. A type II injury shows posterior displacement of the condyles and a disrupted anterior periosteum with an intact posterior periosteal sleeve. A type III injury is a completely displaced fracture with no continuity of the periosteum (Fig. 29–10A). Displacement can be either posteromedial or posterolateral of the condyles.

Type I fractures are treated simply with immobilization. Good functional and cosmetic results can be expected with prompt healing. Type II fractures usually require manipulation. They are often fixed after reduction by percutaneous pinning; traditionally, many were treated with cast immobilization.

It is in the type III fractures that the most severe complications can occur. Type III supracondylar humerus fractures are frequently associated with excessive swelling, and the anterior surface of the fractured humeral shaft can directly

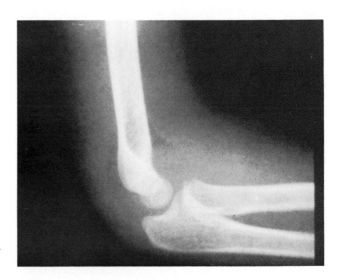

FIGURE 29–9

Lateral radiograph of a child's elbow demonstrating anterior and posterior fat pad signs in the supracondylar region.

injure the brachial artery as well as the radial and median nerves. Similarly, vascular compromise to the forearm and hand secondary to direct injury to the brachial artery and collaterals can result from excessive swelling. Prompt reduction is frequently required to correct the arterial compromise of the extremity. Palpation and Doppler examination of the radial pulse are helpful in assessing these patients. Generally, patients with displaced supercondylar humerus fractures are taken to the operating room, where a general anesthetic is given and closed reduction performed. The adequacy of the closed reduction is measured by the image intensifier. After reduction, the radial pulse and improved signs of perfusion, including capillary refill, color, and turgor are sought. Persistent absence of a radial pulse is not an absolute indication for surgical exploration of the brachial artery unless definite vascular compromise exists. Some researchers report good results with absent radial pulses as long as distal perfusion is adequate. If there is doubt about the quality of perfusion, surgical exploration is performed. There is probably no indication for an arteriogram, because there is minimal morbidity from vascular exploration, and valuable time can be lost in performing the study. In addition, fasciotomies should be performed promptly when required.

Prompt exploration of the artery within 12 hours of the injury has been found to be associated with a 0% incidence of Volkmann ischemia. However, a somewhat increased incidence is seen with exploration between 12 and 24 hours, and a much higher incidence occurs after 24 hours delay.[51] At exploration, the brachial artery can be completely ruptured or in severe spasm. In the past, ligation of the artery was performed with generally good results because of the rich collateral circulation. However, it is currently thought that the brachial artery probably should be reconstructed using microsurgical techniques and vein grafting as required. The brachial artery can also be caught in the fracture site itself. This occurs most commonly in fractures with posterolateral displacement.

In a pooled survey of 7212 supracondylar humerus fractures, there was a 7.7% incidence of neurologic injuries.[77] Radial nerve injuries constituted 41.2% of these injuries, the median nerve was injured 36%, and the ulnar nerve was injured in 22.8%. Radial nerve injuries occur more frequently in posteromedial displacements, when the nerve is tented across the sharp anterior surface of the shaft of the fractured humerus. Similarly, with posterolateral displacement, the median nerve and the brachial artery are tented across the sharp anterior surface of the humerus. Fortunately, these nerve injuries tend to resolve with simple observation, and recommendations suggest that these injuries be observed for 5 months. If no clinical or electromyographic evidence of return of function is present after this period of observation, exploration and neurolysis should be performed.[16] In this study, neurolysis was required in 18 nerve injuries, but only one nerve, a radial nerve, was found to be completely lacerated. All of the neurolysed nerves had excellent recovery.

In displaced supracondylar humerus fractures, adequate reduction and stabilization are required. In the past, closed reduction and immobilization in flexion in a cast were employed; however, this treatment method has become in-

creasingly unpopular as recent published series reveal poor long-term results and a high percentage of early and late complications.[54] Traction, either skin or skeletal, is an old but dependable technique and can be safely performed. Because extreme flexion of the elbow is not required with traction, vascular compromise is rare. Traction does require prolonged hospitalization and considerable time and expertise from the managing physician. Closed reduction and percutaneous pinning under image intensifier control are becoming increasingly popular. Gentle reduction with fixation by smooth pins across the fracture site allows the elbow to be immobilized without extreme flexion, minimizing chances of vascular compromise and subsequent Volkmann ischemia. Additionally, fixation with pins allows for maintenance of the reduction and helps in the prevention of long-term sequelae, such as cubitus varus. Length of hospitalization is minimized with this technique; only a 24-hour period or less is required for observation for compartment syndrome complications. This fixation technique can be performed using either two laterally placed pins or one pin placed through the medial epicondyle and another through the lateral epicondyle (see Fig. 29–10B and C). Despite the proximity of the ulnar nerve to the medial epicondyle, neural injuries with this technique are exceedingly rare. Although open reduction and internal fixation is seldom required, absolute indications for their use include an open fracture and severe vascular compromise, especially if the injury was worsened after closed reduction.[77]

Displaced supracondylar humerus fractures heal promptly and usually require only 3 to 4 weeks of immobilization. However, long-term stiffness frequently complicates recovery. Patients often have hyperextension deformities, as well as a cubitus varus deformity that is believed to be related primarily to inadequate reduction rather than to growth plate injuries.

The much less common flexion-type supracondylar humerus fracture results in anterior displacement of the condyles. Ulnar nerve injury is frequent. Completely displaced fractures often require open reduction and stabilization with pins.

Fractures of the growth plates of the distal humerus are important and often severe injuries. A fracture of the lateral condyle can present as a swollen, painful elbow, similar to the supercondylar humerus fractures; however, the level of swelling and incidence of vascular compromise are lower. Although the short-term complications of lateral condyle fractures are of lesser importance than those of the supracondylar humerus fractures, the long-term complications can be significant because of their intra-articular character. These fractures are either Salter-Harris type II or, less commonly, type IV. The fracture line begins in the metaphysis, passes into the physis, and terminates intra-articularly at the trochlea (Fig. 29–11A). Displacement leads to a step-off in the articular surface with resultant long-term decreased range of motion and potential for osteoarthritis. Again, because much of the young child's distal humerus is not ossified, lateral condyle fractures must be suspected and looked for. Fractures with displacement usually require open reduction and internal fixation with smooth pins (Fig. 29–11B).[4] At the time of surgery, care is taken to prevent injury to the posterior blood supply to the lateral condyles.

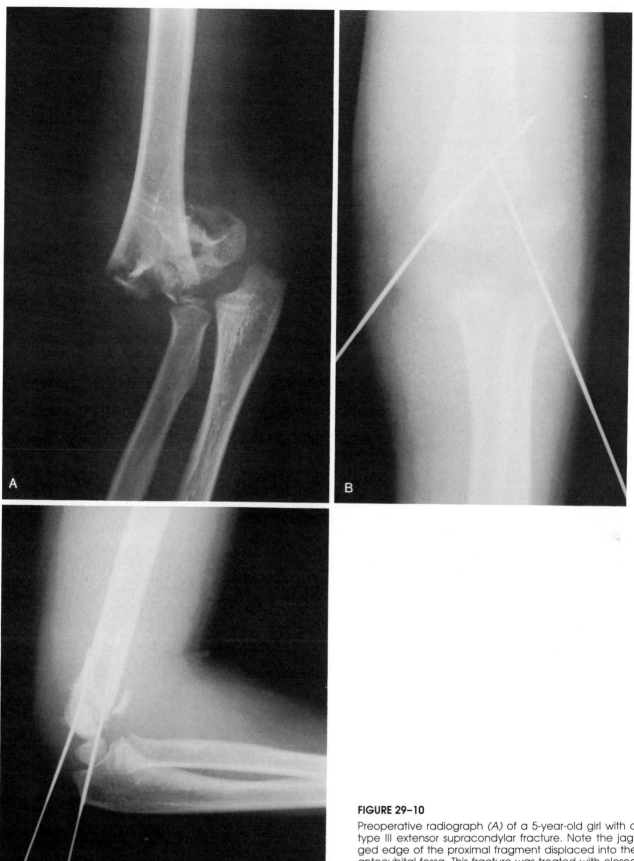

FIGURE 29–10

Preoperative radiograph *(A)* of a 5-year-old girl with a type III extensor supracondylar fracture. Note the jagged edge of the proximal fragment displaced into the antecubital fossa. This fracture was treated with closed reduction and percutaneous medial and lateral pin fixation, as demonstrated on the anteroposterior *(B)* and lateral *(C)* postoperative radiographs.

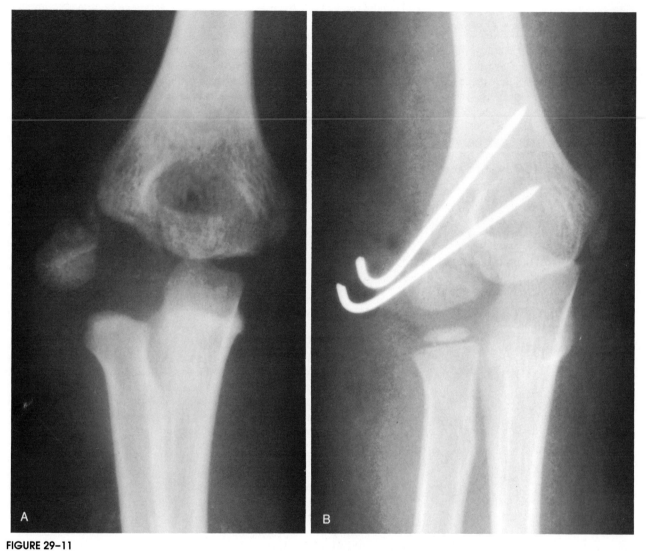

FIGURE 29–11
Preoperative *(A)* and postoperative *(B)* radiographs of a 6-year-old boy with a displaced lateral condyle fracture treated with open reduction and smooth pin fixation.

This fracture is staged I through III: stage I fractures are nondisplaced, stage II fractures are moderately displaced, and stage III fractures are completely displaced and rotated. Long-term complications include non-union, cosmetic deformity of either the cubitus varus or valgus type, and restricted motion and arthritis.

Fractures through the medial condyle are exceedingly rare and are mirror images to those of the lateral condyle. They occur primarily with falls. As in lateral condyle fractures, open reduction and internal fixation is the preferred management.

Fractures can also involve the entire distal humeral physis, with displacement of the entire epiphysis. This rare injury occurs primarily in infants younger than 1 year of age, and should be considered in patients with a swollen and painful elbow, often associated with child abuse. Treatment is usually by closed reduction and frequently percutaneous pinning. If difficulty occurs with the diagnosis, an arthrogram is helpful.

A more common physeal fracture involves the medial epicondyle apophysis (Fig. 29–12). The medial epicondyle serves as the site of attachment of the common flexor group, as well as the pronator teres. It also serves as an attachment to the medial collateral ligaments. Injury to the medial epicondyle is often due to a pulling force applied to the apophysis, resulting in an avulsion. This injury can occur with a dislocation of the elbow, even one that spontaneously reduces, and it is probably this mechanism of injury that results in the occasional incarceration of the medial epicondyle in the elbow joint. Due to their proximity to each other, the ulnar nerve can be injured with avulsion of the medial epicondyle and may sustain further injury with late and progressive instability of the elbow secondary to the loss of the collateral ligaments. The most profound injury to the ulnar nerve occurs with its incarceration within the joint. Although rare, the median nerve also can be incarcerated. Indications for surgical reduction and fixation vary because of excellent results with nonoperative management. Displacement alone is not an indication for surgery, because the apophysis remains extra-articular. Even with non-union of the apophysis, function is generally good. Indications for surgery include incarceration of the apophysis or the ulnar nerve within the joint and valgus instability of the elbow in athletes or other individuals requiring firm stability.

Fractures of the radial head and neck may be seen with falls in the pediatric patient and can be associated with other elbow injuries, including dislocations. These fractures can be either Salter-Harris types I, II, or IV, and most are minimally displaced or angulated. Thus, fractures of the radial head and neck can be treated conservatively with only short periods of immobilization and early active motion. However, when the entire head is severely displaced or angulated, attempts at reduction should be made. Closed manipulation is sometimes successful. It is possible to perform percutaneous manipulation of the fracture fragments using small pins, but care should be taken to avoid injury of the posterior interosseous nerve, which lies in the supinator just distal to the neck of the radius. Open reduction is needed only if significant angulation or displacement exists. Fixation with pins is sometimes required but is difficult. These injuries can frequently be associated with loss of motion, but major vascular and nerve injuries are quite rare. Angulation of less than 30 degrees for radial neck fractures in children probably does not require any active treatment.[68]

Injuries to the olecranon can occur in the pediatric age group, frequently secondary to falls. Closed reduction and immobilization in a cast are possible in stable fractures; however, unstable fractures frequently require some form of internal fixation with pins, wires, or even sutures. The most important consideration in these fractures is ensuring congruity of the articular surfaces.

Dislocations of the elbow can be confused with the more common supracondylar humerus fracture and tend to occur in the older age group with peak incidence at approximately 13 years of age, compared with a peak incidence of supercondylar humerus fractures at 6 years of age. Clinically, a dislocated elbow usually appears to have less swelling than a supracondylar humerus fracture, and the prominence of the dislocation occurs more distally. The normal relation between the epicondyles and olecranon is lost with a dislocation but is preserved with a supracondylar humerus fracture. Diagnosis is confirmed by radiographs. The vast ma-

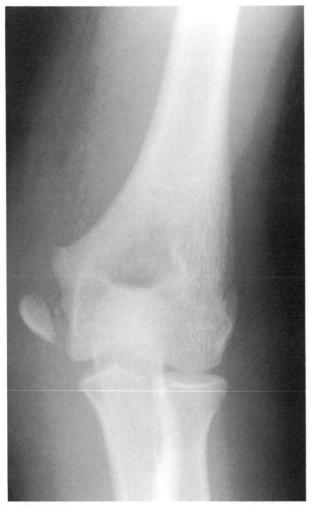

FIGURE 29–12

Radiograph of a 14-year-old boy with a displaced medial epicondyle fracture.

jority of elbow dislocations are of the posterior type. Considerable soft-tissue damage can occur with this dislocation, including disruption of the capsule as well as the brachialis muscle. Medial collateral ligament injury also occurs. The medial epicondylar apophysis can be avulsed, or the ligament can be torn. The lateral collateral ligament is also subject to injury. The collateral arterial system is frequently disrupted by this injury, and such injuries to the brachial artery can result in tissue ischemia distally. Fortunately, brachial artery injuries are rare, because unlike supracondylar humerus fractures, the dislocated distal humerus does not present sharp surfaces that can impale the artery. However, in the process of reduction, the artery can be entrapped within the joint. Owing to collateral compromise from the dislocation, arterial reconstruction is required with brachial artery disruption. Ulnar nerve lesions are the most common neural injury associated with dislocated elbows. All nerve injuries that occur with dislocation tend to resolve with time due to their neuropractic nature.

Prompt reduction is required for dislocated elbows, and most of these can be reduced in a closed fashion. Adequate anesthesia is required, and a general anesthetic is usually necessary for pediatric patients. After reduction, changes in the neurovascular status are noted to ensure that incarceration of the median nerve or other structures has not occurred. Because of the severity of the soft tissue injury that occurs with dislocation of the elbow, restricted motion frequently results. Repeat dislocation is a possibility when there is continued ligamentous compromise.

Dislocation of the radial head can occur with trauma, and it is important to look for an associated fracture of the ulna when assessing a radial head dislocation. It also is important to rule out a congenital or long-term traumatic head dislocation. Radiographic findings that are consistent with a congenital dislocation of the radial head are (1) relatively short ulna or long radius, (2) hypoplastic or absent capitellum, (3) partially defective trochlea, (4) prominent ulna epicondyle, (5) dome-shaped radial head with long neck, and (6) grooving of the distal humerus.[41] Closed reduction of radial head dislocations can be done in injuries that are less than 1 week old; older injuries require an open reduction and usually an anterior ligament reconstruction. The radial head usually must be secured to the capitellum temporarily with a pin. Congenital or chronic traumatic radial head dislocations are usually not amenable to surgical reduction.

One of the most frequent cases of elbow pain in the young child is the so-called nursemaid's elbow. This condition occurs secondary to a longitudinal force applied to the extremity. Classically, the child is pulled or lifted by the hand or forearm, producing pronation and longitudinal pull on the elbow, and the oblicular ligament slips between the radius and capitellum. The child, usually an infant, refuses to move the arm. Swelling is often minimal, and radiographic results are frequently normal. Attempts should be made to elicit a history consistent with this injury. Reduction is usually quite simple. The child's forearm is supinated and the elbow flexed. Usually, a palpable snap can be appreciated with palpation over the radial head. Although the problem can be recurrent, long-term residual problems from nursemaid's elbow are exceedingly rare.

Forearm

Displaced shaft fractures of the radius or ulna are always associated with either a corresponding fracture to the adjacent forearm bone or a proximal or distal dislocation of the radioulnar joint. Because they are rigid bones and the distal and proximal radial and ulnar articulations are nonyielding, a displacement of one bone requires displacement to some degree of the adjacent bone. Thus, when a patient is seen with a fracture of one forearm bone, care must be taken to delineate any injury to the adjacent bone. Displaced or angulated fractures of the proximal ulna are frequently associated with dislocations of the radial head and are called Monteggia fractures (Fig. 29–13). This injury must be investigated with quality anteroposterior and lateral radiographs. A rapid diagnosis is important, because excellent function usually occurs with prompt reduction and appropriate immobilization. Neglected dislocations of the radial head result in its restricted motion and eventual arthritic changes. The radial head can be dislocated posteriorly, laterally, or medially. Usually, the apex of the angulated fracture is in the same direction as the dislocated radial head. Diagnosis requires quality anteroposterior and lateral radiographs, with the radial neck and head aligning with the capitulum.

Most Monteggia fractures in children can be treated with manipulation and closed reduction. Rarely, open reduction and internal fixation are required. Internal fixation of the ulna can often be performed with pins only. If the radial head is not stable on reduction, the annular ligament can be reconstructed using part of the triceps tendon, and the radial head can be pinned to the ulna or to the humerus with a transcapitellar pin. Monteggia lesions can be associated with posterior interosseous or radial nerve injuries. Most of these injuries resolve spontaneously.[50]

Shaft fractures of the pediatric radius and ulna are quite frequent. There are three basic types: torus fractures, greenstick fractures, and complete fractures. Torus fractures are buckle fractures which are caused by compression only.

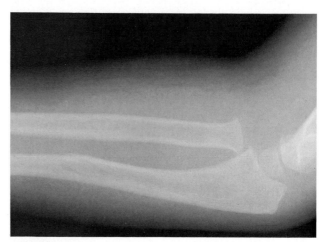

FIGURE 29–13

Radiograph of a 6-year-old boy with a midshaft fracture of the ulna and an anterior dislocation of the radial head (Monteggia fracture).

Greenstick fractures have one intact and one disrupted cortex. In complete fractures, the fragments are unstable, and shortening and angulation are frequent. However, the rotational deformity is often the most difficult to treat, and precise radiographs are required.

Displaced fractures are usually easily diagnosed clinically. Again, films of the proximal and distal joints should be obtained to ensure that the fracture is not associated with a joint disruption. Despite the occasional grotesque appearance of forearm fractures, they are rarely associated with significant neurological or vascular complications. Compartment syndromes, although possible, are also quite rare compared with more proximal fractures (e.g., supracondylar humerus fractures).

Treatment for the torus fracture is simple immobilization for several weeks. This type of fracture heals quickly with minimal residual problems. A greenstick fracture is usually treated with closed reduction if significant angulation is present. Often, there is some associated rotational as well as angular deformity, which should be corrected at the time of reduction. Immobilization is usually in the form of a long arm cast for several weeks.

Treatment for the displaced both-bone forearm fracture is more difficult. Surrounding muscles frequently cause significant shortening of the fracture fragments. Length is usually best restored by application of gentle traction before manual reduction maneuvers. These fractures frequently require a general anesthetic for pain control and relaxation. After a period of traction, reduction is obtained by placing the radius and ulna on end, often in succession. Following manipulation, it is critical to obtain films to look for continued radiographic evidence of malrotation. Radiographically, the diameter of the fragments on both the anteroposterior and lateral views should be the same; differences in diameters are indicative of rotational malposition. It is critical to correct this malposition, because little if any remodelling occurs with growth.[1] Angular deformity will remodel to some extent, but in the older child, it is important to limit angular deformities to prevent loss of supination and pronation.

General principles of reduction for both-bone forearm fractures include placing the distal fragment in line with the proximal fragment. This is usually best performed by noting the position of the biceps tuberosity and distal bony landmarks, such as the ulnar and radial styloid. If the both-bone forearm fracture cannot be reduced adequately or secured with cast immobilization in the older child, open reduction and internal fixation using plates is indicated.

Occasionally in the younger child, neither a complete, greenstick, nor a torus fracture is noted despite significant deformity of the forearm. This plastic deformation occurs due to the child's greater flexibility of the long bones. When applied stress exceeds the elastic limit of the bone, permanent plastic deformation occurs. The amount of deformity may limit rotation of the forearm and can cause a significant cosmetic problem. It is currently believed that very young children can achieve remodeling of this to some extent, but older children may continue to have significant bowing. Plastic deformation can be reduced by applying steady, firm pressure to the forearm to straighten the bowed bone.

Forearm fractures that heal with significant angulation can result in limited supination and pronation. The ability of a child's forearm to remodel after healing with a deformity is dependent on the child's age, the location of the fracture, and the type of deformity. As would be expected, younger children have a much greater potential for remodeling. Because children older than 10 years of age have a lesser potential for remodeling, angular deformities greater than 10 degrees will probably not remodel completely on their own.[19] Fractures in the distal forearm have a greater ability to remodel than proximal fractures, and rotational deformities have a much lower likelihood of being remodeled than either volar-dorsal or radial-ulnar deformities. These facts should be considered before accepting a less-than-perfect closed reduction of a both-bone forearm fracture.

Open reduction, although infrequently required in children with forearm fractures, should be considered when residual deformity will limit forearm rotation. Open reduction can be augmented by internal fixation with pins, plates, or small intramedullary rods.[35, 72]

An unusual complication in fractures of the forearm is a cross-union between the radius and the ulna, a problem that occurs primarily with high-energy–sustained injuries. Cross-union is more common with proximal forearm fractures than with distal fractures. Operative treatment is very difficult, with frequent failure to regain motion.[73]

Distal Radius and Ulna

Fractures of the distal radius and ulna are probably the most common in childhood. It is believed that this is due to the relative weakness of the metaphyseal bone in this area. Fractures of the distal radius and ulna can be classified as torus, greenstick, or complete. The vast majority of these fractures require only protection or a simple closed reduction. It is important that multiple postreduction radiographs be taken to ensure maintenance of reduction for several weeks, because late displacement is not uncommon. Many complete fractures through the distal radius and ulna are physeal fractures, usually of the Salter-Harris types I or II. Closed reduction is the preferred treatment, with care being taken to prevent injury to the physis. This treatment requires adequate anesthesia or sedation and careful technique. Reduction is usually maintained in a long-arm cast, but controversy exists regarding whether reduction should be maintained with supination or pronation. Healing is rapid in children; only 4 to 6 weeks of immobilization are usually required. Fractures of the distal radius and ulna are rarely associated with compartment syndromes or nerve injuries.

Dislocations of the radiocarpal joint or between the carpal bones are extremely rare. The key to diagnosis is careful assessment of the radiographs in a child with significant swelling and deformity of the wrist without the more common distal radius fracture. Dislocations of the distal radioulnar joint are quite rare and require disruption of the dorsal and volar radioulnar ligaments as well as triangular fibrocartilage. If discovered early, treatment is usually closed reduction and immobilization in a long-arm cast with supination of the forearm if the distal ulna is displaced dorsally, or in a long-arm cast in full pronation if the ulna is displaced in a volar direction.

Wrist

Fractures of the scaphoid bone have a different pattern of involvement in children than in the adult. Distal avulsion-type fractures are much more common in the child than the standard mid-waist scaphoid fractures seen in adults.[71] However, waist fractures in the middle of the scaphoid can occur and result in nonunion, as in the adult. Because these fractures are sometimes difficult to identify on initial films, repeat radiographs should be taken 1 to 2 weeks after initial assessment. Pediatric scaphoid fractures are typically non-displaced and can usually be treated in a thumb spica cast with an expected good result. Operative indications include an irreducible fracture and nonunion. Fractures of other carpal bones are exceedingly rare.

Hand

Despite the high frequency of injuries to the child's hand, fractures and dislocations are rare as compared with the incidence in adults. However, most hand fractures in children are stable, and healing is quite rapid.

Most phalangeal fractures can be treated with simple closed reduction and immobilization for approximately 3 weeks. These fractures frequently require plaster immobilization rather than aluminum splints or buddy taping to protect the child from repeat or additional injury and to prevent removal of the immobilization. Although angular deformity can remodel, the rotational deformity does not; it needs to be corrected at the time of reduction. Rotational deformity is best detected by having the child flex his or her fingers and checking the convergence of the flexed fingertips toward the area of the scaphoid. Malrotation is evident by the fractured digit crossing over the adjacent nonfractured digit. Operative indications are few and include a fracture resulting in subluxation of the adjacent joint, commonly seen when there is a fracture of the neck of a phalanx that results in significant rotation of the head of the phalanx.[36] Another indication for surgical intervention is displaced intra-articular fragments. Open reduction with these injuries usually requires fixation with small pins or wires, but occasionally, small screws and plates can be used.

Fractures of the thumb metacarpal, when they are intra-articular at the carpometacarpal joint, usually require open reduction and fixation. This is the children's equivalent of a Bennett fracture and is a Salter-Harris type III injury. Other fractures at the base of the first metacarpal can usually be treated in a closed manner.

Dislocation of any of the interphalangeal, metacarpophalangeal, or carpometacarpal joints can occur, and almost all can be managed with closed reduction and splinting. An exception to this rule is when a dislocation is associated with large fracture fragments that prevent reduction or create instability. Rarely, metacarpophalangeal joint disloca-

tions can be irreducible by closed means (e.g., when the volar plate becomes entrapped between the base of the proximal phalanx and the head of the metacarpal). The surrounding tendons and ligaments prevent reduction as longitudinal traction tightens the surrounding structures around the dislocation. Open reduction by removing the volar plate is usually required.

Complete tears of the ulnar collateral ligament of the metacarpophalangeal joint of the thumb can be associated with nonhealing, as in the adult's gamekeeper's thumb. Healing with cast immobilization is unlikely, and persistent inability to pinch is the usual result. These injuries are best managed by open repair of the ligament or associated avulsion fractures. Dislocations of the carpometacarpal joints are also quite uncommon in children. Dislocations or fracture-dislocations of the ulnocarpometacarpal joints are common in adults but, rarely seen in children. Such injuries require closed or open reduction and pinning.

FRACTURES AND DISLOCATIONS OF THE LOWER EXTREMITY

Hip

Traumatic dislocation of the hip in the child is more common than fracture and tends to occur in two distinct age groups. The first group includes 2- to 5-year-old children in whom dislocation can occur with minimal trauma, such as an insignificant fall, because of their soft, pliable cartilage and generalized joint laxity. The second age group is comprised of 11- to 15-year-old children, in whom dislocation usually occurs secondary to severe trauma such as motor vehicle accidents or sports injuries. Posterior dislocations are seven to 10 times more common than anterior dislocations. In posterior dislocations, the leg is held in flexion, adduction, and internal rotation (Fig. 29–14). For anterior dislocations, the extremity is in extension, abduction, and external rotation.

The primary management of hip dislocations is closed reduction performed in the emergency department. For dislocations that have existed for longer than 12 hours or those that cannot be reduced in the emergency department, closed reduction under general anesthesia should be performed.[13] The most frequent cause of inability to achieve closed reduction of a hip dislocation is soft tissue interposition, which requires an open reduction through a posterior arthrotomy.[47] In cases where there is an ipsilateral hip dislocation and fracture of the femoral shaft, closed reduction may be difficult or impossible, but a traction pin in the trochanteric area may facilitate this procedure. Open reduction is often required with ipsilateral hip dislocations and femur fractures.[6]

The most severe sequela from a hip dislocation is avascular necrosis resulting from disruption of the blood supply to the proximal femoral epiphysis. Delay in reduction of longer than 24 hours appears to be associated with a high degree of avascular necrosis.[52] Occasionally, fractures of the acetabulum or femoral head can be associated with hip dislocation. If after reduction of the hip there is a widening of the medial joint space, a computed tomographic scan is indicated to rule out intra-articular bone fragments.

Hip fractures are extremely rare in children when compared with their incidence in adults. The thick periosteum around the neck of the pediatric femur seems to prevent displacement of the fracture, therefore, children have a higher incidence of mildly displaced or nondisplaced fractures. The subcapital epiphyses ossify at approximately 4 years of age. Studies of the blood supply to the proximal epiphysis show that the vessels of the ligamentum teres are virtually of no importance and contribute very little to the blood supply to the femoral head.[13] The major source of the blood supply to the proximal femoral epiphysis comes from the medial and lateral femoral circumflex arteries.

Unlike in adults, the mechanism of injury of hip fractures in children is usually secondary to severe trauma. Possible complications from hip fractures in children include avascular necrosis, coxa vara, malunion, nonunion, and premature epiphyseal growth arrest. All management efforts attempt to avoid these complications, the most severe of

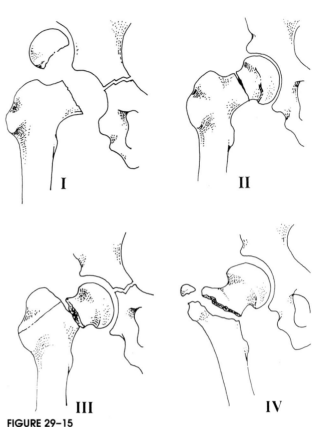

FIGURE 29–15

Schematic representation of the four types of pediatric hip fractures. *I,* Transepiphyseal fracture with dislocation of the femoral head. (This injury can also occur without dislocation of the femoral head.) *II,* Transcervical fracture. *III,* Cervicotrochanteric (basilar neck fracture). *IV,* Intertrochanteric or peritrochanteric fracture.

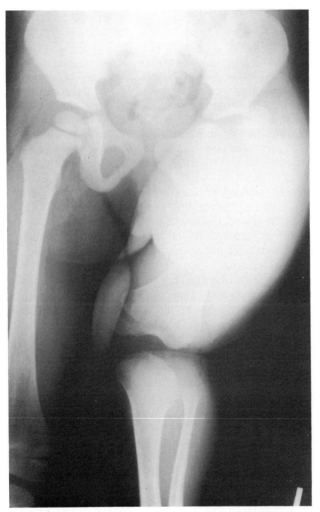

FIGURE 29–14

Radiograph of a 3-year-old girl who sustained a posterior dislocation of the left hip. The distortion of the left femur and tibia is secondary to the flexion, adduction, and internal rotation deformity of the lower extremity.

which is avascular necrosis of the proximal femoral epiphysis. In children, this complication seems to be related to the location of the fracture and the amount of displacement at the time of injury.[12, 46]

There are four basic types of hip fractures in children (Fig. 29–15). A type I injury is a transepiphyseal separation, which accounts for 8% of all hip fractures.[13] Type I fractures are usually associated with severe violence, generally resulting in posterior displacement of the proximal epiphysis with or without dislocation of the femoral head from the acetabulum. Type I fractures of the hip generally occur in young children, although they can occur in the adolescent, in whom they are usually associated with acute slipped capital femoral epiphysis. The long-term results of management of this type injury are poor and may be catastrophic when the femoral head is dislocated from the acetabulum. In transepiphyseal separations in which the femoral head is not dislocated, closed reduction can usually be obtained, but smooth wire fixation is also recommended, along with spica casting. When there is dislocation of the femoral head, an open reduction with internal fixation is usually required. Unfortunately, a high incidence of avascular necrosis and premature growth arrest is associated with this injury.[12, 56]

Type II hip fractures are transcervical fractures that occur

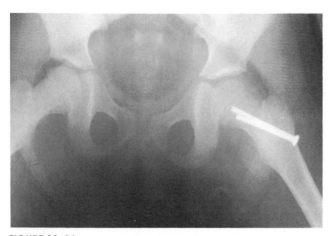

FIGURE 29–16

Radiograph of a 6-year-old girl who sustained a displaced type III fracture of the left femoral neck. This was treated with closed reduction and internal fixation with two cannulated screws.

across the midportion of the femoral neck. Type II fractures are usually displaced and almost never impacted. This is the most common of pediatric hip fractures and accounts for approximately 45 to 50% of these injuries.[13] Management involves closed reduction and internal fixation with pins or screws while attempting to avoid crossing the epiphyseal growth plate with the hardware. If closed reduction cannot be obtained, open reduction and fixation is indicated. There is approximately a 40% avascular necrosis rate associated with this type of fracture.[12, 13]

Type III fractures are the cervicotrochanteric fractures, (i.e., base neck fracture), and they account for approximately 30 to 35% of hip fractures in children.[13] Type III hip fractures occur just proximal to the anterior intertrochanteric line. Management depends on the amount of displacement. With nondisplacement, abduction spica casting can be successful, but close follow-up in the first week or two is necessary to make sure displacement does not occur. In displaced fractures, closed reduction and internal fixation with pins or screws are needed (Fig. 29–16). Although the incidence of avascular necrosis with type III fractures is lower in children, it is higher than that associated with adults, occurs in approximately 20 to 30% of cases, and seems to be related to the amount of initial displacement.[2, 13] Displaced type I, II, and III hip fractures should be reduced as soon as possible to attempt to decrease the incidence of avascular necrosis.

Type IV hip fractures are intertrochanteric or peritrochanteric fractures and represent approximately 10 to 15% of hip fractures in children.[13] They can be treated by skin or skeletal traction with later casting or by open reduction and internal fixation. In older children or children with polytrauma, open reduction and internal fixation is required regardless of the amount of displacement.[29] Type IV fractures have fewer complications than the other types of pediatric hip fractures, and they rarely are associated with avascular necrosis.

Femur

Fractures of the shaft of the femur in children usually result from either direct or indirect trauma. Direct trauma (e.g., when a child's thigh is struck or run over) usually results in a transverse or butterfly-type fracture, often associated with extensive soft tissue damage. Indirect trauma usually results from a rotational force producing a spiral or oblique fracture. These types of fractures can occur with only minimal trauma (e.g., tripping or catching the foot) in the younger child. High-velocity injuries can produce significant displacement of the fracture fragments, with tearing of the periosteum and penetration of the muscle compartments. The amount of initial displacement affects the choice of subsequent management. Open fractures of the femur do occur but are rare in this age group.

Femur fractures are classified according to the level of injury (i.e., subtrochanteric, midshaft, and supercondylar). Subtrochanteric fractures occur 1 to 2 cm below the lesser trochanter, and marked displacement of the proximal fragment can occur from the associated muscle forces. The proximal fragment is usually held flexed, abducted, and laterally rotated, secondary to the pull of the iliopsoas, abductor muscles, and short external rotators, respectively. Marked flexion of the proximal fragment makes control with a spica cast difficult. Initial management in the younger child usually consists of casting for nondisplaced fractures and traction for those that are displaced. Traction in the younger child can be skin traction in the ''90/90 position,'' but in children older than 3 years of age, skeletal traction with a pin in the distal femur is indicated (Fig. 29–17). The traction pin requires placement parallel to the axis of the knee joint with care to avoid the distal femoral physis.[2] When early callus formation is seen, spica casting can be initiated. In the adolescent or multiply injured patient, internal or external fixation is indicated (Fig. 29–18A and B).

Femoral shaft fractures are common in children, and approximately 70% occur in the midshaft area. Management depends on the age of the patient and the presence of other associated injuries. In infants from birth to 2 years of age, immediate spica cast application is usually very effective.[67] Close follow up in the first week or two postinjury is necessary to make sure there is no displacement. Shortening of 1 cm or angulation up to 30 degrees is acceptable in this age group. Most 2- to 10-year-old children can also be treated by early spica casting with the expectation of a good outcome (Fig. 29–19A and B). However, there are two contraindications to early spica casting. The first is excessive shortening of more than 2 to 3 cm on initial radiographs. These injuries would be better managed with a period of skeletal or skin traction until early callus formation is seen. The other contraindication is when there are multiple injuries precluding the use of a spica cast. These patients are managed with external fixation, and good results can be expected (Fig. 29–20A and B).[1, 32]

In children older than 11 years of age, the current trend has been to use more internal fixation and less traction. Traction is still a viable option, but it does require prolonged hospitalization and subsequently is associated with

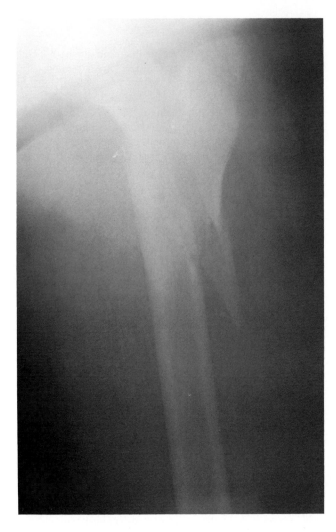

FIGURE 29-17
Radiograph of an 11-year-old boy who sustained a spiral sub-trochanteric fracture of the left femur. This was treated with traction through a distal femoral pin.

more complications.[57] In the adolescent older than 11 years of age, intermedullary fixation such as used in adults provides an excellent means for fixation of the midshaft of the femur [28, 57] (Fig. 29–21A and B). However, care must be taken to avoid injury to the distal femoral physis. Shut down of the greater trochanteric physis is occasionally seen but is usually not a problem if it occurs in this age group. External fixation is also a possible option in the treatment of isolated femur fractures.[3]

There are other indications for operative versus conservative treatment of femur fractures. Children with head injuries or spasticity tend to do better with internal stabilization, and intermedullary fixation is preferable to plate fixation.[67, 78] In the rare case of vascular injury to the femoral artery associated with a femur fracture, internal fixation after vessel repair is the preferred method of management. When the femur fracture is associated with a tibia fracture, this creates a "floating knee"; internal fixation of one or both of these fractures is indicated (Fig. 29–22A, B, and C).[38]

Supercondylar fractures of the femur occur above the level of the origin of the gastrocnemius muscles. The pull of these muscles tend to flex the distal fragment and cause displacement of the fracture. In nondisplaced fractures, cast immobilization seems to be effective. Often these fractures

are unstable, in which case crossed smooth Steinmann pins and a spica cast or external fixation can be employed.[67]

When skeletal traction is indicated for treatment of a femur fracture, the traction pin should be applied through the distal femur. Care must be taken when inserting distal femoral pins to avoid damage to the distal femoral physis and femoral artery. Proximal tibial pins, which are used in adults, can cause epiphyseal damage in the skeletally immature child. The anterior aspect of the proximal tibial physis extends down the front of the tibia and can be injured with traction pins, even if inserted some distance from the physis. Physeal arrest about the knee has been associated with fractures of the femur and tibia that are away from the growth plates. A child with significant lower extremity trauma of the femur or tibia should be observed for 1 or 2 years for potential growth plate arrest.[31]

Knee

Fractures and dislocations about the knee usually result from significant trauma. The majority of the growth of the lower extremity is from the distal femoral and the proximal tibial physes. Injury to either of these structures that causes premature growth arrest in the immature skeleton can lead

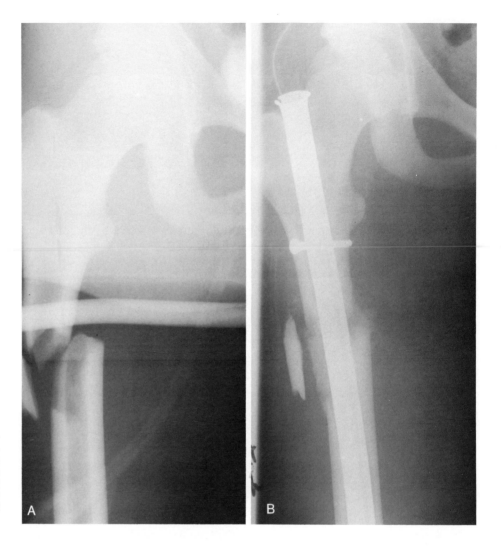

FIGURE 29–18

Preoperative *(A)* and postoperative *(B)* radiographs of a 15-year-old boy who sustained a right subtrochanteric fracture in a motor vehicle accident and was treated successfully with an intermedullary rod and a proximal locking screw.

to significant leg length discrepancy or angular deformity. In addition, vascular injuries or compartment syndromes can be seen with significantly displaced fractures about the knee.

Fractures involving the distal femoral physis can occur in all Salter-Harris types. These fractures can be caused by either indirect or direct injury. The injuring force is applied to the front or side of the knee. If initial films of an injured child's knee are normal but clinical signs suggest an injury to the distal femoral growth plate, stress views may be necessary to reveal the injury.

Salter-Harris type I injuries are typically seen in newborns with birth injuries or in adolescents as nondisplaced separations. The type II injury is the most common, however, and typically occurs in the adolescent. Displacement is usually in the coronal plane and the metaphyseal fragment is either medial or lateral, generally on the side where the epiphysis is displaced (Fig. 29–23A and B). Type II injuries can also have anterior displacement of the distal femoral physis resulting from hyperextension of the knee. In this type of injury, the distal metaphysis is driven into the popliteal fossa with potential injury to the popliteal artery or branches of the sciatic nerve. Type III fractures of the knee occur with displacement of one of the two hemi-epiphyses and can cause substantial incongruity of the articular surface. Type IV fractures are uncommon and involve a fracture line that extends from the metaphysis across the physis into the articular cartilage. Type V injuries can occur in the knee but are seen only retrospectively, when asymmetric growth occurs.

Management of type I injuries usually involves closed reduction and casting. For type II injuries with displacement in the medial or lateral position, closed reduction and application of a long leg cast with the knee in extension is usually adequate. When there is a hyperextension injury with anterior displacement of the epiphysis, closed reduction and casting with the knee in some degree of flexion is recommended. The peroneal nerve may be injured by either lateral or medial displacement of the epiphysis. If the reduction of type II injuries is unstable, percutaneous, smooth, crossed-pin fixation and casting is recommended.[74] If anatomic closed reduction of type III and type IV injuries cannot be obtained, open reduction and internal fixation are indicated. Anatomic reduction and use of internal fixation in unstable type II, III, and IV fractures are the recommended ways to attempt to avoid premature growth arrest.[58] The prognosis for growth arrest cannot always be predicted by the Salter-Harris classification and appears to be related

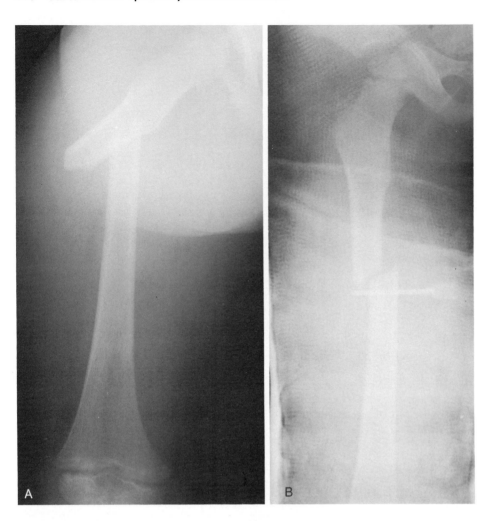

FIGURE 29–19

A, Radiograph of a 3-year-old boy who sustained a proximal shaft fracture of the right femur with a significant overlap. This fracture was treated successfully in a spica cast. *B,* Antero-posterior radiograph of the femur in the spica cast. The needle is placed outside the spica to locate the level of the fracture in case wedging is necessary. This fracture should be observed closely during the first 2 weeks to make sure unacceptable shortening or angulation does not occur.

to the degree of initial displacement of the fracture and the exactness of reduction.[39]

Fractures involving the proximal tibial epiphysis are rare. The most feared complication of this type of fracture is injury to the popliteal artery, which is held by its major branches to the posterior surface of the proximal tibial epiphysis. When a fracture causes posterior displacement of the upper end of the metaphysis, there may be stretching and tearing of the popliteal artery. Fracture separation of the proximal tibial epiphysis can occur by direct or indirect force. Direct force is imposed when a child's leg is run over by the wheels of a vehicle. Indirect force occurs when the lower leg is forced into abduction or hyperextension against a fixed knee.

Most fractures of the upper tibial epiphysis are Salter-Harris type I or II. In type I injuries, the upper tibial epiphysis is displaced laterally or anteriorly, which causes the metaphysis to be placed posteriorly, with the potential for vascular injury. In Salter-Harris type II injuries, the epiphysis is usually displaced laterally, causing the metaphysis to displace medially. Type III and type IV fractures of the proximal tibial epiphysis have also been reported.[11] Treatment of these types of fractures usually consists of closed reduction and application of a long leg cast. However, for unstable injuries, closed reduction and percutaneous pin fixation may be necessary. Open reduction is occasionally

needed for type III and type IV injuries if anatomic reduction cannot be obtained with closed methods.[11] If pulses are impaired, immediate closed reduction is necessary. If pulses are not restored by closed reduction, arteriography and exploration of the artery are necessary. Exploration of isolated peroneal nerve palsy is not recommended, because these injuries generally recover spontaneously.[64]

Avulsion of the Tibial Tubercle

Avulsion of the tibial tubercle is a rare injury that may occur in adolescents. The primary ossification center of the proximal tibial epiphysis forms first; secondary centers of ossification appear in the tibial tubercle later. The patella ligament inserts directly into the developing tubercle, and force applied through this ligament can cause avulsion of the tibial tubercle apophysis. Most of these injuries occur during sports activities with hyperextension or direct blows to the front of the knee.

Three types of tibial tubercle fractures are described (Fig. 29–24).[48] Type I fractures occur through the secondary ossification center at the level of insertion of the patella ligament. Type II fractures occur at the junction of the primary and secondary ossification centers. A type III fracture, which is a variant of the Salter-Harris type III, is a fracture

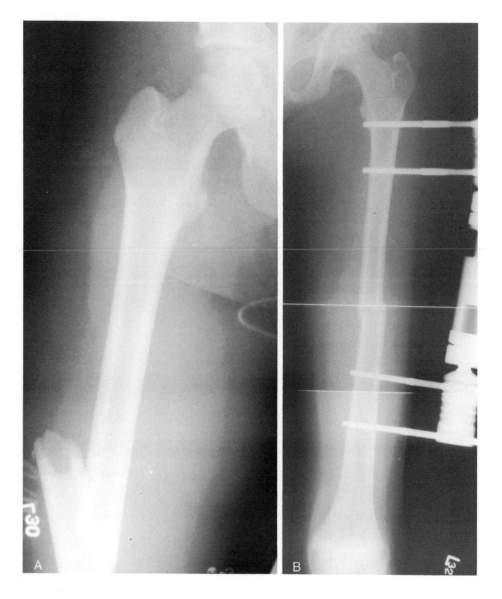

FIGURE 29–20

A, Radiograph of an 11-year-old girl who sustained multiple long bone fractures, including this left femur fracture in an automobile accident. *B,* Because of multiple upper extremity fractures, the left femur fracture was fixed with an external fixator. An alternative method of management here would have been an intermedullary nail.

that propagates upward across the primary ossification center into the knee joint. In all types of tibial tubercle fractures, there is swelling and tenderness at the insertion of the patella ligament, and there may be a joint effusion or hemarthrosis. A lateral film of the knee is preferable for diagnosis of this avulsion injury.

When these injuries are minimally displaced or nondisplaced, the preferred management method is cast immobilization with the knee in extension. Follow-up films are necessary to make sure there is no displacement over the first week or two postinjury. For displaced type II and type III fractures, open reduction and internal fixation are recommended (Fig. 29–25*A* and *B*).[15, 26] A large periosteal flap is usually pulled off with the tibial tubercle and must be sutured to the metaphysis of the tibia. In type III fractures, it is important to reconstruct the congruity of the joint for best results. Type III injury can lead to premature growth arrest of the proximal tibial physis; however, this is usually not a problem, because the injury usually occurs in adolescents who are approaching the end of their growth period.[48]

Fractures of the Patella

Fractures of the patella in children are infrequent, because a surrounding thick layer of cartilage cushions the bone against direct blows. The mechanism of injury in fractures of the patella is usually from a direct blow or sudden contracture of the extensor mechanism. However, there is fracture that is unique to the immature skeleton: a sleeve-type fracture that is seen in younger children. This injury is characterized by avulsion of a small bony fragment from the distal pole of the patella together with an extensive sleeve of articular cartilage. In transverse fractures, the articular cartilage often remains intact, but the fracture gaps interiorly. Management of nondisplaced fractures is by immobilization in a cylinder cast with the knee in extension. If there is displacement of transverse fractures, open reduction with internal fixation is indicated, particularly if a diastasis of more than 4 mm or a step-off in the articular cartilage of greater than 3 mm is present.[59] The sleeve-type fracture may appear benign on films, but if there is marked

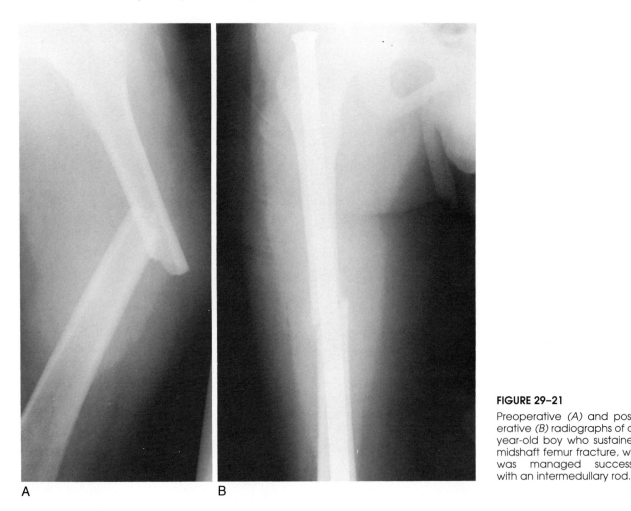

A   B

FIGURE 29–21

Preoperative *(A)* and postoperative *(B)* radiographs of a 12-year-old boy who sustained a midshaft femur fracture, which was managed successfully with an intermedullary rod.

displacement, open reduction and reattachment of the articular sleeve are required.

Patella Dislocation

Dislocation of the patella is a relatively common injury in children and is most commonly caused by falls or sports activities. Direct blows, usually to the medial aspect of the patella, account for only 10% of acute dislocations. In these dislocations, the patella may remain in its dislocated lateral position or may spontaneously reduce with active or passive extension of the knee. Although most of these dislocations reduce spontaneously, they can easily be reduced by extension of the knee and pressure on the lateral aspect of the patella. Follow-up films should be obtained to rule out osteochondral fractures. After an acute patella dislocation, management in a cylinder cast for 2 to 4 weeks is indicated to allow soft tissue healing. If there is evidence of an intra-articular osteochondral fragment, arthroscopic examination and removal of fragments may be necessary.

Fractures of the Tibial Spine

Avulsion of the tibial spine is a relatively rare injury, most commonly caused by athletic or bicycle accidents. The an-

terior cruciate ligament attaches distally to the anterior tibial spine and the anterior horn of the medial meniscus. Injury occurs as the tibia is rotated relative to the femur and forced into hyperextension, resulting in three types of fractures based on the degree of displacement. A type I fracture is minimally displaced, and a type III fracture is completely displaced (Fig. 29–26).[43] Physical findings include pain and effusion of the knee with associated hemarthrosis and reluctance to bear weight. Management of most type I and II fractures of the tibial spine consist of reduction and immobilization with the knee in extension. Occasionally, a tense hemarthrosis will need to be aspirated prior to extending the knee for immobilization.

In type III fractures, the meniscus may be interposed and prevent reduction. If anatomic reduction cannot be accomplished in a closed fashion, open reduction and fixation are indicated.[43] The method of fixation of these types of fractures should avoid crossing the proximal tibial epiphysis, and in one series in which fractures of the tibial spine were completely reduced, some anterior cruciate ligament laxity, although asymptomatic, was noticed.[7]

Tibia

Fractures of the shaft of the tibia and fibula are the most common pediatric orthopedic injury in the lower extremity.

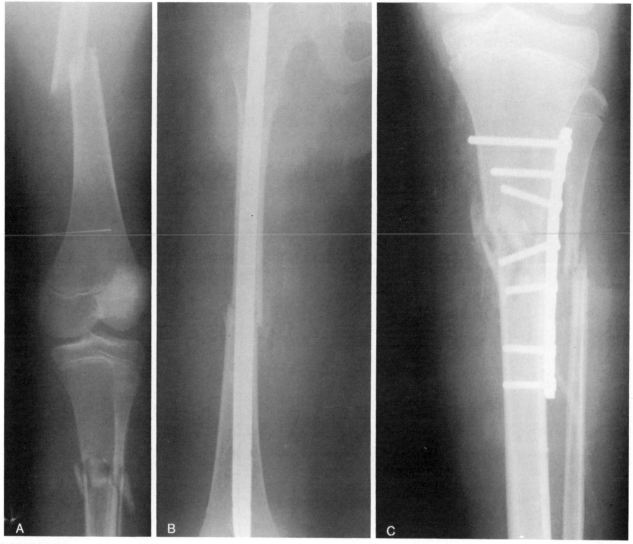

FIGURE 29–22

A, Preoperative radiograph of a 12-year-old girl who sustained epsilateral femoral and tibial fractures in a motor vehicle accident. *B,* Postoperative radiograph of the femoral fracture treated with an intermedullary rod because the injury represented a ''floating knee.'' *C,* Postoperative radiograph of the tibia fracture treated with open reduction and internal fixation with a plate and screws.

Tibial shaft and metaphyseal fractures are usually caused by indirect forces (e.g., rotational twisting injuries) and less frequently by direct trauma. Indirect rotation is associated with an oblique or spiral fracture, whereas direct trauma is usually associated with transverse or butterfly-type fracture. When a fracture of the tibia and fibula is suspected, full-length anteroposterior and lateral films should be taken and must include the knee and ankle joints.

The majority of closed tibia and fibula fractures in children are uncomplicated and can be managed with simple manipulation and application of a long leg cast. The amount of shortening that can be tolerated after closed reduction of a fracture is 5 to 10 mm in the 1- to 5-year-old age group and 0 to 5 mm in the 5- to 10-year-old age group.[21] Up to approximately 10 mm of shortening can be fully or partially compensated by growth acceleration in the tibia.[63] In addition, nearly 10% of angular deformities correct with time;

however, this correction ceases approximately 18 months postinjury.[27] Varus deformities of up to 15 degrees can undergo spontaneous correction, whereas valgus deformities and posterior angulations persist to some degree. Rotational deformities, particularly internal ones, tend to persist.[63] For the rare unstable closed tibia and fibula fracture, two options of management are rigid external fixation or percutaneous K-wire fixation after closed reduction.

Vascular injuries can occasionally occur with tibia fractures, most commonly in the proximal tibial metaphysis where the anterior tibial artery passes through the interosseous membrane. Fractures of the proximal tibial metaphysis can occasionally injure this artery but rarely disturb the posterior tibial artery. Another fracture that may cause injury to the anterior tibial artery occurs in the lower tibia when the foot and distal tibial fragment are displaced posteriorly.

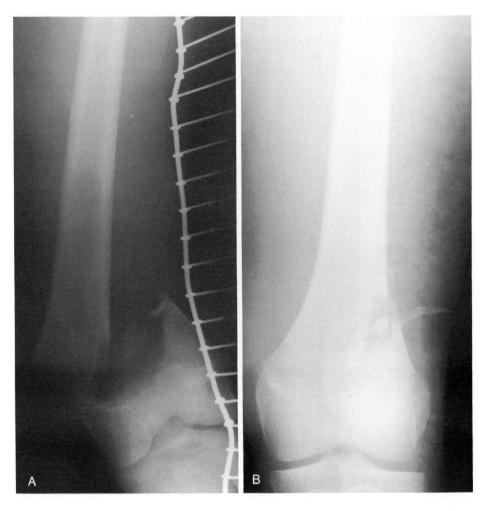

FIGURE 29-23

A, Anteroposterior radiograph of the femur of a 15-year-old boy who sustained a type II epiphyseal fracture of the distal femur in a football injury. *B,* The fracture was successfully treated with closed reduction and application of a long leg cast.

Compartment syndromes should also be ruled out with any closed or open tibia fracture in children. Clinically, pain is out of proportion to the severity of injury, and the most severe tenderness is not over the fracture site, but over the muscle. On palpation, the anterior compartment may be very hard. The dorsalis pedis pulse is usually intact, and the most common sensory deficit is on the dorsum of the foot and is related to injury of the deep peroneal nerve. Compartment pressure measurements can be obtained, and fasciotomy is advised when the tissue pressure rises above 35 to 40 mm Hg.

Management of open fractures of the tibia in children is similar to that in adults: the fracture site should be immediately débrided with irrigation and intravenous antibiotic therapy should be begun. Grade I injuries may be treated with initial débridement and application of a windowed cast. Fractures with instability or significant soft tissue loss can be managed with rigid external fixation. The fixation pins must be placed so that they do not injure the epiphyseal plates.[1] Significant soft tissue injuries should have repeat débridements every 24 to 48 hours until the wound is clean enough for soft tissue coverage, usually by delayed closure, skin grafts, or muscle flaps. Open fractures with vessel injuries should have immediate repair of the vessels and stabilization of the fracture with either internal or external fixation. Grade I open fractures tend to heal without significant complications in children. Grade II and III fractures of the tibia have approximately the same incidence of vascular injury, compartment syndrome, infection, and delayed union in children as in adults. Although delayed union is as common as in adults, non-union is very rare in children.[10] The incidence of delayed union is related to the severity of soft tissue injury, the pattern of the fracture, and

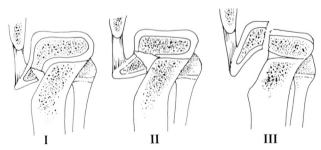

FIGURE 29-24

Schematic representation of the three types of avulsion fractures of the tibial tubercle. Type I injuries represent a fracture at the level of the posterior border of the patella ligament. Type II fractures are at the junction of the primary and secondary ossification centers. Type III injuries have a fracture line that propagates across the primary ossification center into the joint.

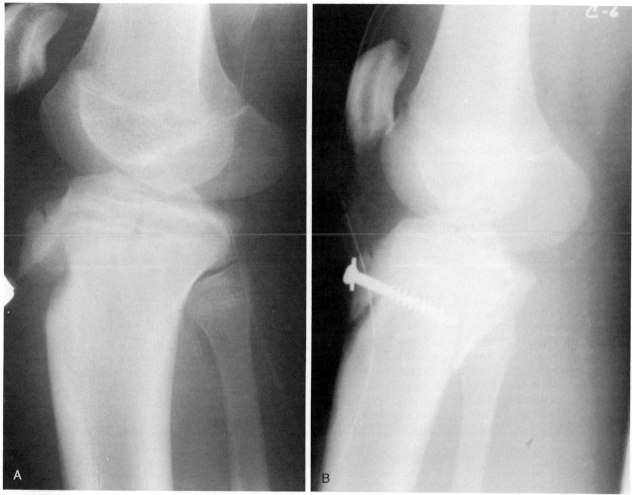

FIGURE 29–25

A, Lateral radiograph of the knee of a 15-year-old boy who was struck on the front of the extended knee during a football game. This resulted in a type III injury of the tibial tubercle. Note the extension across the physis into the knee joint. *B,* Postoperative radiograph showing open reduction and fixation of the tibial tubercle with a screw and washer. Since he is close to the end of his growth, premature growth arrest is not a concern in this patient.

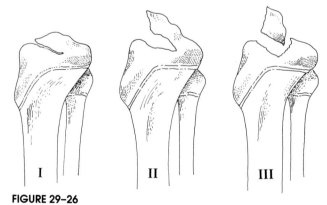

FIGURE 29–26

Schematic drawing representing three types of tibial spine fractures. Type I injuries show minimal displacement; type II injuries have more displacement with a posterior hinge; and type III injuries have complete separation and displacement of the tibial spine.

the amount of segmental bone loss. When débriding open fractures, it is very important to try to preserve as much periosteum as possible for regeneration of any lost bone.

External fixation of tibia fractures is indicated in certain other circumstances, such as for fractures associated with burns or in children with multiple fractures. In addition, external fixation is an appropriate means to fix fractures in the child with a head injury or increased muscle tone and spasticity.[1] Fractures of the tibia and femur on the ipsilateral side, usually involving significant trauma from a motor vehicle accident, create a floating-knee injury, in which fixing at least one of the fractures with rigid internal or external fixation is indicated (see Fig. 29–22*A*, *B*, and *C*).[38]

Another sequela occasionally seen with tibia fractures is progressive valgus deformity with fracture healing, such as that which may occur with proximal metaphyseal fractures in children. The valgus deformity appears to develop during healing and can be accompanied by overgrowth of the tibia; the exact mechanism of this complication is unknown. Although it is alarming to the patient and parents, it does tend to correct somewhat with time, and nonoperative treatment is recommended. However, if the deformity and overgrowth does not correct itself over several years, an appropriately timed epiphysiodesis or osteotomy may be considered. With any proximal tibial metaphyseal fracture, no valgus should be accepted at the time of initial reduction in an attempt to prevent this complication.[5]

Ankle

Injuries to the distal tibial and fibular physis account for approximately 25% of all epiphyseal injuries in children.[21] These injuries can be potentially serious, the most damaging sequela being epiphyseal growth arrest producing angular deformity or shortening. All the Salter-Harris types of epiphyseal injuries can be seen in the distal tibia (Fig. 29–27). In patients older than 14 or 15 years of age, adult patterns of ankle fractures are usually seen. Children's ligaments are stronger than bone, making ligamentous injuries around the ankle unusual in contrast to the common ligamentous injuries seen in adults. Growth plate injury must be eliminated in any child with pain and swelling about the ankle but no fracture noted on radiographic films. Numerous classifications of pediatric ankle fractures have been described, but the Salter-Harris classification appears to be the simplest, for both treatment and prognosis.

Fractures of the fibula in the immature skeleton usually consist of type I or II injuries. Greenstick fractures above the physis in the metaphyseal area are also relatively common, are easy to reduce with closed reduction, and rarely cause problems with growth arrest. Fractures of the distal fibula or fibular physis are usually associated with fractures of the distal tibia.

Type I injuries of the distal tibial physis are found in younger children and children with myelodysplasia or other conditions with comparable neuropathies. Type I fractures can be minimally displaced and are hard to diagnose radiographically, but they can usually be treated with closed reduction without sequelae. If there is severe displacement with adduction and internal rotation of the distal compo-

nent, a localized type V compression growth plate injury can be noted at follow up. Hence, every attempt should be made to accomplish an anatomic reduction using closed methods.

Type II injuries are the most common fractures of the distal tibial physis. This type of fracture extends along the growth plate and into the metaphyseal bone, and the metaphyseal fragment may be either posterior, medial, or lateral, depending on the deforming mechanism. Accompanying fibular fractures are common and usually involve the metaphysis. The site where the fracture propagates from the physis to the metaphysis is a critical area that can result in localized physeal damage and growth plate arrest. Type II injuries can also be managed with closed reduction. However, occasionally, the periosteum can be folded into the fracture gap, preventing anatomic reduction. If reduction cannot be obtained by closed means, open reduction is required, after which fixation with smooth K-wires or cancellous screws while attempting not to cross the growth plate is accomplished. The key to avoiding premature growth arrest is an anatomic reduction by either closed or open methods.[34]

Fractures of the medial malleolus in the pediatric patient may be either type III or IV (Fig. 29–28). This injury is potentially serious because it involves disruption of the articular surface as well as the growth plate, and the type III injuries may be more difficult to diagnose in the young child before complete ossification of the medial malleolus occurs. Both type III and type IV fractures require anatomic reduction to have the best chance to avoid premature growth arrest. Following closed or open reduction, smooth K-wires or screws may be used to hold the reduction in place, trying to avoid the growth plate with fixation measures. If crossing the growth plate is necessary, temporary smooth K-wires are the instruments of choice. Type III and IV injuries of the distal tibia carry a high risk of premature growth arrest.[34] It appears that no more than 2 mm of displacement can be accepted in these injuries.[65]

A rare complex fracture of the distal tibia that occurs in the immature skeleton is the triplane fracture. The fracture line crosses the articular surface, physis, and metaphysis and results in a type IV growth plate injury that may look like a type III injury on the anteroposterior plane and a type II injury on the lateral plane radiographs. The triplane fracture can occur as a two-, three-, and four-part fracture, and often, tomography or limited computed tomographic scan is necessary to delineate the exact type of injury.[66] There may also be an associated fracture of the fibula. The three-part fracture is the most common variety seen (Fig. 29–29).[22] The peak incidence of this injury usually occurs in the 13- to 15-year-old age group in boys and the 12- to 14-year old age group in girls.

The triplane fracture carries a high risk of premature growth arrest.[66] When there is accompanying displacement, exact delineation of the fracture fragments should be done by tomography or computed tomographic scan, and open reduction and internal fixation is often necessary to obtain the best long-term results. Because this fracture does occur late in adolescents, it is more important to align the articular cartilage than the physis itself. Closed reduction can be attempted, but if less than 2 mm of displacement cannot be

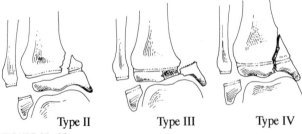

Type II   Type III   Type IV

FIGURE 29–27

Schematic drawing representing three types of distal tibial epiphyseal injuries, all associated with type I injuries of the distal fibula. Type II injuries have propagation of the fracture into the metaphysis, leaving a metaphyseal fragment attached to the epiphysis. Type III injuries fracture across the physis and down into the epiphysis, disrupting the articular cartilage. The type IV injury is a vertical shear fracture crossing the metaphysis, physis, and epiphysis.

is pulled off by the anterior tibiofibular ligament. Markedly displaced fractures can cause a severe step-off in the articular cartilage. Minimally displaced fractures can be treated with cast immobilization. Anatomic reduction must be obtained to restore joint congruity (Fig. 29–31A, B, and C). If this cannot be done by closed methods, open reduction and internal fixation are indicated.[33]

Foot

The child's foot is flexible and resilient, and fractures of the foot are relatively uncommon. If fractures of the foot do occur, most are nondisplaced and require little more than cast immobilization. Most significant foot fractures result from severe direct trauma, such as that sustained in a fall or crush injury. At times, severe soft tissue injury is more significant than the fractures themselves, such as with lawn mower or crush injuries; potential neurologic and circulatory complications must be looked for during the first few days after such trauma. The same forces that can cause injuries in the foot are often transmitted more proximally to the tibia and fibula, which should be carefully evaluated for concurrent injuries.

Although fractures of the talus are uncommon in the child, the most common of these is a vertical fracture through the neck. The mechanism of injury appears to be forced dorsiflexion of the foot and ankle. Major fractures produce obvious pain and swelling at the site of injury, but nondisplaced fractures may be elusive and may be overlooked in light of more significant injuries proximally in the same limb. Standard anteroposterior, lateral, and oblique radiographs usually demonstrate the injury.

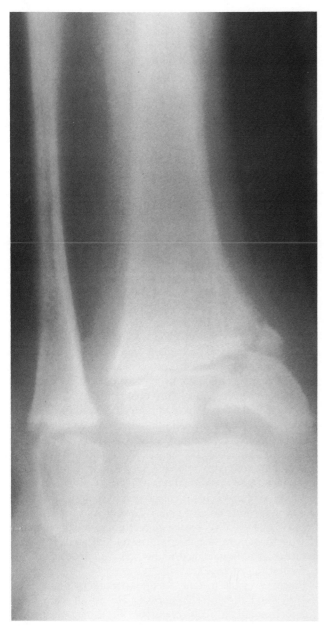

FIGURE 29–28

Anteroposterior radiograph of the ankle of a 6-year-old girl who sustained multiple fractures in a motor vehicle accident. This is a Salter-Harris type IV injury with the fracture crossing from the metaphysis across the physis into the epiphysis. Note the stepoff in both the articular cartilage and the physis. This injury required open reduction and internal fixation.

obtained, open reduction and internal fixation is indicated.[22] The associated fibular fracture may occasionally require internal fixation.

Another injury that occurs in the adolescent is the juvenile "Tillaux-type" fracture (Fig. 29–30). The middle and medial one thirds of the distal tibial epiphyseal growth plate close before the lateral portion, which may stay open for approximately 18 months before complete closure. This time period is when the Tillaux fracture occurs, a type III injury in which the anterior lateral portion of the epiphysis

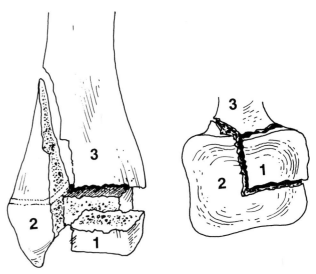

FIGURE 29–29

Schematic representation of a three-part triplane fracture of the distal tibia. This represents a view from the anterior aspect of the ankle and a view looking up on the inferior surface of the distal tibia. Fracture fragment I represents the anterolateral portion of the distal tibial epiphysis. Fragment II represents the remainder of the epiphysis, including the medial malleolus, and the posterolateral spike of metaphysis. Fragment III represents the remainder of the distal tibial metaphysis.

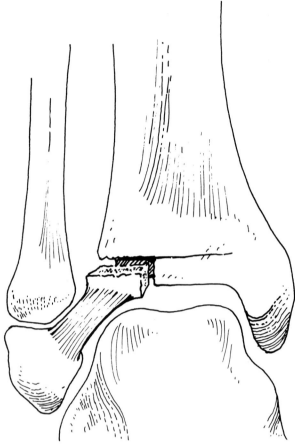

FIGURE 29–30

Drawing of a juvenile Tillaux fracture. This is a Salter-Harris type III injury, which includes avulsion of the anterolateral aspect of the epiphysis by traction through the anterior tibiofibular ligament.

Treatment of nondisplaced fractures initially consists of simple immobilization in a non–weight-bearing cast, which can be converted to a weight-bearing cast when healing begins. Patients with displaced fractures should be taken immediately to the operating room for reduction, and if closed methods produce a stable anatomic reduction, cast immobilization completes the management. If the injury is unstable, percutaneous pin fixation may become necessary, and if closed reduction cannot be obtained, open reduction and K-wire fixation are indicated.[23]

The most significant complication from talus fractures is avascular necrosis of the body of the talus. The blood supply to the body of the talus can be disrupted even in minimally displaced fractures, and occasionally, this injury can go unrecognized until necrosis develops.[37] The most important preventive measure is immediate reduction of displaced fractures with internal fixation if the reduction is unstable.

Fractures of the calcaneus in the skeletally immature patient are unusual and are often less displaced than similar fractures in adults. As with adult fractures, the most common mechanism of injury is vertical compression from a fall. Children have a high incidence of such direct trauma. A 5.4% incidence of associated spine fractures, about one half of that found in adults, can occur and requires attention.[61] Lower-extremity fractures were twice as frequent in children with calcaneus fractures as in adults. Children younger than 7 years of age have a very high incidence of extra-articular fractures, whereas children older than 15 years of age tend to have fractures that extend into the posterior facet. Because many fractures are nondisplaced or extra-articular, they may initially go unrecognized.

Imaging of calcaneus fractures traditionally involves anteroposterior, lateral, and axial views. In older children or those with markedly displaced fractures, a computed tomographic scan may better delineate the type of fracture and the articular involvement.

Os calcis fractures in the younger age group are usually benign and require only conservative treatment, such as below-knee cast immobilization.[76] Nondisplaced intra-articular fractures in the same group can also be treated with non–weight-bearing cast immobilization. Treatment of markedly displaced fractures in younger children and fractures in children older than 15 years of age should be managed the same as for an adult: with possible open reduction and internal fixation.[23]

Injuries to the tarsal metatarsal joint (i.e., Lisfranc joint) can occur in children, particularly in adolescents, in patterns similar to those in adults. The mechanism of injury is an acute plantar flexion force to the forefoot with a rotational component. This type of injury commonly occurs during a fall in which the foot strikes the ground in a tiptoe position, or during a backward fall with the foot pinned to the ground. In displaced injuries, there is often marked soft tissue swelling and ecchymosis. Anteroposterior, lateral, and oblique radiographs of the foot usually can delineate this injury. Associated fractures of the first or second metatarsal base can occur. Management usually consists of closed reduction and cast immobilization, but for displaced fracture dislocations, closed reduction with supplemental K-wire fixation in unstable injuries is indicated.[23, 75] Open reduction is only indicated in the rare case in which closed reduction cannot be achieved.

Fractures of the metatarsals are a relatively common injury in children. These injuries usually result from direct trauma from a falling object or from an indirect mechanism such as those described for tarsal metatarsal injuries. In the severely injured foot, there may be marked soft tissue swelling and ecchymosis accompanying metatarsal fractures. Standard films are generally adequate for diagnosis, and management of the nondisplaced fracture is by cast immobilization. Occasionally, reduction is necessary in displaced fractures. This reduction may require general anesthesia, traction on the toes, and in unstable fractures, percutaneous pinning of the first or fifth metatarsal. Open reduction is rarely necessary but may be indicated for multiple displaced fractures.

Compartment syndromes of the foot, which have received much attention in the adult, can also occur in children with severe injuries to the hindfoot or midfoot. Common injuries associated with compartment syndromes include multiple metatarsal fractures, Lisfranc injuries, and calcaneus fractures. Clinical signs include marked swelling of the foot with the skin tightly stretched. There is often venous congestion of the toes and marked pain in the foot,

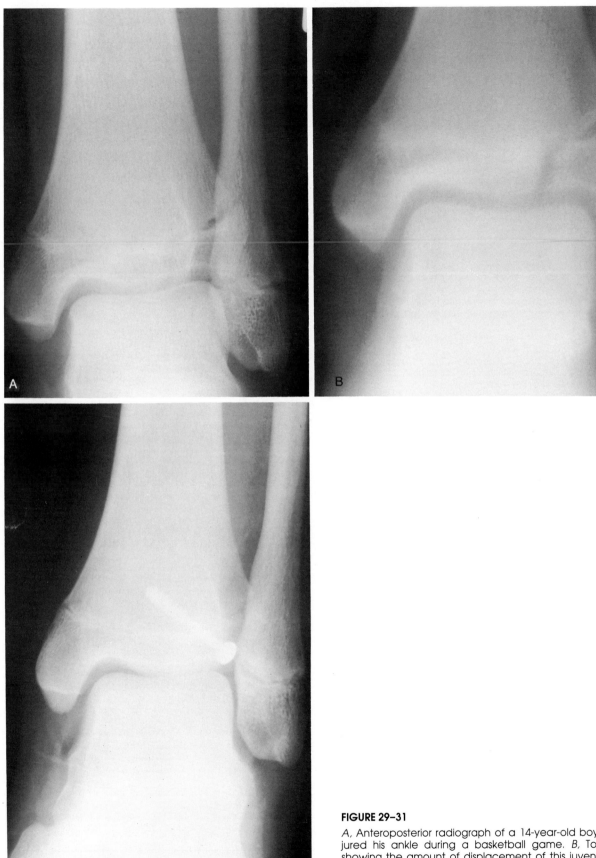

FIGURE 29–31

A, Anteroposterior radiograph of a 14-year-old boy who injured his ankle during a basketball game. B, Tomogram showing the amount of displacement of this juvenile Tillaux fracture. C, Postoperative radiograph showing successful treatment with open reduction and screw fixation.

which is frequently overlooked in the multiply injured patient. Pressure measurements can be made in the different muscle compartments of the foot, and if indicated, fasciotomies can be done through either a dorsal or a medial and lateral approach.

References

1. Alonso JE, Horowitz M: Use of the AO/ASIF external fixator in children. J Pediatr Orthop 7:594–600, 1987.
2. Aronson DD, Singer RM, Higgins RF: Skeletal traction for fractures of the femoral shaft in children: A long-term study. J Bone Joint Surg [Am] 69:1435–1439, 1987.
3. Aronson J, Tursky E: External fixation of femur fractures in children. J Pediatr Orthop 12:157–163, 1992.
4. Badelon O, Bensahel H, Maxda K, et al: Lateral humeral condylar fractures in children: A report of 47 cases. J Pediatr Orthop 8:31–34, 1988.
5. Balthazar DA, Pappas AM: Acquired valgus deformity of the tibia in children. J Pediatr Orthop 4:538–541, 1984.
6. Barquet A: Traumatic hip dislocation in childhood: A report of 26 cases and a review of the literature. Acta Orthop Scand 50:549–553, 1979.
7. Baster MP, Wiley JJ: Fractures of the tibial spine in children. J Bone Joint Surg [Br] 70:228–230, 1988.
8. Behrens F: Knee and leg: Bone trauma. In: Orthopaedic Knowledge Update 3: Home Study Syllabus. Park Ridge, Ill, American Academy of Orthopaedic Surgeons, 1990.
9. Brodeur AE, Silberstein MJ, Graviss ER: Radiology of the pediatric elbow. Boston, GK Hall Medical Publishers, 1981.
10. Buckley SL, Smith G, Sponseller PD, et al: Open fractures of the tibia in children. J Bone Joint Surg [Am] 72:1462–1469, 1990.
11. Burkhart SS, Peterson HA: Fractures of the proximal tibial epiphysis. J Bone Joint Surg [Am] 61:996–1002, 1979.
12. Canale ST, Bourland WL: Fracture of the neck and intertrochanteric region of the femur in children. J Bone Joint Surg [Am] 59:431–443, 1977.
13. Canale ST, King RE: Pelvic and hip fractures. In: Rockwood CA, Wilkins KE, King RE (eds): Fractures in Children. Philadelphia, JB Lippincott, 1984, pp 733–843.
14. Chow JA, Vanbeek AL, Meyers DL, et al: Surgical significance of motor fascicular group of the ulnar nerve in the forearm. J Hand Surg [Am] 10:867–872, 1985.
15. Christie MJ, Dvonch VM: Tibial tuberosity avulsion fracture in adolescents. J Pediatr Orthop 1:391–394, 1981.
16. Cult RW, Osterman AL, Davidson RS, et al: Neural injuries associated with supracondylar fractures of the humerus in children. J Bone Joint Surg [Am] 62:1211–1215, 1990.
17. Dameron TB, Rival DB: Fractures involving the proximal humeral epiphyseal plate. J Bone Joint Surg [Am] 51:289–297, 1969.
18. Dameron TB, Rockwood CA: Fractures and dislocations of the shoulder. In: Rockwood CA, Wilkins KE, King RE (eds): Fractures in Children. Philadelphia, JB Lippincott, 1984, pp 624–653.
19. Daruwalla JS: A study of radioulnar movements following fractures of the forearm in children. Clin Orthop 139:114–120, 1979.
20. DeLee JC: Knee and leg: Bone trauma. In: Orthopaedic Knowledge Update 2: Home Study Syllabus. Park Ridge, Ill, American Academy of Orthopaedic Surgeons, 1987.
21. Dias LS: Fractures of the tibia and fibula. In: Rockwood CA, Wilkins KE, King RE (eds): Fractures in Children. Philadelphia, JB Lippincott, 1984, pp 983–1042.
22. Ertl JP, Barrack RL, Alexander AH, et al: Triplane fracture of the distal tibial epiphysis. J Bone Joint Surg [Am] 70:967–976, 1988.
23. Gross RH: Fractures and dislocations of the foot. In: Rockwood CA, Wilkins KE, King RE (eds): Fractures in Children. Philadelphia, JB Lippincott, 1984, pp 1043–1103.
24. Gustilo RB, Anderson JT: Prevention of infection in the treatment of one thousand and twenty-five open fractures of long bones. J Bone Joint Surg [Am] 58:453–458, 1976.
25. Gustilo RB, Merkow RL, Templeman D: The management of open fractures. J Bone Joint Surg [Am] 72:299–304, 1990.
26. Hand WL, Hand CR, Dunn AW: Avulsion fractures of the tibial tubercle. J Bone Joint Surg [Am] 53:1579–1583, 1971.
27. Hansen BA, Greiff J, Bergmann F: Fractures of the tibia in children. Acta Orthop Scand 47:448–453, 1976.
28. Herndon WA, Mahnken RF, Yngve DA, et al: Management of femoral shaft fractures in the adolescent. J Pediatr Orthop 9:29–32, 1989.
29. Hoekstra HJ, Lichtendahl D: Peritrochanteric fractures in children and adolescents. J Pediatr Orthop 3:587–591, 1983.
30. Hovelius L: Anterior dislocation of the shoulder in teenagers and younger adults: Five year prognosis. J Bone Joint Surg [Am] 69:393–399, 1987.
31. Hresko MT, Kasser JR: Physeal arrest about the knee associated with non-physeal fractures in the lower extremity. J Bone Joint Surg [Am] 71:698–703, 1989.
32. Kirschenbaum D, Albert MC, Robertson WW: Complete femur fractures in children: Treatment with external fixation. J Pediatr Orthop 10:588–591, 1990.
33. Kleiger B, Mankin HJ: Fracture of the lateral portion of the distal tibial epiphysis. J Bone Joint Surg [Am] 46:25–32, 1964.
34. Kling TF, Bright RW, Hensinger RN: Distal tibial physeal fractures in children that may require open reduction. J Bone Joint Surg [Am] 66:647–657, 1984.
35. Lascombes P, Prevot J, Ligier JN, et al: Elastic stable intramedullary nailing in forearm shaft fractures in children: 85 cases. J Pediatr Orthop 10:167–171, 1990.
36. Leonard M, Dubravcik P: Management of fractured fingers in the child. Clin Orthop 73:160–168, 1970.
37. Letts RM, Gibeault D: Fractures of the neck of the talus in children. Foot Ankle 1:74–77, 1980.
38. Letts RM, Vincent N, Gouw G: The "floating knee" in children. J Bone Joint Surg [Br] 68:442–446, 1986.
39. Lombardo SJ, Harvey JP: Fractures of the distal femoral epiphyses. J Bone Joint Surg [Am] 59:742–751, 1977.
40. Lundborg G, Dahlin LB, Danielson N, et al: Nerve regeneration across an extended gap: A neurobiological view of nerve repair and the possible involvement of neuronotrophic factors. J Hand Surg [Am] 7:580–587, 1982.
41. Mardam-Bey T, Ger E: Congenital radial head dislocation. J Hand Surg [Am] 4:316–320, 1979.
42. Merzenich MM, Nelson RJ, Striker MP, et al: Somatosensory cortical map changes following digital amputation in adult monkey. J Comp Neurol 224:591–605, 1984.
43. Meyers MH, McKeever FM: Fracture of the intercondylar eminence of the tibia. J Bone Joint Surg [Am] 41:209–220, 1959, and 52:1677–1684, 1970.
44. Millesi H: Indication, technique, and results of nerve grafting. Handchir Mikrochir Plast Chir (Suppl) 2:10–28, 1977.
45. Millesi H, Meissl G, Berger A: The intrafascicular nerve grafting of the median and ulnar nerves. J Bone Joint Surg [Am] 54:727–749, 1972.
46. Morrissy R: Hip fractures in children. Clin Orthop 152:202–210, 1980.
47. Offierski CM: Traumatic dislocation of the hip in children. J Bone Joint Surg [Br] 63:194–197, 1981.
48. Ogden JA: The uniqueness of growing bones. In: Rockwood CA, Wilkins KE, King RE (eds): Fractures in Children. Philadelphia, JB Lippincott, 1984, pp 1–86.
49. Ogden JA, Tross RB, Murphy MJ: Fractures of the tibial tuberosity in adolescents. J Bone Joint Surg [Am] 62:205–215, 1980.
50. Olney BW, Menelaus MB: Monteggia and equivalent lesions in childhood. J Pediatr Orthop 9:219–223, 1989.
51. Ottolenghi CE: Prophylaxis of Volkmann's contracture in supracondylar fractures of the elbow in children. Rev Chir Orthop 57:517–525, 1971.
52. Pearson DE, Mann RJ: Traumatic hip dislocation in children. Clin Orthop 92:189–194, 1973.
53. Phillips TF, Contreras DM: Timing of operative treatment of fractures in patients who have multiple injuries. J Bone Joint Surg [Am] 72:784–788, 1990.
54. Pirone AM, Graham HK, Krahibich JI: Management of displaced extension-type supracondylar fractures of the humerus in children. J Bone Joint Surg [Am] 70:641–650, 1988.

55. Rang R: Children's Fractures. Philadelphia, JB Lippincott, 1983.
56. Ratliff AHC: Traumatic separation of the upper femoral epiphysis in young children. J Bone Joint Surg [Br] 50:757–770, 1968.
57. Reeves RB, Ballard RI, Hughes JL: Internal fixation versus traction and casting of adolescent femoral shaft fractures. J Pediatr Orthop 10:592–595, 1990.
58. Riseborough EJ, Barrett IR, Shapiro F: Growth disturbances following distal femoral physeal fracture-separations. J Bone Joint Surg [Am] 65:885–893, 1983.
59. Roberts JM: Fractures and dislocations of the knee. In: Rockwood CA, Wilkins KE, King RE (eds): Fractures in Children. Philadelphia, JB Lippincott, 1984, pp 891–982.
60. Salter RB, Harris WR: Injuries involving the epiphyseal plate. J Bone Joint Surg [Am] 45:587–622, 1963.
61. Schmidt TL, Weiner DS: Calcaneal fractures in children: An evaluation of the nature of the injury in 56 children. Clin Orthop 171:150–155, 1982.
62. Seddon HJ: Surgical Disorders of the Peripheral Nerves. Baltimore, Williams & Wilkins, 1972.
63. Shannak AO: Tibial fractures in children: Follow-up study. J Pediatr Orthop 8:306–310, 1988.
64. Shelton WR, Canale ST: Fractures of the tibia through the proximal tibial epiphyseal cartilage. J Bone Joint Surg [Am] 61:167–173, 1979.
65. Spiegel PG, Cooperman DR, Laros GS: Epiphyseal fractures of the distal ends of the tibia and fibula: A retrospective study of two hundred and thirty-seven cases in children. J Bone Joint Surg [Am] 60:1046–1050, 1978.
66. Spiegel PG, Mast JW, Cooperman DR, et al: Triplane fractures of the distal tibial epiphysis. Clin Orthop 188:74–89, 1984.
67. Staheli LT: Fractures of the shaft of the femur. In: Rockwood CA, Wilkins KE, King RE (eds): Fractures in Children. Philadelphia, JB Lippincott, 1991, pp 1121–1163.
68. Steinberg EL, Golomb D, Salama R, et al: Radial head and neck fractures in children. J Pediatr Orthop 8:35–40, 1988.
69. Sunderland S: Nerves and Nerve Injuries. Baltimore, Williams & Wilkins, 1968.
70. Urbaniak JR: Microsurgery for Major Limb Reconstruction. St. Louis, Mosby, 1987.
71. Vahvanen V, Westerlund M: Fracture of the carpal scaphoid in children. Acta Orthop Scand 51:909–913, 1980.
72. Verstreken L, Delrong G, Lamoureux J: Shaft forearm fractures in children: Intramedullary nailing with immediate motion: A preliminary report. J Pediatr Orthop 8:450–453, 1988.
73. Vince KG, Miller JE: Cross-union complicating fracture of the forearm. J Bone Joint Surg [Am] 69:654–661, 1987.
74. Wenger DR: Knee and Leg: Pediatric Aspects. In: Orthopaedic Knowledge Update 3: Home Study Syllabus. Park Ridge, Ill, American Academy of Orthopaedic Surgeons, 1990.
75. Wiley JJ: Tarso-metatarsal joint injuries in children. J Pediatr Orthop 3:255–260, 1981.
76. Wiley JJ, Profitt A: Fractures of the os calcis in children. Clin Orthop 188:131–138, 1984.
77. Wilkins KE: Fractures and dislocations of the elbow region. In: Rockwood CA, Wilkins KE, King RE (eds): Fractures in Children. Philadelphia, JB Lippincott, 1991, pp 509–828.
78. Ziv I, Rang M: Treatment of femoral fracture in the child with head injury. J Bone Joint Surg [Br] 65:276–278, 1983.

Unique and Special Considerations

R. Bruce Davey
K. A. Wallis
K. Perkins
M. Tingay

CHAPTER THIRTY

Thermal and Electrical Injuries

431

EPIDEMIOLOGY

Thermal injuries account for a significant proportion of pediatric trauma, both in total incidence and as a contributor to childhood mortality.[112] As with all forms of pediatric trauma, the management of thermal injuries needs a team approach of dedicated personnel, including nursing staff, therapists, social workers, teachers, surgeons, and physicians, all of whom understand the special needs of children. Support and care of the injured child's parents are also necessary, because a significant burn can traumatize the entire family for a long period.

In the Australian context, all pediatric burn units are located in a major children's hospital, with the associated support of all necessary ancillary pediatric services. The Adelaide Children's Hospital, site of the Paediatric Burns Unit in South Australia, serves a population of 1.3 million. There are approximately 130 new patients admitted per year, with an additional 40 to 50 children per year treated as outpatients.[24, 58]

Scalds account for 70% of these injuries.[40, 85] In the 0- to 2-year-old age group, the commonest injury is a scald due to tea or coffee spilled from a cup, mug, or teapot. The average patient is admitted with a burn that involves 10 to 20% of the body surface area (BSA). With the trend toward early excision and grafting of deep dermal burns, up to 50% of severe burns in this age group are the result of immersion in a hot bath, frequently when an older child turns on the hot water tap when the parent is out of the bathroom.

In the 2- to 5-year-old age group, scalds also account for the majority of burns. Most of these injuries also occur in the kitchen or bathroom, but in this age group, many injuries are caused by other kitchen appliances. Flame burns as a result of the child playing with matches or caused by heaters in the living room also account for a significant number of cases in this age group. In the 5- to 15-year-old age group, scalds account for a lesser proportion of burns, although these types of burns are due to the same sources. Flame burns caused by matches or flammable liquids account for 40 to 50% of admissions in this age group; a majority of these occur outdoors.

In the younger age group, there is a slight predominance of boys; however, there is a marked increase in this male preponderance in the older age group. Burns can affect any socioeconomic age group, but they occur in a significantly higher proportion in the lower socioeconomic groups, particularly in the one-parent family.

A review of all large series shows a similar pattern worldwide, with scalds accounting for up to 70% of cases and the kitchen or bathroom being the commonest location, although the commonest source of hot water varies in differing series.[16, 104, 108] House fires account for less than 7% of burns admissions but have an overall higher mortality due to extensive flame burns in this group. Prevention of burns must be aimed at the source of these thermal injuries.

PREVENTION

Prevention of burns depends on a three-pronged approach.

Education

As the commonest burns occur in children younger than 5 years of age, education must be aimed at the parents of young children.[57] This involves teaching an awareness of the incidence of burns, particularly in the kitchen, and the dangers of the common cup of tea or coffee to the 0- to 2-year-old age group. Education of the older child is important in relation to matches and the dangers of flammable liquids. Teaching by example is important.

Design

The design of kitchens, including kitchen appliances, electrical cords, placement of power outlets, and tap fittings, is particularly important in preventing pediatric burns. Using mugs rather than cups and avoiding the use of tablecloths are part of design as well as education in prevention in the 0- to 2-year-old age group.

Legislation

Legislation and education regarding the flammability of clothing, especially nightclothes, have reduced the incidence and severity of the nightdress flame burn. Design of such nightclothes may be of equal importance to the material used. Legislation regarding the maximum temperature of tap water, use of guards on kitchen stoves, and use of guards on heaters are other examples in which the law may be of value in burn prevention.

FIRST AID

The most obvious first step is to remove the source of thermal injury. This is an obvious step in flame burns, but it must be exercised with care in electrical burns. With scalds, it is important to emphasize the need to remove all clothing, especially thick clothing, as this may absorb hot liquids and be a continuing source of heat.[39] When charred clothes adhere to burned areas, it is better to cut them away if possible rather than to further traumatize the area.

Cold water has long been recommended in the first aid management of burns.[26] Water can be applied locally or by short immersion in a shower or bath. However, the duration of cold water therapy should be restricted to 20 minutes, as recommended by the British Burn Association.[63] This is particularly important in the very young child to prevent the risk of hypothermia. The burned area should then be wrapped in a clean towel or sheet and medical attention sought as soon as possible. If this involves transport to a major burn unit, resuscitation must be commenced before transport if the burn is greater than 10 to 15% of the BSA.

PATHOPHYSIOLOGY

A thermal injury is similar to other forms of pediatric trauma in that it causes damage to tissues with a resultant inflammatory reaction with both local and systemic effects. The severity of the injury depends on the depth of the burn and the surface area involved.

Local Effects

Skin is a specialized tissue that is essential to maintain the internal milieu of the entire body. The skin has an extensive circulation that responds to the external environment as a means of temperature regulation, either by direct heat loss or retention or by fluid loss through sweating. This circulation is also necessary for the high cellular metabolism of the epidermis. Skin is also an essential barrier to bacterial invasion.

Skin is composed of two specialized layers: the epidermis and the dermis. The dermis is composed of two layers: the superficial layer, or stratum corneum, and the germinal layer. The stratum corneum, far from being a layer of dead tissue, is a highly specialized layer consisting of multiple strata of differentiated cells that provide a relatively impermeable layer. Kligman states

the impermeability of the skin largely resides in the stratum corneum. The horny layer is a tough resilient membrane resembling to a surprising degree a sheet of semi-permeable plastic, 'a miracle wrap.' If the function and structure of the stratum corneum is understood, we begin to see the living epidermis in better perspective. Its objective is to die usefully so that its horny shroud forms a renewable wrapping around the body.[60]

The stratum corneum varies in thickness in different areas of the body, with specialization of the horny cells within these areas. The cells of the stratum corneum consist of a tough cell membrane containing a compact fibrous protein, giving a high tensile strength, whereas the layering of the cells creates a graduated permeability. The importance of the stratum corneum, or horny layer, has not been adequately appreciated. With the use of contact media as described later (see Scar Management), it is thought the integrity of the stratum corneum or its substitute is important in the prevention and control of hypertrophy in relation to thermal injuries.[25, 84]

The deep layer of the epidermis is the germinal layer, which provides cells to replace the horny layer. The germinal layer is essential for the regeneration of skin after any form of local trauma, whether thermal, surgical, or of another cause. The melanocytes also reside in the germinal layer. Destruction of the melanocytes results in a loss of pigmentation for a variable period after a burn.

A partial thickness burn causes destruction down to and including the superficial layers of the germinal layer. There is an inflammatory response with capillary hyperemia and mild edema and loss of the horny layer (e.g., sunburn). Regeneration of the epidermis, including the horny layer, results from proliferation of residual cells in the germinal layers. The rapidity of healing depends on the depth of damage to this layer, but healing usually takes place within 7 to 10 days, although the horny covering takes 3 to 4 weeks to mature.

The deep layer of skin is the dermis, which consists of a matrix of collagen and elastic tissue that contains capillaries, nerve endings, sweat glands, hair follicles, and sebaceous glands. A deep dermal burn involves destruction of the germinal epithelium with an increased inflammatory response, with greater edema involving the underlying tissues as well.

Epithelialization can still occur as a result of outgrowth of cells from sweat glands and hair follicles and ingrowth from surrounding epithelium. However, this healing by secondary intention is a delayed process of 2 to 3 weeks with considerable reaction in the deeper dermis, resulting in greater residual scarring and later hypertrophy.

With full thickness burns, there is loss of both epidermis and dermis with a marked inflammatory response. This produces edema of the underlying tissues, but in extensive burns, there is an associated generalized edema. This generalized edema produces significant fluid loss in burns that cover greater than 10% of the BSA in children, with resultant circulatory embarrassment. Owing to capillary damage, there is also a direct loss of circulating red blood cells proportionate to the amount of surface area involved.

Destruction of nerve endings results in an anesthetized wound, and destruction of hair follicles results in lack of hair growth. The latter may be of particular importance in areas such as the scalp and eyebrows.

Healing of a full thickness burn can occur by secondary intention as a result of ingrowth of peripheral epidermal cells. Depending on the size of the area, this can be a very slow process, with marked residual scarring and contracture as a result of changes in the dermal collagen and subcutaneous tissues. Current practice is to preempt these problems by performing early excision and grafting to achieve early healing.

Systemic Effects

In burns that cover more than 10% of the BSA, the inflammatory response locally associated with surface fluid loss is sufficient in children to cause hemodynamic changes. As expected, the greater the injury, the greater the effect associated with a generalized increase in capillary permeability.[2] This results in an increased fluid and protein shift from the vascular to the interstitial space, a decrease in the plasma oncotic pressure, and additional fluid loss.[3, 43] This results in local and generalized edema and increasing hemodynamic changes.[94, 113] Cardiac output is reduced with severe pulmonary edema, compounding the hemodynamic problems. In general terms, all children that have burns that cover more than 10% of the BSA need intravenous resuscitation. An uncommon side effect of thermal injuries is the development of hypertension, which may occur after resuscitation.[18, 28, 87]

Respiratory complications of burns may occur as a result of the onset of pulmonary edema. However, direct injury to the respiratory system can occur as a result of inhalation of smoke (e.g., in house or car fires), with typical thermal injury to the respiratory epithelium, further increasing morbidity and mortality. Respiratory injury can also occur as the result of inhalation of toxic fumes. This risk is becoming greater as a result of the use of plastics in house furniture and car seating.

Renal problems in thermal injuries can be twofold. Peripheral circulatory failure can lead to typical renal effects of shock, such as tubular necrosis. A second effect in deep burns is the release of hemoglobin, leading to a direct tubular effect.

Gastrointestinal effects consist primarily of ileus due to peripheral circulatory collapse. This complication usually resolves in 48 to 72 hours but prohibits oral intake in the early stages in patients with burns that cover more than 20% of the BSA. A second risk is the development of a Curling ulcer, with the added risk of perforation or hemorrhage.[77, 88]

Endocrine disturbances also occur, the most notable being a tendency toward hyperglycemia with a marked resistance to insulin therapy.

Metabolism is also disturbed. Thermal injuries produce a marked catabolic effect, with the basal metabolic rate increasing by up to 50%. This increase is compounded by the demands of the healing tissues and complicated by gastrointestinal disturbances and endocrine changes. Profound psychological problems can also occur both in the child and in the parents.[1]

The management of a burned child is the management not only of the local injury but also of the total patient with the support of surgeons, physicians, and nursing staff. All subspecialties are needed to overcome the associated problems.

ASSESSMENT OF INJURY

The assessment of the severity of a thermal injury is based on a number of factors.

Cause

A knowledge of the causative agent assists in determining the depth of the burn. A flame burn tends to be full thickness, whereas an electrical burn, in addition to being full thickness, may also involve deeper tissues, including tendon, bone, and possibly internal viscera. Scald injuries vary in degree depending on the temperature of the agent and the contact time, and the depth of injury is frequently patchy, making local therapy more difficult.

While taking the history, it is important to be alert to the possibility of nonaccidental injury.[61, 80] Thermal injuries are a common cause of child abuse and must be considered in patients in whom the depth or distribution of injury is unusual or does not match the history.

Depth

Assessment of the depth of injury is based on clinical judgment at the initial examination. The most superficial burn is represented by erythema alone, such as that commonly seen in sunburn. The presence of blisters represents a partial thickness dermal burn, although it may be superficial or deep dermal. This type of burn is the most difficult to assess

early regarding the likelihood of grafting being necessary. A guarded prognosis is advised.

A full thickness burn does not normally blister but is white or charred depending on the agent. Thrombosed vessels may be visible, and the area is anesthetic as a result of destruction of the nerve endings.

Site and Distribution

The site of the burn (e.g., perineal, facial) may determine the need for hospitalization because of the nursing involved. Hand burns also frequently require experienced care because of the risk of loss of function. The distribution of the burn affects the choice of local therapy.

Age and Weight

The age of the patient frequently determines the type of thermal injury, as noted previously. The weight or approximate weight of the patient is necessary to determine the fluid resuscitation requirement.

Associated Injuries or Preexisting Illness

Associated injuries such as smoke inhalation or electrical injuries affects management, as does other preexisting disease (e.g., cardiac, pulmonary, neurologic).

Extent of Body Surface Area

The extent of BSA involved is most important in determining resuscitation and prognosis. There are various charts available to assess the BSA, such as the Lund and Browder system or the rule of nines, but Breckov's Chart (Fig. 30–1) is currently used at the Adelaide Children's Hospital.[69]

It is important to remember that the estimation of BSA injured is only an estimation, usually rounded to the nearest 5% for ease of calculation. A useful exercise is to calculate the nonburned area to check calculation of the BSA.

MANAGEMENT OF MINOR BURNS

Patients who are not immediately hospitalized are classed as having minor burns, usually covering less than 7% of their BSA, that are capable of being adequately dressed. However, a burn that is not well on the way to healing by 10 days after the injury should be considered for grafting.

The objective of treatment of minor burns is to relieve pain, prevent infection, and facilitate healing. Many methods and materials are available, and new materials are promoted regularly. A flexible approach is recommended depending on the site and depth of the burn and the patient's social circumstances.

With all techniques, the burned area must be washed

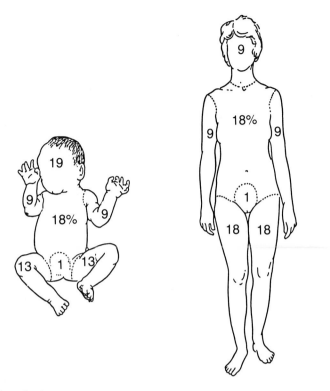

AREA

1. Breckov charts

	Age 1 year	Age 10 + years
Head and neck	19	9
Front of trunk	18	18
Back of trunk	18	18
Each arm	9	9
Each leg	13	18
Genitalia/perineum	1	1

For each year of age over 1, deduct one from the head and add ½ to each leg.

2. For smaller areas, the child's own open hand covers approximately 1% of the surface area.

FIGURE 30-1

Breckov chart. (Courtesy of Adelaide Children's Hospital.)

gently with a warmed aqueous antiseptic solution, and loose skin must be removed. Blisters may be removed, depending on their site and size, the area gently dried, and a suitable dressing applied.

Vaseline Gauze

The time-honored treatment of tulle gras, which is a gauze and crepe bandage, is still a satisfactory method for most burns. It is important to obtain a complete seal of the entire area involved and not to use too bulky a dressing to allow evaporation of exudate through the bandage. The dressing should *not* be changed frequently unless there is evidence of infection (e.g., pain, fever, malodorous discharge, surrounding cellulitis).

Silver Sulfadiazine and Telfa

Silver sulfadiazine (SSD) cream with a nonadherent dressing such as Telfa (Kendall Co., Mansfield, Mass.) may be used as a closed dressing. It also should be left alone for 5 to 7 days unless otherwise indicated.

Opsite

Opsite (Smith & Nephew, Largo, Fla.), an adherent polyurethane semipermeable plastic, is an excellent method of local treatment in selected cases. It produces rapid pain relief, is simple to use, is well tolerated by the patient, and allows for easy inspection of the burn. However, a prerequisite of Opsite therapy is a satisfactory margin surrounding the burn for adhesion of the material. Therefore, Opsite is mainly used on flat areas such as the trunk or limbs. Application of a crepe bandage for 24 to 48 hours is recommended to minimize fluid collection. The burn is inspected every 3 to 4 days, and the Opsite dressing is left in place until complete wound healing has occurred.

Hypafix

A superficial partial thickness burn may be treated well with Hypafix (Smith & Nephew, Largo, Fla.). The burn initially should be treated with tulle gras until exudation ceases; the wound can then be sealed with Hypafix applied directly to the area as an adherent dressing and left for an additional week before inspection. The use of peanut oil 1 hour before inspection facilitates the removal of Hypafix without damaging the healing epithelium. Hypafix can then be reapplied as part of the scar management program. Generally, the less often the dressing is changed, the better. This practice facilitates healing and reduces the risk of infection and the causing of pain to the patient.

RESUSCITATION OF PATIENTS WITH BURNS OF MORE THAN TEN PERCENT OF THEIR BODY SURFACE AREA

Resuscitation involves total management of the patient, with the mobilization of all necessary disciplines in a team approach. The initial resuscitation period is considered to be the first 48 to 72 hours after burn injury.

Airway

An adequate airway is obviously the first essential in management. The history of the injury may suggest inhalation of smoke or noxious fumes or a respiratory tract burn requiring immediate nasotracheal intubation. Physical signs of airway injury include facial burns, singed nasal hairs, burned lips, excessive mucus, or abnormal respiration.

Nasogastric Suction

Extensive burns are associated with a small bowel ileus for the first 24 to 72 hours after the injury; this requires restriction of oral intake. A nasogastric tube should be inserted and antacids given during this period to reduce acidity. The nasogastric tube may be left in situ to allow for gavage feeding of high-calorie, high-protein fluid to supplement oral feeding during the recovery phase. In less severe cases, oral fluids may be given as tolerated.

Indwelling Urinary Catheter

An accurate hourly measurement of urinary output is essential during the fluid resuscitation phase of burn management. All patients who are burned on more than 20% of their BSA should have an indwelling catheter, preferably of the Silastic Foley type.

In patients who have deep burns involving the genital or perineal area, where drainage may be prolonged, a suprapubic catheter should be considered. The minimum expected urine output in a pediatric burn patient is 0.5 to 1.0 ml per kg per hour.

Laboratory Investigation

Hemoglobin estimation, hematocrit, complete blood count, serum electrolytes, and blood glucose determinations are needed as soon as possible after the injury to determine baseline values and at frequent intervals during the resuscitation period. The hemoglobin and complete blood count must be monitored at regular intervals until the patient is discharged from the hospital.

Antibiotics

Tetanus prophylaxis is indicated as necessary in all cases. Aside from fluid loss, the main threat to survival in patients with major burn trauma is the problem of burn wound sepsis. The main organisms involved are *Pseudomonas aeruginosa* and *Staphylococcus aureus*. Streptococcal infection is less of a problem in current practice; therefore, prophylactic use of antibiotics is considered inadvisable.

Bacteriologic swabs should be taken at the time of admission from the burn wound, nose, and throat and should be repeated weekly and before grafting. Swabs should also be repeated if clinically indicated and appropriate antibiotics given intravenously if sepsis is suspected or proved. Early excision of burn eschar with early skin cover reduces the risk of burn wound sepsis, as is discussed later.

Fluid Resuscitation

All fluid resuscitation regimens commence from the time of injury rather than the time of admission to the hospital. This is most important early in the course of treatment, because the greatest fluid loss occurs in the first 8 hours after the injury. Fluid loss decreases by half in the next 16 hours, to one fourth in the next 24 hours. Because of a generalized increase in capillary permeability, there is a loss of sodium and colloid into the interstitial space with a reduction in plasma oncotic pressure. This leads to a significant loss of fluid into the interstitial space, especially in the first 24 hours, with resultant generalized edema. There is also a breakdown of the sodium pump, which leads to a leakage of sodium into the intracellular space and leakage of potassium into the extracellular space. As the patient recovers from the initial shock, there is a return of colloid and sodium to the plasma, followed by diuresis in the 48- to 72-hour period after the injury. These changes are well summarized by Rogenes and Moylan.[96] Fluid replacement is based on the total affected BSA and the actual or estimated weight in kilograms. These estimations must always be regarded as guidelines rather than absolutes and may be modified depending on the patient's progress and results of close monitoring of all parameters. These parameters include pulse, blood pressure, respiration, urinary output, and peripheral circulation in all cases and central venous pressure, temperature, and blood gases in some patients.

At the Adelaide Children's Hospital, the current formula for replacement of fluid, given as serum plasma protein solution, is based on the Muir Barclay formula.[78]

$$\text{ml of fluid/period} = \frac{\% \text{ area of burn} \times \text{child's weight in kg}}{2}$$

Maintenance fluids are given as 3% dextrose in one third normal saline at 80 ml per kg per 24 hours, administered evenly over the total period involved. In severe cases, 2.5% dextrose in half normal saline given at 60 ml per kg per 24 hours is recommended (Table 30–1). These calculations should be included in the case notes, with detailed nursing instructions written out as in Table 30–2.

Other Resuscitation Formulas

There is debate as to the relative merits of the use of colloid solutions in resuscitation.[44, 45, 71, 89] Because of the increased capillary permeability in burned areas, colloid is lost from the vascular compartment into the interstitial space, increas-

Table 30–1
Burns Resuscitation Chart

This Chart Is to Be Used as a Guideline and May Need to Be Varied in Severe Cases or Where Resuscitation is Delayed.

NAME: AGE: WEIGHT:

I. **Muir Barclay Formula for Replacement of Fluid**

$$\text{ml of fluid per period} = \frac{\% \text{ BSA} \times \text{child's weight in kg}}{2}$$

Period 1   0–4 hr from the time of burning
Period 2   4–8 hr from the time of burning
Period 3   8–12 hr from the time of burning
Period 4   12–18 hr from the time of burning
Period 5   18–24 hr from the time of burning
Period 6   24–36 hr from the time of burning

Replacement fluid is given as serum plasma protein solution.

In deep burns of 25% BSA, give one third of the total plasma as whole blood during the second 24-hr period and earlier at the consultant's discretion in patients with very large burns.

A seventh period of 12 hr is used if the patient's clinical state indicates that additional resuscitation is necessary.

II. **Maintenance Fluids**

To be given as 3% dextrose in one-third normal saline IV at 80 ml/kg/24 hr

Calculations

A. Weight in kg   = _____
    % BSA   = _____
    Replacement fluid per period   = _____

B. Maintenance fluid per 24 hr   = _____
    Maintenance fluid per 4 hr period   = _____

    Maintenance fluid per 6 hr period   = _____
    Maintenance fluid per 12 hr period   = _____

III. Expected minimum
      urine output = 0.5 ml/kg/hr in patients younger than 1
                      year of age
                    = 1.0 ml/kg/hr in patients older than 1 year
                      of age

Table 30–2
Nursing Instruction Sheet

Serum plasma protein solution (SPPS) and 3% dextrose in one-third normal saline solution is to be alternated in hourly increments.

First Period (time of burn 4 hr)
SPPS (ml) dextrose in one-third
3% normal saline (ml)
Total (ml)
Rate (ml/hr)

Second Period (4–8 hr)
SPPS (ml) dextrose in one-third
3% normal saline (ml)
Total (ml)
Rate (ml/hr)

Third Period (8–12 hr)
SPPS (ml) dextrose in one-third
3% normal saline (ml)
Total (ml)
Rate (ml/hr)

Fourth Period (12–18 hr)
SPPS (ml) dextrose in one-third
3% normal saline (ml)
Total (ml)
Rate (ml/hr)

Fifth Period (18–24 hr)
SPPS (ml) dextrose in one-third
3% normal saline (ml)
Total (ml)
Rate (ml/hr)

Sixth Period (24–36 hr)
SPPS (ml) dextrose in one-third
3% normal saline (ml)
Total (ml)
Rate (ml/hr)

Plasma and maintenance fluids are to be alternated hourly through each resuscitation period.

Medical Officer's Signature _____

ing the oncotic pressure in this space. The Baxter formula is based on lactated Ringer solution, giving a hypotonic sodium solution with no colloid, whereas the University of Wisconsin formula adds 20 mEq $NaHCO_3$ per liter to restore the solution to isotonic.[4, 5, 96] The availability of colloid solutions is another determining factor. Children seem to tolerate and need colloid more than adults.

However, work by Caldwell and colleagues[17] suggests that hypertonic saline is a more suitable solution for resuscitation in major burns, particularly in cases associated with inhalational injury.[11, 12, 76] Hypertonic lactated saline has the advantage of a high sodium intake with reduced fluid volume and reduces the risk of pulmonary edema. However, the risk of hypernatremia requires very close monitoring of the serum sodium levels.

Blood

Blood is contraindicated in the initial resuscitation period because of the tendency toward hemoconcentration. However, in burns of more than 25% of the patient's BSA, there is an absolute loss of red blood cells in the burned area. Blood is recommended in the recovery phase, in sufficient quantities to return the amount of circulating hemoglobin to normal levels. Blood transfusions are also necessary to replace losses during episodes of débridement and grafting but are preferably given toward the end of the procedures to minimize the total requirements. Blood may also be necessary between such episodes, subject to regular monitoring of hemoglobin levels, especially in the presence of burn wound sepsis.

Pulmonary Edema

Pulmonary edema may occur early in cases of respiratory burns, but it may also occur later as part of the generalized edema. If pulmonary edema occurs, the patient needs nasotracheal intubation with positive-pressure ventilation. Digitalization and diuretics may also be needed; therefore, a team approach using pediatric cardiologists, respiratory physicians, intensivists, and pediatric nephrologists may be necessary in this situation. With current intensive care facilities and the team approach, the prognosis has improved considerably in patients with major burns covering more than 50% of their BSA.

Escharotomy

In circumferential burns, the circulation may be compromised to distal areas, with the potential loss of digits or even more proximal limb structures. This may occur early with full thickness burns or as a delayed effect in deep dermal burns as a result of increasing edema.

The capillary circulation must be constantly monitored, and if in doubt, it is better to do an escharotomy early rather than late. The escharotomy should be down to the fascia, but if no relief is obtained, the fascia should also be divided to give adequate relief.

Escharotomy may also be needed in circumferential burns of the trunk, if respiration becomes compromised, down to and including the deep fascia as necessary.

ANALGESIA AND SEDATION

Immediate analgesia for the burn patient must be given intravenously as the only satisfactory method. It may be given as an initial bolus injection followed by a continuous infusion for the ensuing 48 to 72 hours, depending on the severity of pain. The same technique is also recommended during episodes of surgery.

Regardless of the dressing used, it must be remembered that any change of dressing or associated débridement in a child is a traumatic experience, and sedation is needed. The agent and dosage used for sedation vary depending on the choice of dressing and the unit preference. In some units, all dressings are done with the patient under light anesthesia. This practice disturbs oral feedings but can be overcome by increased nasogastric feedings.

Agents such as ketamine may be used in this context; the use of nitrous oxide (Entonox) without full anesthesia is an alternative in the older child.

Sedation alone may be used if anesthesia is not desired, using chloral hydrate 12 mg per kg in the young child and oral codeine phosphate 1 mg per kg in the older child, given 1 hour prior to dressing. Oral Valium 0.2 mg per kg per dose or acetaminophen (Panadol) may also be used.

Patient-controlled analgesia has become the preferred method of analgesia in cases of extensive burns requiring repeated surgery. The technique may be used in patients 5 years of age or older (i.e., on any child old enough to be taught).

LOCAL THERAPY

The aim of local therapy is to:

1. Prevent infection
2. Facilitate healing
3. Minimize discomfort

The history of burn wound care has been a trial and error progression toward current practice. The main aim of treatment is to reduce or eliminate burn wound sepsis, which has been a major contributor to morbidity and mortality.[86] A wide range of therapies is available, but treatment must be tailored to the individual patient, depending on the patient's age and the site, extent, and depth of the injury. A range of therapies restricted to a reasonable number should be available in each unit for simplicity and ease of nursing management.

The range of materials available for local treatment of burns can be classified as follows:

1. Conventional dressings
2. Topical applications
3. Synthetic dressings
4. Biologic dressings

Conventional Dressings

In less extensive burns, conventional dressings such as a tulle gras gauze and crepe bandage (changed every few days) are recommended, provided a complete seal of the affected area can be achieved. Conventional dressings are a time-honored but satisfactory method that reduces the number of baths and redressings necessary. Conventional dressings are not satisfactory in severe cases because of the lack of control of sepsis.

Topical Applications

These have become popular since the 1960s, when 10% $AgNO_3$ solution was introduced. This agent is effective against *Pseudomonas* organisms, which were the main cause of mortality in severe burns. However, owing to the absorption of $AgNO_3$, which combined with Na^+Cl^1, significant biochemical problems were created.

Sulfamylon cream also was introduced in the 1960s, but as it is painful during application, it is not well suited to pediatric burns. The advent in the late 1960s of SSD, which overcame these problems, has revolutionized the care of major burns.[48] The addition of chlorhexidine has reduced the incidence of bacterial resistance, particularly that of *S. aureus*.[52]

After local cleaning, SSD cream is applied to the affected area, which may then be exposed, covered with degreased tulle gras, or covered with a bandage applied as a closed dressing, depending on the site and extent of injury.

Silver sulfadiazine cream is recommended for extensive burns, for circumferential burns, and in areas in which it is difficult to provide care (e.g., the perineum). However, SSD cream requires daily baths and twice daily applications, and thus the use of more sedation or repeated anesthetics. Silver sulfadiazine cream delays the separation of slough in deep dermal burns; therefore, the use of tangential excision and grafting is recommended for burns that do not heal within 10 days. Due to the difficulty of providing nursing care for facial burns, the use of neomycin ointment as a topical application after daily cleansing is recommended.

Synthetic Dressings

Dressings such as Opsite or Biobrane (Winthrop Pharmaceuticals, Div. of Sterling Drug, Inc., New York, NY) are being used increasingly in pediatric practice. Opsite is a semipermeable adhesive plastic that is particularly useful on the limbs and on small areas, providing a sufficient area of adhesion is available. A technique for the use of Opsite in hand burns has been developed using the Spencer Opsite Applicator, which allows for a sealed dressing without restriction of movement.[105]

A synthetic skin, such as Biobrane, can be used as a primary dressing, for coverage of deep wounds after eschar excision before grafting, for coverage of meshed autografts while awaiting complete healing, and for coverage of extensive skin donor sites.[70, 86]

Biologic Dressings

Biologic dressings include heterograft (i.e., donor or cadaver skin), xenografts (i.e., porcine skin), and amnion, which may be used as a primary dressing or later as a temporary dressing after débridement in extensive burns. Amnion has proved useful in children because it produces immediate pain relief, but it cannot be used across flexures. Amnion is particularly useful on trunk burns, where it can be left in situ for 7 to 10 days, when complete healing will have occurred in partial thickness burns. In deeper burns, amnion can be removed before excision and grafting. Amnion can be used as a true biologic dressing and can be changed daily to cleanse sloughing areas before grafting.

The same techniques can be used with other biologic dressings, such as xenograft or heterograft. The choice of biologic dressing depends on local availability and the physician's experience.

Dressing Techniques in Progress

Cultured Epithelium

Skin culture techniques have moved from the laboratory to the clinical arena. Cultured epithelium should be considered for all extensive burns, to overcome the necessity to re-crop donor sites and thus reduce the time until full skin coverage can be achieved.[31]

Artificial Dermis

Artificial dermis, which consists of a bovine collagen matrix, is also moving out of the laboratory and into the clinical arena. The ultimate marriage of these techniques is at the forefront of management of the major burn.[91, 92]

SPECIAL ANESTHETIC PROBLEMS

The burned child presents a number of problems and challenges to the anesthetist. There may be limited access for intravenous cannulae, and central venous access is frequently required. Burns to the face may interfere with airway management and may indicate thermal damage to the respiratory tract. There is a large rise in extracellular potassium concentration with the use of depolarizing muscle relaxants (e.g., suxamethonium), and the reduction in sympathetic tone that accompanies induction of general anesthesia may produce severe hypotension. Some children must undergo many operations, often several times in 1 week. There is also the problem of face and neck scarring, which may produce airway and intubation difficulties in later stages.

All children who require general anesthesia within 24 hours of a burn should be assumed to have full stomachs and must be intubated. A rapid-sequence intravenous induction is the technique of choice in this situation.

Suxamethonium may be used in the first 24 hours after severe burns, but within a few days, changes in postjunctional physiology contraindicate the use of this drug because of the resultant rise in serum potassium and consequent cardiac arrhythmias.[67] The nondepolarizing muscle relaxants atracurium (0.5 mg per kg) and vecuronium (0.08 mg per kg) have a rapid onset of action enabling children to be intubated in under 2 minutes, an intermediate range of duration, and are easily reversed. These drugs are preferable to D-tubocurarine and pancuronium when anesthesia must last less than 45 minutes. Hypotension is treated by volume replacement, and colloidal solutions are more effective in this situation.

A nasal endotracheal tube is indicated if thermal damage to the upper airway is seen or damage to the lower airway is suspected. The child is not extubated in these cases. Alternatively, a tracheostomy may be performed, especially in patients with facial and severe upper airway damage.

Contraction of neck scars may render laryngoscopy with a rigid laryngoscope impossible. It may be necessary to use a spontaneous breathing technique while a relaxing incision is performed. Blind nasal intubation is an alternative. The use of the flexible fiberoptic bronchoscope is recommended in the older child, and an ultrathin, flexible fiberscope (Olympus PF 27M [Olympus America, Lake Success, NY]) is available and has been used in children as young as 18 months of age.[59]

Hypothermia is a problem when large areas of burn are involved, and its prevention necessitates the heating and humidification of inspired gases, the use of warming blankets, the warming of administered fluids, and raising the temperature of the environment. A room temperature of 26°C to 27°C is a compromise between patient need and staff comfort.

There are a variety of anesthetic methods used for recurrent débridement and skin grafting. Intravenous neurolept analgesia avoids the possible complications associated with repeated intubations. A combination of barbiturate, narcotic, and benzodiazepine, possibly with ketamine and nitrous oxide, is used. Recovery of consciousness may be slow, and side effects such as dreaming and nightmares are common. Neurolept analgesia requires the presence of an anesthetist, and in many centers, general anesthesia remains the preferred method.

Continuous intravenous narcotic administration is also an excellent form of analgesia and can be either patient-controlled analgesia (PCA) in school-aged children or continuous intravenous (CI) infusion in children of any age group.[35, 36, 75] Using either technique, these children should be given intravenous morphine boluses to reach a comfort level before commencing PCA or CI.

Advantages of these techniques are the avoidance of painful intramuscular injections and the prevention of wide swings in analgesic blood levels, and when appropriately prescribed and supervised, they are very safe and can be used in the general ward situation. Patient-controlled analgesia has been reported in burned children 4 years of age and older and offers additional benefits over other methods of administration.[37]

The issue of patient control is very important in burn patients. The patient experiences considerable psychological benefit in being able to control his or her own analgesics, and our experience has shown that children are able to do this extremely well. Patient-controlled analgesia allows for the wide variability in morphine requirements between individual patients. It allows the patient to self-administer analgesics before and during painful procedures such as dressing changes, and with longer-term patients, the development of tolerance to narcotics is easier to manage.[34] Widespread experience with PCA has demonstrated that it is one of the safest ways of administering narcotics. Patients with burned arms may not be able to activate the normal hand trigger; in these cases, a foot-operated trigger is required.

If children are too young for PCA or are unable to use the equipment, then a nurse-managed continuous infusion is preferred. The routine prescription is to add 0.5 mg per kg of morphine into a 50-ml syringe and run it in an infusion pump at up to 5 ml per hour (50 µg/kg/hr). Additional bolus doses are required to cover the additional pain of procedures and dressings.

Morphine is the analgesic drug of choice. The long-term use of pethidine has been associated with the accumulation of a toxic metabolite (i.e., norpethidine), which can cause convulsions. Methadone is a satisfactory alternative if intravenous access is not available. However, procedural pain is not well controlled by methadone. Codeine phosphate (1 mg/kg/4 hr) and paracetamol (15–20 mg/kg/4 hr) are suitable for mild pain.

Entonox (50% nitrous oxide in oxygen) via a demand apparatus has been used in some centers for the control of pain from burn dressing changes. It has the advantages of quick onset and quick offset, and in the majority of patients, it provides profound analgesia at subanesthetic concentrations. It is also controlled by the patient, which accounts for its safety (i.e., the patient must be awake to use it effectively). The use of Entonox must be supervised by an appropriately trained staff member, and protocols for its use must be set in place. The most serious complication of nitrous oxide is the development of bone marrow depression with long-term continuous administration. We avoid this complication by limiting the use of Entonox to no more than 1 hour per day. Longer-term patients (i.e., beyond 2 weeks) are given folinic acid, which may help prevent the development of bone marrow depression.

Regional anesthesia (e.g., caudal, femoral, and brachial plexus blocks), usually in association with general anesthesia, may be useful for initial pain relief following surgery on the limbs and lower trunk. The risk of neural damage with repeated injections limits the usefulness of regional anesthesia, and its use is contraindicated when burns are present at the site of injection. Indwelling catheters may be used to prolong the effects of the block but at the risk of sepsis.

SUBSEQUENT SURGICAL MANAGEMENT

Superficial burns should be healed or nearly healed within 10 to 12 days. If healed, they may require only a moisturizing cream for some period as a protective agent. Burns that are well on the way to healing may be bandaged or dressed with Hypafix and reviewed as necessary, depending on the scar potential.

Full thickness burns and deep dermal burns that have not healed within 10 to 12 days need to be tangentially excised and split skin grafted.[54, 106, 107, 111] This can usually be performed in one session, although occasionally it may be necessary to delay application of skin grafts for 24 hours if there is excessive bleeding. The use of topical thrombin or Por 80 (Por-8-Ornipressin, Sandoz Pharmaceuticals, East Hanover, NJ) may overcome this problem, or the graft may be meshed with minimal stretching.[47, 49]

There are a variety of techniques for fixing grafts in position. They may be simply laid on and the child restrained and sedated for flat areas, or they may be fixed with closed dressings.

Fixation of grafts with Hypafix is the preferred technique in almost all situations.[10] The graft is usually applied as unstretched meshed split skin; the tulle gras is removed, and lightly stretched Hypafix is applied to adhere to the surrounding area or circumferentially on the limbs.

Stapling through the Hypafix may be added for difficult areas such as scalp, groin, or buttocks. The short- and long-term cosmetic results are improved, and this technique considerably reduces the need for splinting or sedation.

In the case of extensive burns where there is a shortage of donor sites, repeated serial excision and grafting is needed. In this situation, priority must be given to reducing the total area involved as rapidly as possible, because the risk of burn wound sepsis is directly proportional to the extent of the unhealed area. In this situation, hands and face assume a lower priority to total cover, whereas with less extensive burns, the face and hands would have priority.

Another possibility in patients with extensive burns is to excise the burned areas early and to provide interim cover with artificial materials such as amnion, Biobrane, allografts, or xenografts until sufficient homografts are available for permanent cover.

SPECIFIC SURGICAL PROBLEMS

Hands

Despite the small BSA involved, burns to the hands may result in a marked functional disability. In extensive burn injuries, the residual hand function is often the most important single factor in rehabilitation.

Deformity may occur in the hands simply as a result of the severity of the burn. This is the case in deep electrical burns; however, in general, thermal injuries are surface injuries and frequently, if deformity occurs, it is secondary to complications in the deeper tissues.

Prolonged inflammation and edema lead to shortening of joint ligaments, adhesions around tendons, and fibrosis within other deep tissues, leading to stiffness and consequent reduced hand function.[7]

The use of topical agents such as SSD minimizes inflammation secondary to infection. In addition, a program of elevation of the hand and early mobilization reduces edema. These techniques, combined with intermittent splinting of the hand in the safe position, prevent deformity.

Surgery

Superficial hand burns heal rapidly without any long-term scarring and deformity and simply require elevation and a protective dressing. With deep dermal and full thickness burns, stiffness and deformity can be best prevented by early débridement and split skin grafting. If the patient's general condition allows, this is best performed 3 to 5 days after the injury, and the débridement is performed tangentially. In deeper circumferential burns, an escharotomy may be required in the early phase after the injury.[65, 100]

When débridement and grafting must be delayed, a continuing program of elevation, mobilization, and splinting should be followed. When splinting, particular attention should be paid to the metacarpophalangeal joints, which should be flexed; the proximal interphalangeal joints, which should be extended; and the thumb, which should be abducted.[30, 56, 98]

When deeper structures such as bone are exposed, repair with a local or distant flap may be indicated. When the burn has healed and skin closure is obtained, the splinting pro-

gram should be continued to prevent deformity from graft contracture. Splinting is combined with the use of elasticized gloves, which are employed to control scar hypertrophy, and other aids such as web spacers. Hand exercises and daily use of the hand are encouraged.

Reconstruction

When the scars have matured, the patient may be left with a number of secondary problems. If skin contractures have not responded to conservative measures, it is best to release these surgically and have the resultant defects grafted. Full thickness grafts, usually taken from the groin, have the advantage of being unlikely to contract and are frequently used in this situation.

Contracture in the web spaces causes syndactyly, which if minimal, responds well to a Z-plasty. If contracture is more advanced, it requires a local flap to reconstruct the base of the web, combined with a skin graft.

Deformity and restricted movement in the metacarpophalangeal and interphalangeal joints may be improved by careful surgical release of the involved ligaments.[7] However, it is frequently not possible to restore full function at this stage. Tendon adhesions are an additional factor limiting restoration of active movement.

In neglected cases, a claw hand deformity with joint stiffness and skin contracture is common, and treatment requires attention to both aspects of this problem. A boutonniere deformity of the fingers may occur if the middle slip of the extensor tendon has become attenuated.[66] Release of a thumb that is adducted as a result of deep contracture in the first web space may prove to be difficult and may often require release of the origin of the adductor pollicis from the third metacarpal and a flap closure of the resultant defect.

Face

Thermal injury to the face presents the surgeon with a number of difficult problems. Because this area is not covered by clothing, it is frequently the only visible area of scarring. Its special features, including the nose, mouth, eyelids, eyebrows, and ears, present healing and long-term reconstructive problems.[79]

The projection of the nose and ears make these structures particularly liable to damage from thermal injury. Mobile structures such as the eyelids and mouth are prone to distortion, not only from injury, but secondary to contractures of the surrounding tissues in the healing phase.

Long-term deformity is a product of the depth of the original burn, loss of tissue (especially in relation to special features), contractures of residual scars, and the degree of scar hypertrophy.

Surgery

Although little can be done in regard to the depth of the burn, contracture and scar hypertrophy can be minimized by preventing delays in healing. If the injury has not healed within 2 weeks, surgical wound closure should be considered. Obvious deep burns should be excised and closed earlier in the course of treatment.

After excision of the burned tissue, repair can be effected by direct closure, the use of local flaps, or the use of a split skin graft, depending on the site and size of the burn. Direct closure and flaps provide the best quality skin; split skin grafts contract and result in a flattening of the facial contour, usually accompanied by some texture and color change. Careful selection of the donor site helps achieve the best color match; the scalp and postauricular skin offer the best match, followed by the neck, upper chest, and arms.[110]

Cosmetic Units

Each burn should be treated on its own merit, but consideration should be given to grafting cosmetic units when the burn damage to the unit is extensive, rather than leaving some areas to heal and grafting adjacent areas.

The forehead and cheeks are typical cosmetic units that may be grafted with split skin. Frequently, this technique results in a very acceptable appearance on the forehead, but the cheek often demonstrates some flattening of contour and obliteration of the angle between the cheek and lateral alar nasae.

A complete graft take is essential if the best cosmetic result is to be attained. Meticulous attention to the grafting procedure is required to achieve this. Frequently, grafts on the face are left exposed to allow continuous monitoring of the graft.

Unfortunately, it frequently is not possible to do much for areas of lost tissue on the ears and nose in the acute phase. Chondritis of the pinnae can be halted by adequate débridement and antibiotics. Tarsorrhaphy may be required to prevent corneal damage.

Scar Maturation

After wound closure has been achieved, the patient enters an intermediate phase in which further gross distortion of facial features can occur from development of contractures of scar hypertrophy.[81] A regimen to control these problems should be commenced at the earliest opportunity. Pressure in the form of a rigid face mask specifically molded for the patient or an elasticized mask and contact media is important in this phase.

Reconstruction

After scar maturation has taken place, usually within 9 to 18 months after the injury, the tissues become more amenable to further reconstructive procedures. Reconstruction of the scarred face and neck may necessitate release of contractures and excision of unsightly scar tissue. Replacement can be achieved with local flap skin when available, or with full thickness grafts or split skin grafts when larger areas are involved.

The technique of tissue expansion has enhanced the use of flap repairs by providing large areas of expanded skin for reconstruction.[74] This has proved to be particularly valuable as a technique to repair extensive burn alopecia.

When the nose has sustained significant damage, a split skin graft to the upper nose may be acceptable, but alar and tip defects are difficult to reconstruct. Smaller defects can be improved by composite grafts from the ear, and larger areas can be repaired using a forehead flap, but the final result is often less than ideal.[38]

Severe burns to the face are frequently associated with a significant loss of tissue from the ear and residual deformity in the long term. Because this deformity can often be disguised by hair, and because of the shortcomings of ear reconstruction, late reconstruction is frequently not attempted. However, late reconstruction is possible using a carved cartilage framework if the remaining postauricular skin is satisfactory.[13]

The mouth and the eyelids are particularly susceptible to deformity produced by contracture, and it is difficult to apply pressure to these areas. When surgical release is required, mucosal flaps are often used to help reconstruct the vermilion.

Tarsorrhaphy is sometimes used in patients in whom extensive contracture of the eyelid is present.[20] Often, repeated release of contractures is necessary. Split skin grafts are preferred on the more mobile upper eyelid, whereas postauricular grafts are more suited for the lower lid.

The eyebrows can be grafted with hair-bearing skin in one or more strips if the subcutaneous tissues are healthy. Alternatively, an island scalp flap based on the superficial temporal arteries and veins can be used.

Neck contractures respond well to Z-plasty if linear or to large split skin grafts if more extensive. However, in the latter, prolonged splinting, contact media, and pressure are required if the best result is to be achieved.

Electrical Burns

Electrical burns constitute a small percentage of burn injuries, but they frequently provide some of the more difficult problems in management.

Classification

Electrical burns may be classified as high-tension (i.e., greater than 1000 volts) and low-tension (i.e., less than 1000 volts) injuries. Low-tension injuries are usually of the contact type, but both types may produce tissue damage due to a flash burn, arcing, or contact.[46] The severity of the injury increases greatly as the voltage rises. Flash burns are treated in a similar fashion to other thermal injuries. Arc burns are caused by current coursing external to the body.[15] This generates temperatures of 3000°C to 4000°C or higher, resulting in tissue damage, which is frequently extensive, at the site of the arc.

Contact or true electrical burns are produced by heat generated by current passing through the body.[90] This heat is maximal where resistance to the passage of the current is greatest, in particular, in the region of dry skin and bones. The severest injury occurs at the sites of entry and exit of the current, which finds passages of least resistance when passing between these points.

Electrical Injury

Examination of an electrical burn reveals a central charred zone of necrosis with complete obliteration of tissues. This area is surrounded by a gray-white zone of necrosis where tissue remains intact. The outer zone of partial coagulation necrosis, which histologically reveals spotty areas of coagulation necrosis and vascular damage, is referred to as the red zone. It is in the red zone that progressive necrosis may occur (Fig. 30–2).[95]

Widespread tissue damage may occur as the current passes through the body.[51] The visible damage to the skin and subcutaneous tissues may be relatively minor compared with the much more extensive underlying damage to muscle, bone, tendons, blood vessels, and nerves. All tissue in the body may be affected, including the kidneys, gastrointestinal tract, nerves, blood vessels, heart, and lungs. In addition, cataracts may develop.

Myohemoglobinemia from muscle destruction, and to a lesser extent, hemoglobinemia, are thought to be the main factors leading to acute renal failure.[8] A high renal output should be maintained from the onset of injury to overcome the destructive renal tubular effects of these products.

Surgery

Fasciotomy is often indicated with limb burns if the deep injury results in constricted swelling deep to the fascia.[99] Early excision of the nonviable tissue is recommended after the patient's general condition has stabilized. This excision is usually performed within 2 or 3 days of the injury. Although early débridement and coverage of the defect with a flap or graft provides the most effective repair, it is believed that if there is any doubt about viability after the initial débridement, that a second-look operation should be performed a few days later before definitive closure. This is preferable to being excessively radical at the time of the initial débridement and is important especially if vital structures such as those in the hand are to be preserved.

Alternatively, the initial débridement may be delayed for a few days. The argument against delay is that without coverage of the débrided injury, progressive destruction of vascularized tissue may occur in the zone of patchy coagulative necrosis.[68]

Flap coverage is essential when deeper structures such as bone and nerves are exposed, as is usually the case in contact burns and some arc burns. Although early surgical débridement is preferred in most cases of electrical burns,

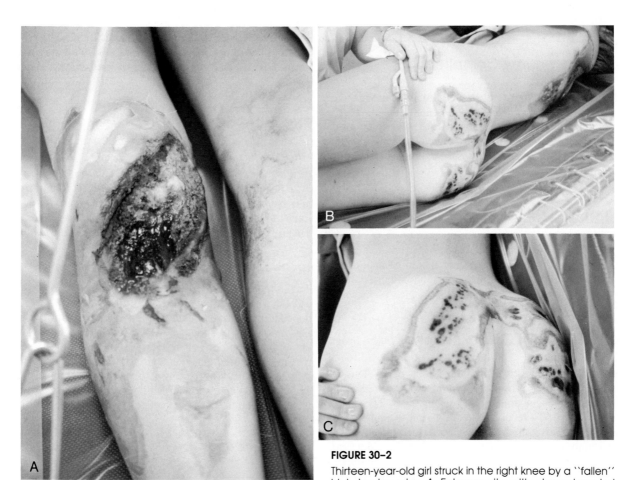

FIGURE 30–2

Thirteen-year-old girl struck in the right knee by a ''fallen'' high tension wire. A, Entrance site with charred central zone of necrosis and surrounding injured but seemingly intact tissue. B, Exit sites at the buttocks and back. C, Buttock injury consistent with classic central charred zone surrounded by gray-white zone of necrosis but intact tissue. A third outer zone of partial coagulation necrosis with histologic changes, referred to as the *red zone.*

some surgeons prefer to conservatively manage the difficult perioral arc burn resulting from children inserting live electrical contacts in their mouths.[27]

After wound closure has been achieved, the same principles of scar management apply as with other burn injuries, although in the limbs complex, reconstruction of nerves, muscle function, and tendons is frequently required.

MANAGEMENT OF COMPLICATIONS

Renal Complications

The initial renal complications are those due to inadequate fluid replacement. As previously stated, replacement formulas are guidelines and should be used as such. If renal output falls below 0.5 ml per kg per hour, fluid replacement must be increased and may need to be supplemented by diuretics such as intravenous furosemide or intravenous mannitol. In extensive deep burns, the release of hemoglobin may be an additional problem if fluid replacement is inadequate. Because of indwelling catheters, urinary tract infection is a possibility and requires antibiotic coverage. For patients that require long-term catheterization, such as those with perineal burns, a suprapubic stab cystostomy catheter may be preferable.

Cardiopulmonary Complications

Patients with inhalational burns require intubation, either nasotracheal or by tracheostomy, depending on the degree of injury, particularly when pulmonary edema complicates management.[55] Digitalization may be required, and the services of a cardiologist, respirologist, and intensivist should be enlisted when necessary.

Metabolic Complications

Hyperglycemia can complicate major burns and require insulin therapy. A metabolic physician should be included in the treatment team, because hyperglycemia in burn patients is frequently insulin resistant.

Gastrointestinal Complications

The initial gastrointestinal problem is that of an ileus, as previously described. However, a more severe complicating problem is the development of a Curling ulcer. The risk of a Curling ulcer is reduced by early oral feeding or by nasogastric feeding, and in some centers, routine antacids are given to prevent such an occurrence.[77, 88] Should a Curling ulcer develop, aggressive medical therapy with cimetidine and antacids should be instituted. If this treatment regimen is unsatisfactory, as very occasionally happens, surgery, preferably vagotomy and pyloroplasty, should be undertaken.

OTHER SUPPORTIVE MEASURES

Nutrition

Thermal injury causes destruction of tissue as well as loss of protein from the circulation. The marked catabolic effect that occurs is only reversed when adequate skin cover is achieved. The patient's basal metabolic requirements may increase by 50% or more.[9] This effect is compounded in the initial stages of injury by adynamic ileus, which requires oral intake to be reduced during the first 48 to 72 hours.

Oral intake should be instituted as soon as possible after this period, and if inadequate, oral intake should be supplemented by nasogastric feeding, which may be given as a continuous infusion.[32, 53] This infusion should consist of a high-protein, high-calorie fluid with vitamin supplements. However, if adequate protein levels cannot be achieved, intravenous nutrition may be used as a supplement.[22]

There is a direct relation between poor nutritional state and increased risk of sepsis in patients with major burns.[23, 29] The more extensive the burn, the greater the nutritional requirement, and the more difficult adequate nutrition is to achieve. Both the intravenous route and oral hyperalimentation are sometimes necessary to overcome this deficiency until adequate skin cover is achieved and the process reversed.

Routine supplements include vitamin B, vitamin C, and iron in all burn patients until discharge from the hospital. A nutritionist is a helpful and necessary part of team management.

Physiotherapy

General

In the acute phase, chest care is the most important aspect of physiotherapy. This is important in all patients with major burns but particularly so with patients who have inhalational burns or in the presence of pulmonary edema. Therapy should be both active and passive when possible.

Local

The important local aspects in the acute stage revolve around positioning, splinting, and movement and exercise, depending on the site and distribution of the burn. Positioning and splinting should be done in conjunction with the nursing staff and orthotist, and movement and exercise are part of continuing management in both the acute and rehabilitation phase. Therapy must be both active and passive, and play and suggestion are an integral part of the management of children.

Psychotherapy

Psychotherapy should be included as part of the normal ward routine. Parents should be encouraged to visit as long as possible or to live-in at the hospital, depending on their social circumstances.

Thermal injuries are traumatic for the child, the parents, and the entire family. All procedures should be performed with minimal distress to all concerned.[6] Parental counseling may be needed both in the acute stage and during long-term management. Parents need to be involved in the management of the patient as much as the situation permits, and they also must be kept fully informed of all aspects of management.[19]

Schooling

In the older child, time should be set aside between nursing and care procedures for schoolwork, both to maintain the child's interests outside the hospital and to facilitate his or her return to normal schooling after hospitalization.

Social Workers

Attention must be given to the social aspects of burns. There is a significantly higher incidence of thermal injuries in lower socioeconomic groups, particularly in the one-parent family; these situations require the services of a dedicated social worker. This is particularly important in cases in which child abuse is suspected or proved.

Orthotic Services

The services of an orthotist may be needed during the acute stage, grafting procedures, and rehabilitation. Splinting may be used to help in the positioning of areas such as the axillae, neck, and knees to prevent contractures and facilitate nursing care. A Bradford frame with mesh nylon netting is useful in the management of circumferential burns of the trunk. The patient may be placed on Zimmer sheeting covering the mesh to facilitate nursing care and allow free circulation of air around the entire trunk. Specially designed baths or beds are also available for patients with this type of injury.

During grafting procedures, various forms of splinting may help with the positioning of grafted areas. However, with the use of Hypafix as a graft retention dressing, the use of splinting in the small child has been considerably reduced. Splinting may be helpful in the rehabilitation phase, particularly with hand burns, but splinting is less frequently due to the use of contact media, as is outlined later.

REHABILITATION

The aim of rehabilitation is to facilitate the return of the child to its normal environment, with particular attention to social aspects, schooling, long-term follow up, and scar management.

Social Aspects

Many of these aspects may have been addressed by the social worker before discharge. Concerns such as socioeco-

nomic factors and housing are important to the family and therefore to overall care. However, acceptance by other members of the family is helped by other children visiting the affected child in the hospital, with counseling provided as necessary.

Self-help groups are also useful. BEES, a group of parents, friends, and burned children, has been developed at the Royal Children's Hospital in Melbourne. Camp Burn is another similar type of group that uses annual camps to help patients and parents adjust. It is much easier to accept a disability when it can be shared with others who are similarly afflicted.

Schooling

In the school-aged group of patients, a significant educational period is lost during hospitalization. Education must be continued as much as possible within the hospital routine; however, the child needs to be accepted back by his or her school peers. It is preferable for the child to return to his or her own class and previous school friends, even though this necessitates extra catch-up study, rather than for the child to have to adjust to a new peer group in another grade.

Before discharge, visits by school friends and teachers should be encouraged, and the school should be visited by a hospital school teacher, physical therapist, and social worker to talk to the class both about the child in particular and burns in general. This opportunity can be used as an education exercise in burn prevention. The peer group may be used in the rehabilitation program.

Follow Up

Follow up is necessary in all burn patients because of the potential for scar hypertrophy. Follow up lasts for a varying period, depending on the depth and extent of the injury.

A designated clinic separate from a general surgical clinic is advisable because of the problems peculiar to burn aftercare. Such a clinic was established at the Adelaide Children's Hospital and has proved most beneficial. It brings together all relevant disciplines and encourages self-help among parents and children who have similar problems. An important aspect of such a unit is to have burn unit nursing staff involved in the clinic to provide continuity of care and also to enable the staff to see long-term results as well as the horrors of the acute burn. This practice has helped the nursing staff to integrate as part of the team, and helps staff to overcome the psychological problems of nursing burn patients.

The other significant advantage of a designated clinic is to monitor various scar management routines to assess the results by close clinical observations. The following scar management program is based on these observations and results.

Scar Management

Scar management programs were slow to develop until the advent of pressure therapy in the mid 1970s. Before this, surgery was limited mainly to excision or revision of small scars and release of contractures.

Larson and colleagues showed that the collagen of hypertrophic scars could be influenced by the use of pressure.[62, 97, 101, 102] This discovery led to the introduction of custom-made antiburn scar pressure garments designed to achieve a pressure higher than that of capillary pressure. These garments were a significant advance, but they required continuing pressure for 23 hours per day—only being removed for bathing—and required up to 2 years of therapy to achieve a mature scar.[64]

Because pressure could not be uniform in all areas, pressure inserts were included in the program.[72] However, with the introduction of silicone gel in 1981, it was shown clinically that pressure was not necessary to control hypertrophy. This has been confirmed by Quinn and colleagues, resulting in the release of a modified Silastic gel in 1986 (Dow Corning).[93]

Since the introduction of silicone gel, an additional range of contact media have been introduced into the current scar management program. These products allow for the use of both pressure and nonpressure therapy programs with a reduction in therapy time, better short- and long-term cosmetic results, and a reduction in the incidence of secondary surgery.[50] The reduction in the use of custom-made pressure garments has also improved the economics of scar management and extended the range of therapy to scars of any size or location.

The current plan of management of scars at the Adelaide Children's Hospital is based on the following[82–84]:

1. Early excision and grafting of obvious full thickness burns and deep dermal burns not healed within 10 days after the injury
2. Early therapy with the appropriate contact media
3. Close observation in a specialized burn review clinic

The current contact media in use at this institution are the following:

1. Contact media with pressure
   Silastic Elastomer (Rolyan)
2. Contact media without pressure
   Spenco Silicone Gelsheet (Spenco)
   Spenco Skin Care Pads (Spenco)
   Tespad (Roval-Barcelona)
3. Adhesive contact media
   Hypafix (Smith & Nephew)
   Adhesive Knit (Spenco)

There is no single ideal contact medium; therefore, it must be emphasized that therapy must be selective, flexible, and individualized to the patient and to the scar. The results should be monitored regularly and therapy changed as necessary, depending on the patient's response and progress.

With the introduction of adhesive contact media in 1985, the use of Hypafix has gradually increased, because this material can be used for graft fixation and then continued immediately as the initial form of scar management, allowing for earlier therapy. Hypafix is currently the material of choice in approximately 50% of patients.[10, 82] Hypafix can also be used in the prevention of hypertrophy of other surgical scars unrelated to burns.

This adhesive, semiporous contact medium is easily applied and has the advantage of remaining in situ for 7 to 10 days before replacement is necessary without restricting normal daily activities such as bathing, showering, or swimming. Hypafix can be removed easily by the application of petroleum jelly or peanut oil and can be easily reapplied by the parent or therapist.

Elastofix is the brand name given to a combination of Hypafix and Elastomer as a two-component adhesive contact medium. Hypafix is applied as detailed previously. A thin smear of Elastomer is applied over the Hypafix to all areas needing more intensive therapy. The addition of Elastomer enhances therapy without the need for retention garments, and the flexibility of therapy remains the same as that for Hypafix.

The mode of action of contact media still requires elucidation. "The mode of action of silicone gel has been shown not to involve pressure, temperature, oxygen tension or occlusion: it is likely to involve both the hydration of the stratum corneum and the release of a low molecular weight silicone fluid."[92] However because neither of these adhesive contact media contains silicone, the answer probably lies in the hydration of the stratum corneum.[25] Davies has shown that there is an increased loss of fluid from burned skin, presumably due to loss of the stratum corneum.[26] By covering the area with a material (i.e., contact media) to reduce water vapor loss, homeostasis is restored. This in turn leads to a reduced capillary ingrowth with a reduction in secondary deposition of scar tissue, presumably due to biochemical mediators. It is suggested that contact media may act as artificial stratum corneum to restore homeostasis.[25, 84]

Secondary Surgery

The need for secondary surgery to revise scars or release contractures has been reduced significantly through the use of contact media. However, surgery is still necessary in selected cases, particularly in the face and hands, but also for late contractures.

Release of Contractures

Because of the potential for scar tissue to contract, especially across flexure surfaces, surgery may be needed early or late in the course of treatment. Another factor is changes that occur due to growth spurts, which may cause a previously satisfactory scar to become tight, especially toward puberty. This is of particular importance in girls, in whom the onset of breast development affects pectoral region scars.[109] All children with significant scars should be followed until at least their midteens to preempt late contracture development.

Revision or Excision of Keloids

Uncontrolled keloids may be excised for cosmetic reasons. Removal is desired mainly in the head and neck area; a difficult area in children is the submental scar. Young children do not tolerate chin straps or face masks well; therefore, the submental scar can be difficult to control, although Hypafix or Spenco Knit has proved useful in this area.

Techniques

Revisional surgery may consist of Z-plasty, W-plasty, or V-Y plasty procedures, if the scar's neighboring skin is soft and pliable or if the procedure involves a limited area.

Inlay Split Skin Graft. When a more extensive release is required or when pliable skin is in short supply, a release of the contracture followed by an inlay split skin graft is advised. The release may be at the level of the flexure crease, or an alternative is to do the release above or below the flexure so that the resultant inlay graft is not placed in the actual flexure. This allows for a greater release of the contracture and facilitates the use of contact media after surgery.

Flap Procedures. Various types of vascularized myocutaneous flap procedures may be used when it is desirable to use normal skin plus subcutaneous tissue to revise a scar. These flaps have been advocated for the neck, face, and hands and in electrical burns in particular.

Tissue Expanders. Tissue expansion using inflatable Silastic implants has become a useful technique. The implant is placed subcutaneously adjacent to the scarred area, and gradual expansion of normal tissue is achieved by serial injection into a Silastic reservoir over a period of weeks. When sufficient expansion has been achieved, the implant is removed, and a flap of normal tissue is rotated to cover an excised scar. This is particularly useful to replace scalp tissue but can be used successfully in other areas as well. Other plastic procedures may be needed depending on the individual needs of the patient.

SUMMARY OF BURN INJURY AND TREATMENT

As can be appreciated, thermal injury is a major cause of morbidity and mortality in children. The management of this form of trauma requires management of the entire patient with a wide range of problems requiring the dedicated attention of surgeons, physicians, varied specialists, nursing staff, therapists, and social workers, a true team approach to therapy both in the short term and the long term. It is important to remember also the support needed for parents and other family members.

As many of these problems are peculiar to the pediatric patient, the personnel involved should include dedicated pediatric-trained staff, preferably within or attached to a pediatric facility with the services of pediatric superspecialties available.

HYPOTHERMIA

Hypothermia is a well-recognized risk in the surgical neonate, especially in relation to transport to a specialized center. This should be preventable by the use of adjuncts such as plastic wraps and space blankets, and transport in a neonatal retrieval warmer. Controlled hypothermia may also be used in the management of certain surgical procedures.

However, accidental hypothermia may also occur in children. The commonest causes are cold-water immersion, accidental exposure to cold weather, or undue exposure during activities such as snow skiing.[14, 33, 41] Children are particularly vulnerable to hypothermia because of their lesser reserves and the ratio of BSA to volume, as well as a tendency to ignore the symptoms of hypothermia and the warnings of their parents.

Pathophysiology

The course of hypothermia has been categorized clinically into three stages based on body temperature.[42]

Responsive Phase

The responsive phase, which lasts from 35°C to 32°C, is characterized by shivering and vasoconstriction with an increase in pulse rate and a tendency to diuresis.

Slowing Phase

In the slowing phase, which lasts from 31°C to 25°C, gross shivering decreases to a fine tremor; there is a fall in blood pressure, pulse rate, and respiration rate; and a slowing of all enzymatic systems occurs. As the patient's temperature falls, tissue oxygen demand decreases in all systems, with a continuing fall in blood pressure, pulse rate, respiration, and significant hypovolemia. Atrial fibrillation occurs between 30°C to 27°C and ventricular fibrillation is likely below 27°C. Volume depletion leads to hemoconcentration, with a tendency to intravascular sludging and microvascular occlusion.

Liver function is impaired, especially the ability to conjugate or detoxify, while the bowel becomes hypomotile. Decreased glomerular filtration may lead to acute tubular necrosis. Cerebral function is depressed with reduced consciousness and a tendency to behavioral disorders.

Poikilothermic Phase

Below 25°C, heat loss becomes that of an inanimate object, and the patient appears to be dead.

Management

A history and full clinical assessment of the patient are necessary. The patient's temperature must be assessed by low-reading clinical thermometers, using the core rectal temperature which is monitored regularly.[73]

Full biochemical assessment, including blood gases, is advisable in severe cases, although the latter need to be corrected to the patient's temperature rather than to normal room temperature.

Passive Warming

Wet clothing is removed and warm dry clothing supplied. In less severe cases, warm clothing plus warm sweetened drinks may be adequate therapy, although a check of temperature is necessary in view of the phenomenon of after-drop.[14, 103]

Active Total Warming

Active total rewarming involves placing the patient in a warm bath or warm environment but carries the risk of peripheral vasodilation and increased hypovolemia and an increased risk of cardiac arrhythmias.

Active Core Warming

Active core rewarming involves rewarming of the trunk by techniques such as immersion in a warm bath with the limbs exposed or more invasive procedures such as warm peritoneal dialysis or cardiopulmonary bypass. The selection of technique depends on the facilities available with appropriate attention given to biochemical and fluid requirements and prevention of after-drop.

Inhalational Warming

Warm moist oxygen is administered through a mask or endotracheal tube. This method rewarms the core without the risk of peripheral vasodilation. The simplicity of the technique makes this the method of choice except in the most profound cases of hypothermia, when it can be used to supplement the previously described techniques.

References

1. Aikawa N, Shinozawa Y, Ishibiki K, et al: Clinical analysis of multiple organ failure in burned patients. Burns 13(2):103–109, 1987.
2. Arturson G, Jonsson CE: Transcapillary transport after thermal injury. Scand J Plast Reconstr Surg 13:9, 1979.
3. Baxter CR: Fluid volume and electrolyte changes of the early postburn period. Clin Plast Surg 1:693, 1974.
4. Baxter CR: Fluid resuscitation, burn percentage and physiologic age. J Trauma 19(Suppl):864–865, 1979.
5. Baxter CR, Shires GT: Physiological response to crystalloid resuscitation of severe burns. Ann N Y Acad Sci 150:874, 1968.
6. Beales JG: Factors influencing the expectation of pain among patients in a children's burn unit. Burns 9(3):174–179, 1983.
7. Beasley RW: Secondary repair of burned hands. Clin Plast Surg 8(1):141, 1981.
8. Bingham HG: Electrical burns. Clin Plast Surg 13(1):75, 1986.
9. Border JR: Acute protein malnutrition in burned patients. J Trauma 19:902, 1979.
10. Boucaut H: Techniques of graft fixation. ANZBA Bulletin, Issue 1, July 1987, pp 16–17.
11. Bowser BH, Caldwell FT: The effects of resuscitation with hypertonic vs hypotonic vs colloid on wound and urine fluid and electrolyte losses in severely burned children. J Trauma 23(10):916–923, 1983.
12. Bowser-Wallace BH, Caldwell FT: Fluid requirements of severely burned children up to 3 years old: Hypertonic lactated saline vs Ringer's lactate-colloid. Burns 12(8):549–555, 1986.
13. Brent B: Reconstruction of the ear, eyebrow and sideburn in the burned patient. Plast Reconstr Surg 55:312, 1975.
14. Budd GM: Accidental hypothermia in skiers. Med J Aust 144(9):449, 1986.
15. Burke JF, Quinby WC, Bondoc C, et al: Patterns of high tension: Electrical injuries in children and adolescents and their management. Am J Surg 133:492–497, 1977.
16. Byrom RR, Word EL, Tewksbury CG, Edlich RF: Epidemiology of flame burn injuries. Burns 11(1):1–10, 1984.
17. Caldwell FT, Bowser BH: Critical evaluation of hypertonic and hypotonic solutions to resuscitate severely burned children: A prospective study. Ann Surg 189(5):546–552, 1979.
18. Cameron JS, Miller-Jones CMH: Renal function and renal failure in badly burned children. Br J Surg 54:132, 1967.
19. Campbell JL, La Clave LJ, Brack G: Clinical depression in paediatric burn patients. Burns 13(3):213–217, 1987.
20. Constable JD, Carroll JM: The emergency treatment of the exposed cornea in thermal burns. Plast Reconstr Surg 46:309, 1970.
21. Cristofoli C, Lorenzini M, Furlan S: The use of Omiderm, a new skin substitute, in a burn unit. Burns 12(8):587–591, 1986.
22. Curreri PW: Nutritional replacement modalities. J Trauma 19:906, 1979.
23. Curreri PW, Richmond C, Marvin J, et al: Dietary requirements of patients with major burns. J Am Diet Assoc 65:415, 1974.
24. Davey RB: The burn clinic. Burns 8:369–371, 1981.
25. Davey RB: Current concepts of burn scar management. ANZBA Bulletin, Issue 1, July 1987, pp 20–21.
26. Davies JWL: Prompt cooling of burned areas: A review of benefits and the effector mechanisms. Burns 9(1):1–6, 1982.
27. de la Plaza R, Quetglas A, Rodriquez E: Treatment of electrical burns of the mouth. Burns 10:49–60, 1983.
28. Douglas BS, Broadfoot MJ: Hypertension in burnt children. Aust N Z J Surg 42:194, 1972.
29. Dudrick SJ: Nutritional therapy in burned patients. J Trauma 19:908, 1979.
30. Edstrom L, Robson MC, Macchiaverwa JR, et al: Management of deep partial thickness dorsal hand burns: Study of operative vs nonoperative therapy. Orthop Rev 8:27, 1979.
31. Eldad A, Burt A, Clark JA, et al: Cultured epithelium as a skin substitute. Burns 13(3):173–180, 1987.
32. Eve MD, Settle JAD: Elemental feeding in severe burns: Monitoring a regime using Vivonex. Burns 5(1):127–135, 1978.
33. Fitzgerald FT, Jessop C: Accidental hypothermia: A report of 22 cases and review of the literature. Adv Intern Med 27:128–150, 1982.
34. Gaukroger PB: Paediatric analgesia: Which drug? Which dose? Drugs 41:52, 1991.
35. Gaukroger PB: Patient controlled analgesia. In: Schechter NL, Berde C, Yaster M (eds): Pain in Infants, Children and Adolescents. Baltimore, Williams & Wilkins, 1992.
36. Gaukroger PB, Tomkins DP, van der Walt JH: Patient controlled analgesia in children. Anaesth Intensive Care 17:264, 1989.
37. Gaukroger PB, Chapman MJ, Davey RB: Pain control in paediatric burns—the use of patient controlled analgesia. Burns 17(5):396–399, 1991.
38. Gonzalez-Ulloa M: Restoration of the face covering by means of selected skin of regional aesthetic units. Br J Plast Surg 9:212, 1956.
39. Gordon PG, Pressley TA: The fire hazard of children's nightwear: The Australian experience in developing clothing fire hazard standards. Burns 5(1):12–18, 1978.
40. Green AR, Fairclough J, Sykes PJ: Epidemiology of burns in childhood. Burns 10(5):368–371, 1984.
41. Hampton WR: Hypothermia in winter and high altitude sports. Conn Med 45:633–636, 1981.
42. Hartnett RM, O'Brien EM, Sias FR, et al: Initial treatment of profound accidental hypothermia. Aviat Space Environ Med 51:680–687, 1980.
43. Harms B, Bodai B, Kramer G, et al: Microvascular transport of fluid and protein in pulmonary and systemic circulations after thermal injury. Microvasc Res 23:77, 1982.
44. Hauben DJ, Mahler D: A burn formula in clinical practice. Ann R Coll Surg Engl 63:293, 1981.
45. Hauben DJ, Mahler D: Fresh frozen plasma, a hypertonic and hyperosmolal solution. Burns 9:68–69, 1982.
46. Hawnmadass ML, Voora SB, Kagan RJ, et al: Acute electrical burns: A 10 year clinical experience. Burns 12:427–431, 1986.
47. Herd AN, Hall PN, Widdowson P, et al: Mesh grafts—an 18 month follow up. Burns 13(1):57–61, 1987.
48. Hermans RP: Topical treatment of serious infections with special reference to the use of a mixture of silver sulphadiazine and cerium nitrate: Two clinical studies. Burns 11(1):59–62, 1984.
49. Higuchi D, Sei Y, Suzuki T, et al: Management of wounds treated by thrombin coagulation. Burns 13(1):75–76, 1987.
50. Hosoda G, Holloway GA, Heimbach DM: Laser Doppler flowmetry for the early detection of hypertrophic burn scars. J Burn Care Rehabil 7(6):496–497, 1986.

51. Hunt JL, Mason AD, Masterson TS, et al: The pathophysiology of acute electric injuries. J Trauma 16:335–340, 1976.

52. Inman RJ, Snelling CFT, Roberts FJ, et al: Prospective comparison of silver sulfadiazine 1 percent plus chlorhexidine digluconate 0.2 percent (Silvazine) and silver sulfadiazine 1 percent (Flamazine) as prophylaxis against burn wound infection. Burns 11(1):35, 1984.

53. Jacobs LS, de Kock M, van der Merwe AE: Oral hyperalimentation and the prevention of severe weight loss in burned patients. Burns 13(2):154–158, 1987.

54. Janzekovic Z: A new concept in the early excision and immediate grafting of burns. J Trauma 10:1103, 1970.

55. Judkins KC, Brander WL: Respiratory injury in children: The histology of healing. Burns 12(5):357–359, 1986.

56. Kalaja E: Acute excision or exposure treatment? Scand J Plast Reconstr Surg 18:95, 1984.

57. Keswani MH: A decade in the field of burn prevention. Burns 5(1):5–7, 1978.

58. Kirkham S: A social survey of thermal injuries in South Australian children. Burns 5(2):199–201, 1978.

59. Kleeman PP, Jantzen JP: Contemporary management of the difficult paediatric airway—introducing the generation of ultra-thin flexible fiberscopes. First European Congress of Paediatric Anaesthesia, Book of Abstracts, Rotterdam, 1986, pp 106.

60. Kligman AM: The biology of the stratum corneum. In: Montagna W, Lobitz WC Jr, (eds): The Epidermis. New York, Academic Press, 1964, pp 387–433.

61. Kumar P: Child abuse by thermal injury—a retrospective survey. Burns 10(5):344–348, 1984.

62. Larson DL, Abston S, Evans EB, et al: Techniques for decreasing scar formation and contracture in the burned patient. J Trauma 11:807, 1971.

63. Lawrence JC: British Burn Association recommended first aid for burns and scalds. Burns 13(2):153, 1987.

64. Leung KS, Cheng JCY, Ma GFY, et al: Complications of pressure therapy for post-burn hypertrophic scars. Burns 10:434–438, 1984.

65. Levine SL, Buchanan RT: The care of burned upper extremities. Clin Plast Surg 13(1):107, 1986.

66. Littler JW, Eaton RG: Redistribution of forces in the correction of the boutonniere deformity. J Bone Joint Surg [Am] 49:1267, 1967.

67. Lowenstein E: Succinylcholine administration in the burned patient. Anaesthesiology 27:494, 1966.

68. Luce EA, Gottleir SE: "True" high tension electrical injuries. Ann Plast Surg 12:321–325, 1984.

69. Lund CC, Browder NC: The estimation of areas of burns. Surg Gynecol Obstet 79:352, 1944.

70. McHugh TP, Robson MC, Heggers JP, et al: Therapeutic efficacy of Biobrane in partial thickness and full thickness thermal injury. Surgery 100(4):661–664, 1986.

71. Mahler D, Baruchin A, Hauben D, et al: Recent concepts regarding the resuscitation of the burned patient. Burns 9(1):30–37, 1982.

72. Malick MH, Carr JA: Flexible elastomer moulds in burn scar control. Am J Occup Ther 34:9, 1980.

73. Marcus P: Laboratory comparison of technique for rewarming hypothermic casualties. Aviat Space Environ Med 49:692–697, 1978.

74. Marks MW, Argenta LC, Thornton JW: Burn management: The role of tissue expansion. Clin Plast Surg 14(3):543, 1987.

75. Mather LE: Pharmacokinetic and pharmacodynamic factors influencing the choice, dose and route of administration of opiates for acute pain. In: Bullingham RES (ed): Clinical Anaesthesiology. Vol. 1. London, WB Saunders, 1983, pp 17–40.

76. Mehrkens HH, Lindner KH, Ahnefeld FW, Nunn T: Fluid resuscitation with hypertonic salt solutions in experimental burn shock. Burns 13(1):53–56, 1987.

77. Moscona R, Kaufman T, Jacobs R, et al: Prevention of gastrointestinal bleeding in burns: The effects of cimetidine or antacids combined with early enteral feeding. Burns 12(1):65–67, 1985.

78. Muir IKF, Barclay TL (eds): Burns and Their Treatment. 2nd ed. London, Lloyd-Luke, 1974, pp 28–31.

79. Neale WN, Billmire DA, Carey JP: Reconstruction following head and neck burns. Clin Plast Surg 13(1):119–136, 1986.

80. O'Neill JA, Meacham WF, Griffin PP, et al: Patterns of injury in the battered child syndrome. J Trauma 13:332, 1975.

81. Parks DH, Baur PS, Larson DL: Late problems in burns. Clin Plast Surg 4(4):547, 1977.

82. Perkins K: The use of semi permeable adhesive backed materials in burn scar management at the Adelaide Children's Hospital. ANZBA Bulletin 1:18–19, 1987.

83. Perkins K, Davey RB, Wallis K: Silicone gel: A new treatment for burn scars and contractures. Burns 9:201–204, 1982.

84. Perkins K, Davey RB, Wallis K: Current materials and techniques used in a burn scar management program. Burns 13(5):406–410, 1987.

85. Phillips W, Mahairas E, Hunt D, et al: The epidemiology of childhood scalds in Brisbane. Burns 12(5):343–350, 1986.

86. Pinnegar MD, Pinnegar FC III: History of burn care: A survey of important changes in the topical treatment of thermal injuries. Burns 12(7):508–517, 1986.

87. Popp MB, Silverstein EB, Srivastava LS, et al: A pathophysiologic study of the hypertension associated with burn injury in children. Ann Surg 193:817, 1981.

88. Prasad JK, Thomson PD, Feller I: Gastrointestinal haemorrhage in burn patients. Burns 13(3):194–197, 1987.

89. Pruitt BA Jr: Fluid and electrolyte replacement in the burned patient. Surg Clin North Am 58:1291, 1978.

90. Pruitt BA Jr, Mason AD Jr: High tension electrical injury. Lancet 3:271, 1979.

91. Purdue GH, Hunt JL, Gillespie RW, et al: Biosynthetic skin substitute versus frozen human cadever allograft for temporary coverage of excised burn wounds. J Trauma 27(2):155–157, 1987.

92. Quinn D, Evans JH, Gaylor JDS, et al: Burn wound dressings—a review. Burns 13(3):218–228, 1987.

93. Quinn KJ, Evans JH, Courtney JM, et al: Non-pressure treatment of hypertrophic scars. Burns 12:102–108, 1986.

94. Roa Romero L, Gomez Cia T: Analysis of the extracellular protein and fluid shifts in burned patients. Burns 12(5):337–342, 1986.

95. Robson MC, Murphy RC, Hoggers JP: A new explanation for the progressive tissue loss in electrical injuries. Plast Reconstr Surg 73:431, 1984.

96. Rogenes PR, Moylan JA: Restoring fluid balance in the patient with severe burns. Am J Nurs 76:1953–1957, 1976.

97. Rose MP, Deitch EA: The clinical use of a tubular compression bandage, Tubigrip, for burn-scar therapy: A critical analysis. Burns 12(1):58–64, 1985.

98. Salisbury RE, Wright P: Evaluation of early excision of dorsal burns of the hand. Plast Reconstr Surg 69:670, 1982.

99. Salisbury RE, Hunt JL, Worden GD, et al: Management of electrical burns of the upper extremity. Plast Reconstr Surg 51:648, 1973.

100. Salisbury RE, Taylor JW, Levine NS: Evaluation of digital escharotomy in burned hands. Plast Reconstr Surg 58:440, 1976.

101. Shakespeare PG, Strange R: Linoleic acid in hypertrophic scars. Burns 9(1):7–12, 1982.

102. Shakespeare PG, van Renterghem L: Some observations on the surface structure of collagen in hypertrophic scars. Burns 3:175–180, 1985.

103. Sherry E, Richards D: Hypothermia among resort skiers: 19 cases from the Snowy Mountains. Med J Aust 144(9):457–461, 1986.

104. Smith RW, O'Neill TJ: An analysis into childhood burns. Burns 11(2):117–124, 1984.

105. Spencer DS, Davey RB: The Spencer Op-Site Applicator, a new technique for treating the burned hand. Burns 13(4):330–333, 1987.

106. Suarez AJ, Hess DM, Hunt JL, et al: Early tangential excision of deep dermal burns with immediate meshed homograft coverage. J Burn Care Rehabil 1:36–39, 1980.

107. Sun YH, Wang XW, Zhang ZM, et al: The tangential excision of extensive or deep burns. Burns 11(1):31–34, 1984.

108. Thomsen M, Bjorn L, Sorensen B: The total number of burn injuries in a Scandinavian population: A repeated estimate. Burns 5(1):72–78, 1978.

109. Trott JA, Hobby JAE: Burns of the female breast: A long term study. Burns 4(4):267–270, 1978.

110. Warpeha RL: Resurfacing of the burned face. Clin Plast Surg 8(2):255, 1981.

111. Xeuwei W, Jiaqu L: Clinicopathologic observations on tangential eschar excision in deep burns. Burns 9(3):174–179, 1983.

112. Yoshioka T, Ohashi Y, Sugimoto H, et al: Epidemiological analysis of deaths caused by burns in Osaka, Japan. Burns 8(6):414–422, 1982.

113. Zetterstrom H, Arturson G: Plasma oncotic and plasma protein concentration in patients following thermal injury. Acta Anaesthesiol Scand 24:288, 1980.

Falls from Heights

The psychomotor development of the child does not occur at an even pace. The child's mastery of bipedal motion precedes his or her intellectual ability to perceive the danger of height; it is therefore little wonder that falls from heights occur particularly often in early childhood. Injuries due to falls represent the cause of trauma in 39% of all accidental childhood injuries reported to the National Pediatric Trauma Registry, followed by motor vehicle accidents, which represent 38%.[9] In contrast to falls from low objects (e.g., beds, tables, stools, bicycles), which occur in both urban and rural settings, the free fall from above a height of one story occurs most often in an urban setting. Because the mortality rate of falls less than 35 feet (i.e., the equivalent of three stories) is usually quite small, the higher incidence of mortalities in the urban setting appears to be directly related to falls from high-rise tenement buildings. It is therefore understandable that there is broad variation in the incidence of death following falls—nationwide, falls are reported to be the cause in approximately 4% of accidental deaths in children, whereas this rate climbs to 13% to 20% of all accidental deaths in the urban childhood population, a rate exceeded only by motor vehicle accidents and fire (Figs. 31–1 and 31–2).[11, 15]

DEMOGRAPHICS OF FALLS

In an analysis of demographic factors contributing to the risk of falls from heights, Bergner and colleagues compared these occurrences in the four boroughs of New York.[3] The two main boroughs of New York City, the Bronx and Brooklyn, showed a marked difference in pediatric mortality resulting from falls, even though both are the site of large ghetto populations. In the Bronx, the inner-ghetto population resides predominantly in high-rise tenements, whereas in Brooklyn, the even larger socioeconomic deprived population is distributed over a large area, predominantly in three- to four-story buildings. Although the number of children in Brooklyn is twice as great as that in the Bronx, the same number of children died as the result of

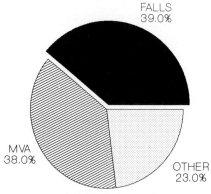

FIGURE 31–1

Mechanisms of injury. Falls constituted 39% of all recorded mechanisms of injuries in the National Pediatric Trauma Registry, followed by motor vehicle accidents (MVA) and other unspecified mechanisms. (From Ramenofsky ML: Pediatric abdominal trauma. Pediatr Ann 16(4):318–326, 1987.)

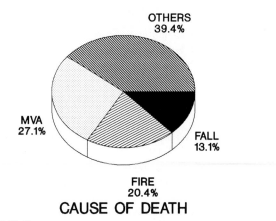

TRAUMATIC DEATH IN URBAN CHILDREN
Brooklyn 1965 - 1974

CAUSE OF DEATH

FIGURE 31–2

A review of 911 traumatic deaths that occurred in Brooklyn between 1965 and 1974 in children younger than 14 years of age indicated that 13.1% died owing to falls from heights, making deaths from falls third behind only deaths due to motor vehicle accidents (MVA) and those due to fire. (From Velcek FT, Weiss A, DiMaio D, et al: Traumatic death in urban children. J Pediatr Surg 12(3):375–384, 1977.)

falls, which strongly suggests that it is the concentration of high-rise buildings that is especially conducive to fatal falls.

Children who were injured or died as a result of falls were predominantly disadvantaged African-Americans or Hispanics.[15] A review of the socioeconomic circumstances of families with children who were injured in falls revealed that 50% of these usually single parents were on welfare.[14] In addition, an unusually high number of prior accidents or a history of siblings having been previously injured from falls was also found. Mental retardation, hyperactivity and past injuries in these children were not uncommon. The deterioration of windows, stairwells, and railings in slum buildings was considered to be an additional contributing factor. The lack of air-conditioners in this socioeconomic group makes the open window an escape area from the heat in the summer, and open windows serve simultaneously as the focal point for neighborly discussions or observation of street activities.[11] In the absence of play areas, other locations such as fire escapes and rooftops function as the site for play and social gatherings, especially for older children. Although most falls are the result of accidents, children also may be pushed or jump while trying to escape beatings or fires.[2]

THE FREE FALL: FACTORS CONTRIBUTING TO INJURY AND DEATH

It is difficult to understand why one child falling out of a second-story window may sustain major injuries whereas another child, having fallen out of a fifth-floor window, may get up and walk away relatively unharmed. Although there are multiple variables that may determine the final outcome of a fall, several major factors usually explain the type of injury sustained or the lack thereof. Reviews of human tolerance to impact of free falls analyzed in detail reveal the following main factors[7, 13]:

1. Velocity or magnitude of force
2. Body orientation
3. Distribution of force
4. Impacted material
5. Duration of impact time

Velocity or Magnitude of Force

The velocity of a falling body depends mainly on the height of the fall and is expressed as the velocity of the body mass at the time of impact: $V2 = 2gh$ (V = velocity, g = acceleration due to gravity, h = height of fall). The increase in velocity during a free fall was first described by Galileo and then calculated with improved accuracy by Newton and Einstein. At sea level, the terminal velocity of a 482-foot fall is 120 miles per hour. In practical terms, a human body's velocity at impact after a fall from the third floor is approximately 35 miles per hour; from the fourth floor, 41 miles per hour; from the fifth floor, 45 miles per hour; and from the sixth floor, 49 miles per hour, eventually reaching the terminal speed of 120 miles per hour, from which it cannot increase, regardless of the height of fall.[8] The velocity is independent of mass; thus a 2-year-old toddler will fall at the same speed as a 200-lb adult. Other factors, such as clothing and body position, also influence velocity, and numerous studies and reports have shown that neither the height of the fall nor increasing velocity absolutely relate to mortality or severity of injuries. Therefore, other factors play important roles in the type and severity of injuries in children who fall from heights.

Body Orientation

The basic orientation of the body at the time impact occurs is usually in one of the following forms:

1. Feet to head
2. Head to feet
3. Buttocks
4. Transverse (prone or supine)
5. Crouch position (hands and knees)
6. Side (right or left lateral)

The patterns of injuries sustained correlate with the directional force of the body orientation. Each position is likely to lead to rather predictable primary and secondary structural body injuries: feet-first impact leads to injury of the feet, ankles, legs, and vertebrae. In the head-first position, the force extends from the head to the shoulder girdle and thorax. In the buttocks-first position, the most likely injuries primarily are sustained in the pelvis and vertebrae, and the secondary impact leads to head trauma. It is possible that the body orientation, more than any other factor, determines

the types of injury sustained from a free fall. In children, it has been postulated that the anatomic relation between the head and body (i.e., the head is relatively larger in proportion to the body than in the adult) may increase their head-to-feet orientation at impact and explain the higher number of skull fractures and central nervous system (CNS) injuries in children.

Distribution of Force

The distribution of force is related to the orientation of the body at impact, the magnitude of the force, and duration of impact time. Theoretically, the greater the area over which the load is applied at the time of impact, the smaller is the load per unit area. A transverse fall, which exposes the largest surface area at impact, should therefore result in the most favorable dissipation and distribution of impact force; however, the body position that leads to the fewest major injuries is when a much smaller surface area, such as the feet, receives the full and only impact. Ten of 12 patients survive falls of more than 100 feet after impact in the feet-first position; this statistic illustrates that the distribution of force alone also is not necessarily a reliable predictor of extent of injury.[13]

Impacted Material

The change of form of the impacted material (i.e., flexing and bending) plays a significant role in the extent of injuries sustained. The relative firmness or elasticity of the impacted material affects the duration of impact. It would seem that impaction on soft material would be preferable to landing on bricks or cement, because the increased resilience of the impacted material deforming in response to the applied force over a relatively long period of time leads to a slower deceleration of the body. In fact, Cummins and Potter reported that only two of six children who fell on grass had a skull fracture (33%), but nine of 13 children who fell on cement or brick (69%) had skull fractures.[5] However, although it appears logical that soft, resilient material should diminish the risk of impact injury, Snyder pointed out that there is no straight-line relation between impact material and injuries.[13]

Duration of Impact Time

A critical factor in both acceleration and deceleration injuries is the duration of time that the force is applied at impact, or the time required to reach the peak form after initial impact. A time duration of less than 0.2 second is considered to be likely to cause significant structural body injuries. Although the resilient qualities of the impacted material affect deceleration, a paradoxical finding has been described wherein major impact with a time duration of less than 0.0006 second may actually increase survival. This underlines the fact that duration of impact time, like the other factors noted previously, is not an absolute predictor of outcome.[13]

FALLS FROM HEIGHTS
1983 - 1987

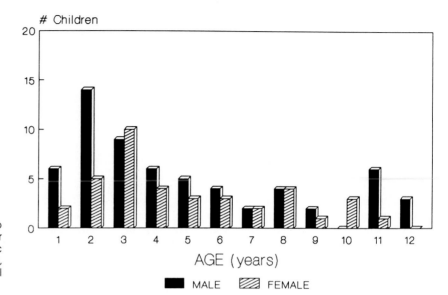

FIGURE 31-3

Between 1983 and 1987, 99 children who had fallen from heights of one story or higher were admitted to the pediatric surgical service in Kings County Hospital, Brooklyn. Males dominated in almost all years.

Other Variables

Good physical condition has been considered to be a major positive factor in the outcome of falls from heights. Trained parachute jumpers, who land with the same impact as untrained jumpers, are less likely to sustain injuries because of their trained and hardened flexible knees and muscles. In contrast, the untrained person, who lands stiff-legged, usually sustains heel injuries. In addition, the intentional or unintentional ability to relax may explain why alcoholics, drugged jumpers, and suicidal jumpers (who actually may enjoy the fall) are less likely to sustain injuries than the apprehensive workman who accidentally falls from a scaffold. Children, who are assumed to be more flexible than adults, have also been reported to have a better survival rate than adults falling from the same height.[2] However, this finding has not been uniform; other researchers have found that the death rate from falls is highest among the very young and the very old.[10]

It should be obvious that an exact evaluation of the contribution of these potential factors to injuries is difficult, because precise information is usually not available in children who have fallen. Although the height of the fall may be known, information concerning impact area, patient condition at the time of the fall, and in particular, the child's body position, which often does not follow the previously outlined neat positions, is usually unknown.

FALLS IN BROOKLYN

As previously stated, falls were the cause of accidental death in 13% of all children under the age of 14 years who were killed in Brooklyn between 1965 and 1974 (see Fig. 31-2). In the present study, we reviewed the outcome of 99

children under the age of 13 years who fell from a height of more than one story (i.e., 12 to 15 feet) and who were admitted to the Pediatric Surgical Service at Kings County Hospital between 1983 and 1987 (Fig. 31-3).

Age and Gender Distribution

More than half of these children were under the age of 4 years; and the largest number was in the 2-year-old age group. Boys, particularly those over the age of 10 years, were predominant, a finding common to all reports.[2, 8, 11, 12, 14] The presumed social role of boys may explain their increasing predominance in the preteenaged and teenaged period. Both age and gender distribution are similar to that of our previous review of traumatic death in urban children—the most likely child to sustain injury from a fall from a height is the boy who is younger than 4 years of age.[2] The number of deaths (5) in the present series is too small to draw any conclusions, but in our previous series of 119 deaths due to falls in Brooklyn, the 2-year-old toddler was most likely to die in a fall from a height.

Height of Fall

Fifty-three percent of all children fell from a height of three stories or higher, but the largest number of falls (32 of 99) occurred from the second floor (Fig. 31-4). Less than 12% of children fell from the fifth and sixth floors. There could be two reasons for the small number of children who fell from floors five and six in Brooklyn: (1) most of these disadvantaged children live in two- to four-story homes, in contrast to the high-rise tenement buildings found in other boroughs of New York; (2) and the effectiveness of the

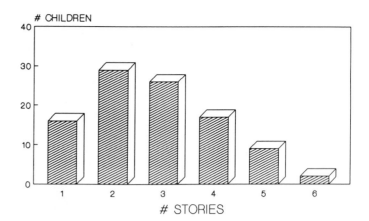

FIGURE 31–4

The figure shows the distribution of the 99 children mentioned in Figure 31–3 and the heights of their falls. Each story is assumed to be between 12 and 15 feet. Although the largest number of children fell from a second-story window, more than half fell three stories or more.

window-fall regulations in New York may have been influential. This regulation mandated window guards in high-rise buildings for all apartments containing children younger than 10 years of age.[14] This law does not apply to private homes or lower-level buildings. Both of these explanations are assumptions only; Sieben and colleagues reported an almost identical distribution in falls from heights, even though they occurred in an area of high-rise tenements before the enforcement of window guards.[11]

Mechanism of Falling

Eighty-eight of 99 children were reported to have fallen accidentally. Of the remaining 11 children, three jumped in suicide attempts, four were pushed (two because of fires), and in four the reason for the fall was unknown. In other series, as many as 23% of falls were nonaccidental, a category that included intentional suicide or foul play. Seventy-four of the 101 children in one study fell out of windows, six fell from roofs, four fell from fire escapes, three fell in elevator shafts, and 12 fell from other elevated structures. The distribution is similar to that in other reports in New York—the toddler is most likely to fall out of a window, whereas the older child is most likely to fall from a fire escape or roof while using it as a play area.[2, 3, 9, 11] Both season and time of day of the falls are similar in all reports—most falls occur during the summer months with a peak in July, and most falls occur during the afternoon.[2]

Mortalities and Injuries

Mortality Related to Height of Fall

There were five deaths; two patients died in the emergency department, and three died after admission (Table 31–1). The deaths occurred after falls from the third, fourth, and fifth stories. Although there appears to be a relation between height and death, with no deaths occurring from falls below the third floor, it should be emphasized that two children who fell from the sixth floor not only survived, but one had only minor injuries (Fig. 31–5). In the Harlem experience of Barlow and associates, no deaths occurred from falls from below the fourth floor.[2] There was a pro-

portional increase in deaths with falls from the fourth to the sixth floor; 50% of those falling from the sixth floor died as a result. Similarly, in a retrospective review of 200 suicide attempts in both adults and children, Reynolds and colleagues found that mortality increased in proportion to height.[10] However, in their review, mortalities also occurred in falls from the first and second floor (5% and 12%, respectively) and increased proportionally from the third floor (10%) to the fourth floor (30%) to the fifth floor (50%) to the sixth floor (65%). Although the mortalities in our series are few, these cases imply that although all falls from heights of three floors or higher are potentially lethal, survival can occur even in falls from as high as the sixth floor.

Major and Minor Injuries

Of the 99 children in our series, 53 sustained major injuries, and 30 had multiple injuries (i.e., more than two injuries in anatomically separate areas, see Table 31–1). Sixteen chil-

Table 31–1

Mortalities and Injuries from Falls (99 children; 5 deaths)

Injuries	Number
Major	53
Minor	16
None or insignificant	25
Multiple	30
Central nervous system	31
Skull fracture	23
Fractures	
Pelvis	6
Vertebra	4
Mandible	4
Ribs	3
Chest	13
Abdomen	3
Lower extremities	
Femur	17
Tibia-fibula	4
Ankle	3
Talus-calcaneus	3
Metatarsal	3
Upper extremities	
Humerus-radius	11
Hand	3

HEIGHT AND INJURY

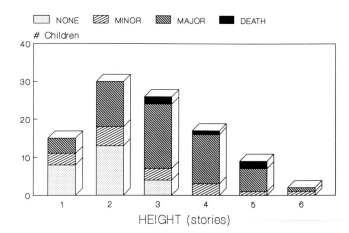

☐ NONE   ▨ MINOR   ▨ MAJOR   ■ DEATH

FIGURE 31–5

Correlating the height of fall and the extent of injury of the 99 children mentioned in Figure 31–3, it is apparent that major injuries increased in proportion to the height of the fall. There were no deaths due to falls from below the third floor.

dren sustained minor injuries, and 25 children suffered either insignificant injuries or no injuries at all. Fractures were the most common injury (61) followed by CNS injuries (31) and skull fractures (23). As in other series, there was no direct relation between skull fractures and CNS injuries.[6] Sixteen children with CNS injuries had no skull fractures, and there were eight children with skull fractures who had no abnormal associated CNS findings. Cummins and Potter emphasized that infants younger than 5 years of age sustained twice the number of skull fractures than adults but had less CNS trauma; they postulated that the flexibility of the skull and its absorption of the applied force explained this occurrence.[5] All deaths, however, were due to brain injuries, and one was associated with exsanguination. There were 30 lower-extremity fractures and 14 upper-extremity fractures. Pelvic fractures occurred in six children and, as with adults, there was a surprising lack of major hemorrhage associated with the pelvic fractures.[1] One child had an associated perineal injury with a rectal tear due to landing and impacting on a fence (Fig. 31–6). Rib fractures occurred in three children. In contrast to other series in which chest injury in children was extremely rare, there were 10 children in our series with chest injuries, including hemopneumothorax, pneumothorax, lung contusions, and one major hemothorax requiring open thoracotomy.[12] The number and type of chest injuries indicate that even though the child's chest is more flexible and rib injuries are not as common as in adults, sudden deceleration can result in parenchymal lung injury, with or without rib fractures. Eleven of these children required thoracostomy tube drainage.

Injuries Related to Height of Fall

Although there were only three abdominal injuries (i.e., two liver injuries and one rectal tear), other researchers have demonstrated that injuries of supporting tissue structures (e.g., the perineum, the mesentery, ligaments) are quite common but often are not diagnosed because of more severe and apparent injuries.[13] Other researchers also found that internal injuries seemingly occurred only in falls of 36 feet or higher and multiple injuries only in falls of 24 feet

or higher.[12] In either situation, it is apparent that abdominal injuries (e.g., liver and kidney injury) are rare in comparison to the occurrence of fractures in most series.[7] We also did not find a direct correlation between height of fall and isolated brain injury, similar to other researchers, who found that among 146 deaths, the severity of brain injury was not related to the height of fall.[6] There also appears to be a direct relation between major and multiple injuries and height of fall. The percentage of major injuries in falls between the second and fifth floor increased proportionately from 26% to 88%. However, one of the two children falling from the sixth floor sustained only a minor injury, emphasizing again that variables rule out an absolute relation between these two factors. Furthermore, a comparison of injuries and death in relation to age showed no direct rela-

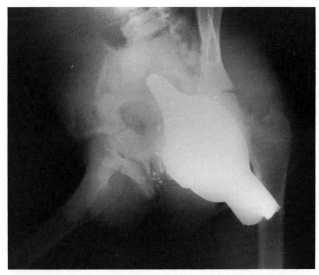

FIGURE 31–6

Radiograph of a 12-year-old boy who fell from a roof four stories high and landed on a picket fence. He arrived in the emergency department with the broken-off fence tip embedded in his pelvis and major pelvic perineal injuries, including a torn rectum, which necessitated a colostomy. Other injuries included a hemopneumothorax and radioulnar fractures.

tion; these findings were shown by other researchers as well (Fig. 31–7).[2]

There are contradictory reports comparing the child's greater propensity to sustain fatal injuries when falling the same distance as an adult. Barlow and associates showed that in falls from the fifth and sixth floors, the pediatric death rate was 55%, whereas adults had a 50% mortality rate with falls from the third and fourth floors.[2] A similar report showed not only a higher percentage of survivors in the 1- to 4-year-old age group, but also fewer injuries.[13] These findings are diametrically opposed to those of Reynolds and associates, who found that the mortality rate was highest in children younger than 5 years of age and in adults older than 51 years of age.[10]

Despite the large number of fractures sustained by children in our series and others, calcaneal fractures are relatively rare in children. Body orientation, which in children is affected by their relatively large head, which may change their center of gravity, is probably different from that generally found in the adult; this could explain the children's greater number of skull fractures and upper extremity fractures, which may be secondary to an attempt at breaking the fall with the hands. In children whose body position was known at the time of impact, feet-first impaction appeared to be well tolerated.[13]

Although vertebral fractures do occur in children as well as in adults, usually as second-impact injuries, cervical fractures are less common in the child than in the adult. There was only one cervical spine fracture in our series. The flexible cartilaginous skeletal structure and thicker layers of subcutaneous fat of the child, which provide better protection to internal structures, are thought to contribute to the child's improved tolerance of falls. Although other researchers have assumed that the flexible chest is the reason for the relative paucity of pulmonary injuries in children who have fallen from heights, our experience does not substantiate this.

It has also been assumed in the past that a child's recuperative power is nearly miraculous, and that most children recover without sequelae from their injuries. It is likely, however, that a lack of follow-up care may be the main reason for this overly optimistic appraisal, because significant CNS sequelae may persist.

Diagnosis and Therapy

Diagnosis and resuscitation of the child who falls from a height is no different from that of any other pediatric trauma victim. It should be stressed, however, that the sudden deceleration that occurs from a fall from a height leads not only to injuries in the primary impact area but also to secondary and tertiary impact injuries, which must be carefully ruled out. If height, impact area, and body position are known, probable sequential injuries can be expected and looked for. Because the number of major or multiple injuries increases in relation to the height of fall, all children who fall from heights of three stories or more can be expected to have major and often multiple injuries and should therefore be transported to the closest trauma center rather than to the nearest available institution. This should not be difficult, because the most likely site of these types of accidents is in an urban setting, where appropriate pediatric trauma facilities should be available.

The frequency of major injuries becomes apparent if the resuscitative or operative measures necessary in the children in our study are considered: six children required early craniotomy, three required laparotomies, and one required a thoracotomy. Eleven children required thoracostomy tubes; 51 children, more than half of whom were intubated,

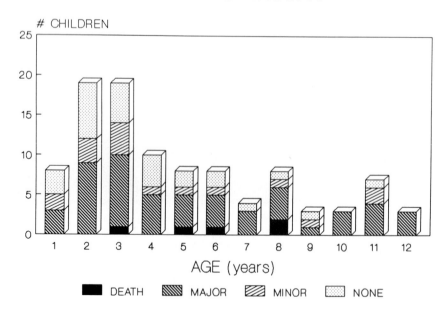

FALLS FROM HEIGHTS
AGE AND INJURY

FIGURE 31–7

A comparison of the injuries and deaths in relation to the age of the 99 children mentioned in Figure 31–3 showed that there is no statistically significant relationship.

were either treated or observed in a pediatric surgical intensive care unit.

An example of a patient who sustained multiple injuries following a fall is shown in Figure 31–6. The abdominal film was obtained on admission from a 12-year-old African-American boy who had fallen off a fourth-story roof while throwing eggs at passing cars. The child landed on the tip of an iron fence, which, fortunately for the child, broke off, and he was admitted with the tip of the fence imbedded in his pelvis. He sustained major perineal, rectal, and pelvic injuries, including sacroiliac separation, hemopneumothorax, and radioulnar fractures. The patient underwent extensive operative correction with colostomies, pelvic-perineal débridement, and external pelvic fixation after a left thoracostomy tube was inserted.

PREVENTION

Our review of traumatic death in urban children in 1977[2] and our recent review revealed similar findings: The most likely child to sustain death or injury from a fall from a height is the young African-American or Hispanic boy living in a ghetto area. The toddler is the most common victim. Because modifying the child's behavior is difficult and socioeconomic circumstances are not likely to change rapidly, other solutions must be sought. One of the most important contributing factors responsible for injuries and deaths due to falls can often be eliminated with minimal cost: the fall from a window. An effective program that has reduced both the morbidity and mortality of falls from windows was instituted through the New York City Board of Health in 1976, leading to the first child accident prevention law of its kind in the nation.[14] This law requires owners of multistory dwellings to provide window guards in apartments in which children 10 years of age or younger reside. The law was preceded by an educational prevention program, "Children Can't Fly," implemented by the New York City Health Department in the Bronx after it was recognized that falls from heights are responsible for at least 12% of all accidental deaths among children younger than 15 years of age. The program was extended to all five boroughs of New York City, and most hospital emergency departments and all police precincts started to monitor the incidence of falls from windows. More than 16,000 free window guards were distributed each year. These window guards were purchased by the New York City Health Department for less than $3 per window guard, and the installation of these guards led to a 50% decline in falls from windows in the Bronx and a city-wide decrease of 31% from the 1973 to 1975 rates. The Harlem experience was even more dramatic, with a 90% decrease in accidental falls.[2] Seventeen full-time window-guard inspectors work under the director of the Window Fall Prevention Program, and in 1986, nearly $1.4 million in fines were levied against violators.[4] Thousands of window fall prevention program flyers were distributed in English, Spanish, Creole, French, Korean, Hindu and Farsi, informing tenants of the code requirement. The decline of mortalities, with 31 fewer deaths in 1987 as in the same period in 1986, has continued. Unexpected resistance has occurred. Some parents have interpreted the law as an indictment of their ability to care for their children and, therefore, have rejected window guards. Other parents removed the window guards because it prevented them from hanging clothing out to dry or it required them to take down plants. However, parents who interfere with the installation of guards can be held liable, and 580 tenants were warned in 1987 that they may have violated the code and may be liable for prosecution because they either refused to allow guards to be installed or removed them.

Our review showed that the number of deaths due to falls from heights in Brooklyn has also declined; however, the number of children admitted to our service with injuries due to falls does not appear to have changed significantly. The reason is probably related to the type of housing available in Brooklyn, which, in contrast to that in the Bronx and Harlem, consists predominantly of two- to four-story buildings, which are not included in the code. When reviewing our statistics, it is apparent that a large number (71 of 99) of children fell from three stories or less, a scenario that is compatible with a small house not under the jurisdiction of the city regulations.

Despite the large number of major injuries, particularly CNS injuries, only five deaths occurred. The positive outcome in the majority of children is reminiscent of the first recorded fall from a window, described in the New Testament of the Bible, Acts, chapter 20, verse 9. Eutychus, one of St. Paul's disciples, fell asleep during one of St. Paul's sermons, which continued past midnight, and fell from a third-story window and was presumed to be dead. St. Paul promptly interrupted his sermon to look after Eutychus, who responded to St. Paul's efforts. He got up and walked away, to the "not little comfort of his friends."

Acknowledgment

The author would like to thank Ms. Janet Runcie, pediatric surgical physician assistant, who compiled the data and analyses of the 99 children who were admitted to the pediatric surgical service after falls from heights between 1983 and 1987.

References

1. Ayuyao A, Samuels H, Al-Sawwaf M, et al: Fall from heights: Injuries and results of management. Presented at the New York Surgical Society, November 11, 1987.
2. Barlow B, Niemirska M, Gandhi R, et al: Ten years of experience with falls from a height in children. J Pediatr Surg 18(4):509–511, 1983.
3. Bergner L, Mayer S, Harris D: Falls from heights: A childhood epidemic in an urban area. Am J Public Health 61(1):90–96, 1971.
4. Cincotti JA: New York gets tough on window guard law. The New York Times, August 25, 1987.
5. Cummins BH, Potter JM: Head injury due to falls from heights. Injury 2(1):61–64, 1970.
6. Goonetilleke UKDA: Injuries caused by falls from heights. Med Sci Law 20(4):262–275, 1980.
7. Gupta SM, Chandra J, Dogra TD: Blunt force lesions related to the heights of a fall. Am J Forensic Med Pathol 3(1):35–43, 1982.
8. Lewis WS, Lee AB, Grantham SA: "Jumpers Syndrome": The trauma of high free fall as seen at Harlem Hospital. J Trauma 5(6):812–818, 1965.

9. Ramenofsky ML: Pediatric abdominal trauma. Pediatr Ann 16(4):318–326, 1987.

10. Reynolds BM, Balsano NA, Reynolds FX: Falls from heights: A surgical experience of 200 consecutive cases. Ann Surg 174(2):304–308, 1971.

11. Sieben RL, Leavitt JD, French JH: Falls as childhood accidents: An increasing urban risk. Pediatrics 47(5):886–892, 1971.

12. Smith MD, Burrington JD, Woolf AD: Injuries in children sustained in free falls: An analysis of 66 cases. J Trauma 15(11):987–991, 1975.

13. Snyder RG: Human tolerances to extreme impacts in free-fall. Aerospace Medicine 34(8):695–709, 1963.

14. Spiegel CN, Lindaman FC: Children can't fly: A program to prevent childhood morbidity and mortality from window falls. Am J Public Health 67(12):1143–1147, 1977.

15. Velcek FT, Weiss A, DiMaio D, et al: Traumatic death in urban children. J Pediatr Surg 12(3):375–384, 1977.

Ann M. Kosloske

Foreign Bodies

Children are naturally curious individuals, and between the ages of 6 months and 3 years, they test new objects, both edible and inedible, by putting them into their mouths. Such objects become foreign bodies when they accidentally fall into the airway or are swallowed. A foreign body is defined as "a mass or particle of material which is not normal to the place where it is found."[27] Aspiration of or swallowing a foreign body is probably the second most common pediatric accident after minor lacerations and contusions in the United States, although there are no statistics to document this. Some children may not even come to medical attention if the aspirated object is coughed out immediately or if the swallowing episode is not observed and the object passes innocuously. Many a parent has been amazed, on changing a diaper, to discover a penny in the stool of an asymptomatic infant. Hospitalization for aspirated foreign bodies is usually brief; most persons who swallow foreign bodies are treated on an outpatient basis. Foreign body accidents are nevertheless serious and potentially fatal. In 1982 in the United States, 341 deaths were reported in children under 5 years of age from choking on food or foreign objects.[2] The majority of fatalities occur in infants younger than 13 months of age who choke on an object that blocks the larynx or upper trachea or in children younger than 4 years of age who asphyxiate from a piece of hot dog.[41, 101] Fatalities represent the tip of the iceberg of this common pediatric calamity.

HISTORY

Perhaps the most ancient reference to foreign body extraction is in the fable of Aesop (600 BC), who told of a crane who placed his head in the mouth of a wolf to remove a bone lodged in the wolf's esophagus.[52] St. Blaise, Bishop of Sebaste (300 AD), saved a boy from suffocation by plucking a thorn from his throat and is revered as the "patron of persons afflicted with throat problems."[52] Paulus Aegineta, in the seventh century, described a method of removing fish bones and other objects caught in the throat. The patient swallowed a soft, clean sponge on a string, which was allowed to expand in the stomach and then was withdrawn.[39] Crude extraction methods for an esophageal foreign body that could not be pushed into the stomach included inserting a finger through the mouth and using forceps, hooks or a probang (a whisklike extractor made of wire or horsehair) passed blindly.[45] Louis Jourdan, in 1819, described esophagotomy via a cervical incision for extraction of impacted esophageal probang foreign bodies.[45] Until this century, a foreign body impacted in the airway or esophagus of a child was often synonymous with death from eventual suppuration or erosion into adjacent vascular structures.

The first real attempt at endoscopic examination was in 1806 by Bozzini, who used a tin tube lighted by a wax candle, with a mirror as a reflector.[9] Modern endoscopy had its beginnings with Kussmaul's demonstration in 1868 of the possibilities of the esophagoscope and the gastroscope. His subject was a professional sword swallower.[45] By 1881, Mikulicz had developed a technique of esophagoscopy and a method of lighting the rigid tube, using a red-hot platinum wire lamp.[45] In 1897, Gustav Killian removed a foreign body from a bronchus, using a primitive bronchoscope. In the early 1900s, Chevalier Jackson elevated bronchoscopy to an art and a science, accumulating an extraordinary amount of personal experience, and founding a school for bronchoesophagology.[50, 51, 57] For nearly a century, endoscopic extractions were by the open tube bronchoscope or esophagoscope. A new era for pediatric endoscopy began in the early 1970s, following the invention by Hopkins of a rod-lens optical system for telescopes, which enabled the development of miniature endoscopes with capabilities never before possible.[31] The first bronchoscopy and esophagoscopy in a neonate, using Hopkins telescopes and fiberoptic lighting, was performed by Gans and Berci at the Cedars of Lebanon Hospital in Los Angeles in January 1970, resulting in the introduction of these instruments into pediatric surgical practice.[34]

MANAGEMENT OF THE CHOKING CHILD

The child who has choked on a piece of food or other foreign object yet can breathe and speak should be taken immediately to a hospital. Back blows or other maneuvers to dislodge the object are necessary only if the object is so large (or the child so small) that it occludes the upper airway, a rare event. If the child is cyanotic and cannot breathe or speak, the adult should quickly look into the back of the throat and remove any visible object that may be caught there; however, blind finger sweeps in the back of the pharynx should be avoided because they may push an impacted foreign body farther down into the airway. Mouth-to-mouth resuscitation is not effective if the upper airway is completely occluded.

The Heimlich maneuver should be carried out in children who are asphyxiating, except in those younger than 1 year of age. The maneuver may be applied in one of two ways: in the first, with the child in a standing or sitting position, the rescuer stands behind the child, wraps both arms around the child, and gives a sharp upward and inward thrust with the fist just above the umbilicus.[90] The thrust may be repeated six to 10 times until the object is expelled. The Heimlich maneuver may also be done with the child supine and the rescuer kneeling beside him. The Heimlich maneuver in small children must be applied gently because of the risk of injury to intra-abdominal organs by upper abdominal thrusts.

Choking infants younger than 1 year of age should be treated initially by a combination of back blows and chest thrusts.[35, 90] The infant is positioned with the head lower than the trunk across the adult's lap and given four brisk back blows with the heel of the hand between the infant's shoulder blades. If breathing does not resume, the infant is turned over and given four brisk sternal compressions.

Controversy concerning the most effective management of the choking child has surfaced, however. The recommendations outlined earlier are those for pediatric basic life support of the 1985 National Conference on Cardiopulmonary Resuscitation and Emergency Cardiac Care.[90] Previously, the Accident and Poison Prevention Committee of the American Academy of Pediatrics had recommended back blows and chest thrusts as the initial treatment for choking children because of the risk of injury to the upper abdominal organs from applying the Heimlich maneuver too roughly, particularly in children younger than 1 year of age.[35, 70] I personally treated a 9-year-old boy who sustained a cervical esophageal perforation after a successful Heimlich maneuver applied by his mother when he was choking on a bologna sandwich. His fever, neck pain, and cervical emphysema resolved completely after a brief hospitalization for antibiotic treatment. The site of perforation was not visible on contrast radiographs or endoscopy. The complication seemed a small price to pay for life, since on two previous occasions I pronounced young children who had choked on hot dogs dead on arrival in the emergency department.

Fortunately, the choking episode is rarely severe enough to require heroic measures at the scene. The child may be wheezing or gagging but can breathe well enough to make it to the hospital, where a variety of ingenious techniques are available for the removal of foreign objects under controlled conditions.

FOREIGN BODIES IN THE AIRWAY

Etiology

Eighty percent of children who aspirate foreign bodies are younger than 3 years of age.[12, 85] Children at this age lack molar teeth to chew nuts finely enough to swallow them, and many, particularly the older ones, are laughing or running with the object in their mouth at the moment of choking.[101] Peanuts and other nuts account for about half of all the foreign bodies aspirated by children throughout the world, documented from the United States, Canada, Australia, Japan, and the former Federal Republic of Germany.[12, 23, 58, 60, 69, 80, 85, 86, 96, 103] In reports from Kuwait and Turkey, however, the majority of foreign bodies aspirated were melon seeds, because in Arab countries, seeds are saved from watermelons and then are dried, salted, and roasted; the kernel is eaten after removal of the shell.[1, 6] After peanuts, other commonly aspirated foreign bodies include small vegetable fragments, pins, toys and plastic fragments, seeds, popcorn, and an infinite variety of objects. Table 32–1 gives the array of tracheobronchial foreign bodies encountered in our own series.

The objects aspirated reflect the environment and the times. Safety pins, which were a common airway foreign body in Jackson's day, are rarely encountered now in the United States, probably owing to the advent of the disposable diaper.[50]

It is generally taught that in an upright patient aspiration of a foreign body is more likely into the right main stem bronchus than the left. Jackson and Jackson explained the right-sided predominance as follows[51]: (1) the greater diameter of the right bronchus, (2) the lesser angle of deviation from the tracheal axis of the right bronchus than that of the left bronchus, (3) the situation of the carina to the left of the midline of the trachea, (4) the action of the trachealis muscles, and (5) the greater volume of air going

Table 32–1

Types of Foreign Bodies Aspirated by 129 Children in New Mexico, 1976–1987

Foreign Body	No. of Children (%)
Peanut or other nut	64 (50)
Husk, seed, bean	24 (19)
Plastic toy or toy fragment	7 (5)
Raw carrot, apple, potato	6 (5)
Popcorn	4 (3)
Stone	3 (2)
Chicken bone	2 (1.5)
Pen or pencil cap	2 (1.5)
Pin	2 (1.5)
Amorphous debris	2 (1.5)
Miscellaneous*	13 (10)
TOTAL	129 (100)

*One each of aluminum foil, cinder, crayon, earring, juniper twig, magnet, orange peel, screw, Styrofoam, thistle, timothy grass, trail mix, tumbleweed tuft.

into the right bronchus on inspiration. However, the Jacksons' series contained a large number of adults with foreign bodies, and recent reports in children have challenged this assumption, because approximately half have shown a left-sided predominance (Table 32–2). Saijo and colleagues' series of 110 cases from Japan showed a right-sided predominance in adults and a left-sided predominance in children younger than 6 years of age, especially in the cases that involved peanuts.[86] Adriani and Griggs's postmortem study showed that both the right and the left main stem bronchi branch from the trachea at an angle of approximately 55 degrees in all children up to 3 years of age.[3] However, this report contradicts Noback's earlier measurements of autopsy specimens of fetal, neonatal, and pediatric airways that showed a greater angulation on the left, averaging 42 degrees from the midsagittal plane, approximately twice the angulation on the right.[74] In personal observations at bronchoscopy in young children, the left main bronchus takes off at an angle similar to the right but then curves sharply laterally. The pediatric airway is exceedingly dynamic, and factors in addition to the bronchial angle from the axis probably determine the final site of lodgment of the aspirated foreign body.

Two thirds of the aspirators of foreign bodies are boys, and this appears not to have changed over the years.[12, 69, 80] Pyman commented that the male predominance was "probably because of their more adventurous and inquisitive natures," although girls may simply be more obedient or better coordinated.[80]

Diagnosis

Emergency "crash" bronchoscopy is rarely necessary in children who have aspirated a foreign body. Usually there is time to take a history, perform a physical examination, obtain radiographs, and prepare the patient for general anesthesia. Only 3 to 6% of children require immediate bronchoscopy because of acute respiratory distress, usually from a laryngeal or tracheal obstruction.[85, 96] However, Vane and associates emphasized the importance of preoperative and

Table 32-2
Anatomic Location of Aspirated Foreign Bodies in Children

Series (Year)	No. of Children	Right Side (%)	Left Side (%)	Larynx, Trachea or Bilateral (%)
Abdulmajid, et al* (1976)[1]	247	173 (70)	32 (13)	42 (17)
Saijo, et al (1979)[86]	89	29 (33)	36 (40)	24 (27)
Cohen, et al (1980)[23]	143	55 (38)	62 (43)	26 (19)
Keith, et al (1980)[58]	33	15 (45)	17 (52)	1 (3)
Rothman and Boeckman (1980)[85]	225	102 (45)	100 (44)	23 (10)
Wiseman (1984)[103]	157	76 (48)	60 (38)	21 (13)
Vane, et al (1988)[96]	119	39 (33)	70 (59)	10 (8)
This series (1988)	129	63 (49)	54 (42)	12 (9)

*Melon seeds (70%) predominated in this series; peanuts and other nuts predominated in all other series.

intraoperative monitoring, because *all* children suffer from some respiratory embarrassment from their aspiration episode, although some may appear to be clinically stable.[96] If the child has a full stomach, it is safer to defer bronchoscopy for a few hours than to risk aspiration of gastric contents under general anesthesia.

Inhalation of a foreign body triggers a violent cough reflex initially, but the child may have ceased coughing before arrival at the hospital. Pyman described the mechanism of a latency period following the inhalation of a foreign body.[80] Surface sensory receptors of the respiratory tract undergo normal physiologic adaptation to prolonged pressure once the foreign body becomes lodged in the airway. Coughing may cease until other sensory receptors are stimulated, either by movement of the foreign body or by production of secretions, which seep up along the airways. The latency period may vary from hours to years. Pyman documented a misleading latency period, which often caused delayed diagnosis, in 10% of his series of 230 children.[80]

On physical examination, the classical physical findings are unilateral decreased breath sounds from decreased aeration of the lung and unilateral rhonchi or wheezes from partial occlusion of a bronchus. Most children are breathing rapidly, however, and often are crying, and the rhonchi and wheezes may be transmitted over both sides of the chest. In a study of 157 children with foreign body aspiration, Wiseman evaluated the clinical triad of wheezing, cough, and diminished or absent breath sounds. Three fourths of the children had one or more of the triad, but the triad was complete in only 39% of the children. Those diagnosed late (after 1 day of aspiration) were more likely to have the complete triad than those diagnosed early (47% vs. 31%).[103]

Chest radiographs should be obtained with frontal views on inspiration and expiration, plus a lateral view. Because only approximately 10% of aspirated foreign bodies are radiopaque, the radiographic diagnosis is based on changes brought about by the unilateral obstruction of a bronchus. The classic abnormality is unilateral emphysema, which may be subtle on the inspiratory view but obvious on the expiratory view (Fig. 32–1). Air is trapped because of the ball-valve effect of an incomplete but a high-grade obstruction of a bronchus. Air enters the affected lung on inspiration but cannot escape on expiration. Unilateral air trapping may also be documented by decubitus views of the chest, in which the dependent lung remains abnormally hyperin-

flated or by chest fluoroscopy. About one fourth of children have atelectasis or infiltrates from total occlusion of a bronchus. Sometimes the radiographic findings are completely normal; however, normal findings do not obviate the need for bronchoscopy if either the history or the physical examination is suggestive of or consistent with foreign body aspiration. Because the radiographic findings depend on unilateral bronchial obstruction, either a tracheal foreign body or bilateral bronchial foreign bodies may be associated with completely symmetric radiographic findings.[71] Furthermore, migration of a foreign body within the airways may produce changing physical and radiographic findings. Hence, when foreign body aspiration is suspected in a child, there is no substitute for a careful history and physical examination; a positive history alone is an indication to proceed with bronchoscopy.

In 10 to 15% of children with foreign bodies in the airway, the aspiration episode was not observed by an adult or a reliable observer. The child presents with unexplained wheezing or pneumonia days or even weeks after aspiration. The adage "all that wheezes is not asthma" is particularly applicable to a 1- or 2-year-old child. Bronchoscopy should be considered for unexplained or persistent wheezing or for pneumonia that fails to clear with appropriate treatment.

The symptoms of laryngotracheal foreign bodies differ from those of bronchial foreign bodies. Esclamado and Richardson evaluated 20 children with laryngotracheal foreign bodies in whom a history of choking was obtained in 90%. The most common presenting symptoms were stridor, wheezing, sternal retractions, and cough. Findings on the chest radiograph were normal in 58%; however, views of the neck suggested the diagnosis in 92%. The normal findings on the chest radiographs led to an initial misdiagnosis of croup in almost half the children. Two thirds of the children with delayed diagnosis had subsequent complications, usually subglottic edema, which required intubation or tracheostomy.[29]

Intervention

Bronchoscopy

Instruments and Anesthesia. Rigid bronchoscopy is the standard treatment for aspirated foreign bodies in children.

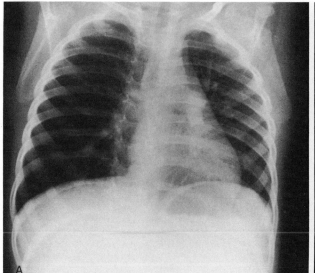
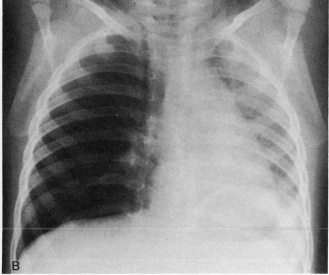
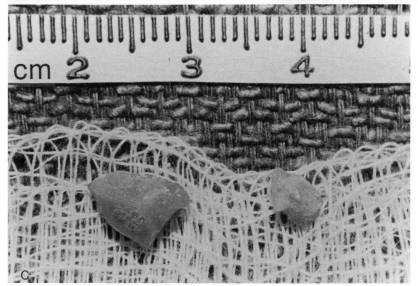

FIGURE 32–1

Peanut aspiration in a 19-month-old boy. The inspiratory posteroanterior view (*A*) shows good aeration of both lungs, but the expiratory view (*B*) shows emphysema on the right, atelectasis on the left, and mediastinal shift to the left. At bronchoscopy, two peanut fragments (*C*) were removed from the right main stem bronchus.

The state-of-the-art instruments for extraction are the pediatric bronchoscopes employing the Hopkins rod-lens system, manufactured by the Karl Storz Company. The Hopkins optical system reverses the traditional arrangement of lenses in a telescope, utilizing instead a glass rod with lens-shaped air spaces. This ingenious telescope has a larger viewing angle, increased light transmission, and exceedingly good resolution.[31] The telescopes have been miniaturized to permit endoscopy in newborn infants, even in premature infants. Endoscopic extraction of foreign bodies is accomplished more accurately because of the excellent view of the object throughout the extraction process (Fig. 32–2). The instrument for extraction, which is passed through the instrument channel or is incorporated into the bronchoscopic sheath, does not impede the view.

Flexible fiberoptic bronchoscopes are now available in small sizes but are not recommended for extraction of foreign bodies from the pediatric airway.[56, 99] Flexible endoscopes have no channel for ventilation, and the most important principle in removal of a foreign body is to maintain an adequate airway while extracting the foreign body atraumatically.[32] Wood and Gauderer suggested that flexible bronchoscopy be performed to screen for foreign bodies in children who have a history of choking or aspiration but inconsistent physical or radiographic findings.[104] This approach, however, has been controversial because two bronchoscopies were then required in infants in whom a foreign body was found. Gauderer has since abandoned this approach (personal communication).

The bronchoscopic extraction of a foreign body is a delicate procedure that should be performed by an endoscopist and an anesthesiologist experienced in the management of the pediatric airway. The first chance to remove a foreign body is usually the best chance.[32] If expert pediatric endoscopy is not available in a community, the child with an aspirated foreign body should be transferred to a center in which such expertise is available.

In preparation for general anesthesia, an intravenous infusion should be begun. An antibiotic, usually penicillin or ampicillin, should be given if the foreign body has been

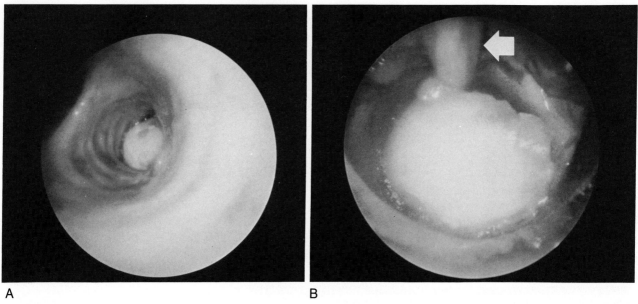

A   B

FIGURE 32–2

A, A peanut in the bronchus intermedius, viewed by the Hopkins telescope, appears six times larger than when viewed through the open tube bronchoscope. *B,* The same peanut in close-up during extraction by a Fogarty catheter (*arrow*) that has been passed beyond the peanut.

present for more than 24 hours or if the child has signs and symptoms of pneumonia. Atropine should always be given before bronchoscopy for foreign body extraction to help reduce secretions, and monitoring devices to be used should include electrocardiogram, blood pressure, and pulse oximeter. Induction of general anesthesia is usually begun using a combination of inhalation agents and oxygen with intravenous muscle relaxants. The bronchoscope is inserted and the extraction procedure begun.

Extraction. The shape and type of foreign body determine the optimal instrument for extraction. For peanuts, the most commonly aspirated foreign body, many endoscopists prefer the optical forceps.[12, 96] This grasping forceps is built into the outer sheath of the bronchoscope, permitting removal of the peanut under magnified direct view. The Fogarty catheter technique is my preference, and that of others, for removal of peanuts and other spherical foreign bodies from the tracheobronchial tree (Fig. 32–3).[59–61, 76] After the catheter is passed beyond the foreign body, the balloon is inflated with just enough saline to draw the peanut into the tip of the bronchoscope, under direct vision. An important feature of the technique is the withdrawal of the telescope and inner sheath back 1 cm into the outer sheath of the bronchoscope to create a protected space to hold the peanut securely during extraction (see Fig. 32–3). The peanut usually comes out intact, even when it has become swollen and mushy after more than 24 hours in the pediatric airway.

Seeds, husks, and other flat foreign bodies with an edge are extracted by forceps. Flat objects grasped by the optical forceps should be rotated to a vertical position to prevent being ''stripped off'' by the vocal cords during withdrawal. Alternatively, objects grasped by the fine foreign body forceps may be sheathed within the tip of the bronchoscope by withdrawal of the telescope and inner sheath about 1 cm

within the outer sheath. Occasionally, the foreign body falls back into the pharynx just as the bronchoscope passes the vocal cords. The endoscopist should insert the laryngoscope quickly and remove the foreign body with Magill forceps. Good communication between the endoscopist and the anesthesiologist is essential throughout the procedure. Whenever the oxygen saturation level falls, attempts at endoscopic removal of the foreign object become of secondary importance to ventilation of the patient; adjustments of the bronchoscopic and ventilation equipment should be made until oxygenation returns to normal, at which time extraction efforts can resume.

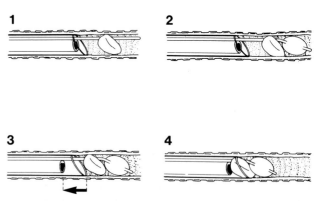

FIGURE 32–3

The Fogarty catheter technique. (1) The catheter is passed beyond the peanut. (2) The balloon is inflated. (3) The peanut is drawn into the tip of the bronchoscope. A small hollow (*arrow*) is created by withdrawal of the telescope about 1 cm. (4) The removal of the peanut between the bronchoscope and the Fogarty catheter. (Reprinted with permission from Kosloske AM: The Fogarty balloon technique for removal of foreign bodies from the tracheobronchial tree. Surg Gynecol Obstet (now J Am Coll Surg) 155:72–73, 1982.)

The Fogarty catheter technique for removal of objects from the airway was first described by Ullyot and Norman in 1968, who demonstrated it in anesthetized dogs.[95] Cases of its successful use were reported in the 1970s, both in an adult and in children using the open-tube bronchoscope and, subsequently, using the new endoscopes with the Hopkins telescopes.[13, 33, 42, 47, 55, 87, 91] Spheric objects are drawn into the tip of the bronchoscope, and beads that are impacted in the airway may be removed after passage of the Fogarty catheter through the hole in the bead.[43, 61, 88, 100] Cohen, however, considered the technique "inappropriate" and "unwarranted" because of a complication in a 19-month-old infant during extraction of a peanut.[24] In this instance the tip of the Fogarty catheter broke off in the right upper lobe and had to be removed under the image intensifier. Other isolated cases of catheters breaking have occurred, probably owing to incorrect usage or a defective product. The catheter and balloon should, of course, be tested before usage. The risk of fragmentation of a peanut with forceps is probably much greater than the risk of a broken catheter. The Fogarty technique has generally proved to be safe and effective, it is easily mastered by students of endoscopy, and is the preferred method of spheric foreign body extraction from the airway by many.[59, 60, 61, 76]

Mantel and Butenandt described an "encasing" technique for removal of crumbly nuts from the airway. With the child under deep relaxation anesthesia, the bronchoscope, with optics drawn back to create a hollow in its tip, was rotated over the foreign body. Then the operating table was tilted head down and the bronchoscope and encased nut were removed. They used the technique "with good results" in 84 of the 224 children in their series.[69] A related technique that used gravity advantageously for removal of small round foreign bodies was reported by Rothman and Boeckman.[85]

Although most foreign bodies are removed successfully from the pediatric airway by forceps or Fogarty catheter, a few objects, such as sharp stones or large screws, may defy extraction by standard methods. Employing the Dormia basket or other grasping forceps may be successful.[56, 60] The ingenuity of the endoscopist and familiarity with the pediatric airway continue to be more important than the type of forceps used.

The Inhalation–Postural Drainage Method

In the early 1970s, a Denver group employed a nonendoscopic method for removal of foreign bodies aspirated into the airways of children. This technique consisted of inhalation of a bronchodilator, followed by a postural drainage–percussion treatment carried out for 5 minutes of every hour throughout the day.[25] They recommended endoscopy if the postural drainage was unsuccessful after 4 days. Although the initial report with this technique was promising (seven out of eight infants coughed out the foreign body), complications in subsequent infants included two cardiopulmonary arrests.[17, 25] Furthermore, a review of 49 children treated by this method showed that it was successful in only 25% of infants.[64] Bronchoscopy returned to favor in Denver after the introduction of the improved pediatric bronchoscopic instruments. The Denver group in 1982 recommended a 24-hour trial of the inhalation–postural drainage technique only for cases involving peripheral foreign bodies and appears to have abandoned the technique completely in favor of bronchoscopy.[20, 26]

Special Methods for Very Large or Very Small Foreign Bodies

Rarely, an object lodged in the trachea is too large to withdraw without risking injury to the vocal cords. A good technique for such situations was described by Swensson and associates, who treated five such children, three of whom had aspirated indwelling tracheal T-tubes (Montgomery tubes). With the ventilating bronchoscope in place, a tracheostomy was performed. The foreign body was grasped with a forceps, brought from the carina to the level of the tracheostomy, and extracted via the tracheostoma with a forceps.[93]

Small peripheral foreign bodies may become impacted in segmental bronchi, beyond the reach of the bronchoscope. A No. 3 Fogarty catheter may be used to dislodge the object, after which it can be grasped by a forceps or other instrument.[33, 42, 55] Even when foreign bodies are out of sight, they may be retrieved endoscopically in most cases. Hight and co-workers described the use of fluoroscopy, endobronchial contrast material, topical vasoactive medications, and diverse retrieval instruments in eight such cases, which obviated the need for either bronchotomy or segmental pulmonary resection.[43]

Long-Term Foreign Bodies

Inhaled foreign objects produce focal bronchitis. The inflammatory reaction is particularly intense with peanuts and other nuts, and if the object is not removed from the airway, distal bronchiectasis and abscess formation may occur. Lobectomy for bronchiectasis, a relatively common pediatric procedure in the 1940s and 1950s, is rarely necessary today, in part because of improved methods of diagnosis and treatment of aspirated foreign bodies in children.[21]

The classic long-term foreign body is the "treacherous timothy grass," which lodges in a bronchus and may go undetected for weeks or months.[49, 54] Grass inflorescences (spiked heads) were distinguished by Hilman and colleagues into two clinical types: the lodging type, in which the grass head remains in the air passages, and the extrusive type, in which the grass head migrates distally by a ratchet effect, penetrating the lung parenchyma, pleural layers, intercostal muscles, and even extruding through the skin of the chest wall.[44] Recurrent pneumonia and hemoptysis are the hallmarks of these long-term foreign bodies. The associated bronchiectasis requires pulmonary resection for cure.[28] Bronchography is helpful in determining the extent of the disease, and wedge resection or segmental resection may be possible for preservation of normal pulmonary parenchyma; lobectomy is not always necessary.

Outcome

Bronchoscopy is usually successful in removing aspirated foreign objects. In Pyman's 1971 series, using the open-tube bronchoscope, 95% of a total of 230 foreign bodies were removed endoscopically; thoracotomy was necessary in only three cases in which the foreign body could not be removed endoscopically; and lobectomy was necessary in five other patients who had prolonged illness due to suppurative lung disease.[80] In three of these five cases, an unsuspected foreign body (grass seed) was found in the specimen. Two other children had an unsuspected foreign body found at autopsy. In series employing newer techniques and the bronchoscopes with the Hopkins rod-lens system, endoscopic failures almost never occur.[55, 69]

Children often have some degree of croup from glottic or subglottic edema following bronchoscopy, particularly if the extraction procedure has been lengthy or difficult. Tracheostomy is rarely necessary in these instances. In Rothman and Boeckman's 25-year experience with 225 children with aspirated foreign bodies, tracheostomy was performed on six patients (2.7%), three of them before removal of the foreign body, and three after endoscopic removal of the foreign body.[85] Tracheostomy is less commonly performed today.[69, 96]

The New Mexico Experience

From July 1976 through December 1987, we treated 129 children in New Mexico who had aspirated foreign bodies. Ninety-four were boys, and 35 were girls. The foreign bodies aspirated are listed in Table 32–1. The anatomic site of lodgment, showing a slight right-sided predominance (70 right vs. 60 left), is depicted in Figure 32–4. Seven children had foreign bodies in two or more sites. The duration from the time of aspiration to bronchoscopy ranged from 1 hour to 8 months, with a median of 26 hours. The children's ages ranged from 6 months to 13 years, with a median of 19 months.

Bronchoscopy was successful in extraction of the foreign body in all but three (2.3%) of the patients. The first failure of bronchoscopy was in an 8-year-old boy who required thoracotomy and bronchotomy for extraction of a pencil cap impacted in a basilar segmental bronchus. A second child required thoracotomy and segmental resection of a bronchiectatic portion of his right lower lobe, secondary to a migrating grass head, which he had aspirated 1 year earlier. The third failure was in a 2-year-old child who underwent two bronchoscopies for four separate fragments of peanut in the airways. A fragment wedged in the left upper lobe orifice could not be removed bronchoscopically, but he coughed the fragment out after the second procedure. One intraoperative complication occurred: a cardiopulmonary arrest from migration of a peanut in the airways during the extraction process resulted in hypoxic brain damage. One death occurred: a 12-month-old boy choked on a large piece of popcorn and suffered a hypoxic cardiopulmonary arrest at home. He was resuscitated in the emergency department, and ventilation was reestablished, but he remained comatose and died several days after removal of the foreign body from his airway.

Because complications in every series are rare, I suggested in 1982 that facility of the extraction procedure be considered.[60] If only one or two passes of the bronchoscope

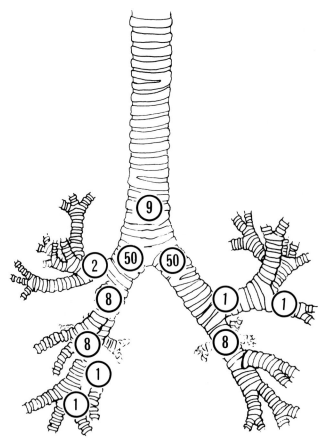

FIGURE 32–4
Anatomic sites of 139 aspirated foreign bodies in 129 children.

is necessary, the procedure is likely to be atraumatic and free of complication. At my medical center, we usually recorded in the operative note the number of passes required for removal of the foreign body. In 91 of 116 such records (78%), the object came out on the first or second pass of the bronchoscope.

After bronchoscopy, children were placed in a mist tent with 30% oxygen. Some experienced a minor degree of croup, but no child required tracheostomy. Those with purulent secretions in the airways were treated by chest physiotherapy to help clear the secretions. One child underwent bronchoscopy a second time 6 weeks later for reevaluation of a large bronchial granuloma that had surrounded the foreign body. At follow-up bronchoscopy, the granuloma had healed completely. In the 128 children who survived, there were no long-term sequelae.

FOREIGN BODIES IN THE GASTROINTESTINAL TRACT

Etiology

Most foreign objects swallowed by children traverse the gastrointestinal tract harmlessly. In 1953, Gross described a series of 766 foreign bodies swallowed by babies and children. Most of them were radiopaque, and their progress (or lack thereof) through the gastrointestinal tract could be followed by radiographs. Approximately one fourth (151) of the objects stuck in the esophagus and had to be removed endoscopically. Once the object reached the stomach, it had a 93% chance of passing unimpeded through the alimentary tract.[38] Coins, usually pennies, are the most common object swallowed by children. Table 32–3 gives the array of gastrointestinal foreign bodies encountered in my own series. Coins predominate in reports from most parts of the world, except in one report from Hong Kong of 343 children in whom fish bones slightly outnumbered coins as the most common esophageal foreign body.[73] This was attributed to the fact that the Chinese consume a considerable amount of fish and eat their fish with chopsticks.

Esophageal Foreign Bodies

The normal esophagus has four areas of anatomic narrowing: the cricopharyngeus (C6), the thoracic inlet (T1), the arch of the aorta (T5), and the diaphragmatic hiatus (T10–11). Swallowed foreign bodies tend to lodge in one of these areas, the great majority in the proximal esophagus between the cricopharyngeus and the thoracic inlet. Because the normal resting esophagus is flattened in the anteroposterior direction, radiographic orientation of a swallowed coin is characteristically flat in the frontal view and displays one edge in the lateral view (Fig. 32–5). A different orientation raises the suspicion of esophageal pathology or location outside of the esophagus.

Esophageal abnormalities, particularly if resulting from previous surgery for esophageal atresia and tracheoesophageal fistula, predispose a person to the retention of foreign

Table 32–3

Types of Foreign Bodies Swallowed by 103 Children in New Mexico, 1976–1987

Foreign Body	No. of Children (%)
Coin:	
penny	32
nickel	4
dime	4
quarter	9
half-dollar	1
unspecified	12
TOTAL COINS	62 (56)
Fruit or vegetable	6 (5)
Pin or needle	5 (4)
Fruit pit	4 (3.5)
Piece of meat	4 (3.5)
Stone	3 (3)
Marble, ball bearing	3 (3)
Tack	3 (3)
Jack	2 (2)
Metal washer	2 (2)
Jewelry	2 (2)
Battery	2 (2)
Food, unspecified	2 (2)
Miscellaneous*	10 (9)
TOTAL	110 (100)

*One each of aluminum tab, aspirin, cardboard, chicken bone, key, Monopoly piece, nail, plastic disk, screw and wing nut, staple.

bodies in the esophagus. The object almost always becomes stuck just above the esophageal anastomosis. Often there is no anastomotic stricture; the foreign body sticks because esophageal peristalsis is markedly diminished or even absent distal to the anastomosis.

Diagnosis

Usually the swallowing episode is witnessed by an adult, and the child is brought to the emergency department. The most common symptoms of an esophageal foreign body are drooling from esophageal obstruction and pain in the neck, probably from peristaltic waves and spasms. Sometimes the child with an esophageal foreign body is able to swallow liquids but spits up solids. Large esophageal foreign bodies may impinge on the airway, causing wheezing, cyanosis, or, rarely, asphyxia, especially in infants younger than 1 year of age. If an esophageal foreign body is suspected, radiographic examinations should include both frontal and lateral views of the chest and neck. It is possible to miss a cervical esophageal foreign body if the neck is not included (Fig. 32–6). If no foreign body is visible in the chest or neck, an abdominal film may identify a radiopaque foreign body that has passed into the stomach or beyond. A barium esophagogram may be helpful in the diagnosis of a food bolus or other nonradiopaque object in the esophagus. Subtle abnormalities may be identified by having the child swallow a piece of barium-soaked cotton or a marshmallow. However, there is the risk of aspiration with a barium esophagogram if the esophagus is completely occluded. In doubtful cases, a tube may be placed in the upper esophagus and small amounts of barium cautiously injected under the fluoroscope. A barium esophagogram should not be performed in children who have severe dysphagia or drooling or a dilated, air-filled esophagus on routine views of the chest. Such children should undergo prompt esophagoscopy.

Occasionally, an esophageal foreign body may go unsuspected and undetected for weeks or months. These are potentially disastrous cases in which erosion of the foreign body through the esophagus produces a paraesophageal inflammatory mass. In the neck, the mass may produce stridor and wheezing, mimicking croup. In the thorax, erosion may produce mediastinal abscess, tracheoesophageal fistula, and even fatal hemorrhage from aorticoesophageal fistula. Such cases have been reported in children from swallowing both sharp objects, such as a nutshell, and smooth foreign bodies, such as coins.[53, 72, 78] Aluminum pop tops from pull-tab cans are notorious problems because aluminum, which is faintly radiopaque, may be missed on routine views of the chest (Fig. 32–7).[16] Eroding esophageal foreign bodies may be missed on endoscopy and barium swallow; the most useful diagnostic study then becomes computed tomography (CT).[89] Remsen and colleagues, in an exhaustive literature review of 321 cases of penetrating foreign bodies, noted that most erosions occurred at the cervical esophageal level. The more distal the site of penetration, the greater the mortality because of the proximity of the thoracic esophagus to the aorta and great vessels. A fistula forms, not from direct penetration by the foreign object but from chronic

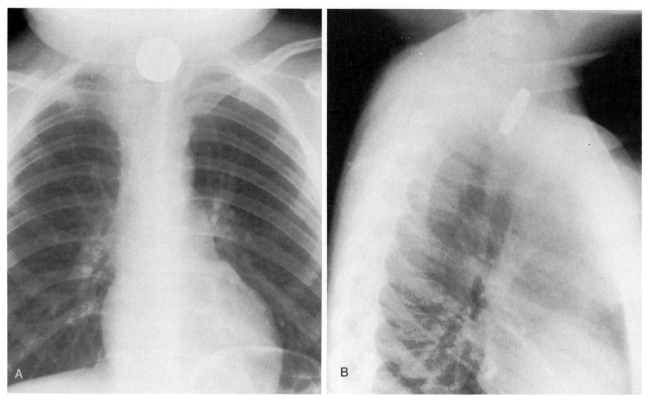

FIGURE 32–5
Two pennies in the esophagus of a 4-year-old boy on frontal view (*A*) and lateral view (*B*). Both coins were removed without difficulty, using the Foley catheter technique.

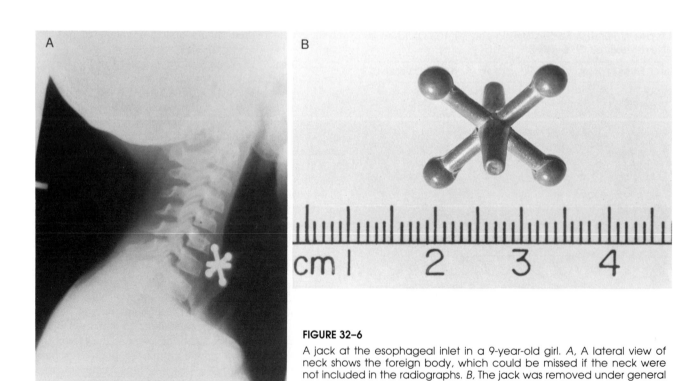

FIGURE 32–6
A jack at the esophageal inlet in a 9-year-old girl. *A,* A lateral view of neck shows the foreign body, which could be missed if the neck were not included in the radiographs. *B,* The jack was removed under general anesthesia, using the laryngoscope and Magill forceps.

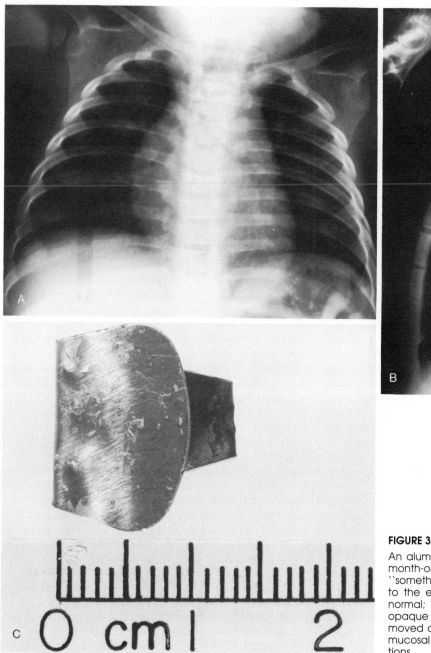

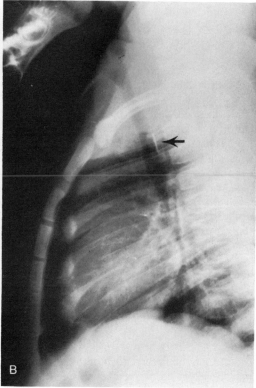

FIGURE 32–7

An aluminum pop tab in the esophagus of a 7-month-old boy, whose mother saw him put "something bright" in his mouth and brought him to the emergency room. *A,* The frontal view is normal; *B,* The lateral view shows a faint radiopaque object (*arrow*). *C,* The aluminum tab removed at esophagoscopy, which showed minor mucosal lacerations. There were no complications.

suppuration.[81] Three fourths of the thoracic erosions were fatal.

Because of the local symptoms of dysphagia and airway compression and the risk of erosion, all esophageal foreign bodies should be removed. They may be extracted or, in some cases, nudged distally into the stomach and allowed to traverse the gastrointestinal tract. Observation of esophageal foreign bodies is never appropriate until they are out of the esophagus.

Methods of Intervention

Esophagoscopy. Esophagoscopy under general anesthesia is the time-honored technique for removal of esophageal foreign bodies. It is certainly the procedure of choice for the removal of all sharp foreign bodies, which must be manipulated under direct vision to avoid esophageal perforation; for foreign bodies of unknown type; and probably for foreign bodies present for more than 48 to 72 hours.

Unless in severe distress from the esophageal foreign body, the child should be prepared for general anesthesia by waiting a few hours for gastric emptying.

The standard instruments for rigid pediatric esophagoscopy are manufactured by the Karl Storz Company and contain the Hopkins rod-lens system. The superb optics of these instruments are, in all respects, superior to those of any flexible instrument on the market.[57] The best views are provided by the endoscopes that have an inside diameter of 4.0 mm and larger and are 30 cm long. An endotracheal tube is placed to secure the airway. The infant's neck is hyperextended, and the esophagoscope is inserted. The instrument is elevated off the upper teeth by the fingers of the left hand and is held like a billiard cue. The endoscope is advanced and positioned above the foreign body, the secretions are suctioned away, and the extraction is carried out. Miniature forceps, balloons, or baskets can be passed through the instrument channel under direct vision, or the central telescope may be removed (sacrificing magnification) to permit introduction of a large forceps through the central open channel.

Coins are usually oriented transversely and, optimally, are grasped through the open tube protective outer sheath to prevent their being stripped off the forceps during withdrawal through the cricopharyngeus. Soft, organic bezoars, marbles, and other spheric objects may be dislodged and drawn into the tip of the esophagoscope, using a Fogarty catheter.[4, 57, 62] If extraction is difficult, small or smooth objects may be pushed down into the stomach, where they may be expected to progress through the gastrointestinal tract. Open safety pins pointing upward are optimally extracted by grasping the spring loop with a forceps, passing the entire pin into the stomach for a ''turnaround,'' and then extracting the pin with the open point downward.[57] After the foreign body is removed, a ''second look'' should be carried out to evaluate the esophageal mucosa and to check for additional foreign bodies.

Rigid esophagoscopy carries an overall risk of perforation near 0.34%, with a reported mortality rate of 0.05%.[84, 89] It remains, in experienced hands, the gold standard for treatment of esophageal foreign bodies.[89]

Flexible fiberoptic endoscopes may also be used for removal of esophageal foreign bodies, particularly small, embedded objects. The foreign body is grasped by appropriate alligator, cup, or tack forceps or grasping wire or basket and is removed with the fiberscope.[57] Smaller objects usually can be withdrawn through the cricopharyngeus without being stripped off the forceps. Flexible esophagoscopy may be carried out under sedation, without general anesthesia, although the pediatric patient is rarely totally cooperative.[7, 57]

Foley Catheter Technique. In 1966, Bigler reported a method of extracting smooth, impacted foreign bodies from the esophagus, using a Foley catheter. He passed the tip of the catheter beyond the foreign body under fluoroscopy, inflated the balloon, and extracted the object by gentle upward traction on the balloon. He recognized a mechanical advantage of distention of the esophagus by inflation of the balloon beneath the foreign body, which tended to free the impacted object with minimal chances for perforation, allowing safe and simple removal.[11] Others have reported favorable experiences with this method, which should be used only in children who are believed to have a normal esophagus.[18, 19, 76, 94]

The Foley catheter technique for extraction has produced controversy, however, particularly in the otolaryngologic literature.[7, 10, 67, 84] The prime objections are, first, that the extraction is an uncontrolled procedure in an unprotected airway. There is a small risk of aspiration and airway occlusion after the object has been dislodged from the esophagus. This complication occurred in the Denver series (WS Davis; personal communication) but was managed without difficulty by quick insertion of a laryngoscope and removal of the coin with forceps. Second, potentially dangerous foreign bodies may be missed. Stool and Deitch described such an instance of unsuspected multiple foreign bodies, in which three pennies, a rubber eraser, and a piece of cloth with string attached were found at esophagoscopy, surrounded by granulation.[92] They cautioned against using the Foley method, which might have missed two of the five foreign bodies or led to perforation.

We have used the Foley catheter technique safely for removal of coins from the esophagus. The method seems particularly appropriate for coins that have been swallowed within a few hours and for children with a full stomach, who might otherwise need hospital admission for preparation for general anesthesia to undergo esophagoscopy. We insist on having the following available in the radiography suite: oxygen, suction, a pediatric laryngoscope, endotracheal tubes, a bag for ventilation, and a pair of Magill forceps. The unsedated child is swaddled and placed on the side, head down, on the fluoroscopy table. A small, well-lubricated Foley catheter is passed through the mouth, and the tip is directed beyond the coin. A contrast medium (3–5 ml) is injected to inflate the balloon, and gentle traction is applied on the catheter. As the coin pops out of the esophagus, the child is turned prone, and usually the coin hits the table. Sometimes Magill forceps are necessary for removal of the coin from the pharynx.

The procedure seems safe if proper precautions are taken. It should never be attempted in a child with respiratory distress, a sharp foreign body, an abnormal esophagus, clinical or radiographic evidence of esophageal perforation, a history of more than a week of lodgment in the esophagus, or an unknown duration of lodgment. If we are not successful after two or three tries, or if we encounter any bleeding, we stop the procedure, and the child is taken to the operating room for esophagoscopy under general anesthesia.

Chemical Methods. In 1945, Richardson reported the use of papain, a proteolytic enzyme, to dissolve esophageal meat impactions.[83] The enzyme is obtained from the leaves and fruit of the papaw tree and is commercially used as a meat tenderizer. Although others have reported similar success, instances of esophageal necrosis from enzymatic digestion of the esophageal wall have occurred, with fatal sequelae.[5, 14, 46] Sharp, in a review of 90 reported cases treated by the papain method, discovered a 3% mortality rate from esophageal perforation and mentioned the technique only to condemn it.[89] I used the papain method once, 15 years ago, to dissolve a meat impaction in the distal esophagus of a 1-year-old girl who had undergone an antireflux procedure a few weeks earlier. There were no com-

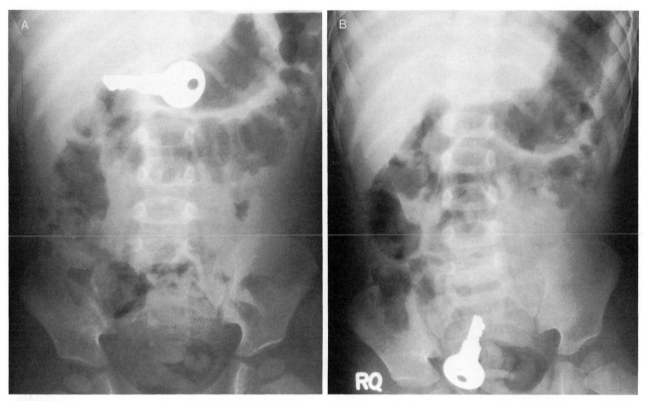

FIGURE 32-8

Uncomplicated passage of a large foreign body through the gastrointestinal tract of a 22-month-old girl. *A,* Key "unlocking" pylorus; *B,* after 24 hours it has moved into the lower intestine and was subsequently passed. She was asymptomatic.

plications, but the technique cannot be recommended for children today.

Other chemical methods have been employed for removal of food impactions from the esophagus. One technique utilized bubbles of carbon dioxide generated by a mixture of sodium bicarbonate and tartaric acid, which was instilled into the esophagus, followed by a column of barium. The procedure was monitored by fluoroscopy and was 100% successful in eight adult patients whose meat impactions were propelled into the stomach.[82] Glucagon, a hormone produced by the pancreatic islet cells, has been used for many years in radiographic procedures on the gastrointestinal tract because of its effect on the relaxation of smooth muscle. An intravenous dose of glucagon has a 50% success rate in dislodging food impactions from the esophagus and does not compromise a subsequent endoscopic procedure.[89] Chemical or fluoroscopic methods that require a cooperative patient should be used with caution in children.

Foreign Bodies in the Stomach and Intestine

General Principles of Management

Once a foreign body reaches the stomach, the chances are better than 90% that it will progress through the alimentary tract without discomfort of any sort and will be eliminated in the stool. In Gross's series of 766 foreign bodies swallowed by babies and children, the passage rate of foreign bodies that reached the stomach was 93%; surgical removal was necessary in 7% of these cases.[38] Long or sharp objects may get stuck at anatomic points of angulation or fixation, such as the "C loop" of the duodenum. Once through the ligament of Treitz, however, there is usually unobstructed movement through the rest of the gastrointestinal tract.[36]

Benson and Lloyd classified foreign objects into three groups.[8] The least dangerous and, fortunately, most common items are rounded or cuboidal foreign bodies, such as coins, small toys, marbles, and closed safety pins. These pass spontaneously and are of little concern. The second group consists of objects with sharp points, such as pins, needles, open safety pins, and tacks. These must be followed to be certain they negotiate the intestinal tract without mishap. The third group consists of long slender objects with relatively blunt points, which produce complications because of their length, such as bobby pins, toothpicks, broom bristles, and most nails (Fig. 32–8). This group has the highest risk of complication and must be followed most carefully.

Pellerin and associates documented the fate of 1250 subdiaphragmatic foreign bodies in children treated over a 17-year period at the Hôpital des Enfants Malades in Paris.[77] They endorsed "conservative management" (observation) of subdiaphragmatic foreign bodies on an outpatient basis. All but 16 (1.3%) of the objects passed spontaneously. Their operative group of 16 children included three with the unusual complication of duodenal fistula to the upper urinary tract from hairpins or sewing needles. In another child, a hairpin migrated transduodenally out the right posterior thoracic wall. The researchers found no need for repeated radiologic examinations during the early days but suggested surgical intervention if the foreign body remained within the duodenum beyond the sixth day of conservative management. The mortality rate in this remarkable series was zero.

Arterial-enteric fistulas may occur from perforation of the duodenum or jejunum by ingested foreign objects that are long and slender. This spectacular complication is usually heralded by massive gastrointestinal hemorrhage. Survivors were reported by Grosfeld and Eng and by Hambrick and co-workers.[37, 40] At operation, the foreign bodies, a whiskbroom bristle and a seamstress's needle, respectively, were removed, and both the arterial and the enteric sides of the fistula were closed.

Management of Ingestion of Alkaline Disk Batteries

Modern times are reflected by a new problem of the electronic age: the ingestion by children of miniature batteries from calculators, watches, cameras, and the like. Some hearing-impaired children have swallowed the batteries from their own hearing aids.[66] Reports of gastrointestinal perforation from these batteries have produced concern and consideration for their operative removal.[98, 102] The mechanism of injury is either from the leakage of alkali out of the battery case or, more likely, from the generation of hydroxyl ions from the tissues as a result of hydrolysis from the electrical current of an intact, active cell.

Litovitz, in an analysis of 56 ingestions of button batteries, found that the battery traversed the gastrointestinal tract without incident in 51 cases. In five cases, the button cell lodged in the esophagus, usually at the level of the cricopharyngeus. The two children who were diagnosed immediately and who underwent endoscopic removal of the battery within 6 hours recovered. Two of the three other children with delayed diagnosis died from the sequelae of esophageal and mediastinal erosion; the third survived after extensive surgery.[65] The only complications from button battery ingestion have occurred when the battery became lodged at one site and failed to progress through the gastrointestinal tract. Thus, careful observation of these children is the management of choice; operative or endoscopic intervention is rarely necessary. Specific recommendations are the following[36]:

1. The child with a history of ingestion should be given nothing by mouth until radiographs document the location of the ingested battery. Emetics should never be given.

2. If the battery is in the oropharynx or esophagus, it must be removed immediately.

3. After removal from the esophagus, observation for possible esophageal stenosis is necessary for 2 to 3 weeks.

4. If the battery is in the stomach or is further along the gastrointestinal tract, it is safe to observe the patient as one would if the patient had ingested a coin or another smooth object. Cathartics may be administered to hasten the transit time.

5. If the intact battery reaches the colon, enemas should be administered to hasten its passage.

6. If the battery fails to progress beyond a specific location in the intestine for 5 to 6 days, cathartics should be administered and an operation considered.

7. Any patient with an ingested battery in the gastrointestinal tract who becomes symptomatic, with signs of localized peritonitis or intestinal obstruction, should have the battery removed.

These recommendations do not represent a departure from the general principles applied to smooth ingested foreign objects in the gastrointestinal tract.[36]

A more aggressive approach was advocated by Ito and colleagues, who used a magnetic device to remove ingested alkaline batteries from the stomachs of 16 Japanese children. He described the method, which did not require general anesthesia, as "easy and safe."[48] Litovitz, director of a national registry that now contains more than 1500 cases of button battery ingestion (TL Litovitz, personal communication), supports the method of observation without intervention once the battery reaches the stomach. There have been only five cases of a perforated esophagus and one of a perforated Meckel diverticulum.[65, 98, 102]

Methods of Intervention

Flexible Fiberoptic Endoscopy. Foreign bodies retained in the stomach or proximal duodenum may be retrieved, using the flexible fiberoptic gastroscope and a forceps, snare, or other device. Christie and Ament used this method for coins retained in the stomach for 10 days to 5 weeks. They recommended general anesthesia for children because of inadequate sedation provided by standard endoscopy drugs.[22]

The Magnet. Equen, in 1945, described the use of an alnico magnet attached to a nasogastric tube to remove an open safety pin from the esophagus under fluoroscopic guidance.[30] Others have used such a magnetic device for retrieving pins, needles, button batteries, and other metallic objects from the stomach or proximal duodenum. A group from Germany successfully used a cylindric vacomax magnet, and a group from Japan favored a powerful rare-earth cobalt magnet.[48, 97] Magnet extraction may be performed without general anesthesia.

Celiotomy. Abdominal exploration for a swallowed foreign body is rarely necessary. Celiotomy is indicated only if there is evidence of (1) a complication, for example, perforation, peritonitis, bleeding, or obstruction that is manifested by abdominal pain and tenderness, fever, vomiting, hematemesis, or bloody stools; or (2) fixation of the foreign body in the duodenum or small intestine for more than 7 days, suggesting potential erosion and fistula formation.[77]

Foreign bodies that might normally pass can become stuck at areas of abnormal narrowing within the gastrointestinal tract. Such obstruction may occur several years after a successful pyloromyotomy or may lead to diagnosis of an underlying abnormality.[68] Fruit pit obstruction has been reported both in adults with narrowing secondary to carcinoma or ileal stricture and in children with congenital or acquired intestinal stenosis.[79] In a personal case, I operated on a 1-year-old girl with acute duodenal obstruction and found a previously undiagnosed malrotation with two recently swallowed dried apricots impacted in the duodenum beneath congenital Ladd bands. After lysis of the bands, the apricots were milked through the intact intestine and subsequently passed in the stool.

Other unique cases of foreign body ingestion that required operation have been reported. Norberg and Reyes treated a 14-month-old boy who ingested a glass Christmas tree ornament and over the next 4 months experienced multiple episodes of gastrointestinal hemorrhage, perforation, abscess, and fistula formation that required multiple operations to manage.[75] Because many children ingest glass fragments that pass through the gastrointestinal tract without doing harm, the investigators attributed the unusual behavior of the foreign body in their case to the thinness of the glass in Christmas tree ornaments, which would have produced razor-sharp, small fragments with little momentum for passage and a predisposition to perforation. Nickel dermatitis occurred in an 8-year-old boy with a history of skin sensitivity who ingested a Canadian quarter.[63] His severe, generalized rash subsided promptly after the quarter was removed from his stomach by celiotomy after endoscopic extraction failed.

Management of Foreign Bodies in Transit

Most swallowed foreign bodies can be managed on an outpatient basis. Our management protocol depends on the nature of the foreign body and the likelihood of its passage. For smooth foreign bodies, such as coins, the parents are told to examine the child's stools carefully for the next 7 days and to call when the foreign body comes out. If it is not seen in 7 days, the child returns for a repeat radiograph of the abdomen. For sharp or long foreign bodies, which are more worrisome, abdominal radiographs every 3 to 5 days are more appropriate. We do not use cathartics after foreign body ingestion because of the theoretic risk that disordered peristalsis might produce intestinal perforation from a sharp foreign body. All of the parents are, of course, told to return immediately if the child vomits or develops abdominal pain, bleeding, or other symptoms. Groff has outlined indications for intervention.[36]

A contrast upper gastrointestinal series may sometimes mobilize a foreign object that appears to be stuck in the upper gastrointestinal tract. If the foreign body is not out of the stomach in 4 weeks, it should be removed by fiberoptic endoscopy under general anesthesia. If the object is fixed in the duodenum or small intestine for more than 7 days and cannot be mobilized with cathartics or a barium meal, celiotomy should be carried out. If the object is fixed in the colon for 7 days, enemas should be administered and are usually successful.

The New Mexico Experience

A pediatric surgical practice is skewed toward swallowed foreign bodies that require intervention (see Table 32–3). Not included on our list are numerous telephone calls over the years from distant emergency departments in which,

after obtaining the essential information about type of foreign body and size of the patient, we reassured the caller that the foreign body beyond the esophagus would almost certainly pass, and as far as we know, it always did. Probably hundreds of other foreign bodies were ingested and passed without the need for a phone call.

Of the 110 swallowed foreign bodies, 93 were located in the esophagus and 17 in the subdiaphragmatic gastrointestinal tract. Of the 93 esophageal foreign bodies, two passed spontaneously into the stomach before any intervention was undertaken. Twenty-nine (28 coins, 1 metal washer) were treated by the Foley catheter method under the fluoroscope and 62 were treated by esophagoscopy. Precautions against and contraindications to the use of the Foley catheter method are described earlier in the chapter. We did not insist on a trial of the Foley catheter method for all coins or smooth foreign bodies; some attending surgeons preferred to proceed immediately to esophagoscopy. The Foley catheter method was successful in removing the foreign body from the esophagus in 26 of 29 instances. Usually, the coin popped out of the esophagus, although on a few occasions, it became dislodged, slipped down into the stomach, and passed through the gastrointestinal tract. There were no complications. The Foley catheter method failed in three children in whom coins were subsequently removed by esophagoscopy without complication.

Sixty-two children underwent esophagoscopy as the initial treatment for their esophageal foreign body. This group of foreign bodies included coins, food impactions, and all of the rough, sharp, or irregular esophageal foreign bodies. The foreign body was successfully removed at esophagoscopy in 61 of the 62 instances. One child required open extraction of an impacted plum pit via a cervical esophagotomy. One complication, an esophageal perforation, occurred during the extraction of a plum pit from a child with a previous esophageal atresia repair. This child underwent thoracotomy for repair of the perforation and made an uneventful recovery.

Fourteen of the 93 episodes of esophageal foreign body impaction occurred in eight children with a history of previous repair of esophageal atresia. A total of 12% of the infants in my medical facility with repaired esophageal atresia went on to develop episodes of foreign body impaction. The objects were usually food items, although an occasional coin or toy found its way into these esophagi as well. Two "repeaters" in the group had three episodes each of esophageal foreign bodies. Both children had no peristalsis in the distal esophagus, predisposing them to food impaction, and neither one chewed food well in spite of our instructions. One additional child with distal esophageal stenosis, probably secondary to reflux, had an impacted food bolus.

During this same period, we treated 17 children with subdiaphragmatic gastrointestinal foreign bodies who were considered at high risk for perforation. All the children were treated by observation initially. Thirteen of the 17 foreign bodies passed without incident; 4 were removed, two because of abdominal symptoms and two because they failed to progress and appeared to be at risk for perforation.

The four children who required intervention for extraction of gastrointestinal foreign bodies were (1) an asymp-

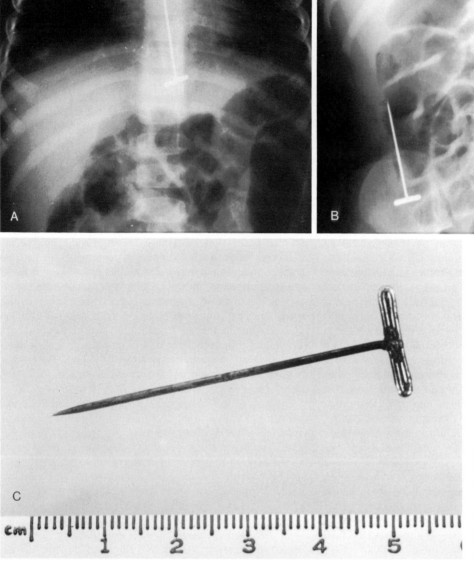

FIGURE 32–9

A, A large craft pin swallowed by a 2-year-old girl. An esophagoscopy at the referring hospital was unsuccessful. *B,* The pin moved distally, and about 18 hours after ingestion she developed acute right-sided abdominal pain and tenderness. At exploration, the pin was inside the cecum. *C,* An appendectomy was performed, and the pin was removed via the appendiceal stump.

tomatic 3-year-old girl with a straight pin stuck in her duodenum, which was removed without anesthesia, using an alnico magnet; (2) a 26-month-old girl who swallowed a formidable T-shaped pin (Fig. 32–9), which was removed by celiotomy because of symptoms; (3) an asymptomatic 6-year-old boy with an AA battery in his stomach for 1 week, which was removed at celiotomy after attempts with a magnet and snare under fluoroscopy were unsuccessful; (4) a symptomatic 9½-month-old boy with a button battery lodged in the pylorus, which was removed without celi-

otomy (Fig. 32–10). There were no complications in these four extraction procedures. All 103 children who swallowed the 110 foreign bodies survived.

PREVENTION

Accidental ingestion of a foreign body is preventable in many instances. Most lay persons are unaware of the danger of feeding peanuts and small particulate foods to young

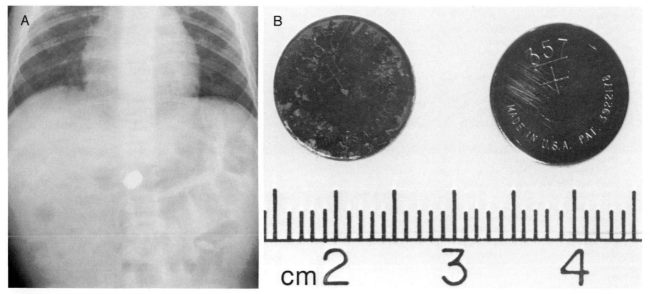

FIGURE 32-10

A, A disk battery at the pylorus of a 9½-month-old boy who began vomiting after ingestion. *B,* The battery, removed under general anesthesia by a combination of the magnet and the esophagoscope, was corroded (left) after about 5 hours in the stomach; an intact battery is shown on the right.

children. The morbidity, mortality, and cost of this calamity might be cut in half if parents would simply slice hot dogs into small pieces for their young children and avoid giving them nuts altogether. Pyman's recommendations addressed the potentially controllable factors in foreign body aspiration[80]:

1. Care should be taken to prevent dangerous items, such as safety pins, coins, and nuts, from being accessible to the young child.

2. In the preparation of food, care should be taken to remove any improper objects, such as egg shells, pits, bone fragments, and the like.

3. As a principle, nutty substances, either in their simple form or as present in "cakes, lollies, biscuits, etc.," should never be given to a child less than 4 years." This statement was based on the fact that of the total 107 inhaled nutty materials in his series, no fewer than 90 (86%) were inhaled by children under the age of 4 years.

4. Care should be taken during eating; laughing, talking, running, fighting, or other boisterous activities should be restrained, especially during the eating of nutty substances.

5. Adults should avoid setting bad examples, such as carrying nails in the mouth.

There is a great need for public education in the hazards and prevention of choking accidents in children.

Governmental mechanisms, properly enforced, can also prevent tragedies associated with the ingestion of foreign bodies.[15] The U.S. Consumer Product Safety Commission is empowered to deal with hazardous toys and other products, not only to mandate their recall but also to prevent their importation. Criminal as well as civil penalties exist for the knowing and willful violation of the Consumer Product Safety Act. Most manufacturers in the United States are keenly aware of product liability; for example,

the design of aluminum cans has been altered so that usually the pop tabs no longer detach from the can. Warning labels on foods that are dangerous to young children (e.g., peanuts, hot dogs, popcorn) have been proposed, similar to warning labels on drugs, cigarettes, or hazardous household products.[41] The role of the physician extends beyond diagnosis and treatment into the arena of public education and activism in the prevention of the accidental ingestion or inhalation of foreign bodies.

References

1. Abdulmajid OA, Ebeid AM, Motaweh MM, et al: Aspirated foreign bodies in the tracheobronchial tree: Report of 250 cases. Thorax 31:635–640, 1976.
2. Accident Facts, 1985 Edition. Chicago, National Safety Council, 1985, p 8.
3. Adriani J, Griggs TS: An improved endotracheal tube for pediatric use. Anesthesiology 15:466–470, 1954.
4. Akel A, McHutchon A: Fogarty catheters and foreign bodies. Anaesthesia 40:920, 1985.
5. Andersen HA, Bernatz PE, Grindlay JH: Perforation of the esophagus after use of a digestant agent. Ann Otol Rhinol Laryngol 68:890–896, 1959.
6. Aytac A, Yurdakul Y, Ikizler C, et al: Inhalation of foreign bodies in children. J Thorac Cardiovasc Surg 74:145–151, 1977.
7. Bendig DW: Removal of blunt esophageal foreign bodies by flexible endoscopy without general anesthesia. Am J Dis Child 140:789–790, 1986.
8. Benson CD, Lloyd JR: Foreign bodies in the gastrointestinal tract. In: Mustard WT, Ravitch MM, Snyder WH Jr, et al (eds): Pediatric Surgery. 2nd ed. Chicago, Year Book Medical Publishers, 1969, pp 825–829.
9. Berci G: History of endoscopy. In: Berci G (ed): Endoscopy. New York, Appleton-Century-Crofts, 1976.
10. Berdon WE: Editorial comment on the preceding paper (by Campbell JB, Quattromani FL, Foley LC). Pediatr Radiol 13:119, 1983.
11. Bigler FC: The use of a Foley catheter for removal of blunt foreign

bodies from the esophagus. J Thorac Cardiovasc Surg 51:759–760, 1966.

12. Black RE, Choi KJ, Syme WC, et al: Bronchoscopic removal of aspirated foreign bodies in children. Am J Surg 148:778–781, 1984.
13. Bonfils-Roberts EA, Nealon TF Jr: Balloon catheter for endoscopic removal of foreign bodies. Ann Thorac Surg 19:196–197, 1975.
14. Brooks JW: Foreign bodies in the air and food passages. Ann Surg 175:720–732, 1972.
15. Buntain WL, Benton JW, Gutierrez JF: Christmas bow tragedies. South Med J 72:1471–1472, 1979.
16. Burrington JD: Aluminum pop tops: A hazard to child health. JAMA 235:2614–2617, 1976.
17. Burrington JD, Cotton EK: Removal of foreign bodies from the tracheobronchial tree. J Pediatr Surg 7:119–122, 1972.
18. Campbell JB, Davis WS: Catheter technique for extraction of blunt esophageal foreign bodies. Radiology 108:438–440, 1973.
19. Campbell JB, Quattromani FL, Foley LC: Foley catheter removal of blunt esophageal foreign bodies. Experience with 100 consecutive children. Pediatr Radiol 13:116–118, 1983.
20. Campbell DN, Cotton EK, Lilly JR: A dual approach to tracheobronchial foreign bodies in children. Surgery 91:178–182, 1982.
21. Campbell DN, Lilly JR: The changing spectrum of pulmonary operations in infants and children. J Thorac Cardiovasc Surg 83:680–685, 1982.
22. Christie DL, Ament ME: Removal of foreign bodies from esophagus and stomach with flexible fiberoptic panendoscopes. Pediatrics 57:931–934, 1976.
23. Cohen SR, Lewis GB Jr, Herbert WI, et al: Foreign bodies in the airway: Five-year retrospective study with special reference to management. Ann Otol Rhinol Laryngol 89:437–442, 1980.
24. Cohen ST: Unusual presentations and problems created by mismanagement of foreign bodies in the aerodigestive tract of the pediatric patient. Ann Otol Rhinol Laryngol 90:316–322, 1981.
25. Cotton EK, Abrams G, Vanhoutte J, et al: Removal of aspirated foreign bodies by inhalation and postural drainage. Clin Pediatr 12:270–276, 1973.
26. Cotton E, Yasuda K: Foreign body aspiration. Pediatr Clin North Am 31:937–941, 1984.
27. Dorland's Illustrated Medical Dictionary. 26th ed. Philadelphia, WB Saunders, 1981, p 180.
28. Dudgeon DL, Parker FB, Frittelli G, et al: Bronchiectasis in pediatric patients resulting from aspirated grass inflorescences. Arch Surg 115:979–983, 1980.
29. Esclamado RM, Richardson MA: Laryngotracheal foreign bodies in children: A comparison with bronchial foreign bodies. Am J Dis Child 141:259–262, 1987.
30. Equen M: The alnico magnet—An aid to bronchoscopy and esophagoscopy. Ann Otol 4:178–182, 1945.
31. Gans SL: Principles of optics and illumination. In: Gans SL (ed): Pediatric Endoscopy. New York, Grune & Stratton, 1983, pp 1–8.
32. Gans SL: Discussion of Wood RE, Gauderer MWL: Flexible fiberoptic bronchoscopy in the management of tracheobronchial foreign bodies in children: The value of a combined approach with open tube bronchoscopy. J Pediatr Surg 19:697, 1984.
33. Gans SL, Austin E: Foreign bodies. In: Holder TM, Ashcraft KW (eds): Pediatric Surgery. Philadelphia, WB Saunders, 1980, pp 116–118.
34. Gans SL, Berci G: Advances in endoscopy of infants and children. J Pediatr Surg 6:199–234, 1971.
35. Greensher J, Mofenson HC: Emergency treatment of the choking child. Pediatrics 70:110–112, 1982.
36. Groff DB III: Foreign bodies and bezoars. In: Welch KJ, Randolph JG, Ravitch MM et al (eds): Pediatric Surgery. 4th ed. Chicago, Year Book Medical Publishers, 1986, pp 907–911.
37. Grosfeld JL, Eng K: Right iliac artery-duodenal fistula in infancy: Massive hemorrhage due to "whisk-broom" bristle perforation. Ann Surg 176:761–764, 1972.
38. Gross RE: Foreign bodies in the alimentary tract. In: Gross RE : The Surgery of Infancy and Childhood. Philadelphia, WB Saunders, 1953, pp 246–252.
39. Gurlt E: Geschichte der Chirurgie. Berlin, H Hirschwald, 1989.
40. Hambrick E, Rao TR, Lim LT: Jejunoaortic fistula from ingested seamstress needle. Arch Surg 114:732–733, 1979.
41. Harris CS, Baker SP, Smith GA, et al: Childhood asphyxiation by food: A national analysis and overview. JAMA 251:2231–2235, 1984.

42. Hendren WH: Pediatric Bronchoscopy. Karl Storz film no. C6010-C1.
43. Hight DW, Philippart AI, Hertzler JH: The treatment of retained peripheral foreign bodies in the pediatric airway. J Pediatr Surg 16:694–699, 1981.
44. Hilman BC, Kurzweg FT, McCook WW Jr, et al: Foreign body aspiration of grass inflorescence as a cause of hemoptysis. Chest 78:306–309, 1980.
45. Hochberg LD: Thoracic Surgery before the 20th Century. New York, Vantage Press, 1960, pp 454–478, 708–722.
46. Holsinger JW, Fuson RL, Sealy WC: Esophageal perforation following meat impaction and papain digestion. JAMA 204:734–735, 1968.
47. Hunsicker RC, Gartner WS Jr: Fogarty catheter technique for removal of endobronchial foreign body. Arch Otolaryngol 103:103–104, 1977.
48. Ito Y, Ihara N, Sohma S: Magnetic removal of alkaline batteries from the stomach. J Pediatr Surg 20:250–251, 1985.
49. Jackson C: Grasses as foreign bodies in the bronchus and lung. Laryngoscope 62:897–923, 1952.
50. Jackson C: Observations on the pathology of foreign bodies in the air and food passages. Based on the analysis of 628 cases. Surg Gynecol Obstet 28:201–261, 1919.
51. Jackson C, Jackson CL: Foreign bodies in the air and food passages. In: Jackson C, Jackson CL (eds): Bronchoesophagology. London, WB Saunders, 1950, p 15.
52. Jackson CL: Ancient foreign body cases. Laryngoscope 27:583–584, 1917.
53. Janik JS, Bailey WC, Burrington JD: Occult coin perforation of the esophagus. J Pediatr Surg 21:794–797, 1986.
54. Jewett TC Jr, Butsch WL: Trials with treacherous timothy grass. J Thorac Cardiovasc Surg 50:124–126, 1965.
55. Johnson DG: Endoscopy. In: Ravitch MM, et al (eds): Pediatric Surgery. 3rd ed. Chicago, Year Book Medical Publishers, 1979, pp 513–517.
56. Johnson DG: Bronchoscopy. In: Welch KJ, Randolph JG, Ravitch MM, et al (eds): Pediatric Surgery. 4th ed. Chicago, Year Book Medical Publishers, 1986, pp 619–622.
57. Johnson DG: Esophagoscopy. In: Welch KJ, Randolph JG, Ravitch MM, et al (eds): Pediatric Surgery. 4th ed. Chicago, Year Book Medical Publishers, 1986, pp 677–681.
58. Keith FM, Charrette EJP, Lynn RB, et al: Inhalation of foreign bodies by children: A continuing challenge in management. Can Med Assoc J 122:52–57, 1980.
59. Kosloske AM: Tracheobronchial foreign bodies in children: Back to the bronchoscope, and a balloon. Pediatrics 66:321–323, 1980.
60. Kosloske AM: Bronchoscopic extraction of aspirated foreign bodies in children. Am J Dis Child 136:924–927, 1982.
61. Kosloske AM: The Fogarty balloon technique for removal of foreign bodies from the tracheobronchial tree. Surg Gynecol Obstet 155:72–73, 1982.
62. Kretschmer KP: Another useful application of the balloon-tipped Fogarty catheter. Am J Surg 122:417, 1971.
63. Lacroix J, Morin CL, Collin PP: Nickel dermatitis from a foreign body in the stomach. J Pediatr 95:428–429, 1979.
64. Law D, Kosloske AM: Management of tracheobronchial foreign bodies in children: A reevaluation of postural drainage and bronchoscopy. Pediatrics 58:362–367, 1976.
65. Litovitz TL: Button battery ingestions: A review of 56 cases. JAMA 249:2495–2500, 1983.
66. Litovitz TL: Battery ingestions: Product accessibility and clinical course. Pediatrics 75:469–476, 1985.
67. McGuirt WF: Use of Foley catheter for removal of esophageal foreign bodies. A survey. Ann Otol Rhinol Laryngol 91:599–601, 1982.
68. Mandell GA, Rosenberg HK, Schnaufer L: Prolonged retention of foreign bodies in the stomach. Pediatrics 60:460–462, 1977.
69. Mantel KM, Butenandt I: Tracheobronchial foreign body aspiration in childhood: A report on 224 cases. Eur J Pediatr 145:211–216, 1986.
70. Mofenson HC, Greensher J: Management of the choking child. Pediatr Clin North Am 32:183–192, 1985.
71. Musemeche CA, Kosloske AM: Normal radiographic findings after foreign body aspiration: When the history counts. Clin Pediatr 25:624–625, 1986.
72. Nahman BJ, Mueller CF: Asymptomatic esophageal perforation by a coin in a child. Ann Emerg Med 13:627–629, 1984.

73. Nandi P, Ong GB: Foreign body in the esophagus: Review of 2,394 cases. Br J Surg 65:5–9, 1978.

74. Noback GJ: The developmental topography of the larynx, trachea and lungs in the fetus, newborn infant and child. Am J Dis Child 26:515–533, 1923.

75. Norberg HP Jr, Reyes HM: Complications of ornamental Christmas bulb ingestion. Arch Surg 110:1494–1497, 1975.

76. O'Neill JA Jr, Holcomb GW Jr, Neblett WW: Management of tracheobronchial and esophageal foreign bodies in childhood. J Pediatr Surg 18:475–479, 1983.

77. Pellerin D, Fortier-Beaulieu M, Gueguen J: The fate of swallowed foreign bodies: Experience of 1250 instances of sub-diaphragmatic foreign bodies in children. Progr Pediatr Radiol 2:286–302, 1969.

78. Poncz M, Schwartz MW: Vocal cord paralysis and mediastinal mass: An unusual esophageal foreign body presentation. Clin Pediatr 17:196–198, 1978.

79. Price JE, Michel SL, Morgenstern L: Fruit pit obstruction: "The propitious pit." Arch Surg 111:773–775, 1976.

80. Pyman C: Inhaled foreign bodies in childhood: A review of 230 cases. Med J Aust 1:62–68, 1971.

81. Remsen K, Lawson W, Biller HF, et al: Unusual presentations of penetrating foreign bodies of the upper aerodigestive tract. Ann Otol Rhinol Laryngol 92(suppl 105):32–44, 1983.

82. Rice BT, Spiegel PK, Dombrowski PJ: Acute esophageal food impaction treated by gas-forming agents. Radiology 146:299–301, 1983.

83. Richardson JR: A new treatment for esophageal obstruction due to meat impaction. Ann Otol Rhinol Laryngol 54:328–348, 1945.

84. Ritter FN: Questionable methods of foreign body treatment. Ann Otol 83:729–733, 1974.

85. Rothman BF, Boeckman CR: Foreign bodies in the larynx and tracheobronchial tree in children: A review of 225 cases. Ann Otol Rhinol Laryngol 89:434–436, 1980.

86. Saijo S, Tomioka S, Takasaka T, et al: Foreign bodies in the tracheobronchial tree: A review of 110 cases. Arch Otorhinolaryngol 225:1–7, 1979.

87. Saw HS, Ganendran A, Somasundaram K: Fogarty catheter extraction of foreign bodies from tracheobronchial trees of small children. J Thorac Cardiovasc Surg 77:240–242, 1979.

88. Saylam A, Yener A, Tanriverdi B, et al: Fogarty balloon catheter. Turk J Pediatr 18:107–109, 1976.

89. Sharp RJ: Esophageal foreign bodies. In: Ashcraft KW, Holder TM (eds): Pediatric Esophageal Surgery. Orlando, Grune & Stratton, 1986, pp 137–149.

90. Standards for cardiopulmonary resuscitation (CPR) and emergency cardiac care (ECC). Part IV: Pediatric basic life support. JAMA 255:2954–2960, 1986.

91. Stein L: Foreign bodies of the tracheobronchial tree and esophagus. Ann Thorac Surg 9:382–383, 1970.

92. Stool SE, Deitch M: Potential danger of catheter removal of foreign body. Pediatrics 51:313–314, 1973.

93. Swensson EE, Rah KH, Kim MC, et al: Extraction of large tracheal foreign bodies through a tracheostoma under bronchoscopic control. Ann Thorac Surg 39:251–253, 1985.

94. Symbas PN: Indirect method of extraction of foreign body from the esophagus. Ann Surg 167:78–80, 1968.

95. Ullyot DG, Norman JC: The Fogarty catheter: An aid to bronchoscopic removal of foreign bodies. Ann Thorac Surg 6:185–186, 1968.

96. Vane DW, Pritchard J, Colville CW, et al: Bronchoscopy for aspirated foreign bodies in children: Experience in 131 cases. Arch Surg 123(7):885–888, 1988.

97. Volle E, Hanel D, Beyer P, et al: Ingested foreign bodies: Removal by magnet. Radiology 160:407–409, 1986.

98. Votteler TP, Nash JC, Rutledge JC: The hazard of ingested alkaline disk batteries in children. JAMA 249:2504–2506, 1983.

99. Weisberg D, Schwartz I: Foreign bodies in the tracheobronchial tree. Chest 91:730–733, 1987.

100. Weisel JM, Chisin R, Feinmesser R, et al: Use of a Fogarty catheter for bronchoscopic removal of a foreign body. Chest 81:524, 1982.

101. Weston JT: Airway foreign body fatalities in children. Ann Otol Rhinol Laryngol 74:1144–1148, 1965.

102. Willis GA, Ho WC: Perforation of a Meckel's diverticulum by an alkaline hearing aid battery. Can Med Assoc J 126:497–498, 1982.

103. Wiseman NE: The diagnosis of foreign body aspiration. J Pediatr Surg 19:531–535, 1984.

104. Wood RE, Gauderer MWL: Flexible fiberoptic bronchoscopy in the management of tracheobronchial foreign bodies in children: The value of a combined approach with open tube bronchoscopy. J Pediatr Surg 19:693–696, 1984.

Animal, Snake, and Spider Bites and Insect Stings

SNAKE BITES

Uniform and consistent treatment guidelines for snake bites are difficult because of the scarcity of controlled studies. Planning such studies is complicated by the variability of envenomation by size and genus of snake, the number of bites, the volume and concentration of injectate, the anatomic location, the adequacy of prehospital care, and the size and state of health of the victim.

Each year 45,000 snake bites occur in the United States, 8000 from venomous snakes and 6000 with envenomation. Snake bites occur most commonly in males, at a 2:1 ratio, usually from May to October and usually on the distal part of an extremity.[60, 73] Outdoorsmen and children in the yard are at greatest risk.[60] The highest incidence of snake bites is in the rural Southeast.[59, 73] Most snake bites could be avoided by the consideration of simple measures when in "snake territory" (Table 33–1).

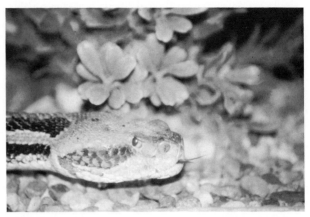

FIGURE 33–1

A rock rattlesnake head showing the typical configuration of a pit viper: an arrow-shaped head, a vertical elliptical pupil, and a pit just anterior to the eye.

Identification

The venomous species in the United States include 15 species of rattlesnake (*Crotalus*); two species of moccasin, the cottonmouth water moccasin and the copperhead (*Agkistrodon*); and pigmy rattlesnakes and massasaugas (*Sistrurus*), all members of the Crotalidae family. In addition, the eastern (*Micrurus*) and the Arizona (*Micruroides*) coral snakes are present. Three percent of snake bites in the United States occur from imported species.

The pit vipers, or Crotalidae, have a vertically oriented elliptical slit pupil, single noncleft ventral plates, fangs, and a characteristic pit anterior to the eye (Fig. 33–1). Harmless snakes, by contrast, have round pupils, no pits, double subcaudal plates, no fangs, and a double row of teeth. All North American pit viper bites can be treated by polyvalent antivenin, obviating the absolute need for identification.[3]

Table 33–1
Prevention of Snake Bites

1. Use caution in areas where snakes are common (rocky ledges, stone or wood piles).
2. Don't put hands or feet into crevices.
3. Don't sit down on or step over logs without visualizing the other side.
4. Look well ahead while walking and carry a walking stick.
5. Wear adequate protective clothing (boots or high shoes).
6. Demonstrate increased awareness during the late evening or the early morning, which are periods of increased snake activity.
7. At night, avoid walking without boots on, and carry a walking stick and a bright flashlight.
8. Don't lie on the ground, especially at night in areas of high snake concentration.
9. Carry a first-aid kit in your backpacking equipment and know how to use it.
10. Don't handle venomous snakes unless experienced.
11. Amateur herpetologists should keep snakes in glass cages with locked tops to prevent accidental bites.
12. Alert children when snakes have been seen in the yard and make them wear shoes.
13. Snakes rarely strike at a distance greater than one half to three quarters of their length; always keep that distance.

However, a Mojave rattlesnake bite may have very serious systemic consequences of lesser local envenomation; thus, species identification is advantageous in its habitat.

The snake controls the position and amount of venom injected. The venom issues from a gland analogous to the human parotid, just posterior to the eye. For the average feeding strike, only 15% of the total venom capacity is injected, although multiple defensive strikes may expend 75%. Children are likely to be stunned by the first strike and may receive multiple bites before they can escape.

The eastern coral snake is a small, shy, burrowing snake that is unable to grasp a digit well enough to envenomate very often. The Sonoran coral snake is rarely encountered by humans. Only 1 to 2% of bites in the United States are from coral snakes, but they can be lethal. Coral snakes are usually 1 to 3 feet in length; have short, fixed fangs; and are colorful, with bands of red, yellow, and black or white and a black nose. Thus, the rhyme "Red on yellow kills a fellow; red on black won't hurt Jack" indicates the difference in stripe pattern between the poisonous coral snake and the nonpoisonous imitators. If the black, amelanistic, and albino forms are considered, the handling of any small snake can be dangerous. Because antivenin must be used without local signs of envenomation, any nonfanged snake should be killed and identified. A killed snake is kept in a bag, away from other potential victims, as the decapitated snake can strike for more than an hour after beheading.[76] If retrieval causes delay, the snake is transported separately. Important body characteristics such as configuration of the eyes, coloring, and length should be sought for noncaptured snakes.

First Aid

If possible, the victim refrains from excitement, exertion, or alcohol consumption and is given nothing by mouth. The injured part is immobilized near atrial level unless that delays definitive treatment. Firm pressure and immobilization of the limb produces low plasma venom levels, and some report victims treated thus fare better than those treated with antivenin alone.[80] This measure reduces shock and retards the spread of venom. Cryotherapy, formerly believed to be helpful, now is believed to increase the risk of amputation and should not be used.[49] Steroids are now contraindicated.

A tourniquet (wide and loosely applied) is believed to reduce central dissemination of venom by approximately 50%.[20] Reported morbidity from tourniquets results from excessively long or tight application. With venous congestion or advancing edema, a second tourniquet is applied proximally before releasing the first. Time must not be wasted searching for a tourniquet as it is better used transporting the victim to a hospital.[67] Coral snake bites are washed only, because no benefit is believed to result from the use of a tourniquet, an incision, or suction.

If the victim is more than 1½ hours from medical help or when the snake is large, rapid and aggressive therapy may be indicated. Immediate use of incision and suction can remove 50% of the venom, although precise incision into the ''venom pool'' is difficult. The incision should parallel the long axis of the limb through the skin bite, subcutaneous tissue, and the fascia if subfascial ecchymosis is present. Cruciate incisions are never used. Extension of the incision past the suction cup leads to excessive bleeding and lowers suction efficiency. Suction applied for 30 minutes extracts 90% of the venom.[49] It should be remembered that the suction fluid contains substances that, when injected into experimental animals, can cause death.[68] Mouth suction can be used as a last resort; it has been suggested that digestive juices neutralize swallowed venom. However, open mouth sores may allow absorption, and tingling of the mouth is often produced in the first aid provider. Hence, mouth suction is not undertaken lightly.

Excision of the bite is no longer performed. When necessary, excision includes the fang marks and a 1-cm margin, but its use should not delay the administration of antivenin. Excision also usually requires a skin graft and to be helpful, should be done within 30 minutes of the bite.

In experiments, five 2-second shocks, 10 seconds apart, using 25 kilovolts with less than 1 milliamp of direct current applied to a bite with the limb grounded next to the bite for 1 to 2 seconds, has been used to treat viper bites.[33] The action is speculative, but contraction of local vessels by electrospasm is believed to confine the venom to the bite area long enough for it to be inactivated. Further substantiation is necessary, and the use of electric shock as a first aid adjuvant seems unlikely.

The most important first aid measure is the rapid transport of the victim to the nearest hospital. The emergency department should be warned that a snake bite victim is enroute (Table 33–2).

Signs and Symptoms

The three cardinal findings of pit viper envenomation are fang marks, pain, and swelling. Prolonged bleeding from one, two, or more fang marks indicates envenomation. An 8-mm interfang distance is unlikely to cause problems; however, an interfang distance of 8 to 12 mm may cause moderate problems, and an interfang distance wider than 12

Table 33–2
First Aid for Pit Viper Bites

1. If possible, capture and kill the snake.
2. Seek identifying characteristics (length, coloration, eye shape).
3. Do not delay transport of the victim to catch the snake; if the snake is caught, keep it in a bag away from potential victims.
4. Avoid excitement, exertion, and consumption of alcohol. Do not take anything by mouth. Immobilize injured part at heart level.
5. Do not use ice, steroids, or antihistamines.
6. Use a loose, wide rubber tourniquet.
7. Consider incision and suction or excision.
8. Transport the victim as rapidly as possible; forewarn hospital if feasible.

mm indicates a large snake is involved and is likely to cause severe problems. The interfang distance is twice the depth of the fang injection.

Pain is immediate and progressive, and hyperesthesia, hypoesthesia, or neurologic change may accompany the pain. Paresthesias include peculiar sensations, formication, and tingling causalgia. Pain is greater after diamondback rattler bites; is less after bites by prairie and other rattlers; and is least after Mojave, copperhead, and massasauga bites. A common complaint following bites by the Southern Pacific rattlesnake is tingling and numbness of the toes, mouth, scalp, fingers, and around the wound.

There may be erythema, advanced pitting edema, cyanosis, necrosis, bullae, hemorrhagic bullae, petechiae, ecchymosis, and discoloration of the skin within several hours and muscle fasciculation within 3 to 6 hours.

Systemic symptoms include weakness, vertigo, diaphoresis, drowsiness, nausea, vomiting, diarrhea, dysrhythmias, hypotension (a grim sign), tachycardia, vascular permeability, increased vascular resistance, decreased cardiac output, poor peripheral perfusion, hemolysis, consumption coagulopathy (another sign of serious envenomation), thrombocytopenia, tremors, fasciculation, mental confusion, euphoria, slurred speech, sialorrhea, ptosis, neurosis, paresthesias, and paralysis. Patients bitten by eastern diamondback rattlesnakes report a characteristic metallic taste in the mouth. Early neurologic symptoms suggest that eastern diamondback, Mojave, cottonmouth, or copperhead bites produce less local reaction than bites by other Crotalidae. In subfascial or vascular injection, local signs are mild compared with early and profound systemic symptoms. Acute myocardial infarction and cerebrovascular accident have occurred after viper bites from coagulopathy and vasculitis.[1]

More than 70% of coral snake bites have insignificant envenomation. Immediate signs of envenomation are slight, as there is little tissue destruction. However, numbness, vomiting, nausea, euphoria, salivation, paresthesias, ptosis, weakness, abnormal reflexes, depression, dyspnea, and respiratory arrest can be found after envenomation.

Venom

Snake venoms are complex mixtures of enzymes and peptides. Some fractions are 20 times more lethal than crude

Table 33–3
Laboratory Studies for Pit Viper Envenomation

Type and cross for blood volume replacement
Hematocrit
Hemoglobin
White blood cell count
Prothrombin time
Partial thromboplastin time
Blood urea nitrogen
Creatinine
Urinalysis
Creatinine phosphokinase (CPK)
Electrolytes

venom. The rich enzyme content distributes throughout animal victims to aid in digestion.[81] *L*-arginine esterhydrolase, phospholipase A, ATPase nucleotides, DNase, RNase, phosphodiesterase, NADase, hyaluronidase, amino-acid esterase, cholinesterases, and anticholinesterases can be found in the venom. Crotoxin causes paralysis, bradykinin release, and direct toxicity to cardiac muscle. The renal lesion is a glomerulonephritis with progressive proliferative endarteritis and cortical necrosis. Necrosis of tubular epithelium results from the direct effect of the toxin, although hypotension and hemoglobinuria also contribute.

Laboratory Studies

Because of the wide effect of the venom, multiple laboratory studies are obtained initially and are studied serially (Table 33–3). Cross-matching blood may be difficult after systemic envenomation. Hematocrit and clotting parameters include partial thromboplastin time, prothrombin time, fibrinogen, and fibrin split products and should be followed closely for several days; these tests should be repeated 4 hours after envenomation.[82] Creatinine phosphokinase evaluation indicates intramuscular injection, a harbinger of rapid systemic absorption. Baseline electrolytes, blood urea nitrogen, creatinine, and urinalysis tests are also important.

Rattlesnake venom induces fibrinolytic activity without causing fibrinogen clotting activity.[7] Copperhead venom does not cause defibrination. Plasma transfusions, fibrinogen infusions, heparin, and epsilon aminocaproic acid used to treat other defibrination syndromes are usually not necessary or useful. Victims with defibrination are hospitalized until coagulopathy reverses. If the patient is young, in good health, has a platelet count higher than 50,000, is without a condition that would be a primary cause of major bleeding, and is without evidence of venom-induced hemorrhagic problems (ecchymosis; discoid hematoma; bleeding gums; or blood in the sputum, urine, or stool), antivenin use is not mandated.

The bacteriology of snake bites includes aerobic and anaerobic bacteria including coliform and clostridial organisms, coagulase negative *Staphylococcus, Bacteroides fragilis, Pseudomonas aeruginosa,* and *Proteus.*[29, 31] This potentially extensive flora results from ingesting small animals that become incontinent and defecate in the snake's mouth with the hypoxia of impending death.

Treatment of Crotalid Bites

On admission, a careful history is obtained and a precise physical examination accomplished. The fang mark characteristics and the extent of hyperesthesia, lymphadenopathy, edema, and erythema are documented, and the proximal extent of each is demarcated. The patient should then be observed at least 6 hours to detail the amount of toxicity.

The degree of envenomation is classified as follows:

1. Zero: Fang marks, no evidence of envenomation
2. Minimal: Local swelling without envenomation
3. Moderate: Swelling to 30 cm; severe pain and ecchymosis beyond the fang marks; vomiting, fever, coagulopathy, or laboratory changes
4. Severe: Marked local reaction to 50 cm with hemorrhagic bullae or impending tissue slough; severe systemic signs such as hypotension, coagulation changes, and rapid swelling

Grading systems do not account for subtle but dangerous systemic manifestations in the absence of local signs, and rating envenomation early in a clinical course can be misleading.[32, 68] In addition, when the species is unknown, therapy should be estimated to be adequate for the worst snake in the area.

Treatment goals are to remove, retard, and neutralize the venom; to minimize local effects; and to prevent infection as necessary. Enzyme-linked immunosorbent assay may eventually identify the snake, but nonspecific cross reactivity currently limits the method.[38] Death from pit viper envenomation is unlikely if more than 2 hours have elapsed after a bite and systemic signs and morbidity are absent or limited; therefore, prevention of complications is preeminent.[40]

Supportive measures include the administration of analgesics to achieve pain relief (Table 33–4). The analgesics should be reduced after therapy begins so effective titration of antivenin can be judged based on the presence of pain. Antibiotics should cover for aerobic and anaerobic organisms such as a second-generation cephalosporin with good anaerobic coverage. In controlled studies, antihistamines and steroids have been shown to be ineffective in preventing swelling or hemorrhage.[32, 74]

Table 33–4
Treatment of Crotalid Envenomation

Antivenin
Analgesics
Antibiotics
Anticonvulsants
Bed rest
Blood products
Immobilize
Intravenous access × 2—central venous line
Nothing by mouth
No steroids, antihistamines, or cryotherapy
Oxygen
Observe at least 6 hours
Sedative
Tetanus immunization
Ventilator

In 1954, Wyeth introduced polyvalent antivenin, and such antivenin therapy is now the cornerstone of management for significantly envenomated snake bite victims.[76] Antivenin is produced by hyperimmunization of horses with four potent crotalid venoms. However, the reduction process fails to remove horse serum albumin, IgG, IgM, and alpha₁ and beta₁ globulins; thus, the incidence of serum sickness is unfortunately high.

The goal of therapy is to completely inactivate the venom as titrated by decreasing pain, decreasing advancement of edema, obliterating ecchymosis, and ablating systemic signs and symptoms. Antivenin is most effective if given within 4 hours of envenomation, less effective after 8 hours, and probably ineffective after 12 hours, except in cases of coral snake envenomation.[8, 56, 68] Antivenin is probably not needed for most bites from copperheads, pigmy rattlers, massasaugas, or very small and young pit vipers in general; however, for bites in young children or debilitated adults it may be necessary. When envenomation by Mojave rattlesnake can be identified definitively, early and more aggressive antivenin therapy is indicated because neurologic manifestations of this snake's venom can be substantial. In addition, bites on the fingers or hands should prompt earlier use of antivenin.

The majority of complications in the treatment of snake bites are attributable to therapy; therefore, persons arriving at an institution 2 hours after being bitten without signs of systemic toxicity may not require antivenin.[7] In one study of persons who exhibited systemic toxicity with nausea and vomiting as the only symptoms, two thirds received no therapy and all recovered without complications.[7] However, when hypotension or bleeding diathesis occurred, two of four died; hence, these two signs of toxicity should prompt aggressive local and systemic management.

Bites of snakes whose venom is predominately neurotoxic do not respond to tourniquet, incision, excision, suction, or fasciotomy. The only useful treatment is specific antivenin. However, antivenin wrongly used can be more dangerous than the snake bite, although acute anaphylactic reactions occur in less than 1% of patients.

One ml of crotalid antivenin neutralizes 1.75 mg of venom. When antivenin is given, the full neutralizing dose must be administered. Pediatric patients require more antivenin for the same relative degree of envenomation. For zero or minimal envenomation, supportive care only should be given. For moderate envenomation by rattlesnake, cottonmouth, or an unknown snake, begin with five vials. For severe envenomation, begin with 10 vials, and for very severe bites, use 15 to 20 vials initially and titrate to a good response.

Two intravenous lines should be started, and epinephrine 1:1000 (0.01 mg/kg to a total of 0.3 to 0.5 ml depending on the size of the patient) should be on hand in a syringe before antivenin testing is done; 0.2 ml of a 1:100 dilution of the antivenin may be given intradermally. The appearance of a wheal with or without pseudopodia, erythema, and pruritus within 15 minutes of injection suggests a positive reaction. When antivenin is strongly indicated for systemic or severe local effects, the antivenin should be given despite positive testing. Reactions may occur despite negative test results, and in some cases with strongly positive

results, antivenin has been infused without reaction.[72] However, the ability to administer a neutralizing dose for the venom may be limited by allergic reactions. In such instances, a process of rapid desensitization is then undertaken, beginning with 0.1 ml of a 1:1000 solution of epinephrine administered intracutaneously. If no reactions occur, antivenin is administered intravenously drop by drop and then more rapidly. Antivenin is temporarily stopped and anaphylactic doses of epinephrine are given if reactions develop. Occasionally an epinephrine drip may be needed.

Injectable medicines cannot prevent tissue necrosis after that process begins. In such instances, excision may be useful. Excision of the bite is useful if it is in a confined area and is done within 2 hours of the injury, preferably within 30 minutes.[40] Excision of fang marks and site of venom injection including skin and subcutaneous tissue should be considered in severe bites and in patients known to be allergic to horse serum if they are seen within 1 hour following the bite. In addition, persons who will not take horse serum for religious reasons may be treated with excision.[26]

When antivenin alone is used as the treatment for pit viper bites, the major amputation rate is 32% for upper extremity bites and 10% for lower extremity bites.[26] Ten to 24% of patients have some allergic manifestations.[32] The complication rate with envenomation of the upper extremities is approximately 30%, including contracture, coagulopathy, tissue necrosis, joint stiffness, or loss of sensitivity.[32] Pathologic conditions should be documented with photographs if permanent damage or amputation seems probable because of sepsis, gangrene, or other complications that are visible.

Information can be obtained from the Antivenin Index Center of the American Association of Zoological Parks and Aquariums in Oklahoma City, Oklahoma ([405] 271–5454), for help with difficult cases.

Complications of Envenomation and Therapy

Persons with the compartment syndrome present with a dusky, ecchymotic, edematous, and tender extremity with dysesthesias, anesthesia, or hypoesthesia, diminished motor function, and pain from passive stretch—signs similar to those of a snake bite. If the two-point discrimination becomes wider, the compartment syndrome is a more likely cause than the effects of venom. The most accurate method to determine the need for fasciotomy is a measurement of intracompartmental pressure. Early open fasciotomy should be performed for signs of compartmental ischemia, particularly in digits, because of their limited capacity to swell. It is better to open a compartment unnecessarily than to allow ischemic contracture to develop.[32] Significant ischemia can occur with intact pulses, but fasciotomy is infrequently needed. Russell believes that fasciotomy is unnecessary as it reflects only an inadequate dosage of antivenin during the early hours of poisoning.[68] However, some patients present many hours after poisoning with evidence of compartment syndrome already present.

Serum sickness occurs in nearly 100% of children who

receive antivenin and in 35 to 85% of adults. Serum sickness usually occurs 3 to 14 days after antivenin injection and manifests itself by fever, malaise, lymphadenopathy, urticaria, arthralgia, plasmacytosis, atypical lymphocytes, and occasional neurotoxicity. A peripheral neuropathy may occasionally be caused by vasculitis affecting the nerve roots, with the most common neuropathy being a C5 and C6 brachial plexus palsy—scapulohumeral paralysis.[84] Although most patients receiving antivenin develop symptoms of serum sickness, virtually all can be treated adequately with appropriate therapy.[69] Forty percent have insignificant symptoms, and 30% present with fever, nausea, vomiting, edema, and arthralgia, which respond readily to antihistamine and steroid therapy. Five percent have more serious reactions that require more intensive therapy, but even these usually have a favorable outcome. The mainstay of therapy is corticosteroid administration aimed at decreasing tissue damage by complement activation.[72] Two mg per kg per day of prednisone tapered over 7 to 10 days is usually appropriate; however, intravenous steroids may occasionally be necessary.

Anaphylactoid reactions may be seen in patients without exposure to foreign protein. When anaphylactoid reactions occur in this circumstance, Sutherland believes there is strong anticomplementary reaction.[79] The antivenin preparation should thus be diluted and infused slowly. In one series, anaphylaxis that was predicted by skin testing did not occur in 12 patients.[53]

Prognosis

Seventy percent of snake bite deaths occur in five states: Texas, Georgia, Florida, Alabama, and California.[49] Rattlesnakes are responsible for 70% of snake bite deaths; the bite of a copperhead as the cause of death is extremely rare.[60] Seventy percent of the deaths occur in boys or men. Deaths are most likely in the untreated, in children, in those belonging to religious cults that specifically exclude treatment, or in those undertreated. Half of all fatalities occur in children younger than 5 years of age.[22] Pulmonary edema is usually found in fatal poisoning with hemorrhage into the lungs, kidney, heart, and retroperitoneum; persistent hypotension and disseminated intravascular coagulation also are found. The pulmonary edema is thought to result from the capillary constriction that is induced by the venom.

In Parrish's nationwide survey, 27% of venomous snake bites were classified grade 0, 37% grade I, 22% grade II, and only 14% grade III or IV.[59] Russell reported that venomous bites treated with prompt intravenous antivenin administration produced no deaths; there were no amputations in his patients, with the exception of those who received cryotherapy before admission.[68]

Treatment of Elapid Bites

Coral snakes are quiet, small, and reclusive. They seize their prey and hold it securely, injecting the venom by a chewing motion. Most bites occur on fingers and toes.

Rapid dislodgment is effective in preventing envenomation, and 73% of such bites result in no envenomation.[64]

Elapid envenomation may be graded as follows:

1. Grade zero: A positive history of a bite with scratches, some local swelling, and no neurologic symptoms
2. Grade I: Moderate envenomation with neurologic findings such as euphoria, nausea, vomiting, paresthesias, ptosis, weakness, paralysis, or dyspnea
3. Grade II: Progression to respiratory paralysis within 36 hours

Marked salivation is almost always present with coral snake envenomation, although symptoms may not appear for 6 to 24 hours after the bite. All coral snake bite victims should be hospitalized at least 24 hours.

A large coral snake can produce 20 mg of dried venom, equivalent to five lethal doses for human adults, which requires 10 vials of coral antivenin for neutralization.[20] It would be quite unusual for a coral snake to inject venom in that amount, and four vials would be the usual maximum dose of antivenin. Once the neurologic manifestations of a coral snake bite develop, they are extremely difficult to reverse. Because of the rapid sequence vomiting that occurs when symptoms begin, a nasogastric tube may be useful.

Coral snake antivenin can be obtained from many state public health departments, and a large supply is available from the U.S. Public Health Service National Communicable Disease Center in Atlanta, Georgia. The same precautions in administration must be observed as are observed in the administration of crotalid antivenin, although with significant envenomation, there is little choice as to whether to use the antivenin should any symptoms occur.

Treatment of Colubrid Bites

Occasionally the bite of a harmless snake may produce swelling, itching, erythema, or other local allergic reactions, which are the result of allergies to snake saliva. Antihistamines relieve most symptoms quickly. The local signs and symptoms might also be secondary to infection or to amphibian skin toxins on the snake's teeth. Ten percent of colubrid snakes possess rear fangs and may cause a low-grade envenomation with mild to moderate local reaction. In addition, certain colubrids in Texas and New Mexico and some imported snakes can cause fibrinolysis. Amateur herpetologists import aodisho, hognose, rat, bull, indigo, boomslang, rough green, blackheaded, black striped, and rednecked keelback snakes, each of which has been implicated in the production of coagulopathy.[56] Even such mild-mannered snakes as the garter snake may occasionally produce envenomation. Platelets may decrease to fewer than 20,000 and stay at that level for 5 to 10 days. Heparin is not useful. Steroids do not help. Antivenin has not been developed. Transfusion of plasma and cryoprecipitate appears to aggravate the condition, and inhibitors of fibrinolysis seem contraindicated. Support of the hematocrit by red blood cell transfusion is the only known therapy at this time.

INSECT STINGS

Hymenoptera include the honeybee, bumblebee, wasp, yellow jacket, yellow hornet, black hornet, ant, and sawfly. More than 100,000 species are in this order, and more bites and stings are inflicted by them than by any other venomous group. Bees are responsible for one half of all Hymenoptera stings. The yellow jacket is most likely to produce anaphylaxis, but there is cross sensitivity of antigens, and one insect bite can trigger an allergic response to any of the others. Only female members can sting, as they are endowed with a canalized ovipositor, which has the dual purpose of injecting venom and depositing eggs. The yellow jacket, wasp, and hornet have stingers contaminated with bacteria, whereas the honeybee is seldom colonized. The stinging apparatus from a bee is barbed, disembowels the insect when engaged, and can rhythmically contract and inject for as long as 20 minutes.

Most deaths from Hymenoptera stings occur near home, during daylight hours, and from April to October.[22] Most deaths occur in adults, but the incidence of generalized severe reaction is greater in children. The sex ratio of such bites is 60:40 male:female.[48]

Reactions

Reactions to Hymenoptera stings include a nonimmunologic direct local tissue response and an immunologic response of a large local reaction, serum sickness, and generalized anaphylactic reaction. Large local reactions persist for more than 48 hours and have both IgG and IgE antibodies to constituents of venom. Seventy percent of persons have skin tests positive to venom. These individuals do not usually have anaphylactic reactions and should be managed only with antihistamines.[27]

Delayed hypersensitivity may herald anaphylaxis with the next sting. A period of relatively frequent stings may predispose to anaphylaxis. Less than 50% of fatalities had histories of problems with insect stings.[48] Some individuals develop increasingly severe reactions with each sting, but the severity of the next sting cannot be predicted. There is a sharp rise in the proportion of serious reactions after age 30.[28] The more rapid the onset of symptoms, the more severe the reaction. Stings of the head and neck cause more serious effects. If constitutional symptoms are going to occur, they generally begin within 30 minutes.

The most frequent types of systemic reactions are urticaria (75%), syncope (65%), and respiratory obstruction (40%). It is estimated that eight out of 1000 people in the United States are allergic to insect stings and 4000 are extremely sensitive.[24, 48]

The amount of venom per sting has been shown to be 0.3 to 0.6 mg; venom contains histamines, serotonin, acetylcholine, formic acid, phospholipase A, hyaluronidase, and meletin.[41] Five hundred stings are necessary to kill by toxicity alone.

Prevention

Being barefoot or wearing abbreviated attire, especially near flower beds, hedges, or garbage cans, is an invitation to a sting. Bright floral patterns and colors, new leather, suede, bright jewelry, perfumes, colognes, lotions, and ointments attract Hymenoptera. In a confrontation, a slow retreat is preferable to a sudden movement or an attempt to destroy the insect. If a person is known to be sensitive, Hymenoptera nests and gathering points near habitations should be located and safely destroyed by individuals who are not allergic or by knowledgeable exterminators. When outside, shoes and clothing of one color, preferably black, gray, or white should be worn. A medical alert tag should also be worn by hypersensitive individuals.

Symptoms

When a sting occurs, there will usually be local pain, although the sting itself may be painless. Anaphylaxis may appear as apprehension, anxiety, confusion, weakness, twitching, spasms, ocular palsy, paralysis, and in some, loss of consciousness. Skin changes include pruritus, petechiae of the skin and mucous membranes, paresthesias, urticaria, and occasional necrosis. Intensive skin flushing, injected conjunctivae, dyspnea, rhinitis, sneezing, cough, bronchospasm, wheezing, constriction of the chest and throat, angioedema, cyanosis, dysphagia, respiratory arrest, dizziness, and a feeling of impending doom are other symptoms. Gastrointestinal symptoms include nausea, vomiting, cramping abdominal pain, diarrhea, and sudden involuntary defecation. Vasodilation, hypotension, cardiac arrhythmias, syncope, and circulatory collapse are cardiovascular signs. Uterine contractions, urinary incontinence, and late serum sickness also occur. Fatal cases manifest glottal and laryngeal edema, pulmonary and cerebral edema, visceral congestion, meningeal hyperemia, and ventricular hemorrhage.

Some reactions occur owing to unknown mechanisms that result in vasculitis, neuritis, or encephalopathy 1 to 2 days after multiple stings.[5] Venom-specific IgE is not found; thus, immunotherapy is not indicated. In multiple bites the total venom load may be sufficient to cause systemic symptoms of diarrhea, vomiting, fainting, edema, muscle spasm, and convulsion.

Subsequent reintroduction of Hymenoptera venom causes antigen-antibody reaction with histamine and other substances released in anaphylactic responses. Skin or radioallergosorbent test (RAST) is necessary to determine the species. Some patients have positive skin test results without detectable antibody, and the antibody response decreases over time. A range of 0.001 to 1.0 μg per ml must be used for skin testing, but neither the dose at which the skin test becomes positive nor the degree of positivity indicates the patient's future risk.[27] Ninety percent of individuals with histories of systemic or large local reactions will have a positive skin test at 1 μg per ml.[27]

Treatment of *Hymenoptera* Stings

The ovipositor is best retrieved with a scalpel, as squeezing or tweezing the barbed stinger may force it deeper or cause it to break off. Local pain may be relieved by lidocaine

(Xylocaine) with epinephrine, and muscle spasms may be relieved by calcium gluconate. Tub baths containing one box of baking soda may help with pruritus. Generalized arthralgia is relieved by methylprednisolone 1 mg per kg (Table 33–5).

Management of the anaphylactic reaction includes the application of a tourniquet proximal to the site, the removal of the stinger, and the administration of epinephrine, 0.1 to 0.3 ml subcutaneously in the area of the bite and 0.1 to 0.3 ml at a distant site. Anorexia, nausea, and vomiting may be treated with intravenous diphenhydramine, 4 mg per kg. Airway support, oxygen, assisted ventilation, sedation, intravenous fluids, antibiotics, pressor agents (preferably an epinephrine drip), and a nasogastric tube to prevent gastropneumonic reflux may be needed. Assuming the Trendelenburg position may be necessary. Theophylline, 7 mg per kg, is given for bronchospam. Serum sickness may occur 10 to 14 days after injury and can be treated with steroids.

Sensitive patients should carry a kit containing tweezers or a blade, a tourniquet, and self-injectable epinephrine. All those who have had a history of severe reaction should be desensitized, guided by specific venom tests. Adults with a history of severe reaction and a positive skin test result have a 50% incidence of reaction to a challenge sting; thus, they must receive immunotherapy.[27]

Fatal reactions in children are rare. Sixty percent of severe reactions in children are urticarial symptoms only, and those children should not receive immunotherapy.[27] In children with a severe anaphylactoid reaction, immunotherapy should be started. Eighty percent of those with large local reactions have positive skin test results or radioimmune-specific RASTs but subsequent systemic reactions only 3 to 10% of the time; therefore, venom immunotherapy is not recommended.[13] Patterns of cross reactivity are unreliable. Individuals should have all skin antigens tested and should be treated with immunotherapy for each positive skin test result. Immunotherapy, although given monthly and indefinitely, is not completely effective.

Table 33–5
Treatment of Hymenoptera Stings

Nonallergic
   Remove ovipositor with scalpel tip
   Wash with soap and water
   Relieve local pain with lidocaine (Xylocaine) with
      epinephrine and hot packs
   Paste of monosodium glutamate
Local—The above plus
   Steroids or calamine lotion
Urticaria
   Intravenous epinephrine or lidocaine
Spasms
   Calcium gluconate
Arthralgia
   Steroids
Anaphylaxis
   Epinephrine
   Airway support
   Sedation
   Pressor agents
   Trendelenburg position
   Nasogastric tube
   Theophylline for bronchospasm

Prognosis

In bites causing severe anaphylaxis, most survivors received treatment within the first hour; 50 victims of fatal anaphylaxis were dead within the first hour and had inadequate or no treatment.[22] Only 6% of children had a systemic reaction after being treated with immunotherapy, and subsequent venom immunotherapy decreased the incidence and probably the severity of systemic reaction.[58]

Treatment of *Solenopsis* Stings

Fire ants (*Solenopsis richteri* and *Solenopsis invicta*) were imported into the United States through Mobile, Alabama, in the early 1920s, and allergic reactions to stings from these ants in the Southeast are as common as those to stings from other *Hymenoptera*. Fire ants are between 2 and 5 mm in length, reddish brown to black, highly mobile, and aggressive creatures that live in colonies. When their nests are disturbed, the ants attack. If left alone, they continue to sting repeatedly. Alkaloids account for most of the venom, which seems to possess hemolytic, bactericidal, insecticidal, and cytotoxic properties. Local reactions result from toxicity to mast cell membranes causing release of histamine with edema, pruritus, erythema, warmth, pain, and burning. There is an immediate erythematous flare, followed by a wheal, and then vesiculation of clear fluid, which becomes cloudy over the next several hours. The pustules are generally sterile. The pustule remains for 3 to 10 days before rupturing or resolving, and fibrotic nodules may form.[25] Therapy has not changed the evolution of the pustules. Reactions that extend 10 cm or greater from the bite site are considered to be exaggerated local response. Yaeger reported 5% had signs severe enough to seek medical care.[83]

Ice, compresses, and meat tenderizer are the only usual means of therapy. Wheezing or hypotension in the child, urticaria, or more severe reaction in the adult should prompt immunotherapy. Although skin tests are useful, RAST is a valid diagnostic test in fire ant allergy.

Treatment of Diptera Bites

The order Diptera includes flies such as the horsefly, deerfly, and sandfly. Many of these blood suckers deposit irritating saliva into the skin. The bite should be cleansed with soap, water, and alcohol and covered with steroid ointment. If the patient is allergic to the bite, epinephrine and steroids may be necessary.

Treatment of Tick Bites

Ticks carry Rocky Mountain spotted fever, Colorado tick fever, tularemia, babesiosis, and Lyme disease.[36, 78] If a tick becomes attached, it should be grasped with tweezers and pulled upward with steady, even pressure.[63] One should not handle the tick with bare hands. After removal of the tick, the bite should be washed with soap and water.

ANIMAL BITES

Eighty percent of the reportable animal bites in the United States each year are inflicted by dogs, the annual incidence being 200 to 1200 per 100,000 population.[50, 57] The apparent increasing incidence is believed due to the growing use of large dogs as protectors. A child is most likely to be bitten by his or her own pet or another dog from the neighborhood that has been provoked. Dog bites are twice as common in males, whereas cat bites are twice as common in females.[45] Fifty percent of dog bites in New York are in persons younger than 20 years of age.[35] In a pediatric practice, 15.4% of the children had been bitten by a mammal, 2.1% more than once.[17] Although no animals were rabid, 20% of the children received rabies vaccine.

Injuries occur most frequently between noon and 10:00 PM during the summer. The extremities are injured in 75% of cases, with facial wounds relatively more common in young children and teenagers.[17, 35, 45] The most typical injury of the face is a crescentic tear extending into the oral commissure. Children with facial bites required revision of the scar in 35% of cases (Fig. 33–2), and one third have been involved in personal injury litigation. Fewer than 10% of bite victims were reimbursed by the dog owner for ex-

penses incurred.[10] In approximately 60% of cases, a specific breed is identified.[45]

In a report of fatal dog attacks, none was by a stray dog, and most victims were younger than 12 years of age.[62] Hemorrhage and shock usually caused death. Witnesses were not present in 50% of attacks, and in those witnessed, the dogs frequently continued to attack until someone intervened. Infants were attacked inside cribs, and most other attacks occurred in the playpen or on the bed or floor. The dogs were usually large in size. In relation to its small registration, the pit bull was responsible for the highest number of deaths.

Children are at higher risk for animal bites because their interaction with household animals may be abusive or may demonstrate inexperience in handling animals, curiosity, recklessness, relative inability to defend themselves, and proclivity for active and aggressive pastimes that excite animals. The facial bites occur because of the child's size and greater tendency to place vulnerable parts of the anatomy at risk.

There are three varieties of human bites: outright bites, striking the teeth of another person, and biting one's own tissues such as the tongue or the lip. Human bites are often associated with heavy alcohol consumption.[51]

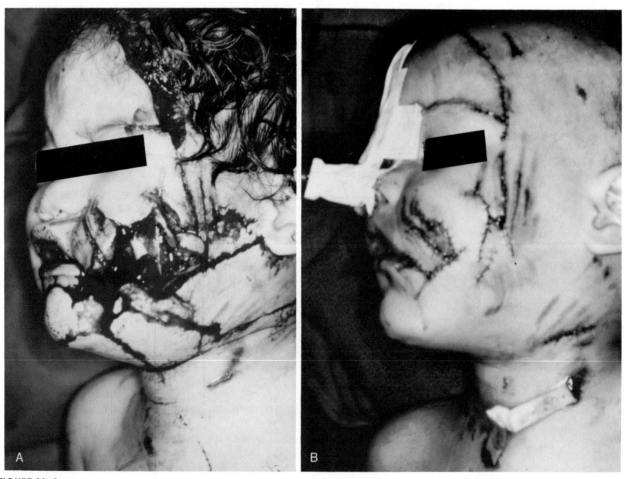

FIGURE 33–2
A three-year-old child who crawled into a neighbor's yard and was attacked by a German shepherd. A, Immediately following injury; B, after repair.

Table 33–6
Prevention of Animal Bites

1. Children should learn rules for interaction with animals, including avoiding strange animals, especially those that are wild, appear sick, or are injured.
2. Notify the health department or police of wild, sick, or injured animals.
3. Do not permit children to break up an animal fight.
4. Make children aware of the danger of mistreating or teasing pets.
5. Alert children to dangerous or nervous animals in the neighborhood.
6. Do not permit children to enter yards or houses that harbor known dangerous animals.
7. Avoid routes where dogs are known to chase bicycles.
8. Have children make friends with pets under adequate adult supervision.
9. Do not awaken a sleeping animal.
10. Do not allow your pets to come into indiscriminate contact with other animals.
11. Do not obtain a pet for a child until the child has sufficient maturity and ability to care for it (4 to 6 years of age).
12. Never hold the face close to an animal.
13. Do not permit a child to lead a large dog.
14. Never tease or pull the tail of an animal.
15. Do not take food from an animal or a toy with which the animal is playing.
16. Do not run, ride a bicycle, or skate in front of a dog.
17. Do not overexcite an animal.
18. Do not keep an animal confined with a short rope or chain, as this may make it aggressive and vicious.
19. Have children avoid a dog raised in a home without children.
20. Do not allow inexperienced children or adults to feed a dog, as they may pull back when the animal starts to take the food.
21. Stop, stand still, and speak softly to dogs.
22. See what the dog is going to do first before making a move.
23. Look for signs of an unsafe dog, such as a rigid body, stiff tail at half mast, shrill and hysterical bark, crouching or slinking position with head lowered, nose close to the ground, a staring expression, or attempts to circle behind you.
24. If a dog tries to circle behind you, pivot slowly, wait until the dog stops moving, then move slowly away. Stop when the dog moves again.
25. Never turn your back on a dog moving toward you.
26. Never touch a strange dog.
27. Never kick a dog or make threatening gestures.
28. Do not hand the dog's owner a package or shake hands while the dog is nearby.
29. Allow the dog to make the first friendship overture.
30. Dogs should be introduced to strangers while being held by collar or tight leash.
31. Enrollment in an obedience school reduces the subsequent likelihood of biting.
32. Do not back an animal into a corner, as it may attack.
33. An injured or dying animal acts more aggressively.
34. Anyone who keeps a pet known to be dangerous should be held strictly liable for any damages caused.
35. Encourage responsible ownership by supporting licensing laws, rabies vaccinations, good pet management, obedience training, spaying and neutering for most pets, and laws mandating leashes or physical restraints for animals in public places.
36. Never adopt wild animals as household pets.
37. Recommend the purchase of small dogs and those with a gentle disposition for children's pets.
38. Long-term efforts may help through applied ethology.

Cats produce narrow, deep puncture wounds and rarely avulsions, and bites from rabbits, guinea pigs, hamsters, and rats are treated the same as those by cats. Rat bites may severely lacerate the face of a baby because the rats are attracted by remnants of food on the face and head. Infants have been attacked by pet European ferrets that also seem attracted to babies. The ferret escapes its cage and attacks the babies in their cribs while the parents are absent or asleep.[54] Multiple severe and even fatal bites have occurred.

Horses, donkeys, burros, zebras, and camels have large, wide incisor teeth, which are responsible for bruising, crushing, and avulsing tissues. The lips are particularly prone to exposure when the child tries to kiss the animal. Soft tissue may be missing from the wound. Fatal fat embolism has occurred following donkey bites.[12] Equine bites are generally débrided and sutured. If the injury is extensive, it should not be closed. Reptile bites such as those by alligators, crocodiles, caimans, and large lizards have a chewing, crushing motion that causes lacerations. Bleeding should be controlled and the wound irrigated extensively; tetanus and antibiotics should then be administered.

Prevention

Prevention of these injuries may result from a number of educational processes (Table 33–6).

Bacteriology

Well-known diseases that are transmitted by animal bite and scratch injuries include pasteurellosis, leptospirosis, erysipelas, bubonic plague, rat-bite fever, sporotrichosis, tularemia, cat-scratch fever, tetanus, gangrene, and rabies. Wound infections also occur. *Bacteroides* and gram-positive and gram-negative aerobic and other anaerobes are found in wounds. Anaerobes are found in 39% of animal bites, 50% of human bites, and 56% of clenched-fist human bite injuries.[30] The same organisms as initial culture are found in 60% of dog bites.[16] In facial bites, infection occurred in only 6%.[75] Five percent of dog bites and 29% of cat bites or scratch injuries produced cellulitis or lymphadenitis.[45] Sixty percent of those with infections had their initial evaluation more than 24 hours after the accident, and one third were already culture positive for *Pasteurella multocida. P. multocida* is a gram-negative facultative anaerobic bacteria found in dog bites within 2 days after the bite. The wound site is inflamed and may drain. One third of those bitten show lymphadenopathy, and one fourth develop low-grade fever. The disease responds to penicillin, but septicemia and osteomyelitis may occur.[42]

Mycotic aneurysms have occurred following dog licks.[21, 61] DF-2 bacillus can cause septicemia, renal failure, diffuse purpuric lesions, hyperpyrexia, and a murmur that suggests endocarditis.[37] It can be preceded by scariform lesions.[44] The two patterns of illness are fulminant shock and intravascular coagulopathy. Previous splenectomy predisposes to a much more serious illness. The organism is usually sensitive to penicillin, erythromycin, clindamycin, and cephalosporin.[37]

The pathogen for cat-scratch fever has not been identified, but it is probably a *Chlamydia*-like organism. A week to 6 months following inoculation, a painless red papule usually develops at the injury site and then pustulates without scar formation. Within 2 weeks, a sterile, regional lymphadenitis may occur that is associated with fever, malaise, anorexia, and fatigue, and patients may present with oculoglandular fever (parotitis, erythema nodosum, thrombocytopenic purpura, or encephalitis). Antibiotics are not indicated. Aspiration or excision may relieve the discomfort of the node, but diagnosis may require biopsy.

Rat bites lead to Haverhill fever caused by *Streptobacillus moniliformis,* an aerobic pleomorphic gram-negative organism isolated from the nasopharynx of rats. An incubation period that lasts for 7 days is followed by fever, chills, pharyngitis, headache, myalgia, and weakness, with diffuse morbilliform rash that involves the palms of the hand and the soles of the feet. Polyarticular migratory arthritis involves small joints of the hands and feet. The disease relapses. Treatment requires penicillin, streptomycin, or tetracycline.

Spirillary rat-bite fever is due to *Spirillum minus* and occurs after a 2-week asymptomatic incubation period with erythema, induration, suppuration, scar formation, lymphangitis, lymphadenitis, fever, chills, myalgia, and macular rash, which resolves after several days but may recur more than once. It is treated with penicillin.

Treatment

Initial therapy includes washing of the area with an antiseptic. The wound is then vigorously débrided of devitalized tissue after using local anesthesia and is copiously cleansed by forceful irrigation. Wounds of the face and slashing wounds found elsewhere can be débrided, irrigated, and closed primarily in the operating room. Puncture wounds are best allowed to heal by secondary intention. Bites near bones are at greater risk for the development of arthritis and osteomyelitis. Baseline radiographs are obtained when periosteal puncture is a possibility. The wound is reexamined in 24 hours. The scar should not be revised earlier than a year following primary closure.[75]

After a human punch injury, the assailant will extend the fingers, causing the dorsal hood to recede proximally and sealing infected material in the joint space. There is often delay in seeking medical attention. A roentgenogram should be examined for air, foreign body, and osteomyelitis. The wound is explored by regional block, and if the inflammatory process has not extended into the joint space, the wound is irrigated extensively. The hand and arm are immobilized, and a bulky dressing is placed. The wound is explored in the operating room if the joint penetration is identified, and meticulous wound débridement and mechanical cleansing as well as intravenous antibiotics are used. *Eikenella corrodens* is a frequent pathogen following human bites. Although data in the literature are conflicting, it seems prudent, particularly with bites of the face and those near joint spaces, with deep bites, and with extensive bites, to provide antibiotic coverage with penicillin and a cephalosporin or to use a penicillinase-resistant penicillin for human, cat, and other mammalian bites.[14, 15]

Tetanus

The clinical manifestations of tetanus are produced by a neurotoxin, tetanospasmin. A sporulated form of the organism is ubiquitous. Suppuration, trauma, and foreign bodies produce local tissue oxidation and an anaerobic milieu for toxin production. Tetanus toxoid should be given if a person has not been immunized or is underimmunized (Table 33–7). Adverse reactions to toxoid include pain, swelling, and erythema. Hypersensitivity may occur with urticaria and angioedema, bronchospasm, and anaphylaxis, but these are very unusual.

Rabies

Seventy percent of reported cases of rabies occur in wildlife.[18] Frequent sources are skunks (the major offender),

Table 33–7

Guidelines for Tetanus Prophylaxis Following Trauma

Primary immunization at 2, 4, 6, and 18 months, at 6 years, and every 10 years thereafter.

	Incomplete Immunization or More Than 10 Years	Complete
Low risk	Tetanus toxoid to complete immunization	Within 10 years no booster
High risk	250–500 units of tetanus immune globulin	More than 5 years Tetanus toxoid
	Tetanus toxoid at a separate site	Tetanus immune globulin if more than 24 hours after the injury

foxes, coyotes, raccoons, and bats, with domestic animals being unusual.[35] Rabies is more likely to be transmitted by dogs whose territory is adjacent to the Mexican border. If a domestic animal is current on immunizations, the risk is very small. Bites of rabbits, squirrels, hamsters, guinea pigs, gerbils, chipmunks, rats, and mice have never been known to produce rabies in humans in the United States.

The rabies virus is usually carried in the saliva. Animal secretions may cause rabies, and bat-infested caves can infect from bat urine and guano. Rabid animals exhibit gait disturbance, excessive salivation, and unusually aggressive behavior. Truly unprovoked attacks by usually placid animals are significant and should alert one to the possibility of rabies.

It is important to obtain information on the rabies pattern in the wildlife in your area from the Centers for Disease Control and Prevention (CDC) or the state or local health department. Raccoons, bats, skunks, and other wild carnivores should be killed immediately and their brains tested by using the fluorescent antibody technique. The head should be prepared by a veterinarian or sanitarian. If the vaccination status of a domestic animal is unknown, the animal must be healthy after 10 days or be killed for signs and the brain examined. If the antibody test is negative, no antirabies treatment is necessary. Dogs and cats are the only species for which an observation of 10 days is known to be adequate, as virus does not appear in the saliva more than 5 days before clinical signs of rabies. No definite observation period exists for other species. Large domestic animals such as horses and cows are confined and observed closely and if any clinical signs of illness develop, they are killed for testing. Brain examination remains the most reliable and rapid means of determining possible infection. If the animal becomes ill during the observation period, it is killed and examined to predict the necessity for treatment. If there is no open wound or if that species does not transmit rabies, treatment is unnecessary. If a possibly rabid animal escapes, vaccination and immunoglobulin must be given. All bat bites should be treated because bats represent a significant reservoir of rabies and may not show encephalitis.

Clinical rabies is likely to progress more rapidly in children, particularly when the wounds are in densely innervated areas close to the central nervous system. The major risk categories for rabies include children younger than 10 years of age, persons with head and neck wounds, persons who received deep lacerations, and persons bitten by animals whose vaccination status is unknown.

Symptoms noted at the onset of clinical rabies are headaches, vertigo, stiff neck, malaise, lethargy, and severe pulmonary symptoms such as wheezing, hyperventilation, and dyspnea; other symptoms are spasm of the throat musculature, dysphagia, drooling, maniacal behavior, convulsions, coma, and paralysis. Death follows if rabies is left untreated. Intensive respiratory support may be necessary. Strict attention is given to airway and pulmonary care; cardiac arrhythmias; seizures; endotracheal intubation (as needed); vigorous suctioning; and close monitoring of blood gases, electrocardiogram, and encephalogram. Occasionally ventriculoperitoneal shunts have been used to relieve pressure. Careful isolation techniques must be enforced to prevent human transmittal of the disease.

Human rabies immune globulin (HRIG) is given on the first and third day of treatment at the rate of 2 ml intramuscularly for every 15 kilograms of body weight. If the bite is in a fleshy part of the body, one half of the HRIG is infiltrated around the wound. This produces immediate antibody protection and is the most important facet of the treatment. An immunized person who is vaccinated using a recommended regimen with human diploid cell vaccine (HDCV) or who has previously demonstrated rabies antibodies should receive two intramuscular doses on days 1 and 3. If rabies antibody is demonstrated, the therapy is discontinued. The HRIG need not be given, although if the patient is immunosuppressed, the full treatment must be given. Full treatment with HDCV requires five 1-ml injections in the deltoid muscle on days 1, 3, 7, 14, and 28.

The vaccine is lyophilized, and each vial is to be recombined with 1 ml of accompanying diluent immediately before injection. The HRIG should not be administered in repeated doses once vaccine treatment has been initiated as the dose may interfere with production of the maximum immunity expected from the vaccine. When postexposure prophylaxis is given to persons who are receiving steroids or who are immunosuppressed, the serum must be tested for rabies antibodies to ensure adequate response. If antirabies antibody can be demonstrated in the serum, treatment can be discontinued after two doses of HDCV. With preexposure, only such factors as a developing febrile illness would contraindicate administration of the necessary immunization.

Immune complex reactions can occur in people receiving HDCV booster doses with an illness characterized by generalized urticaria, arthralgia, arthritis, angioedema, nausea, vomiting, fever, and malaise 2 to 21 days following the booster dose. No illnesses have been reported to be life threatening. Hence, once initiated, rabies prophylaxis should not be discontinued because of local or mild systemic adverse reactions. Such reactions can be managed with anti-inflammatory or antipyretic agents. Local reactions such as pain, erythema, swelling, or pruritus are noted in 25% of recipients and mild systemic reactions such as headache, nausea, abdominal pain, weakness, and dizziness in 20%.[19]

IgA-deficient people have increased potential for developing antibodies to IgA and anaphylactic reactions. Systemic reactions are rare, but epinephrine should be available. Live virus vaccine should not be given within 3 months of HRIG administration because antibodies may interfere with the immune response. Local tenderness, soreness, or stiffness of the muscle may occur at the injection site and may persist for hours. Urticaria and angioedema may also occur.[47]

SPIDER BITES

Latrodectus

Five venomous species of *Latrodectus* are found in the United States.[6] Only the female is dangerous to humans. The most common by far is the black widow spider (*Latrodectus mactans*), and it may reach 1½ cm in length. The spider is black and globular and has a red hourglass marking on the abdomen. The spun web is crude, hidden, and disorganized. Its habitat is rocks, debris, basements, garages, and privies.[39] Most bites occur during spring and summer. The species is prevalent in the South, the Ohio Valley, and the West Coast, but it is found in all states except Alaska. Black widows accounted for 63 deaths in a 10-year period in the United States.[59]

The venom is a complex mixture of proteins that includes alphalatrotoxin, which acts on the presynaptic phase of the neuromuscular junction to cause massive release of acetylcholine. It is one of the most potent of all venoms, but the injected volume is almost always small.

Symptoms

After the bite, there is sudden, intense pain followed by a small wheal and erythema. The most prominent symptoms are generalized muscle spasm and cramps. If bitten on the extremity, the spasm may involve the entire chest or abdomen. Although the abdomen is rigid, it is nontender. Administration of intravenous calcium gluconate, 500 mg per kg per 24 hours, relieves the symptoms. Further progression can include diaphoresis, fever, hypertension (hypertension is probably caused by pain, although the etiology is unknown), ascending paralysis, signs imitative of pneumonia, or myocardial infarction.

Treatment

Careful search may reveal a minute red fang mark with local edema. The wound should be washed. Ice-cold compresses and acetaminophen or an anti-inflammatory drug relieve pain. Muscle spasm, nausea, and vomiting may be treated with calcium or with diazepam (Valium) 0.3 mg per kg up to 10 mg. Respiratory difficulties should be anticipated in children. Children and adults with significant heart disease should be hospitalized. A very rapid onset of symptomatology is often a hysterical response from the victim. Narcotics should not be given, as the effects of the venom may be multiplied. If the victim is pregnant, a tocolytic agent may be necessary. The bite has a mortality of 4%.[76]

There is a lyophilized equine antivenin produced by Merck Sharp & Dohme, and victims with severe symptoms are given 2.5 ml. A person with a strong allergic history should not receive antivenin but should be given supportive care only. Epinephrine should be available and precautions against anaphylaxis instituted before giving the antivenin.

Loxosceles

The medically important brown spiders are *Loxosceles reclusa, Loxosceles unicolor, Loxosceles arizonica,* and *Loxosceles deserta.* The distinguishing mark of *L. reclusa* is the darker violin-shaped band over the dorsal cephalothorax. The spider is native to the South Central United States and is found both indoors and outdoors, under cliffs and overhanging rocks. It is a nocturnal hunter and bites its victims while they are in bed or dressing. The incidence may be decreased by thoroughly vacuuming closets.

The *Loxosceles* venom has a composite poison containing proteases, hyaluronidase, hemolysins, and other cytotoxins that mediate their destruction of the cell wall. Endothelial damage and microvascular thrombosis with local consumptive coagulopathy occur. An aseptic necrosis develops, which may become secondarily infected. Renal failure may result from direct cytotoxic effects or from hemolysis.[52]

When diagnosis is in question, immunologic tests are available but have a lag of 1 to 2 weeks before interpretation of the results can be made. In addition, the bite may go unnoticed because pain may not occur for many hours afterward. Pain becomes prevalent in 2 to 8 hours after injury with erythema, bleb formation, blister formation, irregular areas of ischemia, a zone of hemorrhage with induration, and a surrounding halo of erythema peripherally. The area of central ischemia turns dark, and by the fourteenth day the area sloughs leaving an ulcer that may be open for many months. Only 10% of bites undergo necrosis, but once necrosis occurs, only 10% heal primarily.[23, 66] Occasionally, systemic symptoms (viscerocutaneous loxoscelism) precede local findings. Severe systemic manifestations may occur in small children within 24 to 48 hours with fever, chills, malaise, weakness, nausea, vomiting, joint pain, petechiae, hemolysis, thrombocytopenia, hemoglobinuria, hemoglobinemia, leukocytosis, proteinuria, headache, migratory arthralgia, and a morbilliform rash. Differential diagnosis includes envenomation by ticks, scorpions, kissing bugs, snakes, cutaneous infections, focal vasculitis, emboli, thrombi, fat herniation with infarction, self-inflicted or iatrogenic injections or infusions, and various injuries.[2]

Treatment

After a *Loxosceles* bite, capillary edema and dilation or thickening of vascular endothelium are seen within 18 hours.[65] Local heat appears to alleviate some discomfort.[2] In animal studies, the administration of steroids has not stopped the progression of necrotic lesions and should not be used for this purpose.[9] Antihistamines, low molecular weight dextran, heparin, ethylenediaminetetraacetic acid (EDTA) epsilon, or aminocaproic acid are not agents of proven benefit. Dapsone may reduce tissue necrosis.[66]

It is probably best to allow the eschar to form and then excise it if it is larger than 1 cm in diameter.[4] A 1-cm margin is included, and the lesion can then be grafted 3 to 5 days later. Severe systemic symptoms such as hemoglobinuria should be treated by the administration of fluids to prompt diuresis and to decrease possible renal tubular injury. Exchange transfusion has been used with dramatic effect.[63]

BITES OF OTHER VENOMOUS ANIMALS

Tarantula and Caterpillar

Normally, tarantula bites are not serious. The more serious tarantula bites occur in Central America. The clinical picture is that of local pain, edema, and erythema, which are best treated with topical corticosteroids. Caterpillar bites or stings may cause intensive pain, and with such, analgesics and antihistamines are useful.

Scorpions

Scorpions are cousins of crustaceans. They are found under boards, boxes, and rocks and are largely nocturnal. They have a long, segmented, highly mobile tail with a stinger called a telson. All scorpions are venomous, but stings by the *Centruroides* species, *Centruroides sculpturatus* and *Centruroides guertse* (found in Arizona), may produce severe and even fatal systemic effects. The stings of other such species may produce local swelling, edema, and pain. Death from stings from any species is extremely rare in adults, but substantial morbidity can occur.[77] Death occasionally occurs after stings in infants and children.

Scorpions seek dampness in arid areas and will crawl into moist spaces. While camping in areas in which scorpions are found, a large wet burlap sack spread out overnight will attract them and allow their destruction.

Treatment of the sting consists of the application of a tourniquet and cold compresses to the site. After 5 minutes, remove the tourniquet. If the cryotherapy is continued for 2 hours, the venom will be dissipated adequately, and serious consequences can be avoided. Ammonia inactivates the venom. The site of the sting usually does not swell or become discolored but is hypersensitive to touch. Severe reactions include sialorrhea, convulsions, distended abdomen, cyanosis, and respiratory or cardiac failure. Narcotics are contraindicated, as is epinephrine. Topical steroids can be used for the itching. For apprehension, diazepam (Valium) is recommended. For muscle fasciculations, calcium gluconate is recommended, and for hypersalivation, atropine is recommended. Antivenin is available from the Poisonous Animal Research Laboratory of Arizona State University.

Gila Monsters

The Gila monster, *Heloderma suspectum,* and the beaded lizard, *Heloderma horridum,* are large, corpulent, and largely nocturnal reptiles with lengths up to 55 cm. In a series of 15 bites, 11 occurred with captive specimens, and the others occurred under extreme circumstances.[70] Most bites involve young males in Arizona, with some occurring in New Mexico, Nevada, and Utah. If the reptile chooses to hold fast, it will do so with great vigor for up to 15 minutes, and mechanical means may be necessary to free it from the bitten part. When it bites without some chewing motion, little or no venom is introduced into the wound. The wounds are puncture wounds, although broken teeth may be found in the laceration.

Pain is felt within the first 5 minutes following the bite, intensifies for 45 minutes, and persists for 8 hours or longer. The pain is more severe with larger injections of venom and is described as burning, intense (more than with snake bites), excruciating, or violent. In addition, weakness, faintness, dizziness, shock, cyanosis, diaphoresis, lymph-adenitis, lymphadenopathy, tinnitus, muscle fasciculation, ecchymosis, and slight tissue destruction can occur, but the wound does not become necrotic. No evidence of coagulation defect has been found. Severe periorbital hemorrhage has occurred in a child suspected of being bitten. If signs of envenomation occur, the victim is typed and cross-matched; bleeding and clotting times are obtained; and prothrombin time, hemoglobin, hematocrit, platelet count, complete blood count, and urinalysis tests are administered.

Treatment should include prying the lizard loose, rest, reassurance, and immobilization. The wound should be irrigated thoroughly with lidocaine. Intravenous repletion of fluid and electrolytes and occasional use of pressor drugs may be necessary. Pain can be controlled with aspirin or codeine. Antihistamines and corticosteroids are of no value. Tetanus immunizations should be appropriate. Two antivenins are available, one through the Poisonous Animal Research Laboratory in Arizona and the other through the Venom Poisoning Center at Los Angeles County Hospital, University of Southern California Medical Center.

Fishes

To prevent shark attacks, wire meshing of public beaches and life rafts should be accomplished, and swimmers and bathers should be admonished to avoid swimming with abrasions or bleeding wounds and to avoid urinating in the water.

The catfish is the most prevalent of the poisonous fishes. The dagger sharp dorsal and pectoral fins have venom glands that are toxic to vascular and neural tissues of humans. Treatment consists of incision or débridement of the puncture wounds and cleansing with appropriate antiseptics. Wounds are left open, and broad spectrum antibiotics and tetanus immunization, along with analgesics, may be used.

Stingrays

Approximately 750 people each year in the United States are stung by stingrays while wading in the ocean surf, but only two deaths have resulted from stingray envenomation during a 60-year period.[43] Shuffling the feet while in the surf allows the stingray to escape and prevents injury. If the ray is pinned to the ocean floor, it thrusts the spine into the flesh of the foot, and the sheath surrounding the spine ruptures, releasing venom.[11] Fragments of the sheath may remain within the wound, which is jagged and bleeds freely. Tissues are discolored for several centimeters surrounding the injury. Pain is immediate, severe, and increases to maximum intensity in 1 to 2 hours, lasting 12 to 48 hours. Systemic symptoms include syncope, vomiting, diarrhea, and diaphoresis. Treatment consists of copious irrigation to wash out the toxin and fragments. The venom is inactivated when exposed to heat, so the area of the bite should be placed in water as hot as possible (50°C) for 30 minutes to 1 hour until the pain stops and the wound can be further débrided.[71] Tetanus prophylaxis must be considered. The limb is immobilized and elevated. A similar approach is used for stings from sea urchins, sculpins, and cone shells.

Jelly Fish

The Portuguese man-of-war is a coelenterate found along the southern Atlantic Coast. Its tentacles are covered with thousands of stinging cells, pneumatocytes, that are capable of emitting microscopic organelles, pneumatocysts, which consist of a small sphere containing a coiled hollow thread that when activated by touch uncoils with such force that it can penetrate skin or even rubber gloves. Venom is injected through the thread. The sting produces extreme pain and signs of shock, but deaths have not been reported. Following the sting, there is tightness of the chest and severe muscle spasm; intense, burning pain; weakness; and perhaps cyanosis or respiratory distress. The cornerstone of therapy is to inactivate the pneumatocyte immediately and prevent continuing exposure. Pedicles may be removed by shaving. An alkaline agent such as baking soda is applied to the involved area to neutralize toxins. Antihistamines, analgesics, and corticosteroids may be helpful.

Marine Infection

Atypical mycobacterial infection may be present after handling marine animals or fish. Biopsy and cultures are essential for diagnosis. The synovium of the finger is commonly involved, and carpal tunnel syndrome may result from involvement of the bursae. A presumptive diagnosis should be followed by the administration of isoniazid with ethambutol, rifampin, or both and continued for 18 to 24 months. The causative organisms are *Mycobacterium kansasii, Mycobacterium marinum, Mycobacterium intracellulare,* or *Mycobacterium avium.*[34]

Scorpaenidae

The stone fish, scorpion fish, lion fish, and sculpins have spines with a venom that has an unstable protein with a pH of 6 and a molecular weight of 150,000, produces an intense vasoconstriction, and therefore is self-localizing. It is destroyed by heat, alkali, acid potassium permanganate, and congo red. It is a myotoxin.[46]

Scorpaenidae envenomations are most likely to occur to the hands of aquarists and to cause immediate, intense pain, erythema, pallor, ecchymosis, induration, anesthesia, hyperesthesia, paresthesias, convulsions, paralysis, swelling diaphoresis, dyspnea, chest or abdominal pain, pulmonary edema, cyanosis, generalized weakness, headache, tremors, hypotension, and syncope. Regional lymphadenitis or lymphadenopathy with tissue necrosis and sloughing may occur over a period of several days. Late complications include secondary infections, neuropathies, cutaneous granulomas, and indolent ulcers.[46]

The extremity should be soaked in water as hot as possible for 30 to 90 minutes; the wound should be cleansed; tetanus prophylaxis should be given, if necessary; and systemic reaction should be treated with pressors, fluids, diazepam, methocarbamol, and calcium to relieve the effects of vasoconstriction and muscle cramping. Eighty percent of victims reported complete relief of their symptoms shortly after immersing the envenomated hand in hot water.[46] Pain entirely resolved within 24 hours in all cases. An antivenin can be obtained through the Health Services Department of Sea World in San Diego ([619] 222-6363, extension 2201).[46]

References

1. Aravanis C, Ioannidis PJ, Ktenas J: Acute myocardial infarction and cerebrovascular accident in a young girl after a viper bite. Br Heart J 47:500–503, 1982.
2. Arnold RE: Brown recluse spider bites: Five cases with a review of the literature. JACEP 5:262–264, 1976.
3. Arnold RE: Controversies and hazards in the treatment of pit viper bites. South Med J 72:902–910, 1979.
4. Auer AI, Hershey FB: Surgery for necrotic bites of the brown spider. Arch Surg 108:612–618, 1974.
5. Bachman DS, Paulson GW, Mendell JR: Acute inflammatory polyradiculoneuropathy following *Hymenoptera* stings. JAMA 247:1443–1446, 1982.
6. Baerg WJ: The black widow and five other venomous spiders in the United States. Ark Agr Exp Sta Bull 608:1–43, 1959.
7. Bajwa SS, Markland FS, Russell FE: Fibrinolytic enzyme(s) in western diamondback rattlesnake (*Crotalus atrox*) venom. Toxicon 18:285–290, 1980.
8. Bashir H: The management of snake bite. Med J Aust 1:137–138, 1978.
9. Berger RS, Millikan LE, Conway F: An in vitro test for *Loxosceles reclusa* spider bites. Toxicon 11:465–470, 1973.
10. Berzon DR, DeHoff JB: Medical costs and other aspects of dog bites in Baltimore. Public Health Rep 89:377–381, 1974.
11. Bitseff EL, Garoni WJ, Hardison CD, et al: The management of stingray injuries of the extremities. South Med J 63:417–418, 1970.
12. Bloch B: Fatal fat embolism following severe donkey bites. J Forensic Sci Soc 16:231–233, 1977.
13. Busse WW, Yunginger JW: The use of the radioallergosorbent test in the diagnosis of *Hymenoptera* anaphylaxis. Clin Allergy 8:471–477, 1978.
14. Callaham ML: Treatment of common dog bites: Infection risk factors. JACEP 7:83–87, 1978.
15. Callaham M: Dog bite wounds. JAMA 244:2327–2328, 1980.
16. Callaham M: Prophylactic antibiotics in common dog bite wounds: A controlled study. Ann Emerg Med 9:410–414, 1980.
17. Carithers HA: Mammalian bites of children. Am J Dis Child 95:150–156, 1958.
18. Centers for Disease Control. Rabies surveillance, Atlanta, Georgia. U.S. Department of Health and Human Services, May 1967.
19. Centers for Disease Control. Recommendations of the immunization practices advisory committee (ACIP). Rabies prevention—United States 1984. MMWR 33:393–402, 1984.
20. Christopher DG, Rodning CB: Crotalidae envenomation. South Med J 79:159–162, 1986.
21. Clapp DW, Kleinmann MB, Reynolds JK, et al: *Pasteurella multocida* meningitis in infancy. Am J Dis Child 140:444–446, 1986.
22. Ennik F: Deaths from bites and stings of venomous animals. West J Med 133:463–468, 1980.
23. Fardon DW: The treatment of brown spider bite. Plast Reconstr Surg 40:482, 1967.
24. Frazier CA: Insect stings—A medical emergency. JAMA 235:2410–2413, 1976.
25. Ginsburg CM: Fire ant envenomation in children. Pediatrics 73:689–691, 1984.
26. Glass TG Jr: Treatment of rattlesnake bites. JAMA 247:461, 1982.
27. Golden DBK: Insights in Allergy. St. Louis, CV Mosby, 1986.
28. Golden DBK, Lichtenstein LM: Insect sting allergy. In: Kaplan AP (ed): Allergy. New York, Churchill Livingstone, 1985, pp 507–524.

29. Goldstein EJC, Agyare EO, Vagvolbyi AE, et al: Aerobic bacterial oral flora of garter snakes: Development of normal flora and pathogenic potential for snakes and humans. J Clin Microbiol 13:954–956, 1981.
30. Goldstein EJC, Citron DM, Finegold SM: Role of the anaerobic bacteria in bite-wound infections. Rev Infect Dis 6:S177–S183, 1984.
31. Goldstein EJC, Citron DM, Gonzalez H, et al: Bacteriology of rattlesnake venom and implications for therapy. J Infect Dis 140:818–821, 1979.
32. Grace TG, Omer GE: The management of upper extremity pit viper wounds. J Hand Surg 5:168–177, 1980.
33. Guderian RH, MacKenzie CD, Williams JF: High voltage shock treatment for snake bite. Lancet 2:229, 1986.
34. Gunther SF, Elliott RC, Brand RL, et al: Experience with atypical mycobacterial infection in the deep structures of the hand. J Hand Surg 2:90–96, 1977.
35. Harris D, Imperato PJ, Oken B: Dog bites—An unrecognized epidemic. Bull N Y Acad Med 50:981–1000, 1974.
36. Harwood RF, James MT: Entomology in Human and Animal Health. New York, Macmillan, 1979, pp 371–416.
37. Hinrichs JH, Dunkelberg WE: DF-2 septicemia after splenectomy: Epidemiology and immunologic response. South Med J 73:1638–1640, 1980.
38. Ho M, Warrell MJ, Warrell DA, et al: A critical reappraisal of the use of enzyme-linked immunosorbent assays in the study of snake bite. Toxicon 24:211–221, 1986.
39. Hoelzer DJ, Taylor BD: Animal, insect, and snake bites. In: Erlich FE, Heldrich FJ, Tepas JJ (eds): Pediatric Emergency Medicine. Rockville, Md, Aspen Publishers, 1987, pp 463–468.
40. Huang TT, Lynch JB, Larson DL, et al: The use of excisional therapy in the management of snakebite. Ann Surg 179:598–606, 1974.
41. Itikin I: Bee sting. Am Fam Physician 13:124–126, 1976.
42. Jaffe AC: Animal bites. Pediatr Clin North Am 30:405–413, 1983.
43. Jones RC, Shires GT: Bites and stings of animals and insects. In: Schwartz SI, Shires TG, Spencer FC, et al (eds): Principles of Surgery. 3rd ed. New York, McGraw-Hill, 1979, pp 232–242.
44. Kalb R, Kaplan MH, Tenebaum MJ: Cutaneous infection at dog bite wounds associated with fulminant DF-2 septicemia. Am J Med 78:687–690, 1985.
45. Kizer KW: Epidemiologic and clinical aspects of animal bite injuries. JACEP 8:134–141, 1979.
46. Kizer KW, McKinney HE, Auerbach PS: Scorpaenidae envenomation: A five-year experience. JAMA 253:807–810, 1985.
47. Kjellman H: Adverse reactions to human immune serum globulin in Sweden (1969–1978). pp 143–150, 1980.
48. Light WC, Reisman RE: Stinging insect allergy. Postgrad Med 59:153, 1976.
49. McCollough NC, Gennaro JF: Treatment of venomous snakebite in the United States. In: Minton SA (ed): Snake Venoms and Envenomation. Dekker, New York, 1971, pp 137–154.
50. McGill CW, Amoury RA: Bites. In: Ashcraft KW, Holder TM (eds): Pediatric Surgery. Philadelphia, WB Saunders, 1980, pp 102–111.
51. McKee R, Bryce G: Animal and human bites as an emergency. Health Bull (Edinb) 41:137–140, 1983.
52. Majeski JA, Durst CG: Necrotic arachnidism. South Med J 69:887, 1967.
53. Malasit P, Warrell DA, Chanthavanich P, et al: Prediction, prevention, and mechanism of early (anaphylactic) antivenom reactions in victims of snake bites. BMJ 292:17–20, 1986.
54. Marcus EK: Ferocious ferrets. Pediatrics 79:617, 1987.
55. Minton SA Jr: Venom Diseases. Springfield, Ill, CC Thomas, 1974.
56. Minton SA Jr: Beware: Nonpoisonous snakes. Clin Toxicol 15:259–265, 1979.
57. Mofenson HC, Greensher J: Childhood accidents. In: Hoekelman RA,

Blatman S, Brannel PA, et al (eds): Principles of Pediatrics: Health Care of the Young. New York, McGraw-Hill, 1979, pp 1791–1823.
58. Mueller HL: Maintenance of protection in patients treated for stinging insect hypersensitivity: A booster injection program. Pediatrics 59:773, 1977.
59. Parrish HM: Analysis of 460 fatalities from venomous animals in the United States. Am J Med Sci 245:129–141, 1963.
60. Parrish HM, Carr CA: Bites by copperheads (Ancistrodon contortrix) in the United States. JAMA 201:107–112, 1967.
61. Pestana OA: Mycotic aneurysm and osteomyelitis secondary to infection with Pasteurella multocida. Am J Clin Pathol 62:355–360, 1974.
62. Pinckney LE, Kennedy LA: Traumatic deaths from dog attacks in the United States. Pediatrics 69:193–196, 1982.
63. Pitts RM: Spider bites. In: Randolph JG (ed): The Injured Child. Chicago, Year Book Medical Publishers, 1979, pp 369–375.
64. Pitts WJ: Snakebite. In: Randolph JG, Ravitch MM, Welch J, et al (eds): The Injured Child: Surgical Management. Chicago, Year Book Medical Publishers, 1979, pp 331–367.
65. Ramming KP: Bites and stings. In: Sabiston DC Jr (ed): Textbook of Surgery. Philadelphia, WB Saunders, 1986, pp 284–298.
66. Rees RS, Fields JP, King LE, et al: Do brown recluse spider bites induce pyoderma gangrenosum? South Med J 78:283–287, 1985.
67. Reid HA: Venomous bites and stings. Medicine (3rd series), 1978, pp 341–346.
68. Russell FE: Pressure and immobilization for snakebite remains speculative. Ann Emerg Med 11:701–702, 1982.
69. Russell FE: Snake venom poisoning. Great Neck, NY, Scholium International, 1983.
70. Russell FE, Bogert CM: Gila monster: Its biology, venom and bite—A review. Toxicon 19:341–359, 1981.
71. Russell FE, Lewis RD: Evaluation of the current status of therapy for stingray injuries. In: Buckley EE: Venoms, Publication 44. Washington, DC, American Association for the Advancement of Science, 1956, pp 43–53.
72. Russell FE, Ruzic N, Gonzalez H: Effectiveness of antivenin (Crotalidae) polyvalent following injection of crotalus venom. Toxicon 11:461–464, 1973.
73. Sabback MS, Cunningham ER, Fitts CT: A study of the treatment of pit viper envenomization in 45 patients. J Trauma 17:569–573, 1977.
74. Schottler WHA: Antihistamines, ACTH, cortisone, hydrocortisone and anesthetics in snake bite. Am J Trop Med Hyg 3:1083, 1954.
75. Schultz RC, McMaster WC: The treatment of dog bite injuries, especially those of the face. Plast Reconstr Surg 49:494–500, 1972.
76. Snyder CC, Mayer TA: Animal, snake, and insect bites. In: Mayer TA: Emergency Management of Pediatric Trauma. Philadelphia, WB Saunders, 1985, pp 466–483.
77. Stahnke HL: How to get stung by a scorpion. Desert Mag, August 1960, pp 19, 29.
78. Steere AC, Grodzicki RL, Kornblatt AN, et al: The spirochetal etiology of Lyme disease. N Engl J Med 308:733–740, 1983.
79. Sutherland SK: Serum reactions and analysis of commercial antivenoms and the possible role of anticomplementary activity in de-novo reactions to antivenoms and antitoxins. Med J Aust 23:613–615, 1977.
80. Sutherland SK, Coulter AR: Early management of bites by the eastern diamondback rattlesnake (Crotalus adamanteus): Studies in monkeys (Macaca fascicularis). Am J Trop Med Hyg 30:497–500, 1981.
81. Thomas RG, Pough FH: The effect of rattlesnake venom on digestion of prey. Toxicon 17:221–228, 1979.
82. Van Mierop LHS, Kitchens CS: Defibrination syndrome following bites by the eastern diamondback rattlesnake. J Fla Med Assoc 67:21–27, 1980.
83. Yaeger W: Frequency of fire ant stinging in Lowndes County, Georgia. J Med Entomol 19:366–370, 1982.
84. Young F: Peripheral nerve paralyses following the use of various serums. JAMA 98:1139, 1932.

Michael B. Marchildon
Edward J. Doolin

CHAPTER THIRTY-FOUR

Birth Injuries

ANTENATAL INJURIES

The importance of a protected and homeopathic environment for a developing embryo cannot be overestimated. Nature has always made an attempt to provide this, in the form of an egg, a pouch, or a womb. However, this oasis is itself a living biologic structure susceptible to its own misadventures and to those of the outside world. As a result, the fetus may be exposed to a variety of injuries in its prenatal environment. Although the buffer of the uterus is present, the child and mother function as a unit during gestation, and the fetus is subject to the travels and traumas of the mother. Conversely, the state of pregnancy and the gravid uterus put the mother at certain unique risks, and the fetus may be exposed to varied and sometimes unusual forces.

Uterus versus Fetus

The uterus is a finite space. Although it enlarges to accommodate the growing fetus, the child does not have complete freedom. The term *position of comfort* has been coined to describe the fetal orientation that creates the least stress.[143] Because both the uterus and the fetus are dynamic, position is not fixed but changing, and mishaps leading to injury or deformity can occur during prenatal development. Radiologically, hyperextension of the neck and back, abnormal fetal lie such as transverse or breech presentation, and hyperextension of the limbs have been seen. Terms such as *opisthotonos foetus* and the *flying fetus* have appeared in the literature to describe a specific stressed fetal position.[54, 96] Oligohydramnios, as in the case of posterior urethral valves, can result in a small uterine cavity and cause compression of the fetus. The signs of such compression, including dimpling of the skin and deformities of the extremities, testify to the fact that the uterus can have a mechanical effect on the fetus (FD Stephens, personal communication). Gibberd has outlined the factors that affect fetal attitude, placing more importance on the position of the fetus than on the boundaries of the uterus.[62] He suggests that the most compliant components (the joints) are the most subject to deformity, and radiographic observations support this concept.[62]

The cervical spine may also be subject to malposition. The fetal cervical spine is capable of being extended more than 90 degrees when there is intrauterine stress, putting the child at considerable risk for spinal cord injury; case reports of such injury present at birth have been recorded in several reviews.[10, 23, 153] Healed spinal cord injuries have also been identified in the neonatal period, again suggesting injury in utero.[23] Similarly, pressure on the growing head can result in skull fractures, but this is rare. Although external trauma during pregnancy is an etiologic possibility, ongoing pressure on the fetal head from the sacral promontory or coexistent uterine fibromas have been proposed as causes.[4]

Congenital dislocation of the knee is the most common prenatal orthopedic injury.[43, 106] One case was identified with a prepartum radiograph and confirmed at birth.[46] These infants differ from those suffering trauma transmitted from outside the womb, forces that may produce long bone fractures demonstrable after birth.[25] Bone disease can also predispose the fetus to injury even when only normal stress exists. El Khazen and co-workers reported on successive pregnancies in which fetuses with lethal osteopetrosis and fractures were diagnosed in utero as early as 24 weeks.[49]

Intrauterine Structures versus Fetus

The fetus largely has command of the uterine cavity, but it has to share this space with the umbilical cord, placenta, and amniotic sac, and the relations among these structures of gestation are constantly changing. As co-inhabitants of the uterus, they interact mechanically and mishaps may result. The *amniotic band syndrome* results when a portion of the amniotic sac constricts a limb, causing narrowing or even amputation (Fig. 34-1). Although experimental evidence in animals suggests that this syndrome may be drug induced, such a cause has not been confirmed in humans. A review by Ossipoff and Hall, however, documented a history of significant abdominal injury during gestation in 25% of cases, suggesting that trauma may produce this syndrome by affecting the amnion, chorion, or placenta.[124] Previous uterine injury may also predispose to uterine rupture or may create defects in the uterus itself that ultimately cause direct fetal injury. In one case in which a hernia formed in a uterine scar, the prolapsing umbilical cord incarcerated, causing fetal distress.[14]

Attached to the end of the umbilical cord, the fetus floats freely in its world. Occasionally, the cord and the fetus may intertwine. Nuchal cords are a common finding at birth. Couser and colleagues reported on a fetus that sustained a brachial artery thrombosis because of the tourniquet effect of the cord wrapped around the arm three times.[37] Rarely, the fetus may instigate trauma to itself or the environment. Tuggle and Cook reported on a child delivered by cesarean

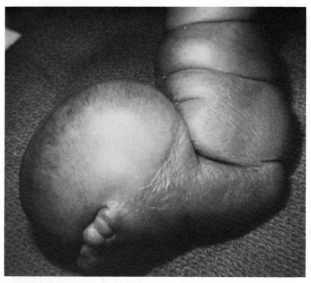

FIGURE 34-1

Amniotic band syndrome with swelling and distortion of the right foot and lower leg.

section who was found to have bloody amniotic fluid and anemia.[158] An isolated laceration of the umbilical cord was present, and the placenta was intact. After careful review, no external force could be implicated, and the cause was believed to be the fingernails of the fetus.

Maternal Blunt Injury

A gravid woman is by no means isolated in today's society. With the increasing number of working mothers, a woman's activity and travel often increase during pregnancy. Although the activity of traveling itself does not affect the outcome of pregnancy, it does put the mother at added risk for injury.[13, 107] The probability of a pregnant woman being involved in a major accident is unknown but is estimated at 6 to 7%.[9] A prospective review revealed that the risk of major injury to a pregnant woman is 9.5% when involved in a vehicular collision, with a resultant maternal mortality rate of 3.4%.[81]

The fetus is also at risk secondary to maternal complications of trauma, such as shock, hypoxia, and sepsis, or by direct injury. Significant fetal morbidity and mortality arise when the usual fetal-maternal relationship is unstable. The detrimental effect of hypoxia and hypoperfusion to the fetus is well documented. Cohn and associates showed that when the uterus is hypoperfused, the fetus became hypoxic, hypercarbic, and acidotic.[33]

In an injured pregnant woman, all methods of maintaining uterine perfusion and oxygenation should be used, maternal blood pressure must be supported by appropriate resuscitation with blood and crystalloid solutions, and the victim should be positioned on her left side to avoid vena caval compression by the gravid uterus. In this setting, the presence of the fetus cannot be ignored. Examination to identify signs of fetal life (heart tones and movement) is mandatory. The presence of vaginal drainage is significant and may indicate uterine injury or amniotic rupture. Use of Doppler ultrasound monitoring and ultrasound imaging helps in the evaluation of fetal viability and diagnosis of injury to the uterus, fetus, and placenta. Haycock recommends that the fetus be monitored for 24 hours, even when no initial injury is documented. She further points out that no direct morbidity to the fetus has been attributed to peritoneal lavage or other maternal diagnostic maneuvers.[79] Hence, these should be performed when deemed necessary during maternal resuscitation and evaluation.

The fetus's microcosm is also subject to direct injury. The two factors that determine risk to the uterus are the stage of gestation and the mechanism of injury. In the first trimester, the uterus is relatively small and immobile; its growth has not yet exceeded the size of the pelvis, so it remains protected within its bony armor.[39] In addition, although the uterus at this stage is much less vascular than later, the embryo and placenta are much lighter and less susceptible to deceleration injury. Three months is the earliest gestational age reported for a uterus to rupture secondary to blunt trauma.[108] Later in the pregnancy, when the uterus enlarges and becomes intra-abdominal, it presents a much more likely target for blunt trauma, such as during a motor vehicle accident. Among early series, no uterine rupture among restrained patients was noted; subsequently, reports documented uterine rupture associated with the use of lap belts.[40, 103, 104, 140] However, controversy has arisen from these observations. Overall, the use of restraints offers a significant reduction in maternal death, from 7.8 to 3.6%, and a statistically insignificant increase in fetal loss, from 14.4 to 16.7%.[40] Some researchers believe that the fetal loss can actually be further reduced if the three-point restraint is used with the belt applied so that it is not directly over the uterus.[79]

In the setting of blunt abdominal trauma, rupture of the uterus is a catastrophic event. Many anecdotal stories describe various successful fetal salvage attempts and unusual final locations of the fetus (thigh, bladder, accidental transabdominal delivery).[26] However, the survival of the fetus is related primarily to the stage of gestation at the time of rupture and the subsequent injuries suffered by the fetus. The literature suggests that immediate delivery of the extruded fetus is warranted; if found alive, the prognosis is good. No successful attempts at restoring the pregnancy are cited or believed indicated.

In blunt trauma situations, the fetus is also subject to direct injury while the uterus remains intact. Primary injuries include intracranial hemorrhage, abruptio placentae, cord rupture, skull fracture, and other skeletal injuries.[35, 145, 149] Any of these injuries may cause fetal death and loss of the pregnancy. Injury to the fetus as a consequence of blunt trauma is not an indication for in utero repair with the intent of preserving the pregnancy; no fetus has survived this type of maneuver. Intervention is limited to emergency delivery of an injured fetus, if it is mature and viable.

A systematic study of minor blunt trauma was compiled by Fort and Harlin.[57] They found the incidence of minor trauma in 210 patients to increase as the pregnancy progressed. However, no increase in fetal loss over that in uninjured control patients was observed.

Penetrating Trauma

Penetrating trauma results in considerably different risks and patterns of injury than does blunt trauma. The uterus is subject to injury by a penetrating missile at any time during gestation, even during the first trimester.[80] In either trauma setting, the approach to maternal injuries does not vary from accepted standards in nonpregnant patients. Decisions regarding maternal celiotomy follow the usual guidelines—the ultimate outcome for the fetus depending on the stage of development, the mechanism of injury, and the state of the mother. Fetal survival of penetrating injury to the uterus has been reported, particularly when stab wounds are involved.[8, 118] Gunshot wounds to the uterus, however, have a higher fetal morbidity and mortality than stab wounds. Buchsbaum reported a 66% fetal mortality rate in such gunshot injuries.[27] Most fetal survivors were infants near term who were delivered by emergency cesarean section and who survived the early delivery and repair of their injuries. Fetal survival has even been reported in the extreme instance of a postmortem cesarean section in a brain-dead mother.[144]

The presence of a penetrating wound to the gravid uterus

does pose a particular problem. In this situation, one must determine the viability of the fetus and consider the possible injuries that it may have sustained. Fetal assessment should begin with auscultatory examination for fetal heart tones. In the difficult setting of an injured pregnant mother, a Doppler ultrasound monitor is particularly useful. Amniocentesis may also be helpful in the less acute situation in which immediate surgery on the mother may not be indicated. Amniotic estriol levels have been reported as a method of determining fetal viability.[108] Blood or meconium in amniotic fluid suggests fetal injury. This information assists in fetal monitoring and in the decision to deliver the baby. As a rule, intervention in a pregnancy in which the fetus is less than 28 weeks' gestation (1000 gm) does little to change the outcome. In these cases, the injured uterus should be approached with the twin intentions of optimizing the recovery of the reproductive organs and preserving the pregnancy if the fetus is viable. Sustained injuries to the uterus should be repaired primarily; if the fetus is viable and uninjured, the pregnancy may progress. If the fetus is dead, spontaneous abortion may be anticipated. The only reason to open the uterus at this stage is if the extent of injury and possibility of infection warrant débridement and evacuation of fetal contents and reconstruction of the uterus.

A dilemma that may face surgeons is a uterus containing a viable (28-week) fetus that has sustained a penetrating injury. In this instance, one must consider the severity of the injury and the degree of fetal maturity. If the fetus is near term and viable, emergency cesarean section with repair of any fetal injuries is appropriate. If the fetus is viable but premature, the uterine injuries should be closed and the pregnancy carefully observed. The fetus sometimes survives with a residual injury.[7] Ongoing fetal monitoring is routinely used.

Invasive Testing

Evaluation of the fetus prenatally is becoming more sophisticated and prevalent, and the demand for these diagnostic techniques is increasing for several reasons. First, the sensitivity of the tests is continually improving while the morbidity of the testing is decreasing, making the liberal use of these approaches more acceptable. Second, options of pregnancy intervention based on the findings are available, including termination of pregnancy, early delivery, cesarean section delivery, and maternal transport. In the future, fetal surgery may also have a definitive role in the management of the developing child. Finally, more women are bearing children later in life. This increases the so-called high-risk maternal population.

Amniocentesis

Amniocentesis was one of the earliest attempts at sampling the products of conception. Any passage of a sharp object into the uterus, even a needle, puts the fetus at risk. Case reports of injury to the umbilical cord and direct fetal injury are well documented.[61, 147, 164] Despite such reports, diagnostic amniocentesis has no statistically demonstrable effect on the overall outcome of pregnancy. When 1040 sampled cases were matched with 992 control cases, no significant difference could be demonstrated.[115] Milunsky's conclusion was to attribute a 0.5% risk of fetal injury but no increased fetal loss to this procedure. He believed this risk could be reduced by ultrasound location of the placenta, by sampling in the middle trimester, and by increasing the experience of the sampling surgeon.[115]

Chorionic Villus Sampling

Certain genetic diseases have predictably poor outcomes, and termination of the pregnancy may be a consideration. These situations require diagnosis early in the pregnancy, and a technique that can accomplish this is chorionic villus sampling. Chorionic material is the greatest mass of zygotic tissue in the first trimester, making it the logical target for biopsy at this time. The three techniques used are aspiration through a transcervical catheter, biopsy with forceps inserted through the cervix, and transabdominal puncture. The most common and serious risk to the fetus is early abortion; initial reports of blind sampling quote a 6% fetal loss. This complication can be reduced with increased experience and by using ultrasonographic guidance. Reports from such experienced centers quote a 3.4% fetal loss.[116] However, these figures include all first-trimester losses and not just those resulting from the procedures.[100] For this reason, the true risk of this technique remains uncertain. The use of an international registry with long-term statistics should yield information accurately establishing its short- and long-term risks.

Fetoscopy

One of the more sophisticated approaches for studying the developing child is fetoscopy. The technique has many capabilities in the area of diagnosis and treatment of the fetus, such as blood sampling and skin or liver biopsies. As with chorionic villus sampling, the principal risk is early fetal loss. Recent reports quote this risk as 4.7%.[94, 167] Most losses result from prolonged leakage of amniotic fluid leading to premature rupture of membranes and spontaneous abortion. This sequence generally occurs within the first week after the procedure. Once this period has passed, long-term survival is expected to be normal.

Spontaneous Uterine Rupture

Abnormalities of structure and position of the uterus or fetus may lead to the catastrophic event of uterine rupture. This event usually occurs during labor, but can happen as early as 22 weeks' gestation. Whether early spontaneous rupture of the uterus is the result of premature labor or is a separate event has not been determined. Although some ruptures occur with no apparent cause, an underlying problem such as previous surgery, trauma to the uterus during delivery, or obstructed labor is associated in most cases. Treatment is immediate delivery of the child with subsequent attention to the uterus.

The diagnosis of uterine rupture is not always obvious.

In one series, 19 of 43 cases were diagnosed postpartum.[170] Hassim and colleagues reported on a fetus that was extruded and carried alive intra-abdominally for 9 weeks.[78] A more acute intra-abdominal delivery was reported by Lalos and colleagues.[98] In another unusual case, the head of the fetus entered the bladder after rupture of the anterior uterus.[78] Although occasional fortuitous recoveries have been reported, delayed recognition of uterine rupture significantly increases fetal loss. The overall fetal mortality rate for complete rupture is 44%.[170]

INTRAPARTUM INJURIES

"The most dangerous journey some people will ever undertake is that from the womb to the outside world."[53] Statistics from 1981 document birth trauma to be the sixth leading cause of neonatal mortality in the United States, numbering 23.8 in 100,000 live births.[160] In addition, for every death secondary to birth trauma, 20 babies suffer major birth injury.[165] Many survivors of birth trauma have poor neurodevelopmental outcomes and permanent handicaps. This discussion of birth trauma is confined to injuries associated with mechanical forces and excludes primary hypoxic-ischemic injury.

Neonatal mortality secondary to birth trauma has decreased by 50% over the past 25 years as a result of regionalization, referral systems, and improved obstetric techniques.[44, 60, 105] However, it is much more difficult to confirm a similar decline in nonfatal birth injuries. Although many researchers suggest that new obstetric knowledge and techniques have resulted in a declining frequency of birth trauma, reliable multicenter studies are not available.[42, 53, 165] The lack of agreement may relate to differing choices of obstetric techniques, particularly the use of midforceps.[44, 99] The overall incidence of mechanical birth trauma, excluding cephalhematoma, is of the order of 7 in 1000 live births.[60, 68] Some investigators note that although the incidence of specific injuries, such as brachial plexus palsies, may not have declined in recent decades, the severity of the injury has definitely decreased.[138]

Risk factors for birth trauma are well known. Large infants (>3500 gm) are at twice the risk for the spectrum of mechanical trauma, whereas flaccid, asphyxiated, premature infants with weaker cranial bones and decreased connective tissue are at extreme jeopardy of head trauma and visceral injury.[44, 68] Prolonged labor presses fetal structures against the maternal pelvic bones, and abnormal fetal presentations, midforceps, and vacuum extraction lead to misdirected forces of labor. Shoulder dystocia increases the risk to the neck and shoulder girdle. Amiel-Tison estimated that nearly half of all significant obstetric traumata injuries are potentially avoidable with recognition and anticipation of risk factors.[6] However, it is difficult to correlate the presence of risk factors into a reliable model for predicting infant injury. In a series of 394 large infants (>4000 gm), Gross and associates were unable to predict which would suffer shoulder dystocia.[70] Workers at the University of Cincinnati developed a risk assessment profile that retrospectively identified 50 to 72% of mechanical birth injuries. The investigators conceded that computer refinement was needed.[99] Conversely, a lack of risk factors in no way precludes injury.

It has long been recognized that intervention and facilitation of delivery could decrease the incidence of birth trauma, whether of mechanical or hypoxic etiology. Initially, such intervention took the form of physical manipulation by the midwife. This was followed by the introduction of obstetric forceps and, most recently, by increased use of the vacuum extractor or cesarean delivery. Because of the known increased incidence of mechanical birth trauma, high forceps have disappeared from obstetric practice in recent years and midforceps are rarely used.[137] Use of midforceps has been reported in 0.8% of deliveries in Cleveland and less than 5% in New York City.[30, 47] In reviewing some 10,000 Montreal deliveries over 2 decades, Cyr and co-workers reported that a dramatic increase in fractures and paralyses occurred in association with increased midforceps use.[44] They concluded that midforceps delivery was a major contributor to serious birth trauma as well as the single most important cause of birth asphyxia in term infants. In 1983, Friedman advocated abolition of midforceps.[59] Cyr and colleagues pointed out, however, that such a policy in Montreal would increase the primary cesarean section rate from 12% to 24%.[44] Several researchers suggest that this increased morbidity is frequently associated with identifiable labor abnormalities that existed before the midforceps procedure, such as fetal distress. Although there is no question that forceps application can result in direct trauma to the facial nerve, the eye, and the cervical spine, it is often difficult to separate the effects of hypoxic-ischemic insults, possibly resulting in encephalopathy or cerebral palsy, from mechanical birth trauma.[42, 53, 59, 161]

Some large series have reported excellent results using the vacuum extractor to facilitate deliveries.[111] Vacuum extractors replaced midforceps at the University of Wisconsin from 1979 to 1984.[24] In comparing vacuum extraction with forceps deliveries, Varner noted less maternal trauma and no difference in cephalhematoma in the vacuum group.[161] As expected, there was a higher incidence of neonatal jaundice in the vacuum extraction group secondary to increased extravasation of blood in the "chignon" (caput succedaneum). For this reason, the technique is not recommended for preterm deliveries but seems a safe alternative to many forceps deliveries and cesarean sections.

High-risk pregnancies, such as those associated with breech presentations or twins, are increasingly being managed by cesarean section. Breech deliveries have a perinatal mortality rate four times that associated with cephalic presentations; they also have the greatest potential for morbidity.[21, 42] Historically, breech presentations are associated with several forms of cerebral palsy and severe mental retardation, particularly in abnormal and low birth weight infants, who more often present in the breech position.[21, 137] Injuries associated with breech deliveries also may have a decreased potential for recovery. In an earlier series of brachial plexus injuries, only 50% of infants with such injuries recovered following breech deliveries compared with 78% after cephalic deliveries.[15] Infants in the breech position who are delivered by cesarean section have an extremely low morbidity and mortality rate.[34] Consequently, in New York City between 1969 and 1977, the cesarean section rate for breech presentations increased from 25 to 75%.[137] Similarly, the increase in cesarean section use for delivery of twins in many institutions has been dramatic; in Montreal, the increase was from 3 to 51% during a 15-year period.[16]

As knowledge and management of potentially threatening perinatal events continue to improve, the focus appropriately turns to the association of morbidity with low birth weight fetuses and neonates.[122] Birth injury today increasingly reflects asphyxial or biochemical injury rather than mechanical trauma, although mechanical trauma remains a major concern for all involved in the care of the neonate. A careful physical examination of a newborn should assess morphologic and neurologic symmetry, cranial nerve function, and active and passive range of motion at each joint, and must include palpation of the scalp and skull as well as examination of the nose and eyes. When a traumatic birth injury is diagnosed, one should suspect the presence of other injuries. This is particularly true in trauma involving the head and neck and the shoulder girdle. If immediate resuscitation is necessary, one should consider birth trauma as one possible cause, particularly in a long and difficult delivery. Although the prognosis with regard to many birth injuries is excellent regardless of therapy, others require early detection and prompt intervention to prevent permanent disability.

Central Nervous System Injury

Mental retardation, spasticity, and epilepsy may sometimes be the result of mechanical birth trauma, but most often no single factor, even asphyxia, can be implicated. In the 1860s, Little associated intrapartum birth trauma with later orthopedic contractures, a condition he named *Little's disease,* now termed *cerebral palsy.*[101, 137] Sigmund Freud in 1893 related precipitous labor, dystocia, and prematurity with cerebral palsy. He concluded that complicated passages through the birth canal and extended labor time were causes of brain damage.[58] Although perinatal asphyxia is generally regarded as the major cause of disability in later life, many reviews of cerebral palsy reveal a high percentage of apparently uneventful deliveries.[83, 137] Large autopsy series of patients diagnosed as suffering birth-related brain damage could confirm birth trauma as the cause of the patient's condition in less than half.[31] We agree with Illingworth that maternal, genetic, and perinatal risk factors are so complex and interwoven that it is simplistic to ascribe all or even most cases of mental retardation or cerebral palsy to birth-related injury.[85]

Head Injuries

Fetal Monitoring and Scalp Trauma

Intrapartum fetal monitoring has become commonplace and is in part responsible for the observed increase in primary cesarean section procedures.[159] Fetal scalp electrodes provide continuous assessment of fetal heart rate. Cordero and Hon reported scalp abscesses in seven of 2003 infants

(0.34%), and cultures of the fluid accumulation were sterile in six of seven, although all infants received antibiotic therapy and drainage of the lesions.[36] Six of the seven affected infants had been previously discharged (at age 3 days) and required readmission (at age 5 to 7 days) for diagnosis and treatment of this complication. Careful examination of areas of electrode placement before discharge, as well as discussion of this potential problem with parents, is essential. Because infection is absent in most cases, the precise pathogenesis is unclear, but liquefying hematoma, fat necrosis, and allergic response to the electrodes have been suggested as possible etiologic factors.

Caput Succedaneum

Caput succedaneum commonly accompanies vaginal delivery and is a self-limited condition. The combination of a large baby and primiparous mother is particularly risky. In caput succedaneum, the infant has a long, narrow head with an edematous, hemorrhagic scalp, overriding of the sutures, and closure of the anterior fontanelle. The swelling may cross the midline or suture lines and occurs over the portion of the scalp that was the presenting part during vertex delivery.[55] Microscopically, an excessive amount of fluid and mild extravasation of blood cells are present between the aponeurotic layer of the scalp and the periosteum.[68, 131, 141, 163] The edema usually recedes in 7 to 10 days, and the ecchymoses may require several weeks for resolution. Aspiration of the area is contraindicated because of the risk of introducing infection. A few infants may develop mild anemia or jaundice.[126] An alopecic "halo" ring on the scalp associated with caput succedaneum with transient or permanent hair loss has been reported in a few infants.[120] This condition is more commonly seen following use of the vacuum extractor (Fig. 34–2).

Cephalhematoma

Cephalhematoma occurs in 0.4 to 2.5% of live-born infants.[60, 68, 169] Risk factors include primiparity, large infants,

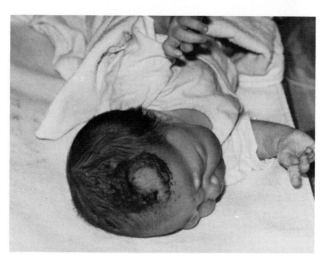

FIGURE 34–2

"Halo ring" scalp injury secondary to vacuum extraction delivery.

male sex, and, especially, forceps deliveries.[141, 163] A comparative study reported cephalhematoma in 32% of midforceps, 3.5% of low forceps, and 1.7% of nonforceps deliveries.[32] The hematoma is generally located over the parietal bone and on the right side, and the lesion is believed to result from shearing forces that produce disruption of small vessels from the skull to the periosteum.[69, 141] Subperiosteal blood accumulates between the calvarial bone and the pericranial membrane. Consequently, the hematoma is sharply demarcated and does not cross suture lines (Fig. 34–3). Diagnosis is often difficult at delivery, since bleeding is generally slow and swelling may not be visible for several hours or even a few days.[53, 55] Eventually, the hematoma becomes surrounded by a slightly elevated ridge, which may give the false impression of a depressed skull fracture. The ridge represents organizing tissue as the hematoma absorbs and may undergo calcium deposition.[131, 141] A true skull fracture, almost always linear, accompanies cephalhematoma in 5 to 25% of cases.[69, 95, 171]

Cephalhematoma is generally benign with spontaneous resorption in a few weeks to a few months, depending on the size of the hematoma. The few hematomas that actually calcify gradually disappear over many months.[163] As they do with caput succedaneum, occasional infants may suffer anemia or hyperbilirubinemia, but infection or more serious complications are uncommon.[42] Roentgenographic and pathologic findings in the area may persist for months or years after disappearance of clinical signs. In rare cases, a neonatal cephalhematoma may be seen in adult life as an asymptomatic mass, the "cephalhematoma deformans of Schuller."[55]

Subgaleal Hemorrhage

The space between the galea aponeurotica and the periosteum is large, extending from the supraorbital ridge along the top of the ears to the nape of the neck. Infrequently, considerable amounts of blood can be lost into this space, occasionally resulting in shock or hyperbilirubinemia. Initially, subgaleal hemorrhage may be confused with caput succedaneum, but the subgaleal hemorrhage often increases in size after birth, is not quickly resorbed, may be accompanied by a significant drop in hematocrit, and can extend into the subcutaneous tissues of the neck.[53, 163]

Vacuum extraction and midforceps procedures may produce a combination of compressive and dragging forces and are believed to be the principal etiologic factors in subgaleal hemorrhage. Therapy consists of transfusion and correction of coagulation deficiencies with fresh frozen plasma, platelets, or vitamin K. Phototherapy may be required for elevated serum bilirubin levels. After the acute phase, resolution generally occurs over 2 to 3 weeks, although a mortality rate as high as 22.8% has been reported.[130, 163]

Skull Fractures

Traumatic injuries to central and peripheral nervous structures have been dramatically decreased as a result of improved obstetric management.[163] The calvarial bones contain less calcium at birth than shortly thereafter, with the degree of calcification being related to the size of the fetus.[131] Although pressure of the bone against the maternal symphysis pubis or sacrum is a possible etiologic factor, skull fractures are almost invariably associated with forceps deliveries.[48, 77, 131] The incidence of skull fractures depends on the diligence of the radiologic examination; figures as high as 10% have been reported.[69] The parietal bone is the most common site of fracture. An overlying cephalhematoma, scalp ecchymoses, or depression may be present. Most fractures are asymptomatic, although seizures, intracranial hemorrhage, and even death can occur in severe injuries.

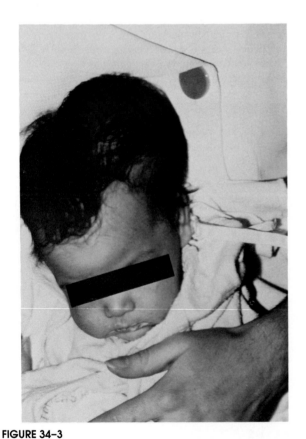

FIGURE 34–3
Left parietal cephalhematoma, not the localization and absence of crossing sutures.

Linear Fractures

The prognosis for linear fractures is generally excellent, with union occurring in 2 months.[53] Intracranial complications are rare. Follow-up skull roentgenograms should be obtained in 3 months to exclude the possibility of development of a leptomeningeal cyst. Such cysts occur secondary to a tear in the dura and may become a focus for seizure activity. They may be heralded by widening of the bony defect or increased transillumination of the region; they always require neurosurgical ablation.[48, 163]

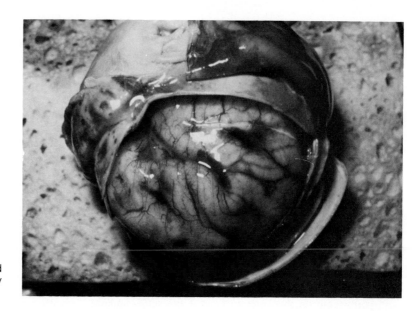

FIGURE 34-4

Postmortem finding of severe subarachnoid hemorrhage and cerebral edema secondary to birth trauma and asphyxia.

Depressed Fractures

Neonatal depressed skull fractures involve no actual break in bone continuity but consist of a buckling inward of the unusually resilient bone, the so-called Ping-Pong fracture.[42, 53, 69] Computed tomography is useful to delineate the fracture and to identify possible associated complications such as intracranial hemorrhage or penetrating bone fragments.[42, 163]

The natural history of depressed fractures is unclear. Spontaneous elevation does occur, although the incidence is unknown.[128, 163] Therapy is controversial, but many depressed fractures can be elevated by thumb compression or use of a breast pump or vacuum extractor.[53, 163] Small fractures (<2 cm) may be observed without surgical treatment.[55] Loeser and associates outlined five indications for direct neurosurgical intervention: (1) bony fragments in the cranium, (2) neurologic deficits, (3) increased intracranial pressure, (4) cerebrospinal fluid (CSF) beneath the galea, and (5) failure of closed manipulation.[102] Antimicrobial therapy to prevent meningeal infection is appropriate if CSF rhinorrhea or otorrhea is present.[55]

Although most skull fractures secondary to birth trauma are benign lesions, occipital osteodiastasis is a rare and deadly variant. In this malady, separation of the squamous and lateral portion of the occipital bone occurs, generally in association with breech delivery. Although cerebellar contusion may be the dominant lesion, massive hemorrhage into the posterior fossa, with death or severe neurologic disability, occurs in most infants.[48, 163]

Intracranial Hemorrhage

The pattern of hemorrhage into the cranial nervous system has changed in the recent past. At present, hypoxia resulting in periventricular hemorrhage, a frequent complication in premature infants, is more common than bleeding secondary to mechanical trauma, although both may be involved in some infants.[141] The adult spectrum of intracranial he-

morrhage has been described in neonates, although differences exist with regard to the frequency and severity of the various types.[55] Symptoms secondary to intracranial hemorrhage may not be apparent until 24 to 36 hours of age. A high-pitched cry, irritability, and convulsions, accompanied by a bulging fontanelle and increased head circumference, are early manifestations.[125] Predisposing factors include prolonged or precipitate labor, cephalopelvic disproportion, use of midforceps or high forceps, and breech delivery. Computed tomography is the most useful diagnostic study.[53]

Subarachnoid Hemorrhage

A high percentage of neonates have some erythrocytes in their CSF. This subarachnoid bleeding is usually minor and rarely of clinical significance.[48, 55, 141] Most infants are asymptomatic, and bloody CSF is usually an incidental finding during a septic workup.[48, 55, 69] Clinically significant subarachnoid hemorrhage is related primarily to asphyxia in preterm infants but may result from trauma alone in full-term neonates (Fig. 34–4). Beginning at around 36 hours of age, affected infants may display a characteristic seizure pattern in which they appear perfectly well between seizures.[53, 60] The presence of seizures adversely affects the generally excellent prognosis, although most infants are normal at follow-up examination.[53, 136] Hydrocephalus and protean neurologic complications may develop in the most severely affected neonates.[160] Supportive therapy consists of attention to clotting parameters, seizure control, and transfusion if necessary.[73, 162]

Subdural Hemorrhage

Neonatal subdural hemorrhage has become a rare entity.[55] Prolonged labor with face and brow presentations may produce excess cranial molding, with fronto-occipital elongation and bleeding.[53] Vaginal breech deliveries are associated with a tenfold increase in subdural hemorrhage.[48, 162] Most infants have no symptoms, although falx or tentorial lacerations can produce major posterior fossa bleeding with brain stem compression and rapid death. Rupture of superficial cerebral veins with bleeding over the cerebral hemisphere is more common. Cerebral contusion may coexist in 20 to 50%, and hydrocephalus is a frequent long-term complication.[162] Therapy for subdural collections depends on the amount of fluid and the presence of increased intracranial pressure. Subdural taps or operative removal of fluid is less commonly required than simple monitoring for fluid resorption.[73, 162] More than half the survivors are normal.[53, 55, 60, 131, 141]

Epidural Hemorrhage

With the decline of high forceps and midforceps deliveries, neonatal epidural hemorrhage has become exceedingly rare, accounting for only 2% of intracranial hemorrhage noted at autopsy.[60, 152] Bleeding occurs in the plane between the bone and periosteum on the inner surface of the skull, making epidural hemorrhage the intracranial analogue of cephalhematoma.[53] The classic fracture of the temporal bone may be absent in 30 to 40% of cases.[53, 152] Arterial bleeding produces rapid deterioration, with signs of increased intracranial pressure in the first hours of life, and requires prompt surgical intervention. Bleeding from major venous sinuses may be accompanied by a prolonged latent phase before symptoms appear.

Spine Injuries

Spine injuries are almost always at the cervical level. Neonatal autopsy series looking specifically for evidence of spinal trauma report an incidence of 10 to 33%.[92, 155] Consecutive series at the same institution 20 years apart reported no change in incidence (25%) but a decrease in severity.[133] Breech, particularly footling, presentations are associated with 70 to 75% of clinical cervical spine injuries.[48, 148] Breech injuries occur at C6–7 or C7–T1 level and involve longitudinal traction on the trunk while the head is still engaged.[55, 82] Difficult vertex deliveries with increased rotation forces may produce high cervical injuries near the occiput (C1–2 articulation). The elasticity of the neonatal spine and supporting tissues is eight times that of the spinal cord itself.[155, 157] Towbin suggested that the spine can be stretched by 2 inches but the spinal cord only by ¼ inch without damage.[155] Accordingly, complete cord transection can occur with an intact dura and no radiologic evidence of bony disruption.[28, 66, 82] If a fracture or dislocation is demonstrated, a severe transection injury of the cord is invariably present.[155] A pop heard during delivery of the head may indicate dural rupture.[155] So-called floppy babies may be diagnosed as having birth asphyxia, amyotonia congenita, myelodysplasia, or Werdnig-Hoffmann disease.[69] The findings on physical and neurologic examination, the birth history, and normal spine roentgenograms generally establish the correct diagnosis.

''Flying fetus'' and ''star-gazing fetus'' refer to an intrauterine presentation involving marked fetal hyperextension that may occur in 5% of breech presentations.[82, 168] This posture makes the neck much more sensitive to stretching and flexion and is associated with a 25% incidence of cervical spinal cord injuries when the infant is delivered vaginally.[22] Injuries are much less common when cesarean section is used, although evidence suggest that some neonates can suffer neck injuries in utero regardless of mode of delivery, as discussed earlier.[9, 20, 23, 29, 55, 153] It is essential that such abnormal presentations be diagnosed before delivery to enable planning for the optimal delivery method.[69] Even with advanced planning, the opisthotonoid posture may persist until 1 to 2 months of age.

The clinical picture and prognosis of cervical injury are related to both the level and the severity of the lesion.[156] Infants with cervical spine injuries may be apneic, though alert and awake. Initial spinal shock may also be irreversible, however, and rapid death can occur. Respiratory failure and superinfection affect most of the early survivors. Urinary retention, constipation, and paralysis of the abdominal musculature with areflexia are sometimes the first observed manifestations of cervical injury. Paraplegia may be noted late in the course. The initial flaccidity of the lower extremities is replaced with spasticity and hyperreflexia, ''triple flexion'' of the lower limbs.[163] As cord edema and hemorrhage subside over weeks or months, some return of function, and occasional startling recoveries, may occur.[31, 55]

Therapy is generally conservative. Any manipulation of the infant, such as endotracheal intubation, must be performed with great care and with the neck immobilized. Support of circulation and body temperature is important initially, and respiratory, bowel, bladder, and skin care are ongoing considerations. Laminectomy and surgical decompression are rarely of benefit. Infants with complete transection have a poor outlook and high mortality. Survivors face late complications of pain, spasticity, autonomic dysfunction, and psychiatric problems.[55]

Birth injuries below the cervical level are uncommon.[84] Neurologic deficits at these levels are most commonly caused by congenital anomalies such as an occult dysraphic state.[155, 163] The prognosis for thoracolumbar traumatic injuries is generally excellent, with function usually recovered in 6 weeks.[41]

Facial Fractures

Facial bone trauma may occur during passage through the birth canal or secondary to forceps application. The proximity of such injuries to the airway, optic nerve and glove, and subarachnoid space makes them of particular importance. In addition, facial trauma may result in cosmetic deformities and functional disability if treatment is inadequate.[53, 55] Union of mandibular fractures occurs in 10 to 14 days. Ankylosis, hypoplasia, malocclusion, and speech and feeding difficulties have been reported in infants in whom reduction and immobilization were delayed.

Subluxation of the nasal septum is the most common facial fracture and may occur in up to 2 to 3% of infants.[42, 67, 89] A careful newborn physical examination involves midline compression of the nasal tip, which results in septal deviation in affected infants. Risk factors include extremes of maternal age, primiparity, and long expulsive time.[5] Such

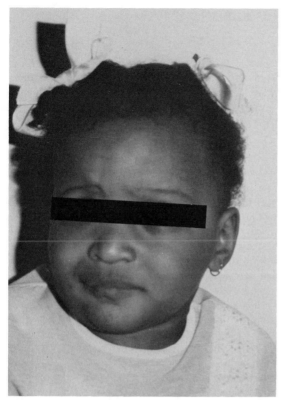

FIGURE 34-5

Two-year-old with persistent left-sided facial palsy secondary to birth trauma.

injuries can produce early respiratory distress, which can worsen with feedings.[141] Early reduction and fixation are essential, since firm union occurs in 7 to 10 days.[88] If necessary, an oral airway can be used to relieve respiratory distress before definitive treatment is begun.[55]

Facial Nerve Injury

Facial nerve palsy represents the most common neurologic manifestation of perinatal trauma.[68, 141, 163] The overall incidence has fallen from 6.4% in 1951 to below 1% in recent years.[42, 44, 99] The incidence of facial nerve injury at a given institution is directly related to the frequency of forceps deliveries, particularly midforceps deliveries.[42, 99] Most commonly, a peripheral nerve injury results from forceps compression of the nerve near its emergence from the stylomastoid foramen or as the nerve tranverses the ramus of the mandible.[53, 55] A mark from the forceps blade may be visible in these areas. The same injury may also result following prolonged pressure by the maternal sacral promontory.[55, 163] About 75% of all facial nerve injuries involve the left side.[163]

A flaccid paralysis on the affected side of the face may be present from birth but usually is noticed on the first or second day of life. At rest, the only signs may be subtle flattening of the nasolabial fold and a persistently open eye secondary to paralysis of the orbicular muscle of the eye. The infant is unable to wrinkle the brow, close the eye

firmly, or move the corner of the mouth. On crying, the mouth is drawn to the opposite side (Fig. 34–5). Liquid may dribble from the mouth during feeding.[42, 55, 68, 163]

In both facial nerve injury and branchial plexus palsies, the pathologic lesion consists of hemorrhage and edema into the nerve sheath. The prognosis is nearly uniformly favorable[163]: spontaneous recovery within 1 to 3 weeks is the rule, although complete recovery may require several weeks or months. Although electrodiagnostic studies may be useful in predicting recovery, they are generally not required. If no recovery or improvement occurs in the first 7 to 10 days, electrodiagnostic testing may differentiate between neuropraxia and nerve interruption or transection. Occasionally, excellent functional recoveries have been reported even with discouraging electrodiagnostic studies. Hence, test results, particularly early in the clinical course, must be interpreted with caution.[53, 55, 68, 163] Uncommonly, continued paralysis may be accompanied by contracture or synkinesis (mass facial motion).[110]

No specific therapy is necessary for most facial palsies. The cornea should be protected with an eye patch and 1% methyl cellulose drops instilled every 3 to 4 hours.[53, 55, 141] No controlled data support the efficacy of massage, electrical stimulation, or surgical intervention.[164]

Vocal Cord Paralysis

Vocal cord palsies secondary to birth trauma are relatively uncommon. Unilateral vocal cord paralysis secondary to recurrent laryngeal nerve trauma may result from excessive head traction during breech delivery or lateral forceps traction in a cephalic presentation. The left nerve is more commonly involved because of its lower origin and longer course in the neck. Bilateral vocal cord paralysis most frequently results from a central nervous system (CNS) injury, such as hypoxia or hemorrhage involving the brain stem.[53, 55]

Infants with unilateral paralysis may have no symptoms at rest, but they exhibit inspiratory stridor and hoarseness when they cry. Direct laryngoscopy to investigate the stridor can establish the diagnosis. Gentle handling and small frequent feedings are recommended to reduce the risk of aspiration. Spontaneous improvement generally occurs, with complete resolution by 4 to 6 weeks, although noisy breathing and the threat of aspiration may persist for up to 1 year.[53, 55, 163]

Immediately after delivery, neonates with bilateral vocal cord paralysis experience respiratory difficulties, including stridor, retractions, dyspnea, and aphonia. Immediate endotracheal intubation is necessary to establish an airway, and most infants require tracheostomy. Some untreated infants have been reported to rapidly develop a pectus deformity of the lower sternum, which is reversible after tracheostomy. Periodic laryngoscopy should be performed to assess possible return of vocal cord function. Recovery is less predictable and may require months or years. If a CNS etiology is involved, reversibility of hemorrhage or edema determines prognosis.[55]

Eye Injuries

Primary injuries to the eye and adnexa occur in 20 to 25% of normal deliveries and 40 to 50% of deliveries with protracted or assisted labor. Serious injuries are present in only 0.25% of live births and are invariably related to forceps use.[48, 87] Pupillary abnormalities can indicate the presence of intracranial hemorrhage or Horner syndrome. Abnormal opening or closure of the eye may be related to Horner syndrome or to facial nerve palsy. Associated findings, such as the presence of a lower or complete brachial plexus palsy (Horner syndrome), severe birth anoxia (CNS), or the use of forceps (facial nerve) may suggest the correct diagnosis.[53]

Subconjunctival and retinal hemorrhages are the most common eye injuries and have been reported in 2.6 to 50% of infants; the most recent figure is 35%.[17, 87, 141] Such hemorrhages are usually resorbed in the first few days of life, so the time of examination greatly influences the findings. The typical retinal hemorrhage is flame shaped, radiates from the disk, and is a benign injury. Rarely, bleeding near the macula may predispose to amblyopia or decreased visual acuity.[87, 129, 141]

Blood in the anterior chamber (hyphema) and vitreous hemorrhage are more serious injuries and usually result from misplaced forceps (Fig. 34–6). Infants with hyphema should be treated to minimize crying or agitation. Secondary hemorrhage or persistence of blood beyond the first week of life may require administration of acetazolamide (Diamox) or surgical removal of blood to reduce the possibility of later development of glaucoma. Large vitreous floaters and an absent red reflex may indicate vitreous hemorrhage. If resolution does not occur within 6 to 12 months, surgical correction should be considered.[55, 87, 141]

Streaky haziness of the cornea is common in newborns and usually results from edema associated with delivery. If such haziness persists beyond 7 to 10 days, rupture of Descement's membrane, the posterior boundary of the cornea, should be suspected. Hyphema and vitreous hemorrhage are frequently associated injuries. Untreated rupture of the Descement membrane can result in formation of a permanent leukoma, a diffuse white opacity of the cornea, and a high incidence of astigmatism, myopia, amblyopia, or strabismus.

Ear Trauma

Most injuries to the ear are related to forceps application and tend to be minor and self-limited. Hematomas of the external ear may require prompt incision and drainage, however. Untreated, a hematoma undergoes organization that results in development of a so-called cauliflower ear.[53, 55]

Sternocleidomastoid Muscle Injury

Several theories have been proposed to explain sternocleidomastoid injury (congenital torticollis), and different infants may have different etiologies. Breech or difficult deliveries may produce hyperextension of the muscle, with disruption of the muscle or fibrous sheath. Hematoma formation is followed by progressive development of scar tissue and muscle shortening.[53, 55] Cramped or distorted fetal positions may also produce torticollis in some infants. Muscle tumors of mature fibrous tissue have been demonstrated on the first day of life, some in infants delivered by cesarean section.[93, 141] An overall incidence of 0.4% has been reported.[141]

Although the characteristic mass in the midportion of the sternocleidomastoid muscle may be present at birth, most such nodules are first palpated at 10 to 14 days of age. The mass is generally 1 to 2 cm in diameter, firm, fixed with the muscle tissue, well circumscribed, and without overlying signs of inflammation. Turning the head to the opposite side facilitates examination. The mass may enlarge during the following few weeks, then regress and disappear over 5 to 8 months. One third of infants with sternocleidomastoid injury have muscle fibrosis and shortening without a palpable mass.[53, 55, 141] The shortened muscle results in head tilt to the affected side, with elevation and rotation of the chin toward the opposite shoulder.

Plagiocephaly consists of flattening of the frontal bone and bulging of the occipital bone on the involved side and the opposite deformity on the contralateral side. It may be present at birth or develop later, and results from the persistent head tilt and unchanging sleeping posture or may be related to the in utero fetal position. Roentgenograms of the

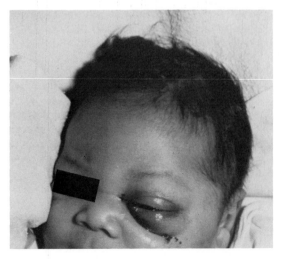

FIGURE 34–6

Newborn infant with left eye injury secondary to forceps use at delivery.

cervical spine and shoulders have been recommended to rule out the other uncommon causes of the clinical symptoms.[53, 55]

Gentle passive stretching exercises are effective. The infant is placed supine, with both shoulders flat, and the head is rotated so that the chin touches each acromion process. The maneuver can be repeated several times each day. In addition, the infant should be stimulated to turn his or her head to the affected side by appropriate positioning of their crib or toys and by placing him or her on the side of the torticollis during sleep. Such therapy should be instituted as early as possible and is successful in 80% of patients.[53, 55] If present, plagiocephaly regresses over months or years.[141] If the neck deformity has not been fully corrected after 6 months of conservative therapy, surgical division of the muscle and fascia colli may be considered. Delayed or inadequate therapy may result in facial hemihypoplasia or permanent skull and cervical spine deformities.[53, 55]

Brachial Plexus Injuries

Brachial plexus palsies were first described by Smellie in his midwifery text in 1764.[50] Erb in 1874 described an obstetric case, localized the anatomy of the lesion associated with his name, and credited Duchenne with the original clinical discussion 2 years earlier.[52] Erb also recognized excessive traction during delivery as the underlying cause. In 1885, Klumpke described sympathetic changes (Horner syndrome) in association with brachial plexus trauma. Risk factors for brachial plexus injuries are summarized in Table 34–1.[50, 65, 163] Most cases involve stretching of the nerve roots that supply the brachial plexus. Disruption of the nerve sheath occurs, with local hemorrhage and edema, as well as compression of nerve fibers. In the most severe cases, there is actual rupture of nerves with loss of continuity or avulsion of roots from the spinal cord, both resulting in irreversible loss of function.[53, 163]

Various types as well as degrees of brachial plexus injury exist. The classic Erb's palsy involves the C5–6 roots and is the most common of such injuries, accounting for 58 to 90% of cases.[48, 50] Affected infants show signs of denervation of the deltoid, supraspinatus, biceps, and brachioradialis. The infant holds the arm loosely and internally rotated at the shoulder with extension of the elbow, pronation of the forearm, and flexion at the wrist (so-called waiter's tip position) (Fig. 34–7). The Moro response is generally de-

Table 34–1
Risk Factors for Brachial Plexus Injuries

Risk Factor	Incidence
Large fetal size (>3500 gm)	56–75%
Abnormal presentation	56%
Breech	14%
Abnormal vertex	42%
Shoulder dystocia	81%
Vertex	51%
Breech	30%
Fetal depression	44%

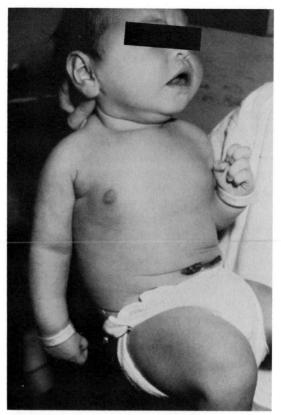

FIGURE 34–7
An infant with Erb's palsy following birth trauma, with the characteristic loose dangling of the arm internally rotated at the shoulder, the elbow extended, the forearm pronated, and the wrist flexed.

creased or absent on the affected side, and biceps and brachioradialis reflexes are absent.[48, 82]

Isolated Klumpke's paralysis is the least common type of brachial plexus injury and involves the lower roots of the brachial plexus, C8–T1. The injury involves the intrinsic muscles of the hand, the flexors of the wrist and fingers (intrinsic minus clawhand deformity), and frequently the sympathetic nerves, with an associated Horner syndrome. In neonates, the classic Horner syndrome of ptosis, miosis, anhidrosis, and enophthalmos may also be associated with delayed pigmentation of the iris for up to 1 year.[48, 163] Klumpke's palsy is associated with sparing of the deep tendon reflexes.

Total brachial plexus palsies (Erb-Duchenne-Klumpke) occur in about 10% of cases, 33% of which have an associated Horner syndrome and may include paralysis of the diaphragm if the C4 root is also involved (5–9%).[48, 82, 163] The entire arm and hand is paralyzed, and no deep tendon reflexes are present. Bilateral brachial plexus injuries are seen in 8 to 23% of infants.[48, 141] The overall incidence of birth-related brachial plexus palsy is 0.38 to 2.5 per 1000 live births. Some reports suggest a recent decline in incidence to below 1 in 1000 births, whereas others report no reduction in recent experience.[48, 82, 138] Even in institutions where there appears to have been a significant decrease in brachial plexus injuries, investigators clearly document an improved prognosis for affected infants.[138]

The most important aspect in evaluating an infant with a suspected brachial plexus injury is a careful joint-by-joint assessment, recording the remaining active musculature.[53] Most researchers agree that electromyography and myelography are seldom useful in the initial phase.[82] Possible associated injuries include cervical spine trauma, fracture of the clavicle (9%), fracture of the proximal humeral epiphysis, torticollis, facial palsy (5–14%), and diaphragmatic paralysis. Accordingly, diagnostic studies should include radiologic assessment of the arm, clavicle, cervical spine, and chest.[48, 82]

The ultimate prognosis depends on the type and severity of the brachial plexus lesion, with Erb's palsy having the highest recovery rate. Infants whose trauma occurred secondary to breech delivery generally have poorer outlooks than those with vertex presentations. Before 1970, full recovery was reported only 7 to 40% of the time.[1, 167] More recent reports have documented complete recoveries in 80 to 95% of affected infants.[50, 65, 75, 138] The neonates who ultimately recover generally show marked improvement in symptoms in the first few months of life. Complete recovery generally occurs by 3 to 6 months of age, although a few patients may require 12 months or more to achieve maximal function. If no clinical improvement occurs by 3 to 4 months, the prognosis is generally poor. Long-term deficits in these patients can include muscle atrophy, joint contractures, and possible impaired limb growth.

Because outlook is excellent in most patients, early therapy should be supportive while allowing spontaneous recovery to occur. The arm should be rested in a sling for 2 to 3 weeks, followed by gentle passive-motion exercises, including abduction and external rotation. Judicious wrist bracing can be considered in some patients. Early surgical intervention, including use of microsurgical techniques, is not advocated, because even nerve roots believed to be avulsed may progressively develop good sensory and motor function.[2, 146, 150] In infants who show no improvement by 3 months—specifically, no return of biceps function—Meyer recommends myelography and electrical studies in consideration of surgical exploration and repair, based on his own experience[114] and large French series by Gilbert and Tassin.[63] He suggests that surgical intervention using intraoperative nerve action potentials can improve the patient's functional classification significantly over that of a nonoperated population.[114] Traditional surgical approaches in patients with long-term disabilities have been aimed at improving shoulder function by anterior tendon release, external rotation osteotomy, or muscle transfer procedures.[64, 91, 138]

Phrenic Nerve Paralysis

Naunyn first described a neonate with unilateral diaphragmatic paralysis in 1902, and the infant had an associated brachial plexus injury.[119] The pathogenesis of the two lesions is similar, with lateral hyperextension of the neck producing stretching or avulsion of the third, fourth, and fifth cervical roots, which supply the phrenic nerve.[42, 55] Phrenic nerve paralysis almost never occurs as an isolated lesion in neonates, generally accompanying either Erb's palsy or total brachial plexus palsy.[53, 164] About 80% of phrenic nerve lesions are on the right side, and less than 1% are bilateral.[163]

Neonates tolerate diaphragmatic paralysis more poorly than do adults or children. The newborn mediastinum is not fixed, and contralateral displacement secondary to paradoxic respiratory movement can be severe, with increased work of breathing, hypoxemia, and hypercarbia. Additional factors include the infant's recumbent posture with decreased vital capacity as his or her weaker intercostal muscles and smaller airways are compromised, increasing the risk of airway obstruction.[163] The infant soon develops respiratory distress, with tachypnea, irregular and labored respirations, and episodes of cyanosis. Dullness and diminished breath sounds are present over the affected side. Breathing is almost completely thoracic, and no bulging of the abdomen occurs with inspiration.[48, 53, 55, 141, 163]

Roentgenograms in the first few days may show little or no elevation of the hemidiaphragm, even in the presence of respiratory distress.[55, 141, 163] Serial films ultimately demonstrate the diaphragmatic elevation, accompanied by a mediastinal shift to the opposite side (Fig. 34–8). Fluoroscopy and ultrasonography are useful diagnostic tools and confirm the paradoxic movement of the affected diaphragm with respiration.[53] Most infants recover spontaneously, although composite series quote a mortality of 10 to 20%, and bilateral paralysis rate of up to 50%.[65, 105] Return of diaphragmatic function generally occurs by age 6 weeks, although several months may be required. If no improvement occurs in the first few weeks of life, recovery of function is unlikely.[42, 48, 55, 128]

Treatment of the affected infant is initially supportive, with administration of oxygen and positioning with the affected side down. More severe cases, particularly cases of bilateral paralysis, may require endotracheal intubation and assisted ventilation. Such infants may also suffer gastroesophageal reflux and severe gastrointestinal symptoms, particularly if the left side is involved, secondary to elevation or even volvulus of the stomach.[68, 141] The risk of aspiration of this population is high, and oral or gavage feedings must be closely monitored.

Most researchers recommend diaphragmatic plication if no improvement occurs within 2 months of supportive therapy or if complications such as pneumonia, respiratory failure, or aspiration are severe and life threatening.[3] Haller and co-workers advocate a therapeutic program using mechanical ventilation followed by weaning with continuous positive airway pressure.[74] Surgical plication is recommended if the child cannot be successfully extubated after 4 to 6 weeks. If paralysis is bilateral, the more severely affected side is plicated. The partial excision or tightening of the diaphragm allows the mediastinum to return to a normal position and appears to produce no long-term pulmonary or chest wall complications.[55] Eventration of the diaphragm may sometimes be confused with diaphragmatic paralysis. Paradoxic movement is generally not present with eventration. Considerations regarding possible surgical therapy are identical for both conditions.

Fractures

Most birth-related fractures consist of either midshaft fracture of long bones, most commonly the clavicle, or epi-

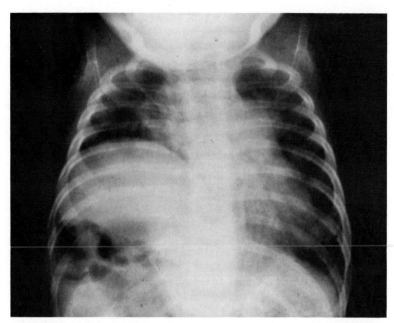

FIGURE 34–8
Right-sided diaphragmatic paralysis secondary to phrenic nerve injury with elevation of the right hemidiaphragm and shift of the mediastinum to the left.

physeal separation of the humerus or femur.[68, 92] Less than 1% of live-born infants are affected. Whereas most clavicle fractures are associated with cephalic presentations, more than 75% of extremity fractures are related to breech deliveries.[42, 135]

Clavicle

The shoulder girdle—including the clavicle, brachial plexus, humerus, and phrenic nerve—is a common site of injury in large, hypotonic infants with shoulder dystocia or in those undergoing difficult delivery of the arm in breech presentation.[53, 99] A high association with fetal asphyxia has also been reported.[99]

Fractures of the clavicle represent 92.4% of obstetric fractures, with most going unrecognized.[109] Such fractures are more common in cephalic presentations and involve the anterior clavicle, which abuts the maternal symphysis. Most clavicular fractures are of the greenstick type and occur at the junction of the middle and lateral third of the bone. In isolated clavicular injuries, signs and symptoms may be slight. The callus is maximal and palpable 1 week after delivery and may be the first sign of a fracture.[141] Arm movement is usually normal. Some infants show pseudoparalysis or an asymmetric Moro response on the affected side, but such symptoms generally suggest the presence of associated injuries. All infants with clavicular fractures should be evaluated for possible brachial plexus, cervical spine, and humerus trauma with appropriate radiographs and examinations.[53, 82]

The prognosis with clavicular fracture is uniformly good, with solid union in 7 to 10 days and return of the bone to normal contour in 2 to 3 months.[141] Reduction or specific therapy is generally not necessary, although some advise using a sling or figure-of-eight bandage for a few days if the infant seems particularly uncomfortable.[53, 82]

Humerus

Proximal Epiphysis. An infant with a long-bone fracture exhibits a tender, swollen extremity that hangs limply and has no voluntary movement (pseudoparalysis). Symptoms and signs are often first noticed the day after delivery. Lack of calcification at ossification centers may make newborn epiphyseal injuries difficult to diagnose. Arthrography may be required in puzzling cases.[53, 135] In an infant with a fracture of the proximal humeral epiphysis, the arm hangs limply with extension and external rotation. The appearance may mimic Erb's palsy, which can coexist. If significant displacement is present, closed reduction is indicated. A Velpeau dressing is applied. Avascular necrosis has never been reported.[53, 82, 125, 142]

Midshaft. Midshaft humeral fractures are often audible at the time of injury. The fracture line is generally diagonal and located in the middle third of the bone, below the insertion of the deltoid.[141] Erb's palsy may be present, depending on the mechanism of injury. The fracture may also produce a radial nerve paralysis with wrist drop, which usually resolves within 6 to 8 weeks.[42, 135] Midshaft fractures result in a limp limb with swelling, crepitus, and motion at the center of the shaft. A Velpeau dressing is adequate therapy. Healing is rapid, with remodeling occurring over 3 years.

Distal Epiphysis. Fractures of the distal humeral epiphysis are uncommon and generally associated with breech delivery.[113] The fractures are typically Salter-Harris type I with complete separation. A deformed, swollen elbow is always present. Gentle reduction of the separation with application of a posterior splint and placement of the elbow in flexion for 2 to 3 weeks should result in full range of motion by 4 weeks.[82, 135]

Femur

Proximal Epiphysis. Historically, Poland first described fractures of the proximal femoral epiphysis in 1898.[11, 123, 127] The fracture is most often confused clinically and radiologically with congenital dislocation of the hip. An infant with congenital hip dislocation generally is pain-free, shows a less severe degree of displacement, and has an abnormal acetabulum. Traumatic obstetric dislocation of the hip has never been described and has never been demonstrated by experimental studies on stillborn infants or animals.[123] Simulated obstetric trauma in these studies consistently resulted in a type I physeal injury.[76] The typical patient is a large infant with a breech, often footling, presentation.

Occasionally, proximal femoral epiphyseal fractures are not recognized until a callus appears, at which point the fracture may be fixed and irreducible. Coxa vara and other long-term complications may then result, although some infants who have had no therapy appear to have excellent results.[123, 154] Therapy consists of closed reduction followed by Bryant traction or a spica cast.[154, 169] If Bryant traction is used, careful observation for possible development of ischemic complications to the limb is essential.[82] The vascular response to a proximal femoral epiphyseal fracture is one of hyperemia; hence, avascular necrosis of bone has never been reported.

Midshaft. Midshaft femoral fractures occur secondary to version maneuvers during difficult deliveries. It is an audible injury, generally recognized at the time of delivery. The extremity is shortened with induration and tenderness of the thigh. Reduction under general anesthesia, with Bryant traction or spica immobilization, is recommended.[86, 135] Immobilization is maintained for 2 to 4 weeks until callus forms.[141] Alignment can be corrected by wedging the cast in the course of therapy.[82]

Distal Epiphysis. Complete fracture of the distal epiphysis of the femur is rare. Closed reduction followed by immobilization in a spica cast for 2 to 3 weeks is recommended. The prognosis is excellent.[11, 135, 139]

Abdominal Trauma

Intraperitoneal and retroperitoneal injuries secondary to birth trauma may not be appreciated until life-threatening complications occur.[51] Although such injuries are uncommon, they should be considered after difficult deliveries, particularly in any newborn infant with pallor, anemia, irritability, and no obvious source of blood loss, or in one who develops shock and abdominal distention.[55] Intra-abdominal organs injured, in decreasing order of frequency, are the liver, adrenal gland, spleen, and kidney.[68] Neonatal asphyxia during delivery is an important factor and can produce visceral congestion and alteration in blood coagulation, resulting in increased susceptibility to injury to these organs.[141]

Liver

The risk of hepatic injury is significantly increased when hepatomegaly, hepatic hemangiomatosis, or coagulopathies are present. Extremes of infant size and breech deliveries are also predisposing factors.[53, 55, 131, 141] Previous studies suggest an incidence of hepatic injuries of 0.9 to 9%, although a recent report from Washington University in St. Louis found only 1 hepatic injury in 10,000 consecutive newborn autopsies.[19, 53, 55]

Subcapsular hematomas are more common than hepatic lacerations. Hematomas caused by abnormal traction forces are generally located in proximity to the support ligaments; those secondary to excess pressure on the costal margin are on the anterior surface.[71] Rupture of the hematoma often occurs after 48 hours of age and can be heralded by shock (Fig. 34–9). The infant may appear normal for the first days of life or may show nonspecific signs associated with loss of blood into the hematoma, including tachycardia, listlessness, poor feeding, falling hematocrit, pallor, and jaundice. A palpable mass or abdominal fullness may be present.[42, 51, 53, 55] Ultrasonography or computed tomography may confirm the presence of an unruptured subcapsular hematoma or may help differentiate hepatic trauma from injuries to the adrenal gland or spleen.[42, 53, 55] Rupture of the hematoma through the Gleason capsule results in free bleeding into the peritoneal cavity and progressive circulatory collapse. Abdominal distention and rigidity may be accompanied by a bluish discoloration of the overlying skin or blood in the scrotum.[42, 55] Uniform opacity of the abdomen, indicating free intraperitoneal fluid, is often seen on abdominal roentgenograms. Paracentesis confirms the presence of free blood in the peritoneal cavity. It is imperative that coagulation defects and volume deficits be corrected before operation. In cases in which severe coagulopathies are present, exchange transfusion can be considered.[45] Surgical hemostasis of the newborn or neonatal liver is often exceedingly difficult, even with modern topical hemostatic agents and suture techniques, and only 11 survivors were reported before 1960. The use of fibrin glue (cryoprecipitate and topical thrombin) has been advocated and may be life saving.[19] In less severe cases, when the infant is hemodynamically stable, supportive therapy, particularly transfusion of blood and blood components, might avoid the necessity for operation, but extremely close monitoring and careful selection is essential in these patients. Unfortunately, as illustrated in Figure 34–9, most infants who die because of hepatic hemorrhage are diagnosed only at autopsy.

Adrenal Gland

The newborn adrenal gland is large. At the time of birth, a major portion of the cortex (inner fetal zone) is undergoing rapid involution, reducing the size of the gland by half in the first few months of life. The involution process results in congestion and loss of supporting structures, making the gland susceptible to birth injury. Approximately 90% of adrenal injuries are unilateral, with 75% occurring on the right side. It is postulated that the direct venous drainage into the inferior vena cava on the right produces significant venous congestion during delivery.[68, 141, 151] Risk factors include macrosomia, breech deliveries, and congenital syphilis. Autopsy series have suggested that the incidence of subclinical adrenal hemorrhage may be much higher than previously suspected.[55]

Symptoms vary according to the degree of hemorrhage. Irritability, lethargy and fever may be present in mild cases, or the full-blown picture of frank shock can occur with severe bleeding. As with liver and spleen injuries, these signs often do not appear until between the second and seventh days of life.[141] Bleeding is generally confined to the retroperitoneum, and up to 30 to 40 ml of blood may be contained in the adrenal capsule[131] (Fig. 34–10).

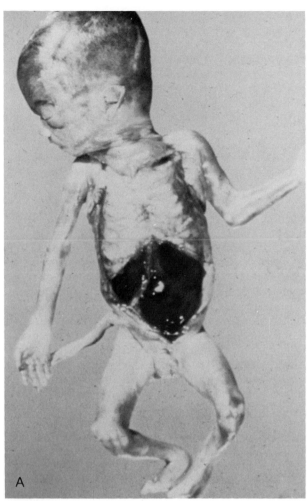

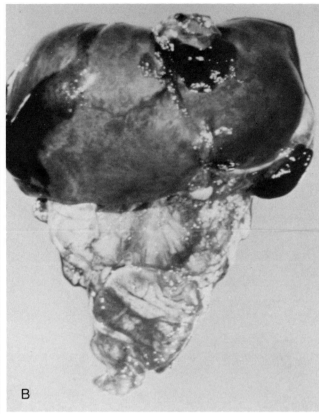

FIGURE 34-9

A, Portmortem photograph of a premature infant who expired secondary to unrecognized disruption of the liver from birth trauma. *B,* Liver of the same infant. Note the residual hematomas, peripheral and subcapsular and central, near the supporting ligaments.

The combination of a falling hemoglobin and a bland mass suggests the diagnosis. Abdominal roentgenograms may reveal anterior displacement of the stomach and duodenum, and serial ultrasonography typically shows characteristic development of cystic components in the area of hemorrhage. Computed tomography, radionuclide scans, and intravenous pyelography may also be useful. Paracentesis generally reveals no free blood within the peritoneal cavity. The differential diagnosis considers the spectrum of flank masses, including neuroblastoma, and analysis of urinary catecholamine levels should be performed. Calcification may occur as early as the twelfth day of life and is generally rim-like as contrasted to the diffuse pattern seen in neuroblastoma.[53, 55, 68, 141] The presence of a calcified adrenal gland on roentgenograms at several years of age may confirm a previously unsuspected neonatal adrenal hemorrhage.

Supportive therapy with restoration of blood volume is generally adequate. Some infants may require surgical exploration and adrenalectomy. Adrenal insufficiency is rare, even with bilateral hemorrhage, although some investigators recommend adrenal function tests after recovery.[53, 55]

Spleen

The high protected location of the spleen in the neonate makes birth injury exceedingly uncommon. As with other intra-abdominal organs, difficult deliveries of large infants may produce traction tears of the capsule with resultant hemorrhage.[51, 68, 131, 141] Infants with coagulopathies or hepatosplenomegaly secondary to erythroblastosis fetalis or intrauterine infections are particularly at risk.

Although splenic rupture is far less frequent than hepatic rupture, the clinical course is similar.[53, 55] Abdominal roentgenograms may reveal displacement of the gastric air bubble or the presence of ascites. As with liver injuries, correction of coagulation defects and restoration of blood volume is essential, but surgery is required in most infants. Patients undergoing splenectomy in the neonatal period are known to be at high risk of developing life-threatening infections later. Accordingly, at operation, every attempt should be made to preserve the spleen, so long as the infant is stable at operation and life-threatening hemorrhage is not present.[72, 112] When splenectomy is required, many researchers recommend autotransplantation of splenic tissue, despite

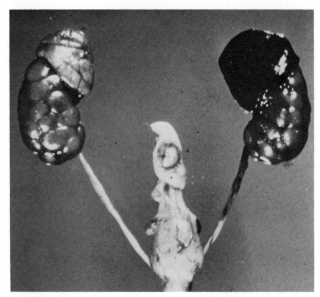

FIGURE 34–10
Autopsy specimen of a left adrenal hemorrhage.

conflicting experimental evidence about the efficacy of this procedure.[134]

Kidney

Renal injuries secondary to birth trauma are exceedingly rare, with only about a dozen cases reported in the literature. Most such injuries are associated with pre-existing anomalies such as hydronephrosis. Signs and symptoms are similar to those of adrenal hemorrhage.[121, 141]

Genital Trauma

Severe genital trauma is rare. Swelling and discoloration of the scrotum or labia majora are invariably associated with breech deliveries. In uncomplicated cases, resolution occurs in 4 to 5 days. When symptoms are more suggestive, neonatal testicular torsion may be suspected. A history of breech delivery and bilateral ecchymoses suggests a traumatic etiology, but some cases may require surgical exploration.[82] Testicular atrophy, scrotal gangrene, and transient hydronephrosis have also been reported in association with birth trauma.[38, 56]

POSTNATAL INJURIES

A wide spectrum of postnatal trauma to the neonate may occur in the delivery room or nursery. Many of these are related to vascular access or blood-sampling procedures and are discussed in other sections of this text.

Pharyngoesophageal Perforation

Iatrogenic perforation of the pharynx or esophagus in the neonate is a well-recognized entity. Attempted endotracheal intubation, often using a stylet, is the most common cause. Traumatic perforations have also been reported secondary to vigorous orotracheal suctioning or passage of orogastric feeding tubes. Most infants who suffer this injury are premature, and intubation is difficult—hence, often traumatic. Blood in the pharynx is commonly seen after the procedure and is a helpful diagnostic clue subsequently.

Krasna and colleagues described three clinical presentations: (1) mimicking esophageal atresia, (2) with right pneumothorax and feeding tube in right chest, and (3) with right-sided infiltrate and an abnormal right extrapleural air collection.[97] Blair and associates noted that in infants with esophageal atresia, a nasogastric tube can pass to a distance of approximately 11 cm before reaching the point of obstruction.[18] Passage of a tube to a distance significantly less or, more commonly, significantly more than 11 cm and with difficulty should lead to questioning the diagnosis of esophageal atresia. The finding of blood on the tube is also exceedingly rare with esophageal atresia but common with esophageal perforation. A chest radiograph may reveal an abnormal position or course of the nasogastric tube, a pneumothorax or pneumomediastinum, subcutaneous air, or an air-fluid level. Additionally, esophageal atresia is suggested by a history of hydramnios. Air-contrast esophagography is usually adequate in studying infants with suspected esophageal atresia. If, however, radiopaque contrast studies are believed indicated in confusing cases, the preferred agent is one of the new low-osmolality, water-soluble formulations.[132]

Although most series contain some infants with iatrogenic esophageal perforation treated surgically, nonoperative therapy has been shown to be safe and efficacious.[18, 90, 117] Krasna and co-workers nonoperatively treated 11 infants, including four with feeding tubes penetrating into their right pleural cavities, with no mortalities related to the esophageal perforations.[97] Infants received broad-spectrum antibiotics, parenteral nutrition, and selective tube thoracostomy. However, neonates suffering esophageal perforation must be monitored closely in an appropriate setting, and clinical deterioration or the development of infectious complications may prompt surgical exploration and mediastinal drainage. Healing in such injuries is rapid and complete within the first few weeks of life. No long-term sequelae have been noted.

References

1. Adler JB, Patterson RL: Erb's palsy: Long-term results of treatment in eighty-eight cases. J Bone Joint Surg [Am] 49:1052–1064, 1967.
2. Alanen M, Halonen JP, Katevuo K, et al: Early surgical exploration and epineural repair of birth brachial palsy. Z Kindenchir 41:335–337, 1986.
3. Aldrich TK, Herman JH, Rochester DF: Bilateral phrenic nerve palsy in the newborn infant. J Pediatr 97:988, 1980.
4. Alexander E, Davis CH: Intrauterine fracture of the infant's skull. J Neurosurg 30:446–454, 1969.
5. Alpini D, Corti A, Brusa E, et al: Septal deviation in newborn infants. Int J Pediatr Otorhinolaryngol 11:103–107, 1986.
6. Amiel-Tison C: Neurologic problems in perinatology. Clin Perinatol 1:33, 1974.
7. Amine AR: Spinal cord injury in a fetus. Surg Neurol 6:369–370, 1976.

8. Avast DC, Jordan GL Jr: Traumatic wounds of the female reproductive organs. J Trauma 4:839, 1964.

9. Baker DP: Trauma in the pregnant patient. Surg Clin North Am 62:275–289, 1982.

10. Ballas S, Toaff R: Hyperextension of the fetal head in breech presentation: Radiological evaluation and significance. Br J Obstet Gynecol 83:201–204, 1976.

11. Baragale RC, Kuhns LR: Traumatic separation of the distal femoral epiphysis in the newborn. J Pediatr Orthop 3:396–398, 1983.

12. Barnett E, Nairn A: A study of foetal attitude. Br J Radiol 38:338–349, 1965.

13. Beach WB: Travel in pregnancy. Am J Obstet Gynecol 54:1054–1057, 1947.

14. Beard RJ, Johnson DA: Fetal distress due to cord prolapse through a fenestration in a lower segment uterine scar. J Obstet Gynaecol Br Commonw 79:763, 1972.

15. Behrman RE, Margurten HH: Birth Injuries in Neonatal-Perinatal Medicine: Diseases of the Fetus and Infant. 2nd ed. St. Louis, CV Mosby, 1977.

16. Bell D, Johansson D, McLean FH, et al: Birth asphyxia, trauma, and mortality in twins: Has cesarean section improved outcome? Am J Obstet Gynecol 154:235–239, 1986.

17. Besio R, Cabellero C, Meehoff E, et al: Neonatal retinal hemorrhage and influence of perinatal factors. Am J Ophthalmol 87:74, 1979.

18. Blair GK, Filler RM, Theodorescu D: Neonatal pharyngoesophageal perforation mimicking esophageal atresia: Clues to diagnosis. J Pediatr Surg 22:770–774, 1987.

19. Blocker SH, Ternberg JL: Traumatic liver laceration in the newborn: Repair with fibrin glue. J Pediatr Surg 21:369–371, 1986.

20. Brans YW, Cassady G: Neonatal spinal cord injuries. Am J Obstet Gynecol 123:918, 1975.

21. Brenner WE, Bruce RD, Hendricks CH: The characteristics and perils of breech presentation. Am J Obstet Gynecol 118:700–712, 1974.

22. Bresnan MJ, Abroms IF: Neonatal spinal cord transection secondary to intrauterine hyperextension of the neck in breech presentation. J Pediatr 84:734, 1974.

23. Bresnan MJ, Abroms IF: Neonatal spinal cord transection secondary to intrauterine hyperextension of the neck in breech presentation. Fetal Neonatal Med 84:734–737, 1974.

24. Brockuizen FF, Washington JM, Johnson F: Vacuum extraction versus forceps delivery: Indications and complications, 1979 to 1984. Obstet Gynecol 69:338–342, 1987.

25. Bucholz R, Mauldin D: Prenatal diagnosis of intrauterine fetal fracture. J Bone Joint Surg [Am] 60:712–713, 1978.

26. Buchsbaum HJ: Accidental injury complicating pregnancy. Am J Obstet Gynecol 102:752–769, 1968.

27. Buchsbaum HJ: Diagnosis and management of abdominal gunshot wounds during pregnancy. J Trauma 15:425, 1975.

28. Byers RK: Transection of the spinal cord in the newborn: Case with autopsy and comparison with normal cord at the same age. Arch Neurol Psychiatr 27:585, 1932.

29. Caterini H, Langer A, Sama JC, et al: Fetal risk in hyperextension of the fetal head in breech presentation. Am J Obstet Gynecol 123:632, 1975.

30. Cesarean Childbirth. NIH Publication No 82-2067, October 1981.

31. Chaney RH, Givens CA, Watkins GP, et al: Birth injury as the cause of mental retardation. Obstet Gynecol 67:771–775, 1986.

32. Churchill JA, Stevenson L, Habhad G: Cephalhematoma and natal brain injury. Obstet Gynecol 27:580, 1966.

33. Cohn HE, Jackson BT, Piasecki AJ, et al: Fetal cardiovascular responses to asphyxia induced by decreased uterine perfusion. J Dev Physiol 7:289–297, 1985.

34. Collea JV, Quilligan EJ: The management of breech presentation. J Reprod Med 23:258, 1979.

35. Conner E, Curran J: In utero traumatic intra-abdominal deceleration injury to the fetus: A case report. Am J Obstet Gynecol 125:567–570, 1976.

36. Cordero L Jr, Hon EH: Scalp abscess: A rare complication of fetal monitoring. J Pediatr 78:533–537, 1971.

37. Couser RJ, Mammel MC, Coleman M, et al: Neonatal brachial artery occlusion from an umbilical cord tourniquet. J Pediatr 104:286–289, 1984.

38. Cromie WJ: Genitourinary injuries in the neonate. Clin Pediatr 18:292, 1979.

39. Crosby WM: Trauma during pregnancy: Maternal and fetal injury. Obstet Gynecol Surv 29:683–699, 1974.

40. Crosby WM, Costilos JP: Safety of lap belt restraint for pregnant victims of automobile collisions. N Engl J Med 284:633–636, 1971.

41. Crumrine PK, Koenigsberger MR, Chutorian AM: Footdrop in the neonate with neurologic and electrophysiologic data. J Pediatr 86:779, 1975.

42. Curran JS: Birth-associated injury. Clin Perinatol 8:111–129, 1981.

43. Curtis BH, Fisher RL: Congenital hyperextension with anterior subluxation of the knee. J Bone Joint Surg [Am] 51:255–269, 1969.

44. Cyr RM, Usher RH, McLean FH: Changing patterns of birth asphyxia and trauma over 20 years. Am J Obstet Gynecol 148:490–498, 1984.

45. Cywes S: Haemoperitoneum in the newborn. S Afr Med J 41:1063, 1967.

46. de Azevido Lage J, Guarniero R, Jabarros TEP, et al: Intrauterine diagnosis of congenital dislocation of the knee. J Pediatr Orthop 6:110–111, 1986.

47. Dierken LJ, Rosen MG, Thompson K, et al: Midforceps deliveries: Long-term outcome of infants. Am J Obstet Gynecol 154:764–768, 1986.

48. Donn SM, Faix RG: Long-term prognosis for the infant with severe birth trauma. Clin Perinatol 10:507–520, 1983.

49. El Khazen N, Faverly D, Vamos E, et al: Lethal osteopetrosis with multiple fractures in utero. Am J Med Genet 23:811–819, 1986.

50. Eng GD: Brachial plexus palsy in newborn infants. Pediatrics 48:18–28, 1971.

51. Eraklis AJ: Abdominal injury related to the trauma of birth. Pediatrics 39:421–424, 1967.

52. Erb W: On a characteristic site of injury in the brachial plexus (reprinted). Arch Neurol 21:433–434, 1969.

53. Faix RG, Donn SM: Immediate management of the traumatized infant. Clin Perinatol 10:487–505, 1983.

54. Falls FH: Opisthotonos foetus. Surg Gynecol Obstet 24:65–67, 1917.

55. Fanaroff AA, Martin RJ: Neonatal-Perinatal Medicine. 4th ed. St. Louis, CV Mosby, 1987, pp 317–342, 495–520.

56. Finan BF, Redman J: Neonatal genital trauma. Urology 25:532–533, 1985.

57. Fort AT, Harlin RS: Pregnancy outcome after noncatastrophic maternal trauma during pregnancy. Obstet Gynecol 35:912–915, 1970.

58. Freud S: Zur Kenntnis der cerebralen Diplegien des Kindesalters (im Anschlerss an die little'sche Krankheit). In: Kassowitz M (ed): Beitrage zur Kinderheilkunde. Leipsiz, Germany, Franz Deuticke, 1893, pp 104–136.

59. Friedman EA: Whither midforceps? Its place in obstetrics today. Contemp Ob/Gyn 21:85, 1983.

60. Gabbe SG, Niebye JR, Simpson JL: Obstetrics: Normal and Problem Pregnancies. New York, Churchill Livingstone, 1986, pp 579–622.

61. Gassner CB, Paul RH: Laceration of umbilical cord vessels secondary to amniocentesis. Obstet Gynecol 48:627–630, 1976.

62. Gibbert GF: The factors influencing the attitude of the foetus in utero. Proc R Soc Med 32:1223–1224, 1939.

63. Gilbert A, Tassin JL: Reparation chirugicale du plexus brachialdens la paralysis obstetrical. Chirugie 110:70–75, 1984.

64. Goddard NJ, Fixsen JA: Rotation osteotomy of the humerus for birth injuries of the brachial plexus. J Bone Joint Surg [Am] 66:257–259, 1984.

65. Gordon M, Rich H, Deutschberger J, et al: The immediate and long-term outcome of obstetric birth trauma. I. Brachial plexus paralysis. Am J Obstet Gynecol 117:51, 1973.

66. Gould SJ, Smith JF: Spinal cord transection, cerebral ischaemic and brain stem injury in a baby following a Kielland's forceps rotation. Neuropathol Appl Neurobiol 10:151–158, 1984.

67. Gray LP: Septal and association cranial birth deformities. Med J Aust 1:557, 1974.

68. Greenwald AG, Shute PC, Shively JL: Brachial plexus birth palsy: A 10 year report on the incidence and prognosis. J Pediatr Orthop 4:689–692, 1984.

69. Gresham EL: Birth trauma. Pediatr Clin North Am 22:317–328, 1975.

70. Gross TL, Sokol RJ, Williams T, et al: Shoulder dystocia: A fetal–physican risk. Am J Obstet Gynecol 156:1408–1418, 1987.

71. Gruenwald P: Rupture of liver and spleen in the newborn infant. J Pediatr 33:195, 1948.

72. Hadley FP, Mickel RE: Conservative surgery in neonatal splenic injury. S Afr J Surg 22:97–101, 1984.

73. Haller ES, Nesbitt RE Jr, Anderson GW: Clinical and pathologic concepts of gross intracranial hemorrhage in perinatal mortality. Surg Obstet Gynecol Surv 11:179, 1956.

74. Haller JA, Pickard LR, Tepas JJ, et al: Management of diaphragmatic paralysis in infants with special emphasis on selection of patients for operative plication. J Pediatr Surg 14:779–785, 1979.

75. Hardy AE: Birth injuries to the brachial plexus: Treatment of defects in the shoulder. J Bone Joint Surg (Br) 63:98, 1981.

76. Harrenstein RJ: Pseudoluxatic Coxae durch abreissen der Femurepiphyse bei den Geburt. Bruns Beitr Z Klin Chir 146:592–604, 1929.

77. Harwood-Nash DC, Hendrick EB, Hudson AR: The significance of skull fracture in children: A study of 1,187 patients. Radiology 101:151, 1971.

78. Hassim AM, Lucas C, Acharva RJ: Fetal survival after partial extrusion into the bladder. Br Med J 1:286–287, 1972.

79. Haycock CE: Saving both mother and fetus. Consultant, January 1982, pp 269–276.

80. Haycock CE: Penetrating trauma in pregnancy. In: Trauma and Pregnancy. Littleton, MA, PSG Publishing, 1985, pp 44–56.

81. Haycock CE: Trauma and Pregnancy. Littleton, MA, PSG Publishing, 1985, pp 34–41.

82. Hensinger RN, Jones ET: Neonatal Orthopaedics. New York, Grune and Stratton, 1981, pp 33–74.

83. Holm VA: The causes of cerebral palsy: A contemporary perspective. JAMA 247:1473–1477, 1982.

84. Hope EE, Bodensteiner JB, Thong N: Neonatal lumber plexus injury. Arch Neurol 42:94–95, 1985.

85. Illingsworth RS: A paediatrician asks: Why is it called birth injury? Br J Obstet Gynaecol 92:122–130, 1985.

86. Irani Rn, Nicholson JT, Chung SMK: Long-term results in the treatment of femoral-shaft fractures in young children by immediate spica immobilization. J Bone Joint Surg (Am) 58:945–951, 1976.

87. Jain IS, Singh, YP, Grupta SL, et al: Ocular hazards during birth. J Pediatr Ophthalmol 17:14, 1980.

88. Jazbi B: Subluxation of the nasal septum in the newborn: Etiology, diagnosis, and treatment. Otolaryngol Clin North Am 10:125, 1977.

89. Jeppssen F, Windfeld I: Dislocation of the nasal septal cartilage in the newborn. Acta Obstet Gynecol Scand 51:5, 1972.

90. Johnson DE, Foker J, Munson DP, et al: Management of esophageal and pharyngeal perforation in the newborn infant. Pediatrics 70:592–596, 1982.

91. Jones BN, Mansek PR, Schoenecker PL, et al: Latissimus dorsi transfer to restore elbow extension in obstetrical palsy. J Pediatr Orthop 4:287–289, 1985.

92. Jones L: Birth trauma and the cervical spine. Arch Dis Child 45:147, 1970.

93. Jones PG: Torticollis in infancy and childhood. Springfield, IL, Charles C Thomas, 1968, p 102.

94. Kanokpungsukdi A, Petrom M, Model B, et al: Diagnostic fetal blood sampling for the hemoglobinopathies: 10 year experience. Eur J Obstet Gynecol Reprod Biol 20:35–41, 1985.

95. Kendall N, Woloskin H: Cephalhematoma associated with fracture of the skull. J Pediatr 41:125, 1952.

96. Knowlton R: A flying foetus. J Obstet Gynecol Br Emp 45:834–835, 1938.

97. Krasna IH, Rosenfeld D, Benjamin BG, et al: Esophageal perforation in the neonate: An emerging problem in the newborn nursery. J Pediatr Surg 22:784–790, 1987.

98. Lalos O, Lundstrom P, Probst FP: Spontaneous rupture of the uterus in the third trimester with a living fetus expelled into the abdominal cavity. Acta Obstet Gynecol Scand 56:153–156, 1977.

99. Levine MG, Holroyde J, Woods JR, et al: Birth trauma: Incidence and predisposing factors. Obstet Gynecol 63:792, 1984.

100. Lilford RJ: Chorion villus biopsy. Clin Obstet Gynecol 13:611–632, 1986.

101. Little WJ: On the influence of abnormal parturition, difficult labors, premature birth, and asphyxia neonatorum, on the mental and physical condition of the child, especially in relation to deformities. Clin Orthop 46:7–22, 1966.

102. Loeser JD, Kilburn HL, Jolley T: Management of depressed skull fracture in the newborn. J Neurosurg 44:62, 1976.

103. McCarty V, Risely DR: Traumatic rupture of the uterus in early pregnancy. J Int Coll Surg 20:228–231, 1956.

104. McCormick D: Seatbelt injury: Case of complete transection of pregnant uterus. J Am Osteopath Assoc 67:1139–1140, 1968.

105. MacDonald PC, Pritchard JA: Williams' Obstetrics. New York, Appleton-Centry-Crofts, 1980, p 5.

106. McFarland BL: Congenital dislocation of the knee. J Bone Joint Surg (Br) 11:281–285, 1929.

107. McFarland RA: Human factors in air transportation. New York, McGraw-Hill, 1953, pp 758–759.

108. McVabey WK, Smith EI: Penetrating wounds of the gravid uterus. J Trauma 12:1024–1028, 1973.

109. Madsen ET: Fractures of the extremities in the newborn. Acta Obstet Gynecol 34:41–74, 1955.

110. Manning J, Adour K: Facial paralysis in children. Pediatrics 1:102, 1972.

111. Maryniak GM, Frank JB: Clinical assessment of the Kobayashi vacuum extractor. Obstet Gynecol 64:31–35, 1984.

112. Matsuyama S, Suzuki N, Nagamachi Y: Rupture of the spleen in the newborn: Treatment without splenectomy. J Pediatr Surg 11:115–116, 1976.

113. Menon TJ: Fracture separation of the lower humeral epiphysis due to birth injury: A case report. Injury 14:168–169, 1982.

114. Meyer RD: Treatment of adult and obstetrical brachial plexus injuries. Orthopedics 9:899–903, 1986.

115. Milunsky A: Risk of amniocentesis for prenatal diagnosis. N Engl J Med 293:932, 1975.

116. Modell B: Chorionic villus sampling. Lancet 1:737–740, 1985.

117. Mollitt DL, Schullinger JN, Santulli TV: Selective management of iatrogenic esophageal perforation in the newborn. J Pediatr Surg 16:989–993, 1981.

118. Moss KL, Schmidt FE, Creech O: Analysis of 550 stab wounds of the abdomen. Ann Surg 28:483, 1962.

119. Naunyn B: Ein Falle von erb'scher Plexuslahmung mit Gleichseitiger sympathicuslahmung. Dtsch Med Wochenschr 28:52, 1902.

120. Neal PR, Merk PF, Norina AL: Halo scalp ring: A form of localized scalp injury associated with caput succedaneum. Pediatr Dermatol 2:52–54, 1984.

121. Newman B, Smith S: Unusual renal mass in a newborn infant. Radiology 163:193–194, 1987.

122. Niswander K, Elbourne D, Redman C, et al: Adverse outcome of pregnancy and the quality of obstetric care. Lancet 1:827–830, 1984.

123. Ogden JA, Lee KE, Rudicel SA, et al: Proximal femoral epiphysiolysis in the neonate. J Pediatr Orthop 4:285–292, 1984.

124. Ossipoff U, Hall B: Etiologic factors in the amniotic band syndrome: A study of 24 patients. Birth Defects 13:117–132, 1977.

125. Oxborn H, Foote WR: Human Labor and Birth. 2nd ed. New York, Appleton-Century-Crofts, 1962, pp 515–519.

126. Pachman DJ: Massive hemorrhage in the scalp of the newborn infant: Hemorrhagic caput succedaneum. Pediatrics 29:907, 1962.

127. Paige ML, Port RA: Separation of the distal humeral epiphysis in the neonate. Am J Dis Child 139:1203–1205, 1985.

128. Painter MJ, Bergman I: Obstetrical trauma to the neonatal central and peripheral nervous system. Semin Perinatol 6:89, 1982.

129. Pajor R, Szabo Z, Poskas E: Control examination at 3 years of age in 227 infants with retinal hemorrhages at birth. Orv Hetil 105:78, 1964.

130. Plauche WC: Subgaleal hematoma: A complication of instrumental delivery. JAMA 24:1597, 1980.

131. Potter EL: Pathology of the Fetus and Infant. 2nd ed. Chicago, Year Book Medical Publishers, 1961, pp 92–111.

132. Ratcliff JF: The use of low osmolality water soluble (LOWS) contrast media in the pediatric gastrointestinal tract. Pediatr Radiol 16:47–50, 1986.

133. Reid H: Birth injury to the cervical spine and spinal cord: A report of 2 cases and review of the literature. Am J Obstet Gynecol 78:498, 1959.

134. Rice HM, James PD: Ectopic splenic tissue failed to prevent pneumococcal septicaemia after splenectomy for trauma. Lancet 1:565–566, 1980.

135. Rockwood CA, Wilkins KE, King RE: Fractures in Children. Philadelphia, JB Lippincott, 1984, pp 175–178.

136. Rose AL, Lambroso CT: Neonatal seizure states: A study of clinical, pathological, and electroencephalographic features in 137 full-term babies with a long-term follow-up. Pediatrics 45:404, 1970.

137. Rosen MG: Factors during labor and delivery that influence brain disorders. In: Freeman JM (ed): Prenatal and Perinatal Factors Associated with Brain Disorders. NIH Publication No 85-1149, 1985, pp 237–261.

138. Rowe MI, Marchildon MB: Pediatric trauma. In: Shoemaker WC, Thompson WL, Holbrook PR (eds): Textbook of Critical Care. Philadelphia, WB Saunders, 1984, pp 914–924.

139. Rutherford Y, Fomufod AK, Gopalakrishmen LJ, et al: Traumatic distal femoral periostitis of the newborn: A breech delivery birth injury. J Natl Med Assoc 75:933–935, 1983.

140. Schoenfield A, Ziv E, Stein L, et al: Seatbelts in pregnancy and the obstetrician. Obstet Gynecol Surg 42:275–282, 1987.

141. Schullinger JN, Driscoll JM Jr: Birth injury. In: Touloukian RJ (ed): Pediatric Trauma. New York, John Wiley and Sons, 1978, pp 137–176.

142. Sherk HH, Probst C: Fractures of the proximal humeral epiphysis. Orthop Clin North Am 6:401–413, 1975.

143. Smith D: Recognizable Patterns of Human Deformities: Identification and Management of Mechanical Effects on Morphogenesis. Philadelphia, WB Saunders, 1981, p 5.

144. Smith GE: Post mortem caesarean section: A case report. J Obstet Gynaecol Br Commonw 80:181–182, 1983.

145. Sokal MM, Katz M, Lell ME, et al: Neonatal survival after traumatic fetal subdural hematoma. J Reprod Med 24:131–133, 1980.

146. Solonen KA, Telerenta T, Ryoppy S: Early reconstruction of birth injuries of the brachial plexus. Pediatr Orthop 1:367–370, 1981.

147. Spinapoulae RX, Wallace D, Kennedy P: Fetal distress secondary to fetal vessel perforation after amniocentesis. J Reprod Med 28:551–553, 1983.

148. Stern WE, Rand RW: Birth injuries to the spinal cord: A report of 2 cases and review of the literature. Am J Obstet Gynecol 78:498, 1959.

149. Stow HM: Rupture of umbilical cord. Am J Obstet Gynecol 46:792–803, 1902.

150. Tada K, Tsuyugucki Y, Kawai H: Birth palsy: Natural recovery course and combined root avulsion. J Pediatr Orthop 4:279–284, 1984.

151. Tahka H: On the weight and structure of the adrenal glands and the factors affecting them in children of 0-2 years. Acta Pediatr 40(Suppl):81, 1951.

152. Takagi T, Nagai R, Wakabayaski S, et al: Extradural hemorrhage in the newborn as a result of birth trauma. Child Brain 4:306, 1978.

153. Taylor JD: Breech presentation with hyperextension of the neck and intrauterine dislocation of the cervical vertebrae. Am J Obstet Gynecol 56:381, 1948.

154. Theodoru ED, Ierodiaconou MN, Mittson A: Obstetrical fracture–separation of the upper femoral epiphysis. Acta Orthop Scand 53:239–243, 1982.

155. Towbin A: Latent spinal cord and brain stem injury at birth. Arch Radiol 77:620–632, 1964.

156. Towbin A: Latent spinal cord and brain stem injury in newborn infants. Dev Med Child Neurol 11:54, 1969.

157. Towbin A: Latent spinal cord and brain stem injury in newborn infants. Dev Med Child Neurol 18:229, 1976.

158. Tuggle AQ, Cook WA: Laceration of a placental vein: An injury possibly inflicted by the fetus. Am J Obstet Gynecol 131:220–221, 1978.

159. Tutera G, Newman RL: Fetal monitoring: Its effect on the perinatal mortality and cesarean section rates and its complications. Am J Obstet Gynecol 122:750–754, 1975.

160. Valdes-Dapena MA, Arey JB: The causes of neonatal mortality: An analysis of 501 autopsies on newborn infants. J Pediatr 77:366, 1970.

161. Varner MW: Neuropsychiatric sequelae of midforceps deliveries. Clin Perinatol 10:455, 1983.

162. Volpe JJ: Neonatal intracranial hemorrhage: Pathophysiology, neuropathology, and clinical features. Clin Perinatol 4:77, 1977.

163. Volpe JJ: Neurology of the Newborn. 2nd ed. Philadelphia, WB Saunders, 1987, pp 638–661.

164. Wang MYW, McCutcheon E, DesForges JF: Fetomaternal hemorrhage from diagnostic transabdominal amniocentesis. Am J Obstet Gynecol 97:1123–1128, 1967.

165. Wegman ME: Annual summary of vital statistics—1981. Pediatrics 70:835, 1982.

166. Whelton J: Development of fetoscopy. Nurs Mirror 160(2):29–30, 1985.

167. Wickstrom J: Birth injuries of the brachial plexus: Treatment of defects in the shoulder. Clin Orthop 23:187–195, 1962.

168. Wilcox HL: The attitude of the fetus in breech presentation. Am J Obstet Gynecol 58:478, 1949.

169. Yasunaga S, Rivera R: Cephalhematoma in the newborn. Clin Pediatr 13:256, 1974.

170. Yussman MA: Rupture of the gravid uterus. Obstet Gynecol 36:115, 1970.

171. Zelson C, Lee SJ, Pearl M: The incidence of skull fractures underlying cephalhematomas in newborn infants. J Pediatr 85:371, 1974.

Carol L. Fowler
William Edmond Fowler
William J. Pokorny

CHAPTER THIRTY-FIVE

Nonaccidental Injuries:
The Physically Abused Child

Although child abuse is largely unrecognized and under-reported, its prevalence is of such concern that the American Academy of Pediatrics has declared it a national crisis.[3] Nonaccidental injuries in children produce at least 2000 to 5000 deaths per year, and the incidence appears to be increasing rapidly.[10] In the period from 1980 to 1985, the annual rate of child abuse increased 11.4% per year, and an overall increase of 31% was seen from 1985 to 1990.[12] In 1990, more than 2.5 million children in the United States were reported to state child protective services (CPS) as possible victims of abuse, an incidence of 39 per 1000 children.[12] However, only 15 to 63% of these cases were able to be substantiated. Although some cases are "unsubstantiated" owing to lack of physical evidence (e.g., fondling), it is dangerous to regard them as unfounded because these maltreated children are at significant risk for further harm; in 9% of these cases, a later incident results in physical harm to the child.[12] Accordingly, many states have three categories for the outcome of investigations for evidence of nonaccidental trauma: positive "evidence," "no evidence," and "no evidence, but reason to suspect."

Child maltreatment is classified as *abuse* (physical or sexual) or *neglect* (physical, educational, emotional). *Physical abuse* is defined as "harm or threatened harm to a child through non-accidental injury as a result of the acts or omissions of the person responsible for the child's care."[47] Nonaccidental injury includes unintentional harm, as in cases of severe physical punishment.[13] *Sexual abuse* is "the commission of any sexual offense with or to a child as a result of the acts or omissions by the child's caretaker."[47] *Neglect* is the "harm that occurs through failure of the caretaker to provide adequate food, shelter, medical care, or other provisions necessary for the child's health and welfare."[47] These types of maltreatment can be further subdivided as listed in Table 35–1. In 1990, 47% of substantiated child maltreatment cases were classified as neglect, 25% as physical abuse, 14% as sexual abuse, 9% as emotional abuse, and 5% as other types of abuse, such as abandonment.[12] Even this classification is artificial, however, as children often suffer more than one type of abuse simultaneously.

DEMOGRAPHICS OF MALTREATMENT

Gender. Although both sexes are maltreated equally, females suffer more abuse overall (13.1 per 1000, or 401,700 per year) than males (8.4 per 1000, or 270,900 per year), largely because of a higher incidence of sexual abuse of females.[13] Females are more likely to suffer injury or impairment, again largely owing to the preponderance of sexual abuse,[13] but no gender differences are noted in neglect.

Age. Among the different categories of abuse, only physical abuse demonstrates a positive correlation with age. Contrary to many published reports, children younger than 2 years of age are the *least* abused group overall and the least physically abused of any age group up to 17 years. Such abuse appears to be greatest in the 12 to 14 year age group.[13] Although young children are not as frequently maltreated as older children, fatalities and serious injuries appear more common in younger than in older children and their injuries are more likely to eventuate in a worse prognosis.[13] However, these age effects are probably attributable to an easier recognition of physical and sexual abuse in older children rather than to any actual difference in incidence.

Age has no relationship to the overall incidence of neglect, although emotional neglect occurs most often in the 15 to 17 year age group.

Race or Ethnicity. There is no significant correlation between race or ethnic group in any category of abuse or neglect.

Table 35–1

Categories of Child Maltreatment

Physical Abuse
Intentional
Nonintentional
Sexual Abuse
Intrusion (e.g., penile penetration whether oral, anal, genital)
Molestation with genital contact (no specific evidence of intrusion)
Other or unknown sexual abuse (e.g., fondling, exposure, allowing child's voluntary sexual activities)
Emotional Abuse
Close confinement (tying or binding and other forms)
Verbal or emotional assault (e.g., habitual belittling or denigrating, repeated threats of maltreatment)
Other or Unknown Abuse
(e.g., attempted physical or sexual assault, withholding food, shelter, sleep)
Physical Neglect
Refusal of health care
Delay in health care
Abandonment
Expulsion (e.g., refusal of custody)
    Other custody issues (e.g., frequently leaving care of child to others for days or weeks)
Inadequate supervision
Other physical neglect (e.g., inattention to home hazards, inadequate hygiene or clothing, leaving child unattended in car)
Educational Neglect
Permitted chronic truancy
Failure to enroll/other truancy (e.g., nonenrollment causing child to miss at least 1 month of school; keeping child at home for nonlegitimate reasons an average of 3 days a month)
Inattention to special educational needs
Emotional Neglect
Inadequate nurturance or affection (e.g., marked inattention to child's needs)
Chronic or extreme spouse abuse (e.g., domestic violence in child's presence)
Permitted drug or alcohol abuse
Permitted other maladaptive behaviors (e.g., chronic delinquency or severe assaultiveness)
Refusal of psychological care
Delay of psychological care (e.g., for severe depression, suicide attempt)
Other emotional neglect (e.g., chronically applying expectations inappropriate for child's age or level of development, overprotection fostering immaturity or overdependence)
Other Maltreatment
General or unspecified neglect (e.g., lack of preventive health care)
Other or unspecified maltreatment (e.g., parent problems, such as prostitution, alcoholism)

Table 35–2
Risk of Maltreatment to Children in Low-Income Families

	No. of Times More Frequent
Maltreatment	7.0
Abuse	4.5
Physical, sexual	4.0
Emotional	5.0
Neglect	9.0
Physical	12.0
Educational	8.0
Emotional	4.5

Family Income. Income has a dramatic relationship to child maltreatment. When families are separated into groups by annual income of more or less than $15,000, significant differences emerge in every category of abuse and neglect (Table 35–2).[13] Children from poorer families are more likely to suffer from all forms of abuse and neglect and to be injured more frequently.

PHYSICAL ABUSE

Physical abuse is the most common form of child maltreatment. In 1986, 311,524 children were physically abused, with an estimated incidence of 4.9 cases per 1000 children.[56] Physical abuse accounts for at least 10% of emergency department visits of children under the age of 5 years,[28] and approximately 715 children died in the United States in 1990 because of physical abuse, with an average age of death being under 3 years.[12] This figure is likely to be a gross underestimate because of probable underreporting and deaths that were erroneously attributed to other causes such as sudden infant death syndrome. The duration of exposure to physical abuse before fatal outcome averages from 1 to 3 years.[28]

Physical Presentation of Physical Abuse

The possibility of physical abuse should be considered in every child who presents with a serious injury.[39] Although injuries suggestive of abuse may occur by accident, a pattern of repeated injuries is always a warning sign of maltreatment.[29]

The physically abused child presents with a number of common findings (Table 35–3). The injury is suspicious if it is unexplained, inadequately explained, implausible, or inconsistent with reason. Also, approximately 20% of siblings of physically abused children have also been abused. Hence, all siblings should be thoroughly examined for abuse as well, although this step is usually unnecessary in cases of failure to thrive.

Bruises. Bruises are the most common indication of physical abuse. Although normally active children are likely to have bruises over bony prominences such as

Table 35–3
Findings Suggestive of Child Abuse

Category	Finding
History	Delay in seeking medical treatment
	History not consistent with injury or development of child
	Changing or discrepant histories told by each parent
	Unexplained injury
Examination	Multiple types of injuries (burns, bruises, fractures)
	Wounds in different stages of healing
	Burn or bruise conforming to shape of object used to inflict injury
	Immersion "stocking-glove" burn
	Wounds involving genitalia, face
Radiographs	Occult fractures
	Multiple fractures of different ages
	Abdominal and head computed tomography

knees, elbows, and chin, bruises over other soft tissue sites are more likely to be intentionally inflicted. Rarely, an underlying coagulopathy is the cause of multiple bruising; therefore, a coagulation profile should be included in the screening of suspected abuse victims.

The color of a bruise is very helpful in estimating the age of the injury (Table 35–4).[60] Immediately after injury, the skin is a reddish color due to capillary rupture. Within the first 24 hours, the bruise changes to a reddish-purple, which darkens over the next 4 days. After this, hemoglobin degradation alters the color to greenish-yellow by days 5 to 7 and then to yellow-brown by days 7 to 10. The bruise fades to a normal skin color within 2 to 4 weeks.

Often the appearance of the bruise suggests its etiology. Multiple oval, indistinct bruises are produced by grabbing and pinching. Slap marks often outline a hand print, whereas strap marks from belts and switches are characteristically long and linear. The bristles of a hairbrush leave multiple punctate bruises, and linear abrasions are made from beating with a comb. Circumferential rope burns are produced from tying extremities with ropes or string. Individual tooth marks can often be distinguished in bites. Bruises over the buttocks and back are usually related to paddling (Fig. 35–1). Contusions of the genital area and inner thighs often are secondary to punishment for toilet training accidents[51] (Fig. 35–2). Lip and facial bruises can be inflicted by trying to force-feed a crying child (Fig. 35–3). Boxing or cuffing of the ear pinna causes bruises (Fig. 35–4) and occasionally perforated tympanic membranes.

Table 35–4
Color of Bruise after Trauma

Time after Trauma	Color
Immediate	Red
1–5 days	Red-purple
5–7 days	Green-yellow
7–10 days	Yellow-brown
2–4 weeks	Normal

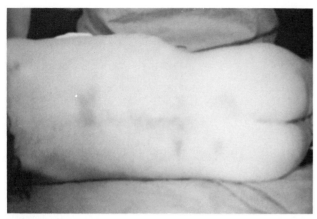

FIGURE 35–1
Multiple bruises and contusions of the back.

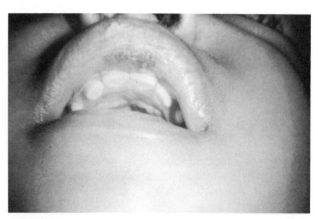

FIGURE 35–3
Contusions of the lip from forced feeding.

The tin ear syndrome is a lethal condition produced by a blow to the ear. Associated are subperichondral hematomas, ipsilateral cerebral edema, and obliteration of the basilar cisterns with hemorrhagic retinopathy.[46]

Occasionally children are reported for suspicion of child abuse who have physical findings unrelated to abuse. Mongolian spots are hyperpigmented areas primarily noted over the sacrum in black infants and other dark-skinned races. These Mongolian spots are sometimes confused with bruising but usually disappear after several months of age, occasionally persisting up to 3 or 4 years.

Burns. Intentional burns are noted in approximately 10% of physical abuse cases and in up to 43% of treated burn injuries.[16] Inflicted burns often show distinctive patterns that may be pathognomonic of the mechanism of injury. Accidental burns are more likely to have indistinct, irregular borders than inflicted injuries. Inflicted burns commonly involve the perineum or buttocks, and most are due to punishment of a child's inability to toilet train.[51] Examples of intentional contact burns are the uniform circular burns formed with a lighted cigarette (Fig. 35–5) and the sharply defined burns produced by a radiator, a hot iron (Fig. 35–6), or a poker (Fig. 35–7). Pathognomonic "stocking-glove" burns occur from emerging extremities into very hot water, whereby a sharp line of demarcation corresponds to the water level.

Both accidental and intentional splashed scald burns are very common. Although it may be difficult to differentiate these, history and physical examination can provide helpful clues. The abused child may have signs of concurrent or past physical abuse or of multiple past incidents (Fig. 35–8). Abusive parents may display certain characteristics, such as those described in Table 35–5. Inflicted burns are more likely to be deeper than accidental burns because a child normally withdraws quickly when hot items are accidentally encountered. The location of the burn is an important feature. Scalds limited to the back may mean that the child was running to escape a parent. In contrast, a common accidental burn results from toddlers pulling hot water down from a stove. Typically a central, severe burn is seen with more superficial splash burns on the face, shoulder, and chest.

The temperature of the water producing a burn can help differentiate intentional from accidental burns because the time required to produce the burn can be deduced. A scald burn develops within 60 seconds of contact at 127°F but

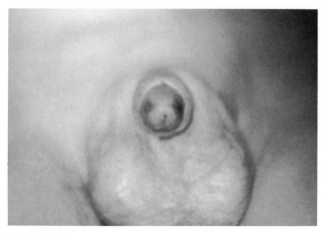

FIGURE 35–2
Bruising of the penis from pinching.

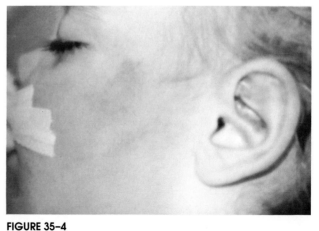

FIGURE 35–4
Multiple slap marks of the face and bruises from boxing of the ears.

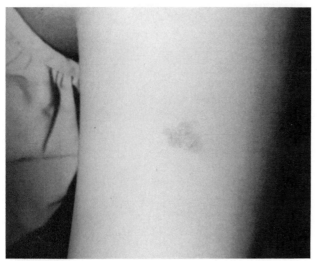

FIGURE 35–5
Several closely approximated cigarette burns.

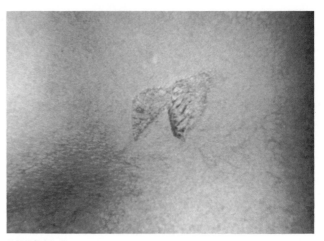

FIGURE 35–7
Hot poker burns.

within 1 second if the water temperature is 158°F.[16] In the absence of a reliable history consistent with producing an accidental severe burn, a deep burn of the palm or plantar surface of the foot suggests intentional injury because of the prolonged exposure required to produce a burn in these thickened areas.

Specific Areas of Abuse and Radiologic Imaging

Radiologic studies are useful in identifying areas of injury and possibly documenting an association between these injuries and child abuse. The most common radiologic findings associated with nonaccidental injury involve fractures and soft tissue trauma (Fig. 35–9).

Fractures

Because fractures are present in 10 to 36% of physically abused patients,[38, 50] a complete skeletal survey for occult

injuries is indicated in children suspected of maltreatment. Reportedly 56% of fractures in infants younger than 1 year of age are the result of abuse[34]; hence, the skeletal survey should include a full evaluation of the skull, spine, chest, and extremities. "Babygrams" should not be done because they cannot reliably detect unsuspected fractures. The skeletal survey is indicated for all children younger than 2 years

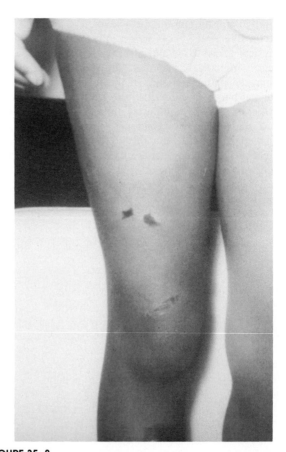

FIGURE 35–8
Multiple lacerations, burns, and contusions of the thigh and leg.

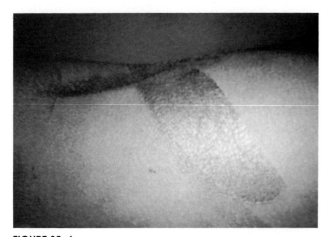

FIGURE 35–6
Iron burn.

Table 35–5
Characteristics of Abusive Parents

1. A parent who gives inadequate or implausible explanations of the injury.
2. A parent who delays seeking medical services following an injury.
3. A parent who is more concerned with the personal inconvenience of taking the child to appointments than with the welfare of the child.
4. A parent who becomes angry or defensive when asked to provide an explanation for the injuries.
5. A parent who becomes angry or defensive when diagnostic tests are discussed or who insists that the tests are not needed.
6. A parent who becomes verbally or physically aggressive toward a child or appears to be overly punitive when the child misbehaves in the office.
7. A parent who overreacts to relatively minor infractions on the part of the child.
8. A parent who is rarely seen or who leaves before the physician arrives.

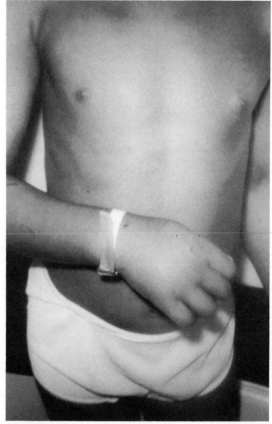

FIGURE 35–9
Swollen hand, indicative of a fracture. Note the multiple lacerations and the cigarette burns on the arm.

of age who have clinical evidence of physical abuse and in infants younger than 1 year of age who have been significantly neglected or deprived.[14, 36, 38] These young infants are more likely to exhibit occult fractures than older children. The skeletal survey is selectively performed in older children who present with signs of physical abuse but is rarely indicated in older children who present with isolated sexual abuse or neglect, as occult fractures are discovered in less than 4% of this group.[38] However, if an area of bone tenderness is present or limited motion of a limb is noted, roentgenograms are indicated; if the initial films are normal, they should be repeated in 2 weeks to look for evidence of bone healing of a missed injury.[36]

Commonly, fractures of differing ages are seen in the abused child (Fig. 35–10). The age of injury can be estimated by correlating the radiographic findings with the known course of normal bone healing. Periosteal new bone growth appears 5 to 10 days following injury; soft callus formation occurs at 10 to 14 days, and hard callus formation is noted 14 to 21 days after injury.[36] By 2 months after the initial injury, the original fracture line is usually obliterated by the callus. Bone remodeling continues over the next 2 to 4 months until the healing process is completed.[31]

Certain patterns of skeletal injury are typical in the child who has been maltreated. Fractures of the extremities most often involve the long bones (77%) and involve the diaphysis four times more often than the metaphysis and epiphysis.[32, 38] Both spiral and transverse fractures are common in nonaccidental injury, spiral fractures typically involving the tibia, femur, radius, or humerus and resulting from strong twisting forces on the extremity (Fig. 35–11) and transverse fractures due to direct blows (Fig. 35–12). Spiral fractures of the diaphysis are more common than transverse fractures in both accidental and nonaccidental injury; however, in the absence of a reasonable history of accidental trauma, spiral fractures should be regarded as having been inflicted in infants and children younger than 2 years of age because of the extreme degree of force required to produce such injuries.[31] Intentional injury should be suspected in the child with spiral fractures and

multiple fractures of different ages. Fractures through the metaphysis and growth plates are virtually diagnostic of intentional injury because of the extreme force necessary to produce them. Bucket-handle (Fig. 35–13), chip, or corner fractures of the metaphysis are classic indications of nonaccidental injury and usually result from violent wrenching or shaking of the extremity.[11] Children younger than 2 years have relatively compliant rib cages; hence, fractures in these areas are difficult to produce unless extreme force is exerted. Therefore, in the absence of major trauma or preexisting bone disease, the presence of rib, sternal, or scapular fractures should be considered evidence of nonaccidental injury.[36] In infants and toddlers, rib fractures are usually posterior or lateral and occur from violent compression of the chest as the child is shaken.[38] In older children rib fractures usually result from a direct blow to the chest. Although these fractures may be subtle immediately after the injury, callus formation will be noted on repeat films 10 to 14 days after the injury (Fig. 35–14).[36] It should also be noted that rib fractures have not been associated with vigorous cardiopulmonary resuscitation.[17] Other occult injuries such as acute nondisplaced fractures and costovertebral junction fractures may be more readily noted with skeletal scintigraphy.[36]

Medical conditions that involve bone can rarely mimic the radiographic findings of nonaccidental skeletal trauma. Among these are nutritional and metabolic defects such as

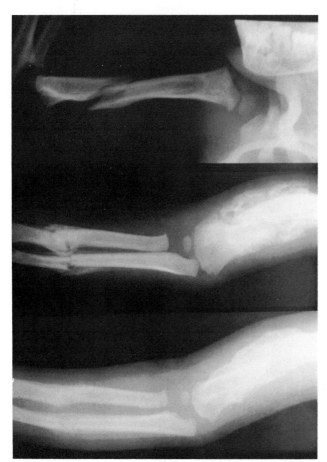

FIGURE 35–10

Multiple fractures of the humerus in various stages of healing.

scurvy, rickets (Fig. 35–15), and secondary hyperparathyroidism; skeletal dysplasias such as osteogenesis imperfecta and infantile cortical hyperostosis; infantile neoplasms such as leukemia, histiocytosis, and metastatic neuroblastoma; congenital disorders like the Menkes kinky hair syndrome and mucolipidosis II; drug-induced skeletal reactions such as those due to hypervitaminosis A, prostaglandin E, or methotrexate; neuromuscular disorders such as cerebral palsy with sensory and motor defects associated with spontaneous fractures; innocent trauma; and infections such as osteomyelitis and congenital syphilis.[36, 45] Birth trauma can result in fractures, but periosteal new bone formation is evident by 2 weeks after birth, which dates the injury.

Head Injury

Head injury is the most common cause of mortality in the abused child. At least 90% of these injuries are in infants younger than 2 years of age, and more than 95% of serious intracranial injuries during the first year of life result from nonaccidental injury.[38, 50] Cerebral injuries are present in more than 50% of infants with inflicted head injury, and diffuse cerebral edema is most commonly noted (Fig. 35–16), with infarction less often resulting from hypoxia due to asphyxia or strangulation or from direct vascular or endothelial damage.[37] Computed tomography (CT) findings

may reveal diffuse decreased density of the cerebral cortex with relative preservation of density in the thalami brain stem and cerebellum, a reversal of the normal brain density pattern.[25] Magnetic resonance imaging (MRI) scans are useful in delineating cerebral contusions, intraparenchymal injury, posterior fossa hemorrhage, and subdural hematomas in the subacute and chronic setting. In acute injury, CT scans are more easily obtained in the unstable patient and better in detecting subarachnoid hemorrhages.[2]

Direct blows to the head can produce skull fractures, often with underlying cerebral injuries. Linear fractures are more common than depressed and comminuted fractures (Fig. 35–17). Skull films are a sensitive radiologic examination to identify the usual fractures; however, cranial CT scans are very useful in demonstrating depressed fractures as well as any underlying cranial trauma.

In small infants intracranial injuries may be due to whip-

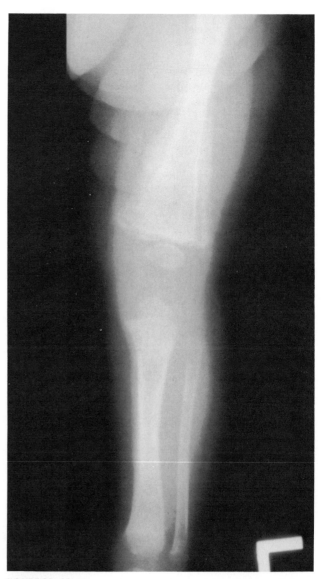

FIGURE 35–11

Diffuse reaction noted in a femur fracture due to a twisting injury.

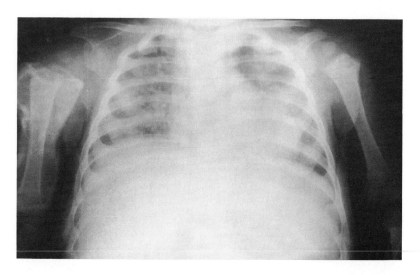

FIGURE 35–12
Right humeral fracture from a direct blow.

lash or to shaken infant syndrome.[7] Rapid acceleration and deceleration of the head during violent shaking of the infant can result in acute subdural hematomas. Although there is no external evidence of head trauma, there may be retinal hemorrhages due to the sudden rise in intracranial pressure and associated grab marks on the trunk from the force of injury application. Long-term posttraumatic sequelae include cerebral atrophy and chronic subdural collections, most readily documented with MRI scans.

Intra-abdominal Injuries

In contrast to the skeletal and cranial trauma typically found in infants, intra-abdominal visceral injuries are most commonly found in children 2 years and older.[11] These visceral injuries are the second most common cause of death in the abused child, with reported mortality rates of 45 to 50%. Usually due to blunt trauma from blows or kicks to the abdomen, external soft tissue injury such as a contusion of the anterior abdominal wall may be the initial most obvious evidence of trauma (Fig. 35–18). Roentgenograms as well as imaging scans such as sonar, CT, or MRI may be needed to identify these associated visceral injuries.

Because of the anatomic location of the duodenum and pancreas in the midabdomen overlying the spine, these organs are particularly susceptible to such blunt injuries. Intramural hematomas of the duodenum primarily affect the fixed third portion where it is compressed against the vertebral column by an intentional blow. Depending on the severity of the hematoma, the clinical presentation can be that of partial or complete duodenal obstruction, appearing from several hours to several days after the initial trauma. Upper gastrointestinal series may reveal either complete duodenal obstruction or the "coiled spring" sign of duodenal hematomas. The CT scans can demonstrate intramural duodenal hematomas also and are particularly useful in patients with potential multiple injuries. Duodenal hematomas usually resolve with nasogastric decompression

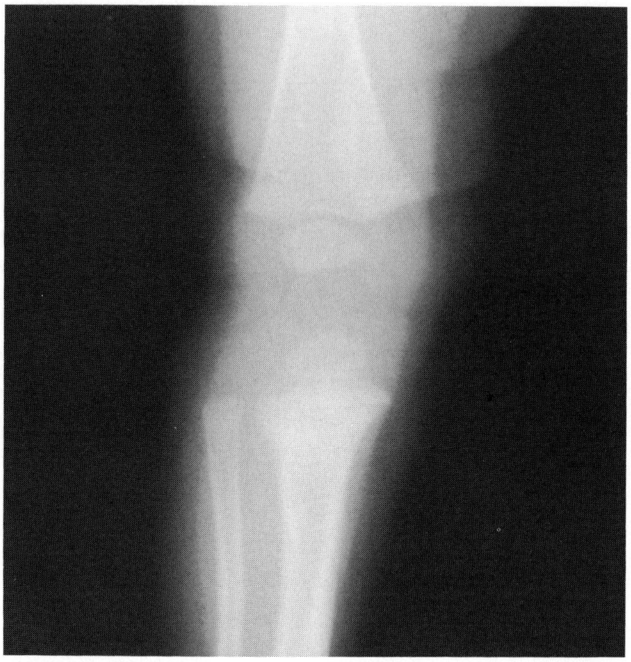

FIGURE 35–13
Bucket-handle fracture of the tibia resulting from a spiral injury.

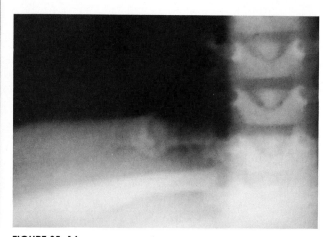

FIGURE 35–14
Healing rib fracture with callous formation.

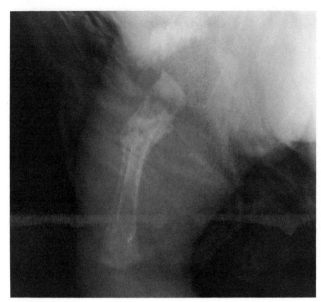

FIGURE 35–15
Femur fracture from rickets may simulate abuse.

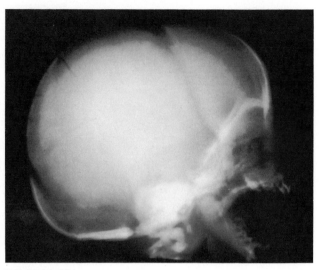

FIGURE 35–17
Skull fracture with widening of sutures due to increased intracranial pressure.

and intravenous alimentation over several days to 2 weeks; however, surgical decompression is indicated for persistent obstruction despite these measures.

In some cases, perforation of the duodenum or proximal jejunum occurs (Fig. 35–19), and because of the retroperitoneal location of the duodenum, gross peritonitis can be absent initially thus delaying diagnosis. Plain films of the abdomen may or may not reveal free air but should be closely inspected for retroperitoneal air. In these situations, prompt surgical exploration is mandatory.

Blunt abdominal trauma also frequently results in pancreatic injury, appearing as acute pancreatitis or pseudocyst formation, and at least half of reported cases of pancreatic pseudocyst in childhood are posttraumatic, with abuse im-

plicated in up to 30% of cases.[43] Ultrasonography and CT scans are helpful in evaluating acute pancreatic injuries, pancreatitis, and pseudocysts (Fig. 35–20). The child with a traumatic pancreatic pseudocyst presents with epigastric or back pain, vomiting, and an upper abdominal mass, and laboratory investigation shows elevated serum and urinary amylase levels. Skeletal lesions from fat necrosis have been reported in association with posttraumatic pancreatitis.[53] Nonoperative management with intravenous alimentation and nasogastric suction is the recommended initial therapy, as many of these traumatic pseudocysts resolve without surgery. However, surgical or percutaneous drainage of pseudocysts is sometimes necessary, although it is usually reserved for persistent or chronic pseudocysts or pseudocysts with complications such as infections, bleeding, or perforations (Figs. 35–21, 35–22).

Hepatic, splenic, and renal injuries occasionally result

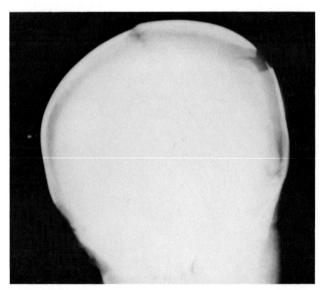

FIGURE 35–16
Skull fracture with diastatic spread from cerebral edema.

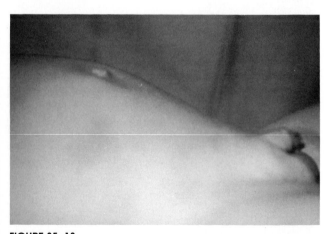

FIGURE 35–18
Multiple inflicted injuries include a bruise from a kick in the left upper abdomen, penile bruising, and abdominal distention from duodenal perforation. Same child as in Figures 35–1, 35–2, 35–4, 35–14, and 35–19.

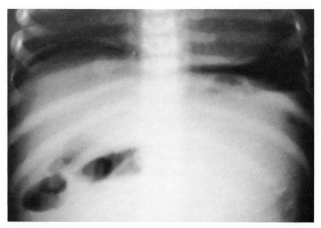

FIGURE 35-19
Same child as in Figure 35-18. Note the free intraperitoneal air from a perforated duodenum secondary to a blow to the abdomen and a healing rib 8 fracture seen just beneath the rim of free air on the patient's right.

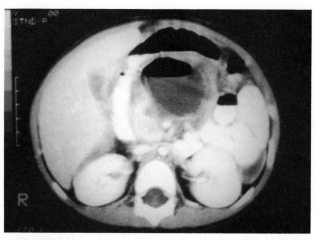

FIGURE 35-21
Pancreatic psuedocyst containing air due to perforation into the colon.

from nonaccidental blunt trauma but are less common than duodenal and pancreatic injuries, and CT is useful in defining these injuries. Occasionally rupture of a distended stomach occurs, most frequently along the greater curvature or anterior gastric wall. Small bowel ischemia, perforations, and mesenteric tears from such blunt abdominal trauma (Fig. 35-23) can also occur.

Intentional penetrating injuries from knives or electric tools are unusual but can occur and may result in bony, vascular, or nerve injuries (Fig. 35-24).

Behavioral Indicators of Physical Abuse

Unlike adults who usually deal with emotions, fears, and stress internally, children typically act out their feelings; thus, certain behavior patterns may indicate abuse, and the continued or repeated occurrence of one or more of these behavior indicators should arouse suspicion of abuse.[58] Examples include preschool children who mimic aggressive behavior they have seen or experienced. Enuresis or encopresis, especially in a child who has been toilet trained previously, social withdrawal, excessive dependence, over-compliance in an attempt to avoid arousing anger, agitation, and hyperactivity are commonly seen. Developmental delays or regression may result. The child may expect nothing in terms of love or affection and may exhibit a flat affect, a lack of curiosity, or a cowering or fear of physical contact or may become extremely frightened when other children cry. He or she may appear afraid of the parents and become frightened or resist going home when they return to the child's presence.

In the latency period of development, such children may begin to exhibit poor peer relationships; extremes of social behavior, such as withdrawal, aggression, or truancy; and signs of depression. Role reversals between parent and child can occur. During this stage, the child might report abuse by a parent.[58]

In adolescence, this aggression and withdrawal may in-

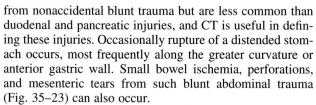

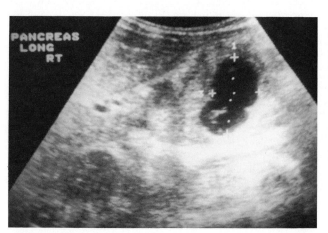

FIGURE 35-20
Ultrasound demonstrating a pancreatic pseudocyst.

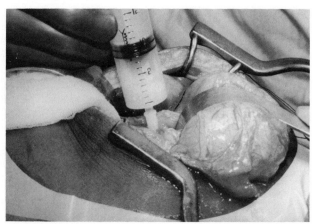

FIGURE 35-22
Localization of the pancreatic pseudocyst by aspiration at an operation to repair the perforation.

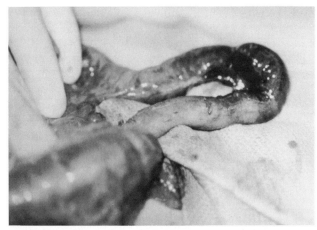

FIGURE 35-23
Devascularized small bowel from a mesenteric defect created by blunt trauma to the abdomen.

crease markedly, and delinquent behavior, truancy, and drug and alcohol use may develop. The adolescent may appear depressed and resist participation in school-related activities, and role reversal becomes more ingrained. The adolescent may exhibit sexual acting-out behavior as a form of seeking affection.

Characteristics of Physically Abusive Families

Abusive families often have traits characteristic of other types of dysfunctional families, such as those of alcoholics. Role boundaries between adults and children are often indistinct. One parent is often distant or absent emotionally or physically. Parents may be depressed or have poor social skills or poor self-esteem. They may not be knowledgeable about normal child development and may make unreasonable demands on their children. Single-parent households, financial stress, overcrowding, inadequate housing, alcohol

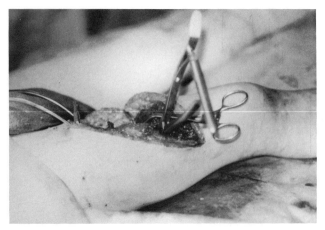

FIGURE 35-24
Intentional deep injury to the thigh from a power saw, involving the femoral vessels, nerve, and femur.

misuse, and social isolation increase levels of depression and tension, anger, and stress and increase the likelihood of maltreatment.[10] Marital relationships are often poor, and parental compromise is lacking. Parents may have lost custody of children previously or may have a criminal history of violence.

The more a child is perceived as being different because of physical or behavioral characteristics, the greater the risk of physical abuse.[39] Unwanted pregnancies and medical conditions that affect the child such as prematurity, congenital defects, frequent illnesses, mental retardation and developmental delays may strain parents financially and psychologically and lead to exaggerated punishment.[5, 39, 40] The risk of physical abuse is also greater among children in large families and in twins.[10, 21]

Parents who were abused as children are more likely to abuse their own children.[10] Up to 90% of mothers who maltreat their children report that they themselves were abused as children. Such parents often display an identifiable set of behaviors in the clinical setting (see Table 35–5).

EFFECTS OF ABUSE AND NEGLECT

Except when functional loss results, the major sequela of abuse stems from the reality that harm occurred as the result of actions or inactions of someone normally expected to care for the child.[55] Normal behaviors such as crying when hungry result in unexpected consequences, and the child's basic sense of security and efficacy is confused and damaged. Maltreated children may fail to develop adequate self-esteem or good interpersonal relationships; they may exhibit deficits in language, motor, and perceptual skills; and severe injuries may result in the loss of physical functions or mental disabilities with retardation. Behavioral and emotional difficulties can emerge at any time, and depression, antisocial behavior, anxiety, aggressiveness, and self-destructive behavior may result. Identity disturbances, borderline and narcissistic personality disorders, and posttraumatic stress disorder are commonly seen.[55] Attachment disorders set the stage for a lifelong pattern of attraction to abusive mates or antisocial behavior such as criminal activities, which may result in incarceration.

SEXUAL ABUSE

Childhood sexual abuse is a problem of enormous proportions in the United States; as many as 38% of females have been sexually abused before their eighteenth birthday.[49] Clinically, boys are seen less often for sexual abuse than girls, but it is unclear whether this represents underreporting of sexual abuse of boys or a true difference in the incidence. Seventy-five percent of reported cases involve the abuse of girls, more than half of whom are younger than 12 years at the time of the first offense.[19, 48] In 1986, 155,900 children were reported as victims of sexual abuse, an incidence of 2.5 per 1000 children.

Medical Evaluation of the Sexually Abused Child

Sexual abuse should be clinically suspected in children with unexplained vulvitis, vaginitis, anal fissures, venereal diseases and warts, or pregnancy.[51] Although only 35% of sexually abused children demonstrated physical evidence of such abuse, a thorough physical examination of the suspected child abuse victim should be performed as well as an assessment of the child's developmental, behavioral, and emotional status.[15] This examination should be performed within 72 hours of the alleged assault if ejaculation is suspected to have occurred. If the child presents after this time, little forensic evidence will exist, and the examination can be scheduled at the earliest time convenient for the child, family, and physician.[3]

Usually the examination is performed in the emergency department; however, depending on age and emotional state of the child, access to the operating room with general anesthesia should be available.[9] The young child is usually more relaxed during the examination with a parent present; however, older children and adolescents may cooperate better alone.

The emergency department must be equipped with the proper equipment for the evaluation of a sexually abused child. A prepackaged rape kit that includes glass slides, sterile cotton applicators, test tubes, saline, urine container, needle and Vacutainer, blood specimen tubes (VDRL and B-HOG), Thayer-Martin medium bottles, gonorrhea culture and Papanicolaou test mailer, comb and sterile package, scissors, and fingernail scraper is available.[9] A pediatric vaginal speculum or a nasal speculum should also be available.

During the physical examination, specific attention should be paid to the mouth, breasts, genitals, thighs, perineum, buttocks, and anus. Any clinical signs of physical trauma such as ecchymoses should be described and photographed. The child's pubic area should be examined and combed for hair or secretions from the assailant. It is preferable to pull samples of the child's head and pubic hair to include the root; however, clipping the samples is less traumatic. Examination of the child's skin and clothing with a Wood lamp may demonstrate areas that contain semen from which appropriate specimens can be obtained. Fingernail scrapings may reveal the assailant's hair, clothing, or secretions if resistance has taken place.

Simple visualization of the external genitalia is performed next. Notes are made of any tears, abrasions, scarring, or distortions of the hymenal opening. The child is alerted and reassured during every step of the examination. In prepubertal children with no evidence of external genital trauma, visualization of the vagina is unnecessary; however, specimens as described previously do need to be collected.[9] In older children and adolescents, use a vaginal speculum or nasal speculum to visualize and collect specimens. In both age groups, examination under anesthesia may be required if any evidence of severe trauma or penetration is present. Small lacerations may not require repair; however deep vaginal and perineal tears require careful evaluation, irrigation, débridement if needed, and reapprox-

imation. Celiotomy is indicated in cases of peritonitis or extensive injury. Treatment of large vaginal hematomas may be selective: Nonexpanding hematomas can be observed only; however, expanding hematomas may require celiotomy with ligation of the anterior hypogastric vessels, or selected embolization with angiography may be considered.[9]

Oral, anal, and pharyngeal swabs are obtained and plated on Thayer-Martin medium for gonorrhea cultures, and a second set of swabs is immediately inspected for the presence of motile sperm.[9] Although motile sperm can be found in the vagina for 2 to 3 hours, nonmotile sperm can persist for 72 hours in the vagina and for 10 to 14 days in the endocervix and can be detected on a Papanicolaou smear or a Gram stain.[52, 54] A third set of swabs is obtained to look for elevated acid phosphatase, which can indicate the presence of semen for up to 12 hours after the incident.[20] Spermatozoa have been detected with no acid phosphatase activity; therefore, acid phosphatase testing should not be the only method used to screen for the presence of semen.[41] A more sensitive and specific test is the detection of P30 by enzyme-linked immunoabsorbent assay.[30] A semen glycoprotein of prostatic origin, P30 can be recovered up to 48 hours after intercourse and is stable in dried specimens.

A technique using monoclonal antibodies allows the positive identification of seminal fluid in forensic specimens as old as 6 months.[27, 41] Mouse antihuman sperm-5 (MHS-5) binds to a sperm-coating peptide secreted by human seminal vesicles in the semen and does not require the presence of sperm. Characterization of deoxyribonucleic acid in a semen or blood sample is highly specific in determining the identity of the perpetrator.[41]

Determination of blood group antigens from residual secretions may be helpful in identifying an unknown perpetrator when ejaculation has occurred, as 80% of individuals secrete blood group antigens in the saliva, semen, and other secretions.[9] The results are then compared to the child's antigens, determined from a sample of the child's saliva, on further evidence obtained.

Medical Treatment of the Sexually Abused Child

Prophylaxis against pregnancy is controversial but should be considered in the postmenarchal victim. In the early period after rape, prophylaxis can be approximately 80% effective with an estrogen combination of ethinyl estradiol and norgestrel (Ovral) if taken within 72 hours after the unprotected coitus. Two tablets are taken immediately, followed by two more tablets 12 hours later.[41]

Prophylactic antibiotics for sexually transmitted diseases are usually not indicated because the risk of acquiring them is very low and the period since the incident may be too long to be effective in preventing the infection. No single agent is effective against all such infections, but antibiotics may be warranted if the history suggests possible exposure. For gonorrhea and syphilis, the recommended coverage in children weighing less than 40 kg is oral probenecid, 25 mg per kg, followed by an intramuscular dose of procaine penicillin, 100,000 U per kg.[9] For larger children, oral probenecid, 1 gm followed in 1 hour by an intramuscular dose of procaine penicillin, 4.8 mU intramuscularly, is recommended. An alternate treatment for children who are allergic to penicillin is tetracycline, 25 mg per kg orally, then 40 to 60 mg per kg per day in four divided doses for 1 week. However, tetracycline should not be used in children younger than 10 years of age because of the possibility of dental staining. In these children, oral erythromycin, 40 mg per kg per day in four doses for 1 week may be used, although its efficacy in treating syphilis in not well established.[9] These children should be closely followed, and repeat gonorrhea culture, Venereal Disease Research Laboratories, and pregnancy tests should be performed after 6 weeks.[9]

Another increasingly important factor in childhood sexual abuse is the acquisition of the acquired immunodeficiency syndrome (AIDS). In one study, sexual abuse was the proven mode of transmission in 4% of children who were infected with the human immunodeficiency virus (HIV).[24]

Behavioral Indicators of Sexual Abuse

Sexual abuse, like physical abuse, may be suspected because of certain behavior patterns exhibited by children who have been sexually abused.[58] Preschool children make sexual advances toward classmates, adults, or toys and use a sophisticated sexual vocabulary; genitals or sexual acts may be depicted in their drawings. Such sexual behavior in a child is recognized as the result and not the cause of molestation, although it may predispose the child to future exploitation.

In the latency phase age, sexual acting out continues, and the child may be depressed, withdrawn, aggressive, or develop poor peer relationships. The child may run away from home, become delinquent, or abuse drugs or alcohol, and school performance may deteriorate rapidly.[58] The child may attempt to reveal the abuse by avoiding the issue, often seeming to be afraid of the perpetrator and to avoid being alone with the person responsible for these feelings.

Adolescents may be extremely self-conscious and refuse to change clothes for gym class. They may regress, retreat into a fantasy world, or dissociate themselves from the situation they find themselves in.

Credibility of the Child

As a rule, children lie to get out of trouble, not to get into it. A child's report of sexual abuse is usually true. In general, the more consistent, vivid, and detailed a child's account, the more believable. A brief examination by simply asking the child the difference between the truth and a lie and whether the child is telling you the truth can begin the process of questioning. Contrary to experience with adults in which a victim's report of a crime and later retraction challenges the credibility of the individual, retraction by children is normal and may be expected. There are five normal reactions of the abused child to these situations, often referred to as the *child sexual abuse accommodation syndrome*[57]:

1. Secrecy—The majority of victims never tell anyone
2. Helplessness—The child feels betrayed and abandoned, is untrusting, and submits to the abuse
3. Entrapment and accommodation—The only option available to the child is to accept the situation
4. Delayed, conflicted, and unconvincing disclosure—The victim usually remains silent until having established a life free of the influence of the parents
5. Retraction—A child is likely to recant because of ambivalence and a sense of obligation to preserve the family[58]

Characteristics of Sexually Abusive Families

Despite the often publicized frequency of abuse of children by strangers, only 5% of all reported cases in 1990 were classified as nonfamilial incidents. In families in which incest occurs, the mother is often nonassertive, dependent, fearful of her husband, and may have no marketable job skills. The marital relationship is often poor, with little sexual interaction. The family is frequently socially isolated and has poor coping skills. Roles between parents and children are often distorted, and the mother-daughter relationship may be characterized by competition or hostility. The perpetrator may feel inadequate in age-appropriate sexual relationships, have poor self-esteem, and seek sexual gratification from children. The abuse most typically begins between the ages of 8 and 12, affects the eldest daughter first, and begins with kissing and hugging before progressing.[22] The majority of sexual abuse incidents are never reported, often because the child may be threatened or wish to protect the mother's feelings. Girls often report the abuse to protect a younger sibling from similar molestation.

The male perpetrator typically appears passive outside of the family and rarely has a police history. He is frequently a rigid disciplinarian and has an intense need to be in control. He is sometimes drawn to such jobs as minister, scout leader, or daycare worker, in which he has access to many children. Perpetrators are either ''fixated'' and have a primary sexual interest in children or ''regressed'' and abuse children when their adult relationships fail. Fixated offenders typically molest boys, and regressed offenders most often molest girls.[23]

The female spouse is often aware of the abuse but because of fear or helplessness attempts to overlook or ignore it. She may view the abuse as preferable to an extramarital affair or as a welcome release from obligatory marital relations; however, she may often express anger or jealousy toward her daughter as well and blame her or see her as a willing participant.

Effects of Child Sexual Abuse

Porter and colleagues identified 10 possible long-term effects of sexual abuse of children.[44] These 10 areas represent a reasonably comprehensive guide to the evaluation and treatment of the sexually abused child (Table 35-6).

The initial consequences of sexual abuse include fear, anxiety, depression, a sense of powerlessness, anger, and inappropriate sexual behavior.[6] Long-term continued depression, sexual dysfunction, poor self-esteem, and impaired ability to trust remain problems.

Generally, younger victims understand the situation poorly despite acquiring a sophisticated but superficial vocabulary, and they may focus more on physical pain. Older victims have more affective reactions, including guilt, anger, and depression. However, the younger the age at which the abuse begins, the greater its impact on the developing personality; the longer and more frequent the abuse is and the closer the blood or emotional relationship between the child and the perpetrator, the more harmful it will be. The impact of the abuse is also greater as the degree of coercion, aggression, and threat by the perpetrator becomes more intense. Most important, nearly all abused children suffer negative consequences, and just one "minor" incident can be as damaging as more frequent and "serious" abuse.[1]

FAILURE TO THRIVE AND NEGLECT

Food deprivation is a type of maltreatment that often results in malnourishment and failure to thrive. Most cases are noted in infants younger than 8 months of age. Such children usually weigh below the third percentile, but their height and head circumference are above the third percentile on regular growth curves.[51] Short stature should not be confused with failure to thrive: children with short stature are small but proportional in height and weight and appear well nourished. The child with failure to thrive because of food deprivation or neglect usually exhibits a rapid gain during hospitalization with proper nourishment and care.

Water deprivation also has been reported. Serum electrolyte abnormalities vary according to the degree and severity of deprivation; however, a hypernatremic dehydration, of varying severity, is usually present.

In general, the causes of failure to thrive have been estimated to be parental neglect in 50% of cases, organic

causes in 30% of cases, and underfeeding due to parental ignorance or other errors in the remaining 20%. Organic failure to thrive includes such things as perinatal insults as well as disorders of the central nervous system and the genitourinary, gastrointestinal, cardiovascular, and pulmonary systems. Interactional causes of failure to thrive include physical or mental illness of the mother; poverty; retardation of the mother or the child; educational limitations of the caretaker parent; early child developmental dysfunctions resulting from mistreatment, neglect, or sexual exploitation; and lack of social support within the family.[26]

Medical care neglect and safety neglect are other important concerns. Parents of children with treatable chronic diseases may refuse or ignore medical recommendations, and court orders may be necessary to hospitalize and treat these children. However, this is a complex issue if the parents' reasons are based on religious or philosophic beliefs. Safety neglect may be due to educational ignorance, as when a toddler is allowed to roam unattended. This situation may be remedied by educating the parents about the importance of constant supervision of young children.[26]

UNUSUAL MANIFESTATIONS OF CHILD ABUSE

Unusual forms of child abuse have been reported, among which is forced feeding of pepper to a child as a form of punishment, resulting in fatal aspiration.[46] Intentional microwave oven burns have also been described. These burn patterns are different from the usual scald burns, and biopsies from these show a characteristic burning configuration.[46] Scald burns produce superficial burns with decreasing damage to the deeper layers of soft tissue. Microwave burns, however, cause deeper tissue with high water concentration, such as muscle, to burn to a greater degree than tissue with a lower water content, such as fat. The wounds are sharply demarcated, full-thickness burns because microwave ovens tend to have hot spots.[46]

Toxic drug ingestion can also be either intentional or accidental, and drug screening is useful to reveal forced or passive cocaine ingestion such as the cocaine-induced seizures that can occur in breast-fed infants of cocaine-addicted mothers and in children with passive inhalation exposure to freebase cocaine use.[46]

Another unusual type of child abuse is referred to as *Munchausen syndrome* or maltreatment by proxy, described by Meadow in 1977.[35] These children have complex, unusual, and often multiple complaints that simulate illness but in reality are induced by a caretaker (usually the mother). The illnesses are atypical and unresponsive to the usual treatments and medications. Usually some very rare disorder is ascribed as the primary diagnosis owing to the unusual manifestations. Features of the disorder are an overattentive mother who will not leave the child and an unstable home environment. In one such case, a child presented with repeated episodes of apnea, and the diagnosis of Munchausen syndrome by proxy was confirmed after suspicious health care workers placed a video recorder in the room and filmed the mother's repeated near strangulations of the child.

Table 35-6
Effects of Sexual Abuse

"Damaged goods syndrome"
Guilt
Fear
Depression
Low self-esteem and poor social skills
Repressed anger and hostility
Impaired ability to trust
Blurred role boundaries and role confusion
Pseudomaturity coupled with failure to accomplish developmental tasks
Self-mastery and control

Reprinted with the permission of Lexington Books, an imprint of The Free Press, a Division of Simon & Schuster, from Porter FS, Blick LC, Sgroi SM: Treatment of the sexually abused child. In: Sgroi SM (ed): Handbook of Clinical Intervention in Child Sexual Abuse. Lexington, Mass, Lexington Books, 1982, pp 109–145. Copyright © 1982 by Lexington Books.

PSYCHOLOGICAL TREATMENT FOR CHILD ABUSE

Without intervention, 5% of abused children are killed and 35% are seriously reinjured.[51] Treatment should be referred to a physician and psychologist or psychiatrist with specialized knowledge of the management of such. It is important to stress that under no circumstance is a child responsible for abuse; it is always the adult who is responsible for any event between a child and an adult. Sexual or seductive behavior on the part of the child should be regarded as a consequence of sexual abuse and not its cause.

Treatment Issues

Child abuse is a family problem, and effective treatment involves the cooperation of a multidisciplinary child abuse task force with representatives from the child protective services, the youth or juvenile court, the family court, the police department, the district attorney's office, the rape crisis center, the hospitals, and the mental health services.[58] Careful management often spares the child from having to repeat statements to different agencies.[59] If the session is videotaped, interview and court evidence is on permanent record and need not be repeated. The task force method also allows a single release of information to be obtained, thus allowing agencies to freely communicate with one another.

The interview process is difficult because of legal evidentiary limits and must be handled by an interviewer with special training in evaluating such children. A thorough physical examination starts the treatment process because in addition to establishing evidence for legal purposes, the examination can provide the basis for referrals. For example, if head injuries are present, the child should be evaluated by a neuropsychologist who can determine the functional implications of the injuries. The physical evaluation can reveal evidence that can form the basis for a court order to the family to attend treatment. Before the physical examination is completed, the physician should answer any questions that the child might have. Children often have naive ideas about cause and effect relationships or think that they are permanently damaged. Reassuring the child that he or she will "soon be all better" or that nothing is "broken inside" often eliminates a great deal of fear.

Assessment by a child psychologist is always indicated to screen for learning disabilities or delays, to evaluate for emotional and personality disorders, and to develop educational remediation plans. Referral to a mental health professional skilled in treatment of abuse should be made for ongoing counseling.

Except in extreme or repeated cases, the aim of the social services department is to reunify the family. After a report of abuse, the child is often removed from the home for reasons of safety and placed with a relative or in foster care. This practice, however, may be psychologically harmful to the child, conveying the message that the child is the wrongdoer. Hence, it is usually more appropriate to have the suspected abuser voluntarily leave the home until treatment is completed. An important factor determining whether a child is to be removed from a home is the extent to which the nonabusing parent believes the child's account of the abuse and will protect the child from repeated assaults.[42] Return of the child to the home is usually a gradual process, with monitoring by CPS. An important sign that return is possible is the demonstration of good, sustained parenting skills as opposed to statements of good intentions. When parents fail to comply with treatment programs, disappear for extended periods, or otherwise seem beyond rehabilitation after a period of 6 months to a year, CPS may legally terminate parental rights and place the child for adoption.[58]

Psychological treatment begins with a complete assessment of the child in all areas of development, including family and peer relationships, school performance, intellect, and emotional status. Treatment may be relatively brief (months) or long-term (years). As a rule, evidence of abuse in one child mandates evaluation of siblings as well. Individual treatment is often supplemented by group treatment in which children learn that others have experienced similar situations.

Important goals in treatment are to help children understand that they are not to blame for the abuse, that it was correct to tell about the abuse, that the perpetrator was responsible for any disruption in the family, and that they are not permanently damaged and to address specific reactions such as guilt, anxiety, phobias, anger, depression, or suicidal ideation. Speakers from agencies such as CPS, the court, and the police or adult survivors of abuse may be invited to explain the specific role of each agency and to discuss what might be expected in the future. Strategies to reduce the likelihood of revictimization are discussed. Sexually abused girls usually prefer female therapists, but there are advantages to using male therapists as well.[18]

Treatment of abusive parents is extremely difficult and involves issues related not only to the abuse of their children but often to their own childhood maltreatment and concurrent substance abuse. Part of the initial evaluation is conducted to determine whether the particular family is likely to respond to treatment.

One major objective is to have the perpetrator accept responsibility for the abusive behavior and to help him or her understand why the behavior was inappropriate. An educational component is very important to help learn about normal child development, parenting skills, and nonphysical means of discipline, such as "time-out." Rebuke or harsh or condescending lecturing is rarely effective. Helping parents to distinguish between feelings and behaviors is important (e.g., anger is a feeling and is normal; abuse is a behavior and is not acceptable). When substance abuse is present, referral to organizations such as Alcoholics Anonymous is indicated. When certain factors are identified as possible contributors to abuse, such as social isolation or financial strains, the parent may be referred to support groups, vocational counseling, or public assistance programs.

Ideally, the abusing parent and the child initially are seen individually with the goal of establishing joint sessions once the perpetrator has accepted full responsibility and the child is comfortable with the idea. The nonabusing spouse needs to address issues such as providing materially for the family, particularly if the perpetrator was the main source of income. If the nonabusing spouse has no job skills or lacks educational qualifications, referral to a Graduate Equivalency Degree program or vocational training, or both, is important. This training helps not only in the short term; should abuse recur, the individual with education and training is more able to achieve independence to leave the situation. Assertiveness training is often indicated. Emotional issues most often involve guilt, anger, betrayal, disgust, denial, or fear that the child is somehow damaged or to blame. If the nonabusing parent was aware of the abuse but did not prevent it, he or she usually has a variety of long-standing personal problems, including an early history of abuse that needs to be addressed. Nonabusing parent support groups are available to help address these issues.

When the perpetrator is someone outside of the family, treatment issues are often less complex, unless the abuse was the result of neglect or inadequate supervision, in which case treatment more closely follows the guidelines for intrafamilial abuse. The parents should be seen together to answer their questions, typically concerning the long-term effect on the child. Parents often experience guilt, view the child as damaged, blame each other, or express extreme hostility toward the perpetrator, including homicidal threats. Helping the parents to express their anger appropriately and to be supportive of the child is vital. The parents' reactions to the abuse may influence how the child views the abuse and reacts in the future.

REPORTING CASES OF SUSPECTED CHILD ABUSE

Although physician recognition of child maltreatment has increased, it is estimated that only 51% of cases were formally reported to CPS in 1986.[13] Despite the requirement by law in all 50 states to report all suspected cases, there is still resistance to mandatory reporting. Some reasons for this include the potential for the report to harm reputations unnecessarily, to produce undue stress on the family, or to discourage offenders from voluntarily seeking treatment. In addition, many fear litigation if abuse is not ultimately proved. However, ''good faith reporting laws'' exist that protect the physician from litigation arising from unproved cases. Furthermore, it is not the physician's function to identify the offender or to prove maltreatment: that is the function of CPS investigators and the court system. The physician who fails to report suspected abuse becomes civilly liable for all damages suffered by the child subsequent to the time of evaluation.

Furthermore, a physician should resist attempting family counseling because the treatment of child abusers is one of the most difficult areas of mental health and carries a low success rate even when it is provided by trained professionals. Naive attempts at counseling by a well-meaning physician endanger not only the health and well-being of the child who is being investigated but perhaps many other children as well. For example, sexual abusers of boys have an average of 150 victims, whereas those of little girls have an average of five.[33]

A verbal report is usually required within 24 hours, followed by a written report within 48 to 72 hours. The appropriate agencies in each state along with their phone numbers and addresses are available from the U.S. Department of Health and Human Services, National Center on Child Abuse and Neglect, P.O. Box 1182, Washington, DC 20013.

COURT TESTIMONY

Physicians who care for abused children should expect to be called into court for testimony sometime during their careers. This should be kept in mind when a child with suspected abuse is first encountered in the emergency department. Because physicians are asked to help determine whether a child's clinical condition is due to accidental or inflicted injuries, the initial medical report should be written clearly and accurately. Most often pediatricians are called as physical abuse experts; however, emergency department physicians and surgeons can also expect to be called as experts in the diagnosis of abuse.

Thorough pretrial preparation is necessary. A pretrial conference with the attorney is mandatory for the physician to know what to expect from the state's attorney to anticipate lines of questioning. Sworn videotaped out-of-court testimony (depositions) can sometimes be used in lieu of live courtroom testimony, especially if the trial is held in a logistically inconvenient location that makes it difficult for the expert witness to be present. Videotaped depositions have the advantage over written depositions that demonstrative evidence can be used to illustrate certain points. It is up to counsel and judge whether this type of deposition is admissible.

In the pretrial period the expert witness should become familiar with all pertinent medical literature regarding the type of injury in question, and all available material concerning the case should be reviewed.[4] The physician must insist on access to complete records of the case, including laboratory and radiologic tests. These details need not be committed to memory, and summary notes may be allowed on the witness stand.[31] Relevant notes and data from the patient's chart may be tagged beforehand for easy referral during testimony. These notes are especially important if long periods of time occur before a case comes to trial.

As outlined by the American Academy of Pediatrics on suggested policies concerning expert testimony, a neutral position should be maintained with thorough and impartial presentation of the facts pertinent to the case.[4] The cross-examining attorney may try to intimidate and undermine the medical expert as much as possible. However, the expert must remain composed and realize that these are legal tactics by the attorney to help win the case.

During interrogation, the physician should testify in a clear, concise fashion, remembering that most of the others present are not medically oriented. Medical jargon should be avoided or the testimony may not be understood. Demonstrative evidence, such as photographs or slides, are indispensable. As always, a picture is worth a thousand words. Good communication with the attorney is necessary, because the attorney helps to develop the expert's testimony. The testimony should not be rushed, and the expert witness should not be intimidated by the examining attorney. If the physician is asked to answer a complex question with a succinct "yes" or "no" response but believes that such an answer would be insufficient or misleading, the physician should state this, and the judge may allow a comprehensive answer without interruption from the attorney.[31]

As it is often impossible for the court system to adhere to prearranged schedules, the physician should request to be on call for testimony. The subpoena lists the date and time that the trial begins, but the physician may not be needed for several days, or perhaps not at all, because many cases are plea-bargained and concluded before or during the trial. In most cases physicians are accommodated and are allowed to continue their normal work schedules and are notified several hours before their testimony is required. If already present in the court before testimony is scheduled, the physician may request to testify out of turn to return to work. The opposing attorney may attempt to subpoena the expert witness and require the witness's presence in court even though the witness is not scheduled to appear on that particular day; physicians should contact the judge to discourage such tactics.[8] Fees for compensations for court testimony vary widely. Advance agreement should be obtained in the pretrial period; otherwise the court can fix the fee.

Acknowledgments

We would like to thank Tag Heister, Department of Psychiatry, University of Kentucky, Lexington; Milton L. Wagner, M.D., Department of Radiology, Texas Children's Hospital and Baylor College of Medicine, Houston, Texas; and Glenn B. Adams, J.D., New Orleans, Louisiana, for their comments and advice on this chapter.

References

1. Adams-Tucker C: Proximate effects of sexual abuse in childhood: A report on 28 children. Am J Psychiatry 139:1252–1256, 1982.
2. Alexander RC, Schor DP, Smith WL Jr: Magnetic resonance imaging of intracranial injuries from child abuse. J Pediatr 109:975–979, 1986.
3. American Academy of Pediatrics Committee on Child Abuse and Neglect: Guidelines for the evaluation of sexual abuse of children. Pediatrics 87:254–260, 1991.
4. American Academy of Pediatrics Committee on Medical Liability: Guidelines for expert witness testimony. Pediatrics 83:312–313, 1989.
5. Ammerman RT: Predisposing child characteristics. In: Ammerman RT, Hersen M (eds): Children at Risk: An Evaluation of Factors Contributing to Child Abuse and Neglect. New York, Plenum Press, 1990, pp 199–221.
6. Browne A, Finkelhor D: Impact of child sexual abuse: A review of the research. Psychol Bull 99:66–77, 1986.
7. Caffey J: The whiplash shaken infant syndrome: Manual shaking by the extremities with whiplash-induced intracranial and intraocular bleedings, linked with residual permanent brain damage and mental retardation. Pediatrics 54:396–403, 1974.
8. Chadwick DL: Preparation for court testimony in child abuse cases. Pediatr Clin North Am 37:955–969, 1990.
9. Cheek JG: Sexual abuse of children. In: Mayer TA (ed): Emergency Management of Pediatric Trauma. Philadelphia, WB Saunders, 1985, pp 435–443.
10. Cohn AH: An approach to preventing child abuse. Chicago, National Committee for Prevention of Child Abuse, 1983.
11. Cooper A, Floyd T, Barlow B, et al: Major blunt abdominal trauma due to child abuse. J Trauma 28:1483–1486, 1988.
12. Daro D, McCurdy K: Current trends in child abuse reporting and fatalities: The results of the 1990 annual fifty state survey. Chicago, National Committee for Prevention of Child Abuse, 1991.
13. Department of Health and Human Services: Child abuse and neglect: A shared community concern. Chicago, March 1989.
14. Ellerstein NS, Norris KJ: Value of radiologic skeletal survey in assessment of abused children. Pediatrics 74:1075–1078, 1984.
15. English KL: Management of sexual abuse of children. Top Emerg Med 3:67–74, 1981.
16. Feldman KW, Schaller RT, Feldman JA, et al: Tap water scald burns in children. Pediatrics 62:1–7, 1978.
17. Feldman KW, Brewer DK: Child abuse, cardiopulmonary resuscitation, and rib fractures. Pediatrics 73:339–342, 1984.
18. Fowler WE: Pre and post intervention preference for and comfort with male vs. female counselors among sexually abused girls attending a structured individual treatment program. Unpublished doctoral dissertation. University of Southern Mississippi, 1991.
19. Fritz GS, Stoll K, Wagner NN: A comparison of males and females who were sexually molested as children. J Sex Marital Ther 7:54–59, 1981.
20. Gomez RR, Wunsch CD, Davis JH, et al: Qualitative and quantitative determinations of acid phosphatase activity in vaginal washings. Am J Clin Pathol 64:423–432, 1975.
21. Gothard TW, Runyan DK, Hadler JL: The diagnosis and evaluation of child maltreatment. J Emerg Med 3:181–194, 1985.
22. Green AH: Overview of the literature on child sexual abuse. In: Schetky DH, Green AH (eds): Child Sexual Abuse: A Handbook for Healthcare and Legal Professionals. New York, Brunner/Mazel, 1988, pp 30–56.
23. Groth AN: The incest offender. In: Sgroi S (ed): Handbook of Clinical Intervention in Child Sexual Abuse. Lexington, Mass, Lexington Books, 1982.
24. Gutman LT, St. Claire KK, Weedy C, et al: Human immunodeficiency virus transmission by child sexual abuse. Am J Dis Child 145:137–140, 1991.
25. Han BK, Towbin RB, DeCourten-Myers G, et al: Reversal sign on CT: Effects of anoxic/ischemic cerebral injury in children. AJR 154:361–368, 1990.
26. Helfer RE: The neglect of our children. Pediatr Clin North Am 37:923–942, 1990.
27. Herr JC, Summers TA, McGee RS, et al: Characterization of a monoclonal antibody to a conserved epitope on human seminal vesicle-specific peptides: A novel probe/marker system for semen identification. Biol Reprod 35:773–784, 1986.
28. Holter JC, Friedman SB: Child abuse: Early case findings in the emergency department. Pediatrics 42:128–138, 1968.
29. Jurgrau A: How to spot child abuse. RN 53:26–33, 1990.
30. Kanda MB, Orr LA: Specimen collection in sexual abuse. In: Ludwig S, Kornberg AE (eds): Child Abuse: A Medical Reference. New York, Churchill Livingstone, 1992, pp 265–278.
31. Kerns DL: Child abuse. In: Mayer TA (ed): Emergency Management of Pediatric Trauma. Philadelphia, WB Saunders, 1985, pp 421–434.
32. Kogutt MS, Swischuk LE, Fagan CJ: Patterns of injury and significance of uncommon fractures in the battered child syndrome. AJR 121:143–149, 1974.
33. Krisa K, Murphy WD, Stalgartis S: Reliability issues in the penile assessment of incarcerants. J Behav Assess 3(3):199–207, 1981.
34. McClelland CQ, Heiple KG: Fractures in the first year of life: A diagnostic dilemma? Am J Dis Child 136:26–29, 1982.
35. Meadow R: Munchausen syndrome by proxy: The hinterland of abuse. Lancet 2:343, 1977.
36. Merten DF, Carpenter BLM: Radiologic imaging of inflicted injury in the child abuse syndrome. Pediatr Clin North Am 37:815–838, 1990.
37. Merten DF, Osborne DRS, Radkowski MA, et al: Craniocerebral trauma in the abuse syndrome: Radiological observations. Pediatr Radiol 14:272–277, 1984.
38. Merten DF, Radowski MA, Leonidas JC: The abused child: A radiological reappraisal. Radiology 146:377–381, 1983.
39. Miles RL, Burns RP: Recognition of the subtle signs of child abuse. J Tenn Med Assoc 83:20–21, 1990.
40. Nakou S, Adam H, Stathacopoulou N, et al: Health status of abused and neglected children children and their siblings. Child Abuse Neglect 6:279–284, 1982.

41. Paradise JE: The medical evaluation of the sexually abused child. Pediatr Clin North Am 37:839–862, 1990.
42. Pelligren A, Wagner WG: Child sexual abuse: Factors affecting victims' removal from home. Child Abuse Neglect 14:53–60, 1990.
43. Pena SD, Medovy H: Child abuse and traumatic pseudocyst of the pancreas. J Pediatr 83:1026–1028, 1973.
44. Porter FS, Blick LC, Sgroi SM: Treatment of the sexually abused child. In: Sgroi SM (ed): Handbook of Clinical Intervention in Child Sexual Abuse. Lexington, Mass, Heath, 1982, pp 1009–1145.
45. Radkowski MR: The battered child syndrome: Pitfalls in radiological diagnosis. Pediatr Ann 12:894–903, 1983.
46. Reece RM: Unusual manifestations of child abuse. Pediatr Clin North Am 37:905–921, 1990.
47. Rhodes AM: Identifying and reporting child abuse. MCN 12:399, 1987.
48. Rogers C, Terry T: Clinical intervention with boy victims of sexual abuse. In: Stuart IR, Green JG (eds): Victims of Sexual Aggression: Treatment of Children, Women, and Men. New York, Van Nostrand Reinhold, 1984, pp 91–104.
49. Russell DEH: The incidence and prevalence of intrafamilial and extrafamilial sexual abuse of children. Child Abuse Neglect 7:133–146, 1983.
50. Schmitt BD, Krugman RD: Abuse and neglect of children. In: Behrman RE, Vaughan VC III, Nelson WE (eds): Nelson Textbook of Pediatrics. 13th ed. Philadelphia, WB Saunders, 1987, pp 79–82.
51. Schmitt LBD, Clemmens MR: Battered child syndrome. In: Touloukian RJ (ed): Pediatric Trauma. 2nd ed. St. Louis, Mosby Year Book, 1990, pp 163–187.
52. Silverman EM, Silverman AG: Persistence of spermatozoa in the lower genital tracts of women. JAMA 240:1875–1877, 1978.
53. Slovis TL, Berdon WE, Haller JO, et al: Pancreatitis and the battered child syndrome: Report of 2 cases with skeletal involvement. AJR 125:456–461, 1975.
54. Soules MR, Pollard AA, Brown KM, et al: The forensic laboratory evaluation of evidence in alleged rape. Am J Obstet Gynecol 130:142–147, 1978.
55. Steele BF: Notes on the lasting effects of early child abuse. Child Abuse Neglect 10:283–291, 1986.
56. Study of national incidence and prevalence of child abuse and neglect. Department of Health and Human Services, 1988.
57. Summit RC: The child sexual abuse accommodation syndrome. Child Abuse Neglect 7:177–193, 1983.
58. Veltkamp LJ, Miller TW: Clinical handbook of child abuse and neglect. Madison, Conn, International Universities Press, 1991. (in press)
59. Wagner WG: Child sexual abuse: A multidisciplinary approach to case management. J Counseling Dev 65:435–439, 1987.
60. Wilson EF: Estimation of the age of cutaneous contusions in child abuse. Pediatrics 60:750–752, 1977.

Bradley M. Rodgers
Gary Wickens Barone

CHAPTER THIRTY-SIX

Farm Injuries

The agricultural industry has become the most hazardous occupation in the United States, surpassing both underground mining and construction. Farming accounts for a fatality rate of 61 per 100,000 workers, 4.5 times the rate of 13 per 100,000 for the entire labor force (Table 36–1).[19] In addition, although the work injury rate for the other two most hazardous occupations (mining and construction) has declined steadily in the past decade, that for agriculture has increased steadily. Rivara noted that the fatality rate from farm machinery accidents increased 44% between 1930 and 1980, but deaths from non–farm machinery accidents decreased over this interval by 79%.[29] In 1980 farm workers suffered an estimated 2000 deaths and 200,000 disabling injuries.[30] Of special importance to physicians caring for children is that nearly 15 to 20% of these deaths and injuries occurred in children and adolescents younger than 19 years of age.[32] Although the rate for childhood household poisonings has shown a fourfold decline during the past 2 decades, the number of children injured in farming activities has continued to increase.

A unique aspect of the agricultural work force is that it is composed of a significant number of children and adolescents who are often exposed at an early age to a hazardous environment of complicated machinery, deep grain bins, large animals, pesticides, and other toxic chemicals. Children and adolescents younger than 19 years of age account for approximately 35% of the 6 million Americans living and working on farms, and 1.2 million are younger than 14 years of age.[32] Many of these children are employed by their families or are members of migrant families working alongside their parents in the fields. In contrast to that for most other industries, there is no federal legislation regulating or protecting minors (children younger than 16 years of age) who work on family-owned farms.

The magnitude of this problem is substantial. It has been estimated that more than 23,000 children are injured per year in farm-related activities and that approximately 300 of these children die from these injuries (Table 36–2). Hansen noted that 14% of the patients hospitalized for farm-related injuries were younger than 15 years of age, yet these children worked fewer total hours on the farm, indicating a

significantly higher injury rate per hour of labor in the younger worker.[16]

Despite this large pediatric work force and the magnitude of the pediatric trauma that it generates, reports documenting the scope of the problem of childhood trauma in the rural environment are few. Our purpose is to review the spectrum of this problem by analysis of (1) the general background of rural trauma to children, (2) the mechanisms of injury, (3) the initial management and triage of rural trauma, and (4) prevention and education strategies.

BACKGROUND AND INCIDENCE

Approximately 300 children die per year and about 23,000 are seriously injured in farm accidents. There is a marked gender difference in accident rates, with 73% of these injuries occurring in males. The rate of injuries increases strikingly with age. The farm accident fatality rate for 15- to 19-year-old males is nearly double that for all younger age groups. Cogbill and colleagues, in a series of 105 children younger than 18 years of age, found a peak age distribution in the early teen years, attributable to the fact that teenagers are expected to start active farm work involving the use of heavy machinery.[9] A second peak of injuries was noted also to occur during the toddler period of 2 to 4 years, which is explained best by the increased activity and curiosity of these children that takes place before the development of mature decision-making practices and protective caution. Injuries are more frequent in most series between May and September, at the time of peak farm activity with planting and harvesting. The western states report the highest accident rate, and the South reports the lowest.

Rivara estimated an injury-to-fatality rate in farm-related trauma of 129 to 1.[29] Ten per cent of the farm-related injuries to persons in his series required hospitalization. Mucha and associates noted that farm-related injuries accounted for 2.2% of the pediatric surgical trauma patients and 1.4% of the trauma mortality in Rochester, Minnesota.[27] Cogbill and co-workers estimated an overall inhospital mortality for farm-related injuries in a series of 105 children of 1% with a long-term disability rate of an additional 10% in the surviving patients.[9] Thirteen patients (12%) in these series also suffered significant hospital morbidity, including pneumonia, severe wound infections, nonunion of fractures, and neuropathy.

Although a wide variety of injuries may be encountered in farm accidents, Cogbill and associates were able to identify certain characteristics of pediatric farm-related trauma. The most commonly injured organ system was orthopedic (44%), followed by neurologic (27%), hand (16%), abdominal (15%), thoracic (14%), and maxillofacial (13%).[9] Also, the type of injuries could often be predicted by the mechanism of injury. Tractor and wagon accidents usually resulted in multiple trauma, with pelvic and long bone fractures and head and thoracoabdominal injuries commonly being seen. Falls from horses principally caused head and upper extremity trauma. Hand and extremity trauma predominated with farm machinery accidents. Animal kicks and assaults usually resulted in maxillofacial fractures, lacerations, and thoracoabdominal injuries.

Table 36–1
Fatality Rate by Industry

Industrial Divisions	Number Employed (thousands)	Number of Deaths	Rate/10⁵
Agriculture	3,300	2,000	61
Mining	1,000	500	50
Construction	5,610	2,500	45
Manufacturing	19,900	1,600	8
Transport/public utilities	5,300	1,500	28
Trade	21,800	1,400	6
Service	24,300	1,800	7
Others	15,590	170	1
Total labor force	96,800	13,000	13

Modified with permission from Kraus JF: Fatal and nonfatal injuries in occupational settings: A review. Am Rev Public Health 6:403–418, 1985. © 1985, by Annual Reviews, Inc.

Table 36–2
Childhood Farm Fatalities

	Age (yr)				
	<5	5–9	10–14	15–19	Total
Average annual no. of deaths					
Male	37	37	66	107	248
Female	14	11	9	4	38
Total	51	48	75	111	286
Annual rate/100,000 population					
Male	14.9	13.9	22.4	30.9	21.5
Female	6.5	4.8	3.6	1.3	3.8
Both sexes	11.0	9.7	13.7	16.8	13.2
Place of death					
Inpatient	14.1%	4.2%	6.7%	6.0%	7.4%
Outpatient	11.0%	9.1%	8.0%	5.4%	7.7%
Dead on arrival at hospital	21.3%	25.2%	20.6%	14.6%	19.1%
Out of hospital	34.5%	46.9%	54.5%	62.1%	52.5%
Other or unknown	19.1%	14.6%	10.2%	11.9%	12.3%

From Rivara FP: Fatal and nonfatal farm injuries to children and adolescents in the United States. Pediatrics 76:567–573, 1985.

MECHANISMS OF INJURY

Overall the most common mechanism of injury in children on farms involves encounters with animals. Next in frequency are accidents related to machinery other than tractors, followed by tractor mishaps, wagon accidents, and falls (Table 36–3). The mechanism of farm-related injuries in children appears to be age dependent. Whereas animal-related injuries and falls from heights predominate in younger children, accidents related to the use of farm machinery and tractors are seen more commonly in teenaged children.

Farm Animals

Despite the fact that in most regions of the United States horses are rarely used for daily transportation or farm work, equestrian activities remain a major recreational activity in rural areas, with an estimated 80 million Americans riding a horse for pleasure at least once a year. Nearly 2 million of these riders are under 20 years of age.[5] In addition, cows and bulls, animals often of a weight equal to a horse, form an important aspect of many farm operations. The handling and management of these large animals is not without risks, and serious injury and death may result from accidents involving them.

Falls, kicks, bites, and assaults by farm animals account for the largest group of injuries in children, and approximately 40% of all farm-related accidents in children occur within this category. Even though injuries by farm animals account for only 2% of the deaths from farm accidents, many of these animal-related injuries result in serious head or maxillofacial trauma or thoracoabdominal injuries. Busch and co-workers reviewed 134 bovine- and equine-related farm injuries, and 30% occurred in children.[6] Thirty-three per cent of all of the injuries in this series were caused by falls from horses, and 13% involved assaults by horses. Although an additional 21% of the patients were injured by a kick from a cow, an equal number suffered injuries by assaults from these animals (Table 36–4). In Cogbill and colleagues's series, 50% of farm animal–related injuries were caused by falls from horses, often resulting in head and upper extremity trauma. Horse and cow assaults accounted for another 40%. These injuries resulted principally in maxillofacial or extremity fractures or serious thoracoabdominal injuries.[9]

The University of Virginia in Charlottesville, Virginia, is located in a rural area of the state that supports year-round equestrian activities. We reviewed the records of 136 pa-

Table 36–3
Farm Accidents in Children

Accident	No. (%) of Children Injured
Fall from horse	22 (21)
Farm machinery	21 (20)
Tractor accidents	17 (7)
Horse assaults	12 (11)
Trailer and wagon accidents	11 (10)
Cow assaults	8 (8)
Fall from building	6 (6)
Other	8 (8)

From Cogbill TH, Busch HM, Stiers GR: Farm accidents in children. Pediatrics 76:562–566, 1985.

Table 36–4
Bovine-Equine Trauma

Mechanism	No. (%) of Patients Injured
Fall from horse	45 (33)
Kicked by cow	28 (21)
Bovine assault	25 (19)
Equine assault	17 (17)
Kicked by horse	11 (11)
Animal-drawn vehicle	8 (8)

From Busch H, Cogbill T, Landercasper J, Landercasper B: Blunt bovine and equine trauma. J Trauma 26:559–560, 1986.

tients 19 years of age or younger who required admission to the University Hospital for equestrian-related trauma over a 14-year interval.[3] These 136 patients accounted for 152 injuries and required a total of 793 days of hospitalization. The largest group of patients—75, or 54%—suffered head or facial trauma, with the majority (79%) of these falling from the mount and suffering closed head trauma. Twenty per cent of this group of 75 children were kicked in the head by the horse, an injury resulting in severe skull and facial trauma. The second largest group of injuries included 57 children, or 41%, who suffered skeletal fractures. The largest percentage of these (66%) suffered extremity fractures, with most occurring when the child fell from the horse. The most serious multiple trauma occurred either when the rider was kicked by the horse or when the horse fell on the rider. A majority of these serious injuries could have been prevented by the use of improved protective helmets or better education about proper barn safety while working around large animals.

All farm animals are potentially dangerous, and children should not be allowed access to livestock without learning respect for them and receiving proper instruction in the handling of large animals. Horses and dairy cows are nervous animals and readily kick when startled. Many animals can bite with enough force to cause serious hand or extremity injury, especially in young children, and can easily cause severe injuries with their weight by stepping on or falling on a child. In addition, any normally docile farm animal may become aggressive and dangerous when protecting its young.

Farm Vehicles

The hazards of farm tractors have been widely recognized since tractors replaced horses as the primary power source on farms. Tractors are the most ubiquitous piece of farm machinery, and they are the most common farm machine that causes fatal injuries involving children, accounting for more than 50% of farm fatalities each year.[29] Tractors also account for about 25% of the nonfatal farm injuries in children, and tractor operators under the age of 14 years are considered about nine times more likely to have accidents than adults.[17] Farming parents often decide that a teenaged child should help on the farm by learning how to operate a tractor. The child is trained by driving around the barnyard and then is sent to operate the vehicle in rough field, often involving uneven terrain.

Tractor accidents commonly result in severe trauma with multiple injuries because the majority of the accidents are due to either being run over (usually young children) or being crushed in rollover accidents (usually teenaged children). Approximately 75% of the tractor-related injuries are secondary to overturns, and this type of accident accounts for the majority of the farm accident deaths.[29] Another 15% of the tractor-related injuries are caused by the power take-off (PTO), and 10% involve either falling from the vehicle or running over individuals. Hansen estimated that there was a 25% chance of death in a tractor overturn.[16] Most tractor accidents are felt to be due to the carelessness or inexperience of the operator. In addition, children are often allowed to ride as passengers on tractors, and many may be seriously injured directly by tractor overturns or by falling off the tractor because they are not properly restrained. Children who fall off of a moving tractor are often run over by the large rear tires of the vehicle.

An additional group of farm vehicle injuries involve accidents related to the use of all-terrain vehicles (ATV).[1] These vehicles initially were marketed for farm work, but their use has spread to more recreational activities by younger individuals.[34] A review of our experience with these injuries at the University of Virginia revealed that children admitted with ATV injuries tended to have multiple and severe injuries, including closed head trauma with basilar skull fractures and blunt abdominal trauma often from hitting the handlebars.[31] Thirty-three per cent of the children admitted required intensive care, and the average length of hospitalization for all of these patients was 20 days. Physicians and the public need to be aware of the significant injury potential of these vehicles and should advocate the use of proper clothing and safety precautions while operating ATVs. The manufacturers of ATVs, in cooperation with the U.S. federal government, have instituted a moratorium on the manufacture and sale of three-wheeled models in this country. Nonetheless, a great number of these vehicles remain in use by young children in rural areas. A few states have enacted legislation regulating the use of ATVs by children and mandating the use of safety equipment and the completion of educational courses before they are used.

CASE 1 (TM: #8–43–89)

This 14-year-old Jehovah's Witness crashed his three-wheeled all-terrain vehicle while riding without a helmet over rough rural terrain. He was found off the vehicle and unresponsive by a friend, an undetermined amount of time following the accident. A local emergency medical team was summoned, and the child was intubated on the scene and taken by ground transportation to a rural Virginia hospital, where he was found to be unresponsive with decerebrate posturing. His vital signs were stable. Thirty minutes later he was transferred via helicopter to the University of Virginia Hospital. A head computed tomography scan revealed multiple intraparenchymal hematomas with intraventricular blood and subarachnoid hemorrhage (Fig. 36–1). There were no abdominal or chest injuries. He underwent bifrontal craniectomy with ventriculostomy. He was discharged to a long-term care facility 2 months following his accident, and 1 year later he is unable to care for himself and is showing little neurologic recovery.

Farm Machinery

Mechanization has greatly improved the productivity of farmers but has also subjected them to the increased possibility of severe and crippling injuries. These types of injuries account for 20% of the trauma to children on farms and include injuries due to corn pickers, PTOs, grain augers, haybalers, and combines.[9] These injuries most commonly involve extremities, which become entangled in the machinery. Most of these injuries are avoidable because they are due to carelessness: placing extremities in jammed machinery, wearing loose fitting clothing that is caught by machinery, or removing the protective safety shielding devices from around the machinery.

The PTO mechanism, which operates off the tractor's power train, is a rotating shaft with coupling devices at both ends (Fig. 36–2). The PTO allows a tractor to power other types of machinery, such as an auger or a haybaler. Injuries from the PTO usually occur when clothing becomes entangled by this shaft, rotating at 500 to 1000 rpm. A child can be injured directly by the rotating shaft, or a PTO can strip the body of clothing and hurl the victim through the air, striking him against other machinery on the ground. Unlike other farm injuries, these injuries tend to occur in the fall and winter months when heavy clothing can become more readily entangled in the rotating shaft of the PTO. On reviewing the experience with PTO injuries at the Mayo Clinic, McElfresh and Bryan noted that 34 of the 49 injuries occurred during the winter months of October to March and involved heavy clothing being worn around the tractor.[23] Ten of the PTO injuries (20%) occurred in children between the ages of 10 and 20 years, and another four (8%) occurred in children younger than 10 years of age. Open fractures and traumatic amputations were common in this series. McElfresh and Bryan noted that if the worker's clothes did not tear from the body, the victim often was killed by this type of accident.[23]

CASE 2 (AB: #65–59–20)

This 15-year-old boy was pulled into the PTO of his father's tractor in November. His coat sleeve was caught in the drive shaft, and he was thrown to the ground forcefully. He suffered transient loss of consciousness and complained of right chest pain on awakening. The farm was about 30 miles from the University of Virginia Hospital, and he was picked up in the field by the university's helicopter. Oxygen was provided in transport. On arrival in the emergency department his vital signs were stable, and he was noted to have subcutaneous emphysema. He had multiple abrasions on his upper extremities and trunk, and he was neurologically intact. A chest roentgenogram revealed a left pneumothorax with fractures of the left seventh and eighth ribs as well as bilateral first and second rib fractures (Fig. 36–3). The mediastinum appeared normal. Chest and abdominal computed tomography scans were normal. He was treated with a tube thoracostomy and was discharged on the sixth day after the accident in stable condition.

The modern grain auger, used to transport grain, is considered to be one of the most hazardous of all pieces of farm equipment. Grain may be fed into it from a hopper, or the lower end may be buried into a pile of grain. A child may become entrapped within the auger directly while operating it, or a small child may be sucked into the auger while curiously investigating a moving pile of grain. Beatty and colleagues noted that 12% of the patients with auger injuries were younger than 16 years of age.[4] Power take-off and grain augers accounted for 50% of the deaths from farm machinery in this series. Using the principle of the Archimedes screw, the 6-inch auger propels grain at 400 feet per minute or about 7 feet per second (Fig. 36–4). A

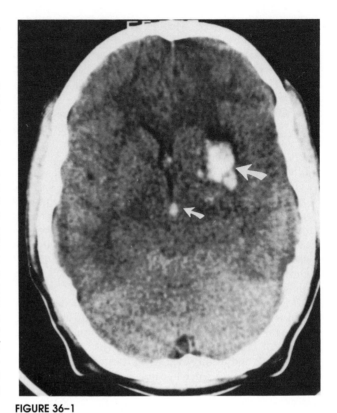

FIGURE 36–1

Transverse computed tomography scan of the head demonstrating intraparenchymal *(large arrow)* and intraventricular *(small arrow)* hemorrhages.

hand, foot, or an entire extremity can easily get caught in the screwlike mechanism and ascend 5 feet before the injured person is even able to react to the danger. Grain auger injuries are usually severe, and traumatic amputations of portions of hands and upper extremities are very common injuries. Letts and Gammon found the grain auger to be responsible for 50% of the traumatic amputations in children under 16 years of age in Manitoba.[22] Although most grain augers are sold with protective shields over the intake, these safety devices are often removed by the farmers because they slow the operation of the machinery (Fig. 36–5). In general, these wounds are very severely contaminated with grain and dirt and contain considerable devitalized tissue.

The roll hay baler is a relatively new addition to the farm. This machine rolls bales of hay, each weighing 850 to 1900 pounds, or about 25 times the weight of conventional rectangular compressed bales. The machine produces a severe wringer-type of injury when an extremity, usually the arm, is caught between the rollers. The degree of tissue damage from a wringer injury depends on the space between the rollers, the peripheral speed of the rollers, the hardness of the rollers, the temperature of the machinery, and how violently the victim struggles to free the extremity. Large modern hay balers are usually driven by tractor PTOs. They produce severe high-energy compression or avulsion injuries to the extremities, often complicated by gross contamination and high frictional heat with deep thermal injuries. The force between the rollers of a modern hay

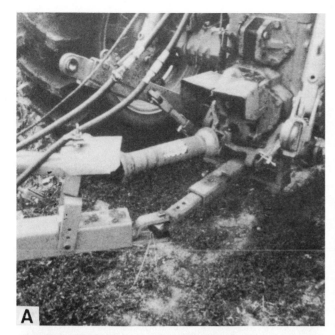

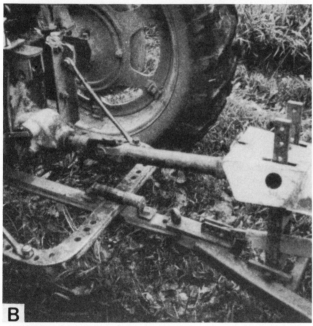

FIGURE 36-2

A, Power take-off protected by a metallic shield coupled to farm machinery. *B,* Power take-off with the protective shield removed. (From McElfresh EC, Bryan RS: Power take-off injuries. J Trauma 13:755–782, 1973.)

baler is between 250 and 1300 pounds. This compares with 15 to 40 pounds force in the commercial wringer washer.[12] Mayba described a "hay balers' fracture," which is a concomitant fracture of the sternum and the T-12 vertebral body caused by an hyperextension injury as these large bales of hay fall on the operator driving the tractor while loading.[25]

Injuries caused by farm machinery often are the most difficult to treat because of their complex nature. They can include elements of laceration, crush, bony fracture, burns,

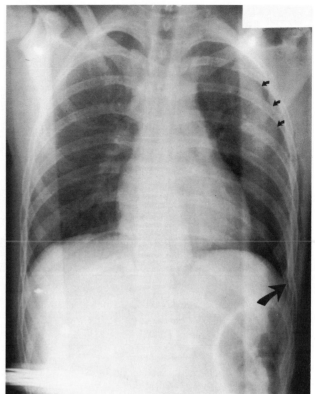

FIGURE 36-3

Anteroposterior chest roentgenogram demonstrating left-sided subcutaneous emphysema. Fractures of the left seventh and eighth ribs *(large arrow)* are evident. A left-sided pneumothorax is present *(small arrows).* The mediastinum appears normal.

amputations, and avulsion. In addition, they often are severely contaminated with manure, grains, grass, soil, and grease. Agger and associates noted the complexity of the bacterial contamination of these injuries and reported a rate of infection of 89% in accidents from farm machinery, whereas the comparable rate for industrial machinery was 33%.[2] Partly because of this extensive soft tissue injury and contamination and partly because of the delay in transport, Koivunen and co-workers reported that the amputation rate for extremities with associated vascular trauma in rural Missouri was almost twice that of the soldiers wounded in the Vietnam War.[18] Injuries due to farm machinery are

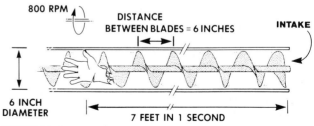

FIGURE 36-4

Functional principles of the Archimedes screw. (From Beatty ME, Zook EG, Russell RC, Kindead LR: Grain augur injuries: The replacement of the corn picker injury. Plast Reconstr Surg 69:96–102, 1982.)

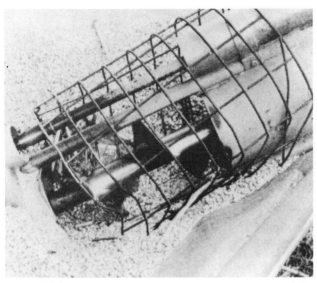

FIGURE 36–5
Grain auger intake covered with a protective wire shield. (Reprinted with permission from Hanson RH: Major injuries due to agricultural machinery. Ann Plast Surg 17:59–64, 1986.)

associated with permanent serious disability in 20 to 60% of the cases because they so frequently involve amputation of hands, feet, or entire extremities.[8]

TRIAGE AND MANAGEMENT OF RURAL TRAUMA

Speed is often considered essential for effective trauma care. The first hour following a critical injury is considered the "golden hour." It is generally agreed that the patient who begins to receive definitive care within the first hour after being injured has a better chance for survival than one treated after a greater delay. For most forms of trauma, mortality doubles for each additional hour of delay in initiating treatment.[26]

Rivara reported that more than half of the children who died from farm accidents did so without ever reaching a hospital or receiving any medical attention.[29] In addition, another 19% died shortly after arrival at a medical facility, and only 7% of those who eventually died lived long enough to receive inpatient care before succumbing to their injuries (see Table 36–2). These data confirm the need for improved resuscitation in the field and for rapid transportation in the management of rural trauma.

Cogbill and Busch noted that the average length of time the victims remained in the field following a tractor rollover accident was more than 1 1/2 hours.[8] It was concluded that this excessive amount of time resulted from several factors that are unique to rural trauma. First, farmers often work alone either early in the morning or late into the evening, and if they become entrapped or are unconscious, they may go undiscovered for hours. Also, extraction of an accident victim from heavy farm equipment may be very difficult and time consuming. Lastly, because of the great distances involved, response and transport times are often very long.

Cogbill and Busch favored the rapid transport of the severely injured patient to smaller but closer rural community hospitals for evaluation and initial resuscitation and subsequent transfer to a designated regional trauma center for definitive care.[8]

Krob and colleagues emphasized the long distances involved in transporting rural trauma victims.[20] In their experience the average time from a motor vehicle accident to definitive care in a rural environment was 2 hours and 20 minutes, and he concluded that the single most important improvement in trauma care for patients in a rural setting would be better education and training of rural trauma care providers, including emergency medical technicians and emergency department physicians. Programs such as the Advanced Trauma Life Support course developed by the American College of Surgeons were supported as an initial and effective step toward achieving this goal. The importance of educating rural health care providers in the resuscitation and evaluation of the trauma victim is underscored also by data provided by Detmer and associates.[10] In a retrospective review of emergency admissions, there was a progressive increase in the frequency of "unacceptable care" as the hospital's emergency trauma capability decreased.

A monumental development in the trauma care system has been the addition of hospital-based helicopters.[24] A review by Leicht and co-workers concerning the impact of helicopter transport on trauma care in rural Pennsylvania summarizes several important points.[21] Helicopter transportation was faster than ground transportation, with the average trip being about 80 miles and involving a wide regional area of 25 community hospitals. Leicht and colleagues concluded that a properly resuscitated patient required about 30 minutes of ground time for the helicopter, whereas an improperly stabilized patient required twice this amount of time.[21] A major source for this delay was failure of the referring physician to have completed an appropriate examination or to have properly stabilized the patient.

Gilmore and associates[13] and Mucha and colleagues[27] reviewed the development of rural trauma systems and stated that because of the long transportation distances involved, properly trained paramedics and physicians are essential for effective trauma care. Advanced Cardiac Life Support and Advanced Trauma Life Support courses are important steps, and improved communication, coordination, and cooperation between the rural community hospitals and the designated trauma centers are absolutely necessary. Evaluating the need for better education in early trauma management, Ramenofsky and co-workers reviewed a series of pediatric trauma victims.[28] The majority of fatal but potentially salvageable cases of trauma had errors made during the early resuscitation and evaluation phases of their care or during transport. Only 17% had fatal errors noted during their definitive care in the hospital (Fig. 36–6).

Haller and associates strongly recommended the formation of regional pediatric trauma centers.[15] In rural areas these could be efficiently incorporated into designated regional trauma centers. Haller and colleagues also felt that improved prehospital care for the pediatric trauma victims was needed and that more complete information regarding the management of pediatric trauma be included in the

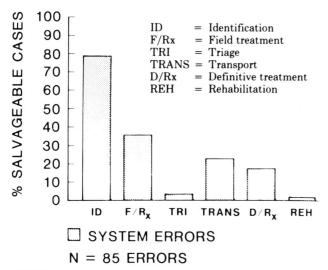

ID   = Identification
F/Rx   = Field treatment
TRI   = Triage
TRANS   = Transport
D/Rx   = Definitive treatment
REH   = Rehabilitation

☐ SYSTEM ERRORS

N = 85 ERRORS

FIGURE 36–6

Frequency of system errors by location in the management of pediatric trauma. (From Ramenofsky ML, Luterman A, Quindlen E, et al: Maximum survival in pediatric trauma: The ideal system. J Trauma 24:818–823, 1984.)

Advanced Trauma Life Support course. In addition, Haller supported the development of a separate but similar advanced pediatric life support course for physicians caring for the multiply injured child.[14]

PREVENTION

Prevention starts with fully identifying the problem. There are very few reports of agricultural-related trauma, fewer yet that specifically evaluate the impact of this trauma on children. Without knowing how frequently farm accidents happen or what kind of trends are occurring, it is very difficult to initiate any type of major prevention program. Rivara concluded that the death and injury rates quoted must be taken as "minimal estimates" of the magnitude of the problem.[29] A good example of this inaccuracy is the possibility of alcohol consumption contributing to agricultural-related trauma, especially in teenagers. Alcohol has been well established as a contributing factor in civilian trauma, especially in motor vehicle accidents. The use of a grain auger, for example, while intoxicated is easily appreciated as a potentially dangerous situation.

Prevention can be addressed through a number of different methods suggested by injury prevention research in related fields. *Education* is an important first step toward prevention. This can start at home, at school, or in the physician's office. Parents must be reminded to keep children away from large animals and to drive tractors and wagons cautiously and well away from children. Parents should be educated about the risks of farm machinery (e.g., PTOs, augers, balers) and its ability to cause severe and often debilitating injuries. Children must be taught respect for farm animals. Young equestrians must be taught the use of protective headgear and safety equipment. As farm children begin to work around agricultural equipment, they should receive formal instruction and training in the opera-

tion of such dangerous machines. Possibly classes, similar to driver education classes, should be included in the curriculum of rural schools to stress the proper operation and safety features of farm equipment. Physicians in a rural environment must learn to use various media modalities for education of their patients. Beatty and co-workers noted that when considerable media attention was directed toward the dangers of operating grain augers the number of serious injuries in Wisconsin declined from 9 in 1979 to 3 in 1980.[4]

For the family car, government-required modifications and improved safety standards have been proved to decrease injuries and mortality. Possibly the same principles can be applied to farm machinery. Currently, however, very few mandatory federal requirements are applicable to the manufacture of off-road vehicles such as tractors, farm wagons, or combines.

Compounding the problem is the fact that most farm machinery is inherently dangerous, a situation often exacerbated by the common practice of farmers of removing or bypassing factory-installed safety devices and covers.[4] Farm equipment and tractor manufacturers have voluntarily developed and installed many optional safety features, but this effort does not appear to have gone far enough. The major mechanism of trauma related to tractors is being crushed when the tractor rolls over, especially while plowing a soft field on a grade. Yet it is still possible to purchase farm tractors without roll bars, crush proof cabs, counterweights, or other roll protective devices. Many of these features are offered as options at additional cost and are not standard safety features. Furthermore farm equipment is very expensive and often infrequently replaced. The average life of a farm tractor is 20 years, and it is not unusual to find older equipment still in use that was built long before the development of these safety features. Most tractor accidents actually involve the use of this older equipment.[17]

Installation of safety devices does not always guarantee their use. Effective shielding is now supplied as standard equipment on PTO units, but this shielding is easily removed and often is never replaced by the farmer (see Fig. 36–2B). Unlike with other heavy industry, there is little enforcement pertaining to the use of safety devices on agricultural equipment. The Occupational Safety and Health Administration has developed strong safety standards for protective devices and regular inspection of farm equipment used by farms employing ten or more nonfamily workers, but these farms account for less than 10% of all American farms.[17] Smaller family farms are exempted from these regulations. There is need for the development of the following:

1. Safer equipment with nonremovable, automatic safety devices
2. Federal regulations to improve safety standards on all farm equipment
3. More comprehensive application of OSHA safety inspections on smaller family farms.

Finally, the legislation regarding child farm labor may need to be changed. The Fair Labor Standards Act of 1938 (Child Labor Bill 102) states that "Minors of any age may be employed by their parents or person standing in the place of their parents at any time in any occupation on a farm owned and operated by their parents or person standing in place of the parent.''[7] This is in stark contrast to restrictions on the employment of minors in other occupations. For most other occupations, 16 years is the minimal age of employment, and minors younger than 18 years are prohibited from hazardous occupations in other industries, even when the minor is employed by the parent. The changing of farm labor laws will be hard to accomplish, and these laws will be difficult to enforce because this double standard is partly economic in origin. Children in nonrural manufacturing industries are viewed as a threat to the adult labor force, while in agriculture children are considered a source of inexpensive labor.

SUMMARY

In summary, although steady progress has been made in the management of pediatric trauma,[11] trauma continues to cause about half the deaths of children older than 1 year of age.[33] Agricultural-related or rural trauma continues to be associated with an especially high morbidity and mortality rate.[29] Progress in the management of rural trauma has been hindered by the wide variety and complexity of the trauma and the great distances involved. Even with the increasing utilization of helicopter transportation, a better functioning rural trauma system needs more paramedics and rural physicians properly trained in the management of trauma and especially pediatric trauma. Prevention starts with better studies to identify the problems and with better education of rural parents and children about the hazards associated with farming activities. The federal government needs to expand its safety regulations covering farm machinery and small farms, and child labor laws may need to be changed to protect children from the severe hazards of farming.

References

1. Adams BE: Trauma caused by three-wheel motor vehicles—An unrecognized epidemic. Ann Emerg Med 15:1288–1292, 1986.
2. Agger WA, Cogbill TH, Busch H, et al: Wounds caused by corn-harvesting machines: An unusual source of infection due to gram-negative bacilli. Rev Infect Dis 8:927–931, 1986.
3. Barone GW, Rodgers BM: Equestrian injuries—A 14 year review. Unpublished data.
4. Beatty ME, Zook EG, Russell RC, Kindead LR: Grain auger injuries: The replacement of the corn picker injury. Plast Reconstr Surg 69:96–102, 1982.
5. Bixby-Hammett DM. Youth accidents with horses. Phys Sportsmed 13:105–108, 1985.
6. Busch H, Cogbill T, Landercasper J, Landercasper B: Blunt bovine and equine trauma. J Trauma 26:559–560, 1986.
7. Child Labor Requirements in Agriculture Under the Fair Labor Standards Act, Child Labor Bill No. 102, U.S. Department of Labor, 1984.
8. Cogbill T, Busch H: The spectrum of agricultural trauma. J Emerg Med 3:205–210, 1985.
9. Cogbill TH, Busch HM, Stiers GR: Farm accidents in children. Pediatrics 76:562–566, 1985.
10. Detmer DE, Moylan JA, Rose J, et al: Regional categorization and quality of care in major trauma. J Trauma 17:592–599, 1977.
11. Eichelberger MR, Randolph JG: Progress in pediatric trauma. World J Surg 9:222–235, 1985.
12. Gainor BJ: Haybaler trauma to the upper extremity: A roller injury. J Trauma 23:1069–1071, 1983.
13. Gilmore KL, Clemmer TP, Orme JF: Commitment to trauma in a low population density area. J Trauma 21:883–888, 1981.
14. Haller JA; Pediatric trauma: The no. 1 killer of children. JAMA 249:47, 1983.
15. Haller JA, Shorter N, Miller D, et al: Organization and function of a regional pediatric trauma center: Does a system of management improve outcome? J Trauma 23:691–696, 1983.
16. Hansen RH: Major injuries due to agricultural machinery. Ann Plast Surg 17:59–64, 1986.
17. Karlson T, Noren J: Farm tractor fatalities: The failure of voluntary safety standards. Am J Public Health 69:146–149, 1979.
18. Koivunen D, Nichols W, Silver D: Vascular trauma in a rural population. Surgery 91:723–727, 1982.
19. Kraus JF: Fatal and nonfatal injuries in occupational settings: A review. Am Rev Public Health 6:403–418, 1985.
20. Krob MJ, Cram AE, Vargish T, Kassell NF: Rural trauma care: A study of trauma care in a rural emergency medical services region. Ann Emerg Med 13:891–895, 1984.
21. Leicht MJ, Dula DJ, Brotman S, et al: Rural interhospital helicopter transport of motor vehicle trauma victims: Causes for delays and recommendations. Ann Emerg Med 15:450–453, 1986.
22. Letts RM, Gammon W: Auger injuries in children. Can Med Assoc J 188:519–522, 1978.
23. McElfresh EC, Bryan RS: Power take-off injuries. J Trauma 13:775–782, 1973.
24. Macione AR, Wilcox DE: Utilization prediction for helicopter emergency medical services. Ann Emerg Med 16:391–398, 1987.
25. Mayba II: Haybalers' fractures. J Trauma 24:271–273, 1984.
26. Morse TS: The child with multiple injuries. Emerg Med Clin North Am 1:175–185, 1983.
27. Mucha P, Farnell MB, Szech JM, et al: A rural regional trauma center. J Trauma 23:337–340, 1983.
28. Ramenofsky ML, Luterman A, Quindlen E, et al: Maximum survival in pediatric trauma: The ideal system. J Trauma 24:818–823, 1984.
29. Rivara FP: Fatal and nonfatal farm injuries to children and adolescents in the United States. Pediatrics 76:567–573, 1985.
30. Simpson SG: Farm machinery injuries. J Trauma 24:150–152, 1984.
31. Stevens WS, Rodgers BM, Newman BM: Pediatric trauma associated with all-terrain vehicles. J Pediatr 109:25–29, 1986.
32. Swanson JA, Sachs MI, Dahlgren KA, Tinguely SJ: Accidental farm injuries in children. Am J Dis Child 141:1276–1279, 1987.
33. Templeton JM, O'Neil JA: Pediatric trauma. Emerg Med Clin North Am 2:899–912, 1984.
34. Trager GW, Grayman G, Harr S: All-terrain vehicle accidents: The experience of one hospital located near a major recreational center. Ann Emerg Med 15:1293–1297, 1986.

David E. Wesson
Michael J. Rieder
Laura J. Spence

Sports and Recreation Injuries

Writing about recreational and sports injuries among children presents several difficulties. There is neither a standard classification of recreational and sport activities nor clear definitions of what activities are included in these categories. For example, bicycles may be used for transportation to and from school and for recreational activities after school and on weekends. Residential swimming pools are designed primarily for recreation, but most drownings in such pools involve toddlers who accidentally fall into them. Children engage in a number of unorganized recreational activities such as fishing, swimming, and pick-up games of football or basketball. Because these activities are unsupervised, it is impossible to determine how much time children spend doing them and therefore how much they are exposed to the risk of injury.

Another problem is the lack of definition of what constitutes an injury. Does an injury require a visit to a hospital or medical treatment either in the hospital or at the playing field? Should we include only injuries for which a formal report is filed or all injuries that require the participant to drop out of the activity for a period of time?

For these reasons, the literature on sports and recreational injuries is difficult to interpret. This difficulty is compounded by the fact that so much of the literature consists of case series treated at specific hospitals or by individual practitioners that the results cannot be generalized to whole populations.

Because of changing behavior and fashion, the types of recreational and sports activities that children and adolescents participate in are constantly changing. A good example is skateboarding, which in the last 10 or 15 years has alternately risen and fallen in popularity.

Despite these problems in interpretation, certain things are clear. Sports and recreation are prominent parts of life in modern Western societies. They include jogging, water sports, and team sports such as soccer. Waller states that at least 2.5 million medically treated injuries and 5000 to 6000 deaths result from sports and recreational injuries each year in the United States.[63] A rational approach to understanding and alleviating these injuries requires better knowledge of their frequency, severity, and distribution. This information can only come from sound epidemiologic research. Prevention is better than cure. People engage in sports and recreational activities primarily to improve their psychological and physical health, in contrast to industrial and transportation activities, which are motivated chiefly by economics. The goal of the physician should be to reduce sports and recreational injuries, first by identifying them and then either by making the activity safer or eliminating it altogether.

In this chapter we present a few basic concepts and facts on the epidemiology of sports and recreational injuries, some examples focusing on the epidemiology of sports and recreational activities, strategies for injury prevention, and a few words about the role of the individual clinician. The treatment of sports injuries is not discussed in any detail.

EPIDEMIOLOGY

Epidemiology is the scientific study of the occurrence, causes, and prevention of diseases. It requires the acquisition of accurate data on the time and place of occurrence and the persons affected. Injuries do not occur randomly; they have definable and correctable causes. Effective surveillance of injuries in populations can detect patterns and changes in patterns. Furthermore, it is necessary to know not just how many people are injured in a particular activity, but how many are exposed to the risk of injury. Data on exposure can help determine the risk of injury to a participant. Some index of the severity of the injuries that result from a particular activity is also helpful. Knowledge of exposure to and severity of injury allows a more rational approach to prevention by identifying dangerous activities in need of modification.

The epidemiology of sports and recreational injuries in children has been reviewed recently by Waller and by Kraus and Conroy.[37, 63] Zaricznyji and colleagues reported that 3% of all elementary school students, 7% of junior high school students, and 11% of high school students in the United States were injured in sporting activities each year.[67] These researchers found that the risk of injury was greater in nonorganized than in organized sports, and that adolescents tended to suffer more severe injuries, especially when playing football. Waller reported that sports and recreational injuries accounted for 7% of spinal cord injuries and 3% of severe head injuries in children each year.[63]

A report from the Hospital for Sick Children in Toronto revealed a 1-year total of 2102 outpatient visits and 123 admissions resulting from sport-related injuries, exclusive of drowning, submersions, bicycle injuries, and playground injuries (Table 37–1).[25] No deaths were reported in this series. Baseball injuries accounted for more outpatient visits and admissions than any other sport, followed by injuries from ice hockey, gymnastics, soccer, football, rugby, and basketball, in decreasing order. Falls from playground equipment led to 451 outpatient visits and 80 admissions, and blows from playground equipment led to 88 outpatient visits and five admissions. Bicycle accidents, which were considered separately from sports injuries, were responsible for 692 outpatient visits, 102 admissions, and one death. During the same year, pedestrians struck by motor vehicles accounted for 244 outpatient visits, 99 admissions, and

Table 37–1

Injuries Causing Hospital Visits and Admissions (In order of frequency)

Visits	Admissions
Falls	Falls
Bumps, blows	Transport
Sports	Sports
Other accidents	Foreign bodies
Transport	Poisoning
Sharp objects	Bumps, blows
Foreign bodies	Violence
Violence	Environmental
Burns, explosions, shock	Self-inflicted injuries
Poisoning	Other accidents
Environmental	Burns, explosions, shock
Self-inflicted injuries	Sharp objects

three deaths. Unfortunately, this type of report does not take into account exposure or severity as reflected in long-term morbidity. In contrast, Mueller quotes several examples indicating that properly designed and executed epidemiologic studies of sports and recreational injuries can lead to effective prevention programs.[43]

Although no single source of data exists on all types of sports and recreational injuries, there are several valuable sources of information on specific aspects of this topic. For example, the reports of the National Electronic Injury Surveillance Systems (NEISS) include data on athletic and recreational injuries in the United States from 1972 to the present. NEISS is the data-collection arm of the United States Consumer Product Safety Commission (CPSC). This data set includes information on injuries that resulted from the use of a consumer product and required medial treatment in a hospital emergency department. The data are entered daily into a central computer system from terminals in selected hospitals across the United States. These hospitals were chosen to provide a statistically valid sample of consumer product–related injuries in the entire population of the United States. Although it has identified some hazardous products associated with recreational use, specifically bicycles and playground equipment, the NEISS has several limitations. In addition to providing no information about injuries that do not require treatment in a hospital, NEISS is limited to injuries involving consumer products, lacks accurate information on the actual activity involved, and does not clearly relate the type of injury to the degree of exposure. Each category in the database involves many different types of activities and thus limits the ability to plan prevention programs. For example, bicycle injuries could be related to transportation to and from school or to organized or nonorganized recreational activities. The NEISS contains little information on severity of injury and no significant information on long-term effects.

Much of the literature on sports and recreational injuries consists of case series, with an emphasis on organized activities such as high school or college football. It is doubtful that these reports reflect the true extent of sports and recreational activities. They generally fail to take an account of exposure and therefore do not allow the calculation of injury rates. The literature often emphasizes fatal or severely disabling injuries and tends to neglect minor injuries that, because of their frequency, could account for significant morbidity in the general population.

Kraus and Conroy estimated that in 1978 there were 6000 deaths in the United States due to athletic, sporting, or recreational activities.[37] Almost 3000 of these deaths involved small-boat occupants or drowning. Motor vehicle nontraffic accidents accounted for more than 800 of these deaths. These researchers also reported that although morbidity data were less reliable than death rates, NEISS estimated that 3.3 million injuries associated with sports and recreational activities occurred during the 12-month period ending in September 1982.

Zaricznyji, in a survey of injuries that occurred during organized athletic activity among school children in Springfield, Illinois, in 1974 to 1975, found that boys suffered twice as many injuries as girls and that the overall rate of injury was 5.9 per 100 students per year.[67] Forty percent of injuries occurred in nonorganized activities. The risk of injury per 100 participants was highest in football at 28.3, followed by wrestling at 16.4, and gymnastics at 13.3. Interestingly, Zaricznyji found that the risk per participant-hour was greatest for track and field. Zaricznyji also found that by far the greatest number of severe injuries occurred in football.[67] This observation has been confirmed by others, including Chambers, and Garrick and Requa.[12, 18] The latter researchers studied high school sports injuries in Seattle in the 1973 to 1974 academic year. The overall injury rate was 39 per 100 participants per year. The highest rates for boys were in football (81 per 100) and wrestling (75 per 100), and for girls the highest rates occurred in gymnastics (40 per 100) and softball (44 per 100).

The topic of injury surveillance systems for sports has recently been reviewed by Damron.[14] Boyce and associates, reporting on a 2-year survey of injuries in an urban school district with 55,000 students in 96 schools, found an injury rate of 49 per 1000 students per year—an incidence of almost one in 20.[9] The injury rate was higher among boys. Athletic activity accounted for 23% of all injuries, and playground or sports equipment was responsible for 14%. Sixty-five percent of injuries occurred on the school playground or in the school gym.

Chambers studied orthopedic injuries in children aged 6 to 17 years involved in athletic activities at a United States military post.[12] He developed an injury index based on number of injuries, number of participants, hours of participation, and length of the athletic season. The injury indices for the most common organized sports were as follows: football, 1.72; basketball, 0.88; gymnastics, 0.85; soccer, 0.29; baseball, 0.14; and swimming, 0. Chambers also found that over the same period, twice as many injuries occurred during unsupervised recreational activities such as tree climbing, running on the school ground, and skateboarding than during organized activities.[12] He recommended that organized soccer and swimming be promoted because of their inherent safety, relative to football and basketball.

SPECIFIC SPORTS AND RECREATIONAL ACTIVITIES

Water Sports

The most serious types of injury resulting from participation in water sports are drowning and hypothermia from immersion, spinal injuries from diving into shallow water, and decompression sickness from scuba diving. Three fourths of all recreational spinal cord injuries occur during swimming. The important predisposing factors are age, exposure, and alcohol use.

In 1983, 2470 children and adolescents up to 19 years of age drowned in the United States. Drowning is the third leading cause of unintentional death from injury in children younger than 5 years of age and the second in children 5 to 10 years of age.[66]

A study by Wintemute and colleagues of drownings in residential swimming pools in Sacramento County between 1974 and 1984 in children from birth to 19 years of age showed that the highest rates occurred among children between 1 and 3 years of age, with another smaller peak occurring in children between 15 and 19 years of age.[66] The latter peak was associated with the use of alcohol in 38% of cases. One third of all drownings in Sacramento County occurred in residential pools. There were 137 drownings among Sacramento County residents over the 10-year study period; however, 36 of these actually occurred in other counties. All were fresh-water drownings; 95% were unintentional, 4% were undetermined, and 1% were homicidal. The average annual rate was five per 10,000 individuals, compared to three per 10,000 individuals for the United States as a whole. The rate was eight per 10,000 boys and two per 10,000 girls. For white children, the rate was five per 10,000, and for black children it was nine per 10,000. One third of all drownings and 58% of drownings in the 0- to 4-year-old age group occurred in residential swimming pools. One half of the drownings occurred at the child's own house or apartment; one third occurred at the residence of a friend, neighbor, or relative (Table 37–2).

None of the victims was recorded as wearing a personal flotation device. In the discussion of their paper, Wintemute and associates stated that child drowning rates in pools were much lower when fencing is required.[66] Pool fencing is required around the property in Sacramento County; however, this practice does not exclude persons already on the premises, in particular, toddlers in the family. They also noted that cardiopulmonary resuscitation (CPR) often started only after emergency personnel arrived. It is quite striking that the drowning rate in public pools, which presumably are staffed by personnel skilled in cardiopulmonary resuscitation is extremely low (see Table 37–2).

Soccer

Soccer is the most popular team sport around the world and one of the safest. According to Pritchett, the frequency of injury and medical cost per player in soccer are 20% and 16%, respectively, of these rates in football.[52] The most significant type of injury is internal derangement of the knee. Nilsson and Roass reported injury rates ranging from 3.6 per 1000 hours of soccer playing for adults, to 13 per 1000 hours for adolescent boys, and to 32 per 1000 hours for adolescent girls.[45] Lingard and colleagues reported only

Table 37–2
Location of Drownings

Location	Number
Residential	57
Swimming pool	49
Bath or shower	9
Other	6
Nonresidential	80
Major river	38
Other river or lake	39
Public pool	3

Adapted from Wintemute GJ, Kraus JF, Teret SP, Wright M: Drowning in childhood and adolescence: A population-based study. Am J Public Health 77(7):830–832, 1987.

one treated injury per 1000 players per week during one soccer season in New Zealand.[38]

Rugby

Rugby has much higher injury rates than soccer. Waller has noted that the literature on rugby reflects a lack of concern for prevention among those associated with the sport.[63] Rugby injuries include lacerations, fractures, concussions, joint dislocations, and soft tissue injuries. Dental injuries are also quite significant. An interesting study from New Zealand proved that mouth guards fitted by dentists could reduce the risk of tooth fracture fourfold.[42] Mouth guards should be considered essential equipment for rugby players.

Football

In contrast to rugby, great efforts have been made to prevent injuries in football. Perhaps as a result, the injury rate per participant has fallen over time and is lower in football than in rugby. The CPSC reports that there are approximately five injuries per game, 0.5 injuries per player per season, and 18 deaths per year due to football injuries. An additional 10 deaths result indirectly from heat exhaustion or heart failure. The CPSC also reports that approximately 300,000 football injuries are treated each year in emergency departments in the United States.[60, 61]

A study conducted in North Carolina by Blyth and Mueller, based on sound epidemiologic principles, covered 43 randomly chosen schools with more than 8700 players during the period from 1968 to 1972.[8] The researchers concluded the following:

1. The injury rate was 0.49 per player per season.
2. More than 95% of injuries resulted in loss of participation for more than 1 day and 35% for more than 7 days.
3. The most frequent cause of injury was a blow from an object, usually a helmet or a shoe. The next most frequent causes were collision with another player, twisting, and collision with an object.
4. The concussion rate varied with helmet make and model.
5. The injury rate could be decreased by limiting contact during training practices.

The NEISS data show that football is the most hazardous organized competitive sport in the United States. For children between 5 and 14 years of age, the injury rate for football is higher than that for baseball and basketball combined.[36] Mueller and Blyth, in a study of fatalities from head and cervical spine injuries in tackle football from 1945 to 1984, reported 433 deaths due to head injuries (most commonly subdural hematomas), 111 deaths due to cervical spine injuries (mostly in high school athletes), and 99 deaths due to other injuries.[44] Most of the players who died were injured while tackling or being tackled. During the period from 1965 to 1974, initial contact during blocking or tackling was usually with the head. The frequency of head and cervical spine injuries rose sharply during this period, peaking in 1968, when there were 36 deaths. In

1976, a rule change made it illegal to butt block, face tackle, or spear. In 1978, a new standard for football helmets was adopted. Since 1969, the National Collegiate Athletic Association has adopted 51 rule changes designed to prevent injuries. Blyth and Arnold reported that the death rate from head and neck injuries in football decreased from 3.4 per 100,000 participants to 0.5 per 100,000 participants during the decade from 1968 to 1978.[7]

As a result of these rule changes, the number of deaths from head and cervical spine injuries in football decreased dramatically during the period from 1978 to 1984. The safest way to make contact in football is with the head up. This practice must be reinforced by proper coaching.

A study by Thompson and associates, based on a literature survey of high school football injuries, suggests the need for a better reporting system.[59] This report identified six significant problems with the literature on football injuries:

1. There is no uniform definition of injury.
2. Injury severity is not clearly defined.
3. Selection criteria vary.
4. There are no uniform methods of data collection.
5. Measuring exposure to injury risk presents difficulties.
6. Control groups for comparisons are lacking.

Albright and colleagues carried out a prospective study of head and neck injuries in college football at one university during the period from 1975 to 1982, when the major rule changes noted previously were made to reduce head and neck injuries.[2] These changes included the banning of blocking and tackling with the helmet or face mask and allowing more liberal use of the hands and arms for blocking. Although the authors documented a decreased injury rate over the study period, they noted a disturbing tendency for repeated neck injuries in individual players. They identified the following factors as important in determining the risk of head and neck injuries:

1. Rules regarding blocking and tackling
2. The amount of contact during practices
3. Coaching that determined the frequency of passing versus running plays and instruction in correct blocking and tackling practices
4. Better communication between coaches and medical staff

Basketball

Severe injuries in basketball are relatively rare. The rate is lower than the rates for football, baseball, wrestling, track and field, and gymnastics, but greater than those for volleyball, swimming, field hockey, golf, tennis, badminton, and cross-country running. Most injuries that occur in basketball are sprains.

Boxing

The goal of boxing is to injure the opponent, primarily through concussion, presumably without permanent dam-

age. The most common injuries are facial contusions and lacerations. In some cases, however, the cumulative effect of repeated injury causes profound neurologic deterioration. A good case could be made for eliminating it from all high school and college programs.

Ice Hockey

Ice hockey has gained tremendous popularity in the United States. Although injuries are frequent, great strides have been made in preventing at least some of them. For example, severe injuries to the eyes caused by stick or puck, which were once common, have been reduced by the compulsory use of helmets and face masks in most amateur leagues.

A report by Tator indicated that in ice hockey, cervical spine and spinal cord injuries, most commonly at the C5 level, seem to be increasing in frequency.[57] Most of these injuries occur during organized games as a result of axial loading from a blow to the head, usually when the player falls head first into the boards with the neck slightly flexed. Half of ice hockey neck injuries are associated with spinal cord injuries, most of which are complete. Tator reports at least four cases per year of quadriplegia in hockey players in Canada. He identified the following as the main factors contributing to injury:

1. An increase over time in the size of players and speed of play
2. Pushing or checking an opposing player from behind
3. Helmets that are designed to reduce impact to the head but that may increase strain on the cervical spine
4. Risk factors, particularly the boards

Tator suggested rule changes to reduce the occurrence of checking from behind and emphasis on conditioning of the neck muscles to strengthen the neck, thereby reducing the risk of neck injury.

Eye injuries in hockey have long been a source of great concern. Pashby reported that 238 eyes had been blinded in Canada in amateur hockey over an 18-year period.[50] Fortunately, no player lost both eyes. Hockey was the source of 37% of sports eye injuries in Canada and 56% of blinding injuries. In the winter of 1974 to 1975, there were 257 injuries and 43 blindings. Between 1986 and 1987, after eye protection had become mandatory throughout amateur hockey, there were only 93 injuries and 18 blindings. None of these blindings occurred in players under 18 years of age. No severe eye injury has been recorded in a player wearing a Canadian Standard Association–approved face protector. Sixty percent of blinding injuries were caused by sticks and 40% by pucks (see Eye Injuries).

Goodwin and associates carried out an epidemiologic study of high school hockey injuries in Minnesota during the 1982–1983 season.[21] They found that the injury rate among 12 varsity hockey teams was 75 per 100 players, and that 41% of the players suffered at least one injury. They estimated that there were 5 injuries per 1000 playing hours. Head and neck injuries accounted for 22% of the total, and concussions accounted for 12%. Nine percent of the players suffered a concussion.

Hastings and colleagues studied hockey injuries in Ontario before the introduction of face masks in 1974.[27] They found that lacerations, contusions, and fractures accounted for more than 70% of all hockey injuries and that the hockey stick was a factor in 41% of injuries. They suggested enforcement of high-sticking rules, the adoption of better shock-absorbing boards, and improved eye protection. Most players in amateur leagues are now required to wear face protectors, but older players and children involved in pick-up hockey may not comply.

Motorcycling and Use of All-Terrain Vehicles and Other Off-Road Vehicles

The family of powered cycles includes minibikes, minicycles, trail bikes, mopeds, motorcycles, and—most recently—all-terrain vehicles (ATVs), introduced to the North American market in 1971. These various motorized vehicles have been defined by Greensher.[22] Minibikes are built on bicycle-style frames, weigh less than 100 lb, have less than 4–horsepower motors, and can travel only at speeds less than 30 miles per hour (mph). Minicycles are miniature motorcycles. Trail bikes are larger than minicycles. Many severe injuries result from illegal use of trail bikes on roads and highways. The American Academy of Pediatrics discourages the use of trail bikes by children younger than 14 years of age. Mopeds are intended for street use and are in effect bicycles with motors. The motor is usually less than 50-cc displacement, and the vehicle is capable of speeds up to about 30 mph. The fact that mopeds are unable to accelerate quickly can make them dangerous to use on busy streets. Motorcycles have been in wide use for many years. In 1985, there were 490,000 injuries and 4500 deaths in the United States among motorcycle riders. A nonhelmeted rider has a five times greater likelihood of receiving a severe or critical head injury. Despite these statistics, some states have recently repealed compulsory helmet laws.

The ATVs are three- and four-wheeled vehicles intended for off-road use and capable of speeds up to 50 mph. In 1985, sales of 780,000 ATVs took place in the United States, and the number of ATVs in use was estimated at 2.5 million. ATVs have large, soft tires, a relatively high center of gravity, and very poor suspension. The three-wheeled types are especially unstable. Most severe injuries in ATV riders result from the loss of operator control. About 40% of ATV deaths in the United States have occurred in children under 16 years of age. In 1986, the CPSC data revealed 86,000 injuries and a cumulative death toll of 696 in ATV riders.[41] The American Academy of Pediatrics' 1987 report included the following information.[3] Since 1982, there were nearly 1000 ATV fatalities in the United States and nearly 300,000 injuries. Approximately half of the fatalities occurred in children younger than 16 years of age and one fourth in children younger than 12 years of age. The Academy urged the federal government to recall ATVs and ban their use. As of December 1987, sales of three-wheeled ATVs had been halted in both the United States and Canada. The American Trauma Society Traumagram identified the following important factors in ATV injuries[51]:

1. Vehicle design
2. Environmental hazards (e.g., trees, fences)
3. Driver factors (e.g., experience, protective equipment, alcohol use)

A 1986 CPSC report included results of public hearings held in several places in the United States.[41] The major findings were the following:

1. Children younger than 12 years of age are unable to operate any size ATV safely.
2. Children younger than 16 years of age are at greater risk of injury and death than adults when operating an adult-sized ATV, owing to poor judgment and failure to operate ATVs within their skill levels.
3. The risk of injury declines with experience.
4. Thirty percent of all fatal ATV accidents were associated with alcohol use.
5. Well-constructed, well-fitted helmets could substantially reduce the number of fatal head injuries in ATV riders.
6. Of three-wheeled ATV accidents, 74% involved tipping or overturning, compared with 59% of four-wheeled ATV accidents.
7. The dynamic stability of four-wheeled ATVs is better than that of three-wheeled ATVs.
8. The handling performance of an ATV is strongly influenced by its suspension system; a properly tuned mechanical suspension for front and rear wheels is better than front-only or tire-only suspended ATVs.

The CPSC task force recommended that the ATV industry should do the following[41]:

1. Cease marketing ATVs intended for use by children younger than 12 years of age
2. Attach warning labels to ATVs intended for use by children younger than 14 years of age, stating that these ATVs are not recommended for use by children younger than 12 years of age
3. Attach a warning label to adult-sized ATVs, stating that they are not recommended for use by children younger than 16 years of age

Pyper and Black reported on orthopedic injuries suffered by children in connection with the use of off-road vehicles in Manitoba from April 1979 to August 1986.[53] There were 233 children in the study: 190 boys and 43 girls ranging in age from 2 to 17 years. Ninety-three of these children were injured riding minibikes or dirtbikes, 72 while riding snowmobiles, 59 while riding three-wheeled ATVs, and nine while riding four-wheeled ATVs. These researchers found that most injuries were caused by loss of control of the vehicle by the operator. There were 352 fractures, 52 major soft tissue injuries, and 186 associated injuries. During the same period, Manitoba had 21 fatal accidents. Haynes and colleagues, in a study of injuries associated with three-wheeled ATVs, concluded that these vehicles were unstable and inherently dangerous.[28] They reported that in 1984 there were 66,956 injuries in the United States associated with ATVs, in contrast to only 33,636 injuries associated with minibikes and 8076 injuries associated with snowmobiles. They recommended that ATV use be restricted to persons older than 16 years of age, that ATV operators be required to wear helmets, and that speed limits be established for ATVs.

The Accident Prevention Committee of the Canadian Paediatric Society has recommended the following[1]:

1. ATVs should be banned for children younger than 14 years of age.
2. There should be compulsory licensing and insurance for all ATVs.
3. Helmet use should be made mandatory.
4. Riding double should not be allowed.

Bicycling

Bicycles top the list of hazardous products, according to the CPSC. It reported that in 1985, there were 108 million pedal cycles in the United States and that the death rate from accidents among adolescents and young adults is rising. The NEISS estimates that up to 1 million bicycle-related injuries occur per year in the United States. Loss of control by the rider is involved in more than 60% of bicycle injuries and violations of traffic rules by the rider in more than 80%.[22] Although head injuries are associated with 75% of bicycle-related deaths, helmet use is still quite low. There have been efforts to establish standards for bicycle helmets. There are two standards, one of the American National Standards Institute, the other of the Snell Memorial Foundation. Bicycle helmets should be required for all children and adolescents.

Skateboarding

Skateboards have risen in popularity throughout North America. *Time* magazine documented three phases in the history of skateboards, beginning with becalmed surfers looking for a replacement through the teen fad and ending with the widespread use of skateboards.[13] More than 20 million skateboards are estimated to be in use in the United States. The sale of skateboard equipment and clothes is a $500-million-a-year business.

Most skateboard injuries involve boys 10 to 14 years of age. The commonest injuries are cuts, abrasions, and fractures, particularly to the forearm.[22] Skateboarders with little experience seem to be at greater risk of injury. The CPSC has made the following recommendations[41]:

1. Never ride in the street.
2. Do not take chances; complicated tricks require careful practice.
3. Only one person per skateboard.
4. Never hitch a ride from a car.
5. Learn how to fall safely.

Greensher and Mofenson have also advised on the use of protective equipment, including helmets, gloves, and elbow and knee pads.[23] These investigators suggest that skate-

boards be prohibited on public streets and recommend that riders stick to clean, smooth surfaces such as those found at skateboard parks.

Playground Equipment

The 1978 NEISS report projected 155,000 playground injuries in the United States, equally divided between home and public playgrounds. Ninety-three percent happened to children younger than 15 years of age. The most common injurious event was a fall. In a review of playground injuries, Fisher and colleagues reported on a pilot Child Playground Injury Prevention Project in New York State.[17] The project began with workshops designed for the general public and those responsible for the purchase, installation, maintenance, and supervision of public playgrounds. These researchers documented improvements in knowledge of playground design and a 22% reduction in injuries at one site.

A study from Australia by Oliver and associates documented a significant playground injury rate in that country as well.[47] These investigators reported that each year, 1% of children between the ages of 2 and 12 years in North Sydney suffered playground injuries requiring hospitalization. Of these injuries, 31% occurred on climbing bars, 26% on swings, 13% on slides, and 11% on trampolines. Body contact with the hard ground was the single, most important direct cause of injury. In their study, one fourth of the injuries were fractures, and one fourth were lacerations. They recommended the following preventive measures to reduce injuries on playground equipment:

1. Ground surfaces should be covered with rubber mats and all exposed concrete eliminated.
2. Swings should have soft rubber seats.
3. Slides should have extended exit chutes.
4. Playground layout should spread out the equipment to remove swings from the direct path between other pieces of equipment.
5. Fences should be installed to prevent preschoolers from wandering off the playground.

Another study by Nixon and colleagues in Brisbane, Australia from 1976 to 1980 concluded that playgrounds were quite safe.[46] Over this 5-year period, Brisbane, with a population of approximately 266,000 children, had no deaths in its playgrounds. The study concluded that although injuries may be frequent, they usually are trivial.

Werner reported on playground injuries and voluntary product standards for home and public playgrounds.[65] He reported that in the United States in 1977, more than 155,000 injuries occurred; swings accounted for most of these, and one half of the injuries were to the head, neck, and face. A CPSC booklet directed at dangers to children aged 3 to 5 years placed playgrounds sixth on the list of hazardous consumer products.[41] The booklet recommends that adults tell children to sit in the center of the swing and never to stand or kneel on the seat, to hold on with both hands, to stop the swing before getting off, and to avoid walking too close to the front or back of the swing. It also recommends that children never push anyone else on a swing and not double up. Children should be instructed to hold on with both hands as they go up the steps of a slide, taking one step at a time; never to try to climb up the sliding surface or the frame; always slide down feet first in a sitting position; and leave the bottom of the slide quickly after their turn. For a climbing apparatus, the CPSC recommended that children be advised to use both hands, to be careful climbing down, and to watch out for other children climbing up.

Baby Walkers

Baby walkers of various designs have been used in the Western world for several centuries, but until recently, only rarely and only by the affluent.[16, 20] These devices have now become so common that it has been estimated that 1 million were marketed in the United States in 1980, and that 55 to 86% of infants in the United States and Canada are placed in walkers before they learn to walk unassisted.[34, 55] The increased use of baby walkers has been accompanied by an increase in reports of injuries associated with them.[16, 20, 29, 31, 35, 39, 54, 55, 61, 64]

Injuries associated with baby walker use follow several well-defined patterns, which can be appreciated by understanding how walkers are used. The most common design in current use is a plastic seat suspended from a plastic platform supported on a steel frame by folding or collapsing metal bars. These rest on a plastic base supported on pivoting wheels with low-friction bearings (Fig. 37–1). The infant is placed in the plastic seat.

Parents put their infants in baby walkers for various reasons; the commonest is to entertain the child by enhancing mobility.[54, 55] An infant of 6 to 8 months, capable of maintaining his or her torso in an erect posture but not of walking unaided, is able to move both easily and quickly in a baby walker, especially on the tiled floors common in contemporary kitchens. Baby walkers are also used as a passive babysitter and as a means to accelerate infants' independent ambulation.[54, 55] This notion has no basis in developmental theory; indeed, in a small but elegant study, Kauffman and Ridenour have demonstrated that infants placed in walkers before they learn to walk unassisted achieve independent ambulation at the same time as those not placed in walkers.[34] Indeed, their results and the observations of Holm and colleagues suggest that infants with neurodevelopmental handicaps such as cerebral palsy suffer deleterious developmental effects if they are placed in a baby walker because of the reinforcement of undesirable reflexes.[32, 34]

Walker injuries are among the commonest injuries in infancy. Studies of private pediatric practices and retrospective reviews of hospital charts indicate that the most frequent injuries have been finger entrapments, dental injuries, abrasions, lacerations, closed head injuries, skull fractures, and hematomas.[16, 31, 35, 39, 55, 61, 64] Most injuries are self-limiting and are treated at home and include minor finger entanglements and abrasions, often due to falls from the walker, collapsing of the walker, or the infant reaching previously inaccessible objects such as door hinges. However, the injuries produced by baby walkers that are most

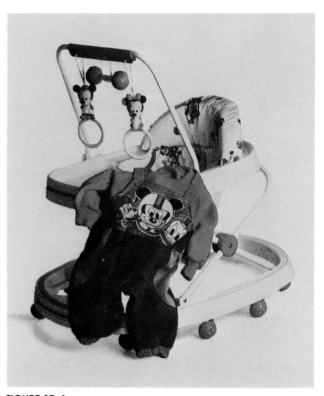

FIGURE 37–1

Commonly used infant walker. Note the plastic base supported on the pivoting wheels with low-friction bearings.

germane to the physician providing acute trauma care are those treated in emergency departments. In these cases, the commonest injury patterns and mechanisms of injury differ from those that occur frequently at home.[20, 54]

Common walker injuries seen in emergency departments are those caused by falls, especially down stairs (Fig. 37–2). Closed head injuries without serious central nervous system involvement are the most common (89%) followed by skull fractures (15%).[54] The latter are typically linear skull fractures that can be managed conservatively; however, depressed and compound skull fractures also occur. The remaining injuries include abrasions and clavicular and forearm fractures.[54] Other walker injuries seen in emergency departments include abrasions and minor closed head injuries sustained in falls through and from baby walkers and finger entrapments.[54, 55] An additional rare but serious injury associated with the use of baby walkers is a burn sustained when infants reach surfaces that are normally inaccessible and pull hot liquids such as tea or coffee on themselves.[39, 54]

Follow-up studies show that up to 65% of infants injured in walkers are placed back in their walkers, even after an injury as serious as a fracture.[54] The parents of infants who have sustained walker injuries should be advised that walker use should be discontinued; this caution may need to be reinforced by the primary care physician. The prevention of baby walker injuries is best accomplished by having the infant's primary caregiver advise parents on the serious risks and limited benefits of walker use. Baby walkers perform no function that cannot be more safely performed by an approved playpen.

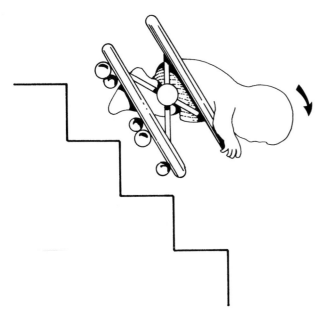

FIGURE 37-2

Depicts infant and walker falling down the stairs. The infant's arms are outstretched, and the head, because of its large size in terms of surface area and relationship to other body parts, is leading the way. Hence, closed-head injuries with frequent skull fractures are common walker-related injuries.

Toy Injuries

Although the value of toys and play in child development has long been recognized, the hazards associated with toys have been less well appreciated. The toy retailing and manufacturing industry is a major sector of the economy; on average, Canadians and Americans spend $150 per child each year for toys. Hasbro, the world's largest toy manufacturer, has had yearly sales figures of $1.2 billion. Total retail toy sales in the United States alone are estimated at $9 billion.[23] Careful appraisal of the durability and suitability of toys is now commonplace.[11]

Toy injuries happen more often than might be expected; in 1983, 594,000 children were treated in hospital emergency departments in the United States for toy-related injuries.[40, 41] Most of these injuries involved bicycles, skates, and skateboards, toys that accounted for most of the 16 fatalities. However, 118,000 injuries resulted from play with other toys. Falling or tripping over toys and being struck by toys were the most common causes of toy-related injury, and choking from ingestion or aspiration of small toys or small parts of toys was the next most frequent source of injury.[40]

Although most toy-related injuries are minor, several points deserve detailed comment. Use of toys by children too young to play with them safely or with parts too small for safe use is a major contributor to toy-related accidents in young children.[23] Developmental levels must be considered when parents purchase toys for their children; a plastic spacecraft with removable rockets and opening doors may be a stimulating toy for a 5-year-old child but a very dangerous one for an 18-month-old child. Strangulation on cords or strings is a potentially fatal event among toddlers and infants; toys for children in this age group must have no loose strings or dangling straps, especially those intended for use in cribs or playpens.[5]

Aspiration of toy parts and choking on ingested toys are major concerns in toddlers and infants. Aspiration was responsible for almost 200 deaths in children younger than 5 years of age in 1982, and several hundred children are estimated to have nonfatal aspirations for every child who dies.[19] Consideration of the developmental issues mentioned previously is important in the prevention of these injuries. The incorporation of small quantities of barium sulfate, a radiopaque substance, into the plastic used to make toys has been shown to be helpful in the diagnosis and management of toy aspirations or ingestions.[19] Adoption of this plastic for toy construction by such major companies such as Mattel Incorporated has been very useful in making the critical differentiation between aspirations and ingestions of small toy parts.[23]

Toy weapons present a major concern for three reasons. Powder firearms such as cap guns have been associated with burns and flash injuries.[56] Toy weapons such as air rifles, BB guns, or bows and arrows that can fire projectiles cause a large number of facial and ocular injuries; of the estimated 818 injuries caused by toy guns in 1980 and 1981, 2.9% required admission to hospital; during the same period, 6.5% of these injuries caused by toy bows and arrows required hospital admission.[56] Eye injuries have included traumatic cataracts, retinal detachment, and sympathetic ophthalmitis, which may be so severe as to require enucleation.[4] BB and pellet guns may have a muzzle velocity of 870 feet per second.[26] Serious abdominal injuries, including perforation of the stomach, jejunum, liver, and pancreas, have been caused by BB and pellet guns.[26] Toys of this nature should be treated with the care that all weapons demand, and only used by older children under close supervision.[4] Children who play with toy guns have on occasion seriously injured themselves or others by mistaking real guns for toys.[4]

The most effective way to reduce the ill effects of these types of injuries is to prevent them. It is unrealistic to expect a ban on the sale or distribution of toy firearms; however, the Committee on Accident and Poison and Prevention of the American Academy of Pediatrics has called for the reduction of muzzle velocity in these toy weapons, regulation of the sale and distribution of air rifles in a fashion similar to that used for firearms, and counseling of parents by pediatricians and primary care physicians on the dangers of having toy firearms in the home.[4]

A little-appreciated hazard associated with toys is hearing loss; commonly used toys such as infant squeaky toys and friction-operated vehicles produce sound levels of up to 100 decibels at a 10-cm distance.[6] Toy firearms such as cap pistols can produce sounds as loud as 150 decibels at 50-cm distances, which exceeds the internationally suggested upper limit of 130 decibels.[6] Sensitivity to loud sounds has been suggested to be greater in children than in adults; these toys may be associated with noise-induced hearing loss.[6]

Toys have also been associated with the transmission of infections; for example, some of them have been shown to be fomites for viruses such as cytomegalovirus.[33]

SPECIFIC TYPES OF INJURIES

Eye Injuries

Pashby reported that ice hockey accounted for more eye injuries and blindings than any other sport. Racquet sports were the second most common cause.[49] Easterbrook, commenting on current methods of eye protection in racquet sports, noted that a squash ball has more kinetic energy than a 0.22-caliber bullet and thus presents a serious danger to the eye.[15] He described eye guards approved by the American Society for Testing and Materials and the Canadian Standards Association and warned against the use of lenseless eye guards, which may be ineffective. Approved models can protect the eye from a squash ball traveling at 90 mph. Polycarbonate lenses are better than plastic lenses, which are less impact resistant, generally thicker, and more easily scratched.

In his report on the prevention of eye injuries in general, Pashby documented a rise in the average age of hockey players with eye injuries from 14 years in 1972 to 26 years in 1981, when mandatory face protectors were introduced into children's leagues.[48] The percentage of eye injuries due to hockey treated at the Hospital for Sick Children in Toronto dropped from 52% in 1973 to 13% in 1978, following the introduction of mandatory eye protectors. Pashby also stated that, "in my view, one-eyed athletes should not play contact sports."[48] In a report from the United States, Vigner estimated that each year, American children suffer more than 100,000 sports-related eye injuries.[62] He added that although there has been much emphasis on hockey and racquet sports, baseball now accounts for most sports-related eye injuries in the United States.

Grin and colleagues conducted a 3-year survey of all children younger than 15 years old admitted to the Wills Eye Hospital in Philadelphia during the period 1983 to 1985.[24] Sports injuries were the most common cause of eye damage, accounting for 45 of the 278 cases. Baseball was involved in 10 cases, tennis in 10, soccer in 7, basketball in 4, hockey in 3, football in 3, and other activities in 8.

Head and Spinal Cord Injuries

Tator and associates reported that sports and recreational activities are an increasing cause of spinal cord injuries in North America, both in absolute and relative terms.[58] They reported 141 cases at two Toronto hospitals during the period 1948 to 1983. Diving accounted for 59% of these injuries. Of these spinal cord injuries, 87% occurred in boys and 38% occurred in the age group from 11 to 20 years. Eighty percent of these injuries were at the cervical level, 8% at the thoracic level, 11% at the thoracolumbar level, and 1% at the lumbosacral level. More than 50% of these spinal cord injuries resulted in the complete loss of motor and sensory function.

Another study of brain and cervical spine injuries incurred by children and adolescents during organized sports revealed that the frequency was quite low compared to injuries incurred in motor vehicle accidents and falls, especially for children under 12 years of age.[10] One half of all spinal injuries and almost all serious injuries occur in contact sports such as football, rugby, and wrestling. Unorganized sports also account for a significant proportion of spinal cord injuries, especially cervical spine injuries in swimming and diving. These investigators reported that diving was responsible for 3 to 18% of all cervical spine injuries in young people. Central nervous system injuries are the cause of the majority of deaths in sports and recreational activities, whereas cervical spine injuries cause most long-term morbidity. The authors stress that spearing in football (i.e., blocking and tackling with the head) can lead to severe axial loading and hyperflexion. Rugby seems to be a significant cause of head and cervical spine injury in Britain, South Africa, and New Zealand. In contrast, soccer has a much lower frequency of head and cervical spine injury. In fact, soccer is the safest of all contact sports for children and probably should be promoted more vigorously in North America. Wrestling has the second highest head and cervical spine injury rate for sports injuries in the United States, whereas baseball has a very low frequency of central nervous system injury.

Hill and colleagues reported on all pediatric neck injuries treated at Columbus Children's Hospital from 1969 to 1979.[30] Among 122 patients, there were 48 strains, 74 injuries to the spinal column, and 27 neurologic deficits. Of the severe cases, diving accounted for 23%, football accounted for 5%, and gymnastics accounted for 7%. These injuries tended to occur at the higher C1 to C3 levels in children younger than 8 years of age.

PREVENTION OF SPORTS AND RECREATION INJURIES

Although important gains have been made in the last few years, everyone must continue to strive to reduce both the frequency and severity of injuries associated with sports and recreational activities. Waller has identified several basic factors in the prevention of sports and recreation injuries[63]:

1. Review of past experience through data registries such as NEISS.
2. Institution of rules governing play.
3. Adoption of standards for health status of participants (e.g., age, size, conditioning).
4. Use of safety equipment.
5. Adoption of standards for the recreational environment.

This conceptual framework provides a useful approach to injury prevention in this field.

In general, children must compete within their own age and developmental or weight category. Appropriate protective equipment must be worn, and rules must be strictly enforced, especially when they are designed to minimize injury.

Notable advances have been made in recent years, for example, the adoption of safety lenses for racquet sports; protective helmets and face masks for amateur hockey players, and changes in the rules for blocking and tackling in high school and college football. All of these measures have led to significant reductions in injury rates and in morbidity and mortality.

The following is a list of recommendations to reduce sports and recreation injuries in children:

1. Promote safe activities such as supervised swimming and soccer, and deemphasize more dangerous ones such as tackle football.

2. Require the use of protective equipment, especially in contact sports. This includes helmets in football, cycling, and hockey; eye and face protectors in football, hockey, and racquet sports; padding in football, hockey, and skateboarding; and mouth guards in rugby.

3. Enforce rules designed to reduce injuries, such as those banning butt blocking and tackling in football and high-sticking, board-checking, and checking from behind in hockey.

4. Instruct football players in safe blocking and tackling techniques, and minimize body contact during practices.

5. Require fences around residential swimming pools, instruct pool owners in cardiopulmonary resuscitation, and warn adolescents about the dangers of alcohol consumption during water activities.

6. Require all children and adolescents to wear bicycle helmets.

7. Ban the use of baby walkers.

8. Prevent infants and small children from using small toys and toys with small parts that could be aspirated.

9. Ban ATV use by children younger than 14 years of age; and require helmet use by all ATV riders.

10. Provide designated skateboard facilities, and discourage their use on public roads and sidewalks.

11. Provide safe playgrounds for children of all ages.

ROLE OF THE CLINICIAN

The role of the clinician in sports and recreation injuries is threefold. The first is to provide medical care for injured participants. Equally important is to identify hazards and to make them known through the medical literature, government agencies, and the media. Finally, the clinician should counsel children and their parents about the hazards of sports and recreation activities to attempt to prevent them from occurring.

References

1. Accident Prevention Committee, Canadian Paediatric Society: Two-, three- and four-wheel unlicensed off-road vehicles. Can Med Assoc J 136:119–120, 1987.
2. Albright JP, McAuley E, Martin RK, et al: Head and neck injuries in college football: An eight-year analysis. Am J Sports Med 13:147–152, 1985.
3. American Academy of Pediatrics Annual Report. Elk Grove Village, Ill, American Academy of Pediatrics, 1987.
4. American Academy of Pediatrics, Committee on Accident and Poison Prevention: Injuries related to "toy" firearms. Pediatrics 79:473–474, 1987.
5. Anonymous: Crib toys caused two infant deaths. Can Fam Phys 32:2585, 1986.
6. Axelsson A, Jerson T: Noisy toys: A possible source of sensorineural hearing loss. Pediatrics 76:574–578, 1985.
7. Blyth CS, Arnold C: The forty-seventh annual survey of football fatalities, 1931–1978. Orlando, Fla, The American Football Coaches Association, 1978, pp 1–17.
8. Blyth CS, Mueller FO: An epidemiologic study of high school football injuries in North Carolina. Chapel Hill, North Carolina, Department of Physical Education, University of North Carolina, 1974.
9. Boyce WT, Sprunger LW, Sobolewski S, Schaefer C: Epidemiology of injuries in a large, urban school district. Pediatrics 74:342–349, 1984.
10. Bruce DA, Schut L, Sutton LN: Brain and cervical spine injuries occurring during organized sports activities in children and adolescents. Clin Sports Med 1:495–514, 1982.
11. Canadian Toy Testing Council: Toy Report 1988. Transmag, Ottawa, 1987.
12. Chambers RB: Orthopaedic injuries in athletes (ages 6 to 17). Am J Sports Med 7:195–197, 1979.
13. Cocks J: The irresistible lure of grabbing air. Time Magazine, June 6:74–75, 1988.
14. Damron CF: Injury surveillance systems for sports. In: Vinger PF, Haerner EF (eds): Sports Injuries. Littleton, Mass, PSG Publishing, 1981, pp 2–25.
15. Easterbrook M: Eye protection in racket sports: An update. Phys Sports Med 15:180–192, 1987.
16. Fazen LE III, Felizberto PI: Baby walker injuries. Pediatrics 70:106–109, 1982.
17. Fisher L, Harris VG, VanBuren J, et al: Assessment of a pilot child playground injury prevention project in New York State. Am J Public Health 70:1000–1002, 1980.
18. Garrick JG, Requa RK: Injuries in high school sports. Pediatrics 61:465–469, 1978.
19. Glasbrenner K: Giving visibility to accidentally swallowed toys (news). JAMA 252:323–324, 1984.
20. Gleadhill DNS, Robson WJ, Cudmore RE, Turnock RR. Baby walkers . . . time to take a stand. Arch Dis Child 62:491–494, 1987.
21. Goodwin GS, Luhmanns S, Finke C, et al: Analysis of severe injuries associated with volleyball activities. Physicians Sport Med 15:75–79, 1987.
22. Greensher J: Non-automotive vehicle injuries in adolescents. Pediatr Ann 17:111–137, 1988.
23. Greensher J, Mofenson HC: Injuries at play. Pediatr Clin North Am 32:127–139, 1985.
24. Grin TR, Nelson LB, Jeffers JB: Eye injuries in childhood. Pediatrics 80:13–17, 1987.
25. Haffey H: The Hospital for Sick Children's injury report. Toronto, Canada, Hospital for Sick Children, 1983.
26. Harris W, Luterman A, Curreri PW: BB and pellet guns—toys or deadly weapons. J Trauma 23:566–569, 1983.
27. Hastings DE, Cameron J, Parker SM, Evans J: A study of hockey injuries in Ontario. Ontario Medical Review 686, 1974.
28. Haynes CD, Stroud SD, Thompson CE: The three wheeler (adult tricycle): An unstable dangerous machine. J Trauma 26:643–648, 1987.
29. Henderson J: Head injuries and baby walkers. Can Med Assoc J 131:1327, 1984.
30. Hill SA, Miller CA, Kosiuk EJ, Hunt MD: Pediatric neck injuries. J Neurosurg 60:700–706, 1984.
31. Hobroyd HJ: Injuries related to baby walkers. Pediatrics 70:147, 1982.
32. Holm V, Harthun-Smith L, Taka W: Infant walkers and cerebral palsy. Am J Dis Child 137:1189–1190, 1983.
33. Hutto C, Little EA, Ricks R, et al: Isolation of cytomegalovirus from toys and hands in a day care center. J Infect Dis 154:527–530, 1986.
34. Kauffman I, Ridenour M: Influence of an infant walker on onset and quality of walking pattern of locomotion. Percept Mot Skills 45:1323–1329, 1977.
35. Kavanagh C, Banco L: The infant walker—a previously unrecognized health hazard. Am J Dis Child 136:205–206, 1982.
36. Kraus JF, Conroy C: Survival after brain injury. Cause of death, length of survival, and prognostic variables in a cohort of brain-injured people. Neuroepidemiology 7:13–22, 1988.
37. Kraus JF, Conroy C: Mortality and morbidity from injuries in sports and recreation. Ann Rev Public Health 5:163–192, 1984.
38. Lingard DA, Sharrock NE, Salmond CE: Risk factors of sports injuries in winter. N Z Med J 83:69–73, 1976.

39. Miller R, Coville J, Hughes NC: Burns to infants using walker aids. Injury 7:8–10, 1975.

40. Morbidity and Mortality Weekly Report: Toy safety—United States, 1983, JAMA 253:187–188, 1985.

41. Morbidity and Mortality Weekly Report: Toy safety—United States, 1984. JAMA 255:312–313, 1986.

42. Morton JG, Burton JF: An evaluation of the effectiveness of mouthguards in high-school rugby players. N Z Dent J 75:151–153, 1974.

43. Mueller F, Blyth C: Epidemiology of sports injuries in children. Clin Sports Med 1:343–352, 1982.

44. Mueller FO, Blyth CS: Fatalities from head and cervical spine injuries occurring in tackle football: 40 years' experience. Clin Sports Med 6:185–196, 1987.

45. Nilsson S, Roass A: Soccer injuries in adolescents. Am J Sports Med 6:358–361, 1978.

46. Nixon J, Pearn J, Wilkey I: Death during play: A study of playground and recreational deaths in children. Br Med J Clin Res 283:6288–6410, 1981.

47. Oliver TI, McFarlane JP, Haigh JC, et al: Playground equipment and accidents. Aust Paediatr J 17:100–103, 1981.

48. Pashby T: Prevention of eye injuries. Can Fam Phys 27:464–469, 1981.

49. Pashby T: Eye protection. Can Fam Phys 32:1491–1496, 1986.

50. Pashby T: Eye injuries in Canadian amateur hockey still a concern. Can J Ophthalmol 22:293–295, 1987.

51. Powers K: ATVs require skill, caution. Traumagram 12:1–3, 1987.

52. Pritchett JW: Cost of high school soccer injuries. Am J Sports Med 9:64–66, 1981.

53. Pyper JA, Black GB: Orthopaedic injuries in children associated with the use of off road vehicles. J Bone Joint Surg [Am] 70:275–284, 1988.

54. Rieder MJ, Schwartz C, Newman J: Patterns of walker use and walker injury. Pediatrics 78:488–493, 1986.

55. Stoffman J, Bass M, Fox AM: Head injuries related to use of baby walkers. Can Med Assoc J 131:573–575, 1984.

56. Tanz R, Christoffel KK, Sagerman S: Are toy guns too dangerous? Pediatrics 75:265–268, 1985.

57. Tator CH: Neck injuries in ice hockey: A recent, unsolved problem with many contributing factors. Clin Sports Med 6:101–114, 1987.

58. Tator CH, Edmonds VE, New ML: Diving: A frequent and potential preventable cause of spinal cord injury. Can Med Assoc J 124:1323–1324, 1981.

59. Thompson N, Halpern B, Curl WW, et al: High school football injuries: Evaluation. Am J Sports Med 15:117–124, 1987.

60. United States Consumer Product Safety Commission 1974 hazard analysis. Football: Activity and related equipment. Bethesda, MD, Bureau of Epidemiology.

61. United States Consumer Product Safety Commission: US consumer products fact sheet, baby walkers. Bethesda, MD, 1979, p 12.

62. Vigner PF: Sports eye injuries: A preventable disease. Ophthalmology 88:108–112, 1981.

63. Waller JA: Recreational activities. In: Waller JA (ed): Injury Control. Lexington, MA, D.C. Health & Co, 1985, pp 361–404.

64. Wellman S, Paulson JA: Baby walker-related injuries. Clin Pediatr 23:98–99, 1984.

65. Werner P: Playground injuries and voluntary product standards for home and public playgrounds. Pediatrics 69:18–20, 1982.

66. Wintemute GJ, Draus JF, Teret AP, Wright M: Drowning in childhood and adolescence: A population-based study. Am J Public Health 77:830–832, 1987.

67. Zaricznyji B, Shattuck LJM, Mast TA, et al: Sports related injuries in school-aged children. Am J Sports Med 8:318–324, 1980.

J. Michael Dean
J. Alex Haller, Jr.

Submersion Injuries

Drowning is a leading cause of death in childhood, and near drowning is associated with significant morbidity.[44, 46, 88, 91, 153, 165, 186, 187] It is unfortunate that although most submersion accidents are preventable, pediatric facilities continue to see victims in emergency departments and intensive care units. In this chapter we describe the epidemiology and pathophysiology of submersion injuries and discuss the clinical presentation and management of these children. The intensive care of these children has achieved some spectacular publicity because of occasional exceptional recoveries from very severe accidents; therefore, we include a detailed discussion of the neurologic aspects and consideration of brain resuscitative therapies for drowning victims.[23–27, 38, 54, 55, 90, 117, 124, 133, 169, 174, 179, 198, 206]

EPIDEMIOLOGY

In the United States approximately 6000 to 8000 people die annually from submersion accidents, and 20 times that number are estimated to drown internationally.[129, 187] The overall incidence of drowning has been estimated as 5.6 drownings per 100,000 population. Drowning is the second leading cause of death for all individuals under 45 years of age, and a large number of these victims are children.[72, 98] There is a male predominance, particularly among teenagers and adults.

In large surveys, swimming pools account for only 13% of the incidents, whereas lakes, ponds, and rivers account for nearly half the deaths. Of the swimming pool accidents, nearly half occur in privately owned pools.[7, 68] Interestingly, nearly a quarter of the deaths occurred while the victim was swimming, with exhaustion as the proximate cause of the accident. The typical drowning victim is found within 30 minutes of the incident, and in more than half of the cases no resuscitation is even attempted. On a global basis, 60% of drowning incidents occur in the summer months (in the Northern Hemisphere; the opposite pattern is seen in Australia), and incidents are clustered on weekends[188] (Fig. 38–

1). Despite the mild weather seen in southern California, a distinct seasonal pattern remains evident (Fig. 38–2), which would suggest that drowning incidents occur while children are playing outdoors without adequate supervision. The problem is not straightforward, however, as the pattern in Salt Lake City (Fig. 38–3) is almost identical, despite markedly different weather patterns. Although the incidence might relate to the timing of the school year, most of the deaths in both locations occurred in children who were under school age (Fig. 38–4). Thus, although there is a definite seasonal pattern, the basis for it is not clear.

The majority of all drowning victims are males under 20 years of age; 40% are under 4 years. As already pointed out, the vast majority of victims seen at two large pediatric centers were under 5 years of age (see Fig. 38–4). In several studies, two groups have been noted to be at particular risk for submersion injuries. The first consists of young male toddlers, who tend to drown in private swimming pools during periods of inadequate supervision.[36, 208] The majority of children in the Los Angeles series had indeed drowned in private swimming pools.[39] The second major risk group is school-aged boys (6 or 7 years old) of lower socioeconomic status (with disproportionate lack of swimming education), who generally drown while swimming in or near unguarded large open bodies of water, such as lakes, ponds, rivers, or irrigation ditches.[95, 170]

It has been estimated that the overall risk of drowning for a child aged 1 or 2 years is 10 times higher than the risk for the general population. Multiple factors contribute to this high drowning rate, including lack of adult supervision, inadequate pool safety barriers, inadequate adult education in water safety and first aid, insufficient number of supervised public swimming areas, and insufficient attention devoted to water safety education in schools.[28, 47, 48, 57, 59, 64, 65, 70, 94, 148, 150, 156] Increased public educational efforts have been advocated by many investigators, and such programs probably exerted a favorable effect on the incidence of submersion accidents in Brisbane.[93, 110, 131, 135, 143, 147, 148, 178, 185, 189] Rowe and colleagues noted that 91% of the chil-

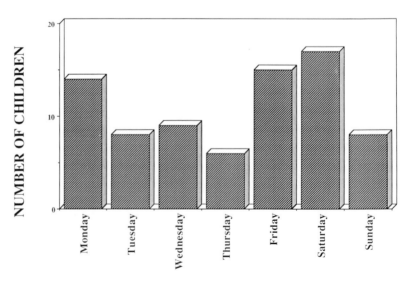

FIGURE 38–1

Distribution of victims of childhood drowning accidents who were patients at Primary Children's Medical Center, Salt Lake City, Utah, according to days of the week, 1982–1987.

DAY OF WEEK

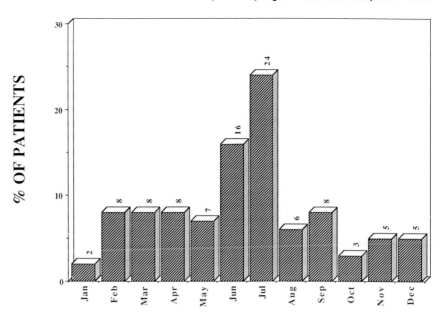

FIGURE 38-2

Distribution of victims of childhood drowning accidents who were patients at Children's Hospital of Los Angeles, Los Angeles, California, according to months of the year, 1975–1977.

dren who were taken to one Miami hospital after submersion were dead on arrival, suggesting that major reductions in drowning mortality might be accomplished only by preventive measures and improved field care.[170]

Analysis of adult drowning statistics have identified several risk factors for drowning in this group, which included some adolescents. Significant blood alcohol levels have been found in 33% of submersion victims in studies from England, Australia, and Finland, and numerous papers have documented the important role of alcohol and other abusive substances in drowning accidents.[1, 16, 17, 19, 28, 29, 31, 35, 45, 67, 78, 89, 105, 106, 108, 109, 114, 146, 157–159, 197, 208] Alcohol increases suscep-

tibility to drowning in several ways. It increases bravado and lowers acceptable behavior standards, thus producing carelessness that could contribute to submersion accidents. Alcohol depresses coordination and promotes a sense of well-being. People who drown with blood ethanol levels of 0.150 gm per 100 ml make clumsy attempts to extricate themselves from the water; with levels of more than 0.300 gm per 100 ml, victims frequently remain motionless in the water and do not struggle or attempt to rescue themselves. Ethanol also depresses hepatic gluconeogenesis, particularly during exercise and fasting, and hypoglycemia may contribute to drowning accidents. Other drugs have also

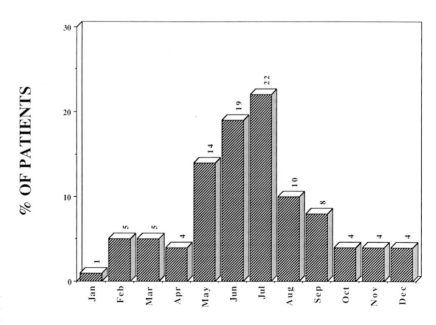

FIGURE 38-3

Distribution of victims of childhood drowning accidents who were patients at Primary Children's Medical Center, Salt Lake City, Utah, according to months of the year, 1982–1987.

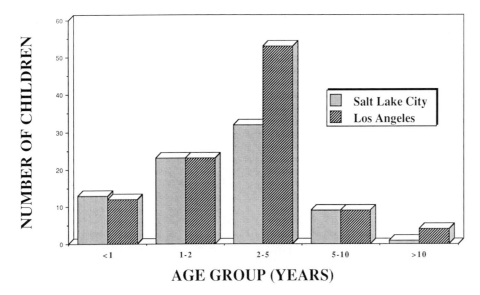

FIGURE 38–4

Age distribution of near drowning victims. Data are combined from Children's Hospital of Los Angeles (1975–1977) and Primary Children's Medical Center (1982–1987).

been implicated, including phencyclidine and glue sniffing.[16, 89] However, the incidence of nonalcohol drug abuse in submersion accidents in unknown.

Drowning often occurs during recreational and sporting activities.[19, 22, 28, 31, 45, 86, 109, 111, 200] Overestimation of skills and resultant exhaustion are the principal causes of drowning in those who drown while swimming.[22] Similarly, exhaustion frequently causes drowning in scuba diving accidents.[190] Among experienced athletes, drowning may occur from hypoxia during underwater swimming after hyperventilation; this has been termed *shallow water blackout*.[11, 33, 34, 193] Medical illnesses such as myocardial infarction have also been implicated, but the frequency of this is unknown. During autopsy it is difficult to differentiate deaths that occurred from other causes while the victim was in the water from those that were caused by the drowning itself. Although several tests (ventricular chloride levels, presence of diatoms in body organs, tympanomastoid hemorrhage) are sometimes used to make this differentiation, none produces conclusive results.[4, 5, 52, 56, 85, 103, 162]

Epilepsy is an important medical condition that may predispose patients to submersion accidents.[10, 92, 136, 141, 144, 145] In one retrospective study from Australia, epileptic children were found to have a fourfold increased incidence of drowning and accounted for 3 to 4% of all drowning victims.[144] It is frequently impossible to determine whether the drowning episodes were related to a seizure, because the histories were inconclusive and the anticonvulsant levels were not always determined at the time of hospital admission.[144] Other handicaps and central nervous system disorders have been anecdotally implicated in submersion accidents, including Friedreich ataxia and Duchenne muscular dystrophy.[18, 73, 77]

Although drowning most often occurs in swimming pools, lakes, and rivers, drownings have also been reported in home recreational facilities such as hot tubs and spas.[127] These pose peculiar problems; spas frequently have uncovered suction devices that can trap body parts underwater. Head and hair entrapment in such devices has been implicated in drowning deaths. Alcohol is frequently consumed in hot tubs, thus increasing the risk of a submersion acci-

dent; the combination of warm water and alcohol has been implicated in several adult and adolescent drowning accidents. During these episodes, the victim falls asleep and drowns without waking. Other unusual sites for drowning accidents include automobiles during flash floods, fermentation tanks, a bitumen tank, and even a water-filled head restrainer in a computerized axial tomography scanner that ruptured.[32, 53, 152, 182]

Young infants and children are frequently victims of bathtub and pail drownings.[17, 83, 149, 176, 205] Bathtub drownings occur most frequently in infants, aged 8 to 9 months, who are left to bathe under the supervision of a sibling who is generally under 4 years of age. The water is generally shallow, and the adult is usually in the home. Because infants can easily sit by themselves at this age, parents are led to believe that they could right themselves and would not drown in shallow water. The young supervisory sibling is not competent to recognize drowning, much less intervene, and is unable to assist the infant in trouble. Pail drownings occur in 9- to 10-month-old infants who are learning to walk. These children fall into pails, often containing cleaning fluid or other liquids, and are unable to extricate themselves. Because of the corrosive nature of many substances found in pails, these submersions have a high mortality rate.

Other factors are involved in the epidemiology of childhood submersion accidents. Carbon monoxide–contaminated air and nitrogen narcosis have been noted in scuba diving accidents. Suicide and nonaccidental trauma of children by adults may take the form of drowning.[21, 151, 177, 183] Frequently the latter is difficult or impossible to prove but may be suggested when the history is atypical or when unusual associated injuries are noted.

PATHOPHYSIOLOGY

Several classification systems have been used to characterize submersion accidents, and disagreements about the terminology used in this field (i.e., drowning vs. near drowning) are not unusual.[116] In our view, the precise definition is not nearly as important as the literature might suggest, because from a clinical standpoint one assumes that the clinician has a patient who is not dead. However, strictly speaking, "drowning refers to death from submersion within 24 hours of the actual incident." All other submersion victims, regardless of eventual outcome, are referred to as "near drowning victims." For clarity of writing, we use the term *drowning* in this chapter to refer to either of the situations mentioned previously because the distinction is highly artificial.

Victims of submersion accidents are frequently divided into groups according to the type of water in which drowning occurs, for example, seawater versus freshwater drowning.[175, 184, 209] This type of distinction intuitively might have importance from the standpoint of fluid and electrolyte changes, and the differentiation is clearly important when evaluating laboratory studies that are based on intratracheal instillation of large volumes of fluid.[66] Clinically, saltwater drownings may have a higher incidence of pulmonary edema than freshwater events, although fresh water appears to cause worse pulmonary damage than sea water.[126, 140, 214] The most dramatic electrolyte abnormalities and renal effects have been reported following saltwater accidents.[130, 137, 213] Experimentally, fresh water is more often associated with ventricular fibrillation, whereas seawater aspiration frequently causes asystole.[12] However, for most purposes the differences between freshwater and saltwater submersion accidents are minor compared with the similarities of the injuries.

Many laboratory studies in this field have dealt with intratracheal instillation of large volumes of fluid and have not addressed the more difficult issue of central nervous system injury.[61, 63] Although early studies concerned themselves primarily with electrolyte changes, blood gas changes, and respiratory problems, these problems are nearly always surmountable in the context of modern pediatric intensive care.[120, 121, 123] The significant neurologic problems supersede these other pathologic processes. In this section, we review the research concerning submersion to show the evolution of our perception of this injury as an initially electrolytic, then pulmonary, and, most recently, a central nervous system insult.

The sequence of events during drowning has been studied extensively in animals as early as the 1930s by Karpovich and Lougheed.[82, 104] Following submersions, there is an initial panic stage during which the animal struggles to surface, and small amounts of water enter the hypopharynx. This water triggers apnea and laryngospasm, and then copious amounts of water are swallowed. The animal struggles violently, gasps, loses consciousness, vomits, and aspirates. In about 10% of animals in these studies, the initial laryngospasm persisted until death, and no aspiration of fluid occurred. These findings coincide fairly well with adult human autopsy material, but data in pediatric drowning are sparse.

Electrolyte Changes

In an attempt to guide therapy, early studies initiated by Swann and colleagues were focused on the fluid and elec- trolyte abnormalities that might accompany drowning accidents.[194, 195] It was commonly thought that large volumes of fluids were swallowed by human victims, followed by large fluid shifts across the alveolus. Experimental models reflected this belief, using direct intratracheal instillation of relatively huge volumes of fluid. These studies demonstrated that large electrolyte, blood volume, and hemoglobin alterations did occur and were highly dependent on the salinity of the drowning medium. Ventricular fibrillation commonly occurred as a terminal event and was believed to be due to the dramatic electrolytic shifts. Swann and colleagues concluded that freshwater drowning caused hemodilution, which resulted in hemolysis and hyperkalemia, hyponatremia, and an elevated circulating blood volume. Seawater ($[NA^+] = 509$ mEq/L) drowning would produce hypernatremia, hemoconcentration, and contraction of circulating blood volume. Therapy predicated on these findings would then consist of intravenous hypertonic saline for freshwater victims and hypotonic solutions for seawater victims.

Subsequent studies in human near drowning victims by Fuller and Modell and associates in the 1960s demonstrated that neither electrolyte imbalance nor hemolysis was a significant problem in these patients, findings that were subsequently confirmed in numerous studies.[56, 121] Data from autopsy findings in human drowning victims also failed to demonstrate life-threatening electrolyte abnormalities.[120] Analysis of these data led to the conclusion that most (85%) human victims aspirate less than 22 ml of fluid per kg of body weight. Although this does not seem surprising, it is important because experiments in dogs that used less than 22 ml of aspirate per kg failed to demonstrate life-threatening electrolyte disturbances in freshwater, seawater, or chlorinated water drownings, although distinct alterations occurred in blood volume, electrolytes, and arterial blood gases.[122, 126] Ventricular fibrillation is also uncommon in human victims who have not suffered concomitant hypothermia, supporting the notion that the *electrolytic shifts noted were not clinically life threatening.*

Pulmonary Abnormalities

The most striking physiologic derangement noted by Modell and colleagues after near drowning in animals was persistent hypoxemia, refractory to supplemental oxygen.[125] This served to refocus attention during the next 2 decades on the primary pulmonary abnormalities that occur in this injury. Fuller had noted that victims could be pulled from the water unconscious, be resuscitated and awaken, only to develop respiratory distress and succumb to hypoxia despite face mask or oxygen tent therapy.[56] Histologic examination of pulmonary tissue revealed alveolar collapse, pulmonary edema, intra-alveolar exudate, and fibrin deposition, a picture reminiscent of infant hyaline membrane disease.[164] The patients who generally survived at this time were those who had aspirated relatively little fluid, perhaps owing to persistent laryngospasm as seen in 10% of the animals studied by Karpovich and Lougheed.

Modell and co-workers demonstrated that hypercarbia, acidosis, and hypoxia routinely occurred after submersion in sea water and fresh water. Despite huge aspirations of as much as 22 ml per kg (intratracheal instillation), hypercarbia and the resultant acidosis were not life threatening and did not persist following resuscitation. In contrast, hypoxia of life-threatening severity occurred following pulmonary aspiration of as little as 2.2 ml per kg, and such hypoxia was persistent unless positive pressure mechanical ventilatory support was provided.[125]

In similar studies dealing with endotracheal tube occlusion, simulating laryngospasm without aspiration, hypercapnia and hypoxia also developed.[125] However, in these instances reversal was possible when the animal was once again permitted to breath. This finding is reasonable, because no significant pulmonary damage occurred from aspirated fluid. In human victims who are submerged without aspiration of fluid, similar rapid clinical improvement is also seen if resuscitation is instituted before serious hypoxic brain damage has occurred.

The persistent hypoxia that develops following fluid aspiration is due to intrapulmonary shunting, which is generally unresponsive to increases of inspired oxygen tension.[87] Analysis of tracheal and pulmonary fluid from dogs after drowning demonstrated elevated surface tension activity.[61] After freshwater drowning, this is due to washout and dilution of surfactant, whereas in seawater aspiration the surfactant is inactivated. This lack of effective surfactant activity leads to alveolar collapse. In addition, proteinaceous fluid accumulates in the alveolar space, and alveolar hemorrhage may occur. Fibrin deposition and hyaline-like membranes develop within several days if the victim survives. As in newborn infants with hyaline membrane disease, this process is highly responsive to positive pressure ventilation with continuous or end-expiratory positive airway pressure. This reverses intrapulmonary shunting and restores oxygenation both clinically and experimentally.[101, 102, 118, 119, 171, 172] Early deaths from pulmonary disease after submersion are now rare because positive airway pressure is routinely employed in these children.

Fatalities from pulmonary complications of submersion certainly occur, however, and generally are related to pulmonary infections and barotrauma. Pneumonia may follow aspiration of contaminated water, may be due to aspiration, or may simply develop after several days of mechanical ventilatory support via an artificial airway that circumvents normal host defenses. Pulmonary interstitial emphysema and pneumothorax frequently occur in patients who drown while scuba diving but also occur in patients who are subjected to very high airway pressures during mechanical ventilation. Tension pneumomediastinum may exacerbate intracranial hypertension.[203]

Chronic pulmonary sequelae of submersion accidents are relatively uncommon.[192] Transient restrictive lung disease has been demonstrated, but it resolved over 4 months.[41, 76] Pediatric patients usually have normal pulmonary status after near drowning, although pulmonary function studies have demonstrated hyperactive airways when challenged with methacholine.[96] This abnormality persists at least for several years and has also been noted in children who did not require ventilatory support during hospitalization after the submersion incident.

Current Viewpoint

We prefer to consider the pathophysiology of submersion injury as four simultaneous processes:

1. Asphyxia, anoxia, and cerebral ischemia
2. Fluid overload
3. Pulmonary injury
4. Hypothermia (and diving reflex)

These four processes occur concomitantly (Fig. 38–5), and it is arbitrary to consider each separately. Although it is clear that near drowning is a considerably more complex problem than mere aspiration of fluid into the lungs, this four-pronged approached to the pathophysiology may assist the reader in understanding the pathophysiology of drowning.

Asphyxia, Anoxia, and Cerebral Ischemia

From the standpoint of the eventual outcome of the child, the most important problem is the extent of anoxic or ischemic central nervous system injury. Submersion injuries involve a variable combination of ischemia and anoxia, and each has its own effect on the affected tissue bed. Ischemia is defined as a decrease of blood flow, and anoxia is defined as the absence of oxygen. The difference is important, because the delivery of blood that contains glucose and other nutrients leads to anaerobic metabolism in the absence of oxygen (anoxic conditions); this may lead to a buildup of lactic acid and other waste products. The continued blood flow also permits the washout of metabolic substances, but intracellular waste substances may continue to increase beyond the washout capability. However, total ischemia stops the delivery of nutrients and the washout of waste products and leads to a rapid shutdown of tissue metabolism. This may result in less buildup of lactate and hence might result in less cerebral edema. In drowning injuries, the duration of asphyxia and anoxia may be significantly longer than the actual period of cardiac arrest and cerebral ischemia, and the exact contributions of each process cannot be estimated very well in the individual victim.

The effects of asphyxia are diagrammed in Figure 38–6.

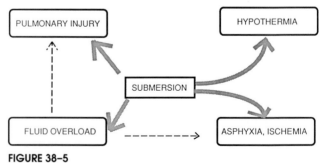

FIGURE 38–5

Pathophysiology of submersion injury.

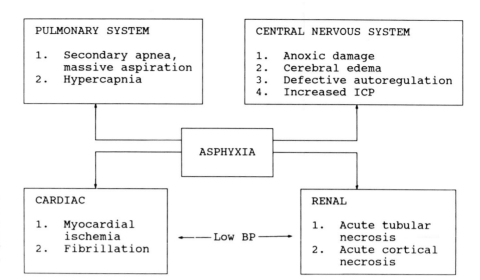

FIGURE 38–6

Pathophysiology of anoxia and ischemia during submersion injury. (Redrawn from Dean JM, Setzer NA: Near drowning. In: Rogers MC (ed): Textbook of Pediatric Intensive Care. Baltimore, Williams & Wilkins, 1987, pp 721–739.)

Oxygen is clearly required for all human tissues; in its absence, one may anticipate damage to the brain, heart, lungs, kidneys, and gastrointestinal tract. The diving seal reflex (see later discussion) is associated with an increased flow of oxygen to the heart and brain at the expense of the peripheral tissues (kidney and gastrointestinal beds).

Anoxia and ischemia affect the brain in numerous ways. Autoregulation is quickly lost, although studies of this in humans are sparse. Death of neurons results in cellular edema and cytotoxic cerebral edema.[50] Generalized cerebral edema leads to an increase of intracranial pressure, which then decreases cerebral perfusion pressure and cerebral blood flow. Although early papers concentrated on respiratory difficulties, later studies have emphasized the common occurrence of intracranial hypertension in children following submersion accidents.[13, 23–27, 38, 115, 133, 174] Intracranial hypertension reduces cerebral perfusion pressure and blood flow, causing further ischemia.

Pulmonary ischemic injury frequently takes the form of adult respiratory distress syndrome, and this has been observed following submersion injuries.[43, 60, 154] A "secondary drowning" phenomenon has also been observed, which reflects not only the primary aspiration injury but also the superimposed ischemic injury.[40, 160] As respiratory failure develops, hypercapnia and hypoxia then worsen the original cerebral insult by dilating the cerebral vasculature and increasing intracranial hypertension.

Cardiac and renal injuries from near drowning are surprisingly uncommon. In the series reported from Los Angeles, no instances of renal failure were encountered, and no instances of long-term myocardial problems were seen.[37, 38] Some patients clearly develop renal failure after submersion, and many patients succumb from hemodynamic collapse early after the injury.[130, 137, 213] However, it is surprising that more frequent permanent myocardial damage is not seen. Myocyte hypercontraction and eosinophilic infiltration have been noted in animal studies of cardiac pathology after drowning.[80]

The diving seal reflex is believed to divert flow away from the gastrointestinal tract, and catecholamine drips, which are commonly employed in the hemodynamic sup-

port of these victims, further increase mesenteric ischemia because of splanchnic vasoconstriction, as with hypothermia. Thus, it is not infrequent to see a profuse bloody diarrhea in children following severe near drowning accidents. Such a finding is almost uniformly associated with fatal injury.

Fluid Overload

The second pathophysiologic process that occurs after drowning accidents is water overload (Fig. 38–7). Although many people have concentrated their attention on the quantity of fluid aspirated into the lungs, few have noted the large quantity of fluid that may be swallowed during immersion.[104] The victim swallows water before aspiration and loss of consciousness, and the stomach is generally filled when the victim is resuscitated. Several clinical aspects become important. First, the victim nearly always vomits during resuscitation, and the potential pulmonary effects of aspirating stomach contents may be worse than the original injury to the lungs. Second, fluid is absorbed via the gastrointestinal tract and may precipitate fluid and electrolyte abnormalities (though generally not life-threatening ones), such as water intoxication with hyponatremia, hypokalemia, and, potentially, hemolysis. These effects are exacerbated by the frequent occurrence of the syndrome of inappropriate antidiuretic hormone secretion (secondary to brain and lung injury). Finally, fluid and water overload contributes to cerebral edema, increasing intracranial hypertension and decreasing cerebral perfusion. This problem is worse with fresh water than with sea water, as the hypertonic solution with sea water would normally decrease cerebral edema.

Pulmonary Injury

The third pathophysiologic process that occurs in submersion injuries is pulmonary damage secondary to aspiration of the drowning medium or stomach contents. Many studies have been conducted in this area, primarily dealing with the types and amounts of fluids aspirated.[14, 15, 30, 81, 132, 202]

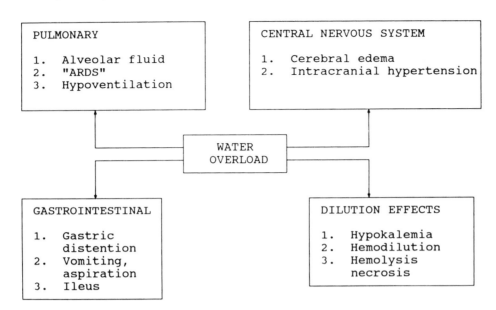

FIGURE 38–7

Pathophysiology of water overload during submersion injury. ARDS, Adult respiratory distress syndrome. (Redrawn from Dean JM, Setzer NA: Near drowning. In: Rogers MD (ed): Textbook of Pediatric Intensive Care. Baltimore, Williams & Wilkins, 1987, pp 721–739.)

Hypothermia and the Diving Reflex

The fourth component of the pathophysiology of drowning is hypothermia (Fig. 38–8). Significant hypothermia (i.e., less than 30°C) is capable of depressing neurologic function and causing the appearance of brain death. Although hypothermia exerts protective effects by reducing cerebral metabolism, the clinician may be misled into declaring the child dead because of the clinical appearance of the child. Thus, it is important to raise the victim's temperature to near normal before making conclusions about brain function.[112, 139] Hypothermia also exerts profound hemodynamic effects, including decreased myocardial contractility and vasomotor tone. Cardiovascular collapse occurs, and vasodilation may be exacerbated during the rewarming phase, causing further hypotension and collapse unless the clinician is fully aware of this process. Severe hypothermia makes cardiac resuscitation impossible, and when arrhythmias cannot be converted the physician should continue resuscitation until rewarming methods raise the temperature above 30°C.

Many papers deal with "cold water" drowning, particularly in reference to dramatic anecdotal survivals after prolonged immersion.[173] This may be confusing. First, most such papers deal with extremely cold water such as is encountered beneath layers of ice. Second, even in warm climates it is possible for water temperature beneath ground level (i.e., in private swimming pools) to be significantly colder than ambient temperature. Third, even moderate water temperatures are much lower than normal body temperature, and the relatively large surface area of the infant and child predisposes pediatric victims to rapid heat loss into the tremendous heat sink provided by hundreds of thousands of gallons of water. Thus, it is possible for a small child to become rapidly hypothermic even in a relatively warm pool in a moderate climate.[6] In the emergency department and in subsequent management, therefore, the victim's temperature should be measured and considered when assessing the neurologic and hemodynamic status of the child.

Many animals undergo profound circulatory changes when submerged.[199] These changes are collectively referred to as the *diving seal reflex*, which maintains blood flow through the heart and brain while markedly decreasing blood flow through nonvital organs and skeletal muscle by vasoconstriction.[71, 191] The blood pressure is maintained, but bradycardia and respiratory inhibition occur. In ducks this reflex is initiated by trigeminal and laryngeal nerve stimulation when the face enters the water and when small amounts of water enter the hypopharynx.[79] Extremely low temperatures exacerbate the response, as does fear. In seals, cardiac output drops from 40 liters per minute to 6 liters per minute during diving, while cerebral metabolism is fully maintained. The diving reflex was demonstrated in a human alligator wrestler in 1940. Subsequent studies by Gooden have demonstrated bradycardia and marked changes in calf and forearm blood flow during submersion, despite constant blood pressure.[62] These changes were dependent on submersion of the face.

On the basis of such observations, investigators have suggested that the diving seal reflex may contribute to the good cerebral outcome, which is occasionally seen following prolonged submersion in cold water. Obviously hypothermia would also lower cerebral metabolism in these patients, which is quite different from what occurs in seals, ducks, and whales.[166] Although this hypothesis (diving reflex in humans) seems attractive, a study in human adults suggests that hypothermia decreases the diving reflex.[69] Early investigators have suggested that the diving reflex might be stronger in children than adults, but a recent study has demonstrated that the converse is true: the diving reflex is very weak in children.[160, 161] Thus, at this point we must

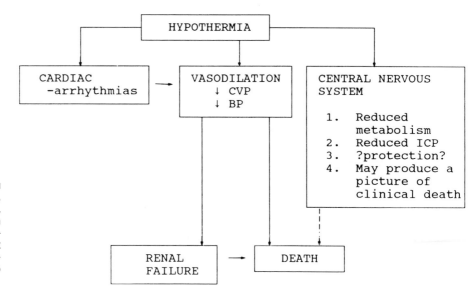

FIGURE 38–8

Pathophysiology of hypothermia during submersion injury. CVP, Central venous pressure; BP, blood pressure. (Redrawn from Dean JM, Setzer NA: Near drowning. In: Rogers MC (ed): Textbook of Pediatric Intensive Care. Baltimore, Williams & Wilkins, 1987, pp 721–739.)

conclude that the diving reflex plays little or no role in the survival of victims of submersion accidents and that prolonged survivals are probably due entirely to the hypothermic protective effects on cerebral metabolism.

CLINICAL PRESENTATION

Following submersion injuries, children generally arrive with one of two presentations. First, and most common, the majority of children reach the hospital facility awake and alert, and many of these children have not suffered a significant injury. Mild aspiration or even severe pulmonary damage may be seen with children in this category, but most of these children have suffered trivial injuries and will do well from all standpoints. The second group suffers cardiac arrest at some point, and these children show a spectrum of pathology that includes severe central nervous system anoxia and ischemia, significant aspiration and interstitial lung disease, adult respiratory distress syndrome, hemodynamic instability, gastrointestinal necrosis, and other facets of multisystem failure. These are the patients who are admitted to the intensive care unit, and it is with these patients that the remainder of this chapter is concerned.

Respiratory Assessment

During the initial assessment of a near drowned child, the clinician must meticulously adhere to the ABCs of emergency management. The goals are no different in this situation than in other emergency situations. The airway must be cleared of vomitus, which is common after these injuries, ventilation must be ensured, and the adequacy of circulation must be maintained. Following emergency stabilization, a specific evaluation of pulmonary status and then of neurologic status is needed.

In the victim who is breathing spontaneously, pulmonary function can be assessed easily by obtaining an arterial blood gas in 40% oxygen. As a general rule of thumb, *a child who cannot maintain a Pa_{O_2} greater than 100 mm Hg in 40% oxygen will require positive pressure ventilatory support and should be intubated.* The astute reader recognizes that this is a poor man's alveolar arterial oxygen gradient (Aa_{O_2}) measurement, and from an arterial blood gas measurement in any inspired oxygen concentration, one can calculate the Aa_{O_2} gradient and make a decision of intubation and respiratory support. An Aa_{O_2} difference of greater than 150 almost always requires medical intervention.

It is worthwhile to point out that a capillary or venous blood gas measurement does not satisfy our requirements in assessing the severity of pulmonary injury. A venous oxygen tension largely reflects the cardiac output and oxygen extraction and may not distinguish a normal and an abnormal Aa_{O_2} gradient if adequate supplemental inspired oxygen is provided.

The radiologic presentation is variable.[39, 211] Drowning victims have been divided into "dry" and "wet," depending on the amount of aspiration that is estimated to have occurred. Estimates of aspiration are as high as 90%, but pediatric data in this regard are sparse. The findings do not correlate well with the eventual central nervous system outcome, and many children with dramatic pulmonary edema respond to therapy and recover completely. Other children may present in a coma and with normal radiographs.[39]

Aspiration often occurs during resuscitation from submersion incidents. In the course of the struggling phase of submersion injury, the victim swallows a large amount of fluid. At resuscitation, particularly when mouth-to-mouth ventilation is provided, the victim vomits. It is difficult to tell from radiographs whether aspiration occurred during the submersion incident itself or during resuscitation; in our experience, it has seemed that a significant portion of aspiration injury occurs during or after resuscitation and could be prevented by judicious placement of a nasogastric tube and stomach evacuation. The implications of aspirating stomach contents are different from those of aspirating distilled water or saline.[63, 212]

Children who have been involved in submersion incidents should nearly always be admitted to the hospital for observation, as at least one fatal case has been described in a child who suffered delayed onset of respiratory failure.[121] It is primarily for respiratory problems that hospital observation is indicated; therefore, the baseline assessment should include a chest radiograph and an arterial blood gas measurement. Admittedly, there is a population of children in whom it is doubtful that a significant submersion incident even occurred (i.e., the child slipped under water, was immediately lifted out, sputtered a few times, and started crying). When the actual incident is doubtful, 6 to 12 hours of emergency department observation seems adequate.

Before concluding this discussion, we want to point out that respiratory system management is not restricted to instances in which lung pathology has been demonstrated. In a child with hemodynamic instability, intubation and ventilatory support are indicated to relieve the myocardium and to allow the clinician to concentrate efforts on other issues. Also, the child in a coma who has a weak or an absent gag reflex clearly needs protection of the airway. Thus, respiratory support may play an integral role in management of submersion victims even if clinical assessment suggests adequate pulmonary function.

Neurologic Assessment

It is extremely important to establish the condition of the central nervous system early in the course of management of these children because early assessment provides the physician with sufficient prognostic information to triage the child to the appropriate facility and possibly to counsel the parents. Efforts to prognosticate victims of submersion incidents have been extensive.[3, 37, 46, 84, 123, 124, 138, 153, 180]

Fandel and Bancalari, reporting their results in children who suffered submersion injuries in the Miami area, found four separate factors that each identified children with 100% mortality.[46] The four factors were (1) a requirement for cardiopulmonary resuscitation in the emergency department, (2) a pH of less than 7.00, (3) coma, and (4) a requirement for ventilatory support. The precise timing of the measurement of pH, the depth of coma, and the rationale for ventilatory support were not further detailed in the paper, but the work did serve as a framework for physicians staffing emergency facilities. Modell and colleagues reported on a larger series that included children and adults and also noted the dire prognosis associated with the necessity for cardiopulmonary resuscitation in these victims.[123] A later paper from the same institution emphasized that nearly all mortality in children was associated with severe coma.[124] Peterson noted that children who required cardiopulmonary resuscitation had a uniformly bad outcome and implied that emergency department physicians should think twice before resuscitating these patients, unless consideration is given to heroic brain resuscitative therapies.[153] Conn and colleagues reported optimistic early results with brain resuscitation in drowning patients, and most researchers advocate an aggressive approach in the emergency department with victims of submersion.[23-27] In summary, a large number of reports correlate a poor outcome with a requirement for cardiopulmonary resuscitation, and most mortality occurs in children with neurologic injury. However, it is notable that few of these studies address the early assessment of drowning patients.

Orlowski constructed a prognostic scoring system after reviewing the experience of four institutions.[138] The score comprised five items: (1) age younger than 3 years, (2) coma on admission, (3) estimated submersion time longer than 5 minutes, (4) failure to receive resuscitation within 10 minutes of rescue, and (5) initial pH less than 7.10. One point was assigned for each item if present, but if information was lacking then no point was assessed. Using this system, most mortality could be identified by a score of 4 or 5. Unfortunately, this system does not separate survivors and nonsurvivors satisfactorily, and correlation with survival would be expected because the parameters are evidence of more severe injury.[37] From our perspective, the main flaw of this scoring system is that absence of information is not handled well, the timing of pH measurement is variable, and the historical information about submersion time and resuscitation is usually unreliable.

The Glasgow coma scale has been used to assess submersion victims and is fairly effective for estimating outcome of these children.[37] When the initial Glasgow coma score is 6 or higher, the outcome is generally good; children who have lower scores have a high probability of mortality. Indeed, based on initial scores, a Glasgow coma score of 6 or higher is associated with a uniformly good outcome. Unfortunately, the Glasgow score does not differentiate the populations well when conducted at the referral (tertiary) institution, and a Glasgow coma score of 3 in the intensive care unit has been associated with a 100% poor outcome.[3, 39]

There are several studies concerning the radiologic assessment of the central nervous system, with various estimates of cerebral edema and injury.[51, 128, 196] In our opinion, these only lend support to the already certain clinical impression. Similarly, electroencephalography, evoked potentials, temperature instability, and absence of spontaneous respirations are of little actual predictive use, because these studies or impressions almost always confirm an obvious clinical picture.[74, 75, 113, 163]

What is the purpose or value of such scoring systems? We believe that submersion victims should be resuscitated aggressively in the emergency department facilities or in the field and that seriously injured children should be transported to an appropriate tertiary facility with a pediatric intensive care unit capable of advanced neurointensive care.[142, 168] Children with a poor neurologic presentation may be candidates for intracranial pressure control or other cerebral resuscitative therapies (see later discussion), but more important, children with an expected good outcome should probably not be exposed to these less than conventional modes of treatment.

GENERAL CLINICAL MANAGEMENT

A child who has been the victim of a submersion incident has suffered a multisystem injury, and the management of this patient must be approached in a system by system manner.[72] Cerebral resuscitation, including issues of intracranial pressure monitoring and barbiturate coma, is distinctly secondary to very compulsive management of the child's respiratory and hemodynamic dysfunctions.

Respiratory Support

The most important body systems that require aggressive support are the respiratory and the cardiac systems, because without these functions it is impossible to devote any attention to the central nervous system.[207] Children who are comatose (i.e., a Glasgow coma score of less than 9) should be intubated, and ventilatory support should be provided. Particular caution must be exercised to avoid aspiration of gastric contents. Arterial blood gas monitoring should guide further support, and an arterial line is usually indicated for convenient sampling access. Conn and associates have suggested that all comatose children receive 100% oxygen for 6 hours, but there is no evidence to support this practice.[25] It does provide assurance that the highest possible oxygenation is provided during this critical period.

Positive end-expiratory pressure (PEEP) is a cornerstone of therapy in submersion victims who have pulmonary injury and has clearly decreased mortality due to respiratory failure following drowning accidents.[2, 43, 84, 101, 102, 154] Although there is debate about the timing of PEEP, we recommend that PEEP be used when indicated by arterial blood gas measurements demonstrating a significant Aa_{O_2} gradient or intrapulmonary shunt. This method of respiratory support can exacerbate intracranial hypertension and can compromise hemodynamic function, and thus we would not use PEEP higher than 5 cm H_2O unless indicated by such measurements. When PEEP requirements exceed 10 to 15 cm H_2O, pulmonary arterial catheterization may be useful for hemodynamic management.[39]

Hemodynamic Support

Hemodynamic management of these children may be very difficult because of the many injuries that have been sustained. For instance, myocardial ischemia during the drowning incident may reduce myocardial contractility; gastrointestinal ischemia may cause third space losses into the gut and lead to hypovolemia; hypothermia may cause vasomotor collapse and distributive shock. Fluid restriction is a standard provision of neurologic care following cerebral edema and may increase the possibility of hypovolemia and shock; this is even more difficult when large amounts of mannitol are utilized as osmotic therapy for intracranial edema. Nearly all seriously ill drowning victims need arterial catheter lines, and we find pulmonary arterial catheterization to be useful in many of these patients. The latter is particularly helpful if high levels of PEEP are necessary because of significant intrapulmonary shunt.

Fluid and Electrolytes

The fluid and electrolyte management of drowning victims is really not different from similar management in any

critically ill patient. The cornerstone of safe fluid and electrolyte management in the face of fluid shifts, hypovolemia, hypothermia, and respiratory instability is frequent monitoring of the patient's clinical status and laboratory measurements. Virtually any fluid and electrolyte disturbance may be encountered, including hyponatremia, hypernatremia, hypokalemia, hyperkalemia, hypocalcemia, hypomagnesemia, inappropriate antidiuretic hormone secretion, diabetes insipidus, hyperglycemia, and hyperosmolality. We emphasize that the only safe avenue of management includes frequent laboratory and clinical assessment of the child.

Gastrointestinal Tract and Nutrition

During a significant submersion incident, with its accompanying ischemia and relative anoxia, it is not surprising that the gastrointestinal tract is adversely affected. This is exacerbated by the diving reflex, which shunts blood away from the skin and gastrointestinal tract.[71, 191] Profuse, bloody diarrhea is often seen following these severe injuries, which both prohibits enteral feeding and also forebodes a poor prognosis. Conservative management usually suffices from the standpoint of the gastrointestinal tract, however, and consists of nasogastric drainage and control of gastric pH.

The nutritional aspects of submersion incidents are not well studied. Children who have obviously good neurologic function generally recover from their accident very quickly and hence do not require sophisticated approaches to nutritional support. The child who has significant lung disease, however, may benefit from aggressive nutritional support, often via total parenteral nutrition. The child with significant central nervous system damage may require prolonged nutritional support. The impact of such support on the central nervous system injury is not known, but there is little evidence that aggressive support greatly affects anoxic encephalopathy.

Other Issues

Steroids and antibiotics are often considered when discussing the management of near drowning victims and deserve comment. Antibiotics are sometimes suggested in the context of aspiration pneumonia, but we are unaware of any published evidence to support this measure. It would seem attractive to treat a child who has drowned in a swamp or similarly contaminated water, but it remains likely that this will only select more exotic and perhaps dangerous forms of bacterial life with which the child may become septic.[60, 97, 99, 181, 204] There are, in fact, several case reports of brain abscess following near drowning accidents, and these cases have uniformly involved unusual organisms.[42, 49, 58] There are no reports concerning the efficacy of antibiotics in the treatment of children following drowning accidents. Our current recommendation is to treat pneumonia when it appears in as specific a manner as possible, utilizing appropriate sampling, culturing, and staining techniques to reach a bacteriologic diagnosis.

Steroids have been utilized in the context of cerebral edema as well as in the context of pulmonary aspiration.[20,

[123, 167, 210, 212] Although steroids are probably efficacious in the setting of cerebral edema surrounding tumors and other masses, there is no evidence whatsoever that steroids are useful for treating cerebral edema following ischemic or anoxic insults. Steroids are also unwarranted from the perspective of aspiration pneumonia. On balance, although there are seemingly few contraindications to the use of steroids, there is little rationale for their use following submersion injuries.

NEUROLOGIC MANAGEMENT

As our understanding of the pathophysiology and treatment of submersion injuries has improved, lowering the mortality rate from electrolyte disturbances and respiratory failure, it has become evident that prognosis is largely related to the injury sustained by the central nervous system. The need for careful neurologic assessment has already been discussed. After the clinician assesses the central nervous system injury to be severe, what management is indicated?

Three categories of intensive care management impinge on central nervous system support. First and most important, good basic intensive care with support of ventilation, oxygenation, and perfusion underlies all other aspects of neurointensive care. Second, intracranial pressure monitoring and control of intracranial hypertension play a role in neurointensive care management; such methods may be helpful in the treatment of submersion injury. Third, various brain resuscitative therapies have been proposed in many contexts, including barbiturates, calcium blockers, hypothermia, cardiopulmonary bypass, and free radical scavengers. Many of these have been suggested or attempted following submersion injury.

Cerebral perfusion pressure is highly dependent on arterial blood pressure; cerebral oxygen delivery is highly dependent on arterial oxygenation as well as on cerebral blood flow. It is worthwhile to emphasize that no experimental therapy can overcome defects in basic support. Discussion of intracranial pressure control or hypothermia is nonsensical unless ventilatory and hemodynamic stability has been accomplished. Thus, from a neurologic standpoint, the first priority remains the airway, ventilation, oxygenation, and perfusion. After these are ensured, we may proceed to more unconventional questions such as intracranial pressure monitoring or barbiturate coma.

Intracranial pressure monitoring has been employed in a wide variety of conditions, including drowning patients.[3, 13, 23–27, 38, 54, 55, 107, 115, 133, 134, 155, 174, 184] The effects of intracranial hypertension include an adverse effect on cerebral blood flow, since cerebral perfusion pressure is calculated as blood pressure minus intracranial pressure. Cerebral herniation may result from significant cerebral edema, and in many circumstances intracranial hypertension control prevents herniation. However, in asphyxial and ischemic injury, intracranial hypertension is usually due to cytotoxic cerebral edema, and an important implication of intracranial hypertension following submersion injury is that a large percentage of the brain cells have been killed. Thus, although there are therapeutic goals for monitoring intracranial pressure and preventing intracranial hypertension (preserve perfusion and prevent herniation), the probability that intracranial pressure control will be possible or helpful is low because of the etiology of the pressure (cytotoxic).

Conn and co-workers published several reports dealing with brain resuscitation of children after near drowning, and intracranial pressure monitoring was an integral part of their management.[23–27] Modell and colleagues have questioned the need for cerebral resuscitation, and results from their series are similar to Conn's results.[117, 124] Dean and McComb noted that patients with intracranial pressure elevation after near drowning had a uniformly bad outcome, and Allman and co-workers have reported further data from the same institution that support the original conclusion.[3, 38] Nussbaum and Galant recommend intracranial pressure monitoring after near drowning, but it is not clear from their paper that intracranial pressure monitoring really contributed more information than the arterial blood pressure measurements.[133] Other individuals have monitored intracranial pressure following submersion, but the data do not clearly demonstrate that such monitoring has been useful or has had an impact on neurologic outcome after drowning. Indeed, a paper from Bohn and associates is quite negative on this issue.[13]

Barbiturates, calcium blockers, and hypothermia have been employed in a variety of cerebral injuries, including drowning. Barbiturates have not been demonstrated to be of any value following near drowning, although barbiturates may have a legitimate role as agents for reducing intracranial pressure in other circumstances. Calcium blockers have not been systematically studied in drowning, though verapamil has been utilized.[90] Calcium blockers do not have an obvious effect in animal models, and it seems unlikely that these drugs will ever be widely used clinically following ischemic cerebral injury. Hypothermia has been used but is associated with no major improvement of prognosis, and it has significantly detrimental effects on immune function and hemodynamic stability.[13] In short, none of the proposed brain resuscitation therapies, including intracranial pressure control, has been shown to have an impact on mortality or morbidity following submersion injuries.

Work in animal models suggests that oxygen radical scavengers may have a beneficial effect on brain function following ischemia. This work seems to have a better basis than that of barbiturates or calcium blockers, and perhaps the next decade will usher in a truly revolutionary drug for this type of injury. Until then, the clinician must maximize basic intensive care, consider intracranial pressure monitoring with a great deal of perspective, and regard more unconventional therapies with skepticism.

PROGNOSIS

The prognosis of children who arrive at the hospital awake is excellent, and most of these children have a normal survival. Children with severe pulmonary injury or aspiration may succumb to respiratory failure, but this outcome is much less common with modern pediatric intensive care. Children with neurologic injury may be stratified according to the initial Glasgow coma score at the initial hospital facility; children with scores higher than 6 generally have a good prognosis. By 6 to 8 hours after the injury, however, significant improvement should have occurred, and continued low Glasgow coma scores are associated with a pessimistic outcome. Even with the worst of examination results, however, including flaccid neurologic presentation, cardiac arrest, and fixed and dilated pupils, a few patients defy the textbooks and recover completely.[60, 179, 198] Such survivals occur at the same relative frequency as survival after cardiac arrest from other causes and are not unique to the drowning injury.[44, 100, 201] This rate of recovery is about 10%, and we suggest that this figure justifies the initial aggressive resuscitation of all near drowned children who reach the emergency facility and at least 6 to 12 hours of aggressive management in the pediatric intensive care unit.

Long-term morbidity from near drowning has not been studied extensively, but there are clearly neuropsychiatric sequelae.[9] Unusual outcomes include the production of the Ondine curse from localized damage to the brain stem.[8] Pulmonary, renal, cardiac, and infectious complications have already been discussed. It is clear that submersion accidents cause significant mortality and morbidity in this nation, and efforts at prevention will continue to be needed to reduce the impact of this injury on our children.

References

1. Able EL, Zeidenberg P: Age, alcohol and violent death: A postmortem study. J Stud Alcohol 46(3):228–231, 1985.
2. Ahnefeld FW, Dick W, Lotz P, et al: The early use of positive end expiratory pressure (PEEP) ventilation in emergency medicine, and some experiments on pigs. Resuscitation 11(1–2):79–90, 1984.
3. Allman FD, Nelson WB, Pacentine GA, et al: Outcome following cardiopulmonary resuscitation in severe pediatric near drowning. Am J Dis Child 140(6):571–575, 1986.
4. Angelini Rota M, Gualdi G, Macchiarelli L: Analysis for diatoms in the diagnosis of drowning. Boll Soc Ital Biol Sper 59(12):1973–1979, 1983.
5. Babin RW, Graves NN, Rose EF: Temporal bone pathology in drowning. Am J Otolaryngol 3(3):168–173, 1982.
6. Barman MR: Hypothermia, in summer? RN 45(6):42, 1982.
7. Barry W, Little TM, Sibert JR: Childhood drownings in private swimming pools: An avoidable cause of death. BMJ 285(6341):542–543, 1982.
8. Beal MF, Richardson EP Jr, Brandstetter R, et al: Localized brainstem ischemic damage and Ondine's curse after near-drowning. Neurology 33(6):717–721, 1983.
9. Bell TS, Ellenberg L, McComb JG: Neuropsychological outcome after severe pediatric near-drowning. Neurosurgery 17(4):604–608, 1985.
10. Beringer GB, Biel M, Lai CW, et al: Submersion accidents and epilepsy (letter). Am J Dis Child 137(6):604–605, 1983.
11. Bernett P, Haas W: Drowning, swimmingpool death and other emergencies related to swimming. Fortschr Med 102(29–30):752–754, 1984.
12. Bhardwaj PK, Mohan M, Rai UC: Electrocardiographic changes in experimental drowning. Indian J Physiol Pharmacol 26(1):85–90, 1982.
13. Bohn DJ, Biggar WD, Smith CR, et al: Influence of hypothermia, barbiturate therapy, and intracranial pressure monitoring on morbidity and mortality after near drowning. Crit Care Med 14(6):529–534, 1986.
14. Brinkmann B, Fechner G, Puschel K: Lung histology in experimental drowning. Z Rechtsmed 89(4):267–277, 1983.
15. Brinkmann B, Fechner G, Puschel K: Ultrastructural pathology of the alveolar apparatus in experimental drowning. Z Rechtsmed 91(1):47–60, 1983.
16. Brunet BL, Reiffenstein RJ, Williams T, et al: Toxicity of phency-
clidine and ethanol in combination. Alcohol Drug Res 6(5):341–349, 1985–1986.
17. Budnick LD, Ross DA: Bathtub-related drownings in the United States, 1979–81. Am J Public Health 75(6):630–633, 1985.
18. Busch DB, Huntington RW 3d, Hartmann HA: Drowning of a Friedreich's ataxia patient. Am J Forensic Med Pathol 8(1):64–67, 1987.
19. Cairns FJ, Koelmeyer TD, Smeeton WM: Deaths from drowning. N Z Med J 97(749):65–67, 1984.
20. Calderon HW, Modell JH, Ruiz BC: The ineffectiveness of steroid therapy for treatment of freshwater near drowning. Anesthesiology 43:642–650, 1975.
21. Caniano DA, Beaver BL, Boles ET Jr: Child abuse. An update on surgical management in 256 cases. Ann Surg 203(2):219–224, 1986.
22. Chao TC: Death in sports and recreation. Ann Acad Med Singapore 12(3):400–404, 1983.
23. Conn AW: Cerebral resuscitation for the near-drowned child. Emerg Med 12:16–25, 1981.
24. Conn AW, Barker GA: Fresh water drowning and near drowning—An update. Can Anaesth Soc J 31(3 Pt 2):S38–44, 1984.
25. Conn AW, Edmonds JF, Barker GA: Near-drowning in cold fresh water: Current treatment regimen. Can Anaesth Soc J 25:259–265, 1978.
26. Conn AW, Edmonds JF, Barker GA: Cerebral resuscitation in near-drowning. Pediatr Clin North Am 26:691–701, 1979.
27. Conn AW, Montes JE, Barker GA, et al: Cerebral salvage in near-drowning following neurological classification by triage. Can Anaesth Soc J 27:201–210, 1980.
28. Copeland AR: Deaths during recreational activity. Forensic Sci Int 25(2):117–122, 1984.
29. Copeland AR: Non-vehicular accidents among teenagers—The 5-year Metro Dade County experience from 1979 to 1983. Forensic Sci Int 27(4):221–227, 1985.
30. Copeland AR: An assessment of lung weights in drowning cases. The Metro Dade County experience from 1978 to 1982. Am J Forensic Med Pathol 6(4):301–304, 1985.
31. Copeland AR: Non-commercial, accidental water transport (boating) fatalities. Z Rechtsmed 96(4):291–296, 1986.
32. Cordes RA, Eagle T: Near drowning: A complication of computerized axial tomography of the head. Anesth Analg 57:359–360, 1978.
33. Craig AB: Causes of loss of consciousness during underwater swimming. J Appl Physiol 16:583–586, 1961.
34. Craig AB: Underwater swimming and loss of consciousness. JAMA 176:255–258, 1961.
35. Davis S, Smith LS: Alcohol and drowning in Cape Town. A preliminary report. S Afr Med J 62(25):931–933, 1982.
36. Davis S, Smith LS: The epidemiology of drowning in Cape Town—1980–1983. S Afr Med J 68(10):739–742, 1985.
37. Dean JM, Kaufman ND: Prognostic indicators in pediatric near drowning: The Glasgow coma scale. Crit Care Med 9:536–539, 1981.
38. Dean JM, McComb JG: Intracranial pressure monitoring in severe pediatric near drowning. Neurosurgery 9:627–630, 1981.
39. Dean JM, Setzer NA: Near drowning. In: Rogers MC (ed): Textbook of Pediatric Intensive Care. Baltimore, Williams & Wilkins, 1987, pp 721–739.
40. Dick AE, Potgieter PD: Secondary drowning in the Cape peninsula. S Afr Med J 62(22):803–806, 1982.
41. Domenighetti G, Genoni L, Buchser E, et al: Restriction of pulmonary capillary volume, delayed sequelae of immersion in fresh water with respiratory distress syndrome. Schweiz Med Wochenschr 112(50):1838–1841, 1982.
42. Dubeau F, Roy LE, Allard J, et al: Brain abscess due to *Petriellidium boydii*. Can J Neurol Sci 11(3):395–398, 1984.
43. Effmann EL, Merten DF, Kirks DR, et al: Adult respiratory distress syndrome in children. Radiology 157(1):69–74, 1985.
44. Eisenberg M, Bergner L, Hallstrom A: Epidemiology of cardiac arrest and resuscitation in children. Ann Emerg Med 12(11):672–674, 1983.
45. Eriksson A, Bjornstig U: Fatal snowmobile accidents in northern Sweden. J Trauma 22(12):977–982, 1982.
46. Fandel I, Bancalari E: Near drowning in children: Clinical aspects. Pediatrics 58:573, 1976.
47. Fergusson DM, Horwood LJ: Risks of drowning in fenced and unfenced domestic swimming pools. N Z Med J 97(767):777–779, 1984.

48. Fergusson DM, Horwood LJ, Shannon FT: Domestic swimming pool accidents to pre-school children. N Z Med J 96(740):725–727, 1983.

49. Fisher JF, Shadomy S, Teabeaut JR, et al: Near drowning complicated by brain abscess due to *Petriellidium boydii.* Arch Neurol 39(8):511–513, 1982.

50. Fishman RA: Brain edema. N Engl J Med 293:706–711, 1975.

51. Fitch SJ, Gerald B, Magill HL, et al: Central nervous system hypoxia in children due to near drowning. Radiology 156(3):647–650, 1985.

52. Foged N: Diatoms and drowning—Once more. Forensic Sci Int 21(2):153–159, 1983.

53. French J, Ing R, Von Allmen S, et al: Mortality from flash floods: A review of national weather service reports, 1969–81. Public Health Rep 98(6):584–588, 1983.

54. Frewen TC, Sumabat WO, Del Maestro RF: Cerebral blood flow, metabolic rate, and cross-brain oxygen consumption in brain injury. J Pediatr 107(4):510–513, 1985.

55. Frewen TC, Sumabat WO, Han VK, et al: Cerebral resuscitation therapy in pediatric near drowning. J Pediatr 106(4):615–617, 1985.

56. Fuller RH: Drowning and the postimmersion syndrome: A clinico-pathologic study. Milit Med 128:22–36, 1963.

57. Gardiner SC, Smeeton WM, Koelmeyer TD, et al: Accidental drownings in Auckland children. N Z Med J 98(783):579–582, 1985.

58. Gari M, Fruit J, Rousseaux P, et al: *Scedosporium (Monosporium) apiospermum*: Multiple brain abscesses. Sabouraudia 23(5):371–376, 1985.

59. Geddis DC: The exposure of pre-school children to water hazards and the incidence of potential drowning accidents. N Z Med J 97(753):223–226, 1984.

60. Genoni L, Domenighetti G: Near drowning in an adult: Favorable course after a 20-minute submersion. Schweiz Med Wochenschr 112(24):867–870, 1982.

61. Giammona ST, Modell JH: Drowning by total immersion. Effects on pulmonary surfactant of distilled water, isotonic saline, and sea water. Am J Dis Child 114:612–616, 1967.

62. Gooden BA: Drowning and the diving reflex in man. Med J Aust 2:583–587, 1972.

63. Greenberg MI, Baskin SI, Kaplan AM, et al: Effects of endotracheally administered distilled water and normal saline on arterial blood gases in dogs. Ann Emerg Med 11:600–604, 1982.

64. Greensher J: Prevention of childhood injuries. Pediatrics 74(5 Pt 2):970–975, 1984.

65. Gustafsson L: Child health services bear the main responsibility for the prevention of accidents among children. Nord Med 97(8–9):219–221, 1982.

66. Halmagye DFJ: Lung changes and incidence of respiratory arrest in rats after aspiration of sea and fresh water. J Appl Physiol 16:41–44, 1961.

67. Halperin SF, Bass JL, Mehta KA: Unintentional injuries among adolescents and young adults: A review and analysis. J Adolesc Health Care 4(4):275–281, 1983.

68. Hassall IB: Drownings in private swimming pools (letter). N Z Med J 95(702):129–130, 1982.

69. Hayward JS, Hay C, Matthews BR, et al: Temperature effect on the human dive response in relation to cold water near drowning. J Appl Physiol 56(1):202–206, 1984.

70. Heiser MS, Kettrick RG: Management of the drowning victim (review). Clin Sports Med 1(3):409–417, 1982.

71. Hochachka PW: Brain, lung, and heart function during diving and recovery. Science 212:509–510, 1981.

72. Hoff BH: Multisystem failure: A review with special reference to drowning. Crit Care Med 7:310–317, 1979.

73. Jackson RH: Accidents and handicap (review). Dev Med Child Neurol 25(5):656–659, 1983.

74. Jacobsen WK, Mason LJ, Briggs BA, et al: Correlation of spontaneous respiration and neurologic damage in near drowning. Crit Care Med 11(7):487–489, 1983.

75. Janati A, Erba G: Electroencephalographic correlates of near drowning encephalopathy in children. Electroencephalogr Clin Neurophysiol 53(2):182–191, 1982.

76. Jenkinson SG, George RB: Serial pulmonary function studies in survivors of near drowning. Chest 77:777–780, 1980.

77. Johnson EW, Reynolds HT, Stauch D: Duchenne muscular dystrophy: A case with prolonged survival. Arch Phys Med Rehabil 66(4):260–261, 1985.

78. Johnstone JR: Alcohol and drowning (letter). Med J Aust 142(3):234–235, 1985.

79. Jones DR: Cardiac receptors in ducks: The effects of their stimulation and blockade on diving bradycardia. Science 91:455, 1940.

80. Karch SB: Pathology of the heart in drowning. Arch Pathol Lab Med 109(2):176–178, 1985.

81. Karch SB: Pathology of the lung in near drowning. Am J Emerg Med 4(1):4–9, 1986.

82. Karpovich PV: Water in the lungs of drowned animals. Arch Pathol 15:828–833, 1933.

83. Kasian GF, O'Farrell NM, Linwood ME: Bathtub near drowning of an infant in a flotation device. Can Med Assoc J 136(8):843–844, 1987.

84. Kaukinen L: Clinical course and prognostic signs in near drowned patients. Ann Chir Gynaecol 73(1):34–39, 1984.

85. Kelemen G: Temporal bone findings in cases of salt water drowning. Ann Otol Rhinol Laryngol 92(2 Pt 1):134–136, 1983.

86. Kizer K: Aquatic rescue and in-water CPR (letter). Ann Emerg Med 11(3):166–167, 1982.

87. Kizer KW: Resuscitation of submersion casualties (review). Emerg Med Clin North Am 1(3):643–652, 1983.

88. Knobel GJ, deVilliers JC, Parry CD, et al: The causes of non-natural deaths in children over a 15-year period in greater Cape Town. S Afr Med J 66(21):795–801, 1984.

89. Kojima T, Une I, Yashiki M, et al: A case of drowning whilst swimming after thinner-sniffing. Hiroshima J Med Sci 31(1):7–9, 1982.

90. Kollar DJ: Cerebral resuscitation by use of verapamil in a victim of near drowning. Am J Emerg Med 2(2):148–152, 1984.

91. Kram JA, Kizer KW: Submersion injury. Emerg Med Clin North Am 2(3):545–552, 1984.

92. Kurokawa T, Fung KC, Hanai T, et al: Mortality and clinical features in cases of death among epileptic children. Brain Dev 4(5):321–325, 1982.

93. Lang-Runtz H: Preventing accidents in the home. Can Med Assoc J 129(5):482, 484–485, 1983.

94. Langley J: Fencing of private swimming pools in New Zealand. Community Health Stud 7(3):285–289, 1983.

95. Langley J, Silva PA: Swimming experiences and abilities of nine year olds. Br J Sports Med 20(1):39–41, 1986.

96. Laughlin JJ, Eigen H: Pulmonary function abnormalities in survivors of near drowning. J Pediatr 100(1):26–30, 1982.

97. Lee N, Wu JL, Lee CH, et al: *Pseudomonas pseudomallei* infection from drowning: The first reported case in Taiwan. J Clin Microbiol 22(3):352–354, 1985.

98. Levin DL: Neardrowning. Crit Care Med 8:590–595, 1980.

99. Leviten DL, Shulman ST: Multiple nosocomial infections: A risk of modern intensive care. Clin Pediatr (Phila) 19:205–209, 1980.

100. Lewis JK, Minter MG, Eshelman SJ, et al: Outcome of pediatric resuscitation. Ann Emerg Med 12:297–299, 1983.

101. Lindner KH, Dick W, Lotz P: Delayed use of PEEP for respiratory resuscitation following standardized near drowning with fresh and salt water. Anaesthetist 31(12):680–688, 1982.

102. Lindner KH, Dick W, Lotz P: The delayed use of positive end-expiratory pressure (PEEP) during respiratory resuscitation following near drowning with fresh or salt water. Resuscitation 10(3):197–211, 1983.

103. Liu C, Babin RW: A histological comparison of the temporal bone in strangulation and drowning. J Otolaryngol 13(1):44–46, 1984.

104. Lougheed DW: Physiological studies in experimental asphyxia and drowning. Can Med Assoc J 40:423–428, 1939.

105. Lowenfels AB, Miller TT: Alcohol and trauma (review). Ann Emerg Med 13(11):1056–1060, 1984.

106. Lynch P: Alcohol associated deaths in British soldiers. J R Army Med Corps 133(1):34–36, 1987.

107. McComb JG: Intact survival rates in nearly drowned, comatose children (letter). Am J Dis Child 140(6):504–505, 1986.

108. MacLachlan J: Drownings, other aquatic injuries and young Canadians. Can J Public Health 75(3):218–222, 1984.

109. Madsen J: Driving accidents in Denmark 1966–80. Ugeskr Laeger 144(8):523–527, 1982.

110. Manciaux M, Jeanneret O: Accidents involving children and adolescents: From epidemiological findings to preventive action. Rev Epidemiol Sante Publique 31(4):433–444, 1983.

111. Marino RV: Primary prevention of aquatic morbidity. J Am Osteopath Assoc 85(6):367–369, 1985.

112. Martin TG: Near drowning and cold water immersion (review). Ann Emerg Med 13(4):263–273, 1984.

113. Mason LJ, Jacobsen WK, Lau CA, et al: Temperature instability as an early predictive factor of brain death in paediatric near drowning victims. Acta Anaesthesiol Belg 36(3):230–233, 1985.

114. Maull KI: Alcohol abuse: Its implications in trauma care. South Med J 75(7):794–798, 1982.

115. Mayer T, Walker ML: Emergency intracranial pressure monitoring in pediatrics: Management of the acute coma of brain insult. Clin Pediatr (Phila) 21(7):391–396, 1982.

116. Modell JH: Drown versus near drown: A discussion of definitions. Crit Care Med 9:351–352, 1981.

117. Modell JH: Treatment of near drowning: Is there a role for H.Y.P.E.R. therapy? Crit Care Med 14(6):593–594, 1986.

118. Modell JH: Near drowning. Circulation 74(6 Pt 2):IV27–28, 1986.

119. Modell JH, Calderwood HW, Ruiz BC, et al: Effects of ventilatory patterns on arterial oxygenation after near drowning in sea water. Anesthesiology 40:376–384, 1974.

120. Modell JH, Davis JH: Electrolyte changes in human drowning victims. Anesthesia 30:414–420, 1969.

121. Modell JH, Davis JH, Giammona ST, et al: Blood gas and electrolyte changes in human near drowning victims. JAMA 203:337–343, 1968.

122. Modell JH, Gaub M, Moya F, et al: Physiologic effects of near drowning with chlorinated fresh water, distilled water and isotonic saline. Anesthesiology 27:33–41, 1966.

123. Modell JH, Graves SA, Ketover A: Clinical course of 91 consecutive near drowning victims. Chest 70:231–238, 1976.

124. Modell JH, Graves SA, Kuck EJ: Near drowning: Correlation of level of consciousness and survival. Can Anaesth Soc J 27:211–215, 1980.

125. Modell JH, Kuck EJ, Ruiz BC, et al: Effect of intravenous vs. aspirated distilled water on serum electrolytes and blood gas tensions. J Appl Physiol 32:579–584, 1972.

126. Modell JH, Moya F, Newby EJ, et al: The effects of fluid volume in sea water drowning. Ann Intern Med 57:68–80, 1967.

127. Monroe B: Immersion accidents in hot tubs and whirlpool spas. Pediatrics 69:805–808, 1982.

128. Murray RR, Kapila A, Blanco E, et al: Cerebral computed tomography in drowning victims. AJNR 5(2):177–179, 1984.

129. Neal JM: Near drowning (review). J Emerg Med 3(1):41–52, 1985.

130. Neale TJ, Dewar JM, Parr R, et al: Acute renal failure following near drowning in salt water. N Z Med J 97(756):3199–3222, 1984.

131. Nixon J, Pearn J, Wilkey I, et al: Fifteen years of child drowning—a 1967–1981 analysis of all fatal cases from the Brisbane Drowning Study and an 11 year study of consecutive near drowning cases. Accid Anal Prev 18(3):199–203, 1986.

132. Noguchi M, Kimula Y, Ogata T: Muddy lung. Am J Clin Pathol 83(2):240–244, 1985.

133. Nussbaum E, Galant SP: Intracranial pressure monitoring as a guide to prognosis in the nearly drowned, severely comatose child. J Pediatr 102(2):215–218, 1983.

134. Oakes DD, Sherck JP, Maloney JR, et al: Prognosis and management of victims of near drowning. J Trauma 22(7):544–549, 1982.

135. O'Connor PJ: Accidental death in Australian children. Aust Paediatr J 19(4):230–232, 1983.

136. O'Donohoe NV: What should the child with epilepsy be allowed to do? Arch Dis Child 58(11):934–937, 1983.

137. Oren A, Etzion Z, Broitman D, et al: Renal involvement following near drowning in the sea. Comp Biochem Physiol A 73(2):175–179, 1982.

138. Orlowski JP: Prognostic factors in pediatric cases of drowning and near drowning. JACEP 8:176–179, 1979.

139. Orlowski JP: Drowning, near drowning, and ice-water submersions (review). Pediatr Clin North Am 34(1):75–92, 1987.

140. Orlowski JP, Abulleil MM, Phillips JM: Effects of tonicities of saline solutions on pulmonary injury in drowning. Crit Care Med 15(2):126–130, 1987.

141. Orlowski JP, Rothner AD, Lueders H: Submersion accidents in children with epilepsy. Am J Dis Child 136(9):777–780, 1982.

142. Ornato JP: Special resuscitation situations: Near drowning, traumatic injury, electric shock, and hypothermia (review). Circulation 74(6 Pt 2):IV23–26, 1986.

143. O'Shea JS, Collins EW, Butler CB: Pediatric accident prevention. Clin Pediatr (Phila) 21(5):290–297, 1982.

144. Pearn J: Epilepsy and drowning in childhood. BMJ 1:1510–1511, 1977.

145. Pearn J: Aquatics for epileptic children. Aust Paediatr J 18(4):255–256, 1982.

146. Pearn J: Drowning and alcohol. Med J Aust 141(1):6–7, 1984.

147. Pearn JH: Secular trends in fatal and disabling child trauma. Aust Paediatr J 21(2):81–84, 1985.

148. Pearn JH: Current controversies in child accident prevention. An analysis of some areas of dispute in the prevention of child trauma (review). Aust N Z J Med 15(6):782–787, 1985.

149. Pearn J, Nixon J: Bathtub immersion accidents involving children. Med J Aust 1:211–213, 1977.

150. Pearn J, Nixon J: Prevention of childhood drowning accidents. Med J Aust 1:616–618, 1977.

151. Pearn J, Nixon J: Attempted drowning as a form of non-accidental injury. Aust Pediatr J 13:110–113, 1977.

152. Pedersen MB, Simonsen J: Accidental death in fermentation tanks: Report of two cases. Med Sci Law 22(4):283–284, 1982.

153. Peterson B: Morbidity of childhood near drowning. Pediatrics 59:364, 1977.

154. Pfenninger J, Gerber A, Tschappeler H, et al: Adult respiratory distress syndrome in children. J Pediatr 101(3):352–357, 1982.

155. Pfenninger J, Sutter M: Intensive care after fresh water immersion accidents in children. Anaesthesia 37(12):1157–1162, 1982.

156. Pitt WR: Increasing incidence of childhood immersion injury in Brisbane. Med J Aust 144(13):683–685, 1986.

157. Plueckhahn VD: Alcohol and accidental submersion from watercraft and surrounds. Med Sci Law 17:246–250, 1977.

158. Plueckhahn VD: Alcohol consumption and death by drowning in adults. A 24-year epidemiological analysis. J Stud Alcohol 43(5):445–452, 1982.

159. Plueckhahn VD: Alcohol and accidental drowning. A 25-year study. Med J Aust 141(1):22–25, 1984.

160. Pratt FD, Haynes BE: Incidence of "secondary drowning" after salt water submersion. Ann Emerg Med 15(9):1084–1087, 1986.

161. Ramey CA, Ramey DN, Hayward JS: Dive response of children in relation to cold water near drowning. J Appl Physiol 63(2):665–668, 1987.

162. Ranner G, Juan H, Udermann H: On the evidential value of diatoms in cases of death by drowning (author's transl). Z Rechtsmed 88(1–2):57–65, 1982.

163. Rappaport M, Maloney JR, Ortega H, et al: Survival in young children after drowning: Brain evoked potentials as outcome predictors. Clin Electroencephalogr 16(4):183–191, 1985.

164. Redmond AD, Mallikarjun TS: Resuscitation from drowning. Arch Emerg Med 1(2):113–115, 1984.

165. Rivara FP: Epidemiology of violent deaths in children and adolescents in the United States. Pediatrician 12(1):3–10, 1983–85.

166. Roberts P: The management of near drowning with hypothermia. N Z Nurs J 75(4):8–9, 1982.

167. Robertson C: A review of the use of corticosteroids in the management of pulmonary injuries and insults. Arch Emerg Med 2(2):59–65, 1985.

168. Robinson MD, Seward PN: Submersion injury in children (review). Pediatr Emerg Care 3(1):44–49, 1987.

169. Rogers MC: Near drowning: Cold water on a hot topic? J Pediatr 106(4):603–604, 1985.

170. Rowe MI, Arango A, Allington G: Profile of pediatric drowning victims in a water oriented society. J Trauma 17:587–591, 1977.

171. Ruiz BC, Calderwood HW, Modell JH, et al: Effects of ventilatory patterns on arterial oxygenation after near drowning with fresh water: A comparative study in dogs. Anesth Analg 52:570–576, 1973.

172. Saenghirunvattana S, Klongkumnuangarn R: Early PEEP in the treatment of a freshwater near drowning patient. J Med Assoc Thai 67(4):258–261, 1984.

173. Samuelson T, Doolittle W, Hayward J, et al: Hypothermia and cold water near drowning: Treatment guidelines. Alaska Med 24(6):106–111, 1982.

174. Sarnaik AP, Preston G, Lieh-Lai M: Intracranial pressure and cerebral perfusion pressure in near drowning. Crit Care Med 13(4):224–227, 1985.

175. Sarnaik AP, Vohra MP: Near drowning: Fresh, salt, and cold water immersion (review). Clin Sports Med 5(1):33–46, 1986.

176. Scott PH, Eigen H: Immersion accidents involving pails of water in the home. J Pediatr 96:282–284, 1980.

177. Shiono H, Maya A, Tabata N, et al: Medicolegal aspects of infanti-

cide in Hokkaido District, Japan. Am J Forensic Med Pathol 7(2):104–106, 1986.

178. Sibert JR: Children's accidents. New hope for prevention. Practitioner 227(1376):205–208, 1983.

179. Siebke H, Breivik H, Rod T, et al: Survival after 40 minutes submersion without cerebral sequelae. Lancet 1:1275–1277, 1975.

180. Simcock AD: Treatment of near drowning—A review of 130 cases. Anaesthesia 41(6):643–648, 1986.

181. Sims JK, Enomoto PI, Frankel RI, et al: Marine bacteria complicating sea water near drowning and marine wounds: A hypothesis. Ann Emerg Med 12(4):212–216, 1983.

182. Singh B: A case report of "drowning" in a bitumen tank. Med Sci Law 22(1):51–52, 1982.

183. Singh B, Ganeson D, Chattopadhyay PK: Pattern of suicides in Delhi—A study of the cases reported at the Police Morgue, Delhi. Med Sci Law 22(3):195–198, 1982.

184. Sirik Z, Lev A, Rauch M, et al: Freshwater near drowning: Our experience in life supportive treatment. Isr J Med Sci 20(6):523–527, 1984.

185. Spyker DA: Submersion injury. Epidemiology, prevention, and management. Pediatr Clin North Am 32(1):113–125, 1985.

186. Statistical Abstract of the United States, Bureau of the Census. US Department of Commerce, 1979.

187. Statistical Abstract of the United States, Bureau of the Census. US Department of Commerce, 1982.

188. Statistical Bulletin (Metropolitan Life Insurance Co.). June 1977, pp 9–11.

189. Stitt VJ Jr: Drowning in North Carolina: How you can prevent unnecessary loss of life. N C Med J 54(6):432–433, 1982.

190. Strauss RH: Medical concerns in underwater sports. Pediatr Clin North Am 29(6):1431–1440, 1982.

191. Stromme SB, Kerem D, Elner R, et al: Diving bradycardia during rest and exercise and its relation to physical fitness. J Appl Physiol 28:614–621, 1970.

192. Strope GL, Stempel DA: Risk factors associated with the development of chronic lung disease in children. Pediatr Clin North Am 31(4):757–771, 1984.

193. Suzuki T, Ikeda N, Umetsu K, et al: Swimming and loss of consciousness. Z Rechtsmed 94(2):121–126, 1985.

194. Swann HG, Brucer M, Moore C, et al: Fresh water and sea water drowning: A study of the terminal cardiac and biochemical events. Texas Rep Biol Med 5:423–427, 1947.

195. Swann HG, Spafford NR: Body salt and water changes during fresh and sea water drowning. Texas Rep Biol Med 9:356–382, 1951.

196. Taylor SB, Quencer RM, Holzman BH, et al: Central nervous system anoxic-ischemic insult in children due to near drowning. Radiology 156(3):641–646, 1985.

197. Tether P, Harrison L: Alcohol-related fires and drownings. Br J Addict 81(3):425–431, 1986.

198. Theilade D: The danger of fatal misjudgment in hypothermia after immersion: Successful resuscitation following immersion for 25 minutes. Anaesthesia 32:889–892, 1977.

199. Tisherman S, Chabal C, Safar P, et al: Resuscitation of dogs from cold water submersion using cardiopulmonary bypass. Ann Emerg Med 14(5):389–396, 1985.

200. Tointon JA: Sports injuries in the services 1969–1980. J R Army Med Corps 180(3):193–197, 1984.

201. Torphy DE, Minter MG, Thompson BM: Cardiorespiratory arrest and resuscitation in children. Am J Dis Child 138:1099–1102, 1984.

202. Torre C, Varetto L, Tappi E: Scanning electron microscopic ultrastructural alteration of the pulmonary alveolus in experimental drowning. J Forensic Sci 28(4):1008–1012, 1983.

203. Tyler DC, Redding G, Hall D, et al: Increased intracranial pressure: An indication to decompress a tension pneumomediastinum. Crit Care Med 12(5):467–468, 1984.

204. Vieira DF, Van-Saene HK, Miranda DR: Invasive pulmonary aspergillosis after near drowning. Intensive Care Med 10(4):203–204, 1984.

205. Walker S, Middelkamp JN: Pail immersion accidents. Clin Pediatr 20:341–343, 1981.

206. Wegener FH, Edwards RM: Cerebral support for near drowned children in a temperate environment. Med J Aust 2:135–137, 1980.

207. White RD: CPR: Basic life support. Clin Symp 34:(6):3–30, 1982.

208. Wintemute GJ, Kraus JF, Teret SP, et al: Drowning in childhood and adolescence: A population-based study. Am J Public Health 77(7):830–832, 1987.

209. Wong LL, McNamara J-J: Salt water drowning. Hawaii Med J 43(6):208, 210, 1984.

210. Wood VM: Steroids in near drowning questioned (letter). JACEP 8:91–92, 1979.

211. Wunderlich P, Rupprecht E, Trefftz F, et al: Chest radiographs of near drowned children. Pediatr Radiol 15(5):297–299, 1985.

212. Wynne JW, Modell JH: Respiratory aspiration of stomach contents. Ann Intern Med 87:466–474, 1977.

213. Yagil Y, Stalnikowicz R, Michaeli J, et al: Near drowning in the Dead Sea. Electrolyte imbalances and therapeutic implications. Arch Intern Med 145(1):50–53, 1985.

214. Yamamoto K, Yamamoto Y, Kikuchi H: The effects of drowning media on the lung water content. An experimental study on rats. Z Rechtsmed 90(1):1–6, 1983.

Walter S. Cain
William D. King

CHAPTER THIRTY-NINE

Chemical Injuries to the Upper Alimentary Tract

The ingestion of certain chemicals may lead to severe damage of the upper alimentary tract. The prevention and treatment of injuries so sustained have long been a challenge and a burden to our society, most significantly to the health professionals and to the families of the afflicted. In this industrialized and inventive society, the chemical agents involved and the forms in which they are presented are numerous. Most commonly, these materials are intended for household cleansing, washing, bleaching, and disinfecting and sometimes for industrial and medicinal purposes. The injurious effects are generally secondary to the extreme basic or acidic contents. In the North American pediatric population, the ingestion of basic materials is prevalent and the event is usually accidental.

Efforts to manage the chemical injuries are preferably targeted toward prevention, because restoration of the significantly damaged structures, particularly the esophagus, has significant limitations. To date, preventive approaches have been rewarded by a general decrease in the severity of the damage sustained. Refinements in treatment seem to have resulted in lowered morbidity and mortality rates.

CHEMICAL AGENTS

A variety of materials when placed in direct contact have the capability of destroying tissue. They have been called *caustics, corrosives,* and *escharotics,* the terms being used interchangeably. The substances are usually further identified as either base or acid on the basis of the hydrogen ion concentration (pH); the injury potential of any substance is directly related to its distance from one of the extremes. The concentrated forms of base materials, usually sodium hydroxide or potassium hydroxide, have been called various names, including caustic sodas and lye.

The caustics appear in a number of domestic products. The base corrosives are seen in a variety of cleansing agents, including drain and oven cleaners, detergents, bleaches, and ammonia. Less frequent but important sources of corrosive injury include batteries, Clinitest tablets, and various medicinal agents. In the household the acids appear most commonly as toilet bowl cleaners. The pH seems to be the most significant factor affecting the damage.[58] Materials with pH levels above 12.0 and below 1.5 are most likely to be associated with severe corrosive injuries. Table 39–1 includes a representative group of caustic agents found on grocery and pharmacy shelves along with their respective hydrogen ion concentrations. The pH was tested in our laboratory with an electronic meter. The container label often did not identify the specific contents, and the pH was never listed.

INCIDENCE

The true frequency of ingestion of corrosive materials remains elusive, but current data suggest that the rate is much higher than the long-reported estimate of 5000 ingestions annually by children younger than 5 years of age.[57] This figure was determined from the report of the National Clearinghouse for Poison Control Centers in 1969 of 500

Table 39–1

Examples of Caustic Agents Available in the United States

Agent	pH
Ammonia	11.80
Bleach	11.43
Battery (disk)	11.60
Clinitest tablet	13.94
Detergent (dishwasher)	11.71
Drain cleaner	13.13
Hair relaxer	13.54
Medications	
Doxycycline	2.00
Emepronium bromide	2.75
Oven cleaner	13.54
Toilet cleaner	1.00

such ingestions when there was an estimated 10% penetrance of population. Since 1984 the American Association of Poison Control Centers National Data Collection System has assumed reporting responsibility, with a resultant increased accuracy and penetrance of population to an estimated 55% during 1986. Based on this figure and the reported 27,992 caustic ingestions by children younger than 6 years of age, approximately 50,000 ingestions occurred in this population group in the United States in 1986.[35] Males were involved twice as often as females.

Two age segments of the population have sustained caustic burns most commonly: children younger than 5 years of age and young adults. Essentially all in the former group are accidental ingestions, whereas many in the latter group are secondary to suicidal intent. Of the 206 cases reviewed at The Children's Hospital of Alabama, 80% were 2 years or younger and 95% were younger than 5 years of age. Ninety-eight percent were reported as unintentional events. Lye or a strong caustic was ingested on 161 (77%) occasions. Ammonia (14), bleach (7), detergents (7), acids (4), and Clinitest tablets (4) were less frequently reported.

PATHOGENESIS

On Ingestion of Alkaline Caustics

On ingestion of materials of significantly high pH, especially those above 11, a series of events occurs that is predictable and that is influenced by several factors. On contact with tissue, in this case mucosa, the process of liquefaction necrosis begins immediately, with a dissolution of surface proteins allowing for the rapid penetration of underlying layers. This process proceeds until the chemicals involved are dissipated. The concentration, quantity, and viscosity of the caustic agent; the exposure time; and the luminal contents before ingestion all influence the depth of injury.

The potency of alkaline corrosives was emphasized by laboratory investigations performed by Krey.[31] With a series of 10-second contacts of the agent to the rabbit esophagus, the following observations were made. A 1 N (3.8%) solution of NaOH produces necrosis of the mucosa and submucosa and encroaches onto the muscularis. A 3 N (10.7%) solution extends the injury into the circular muscle, and a 7 N (22%) solution penetrates the entire thickness of the wall and invades the periesophageal tissues. Ashcraft and Padula had a similar experience and found that potassium hydroxide was more potent.[5]

The oropharynx and esophagus, with their alkaline secretions, are more likely to be injured by base caustics than is the stomach. Nevertheless, the gastric wall is vulnerable to damage when exposed to larger volumes and more potent agents. The pattern of injury is somewhat related to chance but is influenced by the normal sites of external compression, spasm, and regurgitation. A more significant influence on the topography of damage is the physical state of the offending agent. The solid caustics, such as crystals, tend to adhere on first contact with the mucosa, usually in the oral cavity or lips, from which point the diluted chemicals may stream to precipitate irregular patterns of damage. The encased forms, such as batteries, to become clinically significant, lodge at sites of constriction or sluggish motility, where they adhere and cause relatively localized but sometimes severe damage. The liquefied caustics are generally the most injurious, as they tend to pass more freely and bathe all areas circumferentially.

Clinical studies of caustic injuries and their spontaneous repair have served as guides to clinical management. The investigative work of Haller and Bachman defined the pathologic events following significant damage from an alkaline caustic and categorized the damage into three overlapping stages.[26] During the first week, necrosis and inflammation are dominant along with associated bacterial infiltration, all encouraging softening of the esophageal wall, if not perforation. The second phase initiates during the first week with sloughage of tissue, ulceration, and granulation formation as new vessels appear along with fibroblasts and begin the deposition of collagen, glycoproteins, and mucopolysaccharides. The last stage begins during the third week with continual deposition and maturation of collagen to replace the damaged deep layers that have little regenerative capacity. Resurfacing with stratified squamous epithelium without glands is generally rapid. As the collagen organizes, a dense form of connective tissue follows, with associated contracture, with the potential to decrease the lumen and shorten the length of the hollow viscus. These morphologic alterations are associated with dysfunction. Butler and colleagues emphasized that the mature scar is intramural, thin, and not associated with hypertrophied tissue.[10, 11] This lack of substance and loss of elasticity is compatible with the propensity of these injured organs to perforation on bougienage.

The cicatrix of short length must involve 75% or more of the circumference to produce a functionally obstructive site. More lengthy injuries may cause dysfunction with less circumferential involvement. Not infrequently, early motility irregularities are seen to clear spontaneously, suggesting that the inflammatory reaction is a primary contributor. The longitudinal contraction of the esophagus has led to gastroesophageal reflux and sometimes to partial displacement of the stomach into the thorax (Fig. 39–1). Gastric regurgitation has the potential of antagonizing healing of the initial damage and compounding the subsequent cicatrix.

The length of this last maturation phase is influenced by the extent of the initial insult and subsequent antagonists. In the uncomplicated process, collagen, the main source of connective tissue and subsequent wound strength, is completely deposited in 2 to 3 weeks.[44] The tensile strength of the wound is gained as collagen fibrils form and cross-link both intra- and intermolecularly. Further maturation and strengthening occur as the fibers remodel. The completion of this process and the stabilization of the scar probably require 12 months or longer based on clinical experiences.

Among the acute potentials of the extended caustic damage are perforation, fistula formation, mediastinitis, peritonitis, and hemorrhage. These ill-effects may be delayed while the initial damage is augmented by inflammation and infection or manipulation (e.g., endoscopy, bougienage), or a combination of these.

On Ingestion of Acid Caustics

In most series reported from the United States, the ingestion of acidic agents is much less frequent but often is associated with more serious injuries than those seen with alkaline caustics. Although the stomach, with its acid environment, has been more vulnerable to injury by these agents, the oral and esophageal walls are often damaged with the same exposure.[37, 42] Three of the four children who ingested acid in our series subsequently developed severe esophageal stenosis.

The low pH chemicals produce an eschar from a coagulation type of necrosis. The protective coagulum discourages deep penetration, but full thickness damage with perforation readily occurs with the more potent exposures.

The pattern of injury on ingestion of the larger volumes or the concentrated acid materials is somewhat predictable. After coating and injuring the esophagus, the chemical proceeds along the lesser curvature of the stomach. Pylorospasm allows the agent to pool in the prepyloric region, where the most severe damage characteristically occurs. Although prompt perforation may occur, full thickness necrosis and breakdown may follow a latency period of 7 to 10 days. Circumferential damage has often led to pyloric stenosis and obstructive symptoms after a 3-week interval.[37, 49]

Battery-Induced Injuries

Batteries, both the cylindric and the disk types, are apparently ingested often by the pediatric patient as more than 500 cases are reported each year.[34] The disk batteries are particularly hazardous as they may adhere to the esophageal mucosa with breakdown of the container and spillage of the alkaline contents. Focal caustic injuries including stenosis, perforation, fistulas, and death have been recorded.[38, 59] This potential rapidity of deep injury mandates prompt investigation when a battery ingestion, especially the disk type, is reported. If the chest radiograph identifies the battery in the esophagus, immediate esophagoscopy and removal are indicated. Disk batteries rarely lead to complications once they reach the gastrointestinal tract; however they should

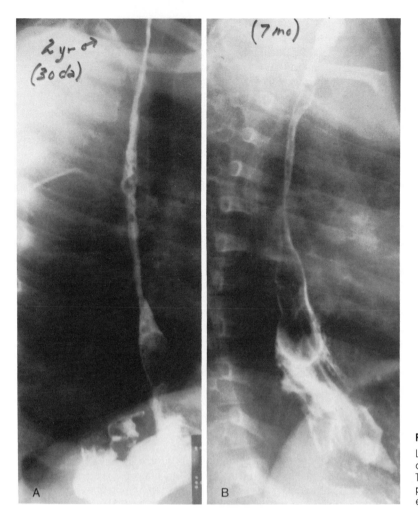

FIGURE 39–1

Lateral views of barium esophagograms at 30 days (A) and 7 months (B) after lye ingestion. The shortening of the esophagus and the displacement of the stomach into the chest is evident.

be followed by radiograph every 4 days and removed if they remain in the same place for 2 days.

Medicine-Induced Injuries

Medications have led to esophageal damage by both direct and indirect routes. Such an event is much more common in adults but is also not infrequently seen in children. Various agents, usually of low pH, have been involved.[8] Although the damage is usually limited to superficial erosion, deeper injuries have been seen. On complaints of retrosternal pain and dysphagia, particularly after a capsule or tablet ingestion, esophagoscopy is indicated to establish a diagnosis and continue appropriate management.

Clinitest Tablets

Clinitest tablets, used for semiquantitative testing for glycosuria, have caused deep localized damage to the esophagus in children. The injury is caused by the excessive heat generated by the chemical reaction as well as the high pH on dissolution. The dissolving tablet is best treated by the immediate ingestion of water and then a chest radiograph and esophagoscopy to assess the damage should the clinical picture suggest a complication.

CLINICAL PRESENTATION

The child who ingests a corrosive material usually experiences immediate oral, if not substernal, pain. On prompt presentation for medical attention, most often the patient presents with ulceration or edema, or both, of the oral mucosa (Fig. 39–2). One or more of the following symptoms are often seen: drooling, dysphagia, vomiting, substernal pain, and epigastric pain. The absence of oral change does not eliminate esophageal injury because the initial presentation has not correlated well with the severity of the esophageal injury. However, the greater the number and persistence of the signs and symptoms, the greater the damage suggested. Increasing pain and evidence of toxicity or even shock suggest mediastinitis, peritonitis, or both.

Although infrequent, respiratory symptoms deserve special attention, as significant laryngotracheal damage may be inflicted. Prompt inspection, cautious intubation, and possibly tracheostomy are indicated. These injuries also imply severe esophageal damage.

The patient may not present for days or even weeks after

the accident, for various reasons. The delayed presentations are often provoked by dysphagia, a manifestation of esophageal obstruction. The initial event may not be identified in this setting.

DIAGNOSIS

The diagnostic challenge includes establishing that a caustic material was ingested, determining the chemical contents, and identifying the anatomic surfaces injured as well as estimating the depth of penetration.

The proof of injury to the pharynx, esophagus, and stomach following caustic ingestion usually depends on endoscopy. However, when a mild acidic or basic agent (pH by measurement between 1.5 and 11.5) is ingested, a significant injury is very unlikely, obviating the need for the procedure. However, when faced with a history of ingestion of a potent material, with or without visible oral damage, direct viewing of the respective mucosal surfaces seems obligatory. In our experience, 9% of those with esophageal injuries exhibited no oral involvement, and 76% of the children with mouth damage had no distal pathologic condition.

As is discussed, radiographs are not used generally in the initial assessment for alimentary tract damage. However, in severe cases, evidence of free air would be diagnostic.

When available, analysis of the offending agent (by pH meter) has been very practical in the assessment of the injury, management, and prognosis.

Endoscopy

Although endoscopy has received increasing acceptance as the mainstay in the acute management of chemical injuries, the usage and expectations have varied. It seems safest to

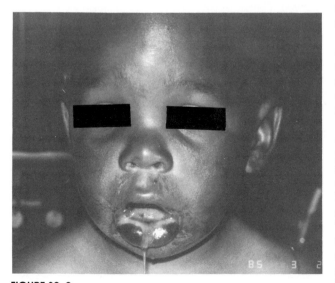

FIGURE 39–2

Acute injury of the lip and tongue from the ingestion of a caustic substance. Associated drooling.

Table 39–2
Grading of Esophageal Injury

Grade	Depth of Injury	Endoscopic Appearance
I (mild or superficial)	Mucosa	Swollen, erythema
II (moderate)	Submucosa	Superficial ulcers
	Muscularis mucosa	Friable, exudate
III (severe or deep)	Submucosa longitudinal muscle	Deep ulcers, loose tissue, bleeding
IV (perforating)	Periesophageal tissue and beyond	Eschar, visible perforation, hemorrhage

have an experienced endoscopist perform the procedure under general anesthesia within 24 hours of the ingestion. Previous experience had been with rigid esophagoscopes, and the inspection was discontinued at the first sighting of injury. Currently, the smaller caliber flexible gastroscopes are used with seemingly increased safety while inspecting the length of the esophagus and the stomach. No perforations have occurred with either approach in our experience. The latter technique allows for a more extensive and accurate assessment of the damage. The very pertinent definition of the depth of injury remains elusive via surface inspection. Separation of the burned areas into superficial, moderate, and deep is probably as accurate and practical as can be expected (Table 39–2).

Radiologic Assessment

Plain radiographs of the chest and sometimes the abdomen are indicated in the initial assessment. Contrast studies of the upper alimentary tract are not included routinely but may be revealing in special situations, for example, if advanced necrosis and perforation are suspected. They are unlikely to identify changes in cases of mild injury, and they demonstrate pathologic conditions inconsistently in cases of moderate damage.

Characteristic plain radiographic findings that are indicative of extension of the pathologic condition beyond the confines of the esophagus or stomach are periesophageal soft tissue thickening and widening of the mediastinum; displacement of the pleural reflection; and free air in the mediastinum, pleural space, or peritoneal cavity.

Contrast studies of the esophagus and stomach performed early are probably best accomplished with propyliodone in peanut oil (Dionosil Oily) (Glaxo Pharmaceuticals, Research Triangle Park, NC) to avoid the potential irritation of the airway and mediastinum. Franken and Martel have highlighted the features that might accompany moderate to severe damage to the esophagus short of perforation.[18, 36] The mildest demonstrable changes may be thickening of the mucosal folds and sluggish motility (Fig. 39–3). Ulcerations are suggested by linear streaking, persistence, and scalloping of the contrast material in the esophageal wall. The dilated, aperistaltic esophagus is seen in the most severe injuries and is compatible with impending perforation (Fig. 39–4). The atonic esophagus usually constricts pro-

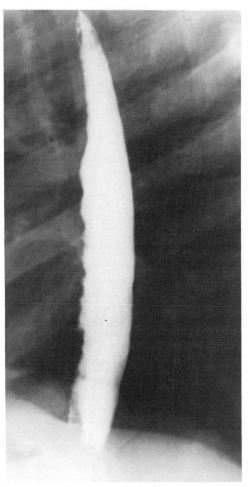

FIGURE 39–3
Barium esophagogram demonstrating mucosal edema and slight dilation. No residue of injury now.

gressively thereafter to severe stenosis (Fig. 39–5). Kuhn and Tunell pointed out the increased accuracy of cine-esophagography in assessing motility, identifying pathologic conditions, and prognosticating.[32]

Barium contrast studies are preferable in the late evaluations. Early evidence of permanent damage is usually present within 3 weeks but may be progressive for lengthy periods thereafter (see Fig. 39–5). The pattern may vary widely, although most commonly the strictures correspond to the normal sites of anatomic pressure.

PREVENTION

The approach to management of an injury that can be so instantaneous and severely destructive must give first priority to preventive measures. In view of the diversity of current products and the marketing of new products that have the chemical potential to be corrosive, a broad-based preventive effort must be made to be effective. As with other health problems, prevention rests on recognition of the principle that interactions among the agent, the host, and the environment determine the injury risk in the population.

When applying this epidemiologic model to corrosive ingestion in children, each of the three factors must be defined and then interventions should be targeted to affect these factors.

1. *Host:* refers to the victim, most commonly an inquisitive, curious, exploring toddler or a preschooler who mouths the environment in an effort to learn
2. *Environment:* the physical as well as the psychosocial surroundings of the child
3. *Agent:* the toxin and its potential harm in the form of the amount of chemical energy it can release

Preventive measures targeted to preschool-aged hosts begin with the recognition that they are high-risk individuals. Measures to change the ingestion behavior of this age group seem unrealistic, as change tends to alter the course of their normal development. As an extension of the child host, the parents, along with the public in general, can be educated to increase their awareness of the importance of poison prevention and of the ingestion behavior of the preschooler. Efforts to educate are already in place in the schools and various media, and the benefits of these efforts are evident.

The physical environment has long been a fundamental point of attack. Investigation has indicated that ingested poisons are usually within easy reach or in "eye contact" of the child.[4] One third or more of the ingestions occurred in the kitchen, where many chemical products were stored at floor level or on a counter top.[4] The obvious intervention is to store these products out of reach, sight, and climbing ability and preferably under lock. Guidelines for poison-proofing the home are available and should be distributed in all health facilities and publicized by the media. A contrary position has been advanced by the work of at least two investigators, who have indicated that the accessibility of the agents is not a very significant cause of the ingestion.[6, 50]

The psychosocial environment and its influence on poison ingestion has received considerable attention and investigation.[47, 60] Live-event stress in the family (e.g., chronic illness, separation, unemployment, death, pregnancy, and relocation of the residence) has correlated with an increased risk of poison ingestion. Data pertaining to family stress and ingestion risk may be helpful in identifying high-risk families. A clinician can use appropriate questionnaires to target the high-risk families and patients before further discussion on safety in the home and poison control.

The most effective interventions in poison control have been those that targeted the agents. The classic example of this was the 65% decline in aspirin poisoning that followed the Poison Prevention Packaging Act of 1970.[12]

Initially, most of the caustic materials available for home use were available in a solid or crystalline form. The liquid form became available in the 1960s. Immediately thereafter there was a distinct rise in the severity of the burns. The cleansing agents often contained sodium hydroxide or potassium hydroxide in concentrations of 30 to 40%. Following the passage of the packaging act of 1970, the concentration dropped in many cases to 5 to 8%, and an associated decrease was noted in the severity of the injuries sustained. Further benefit undoubtedly would be gained by eliminating

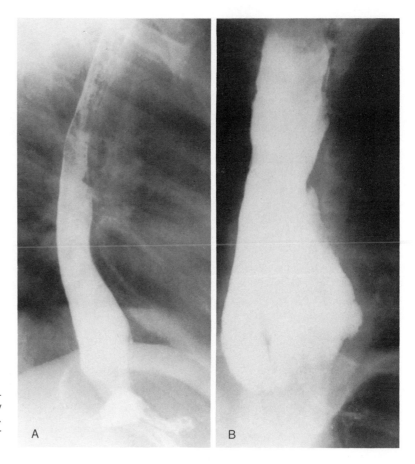

FIGURE 39–4
Barium esophagograms following lye ingestion. *A*, Normal study on day 1. *B*, Day 12 study finds a dilated atonic irregular surfaced organ. Patient expired the following day with an esophagoaortic fistula.

these strong acid and base corrosives for domestic use and replacing them with innovative agents such as "grease-eating bacteria" preparations for opening drains. It is also appropriate to further develop child-resistant containers and to better label them as to harmful contents.

In summary, the model prevention strategy is to address not one but all of the epidemiologic factors involved with the injury in question. It seems reasonable to expect that continued efforts toward prevention of chemical injuries will reap further benefits.

COMPLICATIONS

Stenosis

Cicatrix formation is an inevitable result of the reparative process of a deep burn. The normal maturation process of a circumferential injury includes shortening of the collagen fibers and stenosis. Foreshortening also occurs when the length involved is significant. Six reports with a total experience of 972 caustic exposures in the pediatric population identified 247 burns of the esophagus. Of those sustaining burns, 51 developed stenoses, for an average of 20%.[14, 21, 25, 41, 53, 56] Thus, scar formation represents the most common major complication in the care of these patients. Intense laboratory and clinical investigations have pursued measures to avoid or reduce the cicatrix.

Antibiotics have contributed by reducing the inflamma-

tory process, bacterial translocation, and frank infection.[31, 51] Ampicillin is used until the injury sites have resurfaced. During prolonged usage, an antifungal agent such as mystatin (Mycostatin) is given as a preventive measure.

Antacids are used to neutralize the refluxing gastric contents.

Steroids have received considerable attention in the treatment of corrosive burns for more than 30 years. In 1950, Spain and subsequently others have indicated their favorable influence on inflammation, fibroplasia, collagen synthesis, and suppression of stricture formation.[26, 51, 62] Clinical experience has raised doubts regarding their benefits.[15, 30, 39, 43, 61]

The consensus now is that superficial mucosal burns do not form strictures. All deep or full thickness injuries heal by scarring regardless of the use of steroids, which may actually be detrimental. Currently, the most reasonable use of these agents, if any, is in the presence of moderate burns or laryngeal and tracheal damage, or both. Steroids are contraindicated in the presence of perforation, impending perforation, and active infection. Antibiotics should be given with steroids.

Efforts to selectively control the early development of collagen and, indirectly, its natural tendency to form a firm scar have met with success in animal studies.[11, 22] *Lathyrogenic agents,* namely, B-aminoproprionitrile (BAPN), D-penicillamine, and colchicine, have been shown to interrupt the intermolecular and intramolecular cross-linkages of fragile collagen fibers. This effectively causes a permanent

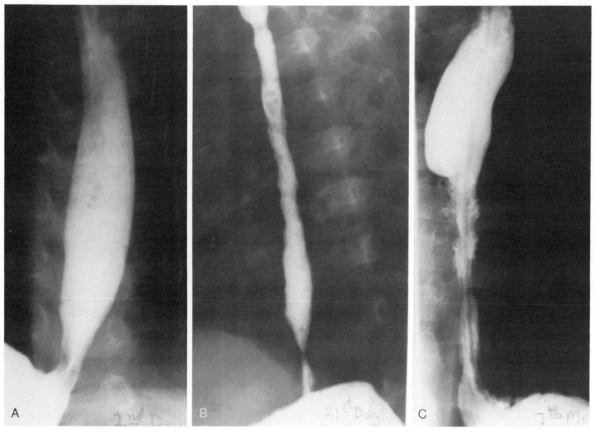

FIGURE 39–5

Maturation of an esophagus that was severely injured by the ingestion of lye. *A,* Dilated, atonic on day 2. *B,* Long, marked narrowing on day 21. *C,* Residual severe stenosis of the distal half following bougienage (7 months). Colon bypass was performed.

change in the physical properties, leading to a softer cicatrix. D-penicillamine (Cuprimine) is available but has not been cleared for use in the management of scar tissue.[22, 44]

Intraluminal stenting of the injured esophagus has resulted in reported clinical successes.[13, 27, 40] The concept has merit, as the Silastic tube prevents opposing granulating surfaces from coating, serves as a template for re-epithelialization, and temporarily prevents contraction of immature collagen until resurfacing is complete, indirectly reducing stenosis. The technique as described by Fell and colleagues has been modified successfully by Reyes and Hill.[17, 46] Experience with selection of patients and clinical application remains limited.

Management of the established symptomatic area of stenosis seems to have no ideal solution. Management is customized, with the mainstays being bougienage, removal or bypass and replacement of the esophagus, and occasional gastric resection.

Dilating a stenotic site leaves much to be desired, because stretching or tearing the cicatrix should encourage more fibrosis; however, it has met with some clinical benefit, and nothing better is currently available. Bougienage has been most successful with strictures of short length and limited depth and circumference (Fig. 39–6). The more severe stenoses offer major challenges and potential for perforation. This has prompted some to encourage

more liberal standards for early replacement of the esophagus.[16, 20, 30]

In practice, the dilations are initiated after identification of stenosis on barium esophagogram 3 to 4 weeks following injury and preferably after re-epithelialization is completed as demonstrated by endoscopy. Because the procedures are unpleasant and carry some risk, a general anesthetic is used on each occasion with the child. Most of those with strictures have had gastrostomies and a nasogastrostomy string (no. 2 silk) passed. This allows for controlled use of Tucker bougies or Plummer dilators and is mandatory for all but the short and minor stenoses. The extent of the dilation on each occasion is individualized, with a desire to make progress but not at the expense of tearing, as suggested by blood on the bougie.

The Maloney tapered mercury bougies are often effective for short and less resistant sites of stricture. Occasionally older children or adolescents have trained themselves to swallow these dilators while sitting upright.

The initial dilations are usually separated by a 4- to 7-day interval. As long as there is a progressive decrease in the degree of stenosis and a lengthening of the necessary interval between dilations, the procedure is continued. Some patients have bougienage intermittently for periods up to 2 years. It remains difficult to determine when it serves the patient's best interest to interrupt this course of

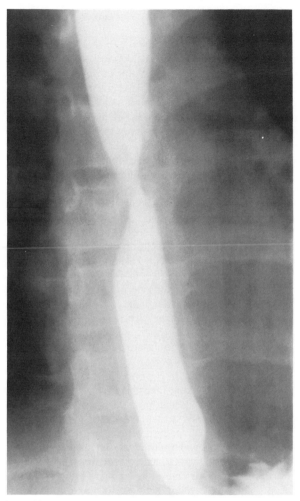

FIGURE 39–6

Short stricture in the central esophagus responded well to bougienage.

action and proceed to replacement or bypass of the esophagus.

The character of strictured sites of the esophagus seldom allows for simple resection and anastomosis. The margins of the respective cut ends of the esophagus must be free of cicatrix; otherwise excessive scarring at the suture line is likely.

Tracheoesophageal Fistula

An extension of the acute inflammatory and necrotic process into the tracheobronchial lumen is a serious complication of corrosive injury. Most often it appears early, during the acute phase, but may appear later, especially in relation to the esophageal bougienage, as was our single experience. Early recognition and proper management are crucial to the salvage of patients with this problem. The addition of a cough to the clinical picture should be viewed with suspicion, particularly when ingested materials and gastric contents are produced. Symptoms of mediastinitis may precede the cough. The diagnosis is confirmed on esophagogram. A

contrast material used for bronchography, such as propyliodone in peanut oil (Dionosil Oily) (Glaxco), is strongly encouraged for this procedure to avoid the antagonism of barium or a water-soluble solution in the airway.

Early excision of the severely injured esophagus may avoid fistula formation, but the selection of candidates for this procedure may be challenging. Untoward experiences on attempted direct repair of these fistulas have highlighted the inflamed and incompetent status of the associated structures.[1, 9] Diversion of the proximal esophagus and gastrostomy are mandatory first steps in the treatment of this fistula. It may then close spontaneously with fibrosis of the adjacent residual esophagus, as was our experience. Continued gastroesophageal reflux in some cases has encouraged the recommendation for division of the distal esophagus also.[9] Esophageal replacement is delayed until optimal conditions are present.

Infections

The acute and long-term changes in the integrity of the gastric and esophageal walls, as well as the associated manipulative procedures, allow infections to be prominent in the clinical courses. Associated esophageal dysfunction also contributes by prompting aspiration, pneumonia, and lung abscess. Included in our experience were mediastinitis (5), cervical abscess (1), and pericarditis (1)—all secondary to perforation—and lung abscess (1) and brain abscess (3).

Brain Abscess

Brain abscess is a rarely reported associate of corrosive injuries.[33] In the absence of additional pathologic conditions, such as a right-to-left intracardiac shunt, the mechanism whereby a cerebral infection may occur secondary to esophageal pathology remains elusive. A consideration is retrograde extension by the "vertebral vein system" (also an explanation for the spread of malignant disease).[7]

Our experience includes three children who developed brain abscesses during the course of multiple dilations of esophageal strictures. Each presented with clinical suggestions of increased intracranial pressure, and each was managed successfully by prompt excisional or drainage operations. Leahy and colleagues presented two similar experiences and recommended that the physician have a high index of suspicion when neurologic changes occur in this clinical setting.[33] Antibiotic coverage (ampicillin) just before and 24 hours after esophageal dilation seems an appropriate prophylaxis and is now our practice.

Carcinoma of the Esophagus

The literature clearly documents an increased occurrence of squamous cell carcinoma in the esophagus that has been injured previously by caustic materials.[3, 28] No correlation has been shown between the severity of the original damage and the potential for malignancy. Some neoplasms have appeared in the esophagus that was considered to be only mildly damaged.[54] There is no documentation of such lesions arising in the organ following procedures that bypassed and placed the esophagus at rest. Therefore, continued antagonism to scarred tissue seems to be the precursor of the malignant change.

Currently, fewer than 180 cases of such lesions are reported. The true incidence secondary to caustic injuries remains unknown. The frequency relative to all carcinomas of the esophagus is below 4%. The latency period between corrosive insult and recognition of the malignancy has varied from 12 to 70 years, with a mean interval of approximately 40 years.[28] The youngest patient reported was 16 years old.[55] The addition to the clinical picture of dysphagia was the most common symptom suggesting the new lesion. Resection was associated with a greater cure rate than that for other esophageal malignancies but has remained less than 10%.

MANAGEMENT

Although individualization of management is appropriate, certain considerations need to be emphasized and should be routine in the initial assessment.

1. History, especially ingestion
2. Physical (toxicity)
3. Examination of the ingested material, especially the pH
4. Discontinue oral intake
5. Initiate ampicillin and prednisone (arbitrary)
6. Endoscopy within 24 hours

Subsequent management is based on the findings obtained in the evaluation steps listed previously.

In the presence of edema and erythema only (mild injury), all treatment is discontinued. As injuries may have been overlooked, the child is seen after a 3-week interval, and in the presence of symptoms, a barium esophagogram is recommended.

The endoscopic recognition of friable mucosa, superficial ulcerations, or thick white exudate (moderate injury) justifies continued inhospital observation, antibiotic coverage, and nonoral nutritional support. Burn injuries in this category represent the most likely benefactors of steroids. Liquid oral intake is reinstituted based on the severity of the initial injury and the clinical performance. Endoscopy is repeated in 14 to 21 days, and on evidence of re-epithelialization full oral intake is initiated. Esophagogastric anatomic and functional statuses are assessed in 3 to 4 weeks with barium studies to determine the need for additional management.

Deep ulcerations, loose tissue, and eschar suggest severe or near full thickness damage with the risk of perforation and adjacent tissue involvement. The child's clinical evaluation and imaging studies are particularly important in the search for complications. A gastrostomy is established, the gastric and abdominal esophageal walls are inspected, and a nasogastrostomy string is passed. Intravenous antibiotics, fluids, and nutritional support are important, as are gastric antacids. Endoscopy and barium studies after 3 weeks identify progress in resurfacing, return of function, and evidence of complications. Bougienage is begun on re-epithelialization.

The presence of full thickness necrosis, perforation, and adjacent structural damage is not always obvious. As the mortality rate is high even in the retrievable cases, early recognition and aggressive management is obligatory. In addition to the obvious, volume and concentration of the offending agent, suicidal intent, clinical instability, and bleeding should alert the physician to a serious penetrating injury. In delayed perforations, atony of the esophagus is suggestive of impending perforation (see Fig. 39–4).

In the absence of overt evidence of these advanced changes, endoscopy may well clarify the status after the administration of general supportive measures. Evaluation of the stomach via celiotomy should follow. Immediate removal of the necrotic structures as well as adequate drainage, diversion of the esophagus, and venting of the stomach or jejunum have improved the results.[29] Simple drainage of necrotic and perforated sites is not considered adequate care. The accompanying intravascular thrombosis and periesophageal edema allow for removal of the afflicted structures with relative ease. The best results reported are associated with nonthoracotomy esophagectomies.[24, 48, 52] Esophageal and gastric replacements are performed on an elective basis.

The normal esophagus performs as a highly coordinated conduit of secretions and ingested materials. Caustic injury may antagonize this function in varying degrees with the destruction of intrinsic musculature and stenosis. Although replacement is occasionally desirable and sometimes mandatory, no other organ reproduces its function. Untoward experiences with the operative procedures and long-term results give cause for careful selection of patients and techniques in the replacement or bypass of the esophagus.

Several absolute indications for esophageal removal and replacement have been mentioned. The decision may be more challenging when the damage is less pronounced. Some factors to weigh in the final determination are length, location, and rigidity of the stenosis; esophageal motility by study and daily performance; required frequency of dilation; complications; and patient and family compliance and attitudes. The presence of multiple, lengthy, or rigid strictures that are resistant to repeat bougienage suggests the wisdom of replacement. Short or even long areas of "soft" stenosis that respond to progressively widening intervals of dilation probably do not justify substitution but rather long-term follow up.

When replacing the esophagus, care should be taken to place the anastomosis in normal unscarred tissue. It is preferable to preserve the upper and lower sphincters to discourage reflux and aspiration. Ideally, resection of the least length or use of the shortest replacement practical is best. With improving skills in microvascular anastomosis, short-segment free jejunal grafts may be applicable in selected cases.[45]

The stomach, jejunum, and colon have been used via various routes (retrosternal, posterior mediastinum in the esophageal bed, or transpleural retrohilar) to replace the esophagus.[2, 19, 23, 48] Although each has its advantages and disadvantages as well as advocates, the multiplicity of clinical challenges encourages the surgeon to be proficient with several technical methods.

Table 39–3
Caustic Injuries, The Children's Hospital of Alabama (TCHA), 1967–1986

Patients	No.	Esophageal Burns	Stenosis	Perforations	Airway Fistula	Vascular Fistula	Brain Abscess
I Treated initially at TCHA	192	44	23	3	1	2	2
II Arrived after 21 days	14	14	14	7	0	0	1
Totals	206	58	37	10	1	2	3

A TWENTY-YEAR EXPERIENCE

Two hundred and six children were treated for the ingestion of caustic materials at The Children's Hospital of Alabama from 1967 through 1986 (Table 39–3). Their ages ranged from 10 months to 16 years; 80% were younger than 2 years, and 95% were younger than 5 years. One hundred and ninety-two had their initial care at this hospital, and the remaining 14 presented approximately 3 weeks after their injury with stenosis.

In a retrospective analysis, 44 of the 192 (23%) initially managed children sustained moderate or severe esophageal injuries, with three suffering gastric injuries in addition. Twenty-three subsequently developed stenoses while receiving a varied combination of supportive measures: antibiotics, steroids, endoscopy, radiologic studies, and gastrostomy. Data surveillance suggests that steroids had little influence on the scarring process. The severity of the injuries sustained appears to be decreasing, as during the first 10 years a 45% significant injury rate was recorded, of which 33% developed stenosis, whereas during the last half of the review the comparable figures were 18% and 6%, respectively. There was a steady increase in children presenting with the history of caustic ingestion over the 20 years. Prompt endoscopy simplified the overall management.

These 44 injuries were also associated with esophageal perforation (3), bronchoesophageal fistula (1), vasculoesophageal fistula (2), brain abscess (2), and lung abscess (1). The 14 children who presented later sustained stenosis (14), perforation (7), and brain abscess (1). All of the perforations occurred later, after 21 days, during a period of bougienage. The two vascular fistulas resulted in death. An aortoesophageal fistula was spontaneous on the thirteenth day. A second child died in his sleep from a communication with the innominate artery on the sixty-third day after the injury, 36 hours after a single dilation. An additional death appeared as a late complication of an esophageal replacement procedure.

References

1. Amoury RA, Krabovsky E, Leonidas J, et al: Tracheoesophageal fistula after lye ingestion. J Pediatr Surg 10:273, 1975.
2. Anderson KD, Randolph JG: The gastric tube for esophageal replacement in children. J Thorac Cardiovasc Surg 66:333–342, 1973.
3. Applequist P, Salmo M: Lye corrosion carcinoma of the esophagus. Cancer 45:2655, 1980.
4. Arena JM: General considerations of poisoning. In: Arena JM: Poisoning. 4th ed. Springfield, Ill, Charles C Thomas, 1979, p 4.
5. Ashcraft KW, Padula RT: The effect of dilute corrosives on the esophagus. Pediatrics 53:226, 1974.
6. Baltimore CL, Meyer RJ: Stress in families of children who have ingested poisons. BMJ 3:87–89, 1975.
7. Batson OV: The function of the vertebral veins and their role in the spread of metastases. Ann Surg 112:138, 1940.
8. Bott SJ, McCallum RW: Medication-induced oesophageal injury. Survey of the literature. Med Toxicol 1:449–457, 1986.
9. Burrington JD, Raffensperger JG: Surgical management of tracheoesophageal fistula complicating caustic ingestion. Surgery 8:329–334, 1978.
10. Butler C, Madden JW, Davis WM, et al: Morphologic aspects of experimental esophageal lye strictures. 1. Pathogenesis and pathophysiologic correlations. J Surg Res 17:232–244, 1974.
11. Butler C, Madden JW, Davis WM, et al: Morphologic aspects of experimental esophageal lye strictures. II. Effect of steroid hormones, bougienage and induced lathyrism on acute lye burns. Surgery 81:431–435, 1977.
12. Clarke A, Walton WW: Effect of safety packaging on aspirin ingestion by children. Pediatrics 63:687–693, 1979.
13. Coln D, Chang JHT: Experience with esophageal stenting for caustic burns in children. J Pediatr Surg 7:588–591, 1985.
14. Crain EF, Gershel JC, Mezey AP: Caustic ingestions. Am J Dis Child 138:863–865, 1984.
15. DiConstanzo J, Noiclere M, Jougland J, et al: New therapeutic approach to corrosive burns of the upper gastrointestinal tract. Gut 21:370–375, 1980.
16. Estrera A, Taylor W, Mills LJ, et al: Corrosive burns of the esophagus and stomach: A recommendation for an aggressive surgical approach. Ann Thorac Surg 41:276–283, 1986.
17. Fell SC, Denize A, Becker MH, et al: The effect of intraluminal splinting in the prevention of caustic stricture of the esophagus. J Thorac Cardiovasc Surg 52:675–681, 1966.
18. Franken EA: Caustic damage of the gastrointestinal tract: Roentgen features. AJR 118:77–85, 1973.
19. Freeman NV, Cass DT: Colon interposition: A modification of the Waterson technique using the normal esophageal route. J Pediatr Surg 17:17–21, 1982.
20. Gago O, Ritter FN, Martel W, et al: Aggressive surgical treatment for caustic injury of the esophagus and stomach. Ann Thorac Surg 13:243, 1972.
21. Gaudreault P, McGuigan M, Chicoine L, et al: Predictability of esophageal injury from signs and symptoms: A study of caustic ingestion in 378 children. Pediatrics 71:767, 1983.
22. Gehanno P, Guedon C: Inhibition of experimental esophageal lye stricture by penicillamine. Arch Otolaryngol 107:145–147, 1981.
23. German JC, Waterston DJ: Colon interposition for the replacement of the esophagus in children. J Pediatr Surg 11:227–234, 1976.
24. Gossot D, Sarfati E, Celerier M: Early blunt esophagectomy in severe caustic burns of the upper digestive tract. J Thorac Cardiovasc Surg 94:188–191, 1987.
25. Haller JA Jr, Andrews HG, White JJ, et al: Pathophysiology and management of acute corrosive burns of the esophagus: Results of treatment in 285 children. J Pediatr Surg 6:578–584, 1971.
26. Haller JA Jr, Bachman K: The comparative effect of current therapy on experimental caustic burns of the esophagus. Pediatrics 34:236–245, 1964.
27. Hill JL, Norberg H, Smith M, et al: Clinical technique and success of the esophageal stent to prevent corrosive strictures. J Pediatr Surg 11:441, 1976.
28. Hopkins RA, Postlethwait RW: Caustic burns and carcinoma of the esophagus. Ann Surg 194:146–148, 1981.

29. Hwang TL, Shen-chen SM, Chen MF: Nonthoracotomy esophagectomy for corrosive esophagitis with gastric perforation. Surg Gynecol Obstet 164:537–540, 1987.

30. Kirsh MM, Peterson A, Brown JW, et al: Treatment of caustic injuries of the esophagus. Am J Surg 188:675–678, 1977.

31. Krey H: Treatment of corrosive lesions in the esophagus. Acta Otolaryngol 102:1–49, 1952.

32. Kuhn JR, Tunell WP: The role of initial cine-esophagography in caustic esophageal injury. Am J Surg 146:804–806, 1983.

33. Leahy WR, Toyka KV, Fishbeck KH Jr: Cerebral abscess in children secondary to esophageal dilatation. Pediatrics 59:300–301, 1977.

34. Litovitz TL: Battery ingestions: Product accessibility and clinical course. Pediatrics 75:469–476, 1985.

35. Litovitz TL, Martin TG, Schmitz B: 1986 annual report of the American Association of Poison Control Centers national data collection system. Am J Emerg Med 5:405–445, 1986.

36. Martel W: Radiologic features of esophagogastritis secondary to extremely caustic agents. Radiology 103:31–36, 1972.

37. Maull KI, Scher LA, Greenfield IJ: Surgical implications of acid ingestion. Surg Gynecol Obstet 148:895–899, 1979.

38. Maves MD, Carithers JS, Birck HG: Esophageal burns secondary to disc battery ingestion. Ann Otol Rhinol Laryngol 93:354–369, 1984.

39. Middelkamp JN, Ferguson TB, Roper CL, et al: The management and problems of caustic burns in children. J Thorac Cardiovasc Surg 57:341–347, 1968.

40. Mills LJ, Estrera AS, Platt MR: Avoidance of esophageal stricture following severe caustic burns by the use of an intraluminal stent. Ann Thorac Surg 28:60–65, 1978.

41. Moazam F, Talbert JL, Miller D, et al: Caustic ingestion and its sequelae in children. South Med J 80:187–190, 1987.

42. Muhletaler CA, Gerlock AJ, deSoto L, et al: Acid corrosive esophagitis: Radiographic findings. AJR 134:1137–1140, 1980.

43. Oakes DD, Sherck JP, Marc JBD: Lye ingestion: Clinical patterns and therapeutic implications. J Thorac Cardiovasc Surg 83:194–204, 1982.

44. Peacock EE: Control of wound healing and scar formation in surgical patients. Arch Surg 116:1325–1329, 1981.

45. Prevot J, Lepelley M, Schmitt M: Small bowel esophagoplasty with vascular microanastomoses in the neck for treatment of esophageal burns in childhood. Progr Pediatr Surg 18:108–117, 1985.

46. Reyes HM, Hill JL: Modification of the experimental stent technique for esophageal burns. J Surg Res 20:65–70, 1976.

47. Rivara FP: Epidemiology of childhood injuries. Am J Dis Child 136:399–405, 1982.

48. Rodgers BM, Ryckman FC, Talbert JL: Blunt transmediastinal total esophagectomy with simultaneous substernal colon interposition for esophageal strictures in children. J Pediatr Surg 16:184–189, 1981.

49. Scher LA, Maull KI: Emergency management and sequelae of acid ingestion. JACEP 7:206–208, 1978.

50. Sobel R: The psychiatric implications of accidental poisoning in childhood. Pediatr Clin North Am 17:653, 1970.

51. Spain DM, Molomut N, Haber A: The effect of cortisone on the formation of granulation tissue in mice (abstract). Am J Pathol 26:720–711, 1950.

52. Stewart JR, Sarr MG, Sharp KW, et al: Transhiatal (blunt) esophagoscopy for malignant and benign esophageal disease: Clinical experience and technique. Ann Thorac Surg 40:343–348, 1985.

53. Tewfik TL, Schloss MD: Ingestion of lye and other corrosive agents—A study of 86 infant and child cases. J Otolaryngol 9:72–77, 1980.

54. Ti TK: Oesophageal carcinoma associated with corrosive injury prevention and treatment by oesophageal resection. Br J Surg 70:223–225, 1983.

55. Tucker JA, Yarington CT: The treatment of caustic ingestion. Otolaryngol Clin North Am 12:343–350, 1979.

56. Tunell WP: Corrosive strictures of the esophagus. In: Welch KJ, et al: Pediatric Surgery. Chicago, Year Book Medical Publishers, 1986, pp 698–703.

57. United States Department of Health and Human Services, Public Health Service: Food and Drug Administration Bulletin, National Clearinghouse for Poison Control Centers, 1982.

58. Vancura EM, Clinton JE, Ruiz, et al: Toxicity of alkaline solutions, Ann Emerg Med 9:118–122, 1980.

59. Votteler TP, Nash J, Rutledge J, et al: The hazard of ingested alkaline disk batteries in children. JAMA 249:2504, 1983.

60. Wadsworth J, Burnell I, Taylor B: Family type and accidents in preschool children. J Epidemiol Community Health 37:100–104, 1983.

61. Webb WR, Koutras P, Ecker RR: An evaluation of steroids and antibiotics in caustic burns of the esophagus. Ann Thorac Surg 9:95–102, 1970.

62. Weisskopf A: Effects of cortisone on experimental lye burns of the esophagus. Ann Otol Rhinol Laryngol 64:681–689, 1952.

Julie A. Long
Arvin I. Philippart

CHAPTER FORTY

Penetrating Injuries

The epidemic of childhood trauma is receiving increasing attention. At least 10,000 children from 1 to 14 years of age die from injuries annually.[1] Blunt trauma accounts for the majority of injuries, but penetrating trauma in this age group also causes significant morbidity and mortality. Penetrating trauma is increasing in frequency in urban areas and is more likely to require surgical intervention than is blunt trauma.

Although only limited statistics on the incidence of penetrating trauma in children are available, the incidence of gunshot wounds (GSW) in all age groups is alarming. Handguns accounted for 31 murders per day in the United States, 50% of all homicides, or a rate of 11 per 100,000 in 1980.[53] In 1981, 630 children under the age of 18 died as a secondary result of handgun injuries. The rate of firearm suicide and homicide has increased in parallel with the increasing availability of firearms from 1946 to 1982 in the United States.[68]

In Detroit in 1983, 1161 people died as a result of accidents, homicide, or suicide. Of these, 505 died as a secondary result of firearm injuries and 100 as a secondary result of other penetrating trauma.[67] In 1986, Detroit had a homicide rate of 59 per 100,000, the highest in the nation, and 365 children under the age of 17 were shot, 43 of them fatally.[62] Although the statistics are less startling for the rest of the country, the national figures reveal an increase in accidental injuries and suicides and homicides in young people (Tables 40–1, 40–2).

As with other epidemics, the medical community has responded to the crisis by efforts to improve the delivery and quality of care. This has resulted in the establishment of trauma centers, new scales for assessing injuries, new applications of technology, and a burgeoning literature. Because a large portion of trauma victims are children and adolescents, pediatric surgeons have an important role in establishing guidelines for the care of young trauma victims, particularly when principles applied to adult patients may not apply. In trauma, as in other areas of pediatric surgery, the infant and young child should not be treated as merely small adults because the mechanisms of injury, resuscitation, and treatment may differ from those applicable to adolescents and adults.

MECHANISMS OF INJURY

Trauma is a normal consequence of the child's actions in the environment. Children are curious, are unaware of hazards, and exercise poor impulse control. Trauma is the negative reinforcement of those characteristics that modifies them over time. The incidence of such trauma is determined by the nature of the child's environment and the availability and maturity of supervision.

Accidental versus Intentional

As in all trauma, the sequelae of penetrating trauma may be minor or significant. Determinants include age of the child, nature of the environment, type of wounding agent, and presence or absence of intent. In the younger child, the preponderance of penetrating trauma is relatively minor and includes lacerations, puncture wounds, and animal bites largely to extremities. Stab and GWSs are infrequent. When they occur, the child is frequently an innocent victim of a hostile act directed against an older family member as a result of either altered relationships in the home or illegal activities. Malevolent intent, with the exception of familial attempted homicide, usually results in random injury patterns, with extremities more commonly involved than the torso. In such circumstances, the intent may be either a warning to an adult or a direct attack on an adult with the child the proximate unintended victim. The most common exception is a GSW of the head in a child that results from playing with an available handgun aimed at the head without intent of injury.

In contrast, penetrating trauma in the adolescent occurs more commonly as a hostile act, is more commonly life threatening, and more frequently involves the torso than the extremities and head. The increased number of adolescents as both consumers and purveyors of street drugs, particularly in large urban areas, has increased the frequency of GSWs in this age group in the last decade. Drug-related income has increased the availability and use of handguns in the teenage population. The patterns of injury and the agents and instigating causes of adolescent penetrating trauma are much more similar to those seen in adults than those common in younger children.

Three additional categories of causes of penetrating trauma deserve mention. In spite of campaigns to increase the safety of children's toys, they are still the source of numerous injuries. Although most of these injuries are simple lacerations or puncture wounds, complications can occur. In a report of two children with head injuries as a

Table 40–1
National Mortality for Children and Adolescents, 1983 (per 100,000 population)

Causes	Total (all ages)	Ages (in years)				
		0–1	1–4	5–9	10–14	15–19
Accidents	39.5	26.1	21.8	12.4	13.0	44.5
Motor vehicle accidents	19.0	5.2	7.5	6.4	6.8	33.2
Other	20.5	20.9	14.3	6.0	6.2	11.3
Suicide	12.1	—	—	0.1	1.1	8.7
Homicide	8.6	5.3	2.3	0.9	1.2	8.5

From Vital Statistics of the U.S. Vol. III: Mortality. U.S. Dept. of Health and Human Services, Public Health Service, National Center Health Statistics, 1983.

Table 40-2
Total Penetrating Injuries in Children and Adolescents, United States, 1983 (per 100,000 population)

	Total Number	Ages (in years)				
		0-1	1-5	5-9	10-14	15-19
Accidents						
Handguns	209	1	8	6	21	31
Other guns	1486	2	32	39	137	230
Suicide						
Handguns	2766	—	—	1	22	139
Homicide	20,191	193	513	144	213	1642
Handguns	980	3	8	10	13	68
Other guns	11,060	4	33	50	96	960
Cutting instrument	4173	3	26	10	40	373

From Vital Statistics of the U.S. Vol. II: Mortality. U.S. Dept. of Health and Human Services, Public Health Service, National Center Health Statistics, 1983.

secondary result of being struck by lawn darts, both patients developed infectious complications after closure of scalp puncture wounds.[23] Although air guns are commonly believed to be innocuous and their sale and use is unrestricted, serious ocular, facial, and abdominal injuries have been reported with their use.[6, 24, 38]

Blunt and penetrating trauma may occur simultaneously. This is most commonly seen with motor vehicular trauma either as a passenger or a pedestrian and is less likely in falls. In such injuries, the sequelae of the blunt injury frequently take precedence over those of the penetrating component.

Suicide

Adolescent suicide is increasing in frequency as is the use of firearms as agents for the suicide. Awareness of this fact is important when the circumstances of injury are poorly understood, as is the frequent nonspecificity of the history in suspected child abuse. From 1970 to 1980, 49,496 people between the ages of 15 and 24 years of age committed suicide.[37] This increase is most notable in young white males. However, for young males and females of all racial groups the proportion of suicide by firearms has increased. Because of the downward age trend in suicide, the years of potential life lost has increased approximately 60% from 1968 to 1984.[36]

The shifting age trends may have an impact on methods of prevention. In a review of prevention strategies for childhood traumatic deaths, Rivara estimated that 60% of suicides and 50% of homicides between the ages of 0 to 14 years old are due to firearms.[49] He commented that prevention by eliminating the source of injury has been effective in other countries and was not associated with an increase in suicides by other means. In a review of firearm use from 1920 to 1982, Wintemute found a positive correlation between increased firearm availability and increased firearm deaths.[68]

Cases from the Children's Hospital of Michigan

A review of activity in the emergency department of the Children's Hospital of Michigan (CHM) in 1986 is intended to provide an overview of the frequency and severity of penetrating trauma in this environment. This facility is the predominant provider of unscheduled health care for the children of Detroit and receives children in transfer from other physicians and institutions in the state. Although an integral part of the Detroit Emergency Medical Service (EMS) network, this emergency department traditionally has not received cases of penetrating trauma in adolescents, who are triaged largely to adjacent adult institutions by the EMS. No attempt has been made to alter this tradition in recognition of the circumstances in which adolescent penetrating trauma occurs and in the interest of maintaining an appropriate environment for a children's hospital.

Penetrating trauma was classified as lacerations, puncture wounds, animal bites, stab wounds, GSWs, and iatrogenic injuries. Of 58,000 patient visits in 1986, 2790 children were seen in the CHM emergency department with penetrating trauma (Table 40-3). Accidental penetrating injuries not clearly falling into other categories were considered lacerations, whereas intentional penetrating injuries were classified as stab wounds. Lacerations accounted for 2327

Table 40-3
Penetrating Injuries, Children's Hospital of Michigan, 1986

Type	No.
Lacerations	2327
Bites	199
Dog	170
Human	21
Other	8
Punctures	225
Stabs	7
Gunshot wounds	32
TOTAL	2790

Table 40–4
Site of Injury for Gunshot Wounds (GSWs) and Stab Wounds (%)

Study	Type of Wound	Head and Neck	Chest	Trunk, Abdomen, Perineum	Extremity
CHM,	GSW and Stab				
n = 39	1986	9 (23)	7 (18)	4 (10)	21 (54)
Ordoz,[43]	GSW				
n = 255	1973–1983	34 (13)	149 (58)	94 (37)	47 (18)
Barlow,[3]	Stab				
n = 75	1969–1982	11 (15)	45 (61)	28 (37)	36 (48)
n = 108	GSW				
	1970–1980	28 (26)	16 (15)	22 (20)	42 (39)

CHM, Children's Hospital of Michigan.

of the injuries. The majority of these were simple injuries treated in the emergency department, after which the patients were discharged. Approximately 1% required hospitalization, general anesthesia, or both for wound closure, including hand lacerations with tendon injuries. One hundred ninety-nine bites, of which 170 were dog bites, 21 were human bites, and eight were other bites (rodent or cat), were treated. Because bites are covered in Chapter 33, they are not extensively discussed here. Puncture wounds, including those with and without a foreign body, numbered 225. Foreign bodies easily palpable or partially protruding were removed in the emergency department. The majority were removed within 24 hours in the outpatient surgery facilities. One child who fell on a chair punctured his abdominal wall and presented with omental evisceration. At celiotomy he had no other significant injuries.

Stab Wounds

Seven stab wounds occurred, six in teenagers. The one injury in a child occurred in an 11-month-old infant who was accidentally stabbed in an altercation between several adults. This child required closure of deep chest lacerations and overnight observation. Of the six stab wounds in adolescents, one was accidental and the others were the result of conflicts. Three received outpatient wound care, and three required hospitalization. A patient with a chest injury received local care and observation, and the others underwent operation. One patient had hand exploration surgery for repair of a nerve and tendon injury, and the other patient had a laparotomy, at which time a bleeding intercostal artery was ligated and a nonbleeding liver injury was noted.

Gunshot Wounds

Thirty-two GSWs occurred, 22 of which were firearm injuries and 10 of which were air gun injuries. Fifteen patients had significant injuries and were treated as outpatients. Of the 16 patients who were hospitalized, four required operations. Two patients required irrigation and débridement of extremity wounds, one patient a craniotomy and partial lobectomy, and one patient a celiotomy for repair of a small bowel injury. One patient, the only mortality, presented dead on arrival from a GSW to the head.

Air gun injuries usually resulted from improper use by older children or teenagers. Of the 10 patients, only one was injured intentionally. Two patients sustained significant injury. One had a pulmonary contusion with effusion and the second a small bowel perforation requiring repair. In a report of air gun injuries, Reddick and colleagues reported that a BB penetrates the skin at a velocity of 350 feet per second and that these weapons can reach muzzle velocities of 400 to 900 feet per second.[48] Nakamura and associates reported four cases of thoracic injury in children from air guns that required surgical treatment.[39] These guns are often the first used by children and may be used in unsupervised settings. Because they are clearly capable of causing serious organ injury, regulation of their sale and distribution appears warranted.

Gunshot or stab wounds were most likely to result in extremity injury (Table 40–4), followed by head and neck, chest and abdominal, and flank injuries. An attempt was made to compare these findings with others' experience; however, several reviews did not quote distribution of injuries. Ordoz and co-workers reported head and neck injuries as most frequent and extremity injuries as least frequent in a review of 255 pediatric GSWs.[43] Barlow and colleagues reported that the extremities were most often injured by gunshots, but the chest was most commonly injured by stabbings.[2, 3] At CHM, 27 children with penetrating wounds were 12 years or older, and 12 were younger than 12 years. However, in other series, adolescents made up more than 80% of the penetrating trauma victims compared with 69% of our patients.[2, 3, 43]

TRANSPORT AND INITIAL EVALUATION

The prehospital evaluation begins with the first person to discover the injury. In small children, this is usually a parent. Common sense indicates whether a serious injury has occurred. A safe maxim is that all penetrating trauma should be evaluated promptly by a physician. In potentially serious trauma, the victim should be transported by the EMS. Delays in initiating treatment account for significant morbidity in penetrating trauma. Lacerations, puncture wounds, and bites are often judged insignificant until infection occurs. In a review of pediatric stab wounds in Harlem, children brought by the EMS presented at an average time of 1 hour, 22 minutes after injury.[3] Notification of EMS accounted for the majority of the delay.

Many researchers have cautioned against elaborate resuscitative efforts at the scene of the accident in pediatric trauma, as resuscitation of pediatric victims is more time consuming outside the hospital environment. Transporters of severely injured children should be urged to keep the victim warm and oxygenated and remember that rapid transport of the victim to the hospital is as important as the ABCs of resuscitation. For these injuries, "snatch and run" should be a guiding principle in the prehospital setting. En route to the hospital, direct pressure should be used over bleeding points rather than tourniquets. Amputated extremities should be wrapped in plastic and placed on ice. Elaborate attempts to clean or débride these or other wounds outside the treatment center are not necessary and may be detrimental.

Pediatric trauma centers will play an increasingly important role in educating the public, physicians, and other hospitals about emergency trauma care in children. Few community hospitals or physicians are prepared to care for pediatric victims of serious penetrating trauma. Within a pediatric trauma center should be a physician designated to receive calls regarding treatment and transfer of trauma victims. A significant role is to counsel the referring physician who may be quite uncomfortable in treating pediatric patients before transfer of the child.

The emergency department evaluation of the patient with serious penetrating trauma can be carried out expeditiously while stabilization and treatment are under way. The airway is usually stable except in cases of facial, neck, or possibly thoracic trauma. While intravenous access is being obtained, blood can be drawn and sent for complete blood count, electrolytes, blood urea nitrogen, amylase, creatinine, and type and crossmatch. Penetrating head trauma usually requires intubation and ventilation for management of intracranial pressure by hyperventilation. In rare cases, uncrossmatched or type-specific blood may be required, although infusion of lactated Ringer solution initially is usually sufficient. A complete physical examination must be performed. All too often significant injuries are missed when a methodic approach is not observed. Obvious but overlooked points include examining all sides of the patient; mentally visualizing the course of the penetrating object, including counting bullet holes and bullets; checking all pulses; completing a neurologic assessment of the central and peripheral nervous systems; and remembering a high association of blunt trauma with penetrating trauma.

Another member of the trauma team should be obtaining a history of the injury from the EMS or family and past medical history of the patient, including a record of immunizations. Tetanus prophylaxis should be administered when appropriate according to the recommendations of the American College of Surgeons Committee on Trauma (Table 40–5). In cases of suspected visceral injury or contaminated open wounds it is appropriate to begin intravenous antibiotics. For contaminated extremity wounds a first-generation cephalosporin is still appropriate, whereas for abdominal injury associated with fecal contamination triple antibiotic therapy or a third-generation cephalosporin is indicated. In the unstable patient with apparent abdominal, thoracic, or head and neck trauma, a chest radiograph may be the only one necessary to identify the unsuspected hemothorax, pneumothorax, or cardiac tamponade. In more stable patients it is advisable to obtain lateral neck films and chest and abdominal films. Other diagnostic radiologic tests are reserved for the stable patient, who constitutes the bulk of pediatric trauma.

Table 40–5
Prophylactic Treatment of Tetanus

| Type of Wound | No. of Patients Immunized or Partially Immunized | Patient Completely Immunized Time Since Last Booster Dose | |
		5*–10 Years	10 Years†
Clean minor	Begin or complete immunization per schedule; tetanus toxoid, 0.5 ml	None	Tetanus toxoid, 0.5 ml
Clean major or tetanus prone	In one arm: Human tetanus immune globulin, 250 units† In other arm: Tetanus toxoid, 0.5 ml, complete immunization per schedule†	Tetanus toxoid, 0.5 ml	In one arm: Tetanus toxoid, 0.5 ml† In other arm: Human tetanus immune globulin, 250 units†
Tetanus prone, delayed or incomplete débridement	In one arm: Human tetanus immune globulin, 500 units† In other arm: Tetanus toxoid, 0.5 ml, complete immunization per schedule thereafter†; antibiotic therapy	Tetanus toxoid, 0.5 ml; antibiotic therapy	In one arm: Tetanus toxoid, 0.5 ml† In other arm: Human tetanus immune globulin, 500 units†; antibiotic therapy

*No prophylactic immunization is required if patient has had a booster within the previous 5 years.
†Use different syringes, needles, and injection sites.
NOTE: With different preparations of toxoid, the volume of a single booster dose should be modified.

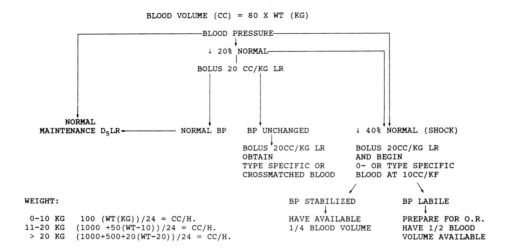

FIGURE 40-1

Recommendations for fluid resuscitation in cases of penetrating trauma. LR, Lactated Ringer solution; D₅, dextrose 5% in water; BP, blood pressure.

RESUSCITATION

Airway

The child arriving in shock, unconscious, or with serious head or neck trauma requires intubation. Emergency tracheostomy is rarely needed in severe facial trauma; because of the increased difficulty in performing tracheostomy in children, it should be undertaken only by experienced surgeons. Needle catheter cricothyroidostomy can be a temporary life-saving maneuver, allowing oxygenation until intubation or tracheostomy can be performed safely.[26, 59] Goldman and associates reported that a small transtracheal catheter can be used in experimentally induced total airway obstruction to maintain normal ventilation if used in conjunction with a Venturi positive pressure device.[20]

Vascular Access and Fluids

Vascular access must be established immediately. Ideally, access is through a large-bore short catheter placed percutaneously in an upper extremity (and also in a lower extremity in cases of serious thoracic injury). If this is not possible, a cutdown should be performed rapidly at either the saphenous vein or the antecubital vein. One advantage of antecubital cutdowns is that if long Silastic catheters are used, they may also serve as central venous pressure monitors. Percutaneous central lines are reserved as a last resort in the emergency setting in the smaller patient because of the increased risk of complications associated with their use or for continued monitoring after initial access has been established. Intraosseous access is rarely utilized initially when patients present in full cardiac arrest for fluid and pharmacologic resuscitation as a cutdown is placed. It is important to remember that the dose of fluids and drugs given by this method is at least as large as that given intravenously, and access to the circulation may be slower.

To calculate volume administration in a child, it is necessary to obtain or estimate the child's weight and calculate the blood volume. A child who presents with hypotension has already lost at least 25% of the blood volume. An initial bolus of 20 ml of lactated Ringer solution per kg is given while blood is being set up. If the patient stabilizes, maintenance intravenous infusion continues, as does the diagnostic evaluation. If the patient remains hypotensive, it is appropriate to give type-specific or O negative blood (Fig. 40–1). Failure to stabilize indicates continued blood loss, and preparation should be made for operative intervention (Fig. 40–2). In children or adults, the discussion of the selective management of penetrating trauma is reserved for the stable patient. Children may be more likely to stabilize, permitting nonoperative approaches.

Emergency Thoracotomy

Sufficient drama and confusion ensues when a trauma victim presents to the emergency department with no vital signs, so that it is important to review past experience of resuscitation of these victims. In a review of 267 adult patients over a 5-year period, Shimazu and Shatney reported a 2.6% long-term survival rate, of which only 1.5% of these patients were functional following resuscitation of patients without vital signs.[57] They were careful to exclude patients who presented with vital signs and deteriorated in the emergency department. The only victims of penetrating trauma who survived underwent thoracotomy in the emergency department (2 of 50). Resuscitating victims with penetrating head and neck trauma was not successful. Shimazu and Shatney believe the only role of emergency department thoracotomy is in resuscitating victims of penetrating chest or heart injuries. Beaver and co-workers reviewed the results of resuscitation and emergency department thoracotomy in 17 pediatric patients who presented with presumed thoracoabdominal injuries and no vital signs and reported that there were no survivors in this series.[4] Multisystem trauma associated with no vital signs on admission is lethal. The resuscitation of victims with single-system involvement, especially central nervous system involvement, is

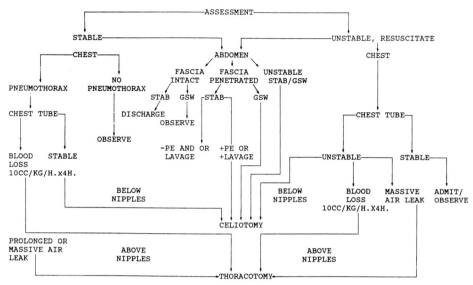

FIGURE 40–2
Management of penetrating torso trauma. GSW, Gunshot wound; PE, physical examination.

occasionally associated with survivors. Rohman and colleagues reported a 33% survival rate in preterminal patients with penetrating cardiac injuries who underwent prompt emergency department thoracotomy.[50] Emergency department thoracotomy should be reserved for the victims of penetrating chest trauma or the rare patient who has reversible injuries who loses vital signs in the emergency department. An established policy cannot limit the tragedy of these injuries in children. It can minimize the emotional response of the hospital personnel and allow proper support and counseling for the victim's family.

DIAGNOSTIC EVALUATION

Radiographs

With the increasing sophistication of diagnostic radiologic studies, the role these studies play in managing penetrating trauma is increasing; in some cases, these studies are replacing surgical intervention. Further diagnostic studies are often indicated for the seriously injured but stable victim. Suspected penetrating trauma of the central nervous system mandates a computed tomography (CT) scan. Bronchoscopy, laryngoscopy, contrast esophagogram utilizing water-soluble agents, and arteriography are advocated for investigating some penetrating neck injuries in adults rather than routine neck exploration for injuries penetrating the platysma. The use of these tests is elaborated on in the discussion of treatment.

When a chest radiograph reveals a widened mediastinum, a CT scan with bolus intravenous contrast or an aortogram is indicated. Aortography is the gold standard for evaluating aortic trauma but in young children requires general anesthesia. In select cases a CT scan with bolus intravenous contrast or digital subtraction angiography may give sufficient information to rule out aortic injury without anesthesia.

Peritoneal Lavage

The most controversial issue in penetrating trauma is mandatory versus selective celiotomy. Historically, the safest management of all penetrating abdominal trauma included exploratory celiotomy.[7] As mortality figures for trauma improved, efforts were focused on minimizing the morbidity. Based on the fact that more than one third of 88 patients undergoing celiotomy for trauma at Kings County Hospital did not require it, Shaftan reviewed another 180 patients, of whom 63% had penetrating trauma. In this study, selective celiotomy was performed for clinical findings of peritoneal irritation or blood in the gastrointestinal tract. Observation of others with penetrating injury and no additional findings was associated with no morbidity or mortality.[55] In a prospective evaluation of 100 patients with stab wounds, de Lacy and colleagues used clinical criteria to determine whether patients required celiotomy after establishing, by local wound exploration, that there was peritoneal penetration. Seventy patients were safely observed, and 30 underwent celiotomy with five having negative results for significant injury. These investigators concurred with Shaftan, that clinical findings discriminated who needed celiotomy, except perhaps in alcoholics.[14] Because of a 70% association with significant visceral injury and omental evisceration, most surgeons consider this an indication for routine abdominal exploration.[8, 22] Demetriades, the most aggressive advocate of selective management of penetrating trauma, does not consider shock, blood on paracentesis, omental evisceration, or free air as absolute indications for celiotomy. If all patients with peritoneal penetration in his series with Rabinowitz of 156 patients had been explored, 28% would have had negative results for significant injuries on celiotomy. By using clinical examination, the incidence of negative laparotomies was 7%, with two patients developing wound infections after delayed operations.[16] Others have advocated wound sinography, local wound exploration, and diagnostic peritoneal lavage combined with physical examination as methods to identify whether patients require celiotomy or observation.[13, 33, 63] Traditional surgical bias claims minimal morbidity associated with a negative celiotomy. However, in an exhaustive review of 1513 operative trauma cases, of 245 without significant injury, Lowe and associates found a mortality rate of 1.6%, a morbidity rate of 19%, and a 3% rate of readmission for adhesive bowel obstruction.[31]

In a classic paper reviewing 2212 patients with penetrating injuries, Nance and co-workers confirmed the safety of selective celiotomy.[40] Although signs of peritoneal injury are the most reliable indication for celiotomy, other studies are advocated to minimize the chance of missed injury. The sensitivity of peritoneal lavage is 96% with a specificity of 88% when the positive criteria are more than 100,000 red blood cells per ml, 500 white blood cells per ml, or elevated amylase.[17] Oreskovich and Carrico recommend local wound exploration in patients with negative physical examinations followed by peritoneal lavage in patients with peritoneal penetration. To eliminate the possibility of missed hollow viscus injury, they recommend lowering the criteria for a positive result on lavage to more than 1000 red blood cells per ml.[44] Most surgeons use the open peritoneal lavage technique and consider more than 100,000 red blood cells per ml; more than 500 white blood cells per ml; elevated amylase; or the presence of bile, bacteria, or stool as a positive criterion.[19, 61] The lavage technique with minimal complications and the easiest application to children is the Lazarus-Nelson percutaneous Seldinger technique. In their original paper, this technique was used on 110 patients by 45 physicians with no morbidity.[30]

Although pediatric surgeons were early advocates of nonoperative management of blunt trauma, enthusiasm has been less for the use of invasive tests to avoid celiotomy for penetrating trauma. Wound sinography and exploration is less well tolerated in children than in adults and still only addresses whether peritoneal penetration, not significant intra-abdominal injury, has occurred. There is some risk that wound exploration and lavage could decrease the value of subsequent physical examination by increasing local tenderness and decreasing cooperation and trust by the younger child. Although Powell and colleagues claimed peritoneal lavage was useful in evaluating children with blunt abdominal trauma, 32% of their patients underwent unnecessary celiotomy and they failed to mention the correlation of physical findings and positive lavage results.[47]

That there is a role for nonoperative management of pediatric penetrating injuries is indicated by a 35% rate of negative celiotomy results in one series of 100 injuries.[58] Tunell and associates reviewed 132 pediatric patients with penetrating abdominal trauma and claimed that 95% of injured patients and 80% of noninjured patients could be identified by physical examination, but they did not comment on the rate of negative celiotomy results.[65] Peritoneal lavage is used infrequently at CHM. In a child, 20 ml per kg of lactated Ringer solution or normal saline should be used. We have reserved the use of peritoneal lavage for the rare patient with equivocal abdominal findings or unexplained hemodynamic instability who requires emergency operation for significant head or chest trauma.

Computed Tomography Scan

Although the utility of the CT scan in evaluating blunt trauma is now established, its role in assessing penetrating trauma is less clear.[28] A major drawback is its decreased sensitivity compared with that of lavage in evaluating hollow viscus injury.[10] Its main usefulness may be in evaluating renal injuries in patients with penetrating flank injuries and otherwise negative abdominal findings. As in its use for blunt trauma, most believe it is necessary to use both oral and intravenous contrast to assess injuries adequately.

TREATMENT OF SPECIFIC ANATOMIC AREAS

Neck

Because of military experience in World War II, a policy of mandatory exploration for neck injuries penetrating the platysma muscle was formulated. This policy has been modified at a number of institutions because of the differences between military and civilian trauma and the high rate of negative results in neck exploration. Advocates of mandatory exploration quote a 1% morbidity and no mortality associated with negative results on exploration and a high rate of significant injury that is present with no clinical findings (17%).[52] Those surgeons opting for selective neck exploration employ early operation for hematomas or hemodynamic instability and further diagnostic evaluation in the patient with negative results on physical examination. Advocates of this approach cite decreased rates of explorations with negative results from 60 to 20%, no increased morbidity, and decreased hospital costs.[5, 35] Although the reported experience of penetrating head and neck injury in children is small, the pattern of injury is similar to that seen in adults, as shown by the Harlem Hospital review of 45 patients.[12] The majority of the injuries were accidental gunshot wounds, but there were seven stab wounds. No deaths were caused by stab wounds, but there was a 16% mortality rate associated with gunshot wounds. No morbidity was caused by a policy of selective exploration.

To safely employ selective neck exploration, diagnostic studies are necessary to assess injuries. For purposes of assigning risk of injury, the neck is divided into three zones: zone 1 below the sternal notch, zone 2 between the sternal notch and the angle of the mandible, and zone 3 above the angle of the mandible. Arch aortography is employed for zone 1 injuries, carotid angiography for zone 3 injuries, and no or selective angiography for zone 2 injuries.[32, 51, 52] Although the vessels in zone 2 are easily accessible, angiography can be helpful for these injuries to plan which side of the neck to explore first and to identify uncommon but troublesome vertebral artery injury. Because arteriography itself is an invasive procedure requiring general anesthesia in children, a CT scan with intravenous contrast or digital subtraction angiography may obviate its need for less suspicious injuries. Other studies useful for patients managed selectively are lateral neck radiographs, esophagogram, and, rarely, esophagoscopy and bronchoscopy. A chest film is the most important study in patients managed operatively or nonoperatively. Although the cost of diagnostic evaluations is high, mandatory exploration results in a 63% rate of negative results on exploration, a longer hospitalization, and increased overall expenditures.[35]

Thoracic

Although thoracic trauma in children is uncommon, in a series of 68 children, Meller and colleagues found that penetrating trauma is more common than blunt trauma, especially in adolescents in urban areas.[34] In their series, in which 60% of the injuries were penetrating, 60% of these were secondary to gunshot wounds. In spite of these figures, the majority of penetrating thoracic injuries do not require thoracotomy.[2, 3, 34, 66] An algorithm for treating these uncommon injuries is necessary. One of the few indications for emergency department thoracotomy is the child with penetrating thoracic trauma who presents with no vital signs or who loses vital signs in the emergency department. Transportable patients with unstable vital signs should be taken to the operating room for resuscitation and thoracotomy. In the remaining patients, evaluation and treatment begin in the emergency department with the insertion of an upper and lower extremity intravenous catheter and the performance of a chest radiograph and a tube thoracostomy for hemothorax or pneumothorax. The subsequent need for thoracotomy is based on a continued blood loss of more than 100 ml per hour, a total blood loss approximating 50% of estimated blood volume, a massive air leak, or a suspected cardiac or esophageal injury. A high index of suspicion, especially for midthoracic injuries, followed by contrast esophagogram is the best way to diagnose often occult esophageal injuries. Findings at thoracotomy in the Meller and co-workers series included bleeding from intercostal and subclavian arteries and vein, bronchopleural fistula, and cardiac injury.

Cardiac

The particular problems of cardiac injury in children have been reviewed by Golladay and colleagues. They state that the smaller pericardial sac can lead to faster hemodynamic decompensation, the likelihood of unsuspected congenital anomalies are higher than that in adults, and the softer thoracic cage and sternum permit penetrating injuries more readily.[21] Penetrating cardiac injuries in infants may be caused by needles puncturing the sternum, ingested sharp objects eroding through the esophagus, and iatrogenic perforation at cardiac catheterization.[45] Historically, cardiac injury from gunshot wounds has been rare in children. However, with the increased use of firearms by teenagers, these injuries can be expected to increase.

Vascular

The special problems of vascular injuries in children are covered in Chapter 19. Commonly, penetrating vascular injury to an extremity appears as an isolated lesion secondary to stab or gunshot wounds. Navarre and associates reviewed 59 cases of major vessel trauma over 17 years, 30% secondary to glass injury.[41] They cautioned against undue optimism regarding nonoperative management. Special considerations remain, such as an increased incidence of complications in popliteal injuries and potential growth impairment, although basic principles remain similar to those of management of adult vascular injuries. In a review of vascular injuries to 118 children who were treated at Johns Hopkins University Hospital over a 10-year period, 22 were due to penetrating trauma and 41 were secondary to iatrogenic penetrating injury. Penetrating trauma was more common in the adolescents, whereas iatrogenic injury was equally distributed throughout all age ranges. Operative intervention was required in 19 of 22 penetrating injuries and in 27 of 41 iatrogenic injuries.[56] In the event of intra-abdominal and extremity gunshot wounds, in most instances exploratory celiotomy should precede repair of the extremity.

Abdominal

The approach to the stable child with a known intra-abdominal injury that requires celiotomy is straightforward. The usefulness of antibiotics in decreasing the infectious complications associated with operations on the gastrointestinal tract is so well established that the only issues that remain are which antibiotics and how long they should be administered.[15] In a prospective randomized trial comparing 12 hours with 5 days of antibiotic therapy, no differences were noted in culture results, trauma-related infection, or nosocomial infection. Patients with colonic injury had significantly more infections than patients with small bowel injury, but the study was designed so that colonic injuries would be equally distributed between the two arms of the study. In two studies comparing different antibiotic protocols for adults with penetrating abdominal trauma, cefoxitin was as effective as a combination of an aminoglycoside and clindamycin.[27, 42] Not surprisingly, therapy with cefamandole was associated with an increased incidence of anaerobic infections.

A midline incision offers the best exposure and most options when exploring a patient for trauma. For infants, a transverse incision may be used but can limit access to the pelvis or chest. After temporarily controlling bleeding and fecal contamination, a careful inventory of all injuries and a plan for repair is made. In the child with multiple organ injury, the most expeditious repair is often the most prudent. In several series, the liver was the most commonly injured solid organ and the small intestine the most commonly injured hollow viscus.[2, 3, 43, 65, 66]

In many patients explored for positive blood on peritoneal lavage, hepatic bleeding has stopped. For those whose bleeding has not, the bleeding can be controlled with packs while the abdomen is explored. The management of specific intra-abdominal organ system injuries is covered extensively in other chapters and therefore is reviewed only briefly here. Splenic injuries are usually amenable to splenorrhaphy in cases of penetrating trauma. If not, partial splenectomy should be employed, with splenectomy reserved for cases of massive disruption of the hilum. The role of heterotopic splenic transplant remains questionable but warrants further investigation.[11, 64]

That the child with serious pancreaticoduodenal injuries may fare better than adults has been reviewed.[46] A variety of techniques from direct repair of duodenal lacerations to duodenal diverticulization to total pancreatectomy are available. Small bowel enterotomies may be closed primarily or in a severely contused segment of bowel resection and enteroenterostomy may be preferred.

The traditional management of colonic injury mandates colostomy. Increasingly, surgeons are suggesting that minor colon injuries may be repaired primarily. Criteria for primary repair over colostomy include operation within 8 hours of injury, a hemodynamically stable patient, less than three injured intra-abdominal organs, and minimal fecal contamination.[60] The advantages of this management include avoidance of a colostomy and a secondary operation, decreased infectious complications, and decreased hospitalization and cost. When these criteria are followed and good clinical judgment is used, morbidity is reduced.

OPERATIVE TREATMENT OF THE UNSTABLE CHILD

In the unstable child with a penetrating injury, skin preparation in the operating room should be wide to provide access to adjacent anatomic areas. For neck injuries, the chest should be included in the event that a sternotomy or "trap-door" incision is necessary. An extremity should also be prepared in case a saphenous vein is needed. Thoracic injuries are more likely to require celiotomy than thoracotomy, but the need for either should not cause surprise.

Anticipation and preparedness has its greatest impact on outcome in dealing with retrohepatic caval injuries. Failure to prepare for this before laparotomy may convert a potentially salvageable injury to a lethal injury. In the face of a penetrating wound to the right upper quadrant in an unstable patient, the equipment and approach should be planned to allow atrial caval bypass to be performed quickly. Either a thoracoabdominal or midline incision from the jugular notch to the symphysis pubis may be used. Our preference is for a midline incision because of its simplicity and speed. Chest tubes of a size appropriate for the child can be modified with side holes cut at the estimated level of the atrium. A cuffed endotracheal tube can also be used for the shunt and may obviate the need for a tourniquet around the inferior vena cava. The shunt is placed according to techniques that have been well described.[54] We agree with Kudsk and co-workers and others who advocate passing the shunt through the atrial appendage rather than the inferior vena cava, thereby avoiding potential bleeding problems associated with a caval venotomy.[29] This approach has the additional benefit of allowing an appropriate adaptor to be attached to the end of the tube to permit the rapid infusion of volume.

In reviewing hepatic venous injuries in children, Coln and colleagues noted that failure to quickly appreciate preoperatively and intraoperatively the seriousness of the liver injury contributed to the mortality in the children surveyed

in his review.[9] Unfortunately, the only factor that identified children with the potential for deterioration was the presence of hemoperitoneum in the face of a liver laceration extending to the retroperitoneum. Because uncontrolled hemorrhage leading to hypothermia and disseminated intravascular coagulation leads to death, there may be a limited role in extreme circumstances for placing packs and performing a second celiotomy when the coagulopathy and hypothermia have been reversed.[18] Others caution against this, stating that the mortality remains unchanged and the septic complications are increased.[25]

EXPERIENCE OF CHILDREN'S HOSPITAL OF MICHIGAN IN DEALING WITH TORSO TRAUMA

The records of all children admitted to CHM with a diagnosis of penetrating torso trauma from 1983 through 1987 were reviewed (Table 40–6). During this 5-year interval, 50 patients were admitted. Their ages range from 11 months to 16 years, with an average of 10.7 years. This average age is somewhat younger than that of other series of pediatric patients and reflects the practices of the referral and triage system in Detroit, where the majority of teenagers with penetrating trauma are taken to adult institutions.

In other respects the CHM patient population matches that of other series. Males predominated with a ratio of 35:15 or 2.3:1.0. Injuries were more common during the summer months and during the evenings when children may be less well supervised (Figs. 40–3, 40–4). Gunshot wounds were most common, resulting in 22 injuries. Knife wounds accounted for 19 injuries, glass shards for eight injuries, and a chair puncture wound for one injury. The average hospital stay for the total series was 6.1 days with a range of from 1 to 49 days.

Attempts were made to categorize the reason for the injury. Twenty injuries were accidental, and in six cases the cause of the injury remained unclear even after inquiries were made. The other 24 injuries were the result of altercations. Eleven children were the victims of violent crimes outside the home. Four were involved in fights. Nine children were assaulted by family members or friends in the home. There were no suicide attempts in our series.

Table 40–7 shows the pathology for all torso injuries including associated injuries and complications. Seventeen

Table 40–6

Torso Trauma, Children's Hospital of Michigan, 1983–1986 (50 patients)

	Chest (n = 22)	Abdomen (n = 32)	Mean
Age (range)	11 mo–16 yr	30 mo–16 yr	10.7 yr
Sex (M:F)	18:4	20:12	35:15
Hospital days			6.1
Instrument			
Knife	19		
Gun	22		
Glass	8		
Other	1		

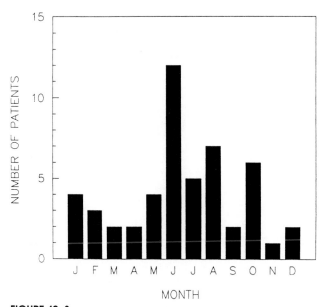

FIGURE 40-3

Torso injuries seen at Children's Hospital of Michigan by month of the year.

patients had chest injuries, 26 patients had abdominal injuries, and seven patients had thoracoabdominal injuries. Of patients with injuries apparently limited to the chest, only three required chest tubes and 13 were managed with repair of the laceration and observation for pneumothorax. One patient with a shotgun blast injury required an arteriogram and an arm exploration to ligate the lateral humeral circumflex artery.

Ten patients with potential abdominal injuries were treated with local wound care either in the emergency department or in the operating room and then were observed. This group included patients with buttock and flank injuries. One patient required examination under anesthesia with proctosigmoidoscopy to exclude rectal injury. There were no complications in this group, and maximum hospital stay was 3 days. Sixteen patients with suspected intra-abdominal injuries underwent celiotomy. Lavage was performed in only one patient, who had a retroperitoneal GSW and required celiotomy. Celiotomy was considered necessary if active bleeding required control, if an omental evisceration was reduced, or if intra-abdominal organs required repair and was justified by operative findings in 12 patients. In the remaining four patients, celiotomy proved to be unnecessary. One of these patients was transferred after a celiotomy elsewhere led to repairs of his aorta, left renal pedicle, liver, kidney, pancreas, and stomach. Concern by the referring surgeon and continued hemodynamic instability after transfer led to re-exploration, at which time no active bleeding was identified. The child subsequently did well.

Of the 12 patients in whom operative findings justified celiotomy, seven had GSWs and five had stab wounds. There were five small bowel injuries; three stomach injuries; two pancreatic injuries requiring drainage; two colonic injuries; two eviscerations; one splenic injury requiring splenorrhaphy; one diaphragmatic injury; one ureteral in-

jury; one isolated bile duct injury; and one combined liver, gallbladder, and common hepatic duct injury. One patient who had had his initial operation at another hospital was operated on again at CHM for a previously unappreciated ureteral transection. Three patients had complications: one rectovesical fistula and two postoperative bowel obstructions. The patient with the rectovesical fistula had had an ileostomy and bladder repair, and his fistula was healed after drainage of a presacral abscess. In both patients with small bowel obstructions, the initial celiotomy was necessary, and both required another operation within 2 months of the original procedure for adhesiolysis.

Five of seven patients with thoracoabdominal injuries underwent celiotomy. Of the two patients in whom celiotomy was not done, one patient had stab wounds to the abdomen, chest, back, and neck and was evaluated by aortogram, esophagogram, and observation. The other patient with chest and abdominal stab wounds had local wound explorations and closure with placement of a chest tube in the operating room. One patient had an unnecessary celiotomy. The other patients were found to have injured colon, small bowel, stomach, and hemopericardium and an actively bleeding intercostal artery. One patient required thoracotomy for repair of the subclavian artery. An additional three patients had chest tubes placed. None of the patients died in this series. A total of five unnecessary celiotomies were performed, one of which was unavoidable because of the clinical situation. In three of the remaining four patients, prior intraperitoneal bleeding had stopped by the time of exploration. One had no intra-abdominal pathologic condition.

In our institution, all patients with injuries suspected of penetrating the abdominal cavity are admitted to the hospital. Patients with stab wounds who receive benign results on abdominal examinations using Shaftan's criteria (i.e., abdominal tenderness, absent peristalsis, or blood in the gastrointestinal tract) are observed overnight; followed with

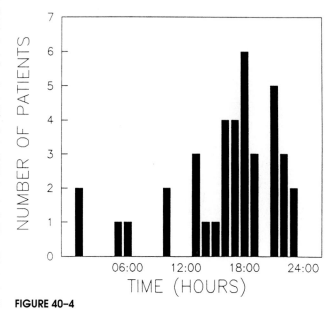

FIGURE 40-4

Time of injury for torso injuries seen at Children's Hospital of Michigan.

Table 40–7
Pathology of 50 Torso Injuries

	Number	Operations	Complications
Head and Neck			
Skull fracture	1		
Superficial	3		
Brachial plexus	1		
Chest		8*	1 unnecessary celiotomy
Wall	16		
Parenchyma	7		
Major vessels	1		
Abdomen		21	Hypoxic
Pericardium/diaphragm	2		Encephalopathy
Liver	9		Footdrop
Gallbladder, CBD	2		
Spleen	1		
Kidney	2		Bile Infection
Ureter/bladder	2		Flank abscess
Pancreas	3		Vesicorectal fistula
Colon	4		
Small bowel	7		2 SBO reoperations
Stomach	5		
Mesentery	1		4 unnecessary
			laparotomies
Major vascular	1		
Flank, abdominal wall	15		
Buttock	2		
Perineum	1		
Extremities		1	Wrist drop
Superficial	7		
Deep	1		
Fracture	1		

*Includes one thoracotomy and eight chest tube operations.
CBD, Common bile duct; SBO, small bowel obstruction.

repeated abdominal examinations, urinalysis, a repeat complete blood count and amylase test; and given liquids the following morning. A social service evaluation is required for all those who have penetrating injuries. If they remain clinically stable, they are discharged. Patients with clinical evidence of peritoneal irritation are explored. Omental evisceration alone is an indication for exploration because of a 70% incidence of major injury associated with this finding, and closure of the wound is facilitated by general anesthesia. Patients with GSWs that are clearly tangential within the abdominal wall are observed overnight following the same protocol described for patients with stab wounds. All GSWs, including air gun wounds, that penetrate the abdominal cavity are explored.

From this review of our recent experience, we conclude that a policy of selective lavage may have spared four of 20 celiotomies. We would agree with others that there is a role for peritoneal lavage in patients with equivocal findings following abdominal stab wounds that penetrate the peritoneum. Our modified approach with patients who have stab wounds that enter the peritoneal cavity is exploration for those with clinical findings of peritoneal irritation and lavage and observation for those without such findings if returns do not mandate celiotomy. This approach is similarly applied to those who have penetrating wounds of the chest below the nipples.

CONCLUSIONS

Penetrating trauma is increasing in frequency and in some urban centers may be more common than blunt trauma.

Victims of penetrating trauma are also more likely to require operative intervention. Although pediatric surgeons were early advocates of selective nonoperative management of blunt trauma, adult general surgeons have pioneered selective celiotomy for penetrating trauma based on findings from peritoneal lavage. These techniques have been used safely in children and will decrease the rate of unnecessary laparotomies when more widely applied.

Although some serious penetrating traumatic injuries are accidental and unavoidable, a large percentage are potentially preventable. Increased home safety with lack of access to knives or loaded guns would have prevented several serious injuries in toddlers and young children in our series. Regulation of air gun sales and use would decrease injuries in the childhood and adolescent age groups. Finally, the widespread availability of handguns has contributed to their increased use in adolescent conflicts and suicides. Children are better able to tolerate significant penetrating injury than adults and have fewer complications and less mortality.

References

1. Baker SP, O'Neill B, Karpf RS: The injury facts. In: The Injury Fact Book. Lexington, Mass, Lexington Books, 1984, p 20.
2. Barlow B, Niemirska M, Gandhi RP: Ten years' experience with pediatric gunshot wounds. J Pediatr Surg 17:927–932, 1982.
3. Barlow B, Niemirska M, Gandhi RP: Stab wounds in children. J Pediatr Surg 18:926–929, 1983.
4. Beaver BL, Colombani PM, Burk JR, et al: Efficacy of emergency room thoracotomy in pediatric trauma. J Pediatr Surg 22:19–23, 1987.

5. Belinkie SA, Russell JC, DaSilva J, Becker DR: Management of penetrating neck injuries. J Trauma 23:235–237, 1983.
6. Blocker S, Coln D, Chang JHT: Serious air rifle injuries in children. Pediatrics 69:751–754, 1982.
7. Bowers WF: Priority of treatment in multiple injuries and summation of surgery of auto trauma. Arch Surg 75:743, 1957.
8. Burnweit CA, Thal ER: Significance of omental evisceration in abdominal stab wounds. Am J Surgery 152:670–673, 1986.
9. Coln D, Crighton J, Schorn L: Successful management of hepatic vein injury from blunt trauma in children. Am J Surg 140:858–864, 1980.
10. Cook DE, Walsh JW, Vick CW, Brewer WH: Upper abdominal trauma: Pitfalls in CT diagnosis. Radiology 159:65–69, 1986.
11. Cooney DR, Dearth JC, Swanson SE: Relative merits of partial splenectomy, splenic reimplantation, and immunization in preventing post-splenectomy infection. Surgery 86:561–569, 1979.
12. Cooper A, Barlow B, Niemirska M, et al: Fifteen years' experience with penetrating trauma to the head and neck in children. J Pediatr Surg 22:24–27, 1987.
13. Cornell WP, Ebert PA, Greenfield LC, et al: A new nonoperative technique for the diagnosis of penetrating injuries to the abdomen. J Trauma 7:307–314, 1967.
14. de Lacy AM, Pera M, Garcia-Valdecasas JC, et al: Management of penetrating abdominal stab wounds. Br J Surg 75:231–233, 1988.
15. Dellinger EP, Wertz MJ, Leonard ES, et al: Efficacy of short-course antibiotics prophylaxis after penetrating intestinal injury. A prospective randomized trial. Arch Surg 121:23–30, 1986.
16. Demetriades D, Rabinowitz B: Selective conservative management of penetrating abdominal wounds: A prospective study. Br J Surg 71:92–94, 1984.
17. Feliciano DV, Bitonda CG, Steed G, et al: Five hundred open laps or lavages in patients with abdominal stab wounds. Am J Surg 148:772–777, 1984.
18. Feliciano DV, Mattox KL, Burch JM, et al: Packing for control of hepatic hemorrhage. J Trauma 26:738–742, 1986.
19. Fischer RP, Beverlin BC, Engrav CH, et al: Diagnostic peritoneal lavage. Fourteen years and 2586 patients later. Am J Surg 136:701–714, 1978.
20. Goldman E, McDonald JS, Peterson SS, et al: Transtracheal ventilation with oscillatory pressure for complete upper airway obstruction. J Trauma 28:611–614, 1988.
21. Golladay ES, Donahoo JS, Haller JA: Special problems of cardiac injuries in infants and children. J Trauma 19:526–531, 1979.
22. Granson MA, Dunovan AJ: Abdominal stab wound with omental evisceration. Arch Surg 118:57–59, 1983.
23. Hanigan WC, Olivero WC, Duffy N, et al: Lawn dart injury in children: Report of two cases. Pediatr Emerg Care 2:247–249, 1986.
24. Harris W, Luterman A, Curreri PW: BB and pellet guns—Toys or deadly weapons? J Trauma 23:567–569, 1983.
25. Ivatury RR, Nallathambi M, Gunduz Y, et al: Liver packing for uncontrolled hemorrhage. J Trauma 26:744–753, 1986.
26. Jacobs HB: Emergency percutaneous transtracheal catheter and ventilation. J Trauma 12:50–52, 1972.
27. Jones RC, Thal ER, Johnson NA, et al: Evaluation of antibiotic therapy following penetrating abdominal trauma. Ann Surg 201:576–585, 1985.
28. Karp MP, Cooney DR, Berger PE, et al: The role of computed tomography in the evaluation of blunt abdominal trauma in children. J Pediatr Surg 16:316–323, 1981.
29. Kudsk KA, Sheldon GF, Lim RC: Atrial-caval shunting (ACS) after trauma. J Trauma 22:81–85, 1982.
30. Lazarus HM, Nelson JA: A technique for peritoneal lavage without risk or complication. Surg Gynecol Obstet 149:889–892, 1979.
31. Lowe RJ, Boyd DR, Folk FA, Baker RJ: The negative laparotomy for abdominal trauma. J Trauma 12:853–861, 1972.
32. Lundy LJ: Experience in selective operations for the management of penetrating wounds of the neck. Surg Gynecol Obstet 147:845–848, 1978.
33. McAlvanah MJ, Shaftan GW: Selective conservatism in penetrating abdominal wounds: A continuing reappraisal. J Trauma 18:206–212, 1978.
34. Meller JL, Little AG, Shermeta DW: Thoracic trauma in children. Pediatrics 74:813–819, 1984.
35. Merion RM, Harness JK, Ramsburgh SR, et al: Selective management of penetrating neck trauma. Arch Surg 116:691–696, 1981.
36. Morbidity and Mortality Weekly Report 35:357–365, 1986.
37. Morbidity and Mortality Weekly Report 36:87–89, 1987.
38. Morgan JC, Turner CS, Pennell TC: Air gun injuries of the abdomen in children. Arch Surg 119:1437–1438, 1984.
39. Nakamura DS, McNamara JJ, Sanderson L, et al: Thoracic airgun injuries in children. Am J Surg 146:39–42, 1983.
40. Nance FC, Wennar MH, Johnson LW, et al: Surgical judgment in the management of penetrating wounds of the abdomen. Ann Surg 179:639–646, 1974.
41. Navarre JR, Cardillo PJ, Gorman JF, et al: Vascular trauma in children and adolescents. Am J Surg 143:229–231, 1982.
42. Nichols RL, Smith JW, Klein DB, et al: Risk of infection after penetrating abdominal trauma. N Engl J Med 311:1065–1070, 1984.
43. Ordoz GJ, Prakash A, Wasserberger J, Balasubramanian S: Pediatric gunshot wounds. J Trauma 27:1272–1278, 1987.
44. Oreskovich MR, Carrico CJ: Stab wounds of the anterior abdomen. Analysis of a management plan using local wound exploration and quantitative peritoneal lavage. Ann Surg 198:411–414, 1983.
45. Pennington DG: Penetrating injuries. In: Golladay ES (ed): Injuries to the Heart and Chest in Children. Mount Kisco, NY, Futura Publishing Co, 1983, pp 201–238.
46. Pokorny WJ, Brandt ML, Harberg FJ: Major duodenal injuries in children: Diagnosis, operative management, and outcome. J Pediatr Surg 21:613–616, 1986.
47. Powell RW, Green JB, Ochsner MG: Peritoneal lavage in pediatric patients sustaining blunt abdominal trauma: A reappraisal. J Trauma 7:6–10, 1987.
48. Reddick EJ, Carter PL, Bickerstaff L: Air gun injuries in children. Ann Emerg Med 14:1108–1111, 1985.
49. Rivara FP: Traumatic deaths of children in the United States: Currently available prevention strategies. Pediatrics 75:456–462, 1985.
50. Rohman M, Ivatury RR, Steichen FM, et al: Emergency room thoracotomy for penetrating cardiac injuries. J Trauma 23:570–576, 1983.
51. Room AN, Christenson N: Evaluation and treatment of penetrating cervical injuries. J Trauma 19:391–397, 1979.
52. Saletta JD, Lowe RJ, Lim LT, et al: Penetrating trauma of the neck. J Trauma 16:579–587, 1976.
53. Schetky DH: Children and handguns. A public health concern. Am J Dis Child 139:229–231, 1985.
54. Schrock T, Blaisdell W, Mathewson C: Management of blunt trauma to the liver and hepatic veins. Arch Surg 96:698–704, 1968.
55. Shaftan GW: Indications for operation in abdominal trauma. Am J Surg 99:657–664, 1960.
56. Shaker IJ, White JJ, Signer RD, et al: Special problems of vascular injuries in children. J Trauma 16:863–867, 1976.
57. Shimazu S, Shatney CH: Outcomes of trauma patients with no vital signs on hospital admission. J Trauma 23:213–216, 1983.
58. Sinclair MC, Moore TC: Major surgery for abdominal and thoracic trauma in childhood and adolescence. J Pediatr Surg 9:155–162, 1974.
59. Spoerel WZ, Narayanan PS, Singh NP: Transtracheal ventilation. Br J Anaesth 43:921–939, 1971.
60. Stone HH, Fabian TC: Management of perforating colon trauma: Randomization between primary closure and exteriorization. Ann Surg 190:430–436, 1979.
61. Thal ER: Evaluation of peritoneal lavage and local exploration in lower chest and abdominal stab wounds. J Trauma 17:642–650, 1977.
62. The Detroit Free Press, October 11, 1987.
63. Thompson JS, Moore EE, Van Duzer-Moore S, et al: The evolution of abdominal stab wound management. J Trauma 20:478–484, 1980.
64. Traub A, Giebink GS, Smith C, et al: Splenic reticuloendothelial function after splenectomy, spleen repair, and spleen autotransplantation. N Engl J Med 317:1559–1564, 1987.
65. Tunell WP, Knost J, Nance FC: Penetrating abdominal injuries in children and adolescents. J Trauma 15:720–725, 1975.
66. Valentine J, Blocker S, Chang JHT: Gunshot injuries in children. J Trauma 24:952–956, 1984.
67. Waller JB, Gaines G: 1983 Data Book. City of Detroit, Office of Epidemiology and Biostatistics, Detroit, Mich, pp 34–353.
68. Wintemute GJ: Firearms as a cause of death in the United States, 1920–1982. J Trauma 27:532–536, 1987.

CHAPTER FORTY-ONE

David B. Reath
Don Larossa

Wound Healing and Traumatic Soft Tissue Defects

The successful recovery of children who are wounded either traumatically or surgically is dependent on satisfactory wound healing, a complex process that begins at the moment of injury. Frequently, this healing process is uncomplicated and efficient and proceeds almost unnoticed. In other instances, the repair and healing of massive soft tissue injuries requires complex reconstructive efforts, such as borrowing tissue from sites near and far from the injury to achieve a closed wound. Recovery from injury is not complete until all wounds are healed.

Successful repair of soft tissue wounds requires the restoration of both form and function. Although one of these may be of relatively greater importance in a specific wound, restoration of both must always be considered and, as much as possible, achieved. Deficiencies in either form or function may result in disfigurement or disability, preventing or delaying a full recovery and return to a normal life.

An important part of the process of wound healing for the parents and child is a basic understanding of what to expect from a healing wound in terms of its appearance and behavior. While the child is still in the hospital, the parents and family should be instructed in basic wound care techniques and taught to assist in this care of the child before and after discharge. This involvement of the family promotes their participation in the recovery of the child from the trauma and is beneficial to all of those involved.

WOUND HEALING

Wound healing is commonly divided into three overlapping phases: the inflammatory phase, the proliferative phase, and the maturation phase. Inflammation begins with wounding, whereas maturation may continue for 1 to 2 years following injury and probably never ends completely. The basic healing process is the same for traumatic or surgical wounds.[5, 7, 9, 19]

Inflammation is a nonspecific response that follows injury of any type. Without inflammation, wound healing cannot be initiated. Normal, acute inflammation is the surgeon's ally. However, prolonged, chronic inflammation may retard, interfere with, or alter normal wound healing.

The inflammatory phase is characterized by changes at both the vascular and cellular levels. At the time of wounding, local tissue disruption allows the entrance of intracellular material into the extracellular space. The immediate vascular response is vasoconstriction. A fibrin clot forms, and with activation of the complement cascade, hemostasis is achieved. However, after 5 to 10 minutes, vasodilation occurs, increasing local blood flow up to tenfold. Under the direction of vasoactive amines and other polypeptides, permeability of the microcirculation increases, compounded by proteolytic enzymes, which alter the vascular membrane and add to the leaking of fluids into the extracellular space. Locally produced prostaglandins also antagonize vasoconstriction and sustain capillary permeability. This increased local blood flow and capillary permeability cause the inflamed wound to appear erythematous and edematous.

The cellular response of inflammation also begins immediately after injury. Initially, leukocytes marginate within the capillaries and enter the wound by diapedesis. Early on, polymorphonuclear leukocytes predominate; their role is one of antisepsis by the ingestion and destruction of bacteria. The more contaminated or dirty a wound is, the greater the presence of polymorphonuclear leukocytes.

Polymorphonuclear leukocytes are short lived; therefore, the macrophage soon becomes predominant within the wound. These cells play a major role in the process of wound healing.[8] Wound healing does not occur in the absence of activated macrophages. These cells continue to enter the wound and are activated by lymphokines, immune complexes, and complement products. In addition to the phagocytosis of wound debris, macrophages modulate fibroblast proliferation and collagen production.

During this period in wound healing, new capillaries, which are both abundant and fragile, are formed by epithelial budding. This process gives the wound its prominent features of erythema and easy bleeding. If excessive amounts of debris, necrotic tissue, bacteria, or blood are present within the wound, the migration of fibroblasts and formation of new capillaries is impeded. In this situation, inflammation of the wound is intensified and prolonged, delaying normal healing.

Usually, most debris is removed by 3 to 5 days postinjury, at a time when new capillaries and fibroblasts are entering the wound. This marks the beginning of the proliferative phase of wound healing, which lasts 2 to 4 weeks. Fibroblasts initially produce a ground substance that is necessary for the proper orientation and aggregation of collagen. By the third day after the injury, collagen can be detected within the wound. Its synthesis is complex and occurs both within the fibroblast and the extracellular milieu.

Tensile strength parallels the collagen content of the wound and peaks at 3 to 4 weeks after the injury. At this time, the collagen deposited in the wound is disarrayed and disorganized. Over the next several months or years, the collagen is reoriented by collagenolysis and continued collagen synthesis. This process constitutes the phase of maturation. Through gradual intermolecular and intramolecular cross-linking, tensile strength continues to rise within the wound, although at a slower rate than during the proliferative phase. At the end of the maturation phase, a scar, which previously was raised and reddened, is now flattened and faded. The time required for scar maturation varies a great deal, depending on both the location of the scar and the individual's own healing process; it may be as long as 2 years.

Wound contraction takes place in all healing wounds and is an active, energy-requiring process mediated by the myofibroblast, the contractible fibroblast. These cells have characteristics of both fibroblasts and smooth muscle cells, as they both produce collagen and actively contract. In addition to shortening the scars of coapted wounds, contraction, along with epithelialization, is responsible for the eventual healing of many wounds that are left open (Fig. 41–1). Epithelialization occurs at the margin of all wounds. The cells mobilize and, through the loss of contact inhibition, migrate away from one another toward the center of the wound. These cells then divide and differentiate to form the normal layers of the skin. This process proceeds more quickly in a moist environment.

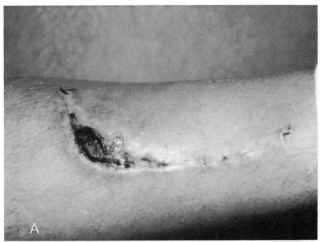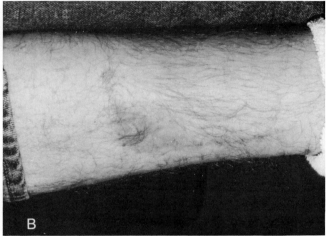

FIGURE 41-1
An open lower leg wound *(A)* that closes over time *(B)* through contraction and re-epithelialization.

TYPES OF WOUND HEALING

Healing by primary intention occurs when the edges of a full thickness wound are coapted or the wound is covered with a skin graft or flap shortly after the creation of the wound. Contraction and re-epithelialization play minor roles in this form of wound healing. The initial strength of the wound is supplied by sutures or tapes used to close the wound.

Wounds that heal without surgical intervention heal by secondary intention. This phenomenon occurs both with uncomplicated wounds left unattended and with large wounds, which, because of soft tissue losses, are not amenable to primary repair. Wound contraction is the most important factor in the healing of these wounds. This contraction decreases the size of all wounds and may allow the apposition of dermal surfaces in smaller wounds. However, in larger wounds, the process is incomplete, and other methods of closure must be employed. Epithelialization and normal collagen production are probably not as important as contraction in healing by secondary intention.

Tertiary intention, or healing by delayed primary closure, involves the coaptation of two granulating surfaces or coverage of a granulating wound with a skin graft or flap. These techniques are appropriate in cases in which delayed closure of the wound is required because of contamination or devitalization. These types of closure do not alter or delay the eventual strength of the wound. A wound closed on the third day after the injury has the same tensile strength on the seventh day as it would if it had been closed primarily.[22]

ACUTE MANAGEMENT OF SOFT TISSUE WOUNDS

The way in which a wound is allowed to heal depends on many factors: the method of wounding, the location and size of the wound, the amount of tissue loss, the tidiness or amount of devitalization of the wound, the functional loss of the wounded body part, and the overall condition of the patient. The mechanism of wounding frequently determines how a wound is allowed to heal. Cleanly incised wounds are most frequently closed and allowed to heal primarily. Crush or bursting injuries may be complicated by large degrees of tissue devitalization and subsequent loss, which interfere with primary closure. Similarly, heavily contaminated or dirty wounds are usually not amenable to primary closure because of the risk of subsequent infection.

The amount and type of tissue loss must be carefully considered. As a result of the loss of skin tension, all incised wounds separate or gape open, giving the initial impression that a certain degree of tissue loss has occurred. If little or no tissue loss has in fact occurred, primary repair is easily accomplished. When large soft tissue deficiencies have been created, primary repair is not possible, and some method of reconstruction must be chosen.

Débridement and Excision

Wound repair begins with the creation of a clean or tidy wound through proper débridement and irrigation. When wounds are created by high-kinetic-energy or crushing forces, significant tissue devitalization occurs. In even minor injuries that are created bluntly, the margins of the wound may have been traumatized to the extent that appreciable soft tissue necrosis may ensue. Proper débridement requires the excision of not only grossly contaminated and devitalized tissues but also marginally viable tissue that is destined to undergo necrosis in the next 36 to 48 hours (Fig. 41–2). It is far better to recognize the impending necrosis of a portion of the wound and débride it than to incorporate it into the repair. The latter occurrence either causes a prolonged inflammatory phase and a poor aesthetic result or leads to wound separation and the possibility of secondary infection.[17, 21]

In complex wounds, good clinical judgment is the best guide to adequate débridement. In areas of relative tissue excess, such as the forehead, cheek, scalp, trunk, and prox-

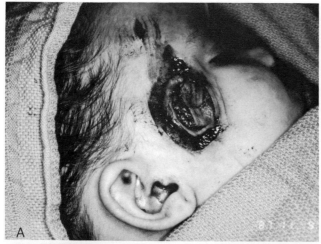
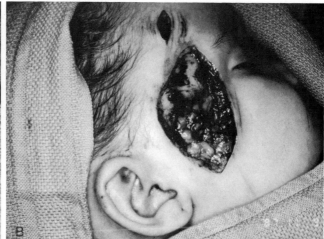
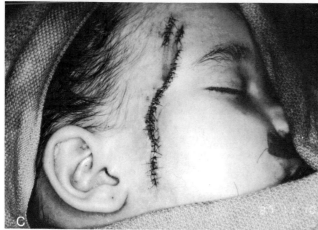

FIGURE 41-2

A large facial wound (A) with significant tissue devitalization is first excised and débrided (B) and then closed (C) with advancement of local skin flaps.

imal extremities, radical débridement can be accomplished with relative impunity. However, when dealing with more specialized soft tissues, such as those of the eyelids, eyebrows, lips, and nose, judicious débridement should be employed to preserve any viable tissue to simplify reconstruction. Occasionally the intravenous injection of fluorescein dye at a dose of 10 mg per kg helps to delineate the extent of tissue devitalization.[18] When injected with this dye, tissue with a healthy blood supply fluoresces under a Wood lamp and provides a guide to the amount of débridement necessary.

Excision of the margins of facial wounds may be appropriate before closure. The contused or devitalized tissues at the wound margins can lead to a more intense inflammatory phase if not excised. In addition, beveled and uneven wound edges may be rendered more favorable for closure if excised (Fig. 41–3A and B). The ultimate result of a properly excised wound is aesthetically far superior to those not treated in this manner. However, if wounds are improperly excised, ultimate reconstruction can be made more difficult or impossible. If doubt exists regarding the advisability of excision in the primary care of facial wounds, they should be closed simply and revised secondarily.

In deep abrasions or explosion injuries, traumatic tatooing may occur. Particulate matter, dirt, or carbon particles may be deeply imbedded in the dermis and, if untreated, become incorporated at that level, leading to a characteristic

and unpleasant appearance. Proper treatment of these wounds requires vigorous scrubbing, dermabrasion, or meticulous excision of all particulate matter and debris when the wound is initially treated. Frequently, this must be done in the operating room with the patient under a general anesthetic. Efforts undertaken to properly treat tatooing are rewarded by the eventual appearance of a clean and well-healed wound. Once tatooed, these particles cannot be removed by simple means, but require full thickness excision of the involved tissues.

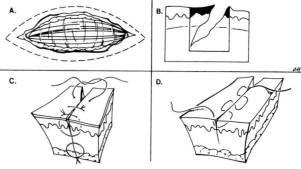

FIGURE 41-3

Proper wound excision creates a smoother (A), straighter wound edge (B) that facilitates closure. C, Layered wound closure. D, Subcuticular pull-out stitch.

Irrigation

After they are débrided and excised, all wounds should be well irrigated before closure. The preferred solutions for irrigation are saline or other balanced salt solutions (e.g., Ringer lactate) because of their low tissue toxicity.[22] Highly caustic irrigants, such as hydrogen peroxide and alcohol, should virtually never be used. In exceedingly contaminated or infected wounds, irrigation with a dilute povidone-iodine solution followed by saline may be appropriate. Irrigation is more effective if it is pulsatile and delivered under pressure. The easiest method of accomplishing this is through the use of a 12-ml syringe and a 22-gauge needle.[13] This instrument can deliver up to 13 pounds per square inch of pressure and has been shown to decrease wound infection. In larger or more contaminated wounds, use of a pulsatile irrigation apparatus, frequently used in orthopedic wounds, has been most effective in delivering large quantities (i.e., 4–6 liters) of irrigant in a pulsatile stream. If a large amount of dirt or foreign material is present in the wound, irrigation, when performed first, may be helpful in determining the extent of tissue devitalization before débridement.

Wound Dressings

The use of topical antibiotics on closed wounds is helpful in keeping the suture lines clean and preventing suture track infection. Closed wounds should be cleansed two or three times daily, and a clear antibiotic ointment should be applied. This method of care is also appropriate for deep abrasions. If wounds, particularly of the extremities, are considered too untidy for closure, serial dressing changes should be undertaken. Wet-to-dry gauze dressing changes are effective in providing serial, modest débridement with each dressing change. In less contaminated wounds, wet-to-wet saline-soaked dressings may be more appropriate, because they allow less tissue disruption. If significant bacterial superinfection becomes a problem, diluted Dakin or povidone-iodine solution can be used. In wounds that are relatively clean but too large for immediate closure, biologic dressings have been helpful. Human allograft skin or porcine xenograft skin used to be the most commonly used biologic dressings. At present, however, a versatile silicone nylon mesh impregnated with highly purified porcine collagen (Biobrane Temporary Biosynthetic Skin Substitute, Woodroof Laboratories, Santa Ana, Calif.) is emerging as the most useful, versatile, and readily available dressing. The use of Biobrane provides temporary wound coverage and allows the reconstructive surgeon a significant amount of time to study a problem wound and plan appropriate reconstruction.

WOUND CLOSURE

Before wound closure, the patient must be assessed carefully for associated injuries. Once closed, the function of the wounded part may not be evaluated as carefully, and associated injuries not previously identified may go undiagnosed for days. In facial injuries, the integrity of such structures as the facial nerve, the parotid duct, and the lacrimal apparatus must be ascertained (Fig. 41–4). Injuries to peripheral nerves and tendons are common in wounded extremities and should be diagnosed before any treatment. After local anesthesia has been injected, it is impossible to evaluate sensory or motor deficits. Appropriate radiographs should be obtained to diagnose associated skeletal injuries. As a general rule, most lacerations should be closed within 8 to 12 hours following injury. This period may be extended up to 18 hours in extremity and truncal wounds or up to 24 hours for facial wounds if the wounds are clean, well débrided, and irrigated and if broad-spectrum antibiotics are used. However, antibiotics need not be routinely used in clean wounds closed in a timely fashion. Tetanus prophylaxis, however, should always be managed adequately.

In patients with wounds that are too heavily contaminated for closure or that present too late for primary closure, open treatment with serial dressing changes and delayed primary closure at 3 days after injury is recommended. Even in extreme cases, most facial wounds can be adequately cleansed to facilitate primary closure as long as major soft tissue losses have not occurred.

When evaluating the injured child, a decision must be made with regard to management under local or general anesthesia. In many cases, local anesthesia supplemented by the intramuscular administration of a sedative, the proper restraint, and the support of a nurse or stalwart family member will allow closure of the wound in the emergency department setting. However, when the child cannot be calmed and restrained properly, when massive wounds are sustained, or when great precision and care is needed to repair the wound and prevent injury to other structures, it is wise to provide general anesthesia.

Clean wounds are routinely closed in a layered fashion (see Fig. 41–3C). Deep stitches of absorbable suture material are placed in the subcutaneous tissues in a buried fashion. The size of the suture (e.g., 5–0, 4–0, or 3–0), varies depending on the location of the injury and the size of the patient. The purpose of deep sutures is to close dead space and reduce the tension on the skin closure. These sutures should be placed judiciously, because excessive suture material in the subcutaneous space may potentiate wound infection.

The skin should be carefully everted and closed with simple stitches of a monofilament, nonabsorbable suture material such as nylon. Fine sutures of 6–0 are used to close facial wounds, whereas larger gauges (i.e., 5–0, 4–0, or 3–0) are used to close wounds of the extremity and trunk. In wounds of the trunk and extremity that are closed under a considerable amount of tension, a subcuticular pull-out stitch of a monofilament suture material such as polypropylene is useful, because this type of suture can be left in place for a longer period of time without the concern of stitch marks (see Fig. 41–3D). The practice of using a subcuticular stitch of absorbable material should be avoided, especially in the face. These sutures incite a greater inflammatory response and may result in a less pleasing aesthetic result.

Facial sutures are removed by 4 to 6 days after the injury

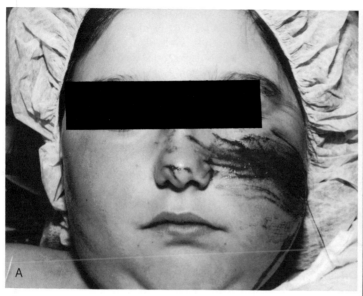

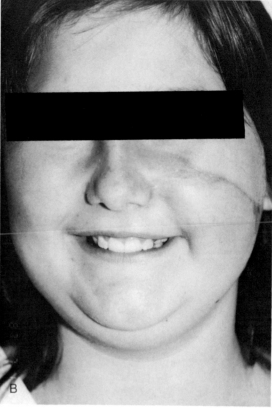

FIGURE 41–4

A, A deep laceration of the left cheek that divided branches of the facial nerve. *B,* Near complete recovery is seen several months after wound closure and nerve repair.

to prevent epithelialization of the suture tracks, which produces stitch marks. Sutures in extremity wounds are usually left in place for 7 to 10 days or even longer. After sutures are removed, the wound may be reinforced with skin tapes if so desired. As previously mentioned, the daily cleansing of the wound and application of an antibiotic ointment produces a cleaner wound and facilitates suture removal.

MANAGEMENT OF SOFT TISSUE LOSSES

Wounds complicated by soft tissue loss frequently require some form of reconstruction. A thoughtful choice of an appropriate form of reconstruction is as important as proper surgical technique in carrying out the chosen reconstruction. Several principles are important in this regard.

As always, the physician must determine the extent of deficit before management. The specific deficiencies in absolute tissue loss and loss of function should be carefully considered so that both may be restored. Through the loss of normal skin tension and traumatic displacement, normal soft tissue elements may come to rest in abnormal positions. These elements must be returned to their normal positions and the wound recreated both as a part of the reconstructive plan and as an aid in properly evaluating the requirements of the defect.

Soft tissue losses should be replaced with similar soft tissues. Skin defects require replacement with skin only, whereas complex defects of skin, muscle, and bone must be replaced with a composite of different tissues. In replacing skin defects, skin of similar color and texture should be chosen from an appropriate donor site to provide a good match with skin adjacent to the defect. Donor sites should also be carefully selected so that they themselves do not create a significant secondary defect. Donor sites that can be concealed in normal skin creases, hidden by shadows, or covered by clothing are preferable to those in plain view.

Complex reconstructive efforts are not without risk of failure. These risks may be lessened if a careful plan is developed and mapped out before reconstruction. Finding out that a certain flap does not adequately reconstruct a defect before its elevation and rotation may save both the patient's hide and the surgeon's. Because even the best laid plans may be subject to failure, a secondary plan should always be available.

If the surgeon is in doubt regarding whether a wound is suitable for closure on the basis of its tidiness and the patient's overall condition, it is prudent to wait. A delay of 1 or 2 days in closing a complex wound or dividing a flap's pedicle usually causes few problems, whereas surgical plans undertaken in haste may fall short of their expectations. Time is the surgeon's ally when defining the exact extent and requirements of a wound.

For the purpose of planning, the reconstructive armamentarium can be organized in a ladder, working from the simplest to the most complex form of reconstruction (Fig. 41–5). Simple methods are usually better than complex methods; however, when simple methods do not suffice, a more complex method must be chosen. When local tissue

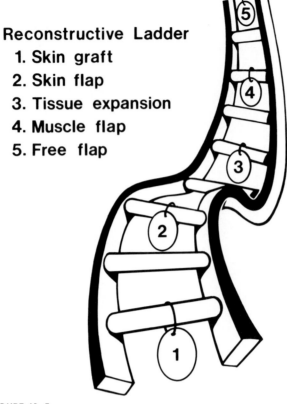

Reconstructive Ladder
1. **Skin graft**
2. **Skin flap**
3. **Tissue expansion**
4. **Muscle flap**
5. **Free flap**

FIGURE 41-5
A reconstructive ladder.

is suitable and available for reconstruction, it should be used in deference to distant tissue. If this is not possible, the surgeon should not hesitate to transfer distant tissue.

Skin Grafts

Skin grafts represent the oldest and most frequently used method of reconstruction. They may either be split thickness, containing epidermis and some of the dermis, or full thickness, containing all the epidermis and dermis. Skin grafts are ideally suited for closing areas where only skin has been lost. The best example of the ideal use of skin grafts is in the treatment of burns, which is thoroughly covered in Chapter 30.

Skin grafts must be revascularized by the recipient bed to heal. Therefore, they can be placed on any vascular bed, such as dermis, muscle, subcutaneous fat, granulation tissue, periosteum, or paratendon. In addition to adequate vascularity, the recipient bed must be clean and contain less than 100,000 bacteria per gram of tissue for reliable healing to ensue (Fig. 41–6A).

Because of the versatility and availability of skin grafts, they must always be considered. The adage ''plan a flap, but do a skin graft'' remains valid. Frequently, skin grafts may make it possible to salvage a failed reconstructive effort or temporarily close a more complex defect and allow the surgeon to operate another day to perform an elective definitive reconstruction.

Split thickness skin grafts may be harvested from virtually any site, and a variety of electric or air-driven dermatomes are currently available for this purpose. Of these, the Padgett Electro-dermatome (Padgett Instruments, Kansas City, Mo.) is favored by many plastic surgeons because of its simplicity and reliability. When these instruments are not available, a hand-held blade such as a Goulian, Watson, or Homby knife is useful (see Fig. 41–6B).

Once harvested, skin grafts may be meshed, allowing for both the expansion of the graft to cover a larger area and the drainage of blood and serum through the graft to prevent a collection of fluid beneath it. However, meshed grafts always retain their meshed or criss-crossed appearance and may not be suitable for areas such as the face, where the smooth appearance of an unmeshed sheet graft is aesthetically superior.

Because skin grafts must heal by an ingrowth of capillaries from the recipient bed, they must be secured to the bed in such a way as to prevent shearing forces and movement. The use of tie-over or bolster dressings, which consist of a layer of nonadherent gauze and mineral oil– or glycerin-soaked cotton, are invaluable in this regard (see Fig. 41–6C).

Splints should also be applied to skin-grafted extremities to prevent movement of adjacent joints. Dressings are left in place or replaced with similar dressings for a period of 5 to 10 days, or until the graft has taken.

Split thickness skin graft donor sites heal by re-epithelialization from their deeper dermal elements. Frequently, these sites, when healed, are darker than the surrounding skin. When small quantities of skin grafts are needed, the buttock, which is concealed in most forms of clothing, can be used as a donor site. When larger quantities of graft are needed, the thighs represent the most useful donor site. As much care must be exercised in the treatment of the donor sites as in the treatment of the skin graft itself. If the donor site is neglected or becomes infected, it can result in an unsightly scar or become an area of full thickness skin loss requiring a skin graft for healing.

A number of different dressing techniques are available for donor sites.[11] If the site is not exceedingly large, a sheet of adhesive polyurethane placed over the entire area provides a neat, pain-free dressing (see Fig. 41–6D). However, this sheet must be carefully placed to prevent leakage of serum about the edges. Larger donor sites can be covered with a single layer of fine-mesh gauze, nonadherent antibiotic-impregnated gauze, or Biobrane. Of these, Biobrane provides the least painful dressing and is currently the preferred wound cover. If the donor site begins to drain turbid or purulent fluid, the dressing should be removed and serial dressing changes with a nonadherent antibiotic-impregnated gauze begun to prevent progression to full thickness skin loss.

Full thickness skin grafts are useful when comparatively smaller defects require a thicker graft or are less prone to contraction, or when the color or texture match of the adjacent skin requires the use of specialized donor sites. Common donor sites include retroauricular, supraclavicular, groin, and infragluteal skin. All such donor sites are closed primarily, which may be advantageous, particularly in infants, in whom the treatment of a secondary donor site may

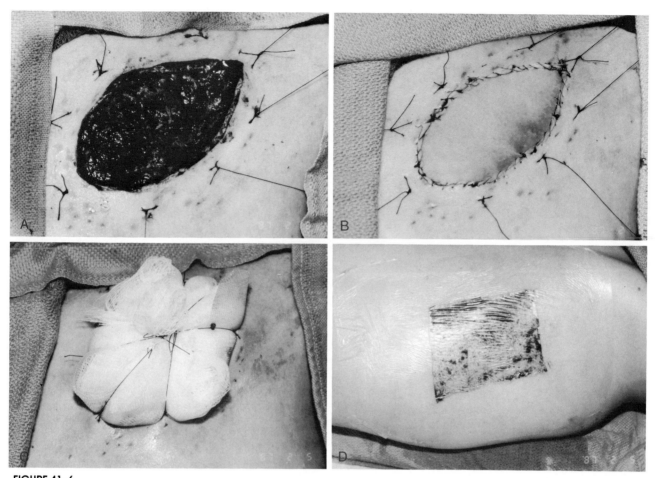

FIGURE 41-6

A, A skin defect of the chest wall prepared for skin grafting. *B,* A split thickness skin graft is placed on the defect and secured with a tie-over dressing *(C). D,* The donor site is covered with a sheet of polyurethane.

be difficult. Because of the match of color and texture, retroauricular and supraclavicular skin are preferred for facial reconstruction.

Once harvested, the full thickness skin graft must be defatted carefully and secured to its recipient site. Some form of bolster or tie-over dressing should be used. Due to its thickness, it is not unusual for the superficial epidermis to slough and subsequently be regenerated during the healing process.

Skin Flaps

Skin flaps consist of skin and subcutaneous tissue only. As a reconstructive tool, they can be used for local reconstruction through advancement, simple rotation, or transposition or as pedicle flaps for more distant reconstruction. Based on their cutaneous blood supply, they are described as either random- or axial-patterned flaps. Random-patterned flaps depend on the dermal-subdermal plexuses of capillaries and can generally be raised in any anatomic location for local wound reconstruction, providing that the length does not greatly exceed the width of the flap. Axial-patterned flaps are based on identifiable cutaneous arteries in specific

anatomic locations. These can be raised with a length several times their width, allowing pedicle transfer to distant sites.

The most commonly used random-patterned skin flap is the simple Z-plasty (Fig. 41-7). In this technique, two adjacent triangular flaps are raised and interposed to lengthen a scar and reorient skin tension. To use a Z-plasty flap, there must be an area of relative skin excess immediately adjacent to the area of relative skin deficiency that is to be reconstructed. Generally, these flaps are more useful in the revision of rather than the primary reconstruction of soft tissue defects. Because they use locally available tissue, skin color and texture match is excellent. In the reconstruction of facial soft tissue losses, advancement flaps can be used (see Fig. 41-2).

Axial-patterned or arterialized flaps are extremely useful as pedicle flaps for the reconstruction of distant wounds. Several such flaps raised from the trunk are the preferred methods of upper extremity reconstruction. The groin flap, based on the superficial circumflex iliac artery, is the workhorse of hand and wrist reconstruction (Fig. 41-8).[5] A distinct disadvantage of this form of reconstruction is the required apposition of the donor and recipient sites during the first stage of transfer. In the case of the groin flap, the arm

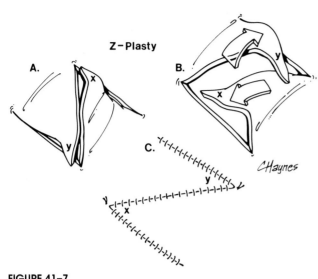

Z-Plasty

A.

B.

C.

CHaynes

FIGURE 41–7
A simple Z-plasty can be utilized to lengthen a scar, the vertical limb in *A*, and reorient skin tension.

must be securely strapped to the trunk to prevent flap or pedicle disruption. After pedicle division, however, the arm can be moved freely and rehabilitated. For the most part, the donor defects of axial-patterned flaps are closed directly and usually can be concealed by clothing.

Muscle Flaps

Muscle or myocutaneous flaps are arterialized flaps that may be required when larger and more complex soft tissue losses have been sustained. Precise anatomic description of the blood supply to most large muscles of the body has provided the reconstructive surgeon with useful muscle flaps in most anatomic locations.[14, 16] Muscle flaps, with or without the overlying skin, are raised from their normal position while taking care not to injure the vascular pedicle and are rotated or transposed into local wounds. In so doing the normal function of the transposed muscle is sacrificed; therefore, the function of this muscle should be expendable if significant donor-site morbidity is to be avoided.

Perhaps the greatest dividend of muscle flaps is the fact that they bring into the reconstructed wound a robust, healthy blood supply, usually outside the zone of injury. This may help to revascularize relatively ischemic elements of a complex wound and add an increased ability to withstand infection. This vascularity is critical in obtaining stable coverage of vascular and orthopedic prostheses and open long-bone fractures. Myocutaneous flaps also obliterate large dead spaces and provide padding in areas of soft tissue deficiency, particularly over bony prominences.

The latissimus dorsi, pectoralis major, and rectus abdominis muscles have been used to restore the function and integrity of full thickness defects of the chest and abdominal walls. Pelvic and thigh wounds are frequently closed with flaps of tensor fasciae latae, gracilis, or a portion of the gluteus maximus muscles. In a paraplegic, the entire

gluteus maximus, an unreplaceable hip extensor, may be used. Severely comminuted and open leg fractures commonly require muscle-flap coverage for extremity salvage. The medial or lateral head of the gastrocnemius and soleus can be used to cover wounds of the proximal and middle third of the leg; however, no reliable local muscle flaps are available for wounds of the distal third of the leg. In these wounds, free tissue transfer is required.

Free Flaps

If local tissue is neither suitable nor available for wound reconstruction, free tissue transfer is used.[4, 12] Free flaps are transferred from a distant donor site to the wound, where microvascular anastomoses between the artery and vein or veins of the flap and local vessels are performed. If the local vasculature is injured, interposition vein grafts allow the anastomoses to be performed outside the zone of injury. The flap vessels are usually not more than 1 to 2 mm in diameter and require microsurgical techniques to perform the anastomoses.

Flaps may be comprised of muscle, skin, bone, or a composite of these, depending on the particular needs of the wound (Fig. 41–9). In most cases, a free myocutaneous flap or a free muscle flap with skin grafts is used. These flaps are most commonly applied to the reconstruction of wounds in the distal one third of the leg. The latissimus dorsi and rectus abdominis muscles are most commonly used for a free tissue transfer; however, numerous other flaps are available, depending on the reconstructive needs of the wound.

Tissue Expansion

Although in many ways less complex than the previous two methods of wound reconstruction, tissue expansion is generally considered a secondary procedure. It was developed in its present form in the late 1970s by Dr. Chedomir Radovan and uses the skin's dynamic ability to stretch and relax as a result of applied tension.[1, 2, 23] The tissue expansion technique involves the placement of an inflatable prosthesis beneath the area of skin to be expanded. Serial injections of saline are added through an injection port. This causes the expander to increase in volume, stretching or expanding the overlying skin. These injections, done on a weekly or biweekly outpatient basis, usually equal about 10% of the total expander volume. When expansion is complete, the expander is removed, and the expanded skin is rotated into the defect to be reconstructed as a random-patterned flap.

Tissue expansion is applicable to most anatomic regions. It is used primarily when adjacent tissue is best suited in quality but deficient in quantity for the reconstruction of a wound. For instance, defects of the scalp should be reconstructed with normal hair-bearing scalp. If local scalp rotation flaps are inadequate to close a scalp wound, expanders may be placed adjacent to the wound and serially expanded (Fig. 41–10). The expanded flaps of normal hair-bearing

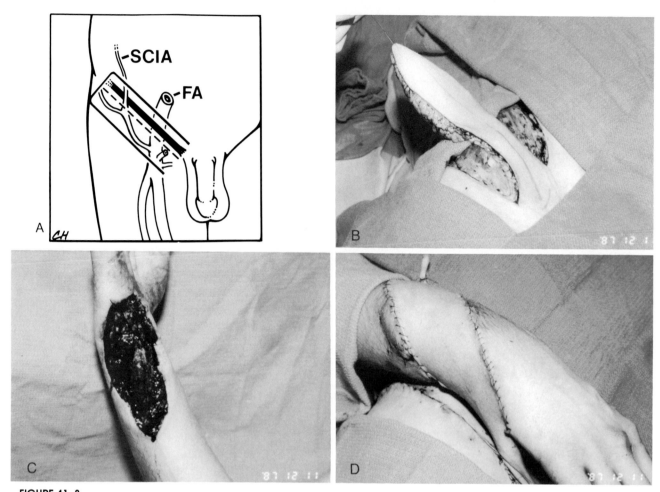

FIGURE 41–8

A, The groin flap is an axial-patterned skin flap based on the superficial circumflex iliac artery (SCIA). In this case the flap is raised *(B)* to cover a distal wrist defect *(C). D,* The flap is inset and remains attached to the groin by its pedicle. FA, Femoral artery.

scalp then are rotated or advanced into the defect, creating a reconstructed scalp that is completely hair bearing.

Tissue expanders have been helpful in scalp and facial reconstruction, extremity reconstruction, chest wall reconstruction, and in the excision of poorly healed wounds or donor sites. Although complications of implant exposure with resultant infection, deflation of the implant secondary to its failure, or skin necrosis from too rapid expansion have occurred, the procedure is generally safe and versatile.[3] It does not create a secondary donor defect and for the most part can be carried out in the outpatient setting. However, tissue expansion is a secondary procedure and is not generally applicable to closure of an acute wound.

COMPLICATIONS

In most children, wound healing is uncomplicated, rapid, and usually occurs faster and with fewer complications than in the adult. Although there is a paucity of hard clinical evidence to support this contention, a few studies have shown that the basic steps in wound healing proceed more quickly in children than in adults.[10, 20, 24]

When wound healing is delayed in children, it is usually related to malnutrition or the use of steroids or chemotherapeutic agents. Although pre-existing illnesses such as diabetes mellitus and arteriosclerosis frequently interfere with adult wound healing, they are seldom seen to complicate pediatric wound healing. Many of the cofactors necessary for collagen formation are nutritionally acquired: ascorbate, α-ketoglutarate, iron, copper, zinc, and magnesium. Additionally, adequate protein and caloric intake is required to synthesize collagen and heal wounds. The vast majority of traumatized children are properly nourished before injury, but if proper nutritional support is not administered after the injury, the child is placed at risk for delayed or compromised wound healing.

Although impairment of wound healing is not commonly seen in children, complications of overhealing are more frequently encountered in the form of hypertrophic scars and occasionally keloid scars. Although both hypertrophic and keloid scars are characterized by exuberant collagen deposition, there are important differences between the two. A hypertrophic scar, although raised and reddened, does not extend beyond the borders of the injury or incision (Fig. 41–11). In addition, as time passes, a hypertrophic scar

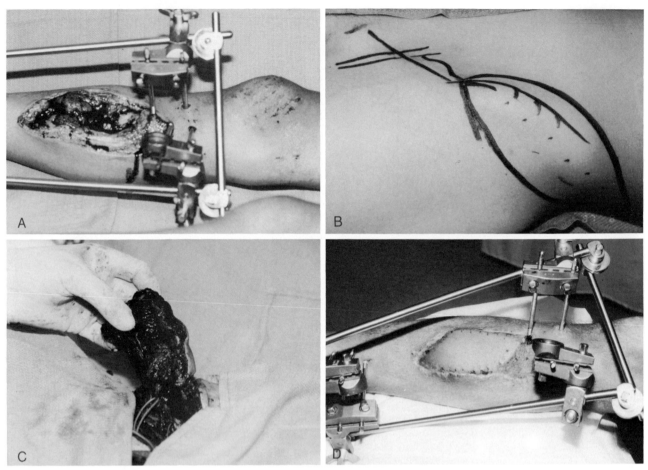

FIGURE 41–9

An 8-cm segmental tibial defect *(A)* required composite reconstruction of bone and soft tissue for which a deep circumflex iliac artery osseocutaneous free flap was designed *(B)*. *C,* The flap is seen raised from the donor area, attached only by the vessels. *D,* Successful reconstruction of both bone and soft tissue is achieved.

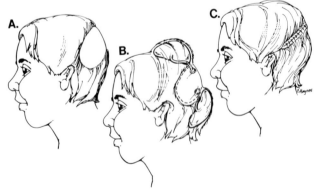

FIGURE 41–10

A, A scalp defect is closed by the placement of two tissue expanders. Once the overlying scalp has been expanded *(B),* the expanders are removed and the scalp flaps are advanced *(C)* for full coverage of the defect with hair-bearing scalp.

tends to regress and improve in appearance without treatment. Keloids, however, extend beyond the boundaries of the previous incision or injury, invade normal skin, and may recur after excision (Fig. 41–12). There also appears to be a genetic or familial predisposition to keloid formation.

The distinction between hypertrophic scars and keloids has significant bearing on their treatment. A hypertrophic scar improves in time without treatment; frequently, the best treatment, at least initially, is observation. This period of observation may extend for months or years. During this time, the parents and child must be reassured frequently. Prolonged inflammation, increased local skin tension, and the patient's own propensity to form hypertrophic scars increase the likelihood of scar hypertrophy.

Keloids generally do not improve without treatment. The simplest form of treatment is intralesional steroid injection with triamcinolone (40 mg/ml). Injections every 4 to 6 weeks, but not to exceed 80 mg every 6 weeks, may result

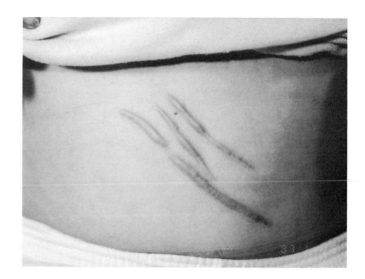

FIGURE 41–11
Hypertrophic scars of a young girl's abdominal wall.

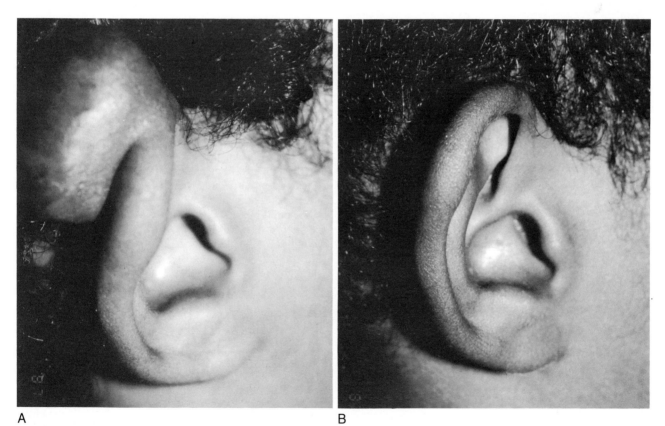

A   B

FIGURE 41–12
A keloid of the helical rim (A) of a young black male that occurred following a trivial injury required excision (B) for successful treatment.

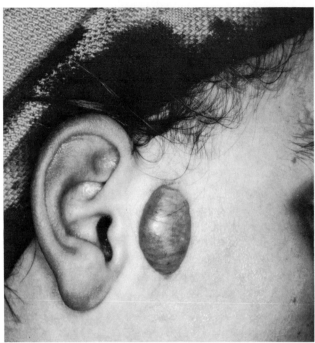
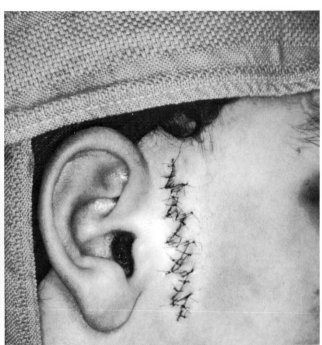

A   B

FIGURE 41–13

A keloid of the preauricular area *(A)* is excised and closed with multiple Z-plasties *(B)*.

in a decrease in keloid size in some individuals[6]; however, local skin atrophy and depigmentation may occur. Frequently, surgical excision of the keloid coupled with intralesional steroid injections is attempted because of either the size of the keloid or failure of other forms of therapy.

Although keloid excision is not always successful in preventing recurrence, several steps may be important in optimizing its potential for success. Surgery should be delayed until the wound is stable, the inflammation has resolved, and the keloid is no longer enlarging. All excessive scar tissue should be excised and normal skin preserved for closure. Attempts should be made to minimize inflammation and tissue destruction. Careful surgical technique and use of a minimum of absorbable sutures are important in this regard. If skin tension seems to have been implicated in keloid formation, it should be locally reoriented with one or more Z-plasties to decrease the tension on the incision (Fig. 41–13). Intralesional triamcinolone injection may be performed at the time of excision or shortly thereafter if keloid re-formation is observed. In some patients, local wound pressure or compression may be helpful in preventing recurrence.

Scars may also become prominent because of wound contraction. Scar contracture because of the tension within the scar may distort normal structures by pulling them out of place. The shortening of circular scars and scars running over normal anatomic curves is very noticeable, creating a seam or indentation. Fortunately, this problem is usually well treated with a Z-plasty or W-plasty. Because the Z-plasty lengthens the shortened scar, the problem of contraction is directly treated (see Fig. 41–7). Proper design of the Z-plasty may also allow for repositioning of displaced elements of the wound.

CONCLUSION

Recovery from injury requires successful wound healing. Although deficiencies in wound healing in the child are uncommon, an understanding of the basic principles of wound healing permits the surgeon to promote optimal wound healing whether the wound is closed primarily or requires some form of reconstruction.

When a child has recovered from injury, he or she will have scars. The scars may be the only reminder or sequelae of the child's trauma, and they will remain with the child for the rest of his or her life. Efforts directed to improving wound healing and the appearance of the resultant scars are far from trivial—They assist in the child's overall recovery and return to normal existence.

References

1. Argenta LC, Martin AH, Iacobuccu JJ: Tissue expansion revisited. Adv Plast Reconstr Surg 4:113–148, 1988.
2. Austad ED: The origin of expanded tissue. Clin Plast Surg 14(3):431–434, 1987.
3. Austad ED: Complications in tissue expansions. Clin Plast Surg 14(3):549–550, 1987.
4. Bank A, Wulff K: Latissimus dorsi free flaps for total repair of extensive lower leg injuries in children. Plast Reconstr Surg 79(5):769–775, 1987.
5. Carrico TJ, Mahrhof AI, Cohen IK: Biology of wound healing. Surg Clin North Am 64(4):721–734, 1984.
6. Cohen IK: Complications of wound healing. In: Greenfield LJ (ed): Complications in Surgery and Trauma. Philadelphia, JB Lippincott, 1984, pp 3–8.
7. Converse JM: Reconstructive Plastic Surgery. 2nd ed. Philadelphia, WB Saunders, 1977.

8. Dieglemann RF, Cohen IK, Kaplan AM: The role of macrophages in wound repair: A review. Plast Reconstruct Surg 68(1):107–113, 1981.

9. Grabb WC, Smith JW: Plastic Surgery. 3rd ed. Boston, Little, Brown and Co, 1979.

10. Grove GL: Age-related differences in healing of superficial skin wounds in humans. Arch Dermatol Res 272:381–385, 1982.

11. Heimbach DM, Engrau LH: Excision and donor site techniques. In: Heimbach DM, Engrau LH (eds): Surgical Management of the Burn Wound. New York, Raven Press, 1984, pp 13–35.

12. Iwaya T, Harii K, Yamada A: Microvascular free flaps for the treatment of avulsion injuries of the feet in children. J Trauma 22(1):15–19, 1982.

13. Longmire AW, Broom LA: Wound infection following high-pressure syringe and needle irrigation. Am J Emerg Med 5(2):179–181, 1987.

14. McGraw JB, Arnold PG: McGraw and Arnold's Atlas of Muscle and Musculocutaneous Flaps. Norfolk, Conn, Hampton Press, 1986.

15. McGregor IA, Jackson IT: The groin flap. Br J Plast Surg 25:3–16, 1972.

16. Mathes SJ, Nahai F: Clinical Atlas of Muscle and Musculocutaneous Flaps. St. Louis, CV Mosby, 1979.

17. Millard DR: Principilization of Plastic Surgery. Boston, Little, Brown and Co, 1986.

18. Myers B: Skin flap viability. Adv Plast Reconstr Surg 7:245–274, 1988.

19. Peacock EE: Wound Repair. 3rd ed. Philadelphia, WB Saunders, 1984.

20. Raekallio J, Viljanto J: Signs of capillary formation in the early phase of wound healing in children. Exp Pathol 23:67–72, 1983.

21. Serafin D, Georgiade NG: Pediatric plastic surgery. St. Louis, CV Mosby, 1984.

22. Theogaraj SD: Complications of traumatic wounds of the face. In: Greenfield LJ (ed): Complications in Surgery and Trauma. Philadelphia, JB Lippincott, 1984, pp 9–26.

23. Versaci AD, Balkovich ME: Tissue expansion. Adv Plast Reconstr Surg 1:94–145, 1984.

24. Viljanto J, Penttinen R, Raekillio J: Fibronectin in early phases of wound healing in children. Acta Chir Scand 147:7–13, 1981.

Critical Care Considerations

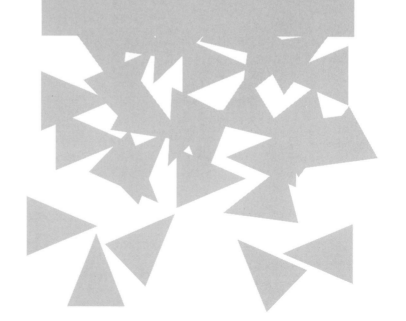

Bradley M. Peterson
Thomas L. Hurt

CHAPTER FORTY-TWO

Vascular Access and Monitoring of the Critically Injured Child

Venous and arterial catheterization play an integral role in the management of the seriously injured child. Knowledge of the relative indications and contraindications as well as the technical proficiency in the placement of venous and arterial catheters is essential tools for the trauma physician. This chapter reviews vascular access and monitoring in the injured child with particular emphasis on the techniques, indications, contraindications, and potential complications of invasive monitoring.

INTRAVENOUS ACCESS

General Principles of Venous Access

Access to the vascular system in critically injured children is an absolute necessity. With the pediatric patient, especially the small child who may be potentially hypovolemic or have physical or anatomic abnormalities, securing an intravenous route can be extremely difficult. Rosetti and colleagues retrospectively studied a 3-year experience at a children's hospital and found that an average time of 7.8 minutes was required to achieve intravenous (IV) access in cases of cardiac arrest, regardless of the cause.[108] In 24% of these cases, access required more than 10 minutes, and in 6%, access was never achieved. Although data are not available, it can be assumed that this delay in establishing an IV line is even greater in hospitals in which the admitting or managing staff is not specialized in the emergency care of children. These times in achieving access are not acceptable for the critically injured child and should be much shorter, and in no patient should venous access be impossible. Skill at securing rapid percutaneous or cutdown venous access via all possible sites is essential to ensure that the pediatric trauma patient receives swift and optimal resuscitation.

Venous access can be acquired either peripherally or centrally, and advantages and disadvantages exist for both methods. Peripheral veins, which are generally visible and easily accessible, are available at several sites. These include the dorsal veins of the hand, the superficial radial veins, the median cephalic and cephalic veins, the median basilic and basilic veins, the brachial veins, and the long saphenous veins (Figs. 42–1 and 42–2).

Although they may not be visible, the long saphenous vein and the brachial vein are constant in their anatomic locations and may be approached percutaneously or by cutdown. The long saphenous vein is at its most predictable point just anterior and superior to the medial malleolus. The brachial vein is located just medial to the brachial artery pulsation and can be cannulated by cutdown or by deep percutaneous venipuncture.[136]

Other advantages of peripheral venous cannulation include avoidance of major cardiothoracic complications, avoidance of central thrombus formation, and the capability of being safely performed in the presence of clotting abnormalities. Disadvantages include small vessel size relative to the deep central veins, difficulty establishing a peripheral IV line in patients with circulatory collapse, potentially low maximal flow rates depending on the vessel size and the size of catheter chosen, and the potential risk of extravasa-

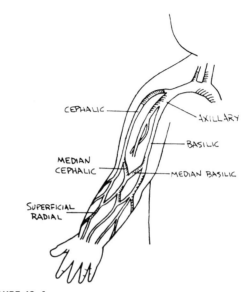

FIGURE 42–1

Veins of the upper extremity.

tion of noxious substances (e.g., epinephrine, dopamine, calcium, bicarbonate, pentothal) into the surrounding soft tissues.[29] Additionally, sodium bicarbonate administered peripherally during shock or full cardiac arrest may have a delayed and shortened effect compared to administration centrally.[122] Complications of peripheral venous catheterizations are relatively minimal and locally include hematoma formation, thrombosis, cellulitis, and phlebitis. Systemic complications include sepsis, thromboembolism, air embolism, and catheter fragment embolism.

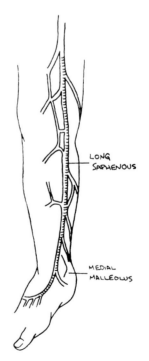

FIGURE 42–2

Course of the long saphenous vein.

Flow Rates

Cannulation site and catheter choice play important roles in the capacity to infuse large volumes of fluid rapidly. Dailey demonstrated that the rate of flow through IV catheters is directly related to the catheter lumen size and the presence of tapering, which is thought to provide turbulence-free flow, and is inversely related to catheter length.[29] This finding correlates well with the Poiseuille theorem for laminar flow, which states: $F = P \subseteq PR^4 / 8VL$, where f = flow, P = pressure gradient at the end of the tube, R = radius, V = viscosity of the fluid, and L = length of the tube. Although this equation predicts linear increase in flow as length decreases, the length-flow relation is actually nonlinear because of turbulence at high flow rates.[104] As an example, a 2-inch 16-gauge Angiocath (Deseret Medical, Inc., Sandy, Utah) under 300 mm Hg pressure allows whole blood to flow at a rate of 216 ml per minute, whereas a 5.25-inch 16-gauge Angiocath under the same conditions allows a flow of only 138 ml per minute.[61] Central access allows for placement of a larger bore catheter; however, unless the proper catheter is chosen, central access does not necessarily provide large-volume infusion capability.

During resuscitation, cannulations of peripheral or femoral veins may be the first choice, because access to jugular or subclavian veins may jeopardize cervical spine stability or force interruption of resuscitation. When large-volume fluid administration is needed, two or three large-bore catheters placed peripherally in the early minutes of the response are recommended.[25] If the patient is in severe shock, our trauma team often places peripheral, femoral, and subclavian catheters simultaneously. In the more stable patient, central venous access can be secured later, if desired. When central venous access is obtained for volume administration purposes only, a short, single-lumen, large-bore catheter allows maximal flow capacity. Multiple-lumen catheters, although useful for other purposes, are not optimal for volume resuscitation. Even though the overall external diameter may be large, the internal diameter of each separate lumen is small, with a subsequent significant restriction in maximal flow rate.

Catheter Types and Insertion Techniques

Three types of catheters are available for use in the pediatric trauma patient. These include the catheter-over-needle type, the catheter-through-the-needle type, and the catheter advanced over a guidewire (i.e., Seldinger technique).[113] It is our practice to use the catheter-over-needle type and the Seldinger technique. The primary reasons for not using the catheter-through-the-needle-type are (1) the relatively small size of catheter able to fit through the large needle, (2) the leakage of blood around the vessel entry site due to the large needle, and (3) the potential for catheter shearing.

In placing a short peripheral venous catheter, a catheter-over-needle setup is generally used. One advantage of this design is that the puncture into the vessel itself is the same size as the catheter and thus limits blood leaking around the catheter.

In placing a central catheter, variations of the catheter-over-wire Seldinger technique are used. Basically, the Seldinger technique involves placement of a needle attached to a non–Luer-Lok syringe into the selected vessel. With gentle traction on the syringe plunger, the vessel is entered. Free-flowing aspirated blood signals entry into the vessel. The syringe is removed, and a guidewire is advanced into the vessel. The guidewire must be at least several centimeters longer than the catheter itself, and direct visualization of the wire must be maintained at all times to ensure that it does not slip under the skin and into the vessel. The flexible end of the guidewire is introduced into the needle. In larger children, a J-tip allows the catheter to move through tortuous vessels. The guidewire should pass easily, and at no time should it be forced, as this may result in perforation of the vessel with positioning of the catheter tip outside the vessel. After the guidewire is in the desired position and the needle is removed, the catheter is introduced over the guidewire and advanced the desired distance. The guidewire is then removed, and the catheter is secured in position. Catheters in position for various lengths of time can be easily exchanged over a guidewire; however, if local or systemic infection is a potential or suspected, an alternate site should be chosen.

Selection of Catheters

Selection of the proper catheter for venous cannulation depends on the site and the indication for insertion. If volume delivery is the objective, then the largest diameter, shortest length catheter possible is the goal. In the small infant, an 18- or 20-gauge catheter can usually be placed into an antecubital fossa vessel. In the young child, a 16-gauge catheter is appropriate, and in the larger child, a 14-gauge catheter can usually be placed. For rapid volume delivery via a central vessel, a large-bore (e.g., 5-Fr in an infant or toddler; 7- or 8-Fr in a school-aged child) single-lumen catheter should be secured. When massive ongoing blood loss is encountered, multiple large-bore catheters should be placed. In the emergency setting, where any delay may be critical, strict adherence to aseptic technique is not always possible. However, after the patient is stabilized, the catheters can be changed in more sterile circumstances, to a new site, if necessary.

A wide variety of multiple-lumen catheters are available. These catheters, although not ideal for volume delivery, are useful in the postresuscitation phase for the simultaneous administration of hyperosmolar total parenteral alimentation and various medications, some of which may be incompatible with each other.

Intraosseous Access: A Temporary Measure

Occasionally, even the most experienced trauma team has difficulty establishing IV access. Medications such as epinephrine, atropine, and lidocaine can be given safely and effectively via an endotracheal tube, but sodium bicarbonate is not well absorbed with this route of administration, and it is caustic to the mucosal surface of the trachea. A temporary access port to the blood system through which all medications, including epinephrine and bicarbonate, can be safely given, is the bone marrow.

There has been renewed interest in the intraosseous route as a method of providing inotropic support as well as volume replacement in a setting in which intravenous access is difficult or impossible.[60, 64, 109] A patient who is severely hypotensive or in shock may have vessels that are poorly distended and nearly impossible to cannulate. In these circumstances, the bone marrow serves as a noncollapsible vein that can be entered fairly easily using a 13-gauge disposable bone marrow needle.[103] Intravenous tubing can be attached directly to the hub.

The most common site of entry is through the medial flat surface of the anterior tibia 2 to 3 cm below the tuberosity. Directed either straight in or at a slightly caudal angle, the needle can be kept away from the proximal growth plate. With a twisting motion, the needle is advanced through the cortex into the marrow. A soft ''pop'' and a release in resistance indicates entrance into the bone marrow. The cortex of the older child may be very hard, and slow, steady pressure with considerable rotatory motion may be needed to enter the marrow space. The cortex of an infant may be fairly soft, and care must be taken to prevent the needle from pushing completely through the marrow space and out the opposite side of the bone. Blood should be obtained on aspiration to verify proper placement. Although fluid administration is limited by virtue of the resistance of flow through the medullary sinuses (i.e., maximal flow rates using pressure bags inflated to 300 mm Hg have been demonstrated to be approximately 2400 ml per hour in adult bones), medications administered intraosseously reach the heart as quickly as medications administered via peripheral veins.[120, 122]

Recognized complications are rare but include localized infection and osteomyelitis, extravasation of noxious substances into the surrounding soft tissue, and disruption of the growth plate if the needle is malpositioned. Definite contraindications to placement of an intraosseous line include a fracture of the involved bone; infection or burn of the overlying skin; previous recent placement of a bone marrow needle, which leaves a defect through which injected substances may leak; and osteogenesis imperfecta. Although the intraosseous route for fluid and pharmacologic resuscitation should only be considered as a final alternative, knowledge of its potential role may be life saving in the setting in which intravenous access is extremely difficult or impossible. Although we have been aware of this route and have only rarely used it during medical resuscitations, we have not found it necessary to use this route in the more than 2000 pediatric trauma cases seen at our regional pediatric trauma center.

ARTERIAL CATHETERIZATION
Principles of Arterial Access

Establishing an indwelling peripheral arterial catheter is not an imperative procedure in the early stages of management of the critically injured child, but it can be extremely helpful. There are two primary indications for placement of an arterial line: (1) the need for continuous measurement of systemic arterial blood pressure with numeric and waveform display and (2) the need for frequent blood gas determinations while causing minimal pain and discomfort to the patient, so that steady-state measurements of the oxygen and carbon dioxide tensions and pH can be obtained. Additional indications include access for atraumatic, accurate blood drawing for frequently monitored laboratory studies; hemodialysis; and continuous arteriovenous hemofiltration.

In comparing indwelling arterial blood pressure readings with those obtained noninvasively, the systolic results measured by indwelling catheters tend to be 5 to 20 mm Hg higher than the noninvasive measurements. The discrepancy increases the farther the catheter is placed toward the periphery. This discrepancy is generally thought to result from changes in the pulse waveform as it proceeds from the heart to the periphery.[23, 57, 106] However, in cases of severe low-flow states, the central systolic pressure is much higher than the peripheral systolic pressure. When indwelling systolic pressure measurements are lower than pressures determined noninvasively, this is almost always due to calibration error or technical problems such as dampening of the waveform by a large air bubble.[85] Systolic discrepancies of greater than 30 mm Hg are usually due to resonance overshoot and can be corrected by insertion of a resonance overshoot eliminator adapter (R.O.S.E., Gould, Inc., Cardiovascular Products Division, Louisville, Colo.). Any patient who requires intravenous inotropic or vasodilatory support to maintain blood pressure requires continuous intra-arterial blood pressure monitoring. This not only helps prevent a potentially erroneous response to falsely low cuff blood pressure readings but also allows second-by-second tracking of changes in blood pressure, which may occur secondary to inotropic or vasodilatory agents.

For an artery to be suitable for indwelling cannulation, it must (1) have adequate collateral circulation to provide blood to the distal tissues, (2) be large enough to provide accurate systemic blood pressure measurements, (3) not be located in an area prone to contamination, and (4) have anatomic integrity to ensure true blood pressure measurements. Some patients with cardiovascular defects may have congenital or surgically acquired shunts or pressure gradients that may affect both the pressure measurements and the oxygen tension.

No medications or hyperosmolar solutions should be administered via peripheral arteries.[42] Attempted cannulation of the femoral vein during resuscitation may accidentally result in cannulation of the femoral artery. This error may be difficult to recognize, because the aspirated blood may appear to be venous. It is important to identify this problem before a potent vasopressor such as epinephrine is injected into the femoral artery.

When placing an arterial catheter in an upper extremity, the nondominant side should be chosen, if possible. This is a precautionary step for the unlikely event that a severe catheter-associated complication occurs, with possible loss of the involved limb or the use thereof.

Complications

Complications that can occur with cannulation of any artery include ischemia with or without tissue necrosis, thrombosis, embolism, hemorrhage, infection, aneurysm, and arteriovenous fistula. Other complications are known to occur, and some of these are described in more detail in the discussions pertaining to each site.

When ischemia occurs, it usually is painful and is manifested by pallor.[4, 70] It can occur distal to or adjacent to the location of the catheter. Ischemia is most commonly the result of thrombosis. Although the incidence of thrombosis is fairly high, ischemia and necrotic complications are infrequent, provided there is adequate collateral circulation. When ischemia does occur, the catheter should be removed.

The incidence of arterial thrombosis increases with the length of time the catheter remains in place, the catheter length, and the catheter diameter.[31, 45] Short, narrow-diameter, nontapered Teflon catheters appear to result in the lowest incidence of thrombosis.[8, 28, 34] The number of puncture attempts before the actual placement of the cannula also influences the incidence of thrombosis.[111] Other factors include low-flow states, vasoconstrictive agents, hypothermia, underlying vasculitis conditions, arteriosclerotic disease, diabetes mellitus, and excessive pressure on the artery to stop bleeding after the catheter is removed.

To help prevent thrombosis and minimize the chance of release of small emboli, a continuous-flush system should be used to maintain catheter patency.[44, 46] Systems that allow a continuous flow of 3.0 ml per hour of flush at 300 mm Hg pressure are available. The flush solution should contain heparin at 1 to 2 IU per ml. These systems allow very accurate propagation of the waveform with accurate pressure measurement.

Embolisms most commonly result from small clots that form at the tip of the indwelling catheter. Air embolism may also occur. Intermittent flushing of the arterial line may result in the release of small emboli.[82] To help prevent this occurrence, the line should be cleared with aspiration of a few milliliters of blood before flushing. Embolization to the brain can occur via any arterial site if care is not taken during flushing. For this reason, gentle flushing with the minimum volume necessary should always be performed.

Significant hemorrhage can occur if any connection in the arterial line becomes disconnected and goes unnoticed. A coagulopathy may allow bleeding to continue at the puncture site. To help prevent hematoma formation or continued oozing after the catheter is removed, pressure should be applied to the insertion site for 10 minutes after removal of the line. The pressure should not be so great as to completely obstruct the pulse, because this may lead to thrombus formation.[24, 132]

Numerous factors contribute to the potential for infection at the site of arterial cannulation.[6, 40, 45] The length of time the catheter remains in place is directly related to the incidence of infection. Catheters placed by cutdown are at greater risk of infection than those placed percutaneously. Failure to conform to aseptic technique may predispose the site to contamination.

Aneurysms and arteriovenous fistulas occur only infrequently. Mathieu and colleagues described a radial artery aneurysm that occurred in a patient who had had an 18-gauge catheter in place for 10 days.[92] Arteriovenous fistulas have been described involving the femoral artery and femoral vein, especially in patients with large catheters.[14, 22]

Selecting Catheters

In selecting the proper catheter for arterial cannulation, the length and gauge depend on the site of insertion and the size of the patient. For cannulation of the peripheral arteries or axillary artery, a 20-gauge, 5-cm catheter is usually adequate in patients of all ages, except the small infant, in whom a 22-gauge, 3-cm catheter may be required. In adults, a 20-gauge catheter, as compared with 18- or 19-gauge catheters, produces the lowest incidence of thrombosis in the radial artery.[8, 31, 34] Because the femoral artery is deep in the large child or adult, a 19- or 20-gauge catheter longer than 5 cm is usually required. Once it is in place, the catheter should always be sutured securely to prevent accidental dislodgement.

Sites of Cannulation, Techniques, and Complications

Our preferred sites for arterial catheterization, in order of preference, are (1) the radial artery, (2) the posterior tibial artery, (3) the femoral artery, (4) the dorsalis pedis artery, and (5) the axillary artery. The temporal artery and the brachial artery can be used, but these should be avoided if at all possible because of the higher risk of serious complications associated with catheterization of these vessels.[11, 19]

Radial Artery

The radial artery, which is a branch of the brachial artery, is the most frequently used artery for indwelling catheterization. The radial artery pulse is palpable along a longitudinal groove at the lateral aspect of the wrist. The pulse of the ulnar artery, the other primary branch of the brachial artery, is palpable at the medial aspect of the wrist. Collateral flow between the vessels is provided by the superficial and deep palmar arches. Mozersky and associates demonstrated by Doppler flow that 12% of hands had either poor collateral flow or an incomplete palmar arch with no collateral circulation at all.[96]

Collateral circulation can be demonstrated using several methods. As early as 1929, Allen described a test to confirm ulnar flow.[3] The modified Allen test, which requires no equipment, serves as the standard bedside test for proof of adequate collateral circulation.[111] Further modifications using a Doppler instrument, pulse oximeter, or plethysmography are very useful in the comatose patient or intraoperatively when patient participation is impossible.[18, 69, 96]

The technique for percutaneous cannulation is the same regardless of the age or size of the patient. An appropriate-sized catheter is chosen, and the patient's nondominant hand is dorsiflexed approximately 45 to 60 degrees. The radial arterial pulse is located just proximal to the head of the radius, and the area is prepped and draped. The use of sterile gloves is optimal. If the patient is awake, 1% lidocaine without epinephrine should be locally infiltrated at the puncture site and to the sides of the artery. At the planned point of insertion of the needle, a full thickness puncture of the skin with a No. 11 scalpel point should be made, with care taken to avoid hitting the artery, to help minimize skin drag and prevent fraying of the catheter tip.

Three methods of cannulation are commonly employed: the transfixation method, the direct-threading method, and the catheter-over-wire method. The transfixation method involves first inserting the catheter-over-needle through the skin puncture at approximately a 45-degree angle with the skin. The needle is aimed at the arterial pulsation. The needle and catheter are quickly thrust through the anterior and posterior vessel walls. The needle is then withdrawn carefully with the catheter still in place. The angle of the catheter is dropped to 30 degrees with respect to the skin, and the catheter is slowly withdrawn. Appearance of a brisk pulsatile blood flow from the catheter hub indicates that the catheter tip is positioned within the lumen of the artery. The catheter is then advanced into the arterial lumen all the way to its hub. If no blood return is achieved upon slow withdrawal of the catheter, the needle is replaced in the catheter and the procedure is repeated.

The direct-threading method differs slightly from the transfixation method. Following the same preparation and using the same type of catheter, the catheter-over-needle is inserted at an angle of approximately 30 degrees through the puncture site and directed toward the arterial pulsation. As soon as brisk blood flow is noted in the hub, the angle is decreased to 10 to 15 degrees, and the needle is advanced another 2 to 3 mm. With the needle held in place, the catheter is advanced over the needle and into the arterial lumen.

The catheter-over-wire method begins with the same preparation. Either a separate 20-gauge needle with a flexible straight wire of appropriate size or a preassembled catheter-with-wire kit can be used. The needle is inserted through the puncture site at a 30-degree angle to the skin and advanced toward the artery. When brisk blood return is noted in the hub, the angle is decreased to 10 to 15 degrees, and the guidewire is inserted into the needle. No resistance should be encountered if the guidewire is properly advanced into the arterial lumen. The catheter is then advanced into the lumen over the wire.

Regardless of the method of cannulation, the catheter should be sutured securely and the hand returned to a neutral position. The site is dressed in a sterile fashion, and extension tubing is connected to the transducer, with care taken to ensure that no air bubbles are in the line.

Complications generally associated with radial arterial cannulation include infection, thrombosis, ischemia, embolism, and necrosis.[89] The potential for infection increases the longer the catheter is in place and if the catheter is placed via cutdown. Thrombosis of the radial artery is quite common; 30% of adult vessels are thrombosed at the time of removal of the catheter.[9] Prolonged ischemia is very rare and is almost always due to persistent thrombosis.[28] Embolism is avoided by careful inspection of the extension set for trapped air and by continuous-flush systems. Necrosis can occur distal to or overlying the insertion site, but digital necrosis is fortunately rare.

Posterior Tibial Artery

The posterior tibial artery extends the full length of the posterior calf and is located most superficially just posterior to the medial malleolus. It is usually larger than the radial artery and thus often easier to cannulate in the small child. Collateral circulation to the distal foot is provided by the branches of the dorsalis pedis artery. Recent puncture of the corresponding dorsalis pedis artery is a relative contraindication to cannulation of the posterior tibial artery.

The technique for percutaneous cannulation of the posterior tibial artery is similar to that of the radial artery but technically is perhaps more difficult. Most of the posterior tibial artery lines we insert are placed by cutdown. Blanching or coldness of the toes indicates inadequate distal flow, and the catheter should be removed.

Femoral Artery

The femoral artery is the continuation of the external iliac artery after it passes beneath the inguinal ligament. The femoral artery passes beneath the inguinal ligament at the midpoint of a line drawn between the anterior superior iliac spine and the symphysis pubis. The femoral nerve lies lateral to the artery, and the femoral vein lies medial to the artery.

Although the radial and posterior tibial arteries are the preferred sites, we often employ femoral artery cannulation when the peripheral circulation is shut down and the need to obtain arterial pressure and blood gas monitoring is urgent. Other indications include continuous blood pressure monitoring in patients whose cardiac output is severely compromised or whose other arterial sites are no longer available.

The techniques of cannulation of the femoral artery are the same as those employed for the radial artery, with the exception that the needle enters the skin at a steeper angle, usually 45 to 60 degrees. The femoral artery is located by palpation. In the adult, the insertion site is approximately 2 cm below the inguinal ligament; in the small child, a site approximately 1 cm below the ligament is chosen. If no pulse is palpable, the previously mentioned landmarks serve as the starting point. When the catheter is in place, it should be securely sutured, because femoral arterial catheters are very prone to accidental dislodgement. If the femoral vein is entered by mistake, the physician may wish to secure this line in place because it serves both as an access portal into the venous system and as a landmark for placement of the arterial catheter.

Complications of femoral arterial cannulation include infection, thrombosis, embolism, hematoma, and arteriovenous fistula. Infection is commonly associated with urinary and fecal contamination. Continuous nursing attention to the dressings to keep them as free as possible from waste products is mandatory. Clear occlusive dressings are helpful in protecting against infection. Following femoral arterial cannulation for cardiac catheterization, the incidence of thrombosis has been reported to range from 1 to 4%.[117] Thrombi may result in release of emboli, with resultant gangrene of the distal extremity. If distal pulses are lost or diminished, the catheter should be removed. Unrecognized retroperitoneal hemorrhage can result if the femoral artery is punctured above the inguinal ligament.[22, 95] Fistulas have been noted between the femoral artery and vein.[14, 22] This is especially true when large catheters, such as those used for cardiac catheterization or angiography, are used.

Dorsalis Pedis Artery

The dorsalis pedis artery is the continuation of the anterior tibial artery over the dorsum of the foot. Collateral flow between this artery and the posterior tibial artery is provided in most individuals by the lateral plantar artery and the main arterial arch of the foot. Approximately 12% of the adult population has an absent dorsalis pedis artery, usually bilaterally.[7, 67] The methods commonly employed for cannulation of the dorsalis pedis artery are the same as those for the radial artery, with the angle of entry being 15 to 30 degrees.

The most common complication of dorsalis pedis cannulation is thrombosis. This occurs in approximately 7% of the arteries cannulated.[135] Identification of thrombus formation serves as a definite contraindication to subsequent cannulation of the corresponding posterior tibial artery.

Axillary Artery

The axillary artery is a continuation of the subclavian artery as it passes by the lateral border of the first rib and enters the axilla. The right subclavian artery arises from the right brachiocephalic trunk and is in direct communication with the right common carotid artery. The axillary artery combines with the axillary vein and the brachial plexus to form a neurovascular bundle within the axillary sheath. The axillary artery becomes the brachial artery when it leaves the axilla.

Our primary indication for placement of an axillary artery catheter is nonavailability of other sites. Even in the presence of severe shock, axillary pulsation can usually be detected, making it a suitable site for cannulation when no other pulses are palpable.

The axillary artery can be cannulated by cutdown or percutaneously in the same manner as the radial artery. The needle is inserted into the artery as high as possible in the axilla at approximately a 30-degree angle to the skin. It is our practice to use a 20-gauge catheter in patients of all ages, except the very small infant, in whom a 22-gauge catheter may be needed.

As a result of the axillary artery's proximity to certain anatomic structures, several unique complications have been noted. Because the axillary artery is quite large, thrombosis is rare. When thrombosis does occur, ischemia is very uncommon because of the extensive collateral circulation that exists between the thyrocervical trunk of the subclavian artery and the subscapular artery, which is a branch of the distal axillary artery.[32] It is possible for small thromboemboli to break off and travel to the radial or ulnar

circulation. In cases of inadequate palmar arch collateral flow, ischemic injury to the hand can occur.

Potential embolic complications are especially important with axillary artery catheters. Because the right brachiocephalic artery joins directly to the right common carotid artery, the possibility exists for catheter tip thrombi or air bubbles to embolize to the brain during flushing. The left axillary artery does not join directly to the left common carotid artery, and for this reason it is generally recommended that cannulation of the left axillary artery be attempted initially, if possible. Flushing of the cannula in either side should be done gently and with minimal volume to help prevent embolization.

Neurologic injury can occur, either secondary to direct injury to the brachial plexus or secondary to nerve compression due to an axillary sheath hematoma.[1] Due to the risk of hematoma formation and pressure injury, cannulation of the axillary artery is relatively contraindicated in the presence of a coagulopathy.

CENTRAL VENOUS CATHETERIZATION

Indications and Contraindications

Central venous catheterization has widespread application, although the potential does exist for abuse of this procedure. Primary indications include (1) the need for venous access in the patient in whom peripheral access cannot be established, (2) placement of large-bore catheters (e.g., 5- and 8-Fr) for rapid massive volume replacement, (3) hemodynamic monitoring, (4) infusion of vasoconstrictive and sclerosing medications, (5) hyperosmolar parenteral nutrition, (6) emergency transvenous pacing, and (7) preoperative preparation of certain patients.

Although there are no absolute contraindications to central venous catheterization, there are relative contraindications to using certain sites in specific patients. In the patient with abnormal coagulation, the internal jugular veins and the subclavian veins should be avoided, if possible. Puncture of the carotid artery may lead to difficult-to-control bleeding with resultant airway or cerebral compromise. Puncture of the subclavian artery may result in bleeding that is difficult to control because of the inability to apply local pressure to the bleeding site. In patients with respiratory compromise, catheterization of the subclavian veins carries the additional risk of a pneumothorax. A site that is traumatized, infected, anatomically abnormal, or thrombosed or was a previous area of surgery should not be chosen.

Complications

A variety of complications are common to all sites and methods of central venous catheterization, including local infection and sepsis, hematoma formation, thrombosis, thrombophlebitis, thromboembolism, vessel perforation, air embolism, and catheter-fragment embolism. Other common but site-specific complications include cannulation of associated arteries, damage of associated nerves, pneumothorax, and hydrothorax.

The incidence of infectious complications, such as cellulitis, septic phlebitis, bacteremia, and septicemia, increases with the length of time the catheter remains in place. Catheters left in place less than 72 hours have an infection rate of only 1 to 2%.[47, 88, 121, 124, 128] The incidence of infection increases thereafter. Venous access accomplished by cutdown carries a higher risk of infection than does percutaneous placement.[114]

Hematoma can occur secondary to perforation of the vein or its adjacent artery. Hematoma is usually not a significant problem, and bleeding can usually be stopped by the application of local pressure. In the presence of a coagulopathy, such bleeding may be difficult to control and may result in shock or hematoma formation compromising adjacent structures.

Thrombotic complications include local and deep phlebitis, thrombosis, and pulmonary thromboembolism. The phlebitis or thrombosis may become infected. The incidence of these complications is related to the length of time the catheter is in place. Clinically recognized thrombosis appears to occur in approximately 1 to 2% of patients in whom catheters are in place for less than 72 hours.[128] Clinically silent partial thrombosis occurs with variable incidence, depending on the detection method used. Incidences from 5% to as high as 90% have been reported for nonocclusive mural thrombi and fibrin sleeves.[2, 5, 17, 37] Despite the high incidence of partial thrombosis, the incidence of recognized pulmonary embolism is low, even though pieces of sleeve thrombosis have been observed to break off during phlebography.[17, 88]

Air embolism can occur via a catheter placed at any site. More commonly, catheters placed centrally, especially intrathoracically, carry a higher risk of associated air embolism.[21] This is especially important in patients with intracardiac right-to-left shunts.

Catheter-fragment embolism can occur at the time of insertion, especially if a catheter-through-the-needle type of cannula is used. Catheters placed via the antecubital fossa or femoral vein can break off at the entry site when an agitated patient bends his or her arm or leg.

Awareness of potential complications helps to limit their occurrence. Complications associated with catheter insertion can be minimized if the procedures are done by experienced personnel. Verification of catheter tip position by x-ray films when indicated and proper attention to catheter-site care can help to minimize additional complications.

Sites of Cannulation, Techniques, and Complications

Central venous catheters are commonly placed in five sites; in our order of frequency of placement, these are the subclavian vein, the femoral vein, the internal jugular vein, the basilic vein in the antecutibal fossa, and the external jugular vein. Various methods of cannulation exist for each site. The subclavian vein may be entered percutaneously by either an infraclavicular or a supraclavicular approach. The femoral vein may be secured either percutaneously or by

cutdown. The internal jugular vein may be approached percutaneously from a central, anterior, or posterior approach or by cutdown. The antecubital fossa vessels and the external jugular vein may be approached percutaneously or by cutdown. Each site and each approach has its own set of indications, contraindications, and complications. The site and approach chosen depend on the unique circumstances at hand as well as the experience of the managing physician.

There are several general principles of catheter placement that are common to all sites. Whenever possible, the site should be prepared and draped in a sterile fashion. This may involve shaving the groin if necessary. In the awake patient, 1% lidocaine should be infiltrated locally into the site. The syringe should be a non–Luer-Lok type to allow easy removal after the vessel has been entered; this helps prevent accidental displacement of the needle position. Very frequently, the vessel is entered and completely traversed without any flash of blood noted in the syringe. If no flash is noted while advancing the needle, gentle suction should be maintained on the syringe while slowly withdrawing the needle. Often, the flash occurs while withdrawing, indicating that the needle tip is positioned within the lumen. If the blood is bright red or if the flow is pulsatile, an artery has probably been entered. Gentle pressure should be applied over the site for 10 minutes if possible before trying again. Once the needle is in position, the flexible end of the guidewire is advanced into the vessel. After the catheter is placed in the proper position, it should be securely sutured. An x-ray film should always be obtained to determine catheter tip location and to exclude early complications.[41]

Desired indwelling catheter length depends on the insertion site, the size of the patient, and the desired position of the catheter tip. If central venous pressure monitoring is desired, placement of the catheter within the thoracic cage is necessary.[54] For all central venous catheters except those placed through the femoral vein, the most desirable location for the catheter tip is in the distal innominate or proximal superior vena cava. Locating the catheter tip in these areas helps to minimize complications.[74, 80, 125] Tip alignment should preferably run parallel with the superior vena cava. Catheters placed from the left side of the chest and inserted a few centimeters short of the ideal location so that the catheter tip impinges on the right lateral wall of the superior vena cava may result in erosion and perforation of the catheter tip through that point.[126] Early recognition of this malposition is important, and the catheter position should be altered.

Although the catheter tip is often positioned in the right atrium and kept there, many researchers believe this to be an unsafe location. Complications reported include irritation of the atrial wall with resultant arrhythmias, migration of the catheter tip to the right ventricle or pulmonary arteries, right atrial perforation with tamponade, and induction of arrhythmias with cardiac arrest, presumably secondary to direct infusion of undiluted medications into the right atrium near the sinus node at suboptimal temperatures.[16, 25, 26, 30, 50, 80, 91, 125] We have not experienced any serious problems with soft catheters (e.g., Silastic and soft polyurethane) positioned in the proximal right atrium in over 500 patients and believe this is a safe position if the catheter is well aligned.

Perfect placement of the catheter tip in the distal innominate or proximal superior vena cava may be difficult. Induction of an isolated arrhythmia (usually a premature atrial contraction) while advancing the guidewire signals position in the right atrium and directs placement. We do not believe that the induction of a brief isolated arrhythmia is a significant risk in most pediatric patients. It is extremely important that a cardiac monitor is operating and that attention is paid to the cardiac rhythm during catheter placement. Measurement of the distance from the site of insertion, following the assumed course of the catheter, to a position 2 cm above the level of the nipples and just to the right of the sternum approximates the proper tip position.

Subclavian Vein

The subclavian vein is our preferred route of venous access. The landmarks are consistent and identifiable, and the awake patient can remain relatively comfortable with the catheter in position. It is the vein of choice for long-term total parenteral nutrition.

The subclavian vein is a continuation of the axillary vein as it crosses over the first rib and extends along the underside of the clavicle. Behind the sternoclavicular joint, the subclavian vein joins the internal jugular vein to form the innominate, or brachiocephalic vein. The subclavian vein contains a single set of valves just distal to the confluence of the external jugular vein. The thoracic duct on the left and a small lymphatic duct on the right empty into the superior aspect of each subclavian vein near the junction of the internal jugular vein. The position of the subclavian vein behind the medial third of the clavicle is relatively immobile owing to fibrous tissue. At the medial third of the clavicle, both the apical pleura and the subclavian artery are posterior to the subclavian vein. The anterior scalenus muscle, which can be 10 to 15 mm thick in the teenager, separates the subclavian vein from the subclavian artery and the brachial plexus.

The subclavian vein can be entered by either an infraclavicular or a supraclavicular approach. Both techniques are comparable in terms of success rate, malposition, and complications.[35, 65] We exclusively use the infraclavicular approach, because the catheter can be secured more comfortably to the chest wall. The patient is optimally placed in a supine 15-degree Trendelenburg position with a roll behind or between the shoulders; however, it is almost always possible to carry out cannulation of the subclavian vein with the patient lying flat. Although it is generally recommended that the head be turned to the side opposite that being cannulated, in our experience, maintaining the head in the midline position, or even turning it somewhat toward the side being cannulated, facilitates proper positioning.[72, 115]

For the infraclavicular method (Fig. 42–3), the operator approaches the patient from the side, just below the shoulder. Surface landmarks include the bend of the clavicle and the suprasternal notch. The length of the catheter to be inserted should be determined prior to inserting the needle. Bending the needle approximately 20 degrees at the distal

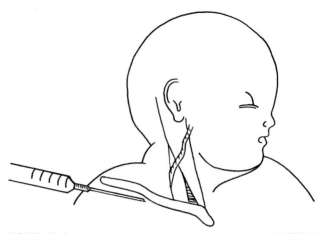

FIGURE 42–3
Infraclavicular approach to the subclavian vein.

third facilitates clearing the clavicle while minimizing the risk for pneumothorax. The needle of the syringe is inserted a few millimeters caudal and a few millimeters medial to the lateral bend of the clavicle. Usually, a 5-ml syringe is used. In the small infant, a 1-ml syringe may be preferred, because it will better allow the needle to be angled under the clavicle. In addition, the smaller negative pressure in a 1-ml syringe will more easily allow free blood flow and recognition of vessel entry. The needle point is walked under the clavicle, and the needle is kept parallel with the surface of the chest. The needle is advanced toward the suprasternal notch with continuous light negative pressure on the syringe, bevel side down and posterior, parallel with the vessel.

When the lumen is properly entered, venous blood will flow easily. If the needle has been advanced to the appropriate depth with no flash of blood, it should be slowly withdrawn with continued negative pressure on the syringe. If no blood appears, the needle should be withdrawn to the edge of the clavicle, redirected slightly cephalad, and advanced again, following the same procedure.

When free flow of venous blood has been achieved, the syringe is removed while holding the needle position steady. The needle is occluded with a finger to prevent air embolism. This is especially important if the patient is breathing spontaneously. In this circumstance, the syringe should be removed at the end of inspiration. If the patient is on a mechanical ventilator, the syringe should be removed at the beginning of the inspiratory phase, although this is seldom truly necessary due to positive-pressure ventilation. The guidewire is advanced to the predetermined length, and the needle is removed. If the guidewire does not pass easily through the needle, repositioning is probably needed.

Proper positioning of the guidewire can often be confirmed by production of a premature atrial contraction. If a premature atrial contraction is not observed and the guidewire encounters resistance after it has been advanced 10 to 15 cm, it is probable that the guidewire is in the ipsilateral internal jugular vein. If this happens, the guidewire should be withdrawn, and the patient's head should be turned to face the operator. The guidewire should then be reinserted through the needle. Alternatively, the needle can be exchanged for an 18-gauge short catheter, which can be advanced into the subclavian vein. This type of catheter is usually short enough to avoid coursing into one of the neck veins, but long enough to remain in the subclavian vein. The guidewire can then be removed, and with the patient's head turned toward the site of entry, the guidewire can be reinserted. After the guidewire is properly positioned, the catheter can be advanced into place. Before advancing the catheter over the guidewire, a vessel dilator may be necessary to facilitate passage of the catheter through the tough fibrous tissues surrounding the vein and between the clavicle and rib.

The landmarks for the supraclavicular approach are the point of insertion of the sternocleidomastoid into the clavicle and the sternoclavicular joint. The operator approaches the patient from the head of the bed. The needle is inserted above the clavicle, just lateral to the insertion of the sternocleidomastoid muscle to the clavicle. The needle is directed toward the contralateral nipple at a 10- to 15-degree angle with respect to the surface of the chest. The jugulosubclavian junction should be entered at a depth of approximately 1 to 3 cm. If the vein is not entered, the needle is withdrawn and redirected at an angle slightly caudal to the contralateral nipple. After the vessel is entered, catheterization continues as described previously.

Regardless of the approach, catheter malposition occurs in approximately 5 to 20% of cases of percutaneous subclavian catheterization.[35, 36, 87] The most common sites of malposition are the ipsilateral internal jugular vein and the contralateral subclavian vein. The most common major complications that occur include pneumothorax, arterial puncture, thrombosis, and infection. Numerous other complications have been reported, including injury to various nerves, hydrothorax, hydropericardium or hemopericardium with tamponade, osteomyelitis of the clavicle, and disruption of the lymphatic ducts. The incidence of pneumothorax has been reported to be between 0 and 5%.[36, 55, 65, 84, 115, 116] Most pneumothoraces are apparent at the time of the procedure, but late-appearing pneumothoraces have been reported. Subclavian artery puncture occurs in approximately 0.5 to 1.0% of cases.[10, 36, 55, 88, 110] This problem is usually easily managed by pressure applied for 10 minutes over the puncture site. In the presence of a coagulopathy, severe hemorrhage may occur. Arteriovenous fistulas may also result.[56, 73] Thrombosis occurs far more frequently than is clinically recognizable. Whereas clinically apparent large-vein thrombosis was reported in approximately 1 to 3% of subclavian vein catheters left in place for variable lengths of time, autopsies on patients who had subclavian vein catheters in place at the time of death revealed an incidence of thrombosis between 20 and 40%.[5, 37, 86, 93, 100, 110]

Information regarding thrombosis due to venous catheterization in children is incomplete. Ongoing studies in our institution reveal a 33% incidence of ultrasound-detectable deep venous thrombi related to 5-Fr polyurethane subclavian vein catheters that have been in place for various lengths of time; using 4-Fr polyurethane catheters, the incidence of thrombi is 24%. Silastic subclavian catheters of various diameters reveal an incidence of catheter-related deep venous thrombosis of only 8%. Clinically evident thrombosis in these patients has been observed in only 2% of cases.

The risk of infectious complications associated with venous catheterization is quite variable and depends on the indication for the catheter. If a strict protocol for changing dressings is followed, subclavian vein catheters in place for total hyperalimentation only can remain for weeks to months with only a 1 to 3% infection rate.[53] In the critically ill patient, the infection rate is higher, with an increase noted after 3 to 5 days of catheterization.[115]

Although it is advisable to change venous catheters regularly to reduce infection, this is not always possible for practical purposes because of nonavailability of sites. In addition, frequent changes repeatedly subject the patients to all the potential complications of insertion. Because of this factor, it is our practice to leave catheters in place longer than the recommended 3 to 5 days; in selected cases, we leave catheters in place for weeks to months.

Femoral Vein

The femoral vein is located just medial to the femoral artery. It is formed from the deep and superficial saphenous veins and becomes the external iliac vein as it passes under the inguinal ligament. One advantage to femoral venous cannulation is that it can be carried out during resuscitation without interrupting chest compressions or airway management. It also avoids most of the major thoracic complications. In the presence of severe abdominal trauma, when the integrity of the inferior vena cava is uncertain, establishment of venous access above the diaphragm is essential, whereas venous access below the diaphragm is contraindicated.

To catheterize the femoral vein, the femoral arterial pulse is located. If no pulsation is palpable, the location of the artery can be estimated by finding the midpoint of a line drawn between the anterior superior iliac spine and the symphysis pubis. In the infant, the femoral vein lies between 0.5 and 1.0 cm medial to the artery. In the large teenager or adult, the femoral vein is approximately 1.0 to 1.5 cm medial to the artery. The needle is attached to a 5-ml syringe, and the skin is entered approximately 1 cm below the inguinal ligament in the infant and approximately 2 cm below the ligament in the teenager. The needle is directed cephalad at a 45-degree angle. In the large teenager, the vessel may not be reached until the needle has penetrated 2 to 4 cm. When a flash of blood is noted, the needle is lowered to an angle more flush with the skin, and the syringe is removed. After the operator is certain that the flow is not pulsatile, the guidewire is advanced into the vein. It is important to select a catheter of adequate length to ensure maintenance of proper position within the vessel. These catheters are very easy to dislodge if they are too short. In the 20-kg child, the catheter should be at least 5 cm long, and in the larger child, it should be at least 8 cm long.

The most common complications of this approach include femoral arterial puncture, infection, and thrombosis. Femoral arterial puncture occurs in approximately 4 to 6% of femoral venous catheterization attempts.[15, 47, 124] This is generally of no consequence with a small hematoma, but retroperitoneal bleeding can occur.[22, 95, 118] If the trauma physician determines that the artery has been cannulated, it may be secured as an arterial line. The occurrence of infection and thrombosis is kept to a minimum if catheters are kept in place less than 72 hours.[47, 124] Other complications include arteriovenous fistula formation, bowel perforation, catheter embolism secondary to extremity movement with catheter breakage, catheter tip malposition with retroperitoneal hemorrhage and puncture of the kidney.[14, 22, 68, 75, 99]

Internal Jugular Vein

The anatomic structures surrounding the internal jugular vein are fairly complex, and knowledge of their relations is necessary to avoid complications associated with faulty penetration by a needle. The internal jugular vein exits from the base of the skull via the jugular foramen and runs within the carotid sheath posterior and lateral to the internal and common carotid artery. The internal jugular vein then runs beneath the sternocleidomastoid muscle and enters the subclavian vein just under the medial end of the clavicle to form the innominate vein. Just before its junction with the subclavian vein the internal jugular vein is located lateral and slightly anterior to the common carotid artery. The right internal jugular vein and the right subclavian vein join to form a nearly straight pathway into the superior vena cava, whereas the left internal jugular vein inserts into the left subclavian vein at a nearly right angle, making passage of a catheter beyond this juncture more difficult. The stellate ganglion and the cervical sympathetic trunk are posterior to the internal carotid artery. The thoracic duct is posterior to the left internal jugular vein, and it empties into the subclavian vein near the internal jugular junction. The right lymphatic duct is much smaller than the thoracic duct, and it empties into the venous system at the junction of the subclavian and internal jugular veins. Iatrogenic disruption of the lymphatic flow therefore is more likely to occur on the patient's left side. As would be expected from the anatomy, malposition of the catheter is more common when the left side is used than the right.[41, 78, 87] In addition, penetration of the right lateral superior vena cava wall with subsequent right-sided hydrothoraces have been reported.[27, 63] For all of these reasons, the right side of the neck is preferred for venipuncture.

Three general approaches to cannulation of the internal jugular vein exist: central, anterior, and posterior. The central approach is the approach we use, and it is generally thought to be the easiest method to learn. For all three approaches, patient positioning and surface landmarks are the same. The patient is placed in a supine, 15-degree Trendelenburg position with the head turned away from the side being cannulated. Landmarks (Fig. 42–4) include the angle of the mandible, the clavicle, the suprasternal notch, the external jugular vein, the carotid pulsation, the two heads of the sternocleidomastoid muscle, and the triangle formed by these two heads and the clavicle.

For the central approach (Fig. 42–5), the triangle formed by the clavicle and the two heads of the sternocleidomastoid muscle is located. This landmark may be difficult to locate in an obese patient. The carotid arterial pulsation

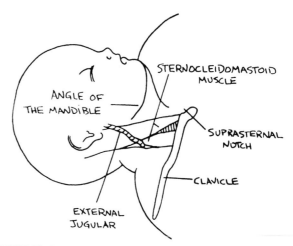

FIGURE 42–4
External landmarks for the internal jugular vein.

may be palpable within the triangle, and it should be retracted medially. A small finder needle is helpful to avoid excess probing or arterial puncture with a large-bore needle. The needle with a syringe attached is inserted at the apex of the triangle just lateral to the carotid artery and directed parallel to the carotid artery, usually toward the ipsilateral nipple at a 45-degree angle to the frontal plane. If the vein is not entered, the needle should be slowly withdrawn with continued gentle negative pressure on the syringe, then redirected 5 degrees more laterally. If additional redirecting is needed, care should be taken never to cross the plane of the carotid artery. When the vessel has been located, the finder needle can either be removed or temporarily left in position. The larger needle and syringe is then inserted through the identical course, and the catheter is then passed the desired length into the vessel in the same manner as for any other site.

The most important landmark for the anterior approach (Fig. 42–6) is the midpoint of the anterior border of the

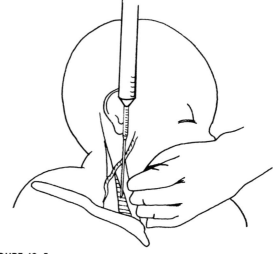

FIGURE 42–5
Central approach to the internal jugular vein.

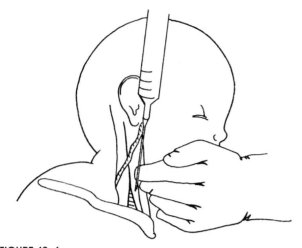

FIGURE 42–6
Anterior approach to the internal jugular vein.

sternocleidomastoid muscle. This landmark corresponds with the point midway between the angle of the mandible and the sternum. The index and middle fingers of the operator's left hand are used to retract the carotid artery medially, and the needle is introduced just anterior to the midpoint of the muscle, approximately 0.5 to 1 cm lateral to the pulsation, depending on the size of the patient. The needle is angled between 30 and 45 degrees with respect to the frontal plane and is advanced parallel to the carotid artery toward the ipsilateral nipple and the junction of the middle and medial one third of the clavicle. If the first attempt is unsuccessful, the angle should be changed 5 degrees laterally and the steps repeated. At no time should the plane of the carotid artery be crossed with the point of the needle.

The most important landmark for the posterior approach is the external jugular vein (Fig. 42–7). The needle is introduced under the sternocleidomastoid muscle just caudal to the point where the external jugular vein crosses the posterior rim of the sternocleidomastoid muscle. This landmark corresponds to a point near the junction of the middle and lower one third of the lateral border of the sternocleidomastoid muscle. The needle is aimed toward the suprasternal notch at a 45-degree angle to the sagittal plane and a 15-degree upward angle in the frontal plane. If this approach is not successful, the next attempt should be redirected slightly more cephalad.

The overall complication rate with internal jugular vein catheterization is low, ranging from 0.1 to 4.2%.[39, 52, 78, 127] The most common complication is carotid artery puncture, which accounts for 80 to 90% of all complications. Arterial puncture is usually without significant sequelae. Application of local pressure for 10 minutes is usually adequate. In the presence of coagulation abnormalities, cannulation of the internal jugular vein is relatively contraindicated. Even in patients with normal coagulation, hematoma formation secondary to arterial puncture has resulted in airway compromise and various nerve compressions including Horner syndrome.[76, 102, 131] Arterial puncture also has led to arteriovenous fistulas and pseudoaneurysm formation.[58, 94, 119] Nu-

merous other complications have been described, including thrombosis, tracheal puncture, cerebrovascular accident, and various otolaryngologic complications.

Antecubital Fossa

Central venous cannulation via the antecubital fossa has the advantage of being safe in the presence of a coagulopathy as well as having fewer thoracic complications associated with placement. Intrathoracic complications of hydrothorax and tamponade can occur later due to movement of the catheter tip secondary to arm motion. Disadvantages of cannulation via the antecubital fossa include a relatively greater time requirement for placement, lower success rate, a relatively high incidence of thrombosis and infection, and a significantly lower flow rate due to the length and smaller gauge of the catheter required. The vessel most commonly cannulated is the basilic vein (see Fig. 42–1). The cephalic and brachial veins may also be used, but cannulation is more difficult, and the success rates are lower.[79] The brachial vein is almost always entered via cutdown, although percutaneous venipuncture can be accomplished.[136]

The basilic vein provides the most direct path from the antecubital fossa to the central venous system.[133] The basilic vein continues directly as the axillary vein in an uninterrupted course to the central venous system. The cephalic vein, although visible and easily entered in the antecubital fossa, is considerably less well suited for central venous catheterization because of its unpredictable anatomy. The cephalic vein frequently enters the axillary vein at nearly a 90-degree angle, making catheter advancement beyond this point very difficult. In a substantial percentage of individuals, the cephalic vein does not empty into the axillary vein at all, but instead drains into the external jugular vein via a network of smaller veins. Other unpredictable anatomic variations make the cephalic vein a very poor choice for central venous cannulation, with only a 30 to 50% success rate on the first attempt.[83, 129] The basilic vein has a 60 to 80% success rate on the first attempt.[83, 98, 129]

When performing central venous cannulation from the antecubital fossa, the right basilic vein should be the first

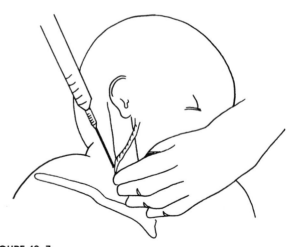

FIGURE 42–7
Posterior approach to the internal jugular vein.

choice due to the shorter length of catheter needed and the greater chance for proper tip positioning. The right brachial vein should be the operator's second choice.

Catheter gauge depends on the size of the patient. It is our practice to use a 22-gauge catheter in the newborn or very small infant, a 19-gauge catheter in the toddler or school-aged child, and a 16-gauge catheter in the older child.

Catheter placement is accomplished using the Seldinger technique. Turning the head toward the side of insertion increases the success rate for proper positioning.[20] A tourniquet is used and then released after the needle has been successfully passed into the vessel.

In the infant, because of the small vessel size, a J-tip wire may be difficult or nearly impossible to advance through the peripheral vessels. In these patients, a straight wire with a flexible tip should be used initially to help guide the catheter into the axillary or subclavian vein and then on into the superior vena cava. In the older patient, a J-tip wire may be used from the start. With the occasional exception of large-build teenagers, our experience with J-tip guidewires used peripherally is uniformly dismal. Straight soft-tipped wires are much more user friendly.

Complications of percutaneous central venous catheterization via the antecubital fossa are primarily thrombotic and infectious in nature. Thrombotic complications are usually restricted to local sterile phlebitis in 5 to 15% of cases.[62, 88, 121, 128] This complication usually resolves after the catheter is removed. Deep venous thrombosis, especially clinically silent small thromboses, occur in as many as 33% of cases, but pulmonary embolism is extremely rare and occurs in less than 0.5% of cases.[88, 128] The incidence of infectious complications is similar to that of shorter polyethylene catheters, with a 1 to 2% complication rate for catheters left in place less than 72 hours.[62, 88, 121, 128]

External Jugular Vein

The external jugular vein begins at the angle of the mandible, crosses at an angle over the surface of the sternocleidomastoid muscle, and then dives deeply to enter the subclavian vein at the medial third of the clavicle. It is a vein with numerous valves and variable size and tortuosity, and it often enters the subclavian vein at a sharp angle, past which it may be difficult to advance a catheter. The main advantages of the external jugular vein include its visibility as part of the surface anatomy, the safety of cannulation in the presence of a coagulopathy, and the avoidance of the risk of pneumothorax. The main disadvantage of the external jugular vein is its anatomic variability and the unpredictable course the catheter may take.

Insertion is accomplished by the Seldinger technique (Fig. 42–8). The arms are at the patient's side, and the head is turned toward the contralateral side. The index finger and thumb of the operator's left hand are used to distend and anchor the vein, and the venipuncture is made midway between the angle of the jaw and the midclavicle. When the free flow of blood is established, the syringe is disconnected, and the guidewire is advanced. Resistance is often met at the subclavian junction, and manipulation at this point may or may not lead to further advancement.

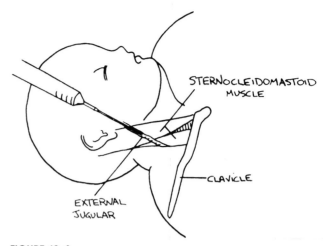

FIGURE 42–8
Cannulation of the external jugular vein.

The overall success rate for proper positioning of catheters in the central venous system via the external jugular vein is only 60 to 70% and is the primary reason why we rarely use this route. In 5 to 15% of patients, the external jugular vein is not identifiable as part of the superficial anatomy, and in up to 10% of cases, venipuncture cannot be performed.[49, 87, 112, 114] Others have reported that use of the J-tip wire improves the success rate to 80 to 90%.[12, 13]

Common complications, such as infection and thrombosis, occur at the same rates as those reported for other sites. Local hematoma has been reported in 1 to 5% of patients, but this generally is of little consequence if recognized before distortion of anatomy occurs.[66, 88, 112] Major complications such as perforation with pericardial tamponade and catheter fragment embolism have been reported.[33, 59] Vessel perforation with hydrothorax has been reported after catheter placement from the left external jugular vein; therefore, we recommend use of the right side initially, if possible.[48]

SPECIALIZED CATHETERS

Pulmonary Artery Catheterization

The first description of balloon-tipped catheters placed into the pulmonary artery was in 1970 by Swan and colleagues.[123] Presently, 5- and 7-Fr quadruple-lumen pulmonary artery catheters are commercially available for children. For measuring cardiac output and for calculation of other hemodynamic parameters, the 5-Fr size is recommended for patients who weigh less than 30 kg. Each catheter is composed of three lumens and a wire. The distal lumen has its port at the tip of the catheter and is used to measure pulmonary arterial and capillary wedge pressures as well as to obtain blood samples. The proximal lumen has its port 10 (in children who weigh less than 12 kg) to 30 cm from the tip of the catheter, depending on the catheter chosen, and is used to measure central venous pressure, to administer fluids or medications, to obtain blood samples, and to inject cold saline used for thermodilution cardiac output determination. The third lumen is used to inflate the balloon, which is located near the tip of the catheter. When inflated, this balloon allows the catheter tip to float into the more distal pulmonary artery to measure the pulmonary capillary wedge pressure. The fourth lumen is actually the wire, which connects the thermistor located near the tip of the catheter to the cardiac output computer. The thermistor continuously measures the temperature of the blood in the pulmonary artery and allows determination of the cardiac output using the thermodilution technique.

Pulmonary artery catheters can be inserted via all sites previously mentioned for central access. Although the differences are not great, we find insertion to be most successful when attempted in the following order: (1) right internal jugular vein, (2) left subclavian vein, (3) left internal jugular vein, (4) right subclavian vein, and (5) femoral veins. This is primarily due to the curves past which the catheter must advance to reach the pulmonary artery. Practical suggestions include shortening the introducer sheath, especially in the infant or small child. If the normal-length introducer sheath is placed in a subclavian vein and is too long, it may be impossible to manipulate the catheter downward into the superior vena cava, and it increases the risk of perforation of the central system if advanced too far. In addition, in the small infant, the final position of the proximal port may be occluded by the sheath. Because insertions via the antecubital fossa or external jugular vein are more difficult owing to the anatomic variability and tortuosity of the vessels, we seldom use these approaches.

There are several rules of thumb to be aware of in pulmonary artery catheter insertion. Before insertion, the thermistor and balloon should be checked for integrity of function. Estimation of the necessary length of catheter insertion should be done. It is important not to use an excessive length of catheter during insertion, because knotting of the catheter can occur, making catheter removal difficult or even impossible.[81] The literature suggests that fluoroscopy may be helpful in cases in which catheter positioning is very difficult. However, almost universally, patients selected for this monitoring requirement are seriously ill or injured and located in a critical care unit in which unnecessary movement or transport is unlikely; therefore, we have found bedside echocardiography to be very helpful, and we have never had to resort to fluoroscopy. Partial inflation of the balloon when it reaches the central circulation often facilitates its passage into the heart. The balloon is fully inflated when it reaches the right atrium. The recommended volume for balloon inflation should not be exceeded, because this may promote rupture of the balloon. When withdrawing the catheter, the balloon should be deflated to minimize the risk of damaging intracardiac or central venous structures. After the catheter has been in place for some time and the tip position has changed to no longer allow wedging, the catheter should not be advanced into the sheath, because bacteria may enter into the blood stream. Special catheter sheaths are now available to allow aseptic manipulation of catheters that have been in place for lengthy periods of time.

Variables that can be directly measured with a pulmonary artery catheter include central venous pressure, pulmonary artery pressure, pulmonary capillary wedge pressure, core body temperature, and right atrial and pulmonary artery blood gas values. Cardiac output can be calculated by means of the Stuart-Hamilton equation (i.e., temperature change integrated over time). Variables that can be derived from pulmonary artery catheter measurements include cardiac index, stroke volume and index, systemic and pulmonary vascular resistances and indices, arterial mixed venous O_2 content, left and right ventricular stroke work indices, left and right cardiac work indices, and intrapulmonary shunt fraction.

The complications associated with pulmonary arterial catheterization are most frequently associated with the insertion process. Bleeding and pneumothorax head this list.[71] Dysrhythmias are frequent but are usually only transient; changing the catheter position usually corrects this problem. Occasionally, an intractable dysrhythmia may require IV drug or electric countershock therapy. Pulmonary arterial catheterization is contraindicated in the patient with a left bundle branch block because of the chance of complete heart block developing if a right bundle branch block is caused during the insertion process. Additional reported complications include pulmonary infarction secondary to prolonged inadvertent wedging, pulmonary artery rupture, valvular damage, and thromboembolism.[38, 43, 51, 71, 101]

Mixed Venous Oxygen Saturation Monitoring

Effective tissue oxygenation is a function of supply and demand. Most efforts in patient care are directed toward the supply side via ventilatory and hemodynamic manipulation. Until recently, recognition of tissue oxygen supply-demand deficit may not have been possible until significant organ dysfunction had occurred. Mixed venous oxygen saturation (SvO_2) monitoring is one way of monitoring the balance between oxygen supply and oxygen demand in the critically ill patient.[130] SvO_2 can be measured continuously by reflection oximetry via fiberoptic channels incorporated into conventional pulmonary artery catheters. The catheter tip is positioned within a proximal pulmonary artery. The emitted light is reflected by the surrounding hemoglobin, and wavelength variation depends on its oxygen saturation. This light signal is then transmitted via the fiberoptic channels to an optical module, where the signal is interpreted and converted into a continuous display. Problems with the monitoring system center around interference with the reception of light and transmission of the signals. Fibrin or clots on the catheter tip, proximity of the tip to a vessel wall, faulty connections, and fiberoptic fracture are recognized causes of faulty signaling. Left-to-right shunt at the cardiac or great vessel level may make interpretation of the SvO_2 in the pulmonary artery more difficult. SvO_2 monitoring can be used with arterial blood gas analysis and hemodynamic indices to estimate the patient's oxygen supply-demand balance. Recognition and correction of tissue oxygenation deficiency can then be carried out earlier in the course of the patient's recovery.

NONINVASIVE MONITORING
Hemodynamic Monitoring

The majority of instruments used to measure systemic blood pressure noninvasively operate on the principle of oscillometry. The accuracy of the values obtained compared to those obtained by invasive measurements depends on several factors. Proper cuff size is required. The arm cuff should cover about two thirds of the upper arm, or two thirds of the thigh if the leg is used. Falsely elevated readings are obtained with cuffs that are too small, and falsely low readings are obtained with cuffs that are too large.[97] Greater discrepancies between cuff pressure and intra-arterial pressure occur in obese patients. The rate of deflation of the cuff influences the measurements obtained: the slower the deflation, the more accurate the results. Optimally, blood pressure cuffs should be deflated at approximately 2 to 3 mm Hg per second.

Noncontinuous blood pressure monitoring can be most easily done using simple sphygmomanometers. When sphygmomanometers are not available, the palpation method of Riva-Rocci or the bounce pressure (i.e., the pressure at which oscillations are first seen) are always useful ways of determining the approximate systolic blood pressure.[107] Listening over the artery with either a stethoscope or Doppler device for Korotkoff sounds allows determination of both the systolic and diastolic blood pressure.[77]

The present-day Dinamap 1846SX (Critikon, Johnson & Johnson Industries, Tampa, Fla.) is an automatic microprocessor-controlled noninvasive blood pressure monitor with the capability of offering continuous cycle readouts of the systolic, diastolic, and mean blood pressures, as well as the heart rate. Readings can be cycled as frequently as every minute or at intervals of up to 90 minutes. This instrument functions via an oscillometric method.[90, 105] A blood pressure cuff is connected to two tubes. One tube is connected to the inflater, and the other tube is connected to a pressure transducer. The cuff is inflated to a pressure greater than the systolic pressure, then deflated at a rate as slow as 5 mm Hg per second if necessary while searching for pulsations. The systolic pressure is the pressure at which oscillations appear. The range of detectable systolic pressures is 30 to 245 mm Hg for both adult and pediatric patients. Mean pressure is a direct reading at the point of maximal oscillation, and diastolic pressure is the pressure at which oscillations return to steady state with no further decrease noted. The range of detectable diastolic pressures is 10 to 210 mm Hg for both adult and pediatric patients.

Pulse Oximetry

Pulse oximetry offers the capability of monitoring a patient's oxygenation and pulse without the need for arterial puncture. Pulse oximeters are useful in the field, resuscitation room, operating room, and intensive care unit. The mechanism is based on the assumption that hemoglobin exists in two main forms in the blood: oxygenated and reduced. Arterial oxygen saturation is the ratio of oxygenated hemoglobin to total hemoglobin. The oximeter measures the absorption of certain light wavelengths that pass through living tissue. Because the wavelengths associated with oxygenated and reduced hemoglobin are known, these two wavelengths are selectively measured to determine the relative concentrations of oxygenated and reduced hemoglobin. Oxygen saturation can then be calculated.

The surface probe of a pulse oximeter can be positioned over any pulsatile vascular bed. Generally, the probe is placed on a digit, but earlobes or the nasal bridge can be used. Not only can oxygen saturation be measured, but the pulse can be determined extremely accurately. The reliability of pulse oximetry is excellent in healthy human subjects.[134]

Some limitations of pulse oximetry exist, but few complications have been reported. Because wavelengths of light are used, the surrounding light can interfere with the ability of the instrument to detect the two specific wavelengths associated with the types of hemoglobin. Environments with bright light, such as direct sunlight, high-intensity lamps, or bilirubin lights, may require simply covering the probe with an opaque material such as a towel or sheet. Because these instruments focus on the blood stream by way of pulse sensation, any condition that diminishes the pulse will diminish the reliability of the oximeter. Shock, hypotension, hypothermia, or the use of vasoconstrictive drugs may prevent accurate readings by pulse oximetry. The probe should not be attached to the same limb as a blood pressure cuff unless only infrequent, intermittent blood pressure readings are taken. Warming the site where the probe is to be placed is helpful only part of the time. Significant levels of dysfunctional hemoglobin (e.g., carboxyhemoglobin, methemoglobin) may interfere with the accuracy of the instrument, because the selected wavelengths only measure the concentrations of oxyhemoglobin relative to reduced functional hemoglobin rather than the concentrations of the dysfunctional hemoglobin. In addition, the pulse oximeter shows a maximum reading of only 100% without any further indication of the exact Pao_2. The potential for unrecognized oxygen toxicity exists if excessively high concentrations of oxygen are administered unnecessarily.

Acknowledgments

The authors wish to thank Evelyn Lizasuain for her secretarial assistance and Nadine Grabowski and Esther Thomas for their artwork.

References

1. Adler DC, Bryan-Brown CW: Use of the axillary artery for intravascular monitoring. Crit Care Med 1:148–150, 1973.
2. Ahmed N, Payne RF: Thrombosis after central venous cannulation. Med J Aust 1:217–220, 1976.
3. Allen EV: Thromboangiitis obliterans: Methods of diagnosis of chronic occlusive arterial lesions distal to the wrist with illustrative cases. Am J Med Sci 178:237–244, 1929.
4. Arthurs GJ: Case report: Digital ischaemia following radial artery cannulation. Anaesth Intensive Care 6:54–55, 1978.
5. Axelsson K, Efsen F: Phlebography in long-term catheterization of the subclavian vein. Scand J Gastroenterol 13:933–938, 1978.
6. Band JD, Maki DG: Infections caused by indwelling arterial catheters for hemodynamic monitoring. Am J Med 67:735–741, 1979.
7. Barnhorst DA, Barner HB: Prevalence of congenitally absent pedal pulses. N Engl J Med 278:264–265, 1968.
8. Bedford RF: Radial arterial function following percutaneous cannulation with 18- and 20-gauge catheters. Anesthesiology 47:37–39, 1977.
9. Bedford RF, Wollman H: Complications of percutaneous radial-

artery cannulation: An objective prospective study in man. Anesthesiology 38:228–236, 1973.

10. Bernard RW, Stahl WM: Subclavian vein catheterization: A prospective study. 1. Non-infectious complications. Ann Surg 173:184–190, 1971.

11. Bjork L, Enghoff E, Grenvib A, et al: Local circulatory changes following brachial artery catheterization. Vasc Dis 2:283–292, 1965.

12. Blitt CD, Carlson GL, Wright WA, et al: J-wire versus straight wire for central venous cannulation via the external jugular vein. Anesth Analg 61:536–537, 1982.

13. Blitt CD, Wright WA, Petty WC, et al: Central venous catheterization via the external jugular vein. JAMA 229:817–818, 1974.

14. Bolasny BL, Killen DA: Surgical management of arterial injuries secondary to angiography. Ann Surg 174:962–964, 1971.

15. Bozzetti F: Percutaneous femoral vein catheterization. Anaesthesia 33:761–762, 1978.

16. Brandt RL, Foley WJ, Fink GH, et al: Mechanism of perforation of the heart with production of hydropericardium by a venous catheter and its prevention. Am J Surg 119:311–316, 1970.

17. Brismar B, Hardstedt C, Jacobson S: Diagnosis of thrombosis by catheter phlebography after prolonged central venous catheterization. Ann Surg 194:779–783, 1981.

18. Brodsky JB: A simple method to determine patency of the ulnar artery intraoperatively prior to radial artery cannulation. Anesthesiology 42:626–627, 1975.

19. Bull MJ, Schreiner RL, Garg BP, et al: Neurologic complications following temporal artery catheterization. J Pediatr 96(6):1071–1073, 1980.

20. Burgess GE, Marino RJ, Peulex MJ: Effects of head position on the location of venous catheters inserted via basilic veins. Anesthesiology 46:212–213, 1977.

21. Campkin TV: Air embolism: Placement of central venous catheters. Anaesthesiology 56:406–407, 1982.

22. Christian CM II, Naraghi M: A complication of femoral arterial cannulation in a patient undergoing cardiopulmonary bypass. Anesthesiology 49:436–437, 1978.

23. Cohn JN: Blood pressure measurement in shock. Mechanisms of inaccuracy in auscultatory and palpatory methods. JAMA 199:118–122, 1967.

24. Colvin MP, Curran JP, Jarvis D, et al: Femoral artery pressure monitoring. Use of the Seldinger technique. Anaesthesia 32:451–455, 1977.

25. Committee on Trauma: Advanced Trauma Life Support. Chicago: American College of Surgery, 1984.

26. Cournand A, Bing R, Dexter L: Report of Committee on Cardiac Catheterization and Angiography of the American Heart Association. Circulation 7:769–774, 1953.

27. Criado A, Mena A, Figueredo R, et al: Late perforation of superior vena cava and effusion caused by central venous catheter. Anaesth Intensive Care 9:286–288, 1981.

28. Crossland SG, Neviaser RJ: Complications of radial artery catheterization. Hand 9:287–290, 1977.

29. Dailey RH: Flow rate variance of commonly used IV units. J Am Coll Emerg Physicians 2:341–342, 1973.

30. Dane TEB, King EG: Fatal cardiac tamponade and other mechanical complications of central venous catheters. Br J Surg 62:6–10, 1975.

31. Davis FM: Radial artery cannulation: Influence of catheter size and material on arterial occlusion. Anaesth Intensive Care 6:49–53, 1978.

32. DeAngelis J: Axillary arterial monitoring. Crit Care Med 4:205–206, 1976.

33. Defalque RJ, Campbell C: Cardiac tamponade from central venous catheters. Anesthesiology 50:249–252, 1979.

34. Downs JB, Rackstein AD, Klein EF Jr, et al: Hazards of radial-artery catheterization. Anesthesiology 38:283–286, 1973.

35. Dronen S, Thompson B, Nowak R, et al: Subclavian vein catheterization during cardiopulmonary resuscitation. Comparison of supra- and infraclavicular percutaneous approaches. JAMA 247:3227–3230, 1982.

36. Eerola R, Karkinen L, Karkinen S: Analysis of 13,800 subclavian catheterizations. Acta Anaesthesiol Scand 29:293–297, 1985.

37. Efsing HO, Lindblad B, Mark J, et al: Thromboembolic complications from central venous catheters: A comparison of three catheter materials. World J Surg 7:419–423, 1983.

38. Elliot CG, Zimmerman GA, et al: Complications of pulmonary artery catheterization in the care of critically ill patients: A prospective study. Chest 76:647–652, 1979.

39. English ICW, Fren RM, Pigott JF, et al: Percutaneous catheterization of the internal jugular vein. Anaesthesia 24:521–531, 1969.

40. Ersoz CJ, Hedden M, Lain L: Prolonged femoral arterial catheterization for intensive care. Anesth Analg 49:160–164, 1970.

41. Fischer J, Lundstrom J, Ottander HG: Central venous cannulation: a radiological determination of catheter positions and immediate intrathoracic complications. Acta Anaesthesiol Scand 21:45–49, 1977.

42. Fleisher G, Ludwin S (eds): Textbook of Pediatric Emergency Medicine. Baltimore, Williams & Wilkins, 1983.

43. Foote GA, Schabel SI, Hodges M: Pulmonary complications of the flow-directed balloon-tipped catheter. N Engl J Med 290:927–931, 1974.

44. Gardner RM, Bond EL, Clark JS: Safety and efficacy of continuous flush systems for arterial and pulmonary artery catheters. Ann Thorac Surg 23:534–538, 1977.

45. Gardner RM, Schwartz R, Wong HC: Percutaneous indwelling radial-artery catheters for monitoring cardiovascular function. Prospective study of the risk of thrombosis and infection. N Engl J Med 290:1227–1231, 1974.

46. Gardner RM, Warner HR, Toronto AF, et al: Catheter-flush system for continuous monitoring of central arterial pulse waveform. J Appl Physiol 29:911–913, 1970.

47. Getzen LC, Pollack EW: Short-term femoral vein catheterization. Am J Surg 138:875–877, 1979.

48. Ghani GA, Berry AJ: Right hydrothorax after left external jugular vein catheterization. Anesthesiology 58:93–94, 1983.

49. Giesy J: External jugular vein access to central venous system. JAMA 219:1216–1217, 1972.

50. Gilday DL, Downs AR: The value of chest radiography in the localization of central venous pressure catheters. Can Med Assoc J 101:363–364, 1969.

51. Golden MS, Pinder T, Anderson WT, et al: Fatal pulmonary hemorrhage complicating use of flow-directed balloon-tipped catheter in a patient receiving anticoagulant therapy. Am J Cardiol 32:865–867, 1973.

52. Goldfarb G, Lebrec D: Percutaneous cannulation of the internal jugular vein in patients with coagulopathies; an experience based on 1000 attempts. Anesthesiology 56:321–323, 1982.

53. Grant JP: Subclavian catheter insertion and complications. In: Grant JP (ed): Handbook of Total Parenteral Nutrition. Philadelphia, WB Saunders, 1980, pp 47–69.

54. Guyton AC, Jones CE: Central venous pressure: Physiological significance and clinical implications. Am Heart J 86:431–437, 1973.

55. Haapaniemi L, Slatis P: Supraclavicular catheterization of the superior vena cava. Acta Anaesthesiol Scand 18:12–22, 1974.

56. Hagley SR: Subclavian arteriovenous fistula from central venous catheterization (letter). Anaesth Intensive Care 13:103–104, 1985.

57. Hamilton WF, Dow P: An experimental study of standing waves in pulse propagated through the aorta. Am J Physiol 125:48–59, 1939.

58. Hansbrough JF, Narrod JA, Rutherford R: Arteriovenous fistulas following central venous catheterization. Intensive Care Med 9:287–289, 1983.

59. Henzel JH, DeWeese MS: Morbid and mortal complications associated with prolonged central venous cannulation. Am J Surg 121:600–605, 1971.

60. Hodge D III: Intraosseous infusions: A review. Pediatr Emerg Care 1(4):215–218, 1985.

61. Hodge D III, Fleisher G: Pediatric catheter flow rates. Am J Emerg Med 3(5):403–407, 1985.

62. Holt MH: Central venous pressures via peripheral veins. Anaesthesia 28:1093–1095, 1967.

63. Iberti TJ, Katz B, Reiner MA, et al: Hydrothorax as a late complication of central venous indwelling catheters. Surgery 94:842–846, 1983.

64. Iserson KV, Criss E: Intraosseous infusions: A usable technique. Am J Emerg Med 4(6):540–542, 1986.

65. James PM, Myers R: Central venous pressure monitoring: Complications and a new technique. Ann Surg 39:75–81, 1981.

66. Jobes DR, Schwartz AJ, Greenhow DE, et al: Safer jugular vein cannulation: Recognition of arterial puncture and preferential use of the external jugular route. Anesthesiology 59:353–355, 1983.

67. Johnstone RE, Greenhow DE: Catheterization of the dorsalis pedis artery. Anesthesiology 44:80–83, 1976.

68. Kalza SA, Cohen EL: Urologic complication associated with Swan-Ganz catheter. Urology 6:716–718, 1975.

69. Kamienski RW, Barnes RW: Critique of the Allen test for continuity of the palmar arch assessed by Doppler ultrasound. Surg Gynecol Obstet 142:861–864, 1976.

70. Katz AM, Birnbaum M, Moylan J, et al: Gangrene of the hand and forearm: A complication of radial artery cannulation. Crit Care Med 2:270–272, 1974.

71. Katz JD, Cronau LH, Barash PG, et al: Pulmonary artery flow-guided catheters in the perioperative period: Indications and complications. JAMA 237:2832–2834, 1977.

72. Kaye W: Venous and arterial catheterization. In: Sprung CL, Grenvik A (eds): Invasive Procedures in Critical Care. New York, Churchill Livingstone, 1985, pp 1–48.

73. Keller FS, Rosch J, Banner RL, et al: Iatrogenic internal mammary artery-to-innominate vein fistula. Chest 81:255–257, 1982.

74. Kellner GA, Smart JF: Percutaneous placement of catheters to monitor central venous pressure. Anaesthesia 36:515–516, 1972.

75. Kjellstrand CM, Merino GE, Mauer SM, et al: Complications of percutaneous femoral vein catheterizations for hemodialysis. Clin Nephrol 4:37–40, 1975.

76. Knoblanche GE: Respiratory obstruction due to hematoma following internal jugular vein cannulation. Anaesth Intensive Care 7:286, 1979.

77. Korotkov NS: A contribution to the problem of methods for the determination of the blood pressure. Rep Imper Milit-Med Acad, St. Petersburg 11:365–367, 1905.

78. Korshin J, Klauber PV, Christensen V, et al: Percutaneous catheterization of the internal jugular vein. Acta Anaesth Scand (Suppl) 67:27–33, 1978.

79. Kuramoto T, Sakabe T: Comparison of success in jugular versus basilic vein techniques for central pressure catheter positioning. Anesth Analg 54:696–697, 1975.

80. Langston CS: The aberrant central venous catheter and its complications. Radiology 100:55–59, 1971.

81. Lipp H, O'Donoghue K, Resnekov L: Intracardiac knotting of a flow-directed balloon catheter. N Engl J Med 284:220, 1971.

82. Lowenstein E, Little JW, Lo HH: Prevention of cerebral embolization from flushing radial-artery cannulas. N Engl J Med 285:1414–1415, 1971.

83. Lumley J, Russell WJ: Insertion of central venous catheters through arm veins. Anaesth Intensive Care 3:101–105, 1975.

84. McCormack T, Lane BE, Tanner WA, et al: Complications of subclavian vein cannulation. Ir Med J 74:373–374, 1981.

85. McIntyre KM, Lewis AJ, eds: Textbook of Advanced Cardiac Life Support. Dallas, American Heart Association, 1983, p 166.

86. McLean-Russ AH, Griffith CDM, Anderson JR, et al: Thromboembolism complications with silicone elastomer subclavian catheters. J Parenter Nutr 6:61–63, 1983.

87. Malatinsky J, Faybik M, Griffith M, et al: Venipuncture, catheterization and failure to position correctly during central venous cannulation. Resuscitation 10:259–270, 1983.

88. Malatinsky J, Faybik M, Samel M, et al: Surgical, infectious and thromboembolic complications of central venous catheterization. Resuscitation 10:271–281, 1983.

89. Mandel MA, Darchot PJ: Radial artery cannulation in 1,000 patients: Precautions and complications. J Hand Surg [Am] 2:482–485, 1977.

90. March GW, et al: The meaning of the point of maximum oscillations in cuff pressure in the indirect measurement of blood pressure. 2. Transactions of the American Society of Mechanical Engineers. J Biomech Eng 28:102, 1980.

91. Marx GF: Clinical anesthesia conference: Hazards associated with venous pressure monitoring. N Y State J Med 69:955–957, 1969.

92. Mathieu A, Dalton B, Fisher JE, et al: Expanding aneurysm of the radial artery after frequent puncture. Anesthesiology 38:401–403, 1973.

93. Maurer AH, Au FC, Malmud LS, et al: Radionuclide venography in subclavian vein thrombosis complicating parenteral nutrition. Clin Nucl Med 9:397–399, 1984.

94. Merino-Angulo J, Cortazar JL, Saez-Garmendia F: Subclavian artery to internal jugular vein fistula following percutaneous internal jugular vein catheterization. Cathet Cardiovasc Diagn 10:593–595, 1984.

95. Morris TR, Bouhoutsos J: The dangers of femoral artery puncture and catheterization. Am Heart J 89:260–261, 1975.

96. Mozersky DJ, Buckley CJ, Haggood CO Jr, et al: Ultrasonic evolution of the palmar circulation. A useful adjunct to radial artery cannulation. Am J Surg 126:810–812, 1973.

97. Nelson WE: Textbook of Pediatrics. 11th ed. Philadelphia, WB Saunders, 1979.

98. Ng WS, Rosen M: Positioning central venous catheters through the basilic vein. Br J Anaesth 45:1211–1214, 1973.

99. Nidus BD, Neusy AJ: Chronic hemodialysis by repeated femoral vein cannulation. Nephron 29:195–197, 1981.

100. Padberg FT, Ruggiero J, Blackburn GL, et al: Central venous catheterization for parenteral nutrition. Ann Surg 193:264–270, 1981.

101. Pape LA, Haffajee CI, Markis JE, et al: Fatal pulmonary hemorrhage after use of the flow-directed balloon catheter. Ann Intern Med 90:344–347, 1979.

102. Parikh RK: Horner's syndrome: A complication of percutaneous catheterization of internal jugular vein. Anaesthesia 27:327–329, 1972.

103. Parrish GA, Turkewitz D, Skiendzielewski JJ: Intraosseous infusions in the emergency department. Am J Emerg Med 4(1):53–63, 1985.

104. Phillip BK, Phillip JH: Characterization of flow in intravenous infusion systems. IEEE Trans Biomed Eng 30:702–707, 1983.

105. Posey JA, Geddes LA, Williams H, et al: The meaning of the point of maximum oscillations in cuff pressure in the indirect measurement of blood pressure. Cardiovasc Res Center Bull 8:15, 1969.

106. Remington JW: Contour changes of the aortic pulse during propagation. Am J Physiol 199:331–334, 1960.

107. Riva-Rocci S: Un nuovo sfigmomano-metro. Gazz med di Torino 47:981–996, 1001–1017, 1896.

108. Rosetti V, Thompson B, Aprahamian C: Difficulty and delay in intravascular access in pediatric arrests. Ann Emerg Med 13:406, 1984.

109. Rosetti V, Thompson B, Miller J, et al: Intraosseous infusion: An alternative route of pediatric intravascular access. Ann Emerg Med 14(9):885–888, 1985.

110. Ryan JA, Abel RM, Abbott WM, et al: Catheter complications in total parenteral nutrition: A prospective study of 200 consecutive patients. N Engl J Med 270:757–761, 1974.

111. Ryan JF, Raines J, Dalton BC, et al: Arterial dynamics of radial artery cannulation. Anesth Analg 52:1017–1025, 1973.

112. Schwartz AJ, Jobes DR, Levy WJ, et al: Intrathoracic vascular catheterization via the external jugular vein. Anesthesiology 56:400–402, 1982.

113. Seldinger SI: Catheter replacement of the needle in percutaneous arteriography: A new technique. Acta Radiol 39:368–375, 1953.

114. Seneff MG: Central venous catheterization: A comprehensive review, Part I. J Intensive Care Med 2(3):163–175, 1987.

115. Seneff MG: Central venous catheterization: A comprehensive review, Part II. J Intensive Care Med 2(4):218–231, 1987.

116. Seneff MG, Rippe JM: Central venous catheters. In: Rippe JM, Irwin RS, Alpert JS, Dalen JC (eds): Intensive Care Medicine. Boston, Little, Brown, and Co, 1985, pp 16–33.

117. Shah A, Gnoj J, Fisher VJ, et al: Complications of selective coronary arteriography by the Judkins technique and their prevention. Am Heart J 90:353–359, 1975.

118. Sharp KW, Spees EK, Selby LR, et al: Diagnosis and management of retroperitoneal hematomas after femoral vein cannulation for hemodialysis. Surgery 95:90–95, 1984.

119. Shield CF, Richardson JD, Buckley CJ, et al: Pseudoaneurysm of the brachiocephalic arteries: A complication of percutaneous internal jugular vein catheterization. Surgery 78:190–194, 1975.

120. Shoor PM, Berryhill RE, Benumof JL: Intraosseous infusion: Pressure-flow relationship and pharmacokinetics. J Trauma 19(10):772–774, 1979.

121. Sorenson TA, Sonne-Holm S: Central venous catheterization through the basilic vein or by infraclavicular puncture? A controlled trial. Acta Chir Scand 141:323–325, 1975.

122. Spivey WH, Malone D, Unger HD, et al: Comparison of intraosseous, central and peripheral routes of sodium bicarbonate during CPR in pigs. Ann Emerg Med 14:1135–1140, 1985.

123. Swan HJC, Ganz W, Forresth J, et al: Catheterization of the heart in man with use of a flow-directed balloon-tipped catheter. N Engl J Med 283:447–451, 1970.

124. Swanson RS, Uhlig PN, Gross PL, et al: Emergency intravenous access through the femoral vein. Ann Emerg Med 13:244–247, 1984.

125. Thomas TV: Location of catheter tip and its impact on central venous pressure. Chest 61:668–673, 1972.

126. Tocino IM, Watanabe A: Impending catheter perforation of superior vena cava: Radiographic recognition. Am J Roentgenol 146:487–490, 1986.

127. Tyden H: Cannulation of the internal jugular vein—500 cases. Acta Anaesthesiol Scand 26:485–488, 1982.

128. Walters MB, Stanger HAD, Rotem CE: Complications with percutaneous central venous catheters. JAMA 220:1455–1457, 1972.

129. Webre DR, Arens JF: Use of cephalic and basilic veins for introduction of central venous catheters. Anesthesiology 38:389–392, 1973.

130. White DM: Completing the hemodynamic picture: Sv0$_2$. Heart Lung 14(3):272–279, 1985.

131. Whittet HB, Boscoe MJ: Isolated palsy of the hypoglossal nerve after central venous catheterization. BMJ 288:1042–1043, 1984.

132. Williams CD, Cunningham JN: Percutaneous cannulation of femoral artery for monitoring. Surg Gynecol Obstet 141:773–774, 1975.

133. Williams PL, Warwick RA (eds): Gray's Anatomy. Philadelphia, WB Saunders, 1980, pp 603–640.

134. Yelderman M, New W Jr: Evaluation of pulse oximetry. Anesthesiology 59:349–352, 1983.

135. Youngberg JA, Miller ED: Evaluation of percutaneous cannulations of the dorsalis pedis artery. Anesthesiology 44:80–83, 1976.

136. Zollinger RW: A useful intravenous access route. Surg Gynecol Obstet 154:725–726, 1982.

Marshall Z. Schwartz
R. Thomas Temes

CHAPTER FORTY-THREE

Organ System Failure in the Injured Child

MULTIPLE ORGAN FAILURE

In the recent past, multiple organ failure (MOF) has emerged from a previously little known entity to one recognized as a leading cause of death following multiple trauma, major surgical procedures or both. Previously, patients who sustained major injury, severe hemorrhage, overwhelming sepsis, or acute cardiopulmonary failure often succumbed in the early postshock or postinjury period. With the evolution of trauma centers, sophisticated intensive care units, improved mechanical ventilation, and sepsis management, patients are routinely salvaged from the initial insult only to develop failure of one or more previously uninvolved organs.

Although MOF has been studied extensively in the adult population, relatively little information on this entity is available that pertains to children. This chapter briefly reviews what is known about the causes, pathophysiology, diagnosis, treatment, and outcome following MOF in children.

Etiology. Multiple organ failure develops most frequently in patients with overwhelming infection, critical illness, and preexisting organ dysfunction. Infection is the most common cause, and although any location is possible, it is usually intraperitoneal. Other causes include shock, hemorrhage, massive transfusion, intraperitoneal contamination from trauma or postsurgical complication, and immune deficits. In patients with preexisting organ dysfunction, MOF almost always involves the previously compromised organ.

Pathophysiology. The pathophysiology of MOF remains incompletely understood. Possible mechanisms include hormonal responses, humoral factors, and altered metabolic states, and shock and sepsis are frequently associated. Common causes of shock are hemorrhage, hypoxia, or anoxia. Criteria for shock in the injured, primarily adults but also applicable to children, have been outlined in Table 43–1. The cardiovascular system of children effectively compensates and maintains vital organ function in mild to moderate shock. However, signs of impending severe shock may be subtle and diagnosis difficult, and because of this the transition from compensated to uncompensated shock is more abrupt in children. Immediate treatment is needed in such situations to prevent organ compromise.

The cardiovascular response varies with the stage of shock. In compensated shock, filling pressures and stroke volumes are low, and the cardiac index is maintained by an increase in myocardial contractility, heart rate, and peripheral resistance. In severe or irreversible shock, these responses may be lost and myocardial performance significantly impaired. The cause of this decreased function is likely to be a cumulative effect of metabolic derangements, altered myocardial metabolism, and circulating cardiodepressants.

In response to shock, a variety of neural and humoral reflexes are activated. Neural reflexes from the hypothalamus are mediated by the sympathetic system and norepinephrine. Epinephrine is released from the adrenal cortex. These substances produce vasoconstriction of most vascular beds with initial preservation of cerebral and cardiac perfusion. Cortisol levels also rise. Vasopressin secretion in-

Table 43–1
Advanced Trauma Life Support Classification of Shock

Class I
15% or less acute blood volume loss
Blood pressure normal
Pulse increased 10–20%
No change in capillary refill
Class II
20–25% loss of blood volume
Tachycardia >150 beats/min
Tachypnea 35–40 breaths/min
Capillary refill prolonged
Systolic blood pressure decreased
Pulse pressure decreased
Orthostatic hypotension >10–15 mm Hg
Urine output >1 ml/kg/hr
Class III
30–35% blood volume loss
All of the above signs
Urine output <1 ml/kg/hr
Lethargic, clammy, and vomiting
Class IV
40–50% blood volume loss
Nonpalpable pulses
Obtunded

creases substantially with hypovolemia, producing peripheral vasoconstriction, renal enhancement of free water absorption, and a secondary increase in intravascular volume. Renal hypoperfusion results in renin release, producing angiotensin-I from angiotensinogen. Angiotensin-I is converted by the lungs to angiotensin-II, a potent vasoconstrictor and stimulator of aldosterone release from the adrenal medulla. These phenomena maintain blood pressure and intravascular volume at the expense of visceral and renal blood flow.

Neural hormones contribute to the shock response. The precise role of endogenous opioids is not known; however, administration of naloxone following experimental septic shock restores mean blood pressure. Other important central nervous system neuropeptides include vasoactive intestinal peptide and thyrotropin releasing hormone. Thyrotropin releasing hormone produces arousal, tachypnea, tachycardia, and hypertension. Its administration improved physiologic parameters and survival in experimental shock induced with leukotriene, anaphylaxis, and platelet activating factor. In contrast, vasoactive intestinal peptide is a potent vasodilator and may produce hypotension. Although it is seen in high concentrations in the central nervous system, its elaboration requires the gastrointestinal tract. The relationship of vasoactive intestinal peptide to shock is not known.

The effects of inflammatory mediators are well described. Histamine and kallikrein-bradykinin are released from circulating mast cells. These substances produce vasodilation and pulmonary hypertension. Platelet aggregates release tissue thromboplastin and vasoactive substances (e.g., serotonin, histamine, and vasoactive amines), which may play a role in the development of increased capillary permeability. Macrophages release leukotrienes and prostaglandins. Leukotrienes depress the cardiac index, produce vasoconstriction, and increase vascular permeability. Inflammation also causes release of oxygen radicals, which produces further cell injury.

Utilization of oxygen is abnormal in patients with MOF. In the uninjured patient, oxygen consumption is independent of delivery. However, children with sepsis, shock, or severe postoperative stress develop a hypermetabolic state with increased oxygen consumption, utilization, and delivery, and survival correlates with their ability to mount a hypermetabolic response. With MOF, the ability to generate this hypermetabolic response is apparently significantly altered or lost. Proposed mechanisms for this include alterations in substrate delivery, oxygen delivery, mitochondrial function, and substrate metabolism.

Diagnosis. In the pediatric population, because of the wide range in patient age and size, diagnosis of organ failure may be difficult. In a review of MOF in a pediatric intensive care unit population, criteria for failure of specific organ systems were established (Table 43–2), criteria that allow objective diagnosis within a given patient population.

Organ failure is detected by impaired function, alterations in organ-specific enzymes, or abnormal histology. The onset of single organ failure or MOF can be rapid and straightforward, or it can be insidious; a latency period of several days between initial resuscitation and organ failure is common. Because organ failure is so often associated with infection, a careful evaluation for a septic focus is mandatory. The peritoneal cavity is the most common site of occult infection, but unfortunately, physical examination is often unreliable in detecting intra-abdominal infection. In one study, only 36% of patients had tenderness and only 7% had a palpable mass. The only suggestion may be nonspecific: hyperglycemia, fever, leukocytosis, and increasing fluid requirements. Evaluation using ultrasound, computed tomography, or other imaging modalities provides the best diagnostic accuracy.

The organs most frequently involved in MOF are the lung, kidney, gastrointestinal tract, liver, and heart (Table 43–3). Failure of the central nervous system, coagulation system, pancreas, and other organs has also been described.

Management. Management of MOF is nonspecific, and mortality unfortunately remains high. Therefore, prophylaxis is the most effective form of therapy. During the immediate postinjury period, rapid correction of shock, early and aggressive intubation and assisted ventilation with positive end-expiratory pressure (PEEP) when indicated, immobilization of fractures, avoidance of technical error, and meticulous sterility are all important.

When organ failure develops, its cause must be sought. Infection is treated with antibiotics, surgical or catheter drainage, and débridement. Other correctable causes of MOF such as hypovolemia, electrolyte imbalance, drug toxicity, and missed injury are sought.

Supportive management includes nutrition, achievement of hyperdynamic cardiovascular parameters, mechanical ventilation, dialysis, and drugs, nearly always in an intensive care setting. Without correction of the underlying cause, supportive therapy is generally unsuccessful.

Outcome. The mortality of patients with MOF is significant. Although pediatric patients have a lower mortality rate than that of adults with similar degrees of illness, the overall mortality rate in pediatric intensive care units is still 10 to 18%. In one pediatric intensive care unit, the mortality rate of children with MOF was 54% but only 0.3% in those

Table 43–2

Criteria for Diagnosis of Failure of Specific Organ Systems

Organ System	Criteria
Respiratory	RR >90/min (infants <12 mo)
	RR >70/min (children ≥12 mo)
	Pao_2 <40 mm Hg (in absence of cyanotic heart disease)
	$Paco_2$ >65 mm Hg
	Pao_2/Fio_2 <250 mm Hg
	Mechanical ventilation (>24 hr if postoperative)
	Tracheal intubation for airway obstruction or acute respiratory failure
Renal	Blood urea nitrogen >100 mg/dl
	Serum creatinine >2 mg/dl
	Dialysis
Gastrointestinal	Blood transfusions >20 ml/kg in 24 hours because of gastrointestinal hemorrhage (endoscopic confirmation optional)
Hepatic	Total bilirubin >5 mg/dl and serum glutamic-oxaloacetic transaminase or lactate dehydrogenase more than twice normal value (without evidence of hemolysis)
	Hepatic encephalopathy ≥ grade II
Cardiovascular	Mean arterial pressure <40 mm Hg (infants <12 mo)
	Mean arterial pressure <50 mm Hg (children ≥12 mo)
	Heart rate <50 beats/min (infants <12 mo)
	Heart rate <40 beats/min (children ≥12 mo)
	Cardiac arrest
	Continuous vasoactive drug infusion for hemodynamic support
Hematologic	Hemoglobin <5 g/dl
	White blood cell count <3000 cells/mm³
	Platelets <20,000/mm³
	Disseminated intravascular coagulopathy (prothrombin time >20 sec or partial thromboplastin time <60 sec in presence of positive fibrin split products assay)
Neurologic	Glascow coma scale <5
	Fixed, dilated pupils
	Persistent (>20 min) intracranial pressure >20 mm Hg or requiring therapeutic intervention

From Wilkinson JD, Pollack MM, Glass NL, et al: Mortality associated with multiple organ failure and sepsis in the pediatric intensive care unit. J Pediatr 111:324–328, 1987.

Table 43–3

Frequency (%) of Specific Organs Failing in Patients with Single Organ Failure and Multiple Organ Failure from Various Causes

System	Reference				
	30	33	34	75	40
Respiratory	100	58	48	97	95
Renal	27	48	45	52	61
Gastrointestinal	5	22	20	—	33
Hepatic	20	84	54	29	33
Cardiovascular	5	—	—	35	59
Coagulation	25	—	—	—	31
Central nervous	—	—	—	32	28

Table 43–4

Mortality (%) by Number of Organs Failing in Single Organ Failure and Multiple Organ Failure from Various Causes

Number of Organs	Reference			
	30	*33*	*34*	*75*
One	30	23	30	10
Two	57	53	60	50
Three	14	79	85	100
Four	73	100	100	—
> Four	100	—	—	—

without MOF. The mortality rate increases with the number of failing organs and approaches 100% with failure of four or more organs (Table 43–4). In survivors, ultimate organ function is good, and therefore aggressive therapy is warranted.

PULMONARY FAILURE

In response to injury or disease at other anatomic sites, total fluid content of the lung increases. This phenomenon, first noted during World War II, is clinically manifested by dyspnea, tachypnea, and cyanosis. Since its first description, this symptom complex has become known by several terms including Da Nang lung, shock lung, pump lung, postperfusion lung, progressive pulmonary failure, adult hyaline membrane disease, respirator lung, and posttraumatic pulmonary insufficiency. In 1967, Ashbaugh and colleagues labeled posttraumatic pulmonary failure as *adult respiratory distress syndrome* (ARDS). Currently, this is the most common term used for this clinical syndrome.

The lung is the most commonly affected organ in single organ failure or MOF (see Table 43–3). Adult respiratory distress syndrome develops in 39% of critically ill patients with hemorrhage or trauma, in up to 40% of patients with intra-abdominal abscess, and in approximately 10% of patients who undergo major surgical procedures. There are approximately 150,000 adult cases of ARDS per year. The incidence in the pediatric population is approximately 1% of all pediatric intensive care unit admissions.

Etiology. Although the causes of ARDS in adults and children is unknown, there is no evidence that causes in children are different from those in adults. Sepsis, usually from gram-negative organisms, is the most common underlying factor in both age groups. In fact, the development of ARDS is uncommon in patients in the absence of sepsis; hence, ARDS may represent an indication of an otherwise occult infection. In children, other causes that may contribute to the development of ARDS include near drowning, near strangulation, multiple trauma, elevated intracranial pressure, and burns.

Pathophysiology. Physiologic abnormalities seen in ARDS include decreased functional residual capacity, decreased pulmonary compliance, and increased pulmonary vascular shunting. These alterations produce hypoxia and an increased work of breathing. Increased pulmonary water from a pulmonary capillary leak causes the early physio-

logic alterations. Multiple factors contribute to this capillary leak, including the release of free fatty acids, lysosomal enzymes, serotonin, histamines, kinins, complement, prostaglandins, leukotrienes, and oxygen-free radicals.

Histologically, the lung parenchyma reveals an accumulation of polymorphonuclear leukocytes, platelet aggregations, fibrin deposition, and microthrombi. With continuation of the process, hyaline membranes form from extravasation of leukocytes, red blood cells, and protein (Fig. 43–1). After approximately 48 hours, type II alveolar cells proliferate. Ultimately, fibroblast, macrophage, lymphocyte, and plasma cell infiltration and proliferation result in pulmonary fibrosis.

Diagnosis. Diagnosis of ARDS is facilitated by a high index of suspicion. In children with previously normal cardiopulmonary function, tachypnea, dyspnea, and hypoxia following acute injury or illness such as major surgery are

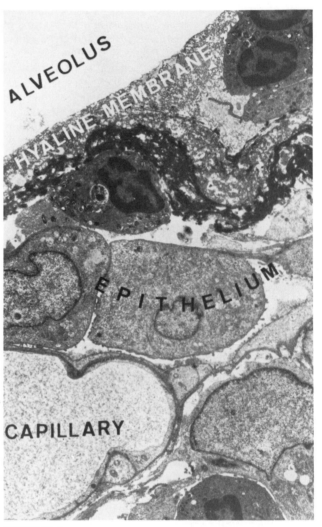

FIGURE 43–1

Electronic micrograph with characteristic findings of adult respiratory distress syndrome. (From Riede UN, Mittermayer C, Horn R, et al: Pathobiology of the alveolar wall in human shock lung. In: Cowley RA, Trump BF (eds): Pathophysiology of Shock, Anoxia, and Ischemia. Baltimore, Williams & Wilkins, 1982, pp 358–371.)

signs of ARDS. The onset is gradual and usually takes 24 to 72 hours. With associated pulmonary trauma, distinguishing ARDS from sequelae of mechanical injury may be difficult. Chest roentgenography reveals progressive development of diffuse alveolar infiltrates, often with sparing of the heart border. Physiologic abnormalities develop, as discussed previously. Acute respiratory distress is more consistent with airway obstruction, aspiration, trauma to the tracheobronchial tree, pneumothorax, flail chest, pulmonary contusion, ruptured diaphragm, or other mechanical injury.

Management. Management is directed at correction of the underlying cause or causes and ventilatory support. Early intubation and application of PEEP may prevent or lessen the severity of ARDS. If ARDS develops, normal tidal volumes of 10 to 15 ml per kg and routine ventilatory rates are usually insufficient. High positive inspiratory pressure and PEEP are often necessary to increase functional residual capacity, overcome decreased compliance, and diminish pulmonary shunting. The PEEP often exceeds 10 cm of water, and under extreme circumstances may exceed 30 cm of water. Maintaining inspired oxygen concentration below 50% minimizes the effects of oxygen toxicity. Oxygen saturations higher than 90% or arterial Po_2 above 65 mm Hg, or both, are acceptable. Volume loading may be required with high PEEP. Wedge pressures of 15 to 18 mm Hg and a cardiac index of 3.0 to 4.5 L/min/m^2 are optimal. Inotropes and vasodilators are sometimes necessary. In addition, paralyzing agents are sometimes used to increase chest wall compliance. Steroids are no longer used to treat ARDS.

Unfortunately, high ventilator pressures and high inspired oxygen concentrations are often necessary. Decreased cardiac index, bronchopleural fistula, pneumomediastinum, pneumothorax, pneumoperitoneum, subcutaneous emphysema, pneumopericardium, and the formation of pneumatoceles are all complications of elevated airway pressure in patients with ARDS. Complications from barotrauma and oxygen toxicity can significantly worsen the prognosis.

Outcome. The mortality rate of from 35 to 74% in adults with ARDS is somewhat lower in pediatric populations. Most pediatric patients who survive ARDS regain normal pulmonary function, but some deficit may persist. One study showed that 33% of pediatric survivors who had normal lung function before ARDS had some functional respiratory deficit after recovering from ARDS. These abnormalities do not have a specific pattern and usually are clinically insignificant. A report in children found outcome correlated with exposure time to inspired oxygen concentrations above 50% and peak inspiratory pressure. Outcome did not correlate with duration of mechanical ventilation.

RENAL FAILURE

Etiology. Acute renal failure (ARF) can be defined as loss of bilateral renal function with or without oliguria. Oliguria is defined as urine output less than 300 ml/m^2 in 24 hours or less than 0.5 ml per kg per hour. Waste products and electrolytes normally excreted by the kidneys accumulate. Although renal failure can be due to many causes, including ischemia, nephrotoxins, or primary par-

enchymal disease, the most common cause in pediatric intensive care units is hypoperfusion from hypovolemia or sepsis.

Acute renal failure is divided into prerenal, parenchymal, and postrenal forms. Prerenal ARF is caused by decreased renal perfusion. Renal blood flow normally represents 20 to 25% of cardiac output; 85 to 95% of flow supplies the renal cortex. Glomerular blood flow is autoregulated and remains constant over a wide range of perfusion pressures by alterations in vascular resistance at the afferent and efferent arterioles. However, when perfusion pressure decreases sufficiently, the renal blood flow and the glomerular filtration rate fall. Prerenal azotemia develops, and with severe or prolonged ischemia renal failure results.

Pathophysiology. The pathogenesis of parenchymal failure is not completely understood. Parenchymal ARF has also been called acute tubular necrosis and vasomotor nephropathy. Histologic evidence of tubular necrosis is found in only a minority of patients. Prolonged and intense prerenal failure with afferent arteriole vasoconstriction and shunting of blood from cortex to medulla (vasomotor nephropathy) is the major predisposing factor for parenchymal renal failure. Other causes of parenchymal ARF include myoglobin and hemoglobin precipitation, intravenous contrast, anesthetics, antibiotics and other drugs, disseminated intravascular coagulation, and direct renal or vascular injury.

Postrenal failure results from obstruction to the flow of urine. In a trauma patient this can occur in pelvic or lower abdominal trauma.

Diagnosis. It may be difficult to distinguish between prerenal and parenchymal ARF. The parameters used to differentiate between these two phenomena are shown in Table 43–5. Unfortunately, in the first 12 to 24 hours, the laboratory features that help distinguish between prerenal and parenchymal ARF may be equivocal. However, once parenchymal ARF is established, the damaged renal tubules are unable to modify glomerular filtration, and urine osmolality is in the approximate range of plasma (300 mOsm/L).

An abrupt cessation of urine output suggests bilateral vascular occlusion or postrenal obstruction. Ultrasound is

Table 43–5

Criteria Useful in Distinguishing Prerenal Azotemia from Oliguric Parenchymal Acute Renal Failure

	Prerenal Azotemia	Oliguric Parenchymal Acute Renal Failure
Specific gravity	>1.015–1.020	1.010–1.014
Sediment	Normal	Casts
Urine sodium	<15–20 mEq/L	>30–40
Urine osmolarity	>400–650 mOsm/L	<300–600
U/P urea	>8–20	<3–14
U/P creatinine	>40	<10–20
U/P osmolarity*	>1.3–1.5	<1.1–1.3
FNa	<1	>1–3
RFI	<1–3	>1.0–2.5

*Osmolarity measurements are not accurate if intravenous contrast, glucose, mannitol, protein, or high urea concentrations are present.

U/P, Urine/plasma ratio; FNa, fractional excretion of sodium (U/P sodium divided by U/P creatinine multiplied by 100); RFI, renal failure index (U/P creatinine multiplied by urinary sodium multiplied by 100).

useful for diagnosis. Other imaging procedures may also be used. These include intravenous pyelography, contrast-enhanced computed tomography, angiography, renal scan, cystoscopy, and retrograde pyelography. Vascular injury and postrenal obstruction must be diagnosed and treated rapidly to prevent progression to ARF.

Renal failure induced by disseminated intravascular coagulation is diagnosed by alterations in coagulation parameters. Elevation of the prothrombin time and partial thromboplastin time, elevated fibrin-split products, thrombocytopenia, and microangiopathic hemolytic anemia suggest the presence of this condition.

Management. The therapy for ARF depends on the cause. When prerenal ARF is present, the treatment is establishment of adequate intravascular volume. Rapid infusions of 10 to 20 ml per kg of crystalloid are used. Invasive monitoring with Foley, arterial, central venous, or Swan-Ganz catheters is often indicated. Vascular injury and postrenal obstruction require operation.

The treatment of parenchymal ARF in its early stage is controversial. If oliguria persists in spite of adequate volume replacement, then hypervolemia may be attempted. Hypervolemia may induce pulmonary edema, and it may be necessary to monitor pulmonary wedge pressure. Diuretics have been used in early acute renal failure, although their use is not universally accepted. Mannitol (1 gm/kg) or furosemide (1–10 mg/kg) may be given intravenously. Diuretics may be beneficial in reversing early acute renal parenchymal failure or in converting oliguric renal failure to nonoliguric renal failure. However, once renal parenchymal failure is established, there is no evidence that diuresis decreases the need for dialysis, the duration of renal failure, or the patient mortality rate. There are risks associated with the use of diuretics. Mannitol may produce hyperosmolality, and furosemide in high concentrations may produce transient or permanent hearing loss. Nephrotoxicity, electrolyte imbalance, and altered urine chemistries are also complications of diuretic use. Visceral vasodilators such as dopamine improve renal blood flow. Intravenous dosages of 2.5 to 5 μg per kg per minute are used.

Following major crush injuries, myoglobin-induced renal failure can occur. To prevent renal tubular myoglobin or hemoglobin precipitation, normovolemia or hypervolemia, alkalinization of the urine, and diuresis are beneficial.

The management of renal failure from disseminated intravascular coagulation involves treatment of underlying factors, such as sepsis. The use of fresh frozen plasma and heparin are controversial. Fresh frozen plasma is useful to replenish consumed coagulation factors, but replacement may fuel continued intravascular coagulation. Following major traumatic injuries, the use of heparin is contraindicated.

Major complications of ARF include hypertension, severe electrolyte imbalance, and hypervolemia. Immunosuppression, coagulopathy, anemia, and stress ulceration also occur. Dialysis, usually peritoneal, is effective for most of these complications.

Outcome. Oliguric ARF generally resolves within 2 weeks. Polyuria develops, followed by recovery of renal function. Mortality is lower in children than in adults and in nonoliguric ARF than in oliguric ARF. In surgical patients, mortality is 25 to 90%, usually from underlying disease or MOF.

GASTROINTESTINAL FAILURE

The gastrointestinal tract is frequently involved in MOF, and injured patients may present in several ways. Most common is gastrointestinal bleeding. Other signs of gastrointestinal failure include perforation, ileus, diarrhea, and enterocolitis.

Etiology. Stress-related gastric bleeding occurs in many adult patients in an intensive care unit setting. Multiple shallow erosions in the fundus and body of the stomach are commonly seen. In infants and children, a single ulceration is more common; the lesion is frequently found in the duodenum, and there is a higher incidence of ulcer perforation. Predisposing conditions in adults include sepsis, burns, trauma, head injury, major surgery, and peritonitis. In the pediatric population, the common predisposing conditions seem limited to head trauma and burns. Certain medications, such as steroids and nonsteroidal anti-inflammatory agents, also may contribute to upper gastrointestinal bleeding.

Pathophysiology. The mechanism of stress ulceration is not known. There is an increase in acid secretion in patients with central nervous system injury mediated by the hypothalamic-vagal pathway and by increased gastrin secretion. However, in sepsis, burns, and trauma, acid hypersecretion is not common. With physiologic stress, the integrity of the gastric mucosal barrier is diminished, and alterations in mucosal blood flow, permeability, and mucus production occur. Breakdown of the mucosal barrier allows back diffusion of hydrochloric acid, and this may produce gastric ulceration. Deficient energy stores, sympathetic-parasympathetic nervous system imbalance, humeral agents, and other endogenous substances are other possible mechanisms.

Diagnosis. Stress-related ulceration most frequently manifests as bleeding. Diagnosis is made with upper gastrointestinal endoscopy. Contrast studies, nuclear medicine scans, and angiography are of less value.

Perforation is evident with free air on radiographs or an acute abdomen on physical examination. Resuscitation and surgery should be performed rapidly.

Management. Prevention is optimal. This requires maintenance of gastric pH above 4.5, either with antacids or H_2 receptor antagonists. Antacids are equal to or more effective than H_2 receptor antagonists but only if the gastric pH is measured frequently and maintained at desired levels.

Conservative management is usually adequate for bleeding. This included intensive monitoring, antacids, intravenous fluids, packed red blood cells, and fresh frozen plasma as needed. A nasogastric tube allows for monitoring of bleeding and iced Ringer lactate or iced saline lavage. Endoscopy is indicated to identify the site or sites of bleeding. If the specific bleeding site is found, electrical or laser cauterization may be used. When gastric lavage or coagulation is unsuccessful in controlling significant bleeding, surgery is performed. Although the use of intra-arterial vasopressors and arterial embolization can be successful, the morbidity and mortality from these procedures in small children and infants may exceed those of surgical intervention.

In a review of seriously ill and injured children who developed upper gastrointestinal bleeding, the majority of patients had a solitary lesion, most often located in the duodenum. Forty per cent required operative intervention. In the group of patients who presented with bleeding alone, vagotomy, pyloroplasty, and oversewing of the ulcer were successful in controlling the bleeding.

Outcome. Perforation associated with stress ulceration is more common in children than in adults. When perforation occurs in children, oversewing of the ulcer has yielded good results, which has not been the case with adults. In children, major gastric resections are unnecessary. Mortality from stress ulceration is 14 to 65%.

HEPATIC FAILURE

Etiology. Improved survival rates in critically ill patients with ARDS or renal failure have allowed recognition of liver failure as part of the MOF syndrome. Liver failure usually occurs in the presence of other failing organs, and sepsis is often the cause. Hepatic failure may be precipitated by preexisting liver dysfunction and by exposure to halothane, certain antibiotics, total parenteral nutrition, and other hepatotoxic drugs (e.g., acetaminophen, anticonvulsants, methyldopa [Aldomet]).

Jaundice is a frequent complication of major surgery, trauma, and massive resuscitation. A transient bilirubin rise of 1.5 mg per dl is seen after uncomplicated surgery, and postoperative jaundice may occur in as many as 20% of patients.

The normal liver is capable of processing large increases in bile pigment with only mild or moderate elevations in serum bilirubin. In trauma, an increased bile pigment load can be caused by free hemoglobin and nonviable red blood cells from transfused blood, crush injury, hematoma absorption, hemolysis, or transfusion reaction. Transient bilirubin elevations can also occur with hypotension, congestive heart failure, and catecholamine release.

Pathophysiology. Hypotension produces diminution in both portal flow and oxygen saturation. In addition, high concentrations of lactate and other anaerobic metabolic products from the gastrointestinal tract are delivered to the liver. Warm ischemia is poorly tolerated and results in hepatocyte damage. This is manifested initially by elevation in cellular enzymes and later by global hepatic dysfunction.

In the first 24 hours following trauma, light microscopy reveals increased intracellular lipids, accumulation of acute inflammatory cells, dilation, and congestion of hepatic veins and sinusoids and compression of liver chords. Electron micrographic changes include mild to moderate alterations in nuclear chromatin, swollen mitochondria, and swollen endoplasmic reticulum. Irreversible injury is best demonstrated by flocculent densities in the mitochondria by electron microscopy. One to 2 weeks after the onset of hepatic failure, inflammation, cellular regeneration, intracellular lipid diminution, and bile inspissation occur. After

3 weeks, chronic inflammation, fibrosis, and bile duct proliferation become evident.

Hepatic failure affects all aspects of liver function. Synthesis of protein and coagulation factors are significantly diminished, and metabolism of bilirubin, glucose, amino acids, and fatty acids is altered. As a result, energy production, detoxification, and bacterial defense by the reticuloendothelial system are also impaired.

Diagnosis. Diagnosis of hepatic failure is by laboratory evaluation of serum bilirubin and liver enzymes. Liver enzymes reflecting hepatocellular insult rise immediately after the injury, and levels correlate with the severity of liver injury. After 3 to 4 days, liver enzyme elevations resolve in the absence of ongoing hepatic injury or failure. Bilirubin peaks occur between the fourth and fifteenth days after injury. Bilirubin levels of 4 to 5 mg per dl are associated with mild hepatic failure and can rise to 10 to 20 mg per dl in severe hepatic failure.

Management. The management of hepatic failure is supportive. Intravascular volume and electrolyte balance must be maintained. Because glycogen stores in the liver are depleted, intravenous glucose is administered. Underlying sepsis or obstruction to bile flow should be excluded. Adequate nutrition is appropriate. Efforts to decrease ammonia production in the gastrointestinal tract by administration of lactulose and neomycin are beneficial.

Outcome. Mortality from hepatic failure is 50 to 100%.

Acute acalculous cholecystitis occurs in adults with MOF or other critical illness. This is also true in children. Cholecystitis associated with trauma is acalculous in approximately 90% of cases and is associated with biliary stasis, obstruction, or infection. Reasons for stasis following trauma include dehydration, anesthesia, mechanical ventilation, narcotics, ileus, total parenteral nutrition, and prolonged bed rest.

The diagnosis of acute acalculous cholecystitis is difficult because gallbladder calculi are absent, and pain is attributed to abdominal trauma or surgery. Despite the absence of stones, ultrasound of the biliary tree is the best diagnostic study and demonstrates an enlarged gallbladder with a thickened wall secondary to edema. Hepatobiliary scanning demonstrates the absence of gallbladder visualization.

Cholecystectomy is the treatment of choice. In patients too ill to undergo general anesthesia, catheter drainage of the gallbladder percutaneously or operatively (under local anesthesia) may be performed.

CARDIAC FAILURE

Etiology. Failure of the myocardium in adults is a common sequela following multiple trauma. Causes include shock, sepsis, or direct myocardial injury. Elevated preload or afterload, acidosis, electrolyte disturbances (e.g., calcium, potassium, magnesium), or tamponade are common causes of myocardial failure after trauma.

Pathophysiology. A peptide referred to as myocardial depressant factor reportedly is released in association with visceral ischemia, sepsis, or both. Myocardial depressant factor is incompletely characterized and has never been proved definitively to play a role in myocardial failure.

Catecholamines, sympathetic or vagal abnormalities, cardiac edema, and alterations in coronary flow have also been suggested as mechanisms for cardiac failure.

Diagnosis. Diagnosis of myocardial injury is made by electrocardiographic changes, echocardiogram, nuclear medicine scans, and abnormal physiologic measurements.

Management. Myocardial failure is managed with cardiotonic drugs and careful fluid and electrolyte balance. If left ventricular failure is profound, an aortic balloon pump or left ventricular assist device can be employed.

Outcome. Mortality from cardiac failure is 75 to 100%.

SUMMARY

Failure of one or more organs simultaneously or in series remains a major cause of morbidity and mortality following multiple trauma. Despite extensive investigation, neither a specific cause nor a definitive treatment of this entity has been identified. The etiology of MOF is likely to include a number of factors. However, sepsis is a frequently associated finding. Although MOF occurs in the pediatric age group following trauma, when injuries are promptly and effectively treated the frequency and severity of MOF is considerably less than that in adults.

At the present time the objective data on MOF in children, especially following trauma, is inadequate. We hope this review provides an impetus for clinical and basic investigation so we may better understand MOF in children in the future.

Selected References

1. Adeyemi SD, Ein SH, Simpson JS: Perforated stress ulcer in infants. Ann Surg 190:706–708, 1979.
2. Ashbaugh DG, Bigelow DB, Petty TL, et al: Acute respiratory distress in adults. Lancet 2:319–323, 1967.
3. Ayres SM: Treatment of the adult respiratory distress syndrome. In: Cowley RA, Trump BF (eds): Pathophysiology of Shock, Anoxia, and Ischemia. Baltimore, Williams & Wilkins, 1982, pp 387–394.
4. Barnes JL, McDowell EM: Pathology and pathophysiology of acute renal failure—A review. In: Cowley RA, Trump BF (eds): Pathophysiology of Shock, Anoxia, and Ischemia. Baltimore, Williams & Wilkins, 1982, pp 324–339.
5. Bartlett RH, Gazzaniga AB, Wetmore NE, et al: Extracorporeal membrane oxygenation (ECMO) in the treatment of cardiac and respiratory failure in children. Trans Am Soc Artif Intern Organs 26:578–581, 1980.
6. Bartlett RH, Gazzaniga AB, Wilson AF, et al: Mortality prediction in adult respiratory insufficiency. Chest 67:680–684, 1975.
7. Baue AE, Chaudry IH: Prevention of multiple systems failure. Surg Clin North Am 60:1167–1177, 1980.
8. Bell MJ, Keating JP, Ternberg JL, et al: Perforated stress ulcers in infants. J Pediatr Surg 16:998–1002, 1981.
9. Bell RC, Coalson JJ, Smith JD, et al: Multiple organ system failure and infection in adult respiratory distress syndrome. Ann Intern Med 99:293–298, 1983.
10. Bland R, Shoemaker WC, Shabot MM: Physiologic monitoring goals for the critically ill patient. Surg Gynecol Obstet 147:833–841, 1978.
11. Border JR, Chenier R, McMenamy RH, et al: Multiple systems organ failure: Muscle fuel deficit with visceral protein malnutrition. Surg Clin North Am 56:1147–1167, 1976.
12. Borzotta AP, Polk HC: Multiple system organ failure. Surg Clin North Am 63:315–336, 1983.
13. Browdie DA, Deane R, Shinozaki T, et al: Adult respiratory distress syndrome (ARDS), sepsis, and extracorporeal membrane oxygenation (ECMO). J Trauma 17:579–586, 1977.
14. Cerra FB, Border JR, McMenamy RH, et al: Multiple systems organ failure. In: Cowley RA, Trump BF (eds): Pathophysiology of Shock, Anoxia, and Ischemia. Baltimore, Williams & Wilkins, 1982, pp 254–270.
15. Cerra FB, Seigel JH, Border JR, et al: The hepatic failure of sepsis: Cellular versus substrate. Surgery 86:409–422, 1979.
16. Champion HR, Jones RT, Trump BF, et al: A clinicopathologic study of hepatic dysfunction following shock. Surg Gynecol Obstet 142:657–663, 1976.
17. Champion HR, Jones RT, Trump BF, et al: Post-traumatic hepatic dysfunction as a major etiology in post-traumatic jaundice. J Trauma 16:650–657, 1976.
18. Chenoweth AI, Dimmick AR: Stress ulcer in infants and children. Ann Surg 161:977–982, 1965.
19. Connor, RC: Heart damage associated with intracranial lesions. BMJ 3:20–31, 1968.
20. Cowley RA, Hankins JR, Jones RT, et al: Pathology and pathophysiology of the liver. In: Cowley RA, Trump BF (eds): Pathophysiology of Shock, Anoxia, and Ischemia. Baltimore, Williams & Wilkins, 1982, pp 285–301.
21. Czer LS, Appel P, Shoemaker WC: Pathogenesis of respiratory failure (ARDS) after hemorrhage and trauma: II. Cardiorespiratory patterns after development of ARDS. Crit Care Med 8:513–518, 1980.
22. Danielson RA: Differential diagnosis and treatment of oliguria in post-traumatic and postoperative patients. Surg Clin North Am 55:697–712, 1975.
23. Draper EA, Knause WA, Wagner DP, et al: Prognosis from combined organ-system failure (abstract). Crit Care Med 11:236, 1983.
24. DuPriest RW, Khaneja SC, Cowley RA: Acute respiratory distress syndrome in children. Radiology 157:69–74, 1985.
25. Effmann EL, Merten DF, Kirks DR, et al: Adult respiratory distress syndrome in children. Radiology 157:69–74, 1985.
26. Eiseman B, Beart R, Norton L: Multiple organ failure. Surg Gynecol Obstet 144:323–326, 1977.
27. Eiseman B, Sload R, Hansbrough J, et al: Multiple organ failure: Clinical and experimental. Am Surg 46:14–19, 1980.
28. Elliott CG, Morris AH, Cengiz M: Pulmonary function and exercise gas exchange in survivors of adult respiratory distress syndrome. Am Rev Respir Dis 123:492–495, 1981.
29. Ellis D, Gartner JC, Galvis AG: Acute renal failure in infants and children: Diagnosis, complications, and treatment. Crit Care Med 9:607–617, 1981.
30. Faist E, Baue AE, Dittmer H, et al: Multiple organ failure in polytrauma patients. J Trauma 23:775–787, 1983.
31. Fanconi S, Kraemer R, Weber J, et al: Long-term sequelae in children surviving adult respiratory distress syndrome. J Pediatr 106:218–222, 1985.
32. Farraris VA: Exploratory laparotomy for potential abdominal sepsis in patients with multiple organ failure. Arch Surg 118:1130–1133, 1983.
33. Fry DE, Garrison RN, Heitsch RC, et al: Determinants of death in patients with intra-abdominal abscess. Surgery 88:517–523, 1980.
34. Fry DE, Pearlstein L, Fulton RL, et al: Multiple system organ failure. Arch Surg 115:136–140, 1980.
35. Fulton RL, Jones CE: The cause of post-traumatic pulmonary insufficiency in man. Surg Gynecol Obstet 140:179–186, 1975.
36. Gehr M, Gross M, Schmitt G, et al: Treatment of acute renal failure. In: Cowley RA, Trump BF (eds): Pathophysiology of Shock, Anoxia, and Ischemia. Baltimore, Williams & Wilkins, 1982, pp 341–357.
37. Glenn F: Acute acalculous cholecystitis. Ann Surg 189:458–465, 1979.
38. Glenney CU, Teres D, Sweet S, et al: The effect of renal and respiratory failure on surgical ICU mortality (abstract). Crit Care Med 7:134, 1979.
39. Gonick HC, Barker WF: Maintenance of renal function following major trauma. Surg Clin North Am 52:783–792, 1972.
40. Goris RJ, Draaisma J: Causes of death after blunt trauma. J Trauma 22:141–146, 1982.
41. Greenhoot JH, Reichenback DD: Cardiac injury and subarachnoid hemorrhage. J Neurosurg 30:521–531, 1969.
42. Grosfeld JL, Shipley F, Fitzgerald JF, et al: Acute peptic ulcer in infancy and childhood. Am Surg 44:13–19, 1978.
43. Holbrook PR, Taylor G, Pollack MM, et al: Adult respiratory distress syndrome in children. Pediatr Clin North Am 27:677–685, 1980.

44. Jones RT, Linhardt GE Jr: Pathology and pathophysiology of the exocrine pancreas in shock. In: Cowley RA, Trump BF (eds): Pathophysiology of Shock, Anoxia, and Ischemia. Baltimore, Williams & Wilkins, 1982, pp 309–324.

45. Kahlstrom EJ: Adult respiratory distress syndrome in children. In: Nussbaum E (ed): Pediatric Intensive Care. Mount Kisco, NY, Futura, 1984, pp 309–324.

46. Klein JJ, Van Haeringen JR, Sluiter HJ, et al: Pulmonary function after recovery from the adult respiratory distress syndrome. Chest 69:350–355, 1976.

47. Lakshminarayan S: Pulmonary function following the adult respiratory distress syndrome. Chest 74:489–490, 1978.

48. Lakshminarayan S, Stanford RE, Petty TL: Prognosis after recovery from adult respiratory distress syndrome. Am Rev Respir Dis 113:7–16, 1976.

49. Lefer AM, Martin J: Origin of myocardial depressant factor in shock. Am J Physiol 218:1423–1427, 1970.

50. Limbird TJ, Ruderman RJ: Fat embolism in children. Clin Orthop 136:267–269, 1978.

51. Long TN, Heimbach DM, Carrico CJ: Acalculous cholecystitis in critically ill patients. Am J Surg 135:31–36, 1978.

52. Lucking SE, Pollack MM, Fields AI: Shock following generalized hypoxic-ischemic injury in previously healthy infants and children. J Pediatr 108:359–364, 1986.

53. Lyrene RK, Truog WE: Adult respiratory distress syndrome in a pediatric intensive care unit: Predisposing conditions, clinical course, and outcome. Pediatrics 67:790–795, 1981.

54. McMenamy RH, Birkhahn R, Oswald G, et al: Multiple systems organ failure: I. The basal state. J Trauma 21:99–114, 1981.

55. Martin LF, Staloch DK, Simonowitz DA, et al: Failure of cimetidine prophylaxis in the critically ill. Arch Surg 114:492–496, 1979.

56. Maxwell LG, Fivush BA, Mclean RH: Renal failure. In: Rogers MC (ed): Textbook of Pediatric Intensive Care. Vol. 2. Baltimore, Williams & Wilkins, 1987, pp 1001–1055.

57. Milley JR, Nugent SK, Rogers MC: Neurogenic pulmonary edema in childhood. J Pediatr 94:706–709, 1979.

58. Mittermayer C, Riede UN: Human pathology of the gastrointestinal tract in shock, ischemia, and hypoxemia. In: Cowley RA, Trump BF (eds): Pathophysiology of Shock, Anoxia, and Ischemia. Baltimore, Williams & Wilkins, 1982, pp 301–308.

59. Moody FG, Cheung LY, Simons MA, et al: Stress and the acute gastric mucosal lesion. Dig Dis Sci 21:148–154, 1976.

60. Moyer E, Cerra F, Chenier R, et al: Multiple systems organ failure: VI. Death predictors in the trauma-septic state—The most critical determinants. J Trauma 21:862–869, 1981.

61. Moylan JA, Evenson MA: Diagnosis and treatment of fat embolism. Annu Rev Med 28:85–90, 1977.

62. Nadrowski L: Paralytic ileus: Recent advances in pathophysiology and treatment. Curr Surg 40:260–273, 1983.

63. Nichols DG, Rogers MC: Adult respiratory distress syndrome. In: Rogers MC (ed): Textbook of Pediatric Intensive Care. Vol. 1. Baltimore, Williams & Wilkins, 1987, pp 237–271.

64. Norton LW: Does drainage of intraabdominal pus reverse multiple organ failure? Am J Surg 149:347–350, 1985.

65. Nunes G, Blaisdell FW, Margaretten W: Mechanism of hepatic dysfunction following shock and trauma. Arch Surg 100:546–556, 1970.

66. Nussbaum E: Adult-type respiratory distress syndrome in children. Clin Pediatr 22:401–406, 1983.

67. Nuytinck JK, Goris RJ: Pathophysiology of the adult respiratory distress syndrome (ARDS) and multiple organ failure (MOF)—A hypothesis. Neth J Surg 37:131–136, 1985.

68. Nuytinckn JK, Goris RJ, Redl H, et al: Post-traumatic complications and inflammatory mediators. Arch Surg 121:886–890, 1986.

69. Orloff S, Potter DE, Holliday MA: Acute renal failure. In: Smith CA (ed): The Critically Ill Child. Philadelphia, WB Saunders, 1977, pp 127–142.

70. Orsmond G: Injuries to children with chronic cardiac disease. In: Mayer TA (ed): Emergency Management of Pediatric Trauma. Philadelphia, WB Saunders, 1985, pp 205–208.

71. Ozawa K, Aoyama H, Yasuda K, et al: Metabolic abnormalities associated with postoperative organ failure. Arch Surg 118:1245–1251, 1983.

72. Perkin RM, Levin DL: Shock in the pediatric patient. Part I. J Pediatr 101:163–169, 1982.

73. Petty TL, Ashbaugh DG: The adult respiratory distress syndrome. Chest 60:233–239, 1971.

74. Pfenninger J, Gerber A, Tschappeler H, et al: Adult respiratory distress syndrome in children. J Pediatr 101:352–357, 1982.

75. Pine RW, Wertz MJ, Lennard ES, et al: Determinants of organ malfunction or death in patients with intra-abdominal sepsis. Arch Surg 118:242–249, 1983.

76. Polk HC Jr, Shields CL: Remote organ failure: A valid sign of occult intra-abdominal infection. Surgery 81:310–313, 1977.

77. Pollack MM, Fields AI, Holbrook PR: Cardiopulmonary parameters during high PEEP in children. Crit Care Med 8:371–376, 1980.

78. Pollack MM, Fields AI, Ruttimann UE: Sequential cardiopulmonary variables of infants and children in septic shock. Crit Care Med 12:554–559, 1984.

79. Pollack MM, Fields AI, Ruttimann UE: Distributions of cardiopulmonary variables in pediatric survivors and nonsurvivors of septic shock. Crit Care Med 13:454–459, 1985.

80. Pollack MM, Yeh TS, Ruttimann UE, et al: Evaluation of pediatric intensive care. Crit Care Med 12:376–383, 1984.

81. Priebe HJ, Skillman JJ, Bushnell LS, et al: Antacid versus cimetidine in preventing acute gastrointestinal bleeding. N Engl J Med 302:416–420, 1980.

82. Riede UN, Mittermayer C, Horn R, et al: Pathobiology of the alveolar wall in human shock lung. In: Cowley RA, Trump BF (eds): Pathophysiology of Shock, Anoxia, and Ischemia. Baltimore, Williams & Wilkins, 1982, pp 358–371.

83. Rogers EL, Perman JA: Gastrointestinal and hepatic failure. In: Rogers MC (ed): Textbook of Pediatric Intensive Care. Vol. 2. Baltimore, Williams & Wilkins, 1987, pp 979–998.

84. Rosenberg IK, Gupta SL, Lucas CE, et al: Renal insufficiency after trauma and sepsis. Arch Surg 103:175–183, 1971.

85. Rotman HH, Lavelle TF Jr, Dimcheff DG, et al: Long-term physiologic consequences of the adult respiratory distress syndrome. Chest 72:190–192, 1977.

86. Sabiston DC Jr (ed): Textbook of Surgery. The Biological Basis of Modern Surgical Practice. 13th ed. Philadelphia, WB Saunders, 1986.

87. Shin B, Mackenzie CF, Cowley RA: Changing patterns of posttraumatic acute renal failure. Am Surg 45:182–189, 1979.

88. Shin B, Mackenzie CF, McAslan TC, et al: Postoperative renal failure in trauma patients. Anesthesiology 51:218–221, 1979.

89. Shoemaker WC, Appel PL, Bland R, et al: Clinical trial of an algorithm for outcome prediction in acute circulatory failure. Crit Care Med 10:390–397, 1982.

90. Shoemaker WC, Appel P, Czer LS, et al: Pathogenesis of respiratory failure (ARDS) after hemorrhage and trauma: I. Cardiorespiratory patterns preceding the development of ARDS. Crit Care Med 8:504–512, 1980.

91. Shoemaker WC, Appel PL, Waxman K, et al: Clinical trial of survivors' cardiorespiratory patterns as therapeutic goals in critically ill postoperative patients. Crit Care Med 10:398–403, 1982.

92. Shulman ST, Grossman BJ: Fat embolism in childhood. Am J Dis Child 120:480–484, 1970.

93. Sibbald WJ, Driedger AA: Pulmonary alveolarcapillary permeability in human septic respiratory distress syndrome. In: Cowley RA, Trump BF (eds): Pathophysiology of Shock, Anoxia, and Ischemia. Baltimore, Williams & Wilkins, 1982, pp 372–387.

94. Siegler RL: Post-traumatic renal failure. In: Mayer TA (ed): Emergency Management of Pediatric Trauma. Philadelphia, WB Saunders, 1985, pp 139–159.

95. Smith PK, Tyson GS Jr, Hammon JW Jr, et al: Cardiovascular effects of ventilation with positive expiratory airway pressure. Ann Surg 195:121–130, 1982.

96. Ternberg JL, Keating JP: Acute acalculous cholecystitis. Arch Surg 110:543–547, 1975.

97. Trey C: Acute hepatic failure. In: Smith CA (ed): The Critically Ill Child. Philadelphia, WB Saunders, 1977, pp 117–126.

98. VanderArk GD: Cardiovascular changes with acute subdural hematoma. Surg Neurol 3:305–308, 1975.

99. Walker L, Eiseman B: The changing pattern of post-traumatic respiratory distress syndrome. Ann Surg 181:693–697, 1975.

100. Weigelt JA, Mitchell RA, Snyder WH III: Early positive end-expiratory pressure in the adult respiratory distress syndrome. Arch Surg 114:497–501, 1979.

101. Weisel RD, Vito L, Dennis RC, et al: Myocardial depression during sepsis. Am J Surg 133:512–521, 1977.

102. Wetzel RC: Shock. In: Rogers MC (ed): Textbook of Pediatric Inten-

sive Care. Vol. 1. Baltimore, Williams & Wilkins, 1987, pp 483–524.

103. Wilkinson JD, Pollack MM, Glass NL, et al: Mortality associated with multiple organ system failure and sepsis in pediatric intensive care unit. J Pediatr 111:324–328, 1987.

104. Wilkinson JD, Pollack MM, Ruttimann UE, et al: Outcome of pediatric patients with multiple organ system failure. Crit Care Med 14:271–274, 1986.

105. Yahav J, Lieberman P, Molho M: Pulmonary function following the adult respiratory distress syndrome. Chest 74:247–250, 1978.

106. Yaster M, Haller JA: Multiple trauma in the pediatric patient. In: Rogers MC (ed): Textbook of Pediatric Intensive Care. Vol. 2. Baltimore, Williams & Wilkins, 1987, pp 1265–1322.

Daniel L. Mollitt

CHAPTER FORTY-FOUR

Immunologic and Infectious Consequences of Childhood Injuries

With the acceptance of trauma as a major surgical "disease," great strides have been made in the resuscitation, treatment, and rehabilitation of injured patients. Despite these advances, sepsis remains a major cause of morbidity and mortality, accounting for more than 75% of nonneurologic deaths in the trauma victim.[19] The causes, characteristics, and pathophysiology of sepsis are unique in the surgical patient, and this recognition has led to increasing interest and research in the area of surgical infectious disease, especially focusing on the trauma patient. The importance of the immune system in responding to trauma has been recognized, and its components and interactions have been progressively characterized.

Trauma-induced alterations in normal immune function have been described and have stimulated attempts at immune therapy. Simultaneously, technologic advances have enhanced our diagnostic capabilities and the therapeutic modalities available to the septic patient. Antimicrobial therapy has been redefined by an increased understanding of pharmacokinetics, microbiology, and mechanisms of resistance and by the introduction of myriad new agents. Supportive care has improved with advances in monitoring, cardiorespiratory support, and clarification of the pathophysiology of adult respiratory distress syndrome and multiorgan failure. The recognition, management, and effective therapy of septic complications is an intricate part of the overall care of the trauma victim that necessitates understanding, integration, and use of these advances in the preventive and therapeutic phases of care.

Although trauma is an epidemic illness of childhood, it has not received the same enthusiastic and intense interest afforded trauma in the adult population. Trauma in children differs in its mechanism, pattern of injury, and physiologic response, but as in the adult, sepsis remains a major complication and a significant cause of morbidity. Within this area, little specific work is available to facilitate care of the injured child. Although advances in treatment of the adult trauma patient cannot be applied uniformly to that of the pediatric age group, much of the information can enhance management and improve survival of pediatric patients. Comprehensive care of the pediatric trauma victim requires a working knowledge of many of the same advances applicable to the adult.

NORMAL HOMEOSTASIS AND INFECTION

Surgical sepsis includes a variety of infectious processes and may be characterized in a number of ways. Despite this diversity, the cause of all infectious processes is an imbalance in the normal homeostasis between the microorganism and the host.

$$\text{Infection} = \frac{\text{Organism}}{\text{Host}}$$

Each component of this association is composed of factors that can render the injured child remarkably resistant to sepsis as long as the balance is maintained. However, a seemingly minor variation can result in the signs and symptoms of infection. An understanding of these factors can clarify the cause of sepsis, identify the child at risk, and enable effective prophylaxis or therapy and the reestablishment of this delicate balance.

Host Resistance

Host resistance to infection depends on local and systemic factors. Local defenses function as physical or specialized cellular barriers, precluding colonization and invasion of potential pathogens (Table 44–1). The intact skin represents the largest local defense because of its relatively impervious nature and because of the antimicrobial effects of fatty acids and other cutaneous glandular secretions.

At the normal body orifices, the epithelial surface progressively changes from a predominantly physical barrier to reliance on specialized cells and their secretions. The mucous lining of the respiratory tract entraps inhaled bacteria and particulate matter, which is cleared proximally by the ciliated respiratory epithelium. Distally, abundant alveolar macrophages actively ingest material that has successfully traversed this mucous barrier. The gastrointestinal tract constantly propels ingested pathogens distally, where they are exposed to gastric acid and digestive enzymes. The abundant resident microflora normally preclude attachment of potential pathogens through their saturation of available binding sites. Similarly, their number, variety, and metabolic interactions inhibit proliferation of exogenous organisms through the successful use of available nutrients.

The urinary tract avoids invasion and microbial growth through the mechanical cleansing action and mild antibacterial properties (i.e., pH, osmolarity, urea content) of urine. The urothelium of the bladder provides a barrier and a specialized lining that hinder bacterial attachment. The female genital tract is protected by the natural acidic environment of the vagina and by the cervical mucous plug.[84]

The systemic defenses are collectively known as the immune system. This complex collection of specialized cells, proteins, and chemical substances functions in self-magnifying reactions that effectively neutralize and dispose of most bacterial, cellular, and chemical threats to the body's homeostasis. Classically, this system has been divided into phagocytic, lymphocytic, and humoral components. The advances of the last decade have elucidated and clarified the

Table 44–1
Local Defenses

System	Defensive Features
Skin	Barrier, antimicrobial secretions
Respiratory tract	Cough reflex, mucous lining, ciliated epithelium, secretory immunoglobulins, alveolar macrophages
Gastrointestinal tract	Salivary enzymes, peristalsis, acid pH, digestive enzymes, secretory immunoglobulins, normal flora
Genitourinary tract	Urinary flow, peristalsis, pH/osmolarity, urethral length, vaginal pH, cervical plug

Table 44-2
Phagocytic Cells

Classification	Types of Cell
Circulating	Neutrophil, monocyte, eosinophil, macrophage
Fixed	Alveolar macrophage, histiocyte, Kupffer cell, microglial cell, nodal macrophage, osteoclast, splenic macrophage

function of these components and have established the intricate associations that exist among them. An effective immune response depends on these coordinated actions, and this response is best viewed in terms of nonspecific or specific reactions.

The initial nonspecific response to bacterial invasion or tissue damage is the inflammatory reaction. The release of vasoactive substances increases capillary permeability, promoting the local tissue accumulation of fluid and immune mediators. The major cellular component of the nonspecific system is the phagocytic cell. These circulating and fixed cells are characterized by their ability to ingest and destroy foreign material (Table 44-2).

The most numerous of the circulating phagocytes is the polymorphonuclear leukocyte (PMN). In response to the inflammatory mediators released with tissue damage, these cells marginate along local blood vessels and adhere to the endothelium. They then leave the intravascular compartment, passing through the junctions between endothelial cells (i.e., diapedesis). Once within the tissue, they actively travel to the site of foreign material. This directed migra-

tion, or chemotaxis, is promoted by numerous chemical attractants that are produced and released with the initial inflammatory reaction. The complement components, C3A and C5A, are particularly powerful chemotaxins, binding to receptors on the PMN membrane, eliciting membrane and intracellular changes that result in directed movement toward the increasing concentration gradient.[66, 175, 206]

Once localized, ingestion (i.e., phagocytosis) requires recognition of the foreign substance, which is facilitated by the process of opsonization or coating of the bacteria. This occurs primarily through the interaction of immunoglobulin with the pathogen. The Fab end of an appropriate immunoglobulin molecule attaches to the bacterial surface, exposing the Fc end for recognition by and binding to specific PMN receptors. The complement component C3B acts as an opsonin in similar fashion.[187]

After bacterial attachment has occurred, a series of complex intracellular alterations takes place within the PMN. Pseudopodia surround the attached microorganism, internalizing it in preparation for digestion.[188] Attachment and internalization trigger metabolic activity within the PMN, which is characterized by increased use of the hexose monophosphate shunt. This ultimately results in the generation of oxygen radicals and unstable reduction products, a process called the respiratory burst (Figs. 44-1, 44-2). These powerful oxidizing agents are released into the phagosome, causing the intracellular lysis of the engulfed target.[18, 63, 93] Target cell lysis can also occur via the oxygen-independent process of degranulation with the release of a variety of bactericidal enzymes, organic acids, and cationic proteins into the phagosome (Fig. 44-3).[62, 63, 130]

Another important cellular component of the nonspecific system is the mononuclear phagocyte or monocyte. Its pri-

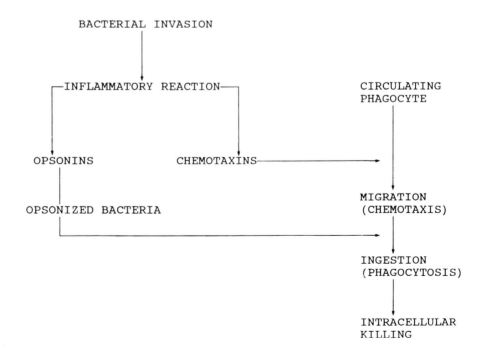

NONSPECIFIC IMMUNE RESPONSE

FIGURE 44-1
Nonspecific immune response.

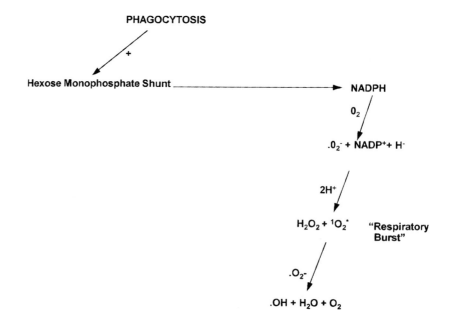

FIGURE 44–2
Oxygen-dependent intracellular killing.

mary significance lies in its role as precursor of the macrophage. Although macrophages may be found circulating throughout the body's tissues, they are most numerous and active in fixed locations (see Table 44–2), where they are responsible for the clearing role of the reticuloendothelial system.[163] In locations in direct contact with the bloodstream, such as the liver and spleen, these phagocytes are remarkably efficient at removing bacteria, foreign material, and debris. This is accomplished through processes similar to those of the PMN.

In addition to its phagocytic role, the macrophage serves as an important source of humoral immunoreactive sub-

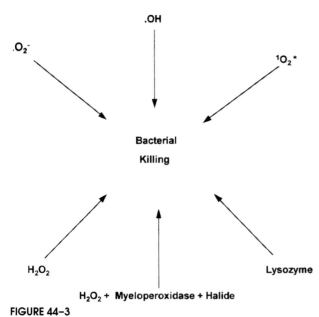

FIGURE 44–3
Methods of intracellular killing.

stances. Fibronectin, an α_2-glycoprotein, is a major opsonin for the reticuloendothelial system and is produced by local macrophages and adjacent cells.[121] The macrophage is the source of interleukin-1 (IL-1), which activates the lymphocyte and is responsible for the systemic signs of sepsis, such as fever and tissue protein mobilization.[166] The macrophage also produces prostaglandin E_2, which functions as an immunosuppressant, modulating local immune interactions.

The macrophage serves as an important link between the nonspecific and specific immune mechanisms. Through methods not yet understood, the macrophage is necessary for antigen processing, enabling recognition by the lymphocyte. The recognition, along with the stimulatory effect of macrophage-produced IL-1, results in lymphocyte activation and ultimately in antibody production.[41]

The major humoral component of the nonspecific immune defense is the complement system, which consists of multiple elements circulating throughout the intravascular and extravascular spaces. Complement activation leads to a cascade of chemical reactions eventuating in target cell lysis. Complement may be activated by the classic (i.e., C1-C4-C2) or alternative (i.e., properdin) pathway. Classic activation requires the participation of antigen-antibody complexes or antibody aggregates. The alternative pathway is readily activated directly by bacterial components. Activation of either results in the cleavage of C3, the central point in the cascade. As each subsequent component is cleaved, an attachment unit and activation enzyme are formed, sequentially cascading through C9 with the ultimate creation of a membrane attack unit and target cell lysis (Fig. 44–4).[69, 115] In addition to cytolysis, complement activation generates numerous immunoreactive substances. C3A and C5A act as anaphylatoxins, inducing mast cell degranulation and release of vasoactive amines, which augment the inflammatory response. C3B promotes phagocytosis through opsonization. C3A, C5A, and C567 function as chemotoxins.[69]

The specific immune defenses are maintained by the thy-

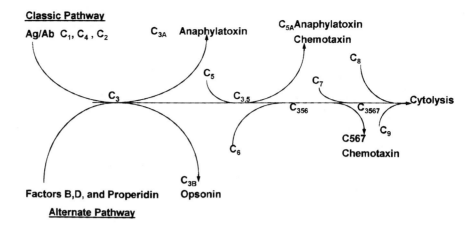

FIGURE 44–4
Complement cascade.

mus-derived lymphocyte, the T cell, and the bursa-derived lymphocyte, the B cell. The T cell is antigen specific and capable of recognizing "self" molecules of the major histocompatibility complex. They are responsible for cell-mediated immunity, modulation of antibody production, and direct cytotoxicity. These functions are maintained by direct cell-to-cell contact and by the production of a variety of immune substances or lymphokines. T cells are specific in their individual roles and are classified according to each capability as helper, suppressor, and effector cells. Each can be differentiated by cell surface markers and can be isolated and identified by monoclonal antibody technology.[79, 152]

The specific system commences defensive action with the presentation of an antigenic substance by the macrophage. With phagocytosis, the macrophage processes the antigen by degrading it into distinct fragments, which are then displayed on the cell surface. This display is accompanied by the production and release of IL-1. With recognition of these antigenic particles by the appropriate helper T (T_H) cell and under the influence of IL-1, two events occur. T cells are stimulated to produce interleukin-2 (IL-2) and to expose a surface IL-2 receptor. Binding of IL-2 to the T-cell membrane results in blastogenesis, the proliferation and differentiation of antigen-specific T-cell clones. This T-cell stimulation is tempered by an inhibitory population of macrophages that produce and release prostaglandin E_2. Stimulated T_H cells promote B-cell proliferation through direct cell contact and release of lymphokines called B-cell growth factor and B-cell differentiation factor. T_H cells also sustain macrophage activity through the stimulatory effects of the lymphokine interferon gamma. Stimulated suppressor T (T_S) cells modulate this activity through inhibitory effects at the macrophage and T_H cell levels (Fig. 44–5).[16, 41, 82, 113, 151]

B cells are characterized by specific antigen cell surface receptors and function as the precursor for the antibody-producing plasma cell. When stimulated, the B cell undergoes a characteristic transformation, resulting in the proliferation of differentiated plasma cells, which are responsible for the production of antigen-specific immunoglobulin that

functions in the opsonization and lysis of bacteria and the neutralization of viruses and endotoxins.

Microbiology

Humans are populated by a large number of normally commensal bacteria. These resident microflora contribute significantly to host resistance through bacterial antagonism. Successful growth of the microflora results in local depletion of the nutrients essential for pathogenic bacteria and decreases the available sites for attachment. Byproducts of resident bacterial metabolism can create an environment

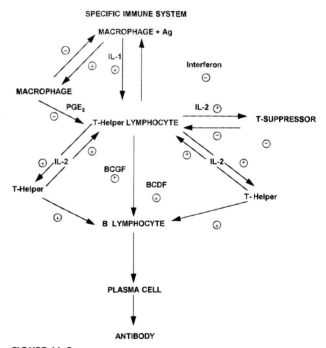

FIGURE 44–5

Specific immune system. Ag, Antigen; IL, interleukin: PGE₂, prostaglandin E₂; BCGF, B cell growth factors; BCDF, B cell differentiation factors.

that restricts the growth of certain exogenous organisms. Several substances produced by these microorganisms have bacteriostatic or bactericidal activity against potentially pathogenic bacteria of a different strain. The gastrointestinal flora play a key role in normal digestion and metabolism. Bacteria modulate the activity of several intestinal enzymes and produce substances that participate in the degradation of bile acids, cholesterol, amino acids, and hormones. The gastrointestinal bacteria also elaborate several substances used by the host, such as essential vitamins.[74, 158]

Despite the usual commensal relation of the resident flora, most organisms represent potential pathogens that must be considered in any infectious process. Although so-called normal flora are subject to a wide degree of variation in type and number, several prominent potential pathogens are consistently found throughout the body (Table 44–3). Coagulase-negative and coagulase-positive staphylococcal species reside in great numbers over the skin, nose, and mouth. *Streptococcus* is recoverable from the nose (e.g., alpha hemolytic and pneumococcus) and mouth (alpha hemolytic and anaerobic). The mouth also contains a variety of Enterobacteriaceae and *Bacteroides* species. The perineum is frequently a reservoir for *Clostridium*. The gastrointestinal flora vary from mainly gram-positive facultative cocci and bacilli proximally to gram-negative Enterobacteriaceae and anaerobes distally. The greatest concentration occurs in the large intestine and invariably includes potential pathogens such as *Escherichia coli, Klebsiella, Enterobacter,* enterococcus, and *Bacteroides,* all of which flourish in large numbers.

Induced Alterations in Host Resistance

For infection to arise, some alteration in the normal balance between the host and the organism must occur. With rare exception, the primary imbalance arises in the host defense mechanisms. This is particularly true in the trauma victim. Trauma and posttraumatic treatment invariably involve disruption of some or all of the local defenses. The mechanisms of injury in the child commonly result in a breach of the cutaneous barrier by way of abrasion, laceration, penetration, or burns. Therapeutic maneuvers such as surgery, intubation, and cannulation further disrupt these physical barriers and provide a direct portal of entry for potential pathogens.

Intubation via the oropharynx or nasopharynx inhibits ciliary activity and blunts the normal cough and gag reflex. Tracheal intubation not only disrupts the normal defenses, but effectively bypasses them, affording easy access to the respiratory system by potential pathogens. Mechanical ventilation can result in desiccation of secretions with inspissation and inability to clear. This reaction inhibits natural defenses and improves the environment for the growth of potential pathogens. Posttraumatic ileus alters the normal bacteriostatic environment of the stomach and upper small bowel and promotes bacterial overgrowth. Intravascular cannulae provide direct access to the circulatory system for the physician and the microorganism. Urinary catheterization bypasses the normal defenses and can promote stasis.

Table 44–3
Potential Pathogens and Normal Flora

Potential Pathogen	Usual Anatomic Site
Staphylococcus epidermidis	Skin, nose, mouth
Staphylococcus aureus	Skin, nose, mouth, gastrointestinal tract
Hemolytic *Streptococcus*	Nose, mouth
Streptococcus pneumoniae	Oropharynx
Anaerobic *Streptococcus*	Mouth
Clostridium perfringens	Skin (perineum)

Enterobacteriaceae
   Escherichia coli
   Klebsiella
   Enterobacter
	Distal gastrointestinal tract

Bacteroides	Mouth, distal gastrointestinal tract
Candida	Mouth, gastrointestinal tract

Alterations of the defense mechanisms induced by trauma extend beyond local defenses. A variety of changes have been described in the nonspecific and specific systemic defenses (Table 44–4).[122] Although trauma results in the release of tissue-injury–derived chemotaxins, phagocyte chemotaxis is consistently depressed and correlates inversely with the extent of injury.[54–56, 109, 111, 112, 196] This depression appears to be caused by injury-induced alterations on the phagocyte membrane rather than intrinsic cellular abnormalities.[59, 217] One alteration is down-regulation of the complement membrane receptors, perhaps secondary to the overabundance of circulating complement fragments released in response to tissue injury.[11, 47, 119, 123, 124, 182, 185] The opsonic capacity of the serum is reduced in the posttraumatic patient, with resulting depression of phagocytosis.[2, 35, 55, 75, 123] Intracellular killing is deficient because of alterations in the membrane trigger mechanism and in the intracellular metabolic pathways needed for microbicidal activity.

Studies indicate that the phagocyte functions normally when removed from the serum of trauma patients, suggesting a depressive alteration in the environment or the presence of a circulating suppressor substance.[45, 60, 98, 99, 100, 118, 180, 181] Although several naturally occurring "stress" hormones can individually affect phagocyte function, laboratory simulation of the hormonal environment characteristic

Table 44–4
Trauma-Induced Immunologic Alterations

Immunologic Changes	Increase (↑) or Decrease (↓)
Nonspecific	
Chemotaxis	↓
Phagocytosis	↓
Intracellular killing	↓
Complement components	↓
Complement fragments	↑
Fibronectin	↓
Specific	
Helper T: suppressor T cell ratio	↓
Mitogen responsiveness	↓
Interleukin-2	↓

of the response to stress and trauma does not result in similar phagocyte derangements, further implicating the presence of one or more unique serum suppressor substances released with injury.[118]

Humoral components of the nonspecific system are altered after trauma. Injury results in complement activation, which results in decreased levels of specific components and an increase in the number of circulating complement fragments.[30–34] The increased level of fragments has been implicated in causing the abnormalities of the phagocyte through modulation of specific membrane receptor sites.[11, 47, 119, 123, 124, 182, 183] Similarly, opsonic fibronectin levels are depressed after trauma, correlating with decreased clearance by the reticuloendothelial system.[7, 51, 157, 164, 168]

The specific system of immune defenses is also affected by trauma. After a major injury, a generalized lymphopenia affects all T-lymphocyte subsets. Much attention has been focused on the ratio of T_H:T_S cells as an index of functional capability. This ratio is shifted toward a preponderance of suppressor cells, suggesting increased inhibition of lymphocyte interactions. It is unclear whether this alteration is caused by a relative increase in T_S cells or a decrease in T_H cells.[9, 10, 23, 107, 133, 143] Lymphocytes have been assessed by mitogen stimulation, an in vitro evaluation of proliferative capability, with findings of decreased responsiveness after trauma.

In the injured child, the greatest deficiency occurs in B-cell responsiveness. This effect appears to be secondary to serum-mediated suppression rather than to intrinsic cellular abnormality.[4, 105, 107, 132, 109] Several investigators have implicated an excess of circulating prostaglandin E_2 in this suppression, but this has not been a consistent finding.[128, 210, 211]

Measurement of other circulating immunoreactive substances has demonstrated increased levels of IL-1 but diminished IL-2 levels after trauma. These decreased levels of IL-2 cannot be correlated with decreased numbers of T_H cells, suggesting a defective cellular response to IL-1 stimulation.[190, 211–213]

Each of the defects elucidated represents an isolated abnormality in what is a spectrum of immune dysfunction precipitated by injury. In most instances, the extent of the alteration correlates directly with the degree of trauma. The most striking abnormalities described have been associated with major burns, but most functional abnormalities have been characterized in in vitro systems, and the clinical significance of any individual defect remains uncertain. Similarly, attempts to identify an abnormality that consistently predicts subsequent septic complications have been unsuccessful. It is clear, however, that major trauma has a profound effect on the immune defenses, which alters the normal homeostasis and significantly increase the susceptibility to sepsis in this setting.

In addition to the abnormalities related to major injury itself, immune dysfunction is associated with a variety of preexistent patient factors and therapeutic maneuvers (Table 44–5). Perhaps the most significant factor is patient age. Immune dysfunction has been described at both extremes of age.[193] In the pediatric population, dysfunction is characterized by a relative immaturity of response that is sufficient to handle minor insults but easily overwhelmed by major or repeated stimulation. The degree of immune adequacy is related to age. It is most immature in the newborn, with a gradual increase in competency associated with growth and development. Many of the abnormalities described in the pediatric age group are similar to those induced by trauma.[8, 12, 37, 80, 90, 116, 148, 184, 185, 195]

The impact of major injury on the fragile immune system of the child is not understood. All of the deficiencies described in postinjury patients have been identified in the adult. Few studies have evaluated immune function in pediatric trauma victims. Although it may be reasonable to assume that a similar response occurs in children, the preexisting immune immaturity may result in an even greater degree of depression and greater susceptibility to sepsis.

Other patient factors may significantly influence immune function. Diabetes and trisomy 21 are associated with phagocytic abnormalities. Immune function is altered in various malignancies, myeloproliferative disorders, inflammatory bowel disease, and sickle cell anemia. Cholestasis, hepatitis, cirrhosis, and uremia can result in a deficient immune response. Protein-losing disorders, such as enteropathy and nephrotic syndrome, are associated with the loss of immunologically important serum proteins. The common pediatric condition of protein-calorie malnutrition profoundly affects immune function.

Within this framework of preexisting patient factors and trauma-related alterations, the pediatric patient is subjected to a variety of vigorous therapeutic measures that may further alter immune function. Anesthetic agents and surgery depress phagocytic and lymphocytic reactions. The cellular immune function is inhibited by a variety of antibiotics, including chloramphenicol, clindamycin, gentamicin, and tetracycline. Morphine, opiates, and psychotropic drugs depress lymphocyte mitogenesis.[85] Steroids have long been used for their immunosuppressant effects. Blood transfusion depresses cellular immune response.[97, 197, 198]

In view of the various immune abnormalities in the trauma patient caused by injury and therapy, it is seemingly remarkable that anyone escapes rapid septic death. However, normal immune defenses are remarkably complex and efficient, and the interactions among the components remain only partially understood. Similarly, the clinical importance of isolated abnormalities continues to be difficult to define, although these abnormalities clearly play a role in the incidence and outcome of sepsis in the trauma victim.

Table 44–5

Factors Affecting Immune Function

Age	Nutrition
Disease	Operation
Diabetes	Drugs
Trisomy 21	Anesthetics
Malignancy	Analgesics
Myeloproliferative disorders	Antibiotics
Inflammatory bowel disease	Psychotropics
Sickle cell anemia	Steroids
Cholestasis	Transfusion
Hepatitis	
Cirrhosis	
Renal failure	
Enteropathy	
Nephrotic syndrome	

Induced Alterations of Microbiologic Factors

In addition to the immunologic alterations induced by trauma, changes in microbiologic factors may be caused by injury and its therapy. With the violation of the natural barriers, normal flora and exogenous organisms are introduced into an otherwise normally sterile environment. The growth of these organisms is enhanced by the debris similarly introduced into traumatic wounds. Dirt, organic matter, and clothing fragments serve as a nidus for bacteria and inhibit effective local immune control. Associated blood, serum, and injured tissue provide ample nutrients for bacterial growth. Penetrating injuries involving intra-abdominal viscera release local flora from the natural inhibitions of their usual environment. The attendant blood, gastrointestinal contents, and tissue damage promote growth and blunt the immune response. Burns destroy the protective barrier and induce local thrombosis, effectively shielding microorganisms from blood-borne defenses.

Introduced microorganisms spread and elude immune defenses to cause disease. Advancement is enhanced by a variety of enzymes and toxic substances elaborated by the organism. Spread throughout tissues is facilitated by enzymes, such as bacterial collagenase, hyaluronidase, and deoxyribonuclease, that cause tissue necrosis and breakdown. Immune mechanisms are thwarted by enzymes such as coagulase and leukocidin. Catalase produced by *Staphylococcus aureus* degrades the normally bactericidal oxygen radical products of the phagocyte. Streptolysin, elaborated by streptococci, inhibits chemotaxis. Certain bacteria are endowed with intrinsic characteristics that facilitate escape from the immune system. Encapsulated organisms such as pneumococcus, *Klebsiella,* and *E. coli* resist phagocytosis, and mycobacteria are capable of inhibiting intracellular killing after phagocytosis.[40]

Bacterial virulence can be enhanced through the interaction of two or more organisms. This phenomenon, known as *synergism,* results in pathogenicity not characteristic of either individual species. The four principal mechanisms of synergism are facilitation of colonization by a second organism, alteration of host resistance, nutritional support, and increased virulence.[108] Viral respiratory infection facilitates the development of bacterial pneumonia through an alteration of the respiratory epithelium, enhancing bacterial adherence and invasion. Infection with the human immunodeficiency virus predisposes the patient to a variety of bacterial illnesses through its effect on the specific immune defenses. The classic surgical infection of mixed aerobic and anaerobic organisms is the result of the nutritional interaction between bacterial species. Bacterial virulence is enhanced through the transmission of drug resistance by gram-negative plasmids, gram-positive bacteriophages, or both. Similarly, the presence of an organism producing extracellular enzymes that inactivate an antimicrobial drug can protect an otherwise sensitive species within the same area.

Unfortunately, the most common factors responsible for alteration of the microbiology of the trauma victim are iatrogenic. With hospitalization and therapeutic measures, the normal flora are rapidly transformed into more virulent, resistant organisms. The widespread, liberal use of broad-spectrum antibiotics promotes resistance and destroys the natural competitive inhibition among organisms, releasing uncommon potential pathogens. The high frequency of resistant organisms in the intensive care unit and the easy access afforded by therapy and monitoring result in rapid recolonization, dramatically increasing the subsequent risk of sepsis. Numerous studies have documented the microbiology of hospital-acquired sepsis, which is characterized by a high incidence of *Staphylococcus epidermidis, Pseudomonas,* enterococcus, and *Candida.*[88] The data are similar for the pediatric age group.[87, 88]

PREVENTION OF INFECTION

The information available suggests that the normal homeostasis between host and organism is invariably altered in the injured child. Some effort seems indicated to restore this balance and prevent septic complications. This effort primarily has involved the use of prophylactic antibiotics. Prophylaxis is the most frequent indication for antibiotics in pediatric surgical patients. Unfortunately, these medications are used inappropriately in as many as 50% of patients.[50] Anti-infective prophylaxis in the injured child should begin not with antimicrobials, but with the basic principles of care. Adequate resuscitation minimizes the metabolic derangements that may profoundly affect cellular function in all systems. Timely therapy of specific injuries lessens the opportunity for the establishment of bacterial contaminants. Attention to detail and technique ensure a local environment less likely to support bacterial growth. Antibiotics may be an added benefit, but only if used in an appropriate manner. It is a misnomer to consider antibiotic use in the pediatric trauma victim as prophylactic; antimicrobials used in this setting are best considered adjunctive, anticipatory, or presumptive. Tissue injury and contamination have occurred before evaluation, and the antibiotics are employed to control rather than prevent bacterial invasion. It follows that the major indication for anti-infective therapy in pediatric trauma is an injury with a high probability of infection, which is determined by the extent of contamination and tissue damage, local flora, and delay in therapy.

Careful consideration should be given to the use of antimicrobials and the specific agent to be employed. Selection should be based on established efficacy against the expected pathogen, and the spectrum of activity should be as limited as possible to accomplish the desired goal. Antibiotics do not sterilize a wound; they limit bacterial proliferation, supplementing effective immune control. Antimicrobials are no alternative to appropriate local wound management. Equally as important in the selection of an antibiotic is the adequacy of tissue levels at the site of contamination. This degree of adequacy is enhanced through intravenous administration, but only after adequate resuscitation.

There is little justification for oral or intramuscular administrations in the trauma victim. Specific indications may require adequate penetration into the cerebrospinal fluid, joint spaces, genitourinary tract, or bone, properties that are not characteristic of all agents. The potential toxicity must

Table 44–6
Antimicrobial Drugs Used for Treating Infections in Children

Agent	Dose	Interval	Adverse Reactions	Comments
Aminoglycosides				
Amikacin	15–30 mg/kg/day	q 8 hr	Ototoxicity (all)	Monitor peak and trough drug levels
Gentamicin	3–7.5 mg/kg/day	q 8 hr	Nephrotoxicity (all)	Monitor urinalysis, blood urea nitrogen, and creatinine levels
Tobramycin	3–6 mg/kg/day	q 8 hr		
Cephalosporins				
First Generation				
Cefazolin	50–100 mg/kg/day	q 8 hr	Rash, anaphylaxis (all)	
Cephalothin	75–125 mg/kg/day	q 4–6 hr		
Second Generation				
Cefamandole	100–150 mg/kg/day	q 4–6 hr	Rash, anaphylaxis (all)	
Ceforanide	20–40 mg/kg/day	q 12 hr	Prolonged PT and bleeding (cefamandole)	
Cefoxitin	80–160 mg/kg/day	q 4–6 hr		
Cefuroxime	70–150 mg/kg/day	q 8 hr		
Third Generation				
Cefotaxime	100–200 mg/kg/day	q 6–8 hr	Rash, anaphylaxis (all)	
Ceftazidime	100–150 mg/kg/day	q 8 hr	Alteration of GI flora, enterocolitis (all)	
Ceftizoxime	150–200 mg/kg/day	q 6–8 hr	Prolonged PT and bleeding (moxalactam)	
Ceftriaxone	50–100 mg/kg/day	q 12–24 hr		
Moxalactam	150–200 mg/kg/day	q 6–8 hr		
Penicillins				
Penicillin G, sodium	100,000–250,000 U/kg/day	q 4 hr	Rash, anaphylaxis	
Antistaphylococcal				
Methicillin	150–200 mg/kg/day	q 6 hr	Rash, anaphylaxis	
Expanded				
Ampicillin	100–300 mg/kg/day	q 4–6 hr	Rash, anaphylaxis (all)	
Azlocillin	300–450 mg/kg/day	q 4–6 hr	Diarrhea, drug fever (ampicillin)	
Carbenicillin	400–600 mg/kg/day	q 4–6 hr		
Mezlocillin	200–300 mg/kg/day	q 4–6 hr		
Ticarcillin	200–300 mg/kg/day	q 4–6 hr		
Miscellaneous				
Chloramphenicol	50–75 mg/kg/day	q 6 hr	Aplastic anemia	Monitor hematologic indices
Clindamycin	25–40 mg/kg/day	q 6–8 hr	Pseudomembranous colitis	
Metronidazole	15–35 mg/kg/day	q 8 hr		
Vancomycin	40 mg/kg/day	q 6 hr	Rash, nephrotoxicity	Monitor serum levels

be considered. Toxicity may be enhanced by the metabolic and physiologic derangements encountered in the trauma patient.

A decision must be made about the length of therapy. Used in preventative or adjunctive modes, antibiotic administration is restricted to the initial treatment period alone. Frequently, a single dose is sufficient, and there is little justification for extending therapy beyond 48 hours. If used in a therapeutic mode, antibiotics are administered for a minimum of 5 days and are discontinued only after signs and symptoms of sepsis have been absent for 36 to 48 hours.

In the pediatric age group the selection of an appropriate agent must take into account established efficacy, safety, and dosage, determinations unavailable for a large number of agents.

The major classes of antimicrobials available for treating pediatric patients include the penicillins, cephalosporins, and aminoglycosides (Table 44–6). The penicillins are beta-lactam antibiotics that inhibit cell wall synthesis, resulting in lysis. After administration, they are widely distributed throughout the body, including the cerebrospinal fluid. Elimination occurs by way of the kidney. The efficacy of the natural penicillins is restricted to the gram-positive cocci. The emergence of staphylococcal resistance resulted in the development of the semisynthetic variety (e.g., methicillin), which is penicillinase resistant and the drug of choice for *S. aureus*. Further alterations of the penicillin molecule led to the introduction of the extended-spectrum penicillins (e.g., ampicillin, carbenicillin), which have increased activity against the gram-negative bacilli and *Pseudomonas*. This increased gram-negative coverage has generally been accompanied by diminished activity against the gram-positive organisms. The exceptions to this are the newer ureidopenicillins and piperazine penicillins (e.g., azlocillin, mezlocillin, ticarcillin), which have broad activity against gram-positive organisms, gram-negative organisms, *Pseudomonas* species, and anaerobes. The chief side effect of all the penicillins is allergic reaction, which ranges from fever and rash to anaphylaxis.[214]

The cephalosporins are also beta-lactam antibiotics with chemical structures and activities similar to the penicillins. Their mode of action is also similar. Distribution throughout the body is adequate, with the exception of the cerebrospinal fluid, in which penetration is quite variable. They are eliminated by the kidney. The cephalosporins are active against many gram-positive and gram-negative organisms. The spectrum of gram-negative activity increases from the so-called first-generation to third-generation drugs, but this is accompanied by diminished gram-positive effectiveness. Activity against *Pseudomonas* and *Bacteroides* species is unsatisfactory. The exceptions are the second-generation cephalosporins, cefoxitin and cefotetan, which are active against *Bacteroides,* but widespread use has resulted in increasing resistance among the susceptible organisms. The toxic effects of the cephalosporins are mostly limited to allergic reactions similar to the reactions to penicillins. Diarrhea and enterocolitis have been associated with the broader-spectrum agents, and prolonged bleeding times are encountered with cefamandole and moxalactam.[191]

The aminoglycosides are molecules of amino sugars linked to a central hexose by glycosidic bond. They are bactericidal owing to irreversible binding to bacterial ribosomes, which inhibits protein synthesis. Serum levels are attained rapidly after intravenous administration, but pulmonary and cerebrospinal fluid levels are poor. The aminoglycosides are eliminated by the kidney. Although they are effective against many gram-positive organisms, their major indications are for gram-negative organisms, including *Pseudomonas*. Anaerobic coverage is inadequate. The major disadvantage of these antimicrobials is their toxicity. Ototoxicity and nephrotoxicity are common effects. The frequency and severity of these adverse reactions, as well as the narrow margin between efficacy and toxicity, necessitate monitoring of serum levels with subsequent adjustment of dosage as indicated.[61]

Several additional antimicrobials have achieved wide usage in treating the pediatric age group. Chloramphenicol is a derivative of dichloroacetic acid. It inhibits protein synthesis by blocking linkages on the messenger RNA-ribosome complex. It is distributed widely throughout the body, including the cerebrospinal fluid. It has a broad, unique spectrum of activity, and it is effective against many gram-positive and gram-negative cocci, *Haemophilus, Salmonella,* and *Bacteroides*. Its use has declined dramatically because of its toxic effect on the bone marrow with resultant pancytopenia. Drug-induced aplastic anemia is uncommon, but it is usually fatal. The use of this drug requires frequent monitoring of blood and platelet counts.[208]

Clindamycin is a derivative of lincomycin, whose mode of action involves binding to bacterial ribosomes, which inhibits protein synthesis. Its major activity is anaerobic, and it is the drug of choice for *Bacteroides* infection. It is also effective against many aerobic gram-positive cocci. Toxicity is related to diarrhea and colitis.[208]

Metronidazole has emerged as the most effective antianaerobic agent available. This small molecule is reduced within bacteria containing nitroreductase, generating highly cytotoxic intermediates. It is widely distributed throughout the body and has good penetration into the major spaces. It is unique in its ability to penetrate abscess cavities in therapeutic levels. Its spectrum of activity is limited to the anaerobic organisms and certain parasites, and its toxicity is minimal.[159]

With the emergence of coagulase-negative *Staphylococcus* and methicillin-resistant, coagulase-positive *Staphylococcus* as prominent pathogens, vancomycin has been increasingly used in the pediatric age group. It is a unique, complex glycopeptide that inhibits the synthesis of certain cell wall components. It is distributed widely throughout the body, with the exception of the cerebrospinal fluid and bile. Its spectrum of activity is limited to the gram-positive and gram-negative cocci, but its efficacy is related to the lack of appreciable staphylococcal resistance. It is the drug of choice for treating *S. epidermidis* and methicillin-resistant *S. aureus* infections. Its major side effect is neurotoxicity, affecting the auditory nerve. Monitoring of serum levels is generally indicated, particularly in patients with renal insufficiency (Table 44–7).[72] Peak and trough levels should be maintained between 25 and 30 μg per ml and 10 μg per ml, respectively.[72]

Soft Tissue Injury

Trauma invariably involves some degree of soft tissue injury. Effective prophylaxis against infection is facilitated by careful preliminary examination, followed by appropriate treatment. Traumatic wounds are classified according to the mechanism of injury, depth, degree of contamination, and length of delay in therapy.

Mechanical soft tissue injury is caused by shear, tensile, or compressive forces acting alone or in combination. Shear forces yield sharp, penetrating injuries with little surrounding tissue damage and little disruption of the defense mechanisms. Tensile force results in stretching and tearing of tissue. The greater force required to induce injury produces greater involvement of the surrounding and adjacent tissue with relatively greater disruption of the defense mechanisms. Compressive injury results in the greatest tissue damage, with significant underlying hemorrhage and edema. This may or may not be accompanied by cutaneous disruption, but it is frequently associated with thrombosis of the local vessels and further tissue necrosis.[42]

Evaluation of wound depth is important in assessing the

Table 44–7
Monitoring Aminoglycoside Therapy

Drug	Peak Level*	Trough Level†
Gentamicin	<6–8 μg/ml	<2 μg/ml
Tobramycin		
Amikacin	<20–30 μg/ml	<8 μ/ml

*The peak level is obtained 30 minutes after intravenous infusion.
†The trough level is obtained immediately before the next dose.

probability of injury to underlying structures and in determining the possibility of endogenous contamination from such an underlying injury. All traumatic wounds are contaminated to a greater or lesser extent. In the absence of predisposing factors, approximately 10 viable organisms must be introduced to cause infection.[206] However, in the presence of foreign material, necrotic tissue, or hematoma, this number is substantially reduced and the probability of infection significantly increased.[142, 155, 156] Even with extensive contamination, there is a latent period of approximately 4 hours between the introduction of the microorganism and commencement of exponential growth and tissue invasion. During this period of acclimation, the microorganisms may remain susceptible to antimicrobial therapy.

Superficial, sharp, penetrating injuries are seldom associated with significant tissue damage or contamination, and they can be adequately treated by débridement, evacuation, and irrigation. With minimal delay, primary closure may be carried out without an increased risk of infection. The therapy of deep penetrating injuries varies only in relation to the possibility of underlying damage. With vigorous local wound preparation, primary closure is acceptable. Blunt soft tissue injuries are associated with various degrees of tissue damage and contamination. Through surgical débridement and mechanical irrigation, an effort should be made to convert these to clean, sharp wounds that are amenable to primary closure. If there has been significant delay or extensive tissue damage, these wounds are best managed by secondary closure after initial débridement and thorough cleansing.

Adjunctive antibiotic therapy is useful in significant blunt soft tissue injuries for which primary closure is employed. Because the usual pathogen is cutaneously derived *Staphylococcus,* a penicillinase-resistant penicillin or first-generation cephalosporin is indicated. It should be administered intravenously, within 4 hours of injury, as a single dose at the time of wound management.

The exception to these guidelines is a soft tissue injury incurred by a bite. In these circumstances, local skin flora and the flora of the oral cavity of the animal species involved are recovered. Local wound care remains vital, and although open treatment is usually advocated, the method of closure should depend on the factors previously elucidated.

The antibiotic choice is based on the circumstances of injury. Human bites are characterized by *S. aureus, Streptococcus,* anaerobic cocci, and *Bacteroides.* Animal bites, in addition to *Staphylococcus* and anaerobic cocci, are frequently associated with *Pasteurella multocida* and *Pseudomonas fluorescens* group. Suitable antibiotic coverage requires combination therapy, because no single agent is effective. A penicillinase-resistant penicillin plus penicillin or amoxicillin plus clavulanic acid (Augmentin) may be used. Either combination is employed in an adjunctive role of short duration.[39, 65, 104, 192]

In addition to the routine antimicrobial measures, all significant soft tissue injuries in children should receive prophylaxis for tetanus. The form of prophylaxis is determined by the condition of the wound (Table 44–8) and the immunization history (Table 44–9).

Table 44–8
Prophylaxis against Tetanus According to Wound Classification

Wound Feature	Tetanus-Prone Wounds	Nontetanus-Prone Wounds
Age of wound	<6 hr	<6 hr
Type	Stellate, abrasion Avulsion	Linear
Depth	1 cm	1 cm
Mechanism	Missile, crush Burn, frostbite	Sharp
Infection	Present	Absent
Devitalized tissue	Present	Absent
Contaminants	Present	Absent

Burn Wound

The leading cause of death of patients with burns is sepsis, and the primary source is the burn wound. Significant burns are associated with loss of the cutaneous barrier, extensive tissue necrosis, and thrombosis of the local blood supply. This combination precludes an effective immune response and promotes bacterial growth. Prophylaxis in this setting is directed at the wound itself and includes ongoing débridement and prompt coverage with topical antimicrobials. There is no role for intravenous antibiotics in the initial management of burns. Superficial burns require no topical antimicrobial therapy unless they occur within an area of ongoing contamination.

Fractures

Skeletal injuries are a frequent component of pediatric trauma. Closed fractures present little or no risk of infection, but the risk of infection with open fractures can be significant. In this setting, the risk of infection correlates directly with the extent of associated soft tissue injury and vascular compromise. The initial therapy is directed at stabilization of the bony fragment, adequate débridement of the damaged soft tissue, and restoration of the blood supply. Internal fixation should be avoided. Antibiotics play a role in the reduction of infectious complications, but contro-

Table 44–9
Prophylaxis against Tetanus According to Immunization History

Immunization Status	Tetanus-Prone Patients		Nontetanus-Prone Patients	
	Td*	TIG†	Td	TIG
Uncertain	Yes	Yes	Yes	No
0 or 1	Yes	Yes	Yes	No
2	Yes	No	Yes	No
3 or more	No‡	No	No§	No

*Td, tetanus and diphtheria toxoids absorbed; in children younger than 7 years of age, use DPT.
†TIG, tetanus immune globulin.
‡Yes, if less than 5 years since last dose.
§Yes, if less than 10 years since last dose.

versy exists regarding selection and duration. As with soft tissue injuries, coverage should be primarily directed at skin flora, and a penicillinase-resistant penicillin or first-generation cephalosporin is sufficient. There is little evidence to support therapy beyond 3 days, and many reports suggest adequate coverage with 24-hour therapy.[27, 28, 76, 138, 139, 160]

Central Nervous System Injury

Antibiotic therapy is not indicated for closed skull fractures. Fractures that may communicate with the sinuses or middle ear (i.e., basilar) traditionally have been considered at risk for cerebrospinal fluid infection, and such patients were routinely administered antibiotics. Few data support the efficacy of this therapy, and it should not be routinely used in these cases.[38, 86, 92] Penetrating central nervous system injury is an indication for antimicrobials, but their use is therapeutic rather than prophylactic. As with other traumatic injuries, adequate initial débridement minimizes infectious complications. Antibiotics should cover the gram-positive cocci and anaerobes, and the antibiotic selected must penetrate the cerebrospinal fluid.

Thoracic Injury

Antibiotic therapy is not indicated for blunt chest injury. Similarly, the need for closed tube drainage of a blunt traumatic pneumothorax or hemothorax is not a specific indication for adjunctive antimicrobials.[103, 189] Tube thoracostomy should be performed in a manner consistent with quality care after local site preparation and using sterile technique. Antibiotics lessen the incidence of empyema after penetrating trauma associated with pleural contamination.[73, 186] They are employed in conjunction with adequate drainage and should be directed against the cutaneous flora. Most studies have used the drugs a minimum of 5 days, although a shorter course may be equally as effective.

A more aggressive approach is required for an esophageal injury. The mediastinum provides little barrier to the rapid proliferation and spread of contaminating microorganisms, and this type of infection is associated with a significant mortality rate. The site of contamination must be controlled and the mediastinum adequately drained. Antibiotics are used in a therapeutic fashion and should provide broad coverage for gram-positive cocci and anaerobes.

Abdominal Injury

In no case is the potential for infection after injury greater than with involvement of the abdomen. The gastrointestinal tract contains the largest collection of potential pathogens in the body. With injury to the hollow viscera, these organisms are released from their normal restraints and proliferate. The accompanying blood, gastrointestinal contents, and injured tissue afford nutrients and protection from the immune defenses. Intra-abdominal abscess is the most frequent sequela. Several studies have documented that the probability of infection after intra-abdominal injury is di-

rectly related to the total number and type of organs injured and to the transfusion requirements. Other important factors include shock and length of the operation.[57, 127, 162]

Antibiotics should be employed for treating any blunt abdominal injury significant enough to warrant surgical exploration and for all penetrating injuries. The agent selected must provide gram-negative and anaerobic coverage. Little difference has been found between appropriate single agents and combination regimens in this case. Whatever agent is selected, it should be initiated after appropriate resuscitation and before surgical exploration. The length of therapy depends on the operative findings and the presence or absence of associated risk factors. If no hollow visceral injury is found, antibiotics are discontinued after the initial dose. For hollow visceral injury and minimal contamination or risk factors, antibiotics are employed perioperatively (i.e., single preoperative and two postoperative doses). For massive contamination or significant risk factors, antibiotics are administered therapeutically and continued for a minimum of 5 days.

SEPSIS

Metabolic Consequences

Despite all attempts at prevention, sepsis invariably intervenes in the course of a significant number of trauma patients. Its manifestations and consequences are systemic and complicated by their appearance in a host already compromised by the stress of injury. Trauma normally results in a series of hormonal and metabolic changes that produce a catabolic response. With an uncomplicated course, these changes stabilize, anabolism ensues, and full recovery occurs. With the intervention of sepsis, the same alterations characteristic of the initial response to injury recur or are magnified.

Sepsis is marked by increased cellular oxygen consumption and hypermetabolism. Infection results in tissue protein degradation and the loss of nitrogen. In the pediatric age group, this occurs at a time normally characterized by positive nitrogen balance to support growth. The metabolism of free amino acids is increased to facilitate gluconeogenesis and the synthesis of hepatic enzymes, lipoproteins, and acute-phase reactants.[21, 25, 26, 52, 144, 145] The increased amino acid levels are needed by the skeletal muscle, where various proteases are activated by IL-1.[21, 48, 58] In the child, this pool is severely limited. Glucose synthesis and release are accelerated, resulting in hyperglycemia.[52, 71] However, the limitation of available stores in the child can prohibit sustained glucose generation, producing hypoglycemia. Paradoxically, a sepsis-induced insulin insensitivity may result in intolerance to exogenous glucose despite relatively high circulating insulin levels.[106]

Ketogenesis is blunted by infection, and there is a rise in the levels of serum triglycerides and free fatty acids.[25, 125] In contrast to states of starvation, fat stores are seldom used as an energy source in the child with acute sepsis. The acid-base balance is disrupted, with an initial respiratory alkalosis secondary to tachypnea followed by the metabolic acidosis associated with sepsis-related hypotension and vascular stasis. Increased aldosterone levels lead to retention of sodium and water.[199] Iron levels drop abruptly secondary to hepatic and reticuloendothelial sequestration, with interruption of erythropoiesis. This can result in a sepsis-associated iron deficiency anemia that is unresponsive to iron therapy.[199] Serum zinc is similarly sequestered, interrupting normal posttraumatic wound healing.

Immunologic Consequences

Infection may disrupt immune function. In the injured child, this occurs at a time when the immune system is already compromised. Many of the immunologic abnormalities elucidated in trauma have also been described in sepsis. Most studies in this area have focused on the phagocyte. Bacterial sepsis is associated with decreased white blood cell adherence and diminished migration, both random and chemotactic.[17, 149, 177, 179, 205] Mobilization of the phagocytic response may therefore be impaired. Phagocytosis in sepsis appears to be intrinsically normal, but it is reduced secondary to serum opsonic deficiency.[3, 91] Defects have also been described in all aspects of bactericidal activity. Generation of unstable oxygen radicals is depressed, and there is decreased activity and release of lysosomal enzymes.[96, 178, 179, 181, 218] Clearance by the reticuloendothelial system is deficient because of diminished levels of fibronectin.[101, 167]

It is unclear whether these sepsis-induced abnormalities represent intrinsic or serum-mediated alterations or merely reflect system exhaustion. Studies of injured pediatric patients suggest that these malfunctions are secondary to an ''overwhelmed'' immune system. The function is normal and appropriate if the bacterial challenge is minimized, but it is reasonable to assume that the susceptibility of the immune system to sepsis-induced dysfunction would be increased in a child recovering from the stress of trauma.

Toxic Consequences

Sepsis leads to the generation of substances potentially detrimental to the human organism.[102] The complement cascade is activated, generating increased levels of circulating fragments. One such fragment, C5A, has been implicated in the pathogenesis of the respiratory distress syndrome and multiple organ failure. Normally considered an anaphylatoxin, this cleavage product also results in neutrophil mobilization, aggregation, and activation. Activation occurs in the form of lysosomal enzyme release. When aggregation and activation take place intravascularly, endothelial cell damage results, increasing leakage in the tissue spaces and disruption of the microcirculation.[29, 83, 131, 137]

Alterations in the metabolism of arachidonic acid, derived from cell wall phospholipids through the action of phospholipase A, have been described in sepsis. This leads to variations in the circulating levels of numerous important eicosanoids, such as prostaglandins and thromboxane. Their normal role appears to be mediation of local inflammation. Prostaglandins function as vasodilators and bronchodilators, inhibitors of platelet aggregation, and membrane stabilizers. The effects of thromboxane are the opposite of those of

prostaglandin, and it is postulated that its function is to act in opposition, balancing vascular tone and flow to the area of inflammation. Although usually undetectable, metabolites of both substances are elevated in sepsis. Chemical inhibition of this increased synthesis in experimental models of septic shock and sepsis-related hyperdynamic states reverses the cardiovascular instability characteristic of severe sepsis, suggesting a role in the pathophysiology of septic shock.[5, 6, 44, 46, 77, 150, 153, 172, 173, 202, 207]

The phagocytic response to infection and inflammation culminates in the production of free radicals that are employed in bacterial lysis. These unstable products of oxygen are extremely toxic, and their activity is nonspecific. With overabundance, cellular damage is incurred beyond that associated with normal bactericidal activity. Similarly, activation of the phagocyte results in the release of the elastase and several leukocytic proteases, all of which can induce structural protein damage.

Diagnosis

Sepsis describes a variety of pathophysiologic processes, each of which is determined by clinical and laboratory parameters. The term is applied to the presence of a known focus of infection, documented bacteremia, and the clinical syndrome of the systemic manifestations of sepsis in the absence of a known focus. The diagnosis of all forms of sepsis in the injured child is facilitated when signs and symptoms are interpreted with a high degree of suspicion against the background of ongoing clinical evaluation and baseline status. As a rule of thumb, sepsis should be considered in the differential diagnosis of any new, unusual clinical finding, abnormality, or alteration in the course of the pediatric trauma patient. This is particularly true in the evaluation of ''nonspecific'' signs, which frequently are the harbinger of full-blown sepsis.

Fever is classically considered one of the primary signs of infection in the surgical patient but requires a certain degree of interpretation when it arises in the pediatric trauma victim. Fever results from the action of IL-1 on the thermoregulatory focus of the hypothalamus.[58] Children tend to have a normally higher body temperature than adults, stabilizing at an adult level at the time of puberty. The circadian rhythm is also more pronounced in children, resulting in a wider swing between extremes of normal. Rectal temperatures as high as 38.5°C (101°F) may be recorded between 5:00 PM and 9:00 PM with lows of 36.1°C (97°F) between 1:00 AM and 6:00 AM.[24] Generation of fever in response to sepsis requires an increase in the metabolic rate. This, combined with stress-depleted energy stores, may prohibit the increased activity necessary to sustain a febrile response. Under these circumstances, it is not unusual for sepsis to result quickly in hypothermia. The tendency for baseline and septic hypothermia is facilitated by increased heat loss because of the large pediatric surface-to-mass ratio and by the immobilization and ''naked'' therapy necessitated by major injury.

The activity of IL-1 on a thermoregulatory focus is nonspecific. IL-1 may be generated by a variety of inflammatory responses in addition to infection. It is not uncommon for fever to be associated with nonseptic processes. This is particularly pertinent in the traumatized child, in whom injury can induce widespread inflammation. Fever has no specific predictive value in the detection of infection in burned children.[136] Similarly, approximately one third of children develop fever within 72 hours of elective operation with no evidence of subsequent sepsis.[216] As a sign of sepsis, fever alone is a nonspecific indicator in the injured child. More useful is a temperature instability, an alteration in baseline value, or an abnormal pattern of change. These should prompt a thorough search for the cause.

Infection may be accompanied by tachypnea and tachycardia. These usually are associated with fever and the resultant increase in metabolic rate, and they are subject to the same vagaries as fever. However, alteration of a previously stable respiratory pattern should prompt an investigation. Similarly, in the child already on ventilatory support, an abrupt change in status or increasing requirements may indicate infection. Sepsis can result in systemic vasodilation, which is signified clinically by a widened pulse pressure, increased fluid requirements, oliguria, and hypotension.

Gastrointestinal function is frequently affected in the septic child and is manifested by abdominal distention, vomiting, and prolonged or renewed ileus. Sepsis-induced platelet dysfunction and thrombocytopenia are suggested by the appearance of ecchymosis and petechiae and by renewed or prolonged bleeding in surgical wounds and sites of cannulation.

Routine laboratory evaluation frequently provides further supportive evidence of infection. Most widely recognized is leukocytosis. This isolated index is less helpful in assessing the pediatric trauma victim in whom an elevated blood cell count accompanies all but the most minimal injuries. As an indicator of sepsis in this circumstance, the leukocyte count is evaluated in terms of persistent leukocytosis, renewed elevation within the normalizing trend, and leukopenia. Blood counts obtained for the investigation of possible sepsis should also include platelet enumeration to detect thrombocytopenia, although thrombocytopenia may accompany repeated blood transfusions.

The acid-base balance may be altered, reflecting the altered physiology of the patient with sepsis. Respiratory alkalosis can be induced by tachypnea, and metabolic acidosis may attend sepsis-induced perfusion abnormalities. In the child, sepsis is frequently associated with alterations in glucose metabolism, which are reflected in serum and urine glucose levels. Hypoglycemia can occur in the critically ill child with insufficient glucose stores to respond to the increased energy requirement. In the child receiving parenteral alimentation, abrupt glucose intolerance reflects the insulin insensitivity of the tissues affected by sepsis. The combination of increased fluid requirements and perfusional alterations associated with sepsis can result in azotemia and an elevation of liver enzymes and bilirubin.

The suspicion of infection necessitates a thorough examination. Although several obvious sites are available in the injured child, evaluation must include possible sources common to the pediatric age group itself. Frequently overlooked areas include the skin (e.g., rash), ears (e.g., otitis), and pharynx (e.g., pharyngitis). All wounds and sites of present and past cannulation should be carefully inspected. The chest and abdomen must be fully examined. Often, this evaluation alone results in the differentiation of infection, precluding the need for a more extensive investigation.

Before any therapy, an attempt to identify the specific pathogen is indicated. Cultures are obtained from any suspicious superficial site. If evaluation suggests a respiratory focus and access to the lower airway is available, sputum is sampled for Gram stain and culture. Blood is obtained peripherally and centrally (if applicable) for aerobic and anaerobic cultures. Urine is similarly sampled. For the rare infant with traumatic injury or children with central nervous system penetration, a spinal tap should be performed.

Despite the most thorough evaluation, a significant number of patients present with the physiologic manifestation of sepsis without an identified focus or bacteremia. Such children with so-called clinical sepsis can present a therapeutic dilemma. Some uniform criteria are necessary to characterize these children, enabling clinical evaluation of the therapy and complications. The published criteria for what is described as the sepsis syndrome are applicable to identified and unidentified infections and provide a useful minimal standard for the diagnosis of sepsis. The criteria include the simultaneous occurrence of two or more of the clinical and laboratory findings of a known site of infection, bacteremia, rectal temperature greater than 38.5°C or less than 35.5°C twice in 24 hours, sustained blood pressure less than 50 mm Hg, a leukocyte count less than 3000/mm³ or greater than 20,000/mm³ or an increase of greater than 3000/mm³ in 24 hours with a "left shift" caused by more than 10% immature granulocytes or more than 60% polymorphonuclear leukocytes (Table 44–10).[206]

SPECIFIC INFECTIONS

Coincidental Infections

Although a high index of suspicion and an aggressive approach is necessary to minimize the morbid consequences of posttraumatic sepsis, admission to the hospital after injury does not preclude the symptomatic onset of the more common infectious diseases of childhood. Lack of appreciation of this fact can easily result in unnecessary diagnostics and therapeutics. Seasonal respiratory illnesses should not

Table 44–10
Clinical Sepsis Syndrome Criteria

Two or more of the following:
  Documented site of infection
  Documented bacteremia
  Rectal temperature >38.5°C or <35.5°C twice in 24 hours
  Sustained blood pressure <50 mm Hg
  Leukocyte count <3000 cells/mm³
  Leukocyte count >20,000 cells/mm³
  Increase in leukocyte count >3000 cells/mm³ with a "left shift" (i.e., 10% immature granulocytes or >60% polymorphonuclear leukocytes)

Modified from Wilkinson JD, Pollack MM, Glass NL, et al. Mortality associated with multiple organ system failure and sepsis in the pediatric intensive care unit. J Pediatr 111:324–328, 1987.

Table 44-11
Most Common Nosocomial Pathogens

Service	Urinary Tract		Wound		Lower Respiratory Tract		Skin		Bacteremia	
	Pathogen	%	Pathogen	%	Pathogen	%	Pathogen	%	Pathogen	%
Medicine	E. coli	32.7	S. aureus	15.7	P. aeruginosa	14.7	S. aureus	29.0	S. aureus	14.7
	Enterococci	14.2	Enterococci	13.4	S. aureus	14.1	Coag-neg Staph.	9.7	Coag-neg Staph.	13.9
	P. aeruginosa	11.1	E. coli	11.1	Klebsiella spp.	13.3	P. aeruginosa	8.9	E. coli	10.7
	Klebsiella spp.	8.2	P. aeruginosa	10.8	Enterobacter spp.	9.2	Enterobacter spp.	7.5	Klebsiella spp.	10.6
	Proteus spp.	8.0	Enterobacter spp.	8.0	E. coli	7.5	E. coli	7.1	P. aeruginosa	7.5
Surgery	E. coli	28.6	S. aureus	19.6	S. aureus	15.6	S. aureus	19.2	Coag-neg Staph.	13.1
	P. aeruginosa	16.2	Enterococci	11.3	Klebsiella spp.	12.4	Enterococci	13.5	S. aureus	12.0
	Enterococci	14.4	E. coli	10.9	Enterobacter spp.	11.4	P. aeruginosa	10.0	Enterobacter spp.	10.3
	Klebsiella spp.	7.3	P. aeruginosa	9.0	S. aureus	11.1	Coag-neg Staph.	8.9	Enterococci	9.6
	Proteus spp.	7.1	Coag-neg Staph.*	8.4	E. coli	6.9	E. coli	8.0	E. coli	8.8
Pediatrics	E. coli	38.6	S. aureus	28.8	Klebsiella spp.	16.7	S. aureus	35.2	Coag-neg Staph.	18.0
	Candida spp.	16.9	Coag-neg Staph.	16.4	P. aeruginosa	13.0	Coag-neg Staph.	14.8	S. aureus	12.4
	P. aeruginosa	10.8	E. coli	8.2	S. aureus	13.0	Enterococci	8.0	Klebsiella spp.	10.1
	Enterococci	8.4	P. aeruginosa	6.8	Candida spp.	7.4	E. coli	6.8	E. coli	9.0
	Klebsiella spp.	8.4	Enterococci	6.8	E. coli	3.7	Candida	6.8	Candida	6.7
			Klebsiella spp.	6.8			P. aeruginosa	6.8		

*Coagulase-negative *Staphylococcus*.

be confused with pneumonitis nor common viral exanthems misinterpreted as allergic reaction or evidence of inflammation. Frequently, the issue can be clarified by a careful history obtained from the family.

Pharyngitis and otitis media are commonly encountered causes of infection in the pediatric age group and should be considered in the evaluation of possible sepsis in the injured child. Pharyngitis is an inflammatory illness of the mucous membranes of the throat, including the tonsils. It is primarily of viral origin, but the major bacterial pathogen is group A *Streptococcus*. The onset is acute and usually accompanied by fever. Aside from the expected sore throat, symptoms may range from headache to abdominal pain. Viral disease is self-limited and requires only symptomatic therapy. Antibiotics are indicated for streptococcal pharyngitis because of the possibility of cardiac sequelae (e.g., rheumatic fever). The possibility of this complication necessitates a definitive diagnosis based on a throat culture. With documentation of streptococcal infection, the treatment is a single intramuscular dose (50,000 U per kg) of benzathine penicillin.

Otitis media may be coincidental or nosocomial in the pediatric trauma patient. The cause is dysfunction of the eustachian tube, a normally patent, unidirectional valve draining the middle ear. Obstruction can accompany any inflammatory processes of the nasopharynx or oropharynx with secondary bacterial infection. Intubation via these routes predisposes the patient to eustachian tube dysfunction and can result in otitis media. The most common bacterial pathogens are *Streptococcus pneumoniae* and *Haemophilus influenzae*. Antibiotic therapy is indicated to minimize the damage to the middle ear and to avoid the potential complications of acute mastoiditis and facial nerve paralysis. The most commonly employed drugs include ampicillin and trimethaprim-sulfamethoxazole.

Nosocomial Infections

Nosocomial infections are infections occurring during hospitalization unless the patient is intubated on admission. These are differentiated from surgically related infections, which arise in tissues, organs, or cavities exposed or manipulated during an operative procedure. The exception is wound infection, which, although it fulfills the criterion for surgically related infection, has classically been considered nosocomial.

As in the adult, nosocomial infection accounts for most of the septic problems encountered in hospitalized children, although the overall rate of nosocomial infection is lower in the pediatric service than adult services. Among pediatric wards, the highest rate is encountered in the neonatal and pediatric intensive care units. Characteristics of pediatric nosocomial infection include a higher incidence of secondary bacteremia and an equal incidence of gram-positive and gram-negative pathogens (Table 44–11). The lower respiratory tract is the most common site of pediatric nosocomial infection (Table 44–12).[87, 88]

Wound Infections

Because of the nature of the indications for surgery in the injured patient, most surgical wounds are best classified as contaminated or dirty. The incidence of wound infection in this setting ranges from 15 to 40%, and the surgical wound becomes a prime suspect in the septic trauma victim. In the

Table 44-12
Nosocomial Infections According to Site

Site	Percentage of Adult Patients	Percentage of Pediatric Patients
Urinary tract	41	16
Surgical wound	18	10
Lower respiratory tract	16	30
Cutaneous sites	6	17
Bacteremia	7	13
Miscellaneous	12	32

child, the most frequent pathogen recovered is coagulase-positive and coagulase-negative *Staphylococcus,* occurring in almost 50% of infections. Enteric gram-negative infection occurs much less frequently. The cause often can be accurately determined by the characteristics of the infected wound itself (Table 44–13).

Wound infection with *S. aureus* generally arises within 4 to 7 days of the operative procedure. It is characterized by marked induration and erythema and associated with significant localized tenderness. Cellulitis is usually restricted to the immediate peri-incisional area. With progression, fluctuance develops rapidly with the formation of a wound abscess. The purulent discharge is thick, creamy, and white to yellow. There is seldom an associated odor. Treatment consists primarily of wound drainage, débridement, and packing of the abscess cavity. Antibiotics are unnecessary unless infection is accompanied by significant evidence of septicemia. Infection with *S. epidermidis* is similar in nature, although its clinical manifestations are delayed and milder, and suppuration, if present, is of a lesser degree. Treatment is the same as for *S. aureus.*

Wound infection caused by enteric gram-negative rods occurs 7 to 14 days after surgery. The most frequently involved organism is *E. coli.* Local signs of wound cellulitis are characteristically overshadowed by symptoms of systemic toxicity. Abscess formation is much less prominent, and the drainage is seropurulent. A foul odor may accompany the wound discharge. Although seldom recovered from culture, anaerobes are presumed to be present by the nature of the contamination necessary to cause gram-negative wound infection. Treatment includes local wound drainage. Appropriate antibiotics are employed against significant systemic toxicity. A cephalosporin with appropriate gram-negative coverage is usually sufficient.

Group A streptococcal wound infection is uncommon in the child but deserves mention by virtue of its unusual clinical picture. It is marked by the development of high fever and striking systemic signs within 48 hours of surgery. The incisional site is characterized by rapidly spreading cellulitis and lymphangitis. Drainage, if present, is serous to serosanguineous. Treatment is high-dose penicillin, which should be instituted if streptococcal infection is suspected. Formal wound drainage is usually unnecessary.

Lower Respiratory Tract Infections

Community-acquired pediatric pneumonitis is a viral illness. Bacterial pneumonia accounts for 10% or fewer of these cases and predominantly involves gram-positive cocci or *Haemophilus.* Hospital-acquired pneumonia in the child is generally caused by gram-negative organisms or *Pseudomonas.*[88] Infection is secondary to colonization caused by airway control and manipulation and, with intensive care, recolonization occurs rapidly. Abnormal colonization alone has no pathologic significance, but with continued compromise of local and systemic defenses, distal invasion and infection can occur. Distal invasion is facilitated by poor pulmonary toilet, hypoventilation, atelectasis, pulmonary edema, and pulmonary parenchymal injury. The difficulty lies in differentiating colonization from infection. An ag-

Table 44–13
Characteristics of Wound Infection

Pathogen	Incubation (days)	Local Signs	Toxicity	Drainage
Staphylococcus aureus	4–7	Cellulitis, pain, abscess formation	Minimal	Purulent
Enteric gram-negative organisms	7–14	Induration, edema	Moderate to marked	Seropurulent
Group A *Streptococcus*	1–2	Rapidly spreading cellulitis, lymphangitis	Marked	Serous Serosanguineous

gressive approach is warranted in the diagnosis and treatment of pediatric nosocomial pneumonia, because each of the three major pathogens recovered (i.e., *Klebsiella, Pseudomonas, S. aureus*) are characterized by a severe course, rapid progression, and extensive necrosis of lung tissue. The mortality rate is accordingly high.

The diagnosis of pneumonia in the injured child is best made on the basis of a change in clinical and radiographic pulmonary status. Routine surveillance cultures may provide information about the extent of disease and the possible pathogen. They are most useful when clinical and radiographic signs accompany a change in the airway flora. However, the overall correlation between these cultures and documented pathogens is less than 50%.

More invasive diagnostic measures, such as transtracheal aspiration and percutaneous biopsy, have only limited applicability in children. Flexible fiberoptic bronchoscopy has proved useful in the diagnosis and therapy of pediatric pneumonia. Performed at the bedside, this technique enables distal airway sampling for culture and pulmonary toilet. If pleural effusions accompany signs of respiratory infection, thoracentesis is indicated for culture. Regardless of the method used to obtain a specimen, a Gram stain is performed to assist the initial antibiotic selection.

Therapy consists of ventilatory support and aggressive pulmonary toilet. Effusions should be drained by thoracentesis. Tube thoracostomy is indicated for a rapid recurrence, and the development of empyema necessitates tube drainage. Initial antibiotic therapy is guided by results of the Gram stain. For gram-negative bacilli or *Pseudomonas,* the combination of an aminoglycoside and one of the expanded penicillins is indicated. A penicillinase-resistant penicillin or vancomycin is substituted in gram-positive disease. Therapy is altered on the basis of the clinical response and final culture results.

Urinary Tract Infections

The cause of pediatric nosocomial urinary tract infection is almost invariably urethral catheterization for monitoring. The catheter effectively bypasses the local defense mechanisms and provides direct access to the urinary tract for potential pathogens. The most frequent organism recovered, *E. coli,* is probably of perineal origin.[88] Diagnosis is based on suspicion, because the usual clinical symptoms of frequency, urgency, and dysuria are negated in the presence of an indwelling catheter. Similarly, pyuria correlates poorly with urinary tract infection in all children, but particularly in the case of an indwelling catheter. Confirmation of infection is determined by an adequately obtained quantitative urine culture. The criteria for defining infection depend on the method of urine collection (Table 44–14). The best method is suprapubic aspiration, although it is seldom used beyond the neonatal period. More than 100 colonies of a single organism per 1 ml of urine obtained in this fashion is considered a positive result. This number increases to 50,000 colonies for a catheterized specimen and 100,000 colonies for a "clean catch." The presence of more than one organism, low colony count, or the recovery of *S. epidermidis* indicates possible contamination.[14] Infection is treated by the maintenance of a high urinary flow and an aminoglycoside, ampicillin, or trimethoprim-sulfamethoxazole.

An exception to these guidelines is the recovery of *Candida* from a urinary culture. Although an uncommon pathogen in the urinary tract of normal children, *Candida* is second only to *E. coli* as the most frequent organism recovered in nosocomial urinary tract infections. Predisposing factors include immunosuppression, antibiotic therapy, and an indwelling catheter—factors characteristic of the critically injured child. The diagnosis is confirmed by recovery of more than 10,000 colonies per 1 ml of urine.

Treatment consists of removal or changing of the catheter. This alone is frequently curative. If candiduria persists, and the infection is localized to the bladder, irrigation is performed with 100 to 300 ml of a 15% solution of amphotericin B (15 mg/100 ml of D5W). The irrigant is left in place for 30 to 60 minutes, and irrigation is repeated three to four times daily for 3 to 5 days. Oral therapy with flucytosine (50–100 mg/kg per day divided every 6 hours) is also effective. If the site of infection is unknown or the child is immunocompromised, systemic antifungal therapy is indicated. Flucytosine is given as previously described for 7 days. For intravenous therapy, amphotericin B (0.5 mg/kg per day) is administered once daily for 5 to 10 days. In cases of significant renal involvement or systemic sepsis, the combination of flucytosine and amphotericin should be used and the length of therapy extended.[14]

Lines and Monitors

All injured children at some time during the course of their hospitalization are cannulated for the administration of

Table 44–14
Criteria for the Diagnosis of Pediatric Urinary Tract Infections

Type of Sampling	Positive Culture Results
Suprapubic aspiration	>100 colonies/ml of urine, single organism
Catheterized	>50,000 colonies/ml of urine, single organism
Clean catch	>100,000 colonies/ml of urine, single organism

fluids and medications, and they are subjected to invasive monitoring techniques. Although these modalities have greatly aided the support and treatment of the trauma victim, they have also been a significant source of septic complications. Approximately one third of all intravenous catheters are culture positive on removal. This colonization bears little correlation with the presence of phlebitis.[49, 120] The incidence increases with the length of time the lines are used, and contamination is greater in lines placed by surgical cutdown.[49, 120, 140] The organisms recovered usually are skin flora. The exact relation between colonization and infection is more difficult to ascertain. Colonization has been associated with as many as 30% of cases of local infection and with 2 to 10% of bacteremia cases.[78, 110, 140, 174] One study reported that 9% of positive blood cultures occurred in adult patients with no identifiable source of infection other than an intravenous catheter.[174]

The data are similar for arterial lines. The incidence of local infection is increased significantly in lines inserted by cutdown and in those in place longer than 4 days.[20] The local infection rates vary from 0 to 20% and have associated bacteremia in as many as 30% of these patients. Location of the catheter does not appear to be a major factor.[176] In contrast to intravenous catheters, the likely pathogens have included gram-negative organisms, yeast, and gram-positive cocci.[64]

Lines placed into the central venous system are at risk for contamination from cutaneous organisms and unassociated bacteremia. Lines inserted in areas of active infection become colonized with the same organisms in as many as 50% of cases.[114] They may serve as a source of primary bacteremia and continued seeding in established infection. In severely burned patients, central venous lines are associated with a 30% incidence of suppurative thrombophlebitis.[147] Catheters that traverse the heart (e.g., pulmonary artery catheter) may become colonized and induce valvular trauma, increasing the possibility of infective endocarditis. An autopsy study after pulmonary artery catheterization found a 3% incidence of endocarditis.[161]

Sepsis should prompt suspicion of all sites of cannulation. Venous and arterial lines should be inspected carefully, and blood is obtained through the catheter for culture. Simultaneous peripheral blood cultures are frequently of value in differentiating contamination from bacteremia. In cases of positive blood culture results or ongoing sepsis, all central lines are removed. Under ideal circumstances, they should not be replaced until the focus of infection is controlled and the blood stream sterilized. However, many of these children require the ongoing presence of a central line, and in these circumstances, evidence suggests that replacement via a guidewire (i.e., Seldinger technique) may be effective in removing the focus of central line sepsis.[13] Similarly, antibiotic therapy administered through the existing catheter may be equally as effective in controlling sepsis, although the incidence of recurrent infection is increased.[146]

Intra-abdominal Infections

The peritoneal cavity is a normally sterile, potential space containing only a few milliliters of fluid. This condition is maintained by the semipermeable nature of the mesothelial lining and a defined circulation. Through the forces of gravity, peristalsis, and diaphragmatic motion, peritoneal fluid normally courses from the central areas to the lateral gutters and then to the subdiaphragmatic spaces. Fenestrated lymphatics within the mesothelium beneath the diaphragm absorb excess fluid, promoting continued flow. The circulation maintains the peritoneal cavity and serves as an important local defense mechanism, effectively clearing limited amounts of bacteria or cellular debris introduced. Bacteria injected into the peritoneal space can be recovered from the lymphatics within 6 minutes.

With mesothelial irritation, as accompanies the spillage of gastrointestinal contents, there is the exudation of fluid and plasma, containing opsonins and phagocytic cells, into the peritoneal cavity. Additional cells are mobilized through activation of the complement cascade, generating potent chemotactic factors. These mechanisms localize the nonspecific immune defenses at the site of contamination. Fibrinogen within the exuded fluid isolates the site of contamination and entraps bacteria.

Although these processes preclude the development of significant infection, each is self-limited and easily overcome by the pathophysiology of substantial injury. Initial lymphatic absorption of large quantities of pathogens overwhelms the reticuloendothelial system and results in the systemic manifestations of sepsis. With ongoing irritation, ileus, hypoventilation, and abdominal wall rigidity impair peritoneal circulation and further absorption. The continued outpouring of fluid dilutes the various opsonins, chemotaxins, and phagocytic cells, hindering the immune response. Fibrin localization effectively shields bacteria from the immune defenses. The result is a clinical syndrome of peritonitis.[170, 171]

Peritonitis or its potential from penetrating trauma generally presents little diagnostic difficulty. Therapy consists of resuscitation, antibiotics, and control of the source of contamination. Fluid is exuded into the inflamed peritoneal cavity at the expense of the intravascular space, rendering these patients hypovolemic. In the child, initial fluid resuscitation should be with nonglucose-containing crystalloids delivered as bolus therapy (10–20 ml/kg) until a response is obtained. Subsequent therapy is usually guided by monitoring central venous pressure and urinary output. Abdominal distention and rigidity may compromise respiration, necessitating ventilatory support. Ileus leads to intestinal distention and vomiting, requiring nasogastric intubation. Antibiotic therapy is based on the gastrointestinal flora and should provide broad gram-negative and anaerobic coverage. Emergent surgery is indicated to remove and control contamination.

The most common infectious complication of bacterial peritonitis is abscess formation. Abscesses form, in part, through the intrinsic defense mechanisms of the peritoneal cavity. Fibrin deposition entraps pathogenic bacteria, leukocytes, and macrophages. Unable to reach the bacteria, these cells soon die, releasing their lysosomal and proteolytic enzymes, adding to the tissue destruction and the creation of an abscess cavity. The hypertonicity of the abscess contents results in the influx of fluid, gradually enlarging the cavity and facilitating extension. The organizing fibrin wall prevents antibiotic penetration, effectively shielding the microorganisms from the immune defenses and therapeutic medications. Bacterial growth is enhanced through synergism; enteric aerobes lower the local oxygen tension and pH, creating an environment in which anaerobes thrive and become the prominent pathogens. Within 5 to 10 days, this enlarging abscess has become a source of renewed sepsis.[22, 36, 126, 171]

Intra-abdominal infection is a biphasic process. The initial sepsis and mortality is related to absorption of gram-negative bacilli and their toxic products in peritonitis. With localization, morbidity is secondary to the activity of the anaerobes in abscess formation.[134, 135, 200, 201]

The diagnosis of intra-abdominal abscess is based on a knowledge of the circumstances under which they occur, of the pathophysiology, and on a high index of suspicion. The distinction and magnitude of clinical signs and symptoms are modified by the usual antimicrobial therapy and postoperative state encountered in most patients with this complication. This often delays the diagnosis and increases the mortality rate.[141] Most patients with intra-abdominal abscess are characterized by persistent low-grade fever and leukocytosis. Localized tenderness is apparent in approximately one third of patients.[70] Additional findings are insidious and related to the abscess location. With a subphrenic collection, there may be basilar pulmonary infiltrates, atelectasis, or effusion resulting in diminished breath sounds. The involved diaphragm is frequently elevated with limited excursion. With pelvic localization, diarrhea may occur secondary to rectal irritation. A palpable mass is usually revealed on rectal examination. Interloop gutter abscesses can present with renewed or prolonged ileus.

Radiography can provide supportive evidence in the form of thoracic abnormalities as described earlier and as a mass lesion, air-fluid level, or the mottled soap-bubble appearance of an established intra-abdominal process.[70] Axial computed tomography (CT) is the most reliable radiographic technique for the documentation and localization of intra-abdominal abscess. Its accuracy approaches 90% in most large series.[53, 95, 117, 129, 154, 165] Similar accuracy has been reported with ultrasonography, but this technique requires greater technical and interpretive expertise.[81, 94, 117, 129, 189] Radionuclide procedures, such as gallium and labeled leukocyte scans, have proved to be of limited value.[15, 43] Usually, the diagnosis of intra-abdominal abscess is a clinical one, and the failure of laboratory documentation should not preclude appropriate therapeutic maneuvers in suspect cases.[215]

The therapy for intra-abdominal abscess is drainage. Antibiotics are employed solely to treat the surrounding cellulitis and bacterial seeding. They have minimal effect against the abscesses themselves. The methods of abscess drainage have changed over the last decade with the establishment of the efficacy of nonoperative alternatives. Although surgical exploration remains the standard if the abscess cannot be accurately localized or there is a possibility of multiplicity, percutaneous drainage has proved to be an acceptable alternative in the isolated, localized case.[1] Drainage is performed under CT or ultrasound guidance with placement of a dependent catheter. The specific criteria for attempted percutaneous drainage include a well-defined and unilocular collection, a safe access route, and the aspiration of purulent material on initial needle puncture. Under these conditions, successful resolution of the abscess may be obtained in approximately 85% of adult cases, with an acceptable morbidity rate of 8 to 15%.[89, 194] Similar results should be obtainable with the availability of pediatric expertise.

The inability to use percutaneous drainage, for whatever reason, necessitates prompt operative treatment. In the case of an unknown location or multiple sites of infection, wide exploration is indicated. A more limited or extraperitoneal procedure should be performed if preoperative documentation and localization are successful. This avoids further peritoneal contamination from drainage.

Septic Shock

Septic shock describes an infection-induced, generalized hypoperfusion with decreased delivery and consumption of oxygen and other metabolites by the peripheral tissues. Although generally associated with gram-negative sepsis in adults, it may be secondary to a variety of different pathogens in children. In its initial phase, septic shock is characterized by diffuse vasodilation and decreased peripheral vascular resistance, which is manifested clinically by a flushed appearance (i.e., "warm" shock). Despite compensatory tachycardia and increased cardiac output, hypotension is generally present. The vasodilation is accompanied by a relative hypovolemia with a diminished cardiac preload and a redistribution of blood flow, which is reflected in hypoxemia, oliguria, and altered mental status. With progression, generalized capillary leak ensues, resulting in peripheral and pulmonary edema, exacerbating the hypoperfusion and hypoxemia. The subsequent release of endogenous catecholamines precipitates intense vasoconstriction and increased peripheral resistance, which may transiently normalize blood pressure at the further expense of peripheral perfusion (i.e., "cold" shock). Ultimately, intractable metabolic acidosis and myocardial depression ensues with dropping cardiac output and death.

Successful management of the child with septic shock depends on effective treatment of the sepsis and intense supportive measures. Accurate monitoring is mandatory and necessitates a minimum of an arterial line, a central line or pulmonary artery catheter, and bladder catheterization. The goal of therapy is to maximize perfusion and oxygen delivery (Fig. 44–6). Endotracheal intubation and ventilatory support is undertaken to optimize oxygen saturation. Hypovolemia and diminished preload are corrected with crystalloid therapy to achieve and maintain a central venous pressure of at least 10 or a pulmonary wedge pressure of at least 12. Blood is administered as indicated to normalize the hematocrit and oxygen-carrying capacity. Acid-base and electrolyte abnormalities, particularly calcium, are corrected. If perfusion remains inadequate after these maneuvers, vasoactive support, inotropic support, or both are indicated. During the initial phase of vasodilation, dopamine may be employed at low dosage (2–4 µg/kg per minute) to correct abnormalities in the distribution of blood flow. If further support is necessary, dobutamine (2–20 µg/kg per minute) is used to improve myocardial contractility. In appropriate circumstances, dobutamine may be combined with low-dose dopamine to achieve the potential benefits of improved cardiac output and redirection of the flow to more vital areas. Vasodilators may be helpful for vasoconstriction. They should only be employed when the blood pressure is normal and associated with an increased left ventricular filling pressure. Under these circumstances, nitroprusside (0.5–10 µg/kg per minute), carefully titrated, can maximize tissue perfusion.[67, 68, 169]

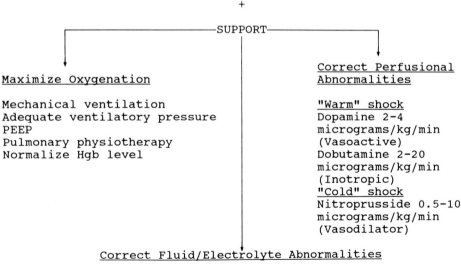

FIGURE 44–6

Management of septic shock. PEEP, Positive end-expiratory pressure; Hgb, hemoglobin; CVP, central venous pressure; PWP, pulmonary wedge pressure; HCT, hematocrit; Ca, calcium; pH, acid-base scale.

Multiorgan Failure

The potential consequence of sepsis-induced hypoperfusion and hypoxemia is organ system failure. In the adult trauma patient, sepsis-related multiorgan failure accounts for most late deaths. A similar pathophysiology has been described in the pediatric patient, although characteristic differences are apparent. Organ system failure is defined on the basis of physiologic and therapeutic data pertinent to one of several accepted organ systems. The pediatric criteria are outlined in Table 44–15. In the child, as in the adult, mortality is directly related to the total number of systems failed, and approaches 80 to 90% with four-system involvement. Pediatric mortality is greatest with simultaneous organ system involvement rather than progressive failure. The respiratory and cardiovascular systems are the most frequently involved systems in children, among whom there is a relatively low incidence of renal failure. Sepsis can be identified as the inciting process of more than 50% of pediatric cases of multiorgan failure.[203, 204]

Table 44–15
Criteria for Failure of Specific Organ Systems

Organ System	Criteria
Cardiovascular	MAP <50 mm Hg HR <40 beats/min Cardiac arrest Continuous vasoactive drug infusion for hemodynamic support
Respiratory	RR >70/min Pao_2 <40 mm Hg (in absence of cyanotic heart disease) $Paco_2$ >65 mm Hg Pao_2/Fio_2 <250 mm Hg Mechanical ventilation (>24 hr if postoperative) Tracheal intubation for airway obstruction or acute respiratory failure
Neurologic	Glasgow coma scale <5 Fixed, dilated pupils Persistent (>20 min) intracranial pressure >20 mm Hg or requiring therapeutic intervention
Hematologic	Hemoglobin <5 gm/dl Leukocytes <3000 cells/mm³ Platelets <20,000/mm³ Disseminated intravascular coagulopathy (PT >20 sec, or a PTT >60 sec in presence of positive FSP assay)
Renal	BUN >100 mg/dl Serum creatinine >2 mg/dl Dialysis
Gastrointestinal	Blood transfusions >20 ml/kg in 24 hr because of GI hemorrhage
Hepatic	Total bilirubin >5 mg/dl and SGOT or LDH more than twice normal value (without evidence of hemolysis) Hepatic encephalopathy

MAP, Mean arterial pressure; HR, heart rate; RR, respiratory rate; Pao_2, partial pressure of oxygen; $Paco_2$, partial pressure of carbon dioxide; Fio_2, fraction of inspired oxygen; PT, prothrombin time; PTT, partial thromboplastin time; FSP, fibrin split products; BUN, blood urea nitrogen; LDH, lactate dehydrogenase; SGOT, serum glutamic-oxaloacetic transaminase.

References

1. Aeder MI, Wellman JL, Hagga JR, et al: Role of surgical and percutaneous drainage in the treatment of abdominal abscesses. Arch Surg 118:273–280, 1983.
2. Alexander JW, Hegg M, Altemeier WA: Neutrophil function in selected surgical disorders. Ann Surg 158:447–458, 1968.
3. Alexander JW, McClellan MA, Ogle CK, et al: Consumptive opsoninopathy: Possible pathogenesis in lethal and opportunistic infections. Ann Surg 184:672–678, 1976.
4. Alexander JW, Ogle CK, Stinnett JD, et al: A sequential, prospective analysis of immunologic abnormalities and infection following severe thermal injury. Ann Surg 188:809–816, 1978.
5. Almqvist PM, Ekstrom B, Keunzig M, et al: Increased survival of endotoxin-injected dogs treated with methylprednisolone, naloxone, and ibuprofen. Circ Shock 14:129–136, 1984.
6. Almqvist PM, Keuznig M, Schwartz SI: Treatment of experimental endotoxin shock with ibuprofen, a cyclooxygenase inhibitor. Circ Shock 13:227–232, 1984.
7. Altura B, Hershey SG: RES phagocytic function in trauma and adaptation to experimental shock. Am J Physiol 215:1414–1418, 1968.
8. Ambruso DR, Altenburger KM, Johnson RB Jr: Defective oxidative metabolism in newborn neutrophils: Discrepancy between superoxide anion and hydroxyl radical generation. Pediatrics 64(suppl):722–725, 1979.
9. Antonacci AC, Good RA, Gupta S: T-cell subpopulations following thermal injury. Surg Gynecol Obstet 155:1–8, 1982.
10. Antonacci AC, Reaves LE, Calvano SE, et al: Flow cytometric analysis of lymphocyte subpopulations after thermal injury in human beings. Surg Gynecol Obstet 159:1–8, 1984.
11. Antrum RM, Solomkin JS: Complement activation products and monocyte migratory function in trauma. Curr Surg 42:301–303, 1985.
12. Arenson EB, Epstein MB, Seeger RC: Monocyte subsets in neonates and children. Pediatrics 64(suppl):740–744, 1979.
13. Armstrong CW, Mayhead CG, Miller K, et al: Infectious complications of hyperalimentation (abstract 861). Twenty-first Interscience Conference on Antimicrobial Agents and Chemotherapy, Chicago, November, 1981.
14. Arnold W: Urinary tract infections. In: Steele RW (ed): A Clinical Manual of Pediatric Infectious Disease. East Norwalk, Conn, Appleton-Century-Crofts, 1986, pp 231–248.
15. Ascher NL, Ahrenholz DH, Simmons RL, et al: ¹¹¹Indium autologous tagged leukocytes in the diagnosis of intraperitoneal sepsis. Arch Surg 114:386–392, 1979.
16. Ashuson GL: An overview of T-suppressor cell circuits. Ann Rev Immunol 4:37–68, 1986.
17. Atik M: Granulocyte adherence assay in acute infection as a reflection of the host resistance. Surg Gynecol Obstet 149:879–880, 1979.
18. Babior B: Oxygen dependent microbial killing by phagocytes. N Engl J Med 298:659–668, 1978.
19. Baker CC, Oppenheimer L, Stephen B, et al: Epidemiology of trauma deaths. Am J Surg 140:144–150, 1980.
20. Band JD, Maki DG: Infections caused by arterial catheters used for hemodynamic monitoring. Am J Med 67:735–741, 1979.
21. Baracos V, Rodeman HP, Dinarello CA, et al: Stimulation of muscle protein degradation and prostaglandin E_2 release by a leukocytic pyrogen: A mechanism for increased degradation of muscle protein during fever. N Engl J Med 308:545–552, 1983.
22. Bartlett JG: Intraabdominal abscesses: Pathogenesis and antibiotic selection. In: Simmons RL (ed): Topics in Intraabdominal Surgical Infection. East Norwalk, Conn, Appleton-Century-Crofts, 1982, pp 49–64.
23. Bauer AR Jr, McNeil C, Trentelman E, et al: The depression of T lymphocytes after trauma. Am J Surg 136:674–680, 1978.
24. Bayley N, Stolz HR: Maturational changes in rectal temperatures of 61 infants from 1 to 36 months. Child Dev 8:195–206, 1937.
25. Beisel WR: Metabolic effects of infection. Prog Food Nutr Sci 8:43–75, 1984.
26. Beisel WR, Rapoport MI: Inter-relations between adrenocortical functions and infectious illness. N Engl J Med 280:541–546, 569–604, 1969.

27. Benson DR, Riggins RS, Lawrence RM, et al: Treatment of open fractures: A prospective study. J Trauma 23:25–30, 1983.

28. Bergman BR: Antibiotic prophylaxis in open and closed fractures. Acta Orthop Scand 53:57–62, 1982.

29. Bjork J, Hugli TE, Smedegard G: Microvascular effects of anaphylatoxins C3a and C5a. J Immunol 134:1115–1119, 1985.

30. Bjornson AB, Altemeier WA, Bjornson HS: Host defense against opportunist microorganisms following trauma. II. Changes in complement and immunoglobulins in patients with abdominal trauma and in septic patients without trauma. Ann Surg 188:102–108, 1978.

31. Bjornson AB, Altemeier WA, Bjornson HS: A model for studying the role of complement and immunologlobulins in opsonization of opportunist microorganisms. Ann Surg 189:515–527, 1979.

32. Bjornson AB, Altemeier WA, Bjornson HS: Complement, opsonins, and the immune response to bacterial infection in burned patients. Ann Surg 191:323–329, 1980.

33. Bjornson AB, Altemeier WA, Bjornson HS, et al: Host defense against opportunist microorganisms following trauma. I. Studies to determine the association between changes in humoral components of host defense and septicemia in burned patients. Ann Surg 188:93–101, 1978.

34. Bjornson AB, Bjornson HS, Altemeier WA: Reduction in alternative in complement pathway mediated C3 conversion following burn injury. Ann Surg 194:224–231, 1981.

35. Bjornson AB, Bjornson HS, Altemeier WA: Serum-mediated inhibition of polymorphonuclear leukocyte function following burn injury. Ann Surg 194:568–575, 1981.

36. Bjornson HS: Bacterial synergy, virulence factors, and host defense mechanisms in the pathogenesis of intraabdominal infections. In: Simmons RL (ed): Topics in intraabdominal surgical infection. East Norwalk, Conn, Appleton-Century-Crofts, 1982, pp 65–78.

37. Blaese RM, Poplack DG, Muchmore AV: The mononuclear phagocyte system: Role in expression of immunocompetence in neonatal and adult life. Pediatrics 64(suppl):829–833, 1979.

38. Brawley RW, Kelley WA: Treatment of basal skull fracture with and without CSF fistulas. J Neurosurg 26:57–61, 1967.

39. Brook I: Microbiology of human and animal bite wounds in children. Pediatr Infect Dis J 6:29–32, 1987.

40. Brubaker RR: Mechanisms of bacterial virulence. Pediatr Surg 39:21–50, 1985.

41. Bukower I, Steicher HZ: The mononuclear phagocyte as antigen presenting cell. Pediatr Ann 16:395–401, 1987.

42. Bunkis J, Walton RL: Wounds. In: Runkey DD, Lewis FR (eds): Current Therapy of Trauma. 2nd ed. St. Louis, CV Mosby, 1986, pp 136–137.

43. Caffee HH, Watts G, Mena J: Gallium citrate scanning in the diagnosis of intraabdominal abscess. Am J Surg 133:665–669, 1977.

44. Carmona RH, Tsao TC, Trunkey DD: The role of prostacyclin and thromboxane in sepsis and septic shock. Arch Surg 119:189–192, 1984.

45. Carpenter AB, Boykin JV Jr, Crute SL, et al: The acridine orange fluorochrome microassay: A new technique for quantitation of neutrophil function in burned patients. J Trauma 26:389–392, 1986.

46. Casey LC, Fletcher JR, Zmudka MI, et al: The role of thromboxane in primate endotoxin shock. J Surg Res 39:140–149, 1985.

47. Christou NV, McLean APH, Meakins JL: Host defense in blunt trauma: Interrelationships of kinetics of energy and depressed neutrophil function, nutritional status, and sepsis. J Trauma 20:833–841, 1980.

48. Clowes GHA Jr, George BC, Villee CA Jr, et al: Muscle proteolysis induced by a circulating peptide in patients with sepsis or trauma. N Engl J Med 308:545–552, 1983.

49. Collins RN, Braun PA, Zinner SH, et al: Risk of local and systemic infection with polyethylene intravenous catheters. A prospective study of 213 catheterizations. N Engl J Med 279:340–343, 1968.

50. Committee on Infectious Diseases, Committee on Drugs, Section on Surgery: Antimicrobial prophylaxis in pediatric surgical patients. Pediatrics 74:437–439, 1984.

51. Cuddy BG, Loegering DJ, Blumenstock FA, et al: Hepatic macrophage complement receptor clearance function following injury. J Surg Res 40:216–224, 1986.

52. Curnow RT, Rayfield EJ, George DT, et al: Altered hepatic glycogen metabolism and glucoregulatory hormones during sepsis. Am J Physiol 230:1296–1301, 1976.

53. Daffner RH, Halber MD, Morgan CL, et al: Computed tomography in the diagnosis of intraabdominal abscesses. Ann Surg 189:29–33, 1979.

54. Davis JM, Dineed P, Gallin JI: Neutrophil degranulation and abnormal chemotaxis after thermal injury. J Immunol 124:1467–1471, 1980.

55. Deitch EA, Dobke M, Baxter CR: Failure of local immunity: A potential cause of burn wound sepsis. Arch Surg 120:78–84, 1985.

56. Deitch EA, Landry KN: Neutrophil subpopulations change after thermal injury. J Trauma 26:534–537, 1986.

57. Dellinger EP, Oreskovich MR, Wertz MJ, et al: Risk of infection following laparotomy for penetrating abdominal injury. Arch Surg 119:20–27, 1984.

58. Dinerallo CA: Interleukin-1. Rev Infect Dis 6:51–95, 1984.

59. Donabedian H, Gallin JI: Deactivation of human neutrophil chemotaxis by chemoattractants: Effect on receptors for the chemotactic factor f-MET-LEU-PHE. J Immunol 127:839–844, 1981.

60. Duque RE, Phan SH, Hudson JL, et al: Functional defects in phagocytic cells following thermal injury: Application of flow cytometric analysis. Am J Pathol 118:116–127, 1985.

61. Edson RS, Keys TF: The aminoglycosides: streptomycin, kanamycin, gentamicin, tobramycin, amikacin, netilmicin, sisomicin. Mayo Clin Proc 58:99–102, 1983.

62. Elsbach P: Degradation of microorganisms by phagocytic cells. Rev Infect Dis 2:106–128, 1980.

63. Elsbach P, Weiss J: Oxygen-dependent and oxygen-independent mechanisms of microbicidal activity of neutrophils. Immunol Lett 11:159–163, 1985.

64. Ersoz CJ: Prolonged femoral arterial catheterization for intensive care. Anesth Analg 49:160–164, 1970.

65. Feder HM Jr, Shanley JD, Barbera JA: Review of 59 patients hospitalized with animal bites. Pediatr Infect Dis J 6:24–28, 1987.

66. Fernandez HN, Henson PM, Otani A, et al: Chemotactic response to human C3a and C5a anaphylatoxins. I. Evaluation of C3a and C5a leukotaxis in vitro and understimulated in vivo conditions. J Immunol 120:109–115, 1978.

67. Fiser DH: Infectious disease emergencies. In: Steele RW (ed): A Clinical Manual of Pediatric Infectious Disease. East Norwalk, Conn, Appleton-Century-Crofts, 1982, pp 37–41.

68. Fiser DH: Infectious diseases. In: Berman IS (ed): Problems in Critical Care. Philadelphia, JB Lippincott, 1987, pp 296–299.

69. Frank MM: The complement system in host defense and inflammation. Rev Infect Dis 1:483–501, 1979.

70. Fry DE, Garrison RN, Heitsch RC, et al: Determinants of death in patients with intraabdominal abscess. Surgery 88:517–523, 1980.

71. George DT, Rayfield EJ, Wannemacher RW Jr: Altered glucoregulatory hormones during acute pneumococcal sepsis in the rhesus monkey. Diabetes 23:544–549, 1974.

72. Geraci JE, Hermans PE: Vancomycin. Mayo Clin Proc 58:88–91, 1983.

73. Glover FL, Richardson JD, Fewel JC, et al: Prophylactic antibiotics in the treatment of penetrating chest wounds. J Thorac Cardiovasc Surg 74:528–536, 1977.

74. Gorbach S: Function of normal human microflora. Scand J Infect Dis Suppl 49:17–30, 1986.

75. Grogan JB: Altered neutrophil phagocytic function in burn patients. J Trauma 16:734–738, 1976.

76. Gustilo RB, Anderson JT: Prevention of infection in the treatment of one thousand and twenty-five open fractures of long bones. J Bone Joint Surg 58:453–458, 1976.

77. Halushka PV, Reines HD, Barrow SE, et al: Elevated plasma 6-keto-prostaglandin FL alpha in patients in septic shock. Crit Care Med 13:451–453, 1985.

78. Harbin RI, Schaffner W: Septicemia associated with "scalp-vein" needles. South Med J 66:638–640, 1973.

79. Hayward AR: T lymphocytes: An update. Pediatr Ann 16:391–394, 1987.

80. Hayward AR, Lydyard PM: B cell function in the newborn. Pediatrics 64(suppl):758–764, 1979.

81. Heevel JG, Boetes C, Van der Werken C, et al: Dewaarde van echografie voor de diagnostiek van intra-abdominale abcessen. Ned Tijdschr Geneeskd 128:546–548, 1984.

82. Homaoka T, Ono S: Regulation of B cell differentiation: Interaction of factors and corresponding receptors. Ann Rev Immunol 4:167–204, 1986.

83. Horn JK, Goldstein IM, Flick MR: Complement and endotoxin-induced lung injury in sheep. J Surg Res 36:420–427, 1984.

84. Howard RJ: Host defense against infection—Part I. Curr Probl Surg 27:268–275, 1980.

85. Howard RJ, Simmons RL: Acquired immunologic deficiencies after trauma and surgical procedures. Surg Gynecol Obstet 139:771–782, 1974.

86. Ignelzi RJ, Vanderarh GD: Analysis of treatment of basilar skull fracture with and without antibiotics. J Neurosurg 43:721–726, 1975.

87. Jarvis WR: Epidemiology of nosocomial infections in pediatric patients. Pediatr Infect Dis J 6:344–351, 1987.

88. Jarvis WR, White JW, Munn VP, et al: Nosocomial infection surveillance, 1983. MMWR 33:9SS–21SS, 1985.

89. Johnson WC, Gerzof SG, Robbins AH, et al: Treatment of abdominal abscesses. Comparative evaluation of operative drainage versus percutaneous catheter drainage guided by computed tomography or ultrasound. Ann Surg 194:510–520, 1981.

90. Johnston RB Jr, Altenburger KM, Atkinson AW Jr, et al: Complement in the newborn infant. Pediatrics 64(suppl):781–786, 1979.

91. Kellerman JS, Brown GL, Lamont PM, et al: Characterization of neutrophil iodination for the assessment of phagocytic and opsonic function in septic patients. Am J Surg 150:301–305, 1985.

92. Klastersky J, Sadeghi M, Brihave J: Antimicrobial prophylaxis in patients with rhinorrhea and otorrhea: A double blind study. Surg Neurol 6:111–114, 1976.

93. Klebanoff SJ: Mycloperoxidase-halide-hydrogen peroxide antibacterial system. J Bacteriol 95:2131–2138, 1968.

94. Knochel JQ, Koehler PR, Lee TG, et al: Diagnosis of abdominal abscess with computed tomography, ultrasound and ¹¹¹In leukocyte scans. Radiology 137:425–432, 1980.

95. Koehler PR, Knochel JQ: Computed tomography in the evaluation of abdominal abscesses. Am J Surg 140:675–678, 1980.

96. Konn G, Himal HS: Leukocyte lysosomal function in sepsis. Surg Gynecol Obstet 159:457–460, 1984.

97. Krob MJ, Shelby J: Immunosuppressive effects of burn injury and nonspecific blood transfusion. J Trauma 26:40–43, 1986.

98. Lanser ME, Brown GE, Mora R, et al: Trauma serum suppresses superoxide production by normal neutrophils. Arch Surg 121:157–162, 1986.

99. Lanser ME, Mao P, Brown GE, et al: Neutrophil chemiluminescence and opsonic fibronectin levels following blunt trauma. J Surg Res 41:264–273, 1986.

100. Lanser ME, Mao P, Brown GE, et al: Serum mediated depression of neutrophil chemiluminescence following blunt trauma. Ann Surg 202:111–118, 1985.

101. Lanser ME, Saba TM: Opsonic fibronectin deficiency and sepsis: Cause or effect? Ann Surg 195:340–345, 1985.

102. Larsen GL, Henson PM: Mediators of inflammation. Annu Rev Immunol 1:335–359, 1983.

103. LeBlanc KA, Tucker WY: Prophylactic antibiotics and closed tube thoracostomy. Surg Gynecol Obstet 160:259–263, 1985.

104. Lindsey D, Christopher M, Hollenbach J, et al: Natural course of the human bite wound: Incidence of infection and complications in 434 bites and 803 lacerations in the same group of patients. J Trauma 27:45–48, 1987.

105. Lobe TE, Stein M: The effects of trauma on cell mediated immunity (CMI) in childhood. Pediatr Res 20:181A, 1986.

106. Long CL, Kinney JM, Geiger JW: Nonsuppressibility of glucogenesis by glucose in septic patients. Metabolism 25:193–201, 1976.

107. McIrvine A, O'Mahony JB, Saporoschetz I, et al: Depressed immune response in burn patients: Use of monoclonal antibodies and functional assays to define the role of suppressor cells. Ann Surg 196:297–304, 1982.

108. Mackowiak PA: Microbial synergism in human infections (2nd of 2 parts). N Engl J Med 298:83, 1978.

109. Maderazo EG, Albano SC, Woronick CL, et al: Polymorphonuclear leukocyte migration abnormalities and their significance in seriously traumatized patients. Ann Surg 198:736–742, 1983.

110. Maki DG, Drinka PJ, Davis TF: Suppurative phlebitis of an arm vein from a "scalp vein" needle. N Engl J Med 292:1116–1117, 1975.

111. Manktelow A, Meyer AA: Lack of correlation between decreased chemotaxis and susceptibility to infection in burned rats. J Trauma 26:143–148, 1986.

112. Meakins JL, McLean APH, Kelly R, et al: Delayed hypersensitivity and neutrophil chemotaxis: Effect on trauma. J Trauma 18:240–247, 1978.

113. Melchers F, Anderson J: Factors controlling the B-cell cycle. Annu Rev Immunol 4:13–36, 1986.

114. Michel L: Microbial colonization of indwelling central venous catheters: Statistical evaluation of potential contaminating factors. Am J Surg 137:745–748, 1979.

115. Miller-Eberhard HJ: The membrane attack complex of complement. Annu Rev Immunol 4:503–528, 1986.

116. Miller ME: Phagocytic function in the neonate: Selected aspects. Pediatrics 64(suppl):709–712, 1979.

117. Moir C, Robins RE: Role of ultrasonography, gallium scanning, and computed tomography in the diagnosis of intra-abdominal abscess. Am J Surg 143:582–585, 1982.

118. Moon B, Girotti MJ, Wren SF, et al: PMN superoxide radical production following a metabolic-endocrine simulation of trauma. Ann Surg 203:246–249, 1986.

119. Moore FD Jr, Davis C, Rodrick M, et al: Neutrophil activation in thermal injury as assessed by increased expression of complement receptors. N Engl J Med 314:948–953, 1986.

120. Moran JM, Atwood RP, Rowe MI, et al: A clinical and bacteriologic study of infections associated with venous cutdowns. N Engl J Med 272:554–560, 1965.

121. Mosesson MW, Amrani DL: The structure and biologic activities of plasma fibronectin. Blood 56:145–158, 1980.

122. Munster AM: Immunologic response of trauma and burns. Am J Med 76:142–145, 1984.

123. Nathenson G, Miller ME, Myers KA, et al: Decreased opsonic and chemotactic activities in sera of postburn patients and partial opsonic restoration with properdin and properdin convertase. Clin Immunol Immunopathol 9:269–276, 1978.

124. Nelson RD, McCormack RT, Fiegel VD, et al: Chemotactic deactivation of human neutrophils: Evidence for nonspecific and specific components. Infect Immun 22:441–444, 1978.

125. Neufield HA, Pace JA, Kaminski MY, et al: A probable endocrine basis for the depression of ketone bodies during infections or inflammatory state in rats. Endocrinology 107:596–601, 1980.

126. Nichols RL: The role of anaerobes in intraabdominal surgical infections. In: Simmons RL (ed): Topics in Intraabdominal Surgical Infection. East Norwalk, Conn, Appleton-Century-Crofts, 1982, pp 27–48.

127. Nichols RL, Smith JW, Klein DB, et al: Risk of infection after penetrating abdominal trauma. N Engl J Med 311:1065–1070, 1984.

128. Ninnemann JL, Stockland AE: Participation of prostaglandin E in immunosuppression following thermal injury. J Trauma 24:201–207, 1984.

129. Norton L, Eule J, Burdick D: Accuracy of techniques to detect intraperitoneal abscess. Surgery 84:370–378, 1978.

130. Odeburg H, Olsson I: Antibacterial activity of cationic proteins from human granulocytes. J Clin Invest 56:1118–1124, 1975.

131. Olson LM, Moss GS, Baukus O, et al: The role of C5 in septic lung injury. Ann Surg 202:771–776, 1985.

132. O'Mahony JB, Palder SB, Wood JJ, et al: Depression of cellular immunity after multiple trauma in the absence of sepsis. J Trauma 24:869–875, 1984.

133. O'Mahony JB, Wood JJ, Rodrick ML, et al: Changes in T lymphocyte subsets following injury: Assessment by flow cytometry and relationship to sepsis. Ann Surg 202:580–586, 1985.

134. Onderdonk AB, Bartlett JG, Louie TJ, et al: Microbial synergy in experimental intraabdominal abscess. Infect Immun 13:22–26, 1975.

135. Onderdonk AB, Weinstein WM, Sullivan NM, et al: Experimental intraabdominal abscesses in rats: II. Quantitative bacteriology of infected animals. Infect Immun 10:1256–1259, 1974.

136. Parish RA, Novack AH, Heimbach DM, et al: Fever as a predictor of infection in burned children. J Trauma 27:69–71, 1987.

137. Parker M, Ognibene F, Natanson C, et al: Elevated C5A levels in patients with septic shock. Crit Care Med 13:303–307, 1985.

138. Patzakis MJ, Wilkins J, Moore TM: Considerations in reducing the infection rate in open tibial fracture. Clin Orthop 178:36–41, 1983.

139. Patzakis MJ, Wilkins J, Moore TM: Use of antibiotics in open tibial fractures. Clin Orthop 178:31–35, 1983.

140. Peter G, Lloyd-Still JD, Lovejoy FH: Local infection and bacteremia from scalp vein needles and polyethylene catheters in children. J Pediatr 80:78–83, 1972.

141. Pitcher WD, Musher DM: Critical importance of early diagnosis and treatment of intraabdominal infection. Arch Surg 117:328–333, 1982.

142. Polk HC Jr, Lopez-Mayor JF: Postoperative wound infection: A prospective study of determinant factors and prevention. Surgery 66:97–103, 1969.

143. Polk HC Jr, Wellhausen SR, Regan MP, et al: A systematic study of host defense processes in badly injured patients. Ann Surg 204:282–299, 1986.

144. Powanda MC: Change in body balance of nitrogen and other key nutrients: Description and underlying mechanism. Am J Clin Nutr 30:1254, 1977.

145. Powanda MC, Beisel WR: Hypothesis: Leukocyte endogenous mediator/endogenous pyrogen/lymphocyte-activating factor modulates the development of nonspecific and specific immunity and affects nutritional status. Am J Clin Nutr 35:762–768, 1982.

146. Prince A: Management of fever in patients with central vein catheters. Pediatr Infect Dis 5:20–24, 1986.

147. Pruitt BA: Diagnosis and treatment of cannula-related intravenous sepsis in burn patients. Ann Surg 191:546–554, 1980.

148. Quier PG, Mills EL: Bactericidal and metabolic function of polymorphonuclear leukocytes. Pediatrics 64(suppl):719–721, 1979.

149. Regel G, Nerlich ML, Dwenger A, et al: Phagocytic function of polymorphonuclear leukocytes and the RES in endotoxemia. J Surg Res 42:74–84, 1987.

150. Reines HD, Halushka PV, Cook JA: Plasma thromboxane levels are elevated in patients dying with septic shock. Lancet 2:174–175, 1982.

151. Rich RR, El Mosby MN, Fox EJ: Human suppressor T cell: Induction, differentiation and regulatory functions. Hum Immunol 17:369–387, 1986.

152. Roamin PL, Schlossman SF: Human T-lymphocyte subsets: Functional heterogenecity and surface recognition structures. J Clin Invest 74:1559–1565, 1984.

153. Robinson DR: Prostaglandins and the mechanisms of action of antiinflammatory drugs. Am J Med 75:26–31, 1983.

154. Robinson JG, Pollock TO: Computed tomography in the diagnosis and localization of intraabdominal abscess. Am J Surg 140:783–786, 1980.

155. Robson MC, Lea CE, Dalton JB, et al: Quantitative bacteriology and delayed wound closure. Surg Forum 19:501, 1968.

156. Roettinger W, Edgerton MT, Kurtz LD, et al: Role of inoculation site as determinant of infection in soft tissue wounds. Am J Surg 126:354–358, 1973.

157. Rogers FB, Sheaff CM, Nolan PJ, et al: Fibronectin depletion and microaggregate clearance following trauma. J Trauma 26:339–342, 1986.

158. Rolfe RD: Interactions among microorganisms of the indigenous intestinal flora and their influence on the host. Rev Infect Dis Suppl 6:73–79, 1984.

159. Rosenblatt JE, Edson RS: Metronidazole. Mayo Clin Proc 58:154–157, 1983.

160. Roth AI, Fry DE, Polk HC Jr: Infectious morbidity in extremity fractures. J Trauma 26:757–761, 1986.

161. Rowley KM: Right-sided infective endocarditis as a consequence of flow-directed pulmonary-artery catheterization. A clinicopathological study of 55 autopsied patients. N Engl J Med 311:1152–1156, 1984.

162. Rush DS, Nochols RL: Risk of infection following penetrating abdominal trauma: A selective review. Yale J Biol Med 59:395–401, 1986.

163. Saba TM: Physiology and pathophysiology of the reticuloendothelial system. Arch Intern Med 126:1031–1052, 1970.

164. Saba TM, McCaffety MH, Lanser ME: Depressed reticuloendothelial function in the surgical patient. Infect Surg 1:124–131, 1983.

165. Saini S, Kellum JM, O'Leary MP, et al: Improved localization and survival in patients with intraabdominal abscesses. Am J Surg 14:136–142, 1983.

166. Schmidt J: Purification and partial biochemical characterization of normal human interleukin-1. J Exp Med 160:772–787, 1984.

167. Scovill WA, Saba TM, Blumenstock FA, et al: Opsonic alpha$_2$ surface binding glycoprotein therapy during sepsis. Ann Surg 188:521–529, 1978.

168. Scovill WA, Saba RM, Kaplan JE, et al: Disturbances in circulating opsonic activity in man after operative and blunt trauma. J Surg Res 22:709–16, 1977.

169. Shaffner DH Jr, Aronoff SC: The management of septic shock. In: Gellis SS, Kagan BM (eds): Current Pediatric Therapy. Philadelphia, WB Saunders, 1986, pp 620–624.

170. Simmons RL, Ahrenholz DH: Pathobiology of peritonitis: A review. J Antimicrob Chemother 7:29–36, 1981.

171. Simmons RL, Ahrenholz DH: Therapeutic principles in peritonitis. In: Simmons RL (ed): Topics in Intraabdominal Surgical Infection. East Norwalk, Conn, Appleton-Century-Crofts, 1982, pp 1–27.

172. Simpkins CO, Alailima ST, Tate EA, et al: The effect of enkephalins and prostaglandins on O$_2$ release by neutrophils. J Surg Res 41:645–652, 1986.

173. Slotman GJ, Quinn JV, Burchard KW: Thromboxane interaction with cardiopulmonary dysfunction in graded bacterial sepsis. J Trauma 24:803–810, 1984.

174. Smits H, Freedman LR: Prolonged venous catheterization as a cause of sepsis. N Engl J Med 276:1229–1233, 1967.

175. Snyderman R: Regulatory mechanisms of a chemoattractant receptor on leukocytes. Fed Proc 43:2743–2748, 1984.

176. Soderstrom CA, Wasserman DH, Cowley RA, et al: Arterial monitoring catheters: A prospective study of use and complications. Crit Care Med 9:203, 1981.

177. Solomkin JS, Bauman MP, Nelson RD, et al: Neutrophils dysfunction during the course of intraabdominal infection. Ann Surg 194:9–17, 1981.

178. Solomkin JS, Brodt JK, Antrum RM: Suppressed neutrophil oxidative activity in sepsis: A receptor-mediated regulatory response. J Surg Res 39:300–304, 1985.

179. Solomkin JS, Brodt JK, Zleman FP: Degranulation inhibition: A potential mechanism for control of neutrophil superoxide production in sepsis. Arch Surg 121:77–80, 1986.

180. Solomkin JS, Cotta LA, Brodt JK, et al: Neutrophil dysfunction in sepsis. III. Degranulation as a mechanism for nonspecific deactivation. J Surg Res 36:407–412, 1984.

181. Solomkin JS, Cotta LA, Brodt JK, et al: Regulation of neutrophil superoxide production in sepsis. Arch Surg 120:93–98, 1985.

182. Solomkin JS, Jenkins MK, Nelson RD, et al: Neutrophil dysfunction in sepsis. II. Evidence for the role of complement activation products in cellular deactivation. Surgery 90:319–327, 1981.

183. Solomkin JS, Nelson RD, Chenoweth DR, et al: Regulation of neutrophil migratory function in burn injury by complement activation products. Ann Surg 200:742–746, 1984.

184. Stiehm ER, Winter HS, Bryson YJ: Cellular (T cell) immunity in the human newborn. Pediatrics 64(suppl):822–828, 1979.

185. Stites DP, Pavia CS: Ontogeny of human T cells. Pediatrics 64(suppl):795–802, 1979.

186. Stone HH, Symbas PN, Hooper CA: Cefamandole for prophylaxis against infection in closed tube thoracostomy. J Trauma 21:975–977, 1981.

187. Stossel TP: Phagocytosis. N Engl J Med 290:717–723, 1974.

188. Stossel TP: Phagocytosis. N Engl J Med 290:774–781, 1974.

189. Taylor KWJ, Wasson JFM, deGraaff C, et al: Accuracy of grey-scale ultrasound diagnosis of abdominal and pelvic abscesses in 220 patients. Lancet 1:83–84, 1978.

190. Teodorczyk-Injeyan JA, Sparkes BG, Mills GB, et al: Impairment of T cell activation in burn patients: A possible mechanism of thermal injury-induced immunosuppression. Clin Exp Immunol 65:570–581, 1986.

191. Thompson RL, Wright AJ: Cephalosporin antibiotics. Mayo Clin Proc 58:79–87, 1983.

192. Trott A: Care of mammalian bites. Pediatr Infect Dis J 6:8–10, 1987.

193. Van Epps DE, Goodwin JS, Murphy S: Age-dependent variations in polymorphonuclear leukocyte chemiluminescence. Infect Immun 22:57–61, 1978.

194. VanSonnenberg E, Ferrucci JT Jr, Mueller PR, et al: Percutaneous drainage of abscesses in fluid collections: Technique, results, and applications. Radiology 142:1–10, 1982.

195. Wara DW, Barrett DJ: Cell-mediated immunity in the newborn: Clinical aspects. Pediatrics 64(suppl):822–828, 1979.

196. Warden GD, Mason AD Jr, Pruitt BA Jr: Evaluation of leukocyte chemotaxis in vitro in thermally injured patients. J Clin Invest 54:1001–1004, 1974.

197. Waymack JP, Gallon L, Barcelli U, et al: Effect of blood transfusions on immune function. III. Alterations in macrophage arachidonic acid metabolism. Arch Surg 122:56–60, 1987.

198. Waymack JP, Gallon L, Barcelli U, et al: Effect of blood transfusions on macrophage function in a burned animal model. Curr Surg 43:305–307, 1986.

199. Weinberg ED: Iron and susceptibility to infectious disease. Science 184:952–956, 1974.

200. Weinstein WM, Onderdonk AB, Bartlett JG, et al: Antimicrobial

therapy of experimental intraabdominal sepsis. J Infect Dis 132:282–286, 1975.

201. Weinstein WM, Onderdonk AB, Bartlett JB, et al: Experimental intraabdominal abscesses in rats: I. Development of an experimental model. Infect Immun 10:1250–1255, 1974.

202. Whittle BJR, Moncada S: Pharmacologic interactions between prostacyclin and thromboxanes. Br Med Bull 39:232–238, 1983.

203. Wilkinson JD, Pollack MM, Glass NL, et al: Mortality associated with multiple organ system failure and sepsis in the pediatric intensive care unit. J Pediatr 111:324–328, 1987.

204. Wilkinson JD, Pollack MM, Ruttimann UE, et al: Outcome of pediatric patients with multiple organ system failure. Crit Care Med 14:271–274, 1986.

205. Wilkinson PC: Leukocyte locomotion and chemotaxis: Effects of bacteria and viruses. Rev Infect Dis 2:293–318, 1980.

206. Wilkinson PC: Random locomotion, chemotaxis and chemokinesis. Immunol Today 6:273–278, 1985.

207. Williams TJ: Interactions between prostaglandins, leukotrienes, and other mediators of inflammation. Br Med Bull 39:239–242, 1983.

208. Wilson WR, Cockerill FR III: Tetracyclines, chloramphenicol, erythromycin, clindamycin. Mayo Clin Proc 58:92–98, 1983.

209. Wolfe JHN, Saporoschetz I, Young AE, et al: Suppressive serum, suppressor lymphocytes, and death from burns. Ann Surg 193:513–520, 1981.

210. Wolfe JHN, Wu AVO, O'Connor NE, et al: Anergy, immunosuppressive serum, and impaired lymphocyte blastogenesis in burn patients. Arch Surg 117:1266–1271, 1982.

211. Wood JJ, Grbic JT, Rodrick AJ, et al: Suppression of interleukin 2 production in an animal model of thermal injury is related to prostaglandin synthesis. Arch Surg 122:179–184, 1987.

212. Wood JJ, O'Mahoney JB, Rodrick ML: Abnormalities of antibody production after thermal injury. Arch Surg 121:108–115, 1986.

213. Wood JJ, Rodrick ML, O'Mahoney JB, et al: Inadequate interleukin 2 production: A fundamental immunological deficiency in patients with major burns. Ann Surg 200:311–320, 1984.

214. Wright AJ, Wiklowske CJ: The penicillins. Mayo Clin Proc 58:21–32, 1983.

215. Wright HK, Dunn E, MacArthur JD, et al: Specific but limited role of new imaging techniques in decision-making about intraabdominal abscesses. Am J Surg 143:456–459, 1982.

216. Yeung RSW, Buck JR, Filler RM: The significance of fever following operations in children. J Pediatr Surg 17:347–349, 1982.

217. Yurt RW, Shires GT: Increased susceptibility to infection due to infusion of exogenous chemotaxin. Arch Surg 122:111–116, 1987.

218. Zimmerman JJ, Shelhamer JH, Parrillo JE: Quantitative analysis of polymorphonuclear leukocyte superoxide anion generation in critically ill children. Crit Care Med 13:143–150, 1985.

John R. Wesley
Arnold G. Coran

Nutritional Management in Pediatric Trauma

The nutritional management of the pediatric trauma victim represents a different and sometimes more complex therapeutic problem than does support of the injured adult. In addition to the metabolic demands imposed by the traumatic event, special consideration must be given in the pediatric patient to the smaller body size, the highly variable fluid requirements, rapid growth, and, in the newborn, the immaturity of certain organ systems. These factors, plus the low caloric reserves in the young child, make adequate nutrition particularly important. Furthermore, because the traumatized child is usually otherwise healthy with no underlying debilitating disease, his or her nutritional support may be overlooked in the initial days of management. Consequently, the pediatric patient whose nutritional needs are not met can very rapidly develop protein-calorie malnutrition. That this is indeed a problem is clear from a nutritional survey in a large pediatric referral center, which demonstrated that one third of the hospitalized patients had evidence of acute malnutrition.[41] Even a relatively short period of inadequate nutrition can result in decreased host resistance, increased risk of infection, and poor wound healing, which in turn contributes appreciably to morbidity and mortality in infants and children recovering from accidental trauma and associated corrective surgical procedures. Whereas the nutritional requirements of teenagers do not differ significantly from those of adults, the requirements of infants and young children are very different. This chapter focuses on the nutritional requirements, assessment, and support of the pediatric age groups most often involved in trauma—the toddler, young child, and teenager. Emphasis is placed on basic nutritional requirements, the metabolic response to trauma, nutritional assessment, indications for initiating nutritional support, techniques of administration, monitoring, and the complications associated with both enteral and parenteral nutrition.

BASIC NUTRITIONAL REQUIREMENTS

When a patient is recovering from major trauma, he or she frequently cannot or will not eat or drink sufficient amounts to supply ongoing energy needs. These patients quickly use up readily available glucose and glycogen stores and pirate fat and protein stores, to the detriment of visceral and somatic muscle function and immune defenses. Most otherwise healthy older children and teenagers can tolerate this form of energy deficit-spending for 5 to 7 days, after which time increased muscular weakness and impaired host defenses begin to cause clinical problems. Infants and younger children have a shorter time period during which they can tolerate lack of nutritional support. Managing physicians must recognize the problem, estimate or measure the patient's nutritional needs, provide calorie and protein support in the right mix by the most efficient route, and monitor whether or not these efforts are effective. The discussion that follows includes a review of useful nutritional physiology and facts.

Water

Infants have a higher water content than adults (70–75% of body weight versus 60–65%); therefore, the water require-

ments of infants and small children per unit of body weight are greater. The healthy infant consumes water at a daily rate of 10 to 15% of body weight, in contrast to only 2 to 4% in the teenager and adult. In infants who are in good health, only 0.5 to 3% of fluid intake is retained; approximately 50% is excreted through the kidneys, 3 to 10% is lost through the gastrointestinal tract, and 40 to 50% is insensible loss.

Calories

The caloric requirements for infants and children at different ages are outlined in Table 45–1. Energy requirements are often increased by periods of active growth and extreme physical activity. In addition, major trauma or surgical stress increases the caloric requirements as follows: 12% increase for each degree of fever above 37°C, 20 to 30% increase with a major operation, 40 to 50% increase with severe sepsis, and 50 to 100% increase with major burns. In establishing a daily caloric budget for hospitalized patients, the physician should approximate the distribution of kilocalories according to that found in a well-balanced diet: protein, 15%; carbohydrate, 50%; and fat, 35%.

Carbohydrates

The three sources of energy are carbohydrate, fat, and protein. Carbohydrate, including ketones and alcohol, is the most important immediate energy source, but it is in the shortest supply. The total carbohydrate reserve in the average 70-kg man is only 2400 calories, distributed approximately equally between the liver and skeletal muscle. This carbohydrate reserve is stored primarily as glycogen, and in the infant, accounts for approximately 10% of body weight. The liver and muscle mass is proportionately much smaller in the child than in the adult; therefore, the infant's and young child's carbohydrate reserve is significantly smaller. Glycogen is converted to glucose within the liver and is then metabolized throughout the body, either aerobically to carbon dioxide and water (38 mol of adenosine triphosphate/mol of glucose) or anaerobically to lactic acid (2 mol of adenosine triphosphate/mol of glucose). Aerobic metabolism of carbohydrates supplies 3.4 calories per gram hydrous, requires 1 liter of oxygen for each 5 kcal produced, and gives off a volume of carbon dioxide equal to the volume of oxygen consumed for a respiratory quotient

Table 45–1

Estimated Calorie and Protein Requirements for Infants and Children

Age (y)	Kilocalories (kcal/kg body weight)	Protein (gm/kg body weight)
0–1	90–120	2.0–3.5
1–7	75–90	2.0–2.5
7–12	60–75	2.0
12–18	30–60	1.5
>18	25–30	1.0

(RQ) of one (RQ = ratio of CO_2 produced to O_2 consumed).

Fat

Fat is the major source of nonprotein calories for the human body. Reserves total 140,000 calories in the average 70-kg man. Because young children and rapidly growing adolescents frequently have less fatty tissue than adults, their energy stores are proportionately reduced. Fat is the most efficient energy source per unit of weight, providing 9 kcal per gram and 4.7 kcal per liter of oxygen consumed, with an RQ of 0.7. This is the lowest RQ of the three energy sources, and therefore it results in the least amount of carbon dioxide and respiratory work per unit of energy produced. This is an important fact to consider in setting up a calorie budget for a patient with incipient respiratory failure or in a patient having difficulty being weaned from a respirator.[41] The triglycerides are the most abundant of the dietary fats and contain both saturated and unsaturated long-chain fatty acids. These vary in length from 4 to 24 carbon atoms, most often containing 16 to 18 carbon atoms. Linoleic acid has an 18-carbon chain with two double bonds, cannot be synthesized in the human body, and therefore, is classified as an essential fatty acid. It must be supplied as at least 2 to 4% of the daily administered kilocalories to avoid a deficiency syndrome characterized by hair loss, mental aberrations, and a dry, flaky, erythematous skin rash. In general, fat intake should not exceed 50% of the total caloric load to avoid the fat overload syndrome.

Protein

The protein requirement in infants and children is based on the combined needs of maintenance and growth. Protein makes up 13% of body weight in an infant, compared with 20% in the adult. Most of the increase in body protein occurs during the first year of life; this is reflected in the major protein requirements that exist during infancy. Protein provides 4.1 kcal per gram and 4.5 kcal per each liter of oxygen consumed, with an RQ of 0.8. In normal protein metabolism, there is an ongoing excretion of nitrogen equivalent to approximately 50 gm of protein per day in the adult; this excretion is matched by a comparable protein intake. Protein synthesis and breakdown occur simultaneously, approximating 300 gm a day in the adult, with most endogenous amino acids being recycled into new protein. This protein flux is most conveniently measured as nitrogen flux, and during trauma or critical stress, the rate of protein catabolism generally increases while intake stops, resulting in a condition commonly referred to as negative nitrogen balance.

Body protein is not intended to be an intrinsic energy source, because all body proteins are contained in structural elements whose integrity must be preserved for normal organ function, enzyme elaboration, and antibody production. Nevertheless, it appears that a traumatic event, whether planned or accidental, results in an obligatory catabolism of a variable amount of protein during the first 24 to 48 hours after the event.[33] This protein breakdown is necessary to produce more glucose through the gluconeogenic pathway when other carbohydrate stores have been exhausted. The presence of a negative nitrogen balance does not mean that protein synthesis stops or slows down. On the contrary, synthesis of new cells, collagen, coagulation factors, inflammatory cells, antibodies, and a multitude of other biologic proteins occurs at an accelerated rate during critical stress.

Amino acids derived from the breakdown of muscle tissue or visceral proteins become the building blocks for protein in healing tissues and host defense mechanisms. A traumatic or surgical wound is a privileged site for approximately 14 days, during which time the protein building blocks are diverted from other visceral and somatic sites in favor of wound healing. If exogenous sources of energy and protein have not been reestablished after this period of time, the wound loses its privileged status and becomes a source for needed energy, along with other protein matrices in the body. Left unchecked, this catabolism may lead to wound dehiscence and disastrous infectious complications.

A large part of the goal of nutritional management is to provide an energy source so that endogenous proteins are not required for energy and to supply exogenous proteins so that all of the needs of protein synthesis can be met without breaking down the patient's own vital protein structures. In this regard, the amino acid composition of protein administered to infants and children is important in determining its nutritional value. Of the 20 amino acids identified in mammalian physiology, nine are essential in infants and children; two additional amino acids may be essential in the premature infant (Table 45–2). All of the essential amino acids must be present in the diet simultaneously for the formation of new lean body tissue. The absence of a single essential amino acid will result in a negative nitrogen and protein balance.

Providing a balanced energy source early in the course of recovery can minimize somatic and visceral protein catabolism, resulting in a protein-sparing effect. A number of investigators have studied this effect clinically and experimentally and have found that nitrogen sparing is achieved when the total nonprotein-calorie to gram-nitrogen ratio is 150:1 to 300:1.[6, 35] Not only does the appropriate amount of administered fat and carbohydrates spare the continued breakdown of body protein for energy needs, but after an initial period of obligatory protein breakdown, it also allows the administered intravenous or enteral protein to be anabolized as new lean body mass.

Table 45–2
Essential Amino Acids

Threonine	Phenylalanine
Leucine	Tryptophan
Isoleucine	Histidine*
Valine	Tyrosine†
Lysine	Cystine†
Methionine	

*Essential only in infancy.
†May be essential in the premature baby.

A sufficient supply of carbohydrate appears to be the most important factor in achieving a protein-sparing effect. Hypocaloric infusions of glucose (5% dextrose in water or 5% dextrose in normal saline) are administered to provide fluid requirements and initially help stave off some protein catabolism, but are inadequate energy sources for even a short period of 2 to 3 days. Higher concentrations of glucose have proved effective, but they must be administered by central venous infusion. When given by continuous drip with the appropriate amount of intravenous protein, this will result in effective protein-sparing. However, as noted previously, any energy source devoid of fat for 2 to 3 weeks may lead to the development of hair loss, mental depression, and a seborrheic-type dermatitis on the face and intertriginous zones. These are the signs and symptoms of fatty acid deficiency, and the patient must have approximately 4 to 10% of his or her daily caloric requirement in the form of fat containing linoleic acid to avoid this complication. Because fat is such an efficient source of calories, clinicians have investigated using it as the sole source of energy and protein sparing.[27, 34] An elegant study by Brennan and colleagues showed that the protein-sparing effect was actually due to the glycerol in which the lipid was suspended plus the esterified glycerol in the triglyceride.[7] However, other studies have shown that intravenous fat is protein sparing both in children and adults.[6, 11, 12, 33, 34] Fat given in disproportionately large quantities becomes a very expensive source of carbohydrate. The same can be said with respect to protein. Given alone in sufficient quantities, solutions of intravenous protein spare the host's lean body mass from being consumed for energy needs. However, this occurs only because the intravenous protein is itself transaminated in the liver and broken down into a very expensive source of carbohydrate. Therefore, a balanced mixture of carbohydrate, fat, and protein is the most effective means of providing a patient's energy and protein repletion requirements while minimizing the catabolism of his or her lean body mass. The exact balance depends on the specific patient's needs. For example, an adult requires only enough fat to prevent essential fatty acid deficiency (2–10%), whereas an infant requires much more fat (35–50%) due to the rapidly growing central nervous system and the need for nerve sheath myelinization.

Electrolyes, Vitamins, and Trace Elements

Administering a well-balanced nutritional regimen can be likened in some respects to taking off in an airplane. The success of the effort is dependent on careful attention to detail, and a diligent pilot has a check list to ensure that no important steps are omitted. The major components of a nutritional regimen—carbohydrate, fat, and protein—require the presence of vitamin catalysts and trace element cofactors to drive the metabolic machinery and achieve the desired anabolic effect. The absence or deficiency of even one small component may result in patient deterioration and failure of an otherwise carefully designed nutritional program. Attention therefore must be given to an adequate supply of daily electrolytes, keeping in mind that potas-

sium, calcium, magnesium, and phosphorus are utilized in increased amounts by a patient during tissue anabolism (Table 45–3). Increased amounts of calcium and phosphorus are particularly important because of the rapid skeletal growth rate of a young child. Likewise, the infant and young child require more vitamins per kilogram of body weight than the adult, and a hypermetabolic patient catabolizes vitamins more rapidly than a normal one. Although fat-soluble vitamin (i.e., A, D, K, and E) stores are plentiful, and deficiencies tend to develop slowly in an otherwise healthy patient, water-soluble vitamins (i.e., B, C, and folic acid) must be replenished frequently, and the critically ill trauma patient may reach a deficiency state in a relatively short time. In addition, there is some evidence that high doses of vitamins A and C may be beneficial to patients with injuries.[24] A specially convened American Medical Association panel published recommendations for vitamin dosages with parenteral nutrition for adults and children. These are listed in Table 45–4.[44]

Trace elements are also important in establishing adequate nutrition; zinc, copper, fluoride, chromium, manganese, and selenium have known metabolic functions. Silicon, boron, nickel, aluminum, arsenic, tin, molybdenum, vanadium, and strontium are also required by the body, but their specific metabolic functions and the amounts needed are not well known. Trace element deficiencies were seldom seen in patients receiving protein hydrolysate in the early days of total parenteral nutrition because of the myriad of trace elements accompanying the relatively impure biologic protein mixture. Because of patient allergic reactions to the antigens in these biologic protein solutions, synthetic amino acids were developed, which are largely free of trace element contaminants. This has in turn necessitated the addition of trace elements to total parenteral nutrition solutions, and it will not be long before additional trace elements, such as molybdenum and nickel, are added to the list in Table 45–5.[50]

METABOLIC RESPONSE OF INFANTS AND CHILDREN TO TRAUMA AND SURGICAL STRESS

The traumatized patient undergoes a well-described metabolic response to the stress of the event or the operation to correct the injury, which in turn affects nutritional requirements and management. In 1959, Francis D. Moore analyzed data based on a collected series of adult patients undergoing various types of operations and described the metabolic response to surgery in his classic textbook.[42] At that time, based on the initial work by Rickham in 1957, it was thought that infants responded quite differently than adults to the stress of trauma and surgery.[48] However, a subsequent extensive study on postoperative neonatal metabolism by Knutrud in 1963 demonstrated only quantitative differences between infants and adults.[36]

The metabolic response to surgery or severe trauma can be divided into four phases, collectively referred to as the phases of surgical convalescence: (1) adrenergic-corticoid phase; (2) corticoid withdrawal phase; (3) spontaneous an-

Table 45-3

Recommended Ranges for Electrolyte Supplements for Pediatric and Adolescent (Adult) Patients on Total Parenteral Nutrition

Electrolyte	Infant Range (<10 kg)	Pediatric Range (10-30 kg)	Adolescent Range (<30 kg)
Calcium	0.5-3.0 mEq/kg/day	5-20 mEq/day	10-15 mEq/day
Magnesium	0.5-1.0 mEq/kg/day	4-24 mEq/day	8-24 mEq/day
Potassium	2-4 mEq/kg/day	20-240 mEq/day	90-240 mEq/day
Sodium	2-4 mEq/kg/day	20-150 mEq/day	60-150 mEq/day
Acetate	2-8 mEq/kg/day	20-120 mEq/day	80-120 mEq/day
Chloride	4-12 mEq/kg/day	20-150 mEq/day	60-150 mEq/day
Phosphorus	0.5-1.0 mmol/kg/day	6-50 mmol/day	30-50 mmol/day

abolic phase; and (4) the fat-gain phase. The length of each phase is directly related to the severity of the injury and the avoidance of complicating factors such as sepsis, shock, and malnutrition. The first phase begins immediately following the traumatic event, with a marked increase in the output of catecholamines, antidiuretic hormone, glucocorticoids, and mineralocorticoids. The increase in antidiuretic hormone leads to early water retention. The increase in mineralocorticoid output, especially aldosterone, along with marked catecholamine excretion, leads to an increase in protein breakdown with an elevation of the urinary nitrogen level. A measure of the catabolic effect is found in the potassium-to-nitrogen ratio in the urine, which is normally 3 mEq of potassium for every gram of nitrogen excreted. This ratio increases in the early postoperative period to 6 mEq of potassium per gram of nitrogen excreted. Depending on the degree of trauma, phase one generally lasts for 36 to 72 hours postinjury.

Phase two is characterized by a return to normal of adrenal steroid output and catecholamine production. This phase usually begins on the third to fourth postoperative day, and lasts 2 to 3 days. As body homeostasis is reestablished at the site of tissue injury, third space fluid losses begin to be reabsorbed, and the levels of antidiuretic hormone and aldosterone return toward normal. A water diuresis then ensues, accompanied by an increase in sodium excretion and a decrease in potassium and nitrogen excretion in the urine.

During phase three, protein synthesis begins. Provided that there is a source of energy and protein building blocks, nitrogen balance changes from negative to positive. This is the beginning of the anabolic phase of recovery, marked by an increase in the patient's strength, activity, and incremental increases in weight, usually due to the synthesis of new protein. Phase three usually begins on postoperative days 5 to 7 and lasts several weeks.

The fourth phase of convalescence is called the fat-gain phase. This phase usually begins when the patient is more active and ambulatory and is receiving oral nutrition. Most of the body weight increase during this phase is due to the accumulation of fat, which may last up to several months in cases of severe trauma. Progression through these four phases is frequently more rapid in the infant and young child than in the adult.

An important difference between the adult and pediatric patient is that the infant and young child have a more severe negative calcium and phosphorus balance than does the adult because of the child's rapidly growing skeleton. In addition, the normal adult requirement of 150 to 300 nonprotein kilocalories for every gram of nitrogen administered probably tends toward the higher range in children under conditions of stress and trauma, although the exact ratio is not known. Clinical studies have indicated that for the infant, this ratio is probably in the range of 230 to 1 after major surgery.[6]

Table 45-4

Recommended Daily Vitamin Supplements for Pediatric and Adolescent (Adult) Patients on Total Parenteral Nutrition According to AMA Guidelines

Vitamin	Pediatric Amount/Day	Adolescent Amount/Day
Ascorbic acid	80 mg	100 gm
Vitamin A	2300 IU	3300 IU
Vitamin D	400 IU	200 IU
Thiamine HCl (B$_1$)	1.2 mg	3 mg
Riboflavin (B$_2$)	1.4 mg	3.6 mg
Pyridoxine HCl (B$_6$)	1 mg	4 mg
Niacinamide	17 mg	40 mg
Pantothenic acid	5 mg	15 mg
Vitamin E	7 IU	10 IU
Biotin	20 μg	60 μg
Folic acid	140 μg	400 μg
Cyanocobalamin (B$_{12}$)	1 μg	5 μg
Phytonadione (K$_1$)	200 μg	1 mg

From Nutrition Advisory Group. American Medical Association: Guidelines for multivitamin preparations for parenteral use. December 1975, Table 1, p 19.

Table 45-5

Recommended Daily Trace Element Supplements for Pediatric and Adolescent (Adult) Patients on Total Parenteral Nutrition

Element	Pediatric Amount (μg)	Adolescent Amount (μg)
Zinc sulfate	300.0	5.0
Copper sulfate	20.0	1.0
Manganese sulfate	10.0	0.5
Chromium chloride	0.2	0.010
Selenium as selenious acid	1.2	0.060

From Shils ME: AMA Department of Foods and Nutrition: Guidelines for essential trace element preparations for parenteral use: A statement by an expert panel. JAMA 241:2051-2054, 1979. Copyright 1979, American Medical Association.

Nutritional Assessment and Monitoring

Nutritional assessment should be a fundamental part of the total evaluation of any traumatized patient, particularly when the injuries are extensive. A severely malnourished patient is usually easily recognized, even without anthropometric measurements and serum chemistries. However, patients in a state of moderate malnutrition are often a challenge to the physician's diagnostic skills. Early identification of patients at risk of progressing to severe nutritional depletion is the first important step in providing proper nutritional therapy. Fortunately, most injured pediatric patients are reasonably well nourished at the time of trauma, and nutritional support is prophylactic for the anticipated stress of the traumatic event, recovery process, and ongoing growth requirements rather than therapeutic for preexisting chronic deficiencies. Establishing simple baseline nutritional measures, such as height, weight, head circumference, albumin, and total protein, provides direction for nutritional management. A complete nutritional assessment should include evaluation of risk factors, diet history, clinical examination including basic anthropometric measurements and laboratory data, energy requirements, and if available, indirect calorimetry. Traumatized patients who are allowed to slip into a state of malnutrition experience impaired wound healing, compromised immune status, and increased morbidity and mortality.

The evaluation of risk factors centers around the initial traumatic event. Large, open wounds indicate the risk for protracted nutrient losses and increased metabolic needs. Similarly, the presence of extensive burns, blunt closed trauma, and the onset of fever produce increased metabolic requirements. Recent loss of 10% or more of usual body weight and the anticipation of nothing by mouth for longer than 7 days on simple intravenous solutions are also indications to initiate formal nutritional support.

Diet history is important in assessing a patient's nutritional status. Prior consumption of a special diet, changes in taste, appetite, or poor intake before the traumatic event may indicate a significantly altered nutritional status. The clinical examination is very important in assessing the patient's nutritional state and potential need for nutritional intervention. The assessment of vascular and gastrointestinal injuries has a direct bearing on the type and form of nutritional support that is required. An important question in every instance is whether the gastrointestinal tract will be functional in 24 to 48 hours. For example, a large retroperitoneal hematoma or spinal cord injury would be expected to result in a prolonged ileus, and parenteral nutrition would be expected to be needed during the recovery period.

Assessment Indices

Because every molecule of protein in the body performs a vital function and protein is not stored in the body, protein depletion indicates nutritional impairment. The protein status directly affects the patient's ability to respond to stress, especially when fat or glycogen stores are also depleted. Therefore, nutritional assessment focuses on the protein compartments, both somatic (muscle proteins) and visceral (all other proteins). Several indices may be measured for each protein compartment. No single test or measurement adequately defines a patient's nutritional status; therefore; reliance on a single factor is not appropriate. Individual serum chemistries, however, are useful in noting potential toxicities or deficits, and trends are useful in assessing overall nutritional status. It is not necessary that every patient undergo all available tests (Table 45–6).[54]

Weight

Weight is one of the most easily obtained and useful indicators of nutritional status. Weight loss often reflects the use of body protein (i.e., muscle and organ tissue) as a metabolic fuel, and it occurs quickly when caloric intake in a traumatized patient is severely restricted. The patient's current weight should be used in conjunction with his or her usual weight, recent weight changes, and ideal weight for height when evaluating nutritional status.

Triceps Skin Fold

The triceps skin fold measurement is a good indicator of body fat (i.e., calorie) reserves, because approximately 50% of adipose tissue is located in the subcutaneous area.

Midarm Muscle Circumference

The measurement of midarm muscle circumference reflects both the adequacy of caloric support and the muscle mass. The midarm circumference is measured; then the contribution of the underlying fat tissue (i.e., triceps skin fold) is subtracted by the formula in Table 45–6.[54] It must be remembered that measurements of arm muscle circumference are estimated, because the thickness of the humerus is not taken into account, and the upper arms are not perfectly round. The formula assumes these factors. Furthermore, fat compressibility varies, with greater compressibility occurring in girls and obese patients.

Visceral Protein

Enzymes, clotting factors, albumin, globulin, transport proteins, and visceral organ cell structures are all composed of the visceral (i.e., nonmuscle) proteins. Visceral protein deficits adversely affect the patient's ability to mount an immune response and to heal wounds. Deficits in serum albumin and transferrin reflect an impairment in hepatic synthesis due to a limited substrate supply. Because serum albumin has a half-life of 20 days, it is not a sensitive indicator of malnutrition or protein repletion. Transferrin, a carrier protein involving iron metabolism with a 9-day half-life, is a much better indicator of protein status, although it is more expensive to measure, is not as readily attainable, and it is not useful in septic patients or patients with iron deficiency. The total lymphocyte count provides a general guide to the patient's ability to respond to infection. Lymphocytes are rapidly destroyed, and protein is required for

Table 45–6
Nutrition Assessment Indices

Assessment Parameters	Degree of impairment				Comments/Calculations/Limitations
	Normal	*Mild*	*Moderate*	*Severe*	
Weight	<10%	10–20%	20–30%	>30%	Should be done daily at the same time, on the same scale, and with similar clothing. The average adult on full TPN is expected to gain 110–220 gm/day (¼–½ lb) when the goal is repletion. $$\% \text{ Weight loss} = \frac{\text{Usual weight} - \text{Current weight}}{\text{Usual weight}}$$ Limitation: Weight change may reflect increased or decreased hydration and not change in lean body mass.
Creatinine/height index		5–15%	15–30%	>30%	A urine specimen is collected for 24 hr. $$\text{Creatine/height index} = 1 - \frac{\text{Total actual urinary creatinine}}{\text{Total ideal urinary creatinine}} \times 100$$ Limitation: May be falsely low secondary to altered renal function.
Triceps skin fold (TSF) (mm)	Male: 12.5–11.3 Female: 16.5–14.9	11.3–10.0 14.9–13.2	10.0–7.5 13.2–9.9	<7.5 <9.9	Calipers are used to measure the skin fold. Midway between the acromion process of the scapula and the olecranon process of the ulna, a fold of skin on the posterior aspect of the nondominant arm is grasped and gently pulled away from the underlying muscles. This is measured in mm. Limitation: Not accurate in the obese or geriatric patient. Plastic calipers should not be used. This is not a sensitive parameter.
Midarm muscle circumference (cm)	Male: 25.3–22.8 Female 23.2–20.9	22.8–20.2 20.9–18.6	20.2–15.2 18.6–13.9	<15.2 <13.9	Midarm circumference is measured at a point halfway between the acromion process of the scapula and the olecranon process of the ulna. Arm muscle circumference (cm) = midarm circumference − (0.314 × TSF (cm)) Limitation: Not sensitive to short-term changes.
Albumin	3.5	3.5–3.0	3.0–2.5	<2.5	Albumin comprises over 50% of the visceral protein and has a half-life of 20 days. A serum level below 3 gm/dl is associated with increased morbidity and mortality. Limitation: Due to long half-life of about 20 days, visceral depletion and repletion will not be detected rapidly. Serum levels may be affected by hepatic and renal disease, congestive heart disease, and chronically draining wounds.
Transferrin	450–200	200–180	180–160	<160	Transferrin, a carrier protein involved in iron metabolism, is a more sensitive indicator of visceral protein deficit than albumin, because its half-life is approximately 9 days. Limitation: Expensive and modified in the presence of hepatic and renal disease, congestive heart failure, and chronically draining wounds.
Total lymphocyte count	>1800	1800–1500	1500–900	<900	Provides a general guide to the patient's ability to respond to infection. Depressed in patients with protein-calorie malnutrition. $$\text{Total lymphocyte count} = \frac{\% \text{ lymphocytes} \times \text{whole blood cells}}{100}$$ Limitation: Many factors other than protein-calorie malnutrition will cause a decrease in total lymphocyte count, such as chemotherapy, sepsis, and trauma.

Table continued on following page

Table 45–6 *Continued*
Nutrition Assessment Indices

Assessment Parameters	Degree of impairment				Comments/Calculations/Limitations
	Normal	*Mild*	*Moderate*	*Severe*	
Skin test antigens	>15	15–10	10–5	5–0 (anergy)	A test of cellular immune function. The test antigens are injected intradermally and the area of induration is measured in mm after 24 and 48 hr. Induration of 0–5 mm indicates failure of the patient to respond to foreign protein (anergy), or lack of previous exposure to antigen.
					Limitation: Factors other than malnutrition may affect induration, such as chemotherapy, medications, and sepsis.
Urine urea nitrogen (UUN)	The values must be used in conjunction with the amount of nitrogen that has been ingested and incorporated into a nitrogen balance profile.				A 24-hr collection of urine is reported in mg/dl. This value is then converted into gm/L by moving the decimal point to the left two places. The total volume of urine excreted in the 24-hr collection period is multiplied by this value to give grams of UUN excreted.
Nitrogen balance	Repair of significant protein deficits can only occur if the nitrogen balance is significantly positive. A near neutral or 0 balance indicates that no change in the patient's nutritional status is likely to occur. If no deficit exists, maintaining a 0 nitrogen balance is desirable as a goal of therapy. A large negative nitrogen balance parallels a continuing and increasing deficit in the protein compartments.				

Skin Test Antigen / Dilutions / Inject (under Skin test antigens comments):

Skin Test Antigen	Dilutions	Inject
Mumps	Undiluted	0.1 ml
PPD	5TU	0.1 ml
Candida albicans	1:1000 or 10 PNU/ml	0.1 ml

(Nitrogen balance comments/calculations:)

Oral and Enteral Intake
$$\frac{\text{Protein intake in gm}}{6.25} - (\text{UUN} + 3) = \text{Nitrogen balance}$$

IV Intake
$$(\text{gm nitrogen/L} \times \text{Number of L/day}) - (\text{UUN} + 3) = \text{Nitrogen balance}$$

IV and Oral Intake
$$(\text{gm nitrogen/L} \times \text{Number of L/day}) + \left[\frac{\text{Protein intake in gm}}{6.25}\right] - (\text{UUN} + 3) = \text{Nitrogen balance}$$

A constant of 3 is added to cover the excretion of nonurea nitrogen and of that lost through skin and intestinal contents.
Limitation: Not accurate in patients with fistulas, burns, or draining wounds.

From Wesley JR, Khalidi N, Faubian WC, et al: The University of Michigan Hospital Parenteral and Enteral Nutrition Manual. 4th ed. North Chicago, Ill, Abbott Laboratories, Hospital Products Division, 1986.

the formation of new cells. Consequently, the absolute lymphocyte count is a useful measure of the status of protein reserve.

Protein is also required for synthesizing the cells and mediators involved in the response to various skin antigens. Although skin-test reactivity is a manifestation of lymphocyte-mediated immunity, the reactivity is probably a measure of the general status of host defenses rather than lymphocyte activity itself. Many chronically and acutely malnourished patients convert from a reactive state so anergy and reactivity can be restored by nutritional repletion, thereby making these various skin tests an indirect measure of nutritional status. Christou and colleagues showed that neutrophil chemotaxis, or the lack of it, correlates with cutaneous sensitivity to recall antigens, suggesting that other immunologic tests may also be indirect measures of the patient's nutritional state.[10]

Measurement of a patient's nitrogen balance is a useful means of determining daily nitrogen requirements as well as the effectiveness of ongoing nutritional therapy. The goal for growth or repair is a daily positive balance of 4 to 6 gm in the adolescent or adult and proportionately less in the infant and small child. A 24-hour urine collection is necessary, which makes the balance study somewhat difficult to obtain, and protein intake, whether enteral or parenteral, must be accurately recorded.

Metabolic Rate

Metabolic rate or energy requirements for traumatized patients can be calculated either by the use of nomograms or by respirometry and indirect calorimetry. Nomograms usually provide an estimated basal energy expenditure (BEE) based on age, height, and weight and allow computation of energy expended due to additional factors that may alter BEE, such as postoperative stress, multiple trauma, fever, and severe infection. Table 45–1 and Figures 45–1 through 45–3 are examples of nomograms currently in use.

Although a number of previous studies on nutritional requirements during health and disease have been based on

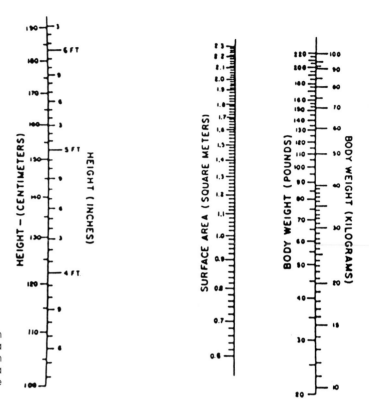

FIGURE 45-1

Nomogram for surface area. Surface area based on height and weight. To determine body surface area from the height on the left-hand scale and weight on the right-hand scale, connect these points with a straight edge and read surface area from the middle scale.

estimated energy expenditure, actual measurement is much more accurate and is becoming an important aspect of critical care management. The most commonly used method of measurement of energy expenditure is indirect calorimetry. In this method, the amount of oxygen absorbed across the lung is assumed to be exactly equal to the amount of oxygen consumed in metabolic processes. This is the basic assumption of the Fick equation and the reason why oxygen consumption is a valid measure of metabolism, even in patients with abnormal lung function. The energy released by oxidation of various food substrates is known from direct measurements; therefore the metabolic rate measured in cubic centimeters of oxygen per minute can be converted to calories per hour or per day if the substrates are known. For practical purposes, a conversion factor of 5 kcal of energy per liter of oxygen consumed is a reasonable approximation. This slightly overestimates the metabolic rate, but it is a much more accurate approximation of the patient's metabolic rate than a number derived from a chart or a table. We have developed a method of closed-circuit, water-sealed indirect calorimetry for infants breathing spontaneously that has demonstrated a much wider range of energy expenditure for infants of similar weight and gestational age than that calculated by nomograms and tables.[17, 18] We have found that commonly used nomograms may underestimate energy expenditure by as much as 70%.[39]

Respirometry is easy to perform in patients who are not intubated and are breathing spontaneously. However, many critically ill patients are intubated and on mechanical ventilators, which can complicate the techniques of respirometry. We have recently tested a miniature indirect calorimetry device that can be interposed between the patient's pressure-limited respirator and endotracheal tube and greatly simplifies the problem of measuring oxygen consumption and carbon dioxide production in infants maintained on pressure-limited respirators.[30]

Oxygen consumption can be obtained (1) by measuring direct volumetric change in a closed-circuit rebreathing spirometer system with carbon dioxide absorber, (2) by measuring the volume and composition of exhaled gas and knowing the composition and volume of inhaled gas, and (3) by measuring the oxygen content of arterial and mixed venous blood and cardiac output and then calculating oxygen consumed by peripheral tissues using the Fick equation. The last method requires pulmonary artery catheterization, but it may become more practical as miniature oximeters are added to smaller Swan-Ganz catheters.[32] Mixed expired gas analysis is the easiest method for use in normal subjects, but it is not suitable for patients on supplemental oxygen or on mechanical ventilators because of minor variations in the inspired volume and oxygen concentration during the respiratory cycle. Direct volumetric spirometry is the best method for measuring oxygen consumption and also lends itself to simultaneous measurement of carbon dioxide production using an infrared capnometer. With measurement of oxygen consumption and carbon dioxide production, the respiratory quotient can be determined and caloric expenditure calculated using the Weir equation.[17, 55]

The previously described methods of nutritional assessment are used to classify the nutritional status of patients at the time of injury, operation, or critical illness. Baker and associates have shown that a careful clinical examination is as accurate as more complex and expensive laboratory and

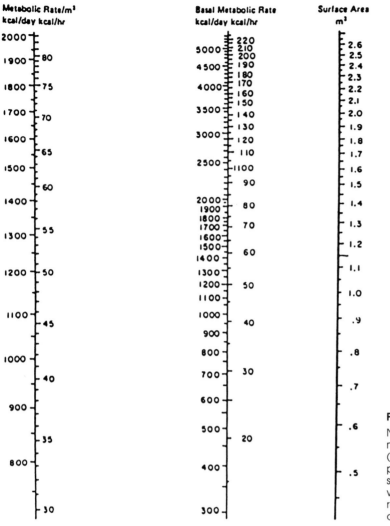

FIGURE 45–2

Nomogram for metabolic rate. To predict daily metabolic requirements, determine surface area (right-hand scale) and metabolic requirements per m² body surface for age and sex (left-hand scale) (see Fig. 45–1). By connecting these points with a straight edge, the predicted daily or hourly requirements may be determined from the middle scale.

anthropometric measurements in identifying malnutrition in stressed patients.[2] In another excellent study, Forse and Shizgal measured body cell mass, the gold standard measurement of nutritional status, and found that the depleted state could not be reliably detected based on weight-height ratio, triceps skin fold, midarm circumference, albumin, total protein, hand strength, or creatinine-height ratio.[22] Actual measurement or estimation of metabolic rate is the best method of following the nutritional status in a critically ill patient.

In summary, the estimation or measurement of metabolic rate and cumulative energy balance is gaining an important place in the management of the critically ill patient. At the very least, daily energy balance should be estimated, and at best, metabolic rate and cumulative caloric balance should be measured daily. A diagrammatic representation of such balance measurement is shown in Figure 45–4. The intake is plotted from the baseline up, and the output or caloric expenditure is plotted from the top of the intake line down. Therefore, positive balance appears as a deviation above the baseline and negative balance as a deviation below the baseline. By totaling the daily positive or negative balance in a running fashion, the cumulative caloric balance can be determined. Bartlett and colleagues have determined that acutely ill adult patients with caloric deficits greater than 10,000 calories had a much higher mortality than patients with positive caloric balance.[3] Similar studies have yet to be done in infants and children.

ADMINISTRATION OF ENTERAL AND PARENTERAL NUTRITION

A patient in a state of good health before accidental trauma or the need for major surgery can sustain a 5- to 7-day interval of no significant energy intake without serious systemic consequences, provided that adequate nutritional support is initiated thereafter. However, it is easier to preserve lean body mass than to make up for its catabolism and deficiency. Therefore, nutritional support of the critically ill child is essential to avoid the added problems of severe nutritional depletion. The type of nutritional support depends on the form and extent of stress affecting the individual child. From the standpoints of the physiologic efficiency of utilization and the economy of administration, enteral feedings are preferable and should be the first choice in

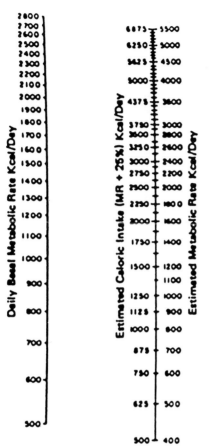

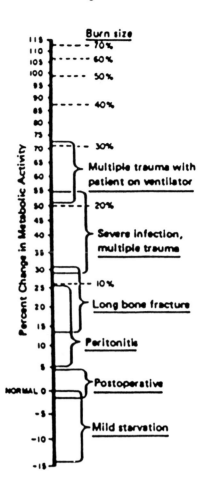

FIGURE 45-3

An estimate of energy requirements for critically ill patients.

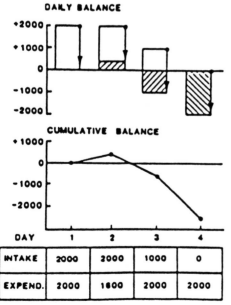

FIGURE 45-4

Measurement of cumulative energy balance.

patients with adequate function of the gastrointestinal tract.[31, 46] However, if the nutritionally compromised patient is unable either to accept or absorb enteral feedings, then total parenteral nutrition (TPN) is required.

Enteral Nutrition

Enteral feedings are begun after the resolution of posttraumatic or postoperative ileus, which is manifested by disappearance of the bilious green color of the gastric aspirate, a decrease in the volume of the gastric aspirate, and by the passage of stool. The return of bowel sounds is a helpful sign in the older child and adolescent, but this sign is not as sensitive or reliable in determining the disappearance of ileus in the infant. Small volumes of sugar water or dilute formula are administered to the infant or small child by mouth or nasogastric tube. In the older child and adolescent, clear liquids are given in a similar fashion, remembering that the stressed and recovering gastrointestinal tract tolerates increases in volume much more readily than increases in osmolarity. As the patient is advanced through progressive stages of increased concentration of formula or liquids and solids toward normal feeding, inability to tolerate increased osmolarity, if it occurs, is usually manifested by cramps and diarrhea. Inability to tolerate increased volume is usually evidenced by vomiting or increased residuals in the nasogastric tube.

With the emphasis on enteral feeding early in the patient's hospital course, nasogastric tubes are frequently used for the feeding of blenderized food or commercial formulas. However, these relatively hard rubber and plastic tubes are not well tolerated and frequently cause esophageal and gastric irritation with intermittent bleeding and nasopharyngeal discomfort. A new generation of feeding tubes using softer materials (e.g., silicone rubber), and built-in lubricant (e.g., hydromer) in smaller caliber tubes that stretch more easily is available. Some of these tubes have mercury weights that make their passage into the duodenum or proximal jejunum more certain. For example, the Dobbhoff feeding tube and the Nutriflex and Entriflex tube (Biosearch, Raritan, NJ) are much better tolerated by patients than the stiffer sump nasogastric tubes used for gastric decompression. If a patient undergoes abdominal surgery and difficulty or prolonged delay in oral feeding is anticipated, surgical placement of a feeding gastrostomy or jejunostomy alleviates the discomfort to the nasal or oral passages altogether. Recent proponents of the feeding catheter jejunostomy have emphasized placement during surgery, employing the prescribed catheter insertion technique. These investigators cite the rapidity with which feedings can be initiated, frequently within the first 24 hours after major abdominal surgery.[19, 46]

A host of commercial formulas are available for routine and specialized enteral feedings, and new ones appear on the market each year. Because it is difficult to keep up with and remember the characteristics, applications, and relative advantages of this plethora of formulas, we have altered the table initially developed by Steffee by grouping the formulas according to gastrointestinal function, with those requiring an intact gastrointestinal tract on the left and moving right as gastrointestinal function decreases, so that elemental diets requiring very little metabolic work for digestion are located on the far right (Fig. 45–5).[51] Generally, critically ill and severely stressed patients frequently have an

acquired lactase deficiency, and a lactose-free diet is a good starting point for enteral feeding. Patients who have sustained traumatic loss of significant portions of the gastrointestinal tract with the creation of stomas or development of fistulas that preclude oral feeding can be fed by cannulating the fistula or stoma and sliding a feeding tube distally. An elemental diet, which can be fully absorbed in as little as 30 to 40 cm of small intestine, can then be infused. Likewise, the drainage from a proximal fistula can be re-fed by this route, considerably easing the task of fluid and electrolyte replacement.

Administration of an enteral feeding regimen is more certain of success when a few simple guidelines are observed. As indicated previously, the gastrointestinal tract generally tolerates increased volume more readily than increased osmolarity, and cramps, diarrhea, and subsequent poor absorption can be avoided by initiating one-fourth or one-half strength formula and advancing gradually. Administration of formula by continuous drip is better tolerated than by bolus feeding, and the threat of gastroesophageal reflux, vomiting, and subsequent aspiration is thereby greatly reduced. Care must be taken to see that the enteral formula does not become contaminated, either during preparation or while hanging at the bedside. Expiration time should be observed and a low threshold maintained for obtaining fresh formula. The use of pectin, Metamucil, Lomotil, paregoric, and Imodium in patients with short bowel syndrome often permits enteral feeding to succeed when almost certain failure would result without the use of one or more of these agents. The concept of gradually advancing and fine tuning the diet is the key to ultimate success in these often complicated patients.

Once the decision has been made to begin nutritional support by feeding tube, the risk of aspiration determines whether the tube should be placed in the stomach or jejunum. Gastric feeding is always preferable, because it enables normal digestive processes and hormonal responses to occur; provides for easier tube insertion; allows tolerance of larger osmotic loads with less frequent distention, cramping, or diarrhea; and results in a lower likelihood of the dumping syndrome compared with jejunal feedings. Trans-

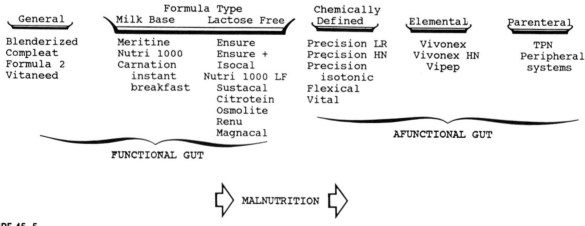

FIGURE 45–5

Enteral formulas. (Adapted from Steffee WP, Krey SH: Enteral hyperalimentation of the cancer patient. In: Newell GR, Ellison NM (eds): Nutrition and Cancer: Etiology and Treatment. New York, Raven Press, 1981, pp 7–31.)

pyloric tube placement is indicated in patients who have a high risk of aspiration, such as those with delayed gastric emptying, gastroesophageal reflux, or a depressed gag reflex secondary to coma. Verification of the location of the tube is mandatory before beginning enteral tube feedings. Simple insufflation of air into the tube is insufficient, because auscultation over the stomach can pick up sound transmitted by a tube inadvertently placed into the bronchial tree. Many of the newly developed and specialized enteral feeding tubes are small enough to pass through the vocal cords and trachea with minimal interference with phonation or respiration. Enteral solutions delivered into the lung through a misplaced tube can cause pneumonia and death. The simplest means of confirming tube placement is by aspirating gastrointestinal contents using a small syringe. Gentle aspiration is important, because small-bore, soft tubes tend to collapse with negative pressure. If gastric or intestinal contents cannot be aspirated through the tube, then roentgenographic confirmation is mandatory. Most of these tubes are radiopaque, and a simple plain radiograph of the abdomen is sufficient.

If transpyloric tube feedings are required, a mercury-weighted tube (e.g., Dobbhoff, Enteroflex, Flexiflo) is passed into the stomach, and the patient is turned with the right side down to assist the passage of the weighted tip through the pylorus into the duodenum by gastric peristalsis. If the tube does not pass into the duodenum after 8 to 24 hours, metoclopramide may be given to stimulate gastric emptying. Alternatively, the tube can be manipulated into the duodenum under fluoroscopic control using a stylet or well-lubricated arteriography guidewire.[37] The optimal location for a transpyloric feeding tube is with the tip located just distal to the ligament of Treitz.[28] This position assures minimum reflux through the pylorus during the administration of feedings.

A tube gastrostomy offers a more secure and manageable access site for enteral nutrition when long-term alimentation (i.e., more than 8 weeks) is anticipated, as in patients with severe head trauma. If abdominal exploration is required in the course of treatment of the traumatized patient, a gastrostomy tube may be placed at that time. Initially, the tube provides gastric decompression during the healing and recovery phases, and subsequently enables enteral tube feeding to be administered.

The safety and utility of gastrostomy in pediatric surgery patients has been well documented.[5, 38] The potential mortality and high morbidity if the tube gastrostomy is not correctly performed has also been described.[23, 29] Fewer children undergo abdominal exploration for blunt trauma today than previously; therefore, the decision to place a feeding gastrostomy or catheter jejunostomy is usually a primary one made later in the course of the patient's recovery. When considering operative placement of a feeding gastrostomy, the physician should always evaluate the patient for gastroesophageal reflux, which, if present, frequently is made worse by the addition of the gastrostomy tube.[9] This is particularly important in the case of brain-damaged children, for whom uncontrolled reflux is particularly dangerous.[53]

The easiest and safest technique for performing a gastrostomy is the Stamm technique.[49] When done as a primary procedure, it can be performed through a small midline or paramedian incision. A tube is inserted within two or three concentric pursestring sutures and brought out through a separate stab-wound incision. The Pezzer mushroom catheter with two added holes has the advantage over a Malecot of a firm solid flange, which aids in approximation and fixation of the stomach to the underside of the anterior abdominal wall and is less likely to be accidentally dislodged. Both catheters are superior to the Foley catheter, because the inflated Foley balloon frequently fatigues and leaks after 10 to 14 days.

Additionally, the percutaneous endoscopy technique for placing a feeding gastrostomy tube without the need for celiotomy is also available for children.[4, 25] Performed with the aid of a flexible fiberoptic endoscope in experienced hands, it has proved safe and effective in selected patients. An additional improvement in the gastrostomy tube for use later in the course of treatment is the gastrostomy button, which is a nonreactive Silastic valve placed in a previously constructed tube site. The button lies almost flush with the abdominal wall and can be easily capped off between uses.[26]

When an abdominal exploration is required during early treatment of the traumatized pediatric patient, catheter jejunostomy has reportedly provided an early and relatively safe postoperative route for enteral nutrition. However, we prefer a combination of early parenteral nutrition followed by nasogastric tube feedings later, if necessary. Alternatively, when we prefer jejunal feedings because of gastroesophageal reflux or poor gastric motility, we place a jejunal tube via a previously placed Stamm gastrostomy. The jejunal tube can be inserted through the gastrostomy stoma, with accurate placement of the tip under fluoroscopy or with the aid of flexible endoscopy.[43]

The rapid development of technology and enteral pharmacology has resulted in increasingly more effective enteral nutrition with better absorption and fewer side effects than possible a few years ago. Enteral feeding is possible in most traumatized patients earlier than previously recognized; it can provide protein and other special nutrients equivalent to that supplied by TPN and can be furnished at a greatly reduced cost. Nasoenteric tube feedings are appropriate for most situations in which oral feeding is slow to return. Gastrostomy is most useful for long-term enteral feeding, and catheter jejunostomy, when appropriate, has the advantage of providing a route for enteral support during the recovery phase of postoperative ileus at reduced risk of aspiration because of infusion beyond the pylorus. The use of fluoroscopy and flexible endoscopy aids in the placement of feeding tubes at various sites in the gastrointestinal tract, often avoiding the need for additional surgery, and hastening the transition from parenteral nutrition to full enteral support.

Total Parenteral Nutrition

Total parenteral nutrition is a carefully balanced system of intravenous feeding developed to meet the requirements of infants and children threatened by catabolic or nutritional deficits because feeding via the gastrointestinal tract is hazardous, inadequate, or impossible. The restoration and maintenance of adequate nutrition is crucial for the successful recovery of infants and children from severe trauma. In infants and small children, TPN is indicated if there is inadequate nutrition for 4 or 5 days. In older children, the tolerable period of inadequate nutrition may be longer, depending on the nutritional status of the patient before the traumatic event. The benefits of TPN in reducing the risks of malnutrition must be weighed against the risks of serious complications, especially sepsis. As stated earlier, TPN should not be used when nutrition is possible by enteral means.

Although TPN can be administered by peripheral vein, this route is sometimes limited by considerations of the high osmolality of the solution and the large volumes necessary to achieve adequate calories. In infants and small children, the cephalic, external jugular, inferior thyroid, and facial veins can be used for central venous access through the appropriate neck incision. A Silastic catheter is preferred because of its flexibility and low thrombogenicity. The deep inferior epigastric vein has been successfully used in children as an access site for inferior vena cava infusion and it can also be used in the adolescent when no other access site is available.[21]

The development of miniature peel-away sheaths has enabled the percutaneous introduction of Silastic catheters. The infraclavicular approach is the preferred route in older children and young adults, because of both the technical ease of insertion and patient comfort. A specific protocol should be followed at the time of insertion to help ensure successful access from the technical standpoint.[54] Insertion of a central line for parenteral nutrition is a surgical procedure and requires the use of strict aseptic technique. Parenteral nutrition is never an emergency; therefore, catheter insertion should be done under well-controlled circumstances. After insertion, the site should be dressed using a standard dressing protocol.[54] Sterility of the catheter-skin junction and an occlusive dressing in place at all times are keys to catheter longevity. A chest roentgenogram immediately after placement or placement with fluoroscopy ensures correct position before initiating infusion of the parenteral nutrition.

Composition of Solutions

Commercial preparations for parenteral nutrition are currently limited to glucose (5–45%) and fat (10–20%) as energy sources, with amino acids or peptide solutions (2–10%) as protein sources. Both parenteral and enteral tube feedings are planned so that total energy requirements can be met through fat, carbohydrate, or both. All protein administered should be available for anabolic processes. Consequently, one of the most important considerations in calculating a daily caloric budget is that the sum of the nonprotein calories should be sufficient to provide a total nonprotein-calorie–to–gram-nitrogen ratio of 150:1 to 300:1. Provided that the total number of calories is sufficient for the patient's energy requirements, this range achieves the optimal utilization of the administered amino acids.

Seven standard TPN formulas have been developed at the University of Michigan. These formulas cover the nutritional needs of 85 to 90% of patients requiring parenteral nutrition.[54] The composition of the five standard nutrition formulations available for adolescent and adult patients is shown in Table 45–7, and the protocol for ordering the solutions is presented in Figure 45–6. The most commonly administered solution is the mixed amino acid formulation, and that, along with the same formulation with low potassium and added sodium and the mixed amino acid peripheral formulation, are designed to be administered with fat emulsion to increase their respective nonprotein-calorie–to–gram-nitrogen ratios into the effective range. In the event that these standard solutions are inappropriate for the adolescent patient's requirements, a nonstandard order form is provided (Fig. 45–7) together with a protocol for calculating the necessary additives (Table 45–8).

For pediatric patients weighing between 10 and 30 kg, an order sheet is provided outlining the standard central formulation, the standard peripheral formulation, and a protocol for making up a nonstandard formulation (Fig. 45–8 and Table 45–9). The standard central pediatric formulation contains 35 gm of nitrogen per liter with a nonprotein-calorie–to–gram-nitrogen ratio of 155:1, and the standard peripheral pediatric formulation contains 20 gm of nitrogen per liter with a nonprotein-calorie–to–gram-nitrogen ratio of 85:1. The latter solution is designed to be administered with an intravenous fat emulsion to move the nonprotein-calorie–to–gram-nitrogen ratio into the effective range. An additional advantage accrues from the concurrent piggyback infusion of a fat emulsion with the peripheral solution, in that the sclerosing properties of the high osmolar peripheral solution are offset by the mechanical protective effect that the fat emulsion appears to have on the vascular endothelium, providing increased longevity for peripheral veins. When setting up a nonstandard formulation, care must be taken not to exceed the calcium phosphate precipitation factor, which is less than or equal to 30 mEq per liter (see Table 45–9), and that none of the critical additives is omitted. In this regard, the order form serves as a check list and is a valuable aid in avoiding errors of omission.

Figure 45–9 displays the protocol order form for setting up the daily caloric budget for neonatal and infant patients weighing less than 10 kg. Because such wide differences exist among sick infants, and because their tolerance to excess and deficiency is so much less than the tolerance of a child or adolescent, we have not established a standard formulation; rather, Table 45–10 summarizes the protocol for calculating the additives for each individual infant based on weight.

The infusion of central parenteral nutrition is started at half-strength on the first day to allow the patient to adapt to the osmotic load, thus preventing osmotic diuresis and hypertonic dehydration. Three-fourth strength solution is infused on the next day. When the patient develops tolerance, as indicated by appropriate blood-sugar levels and diminished glucosuria, full-strength solution is administered. Exogenous insulin is generally not required for nondiabetic children. Any abnormal electrolyte losses should be taken into account and additional electrolytes added to the infusate. In general, gastrointestinal losses should be replaced by

Table 45–7
Standard Parenteral Nutrition Formulations

Designated are the contents of each standard parenteral nutrition solution. Multivitamin with biotin B$_{12}$ and folic acid (2 ml) will be added to the first bottle of the day. Trace elements (1 ml) will be added daily to the first bottle of the day except in the essential amino acid formulations or when requested. Regular human insulin will be added if ordered. Vitamin K will be added to the first bottle weekly unless otherwise requested. Physicians may request additions to the standard parenteral nutrition solution, but only phosphate salts (i.e., potassium or sodium) may be deleted. When reduction of other electrolytes is desired, physicians must write the detailed order on the nonstandard form.

Mixed Amino Acid Formulation

Amino acids (4.25%)	42.5 gm
Dextrose (25%)	250 gm
Calcium	4.5 mEq
Magnesium	5 mEq
Potassium	40 mEq
Sodium	35 mEq
Acetate	74.5 mEq
Chloride	52.5 mEq
Phosphorus	12 mM
Heparin sodium	1000 U

Volume: 1050 ml Caloric Value: 1020 kcal
Approx. Osmolarity: 1825 mOsm

Mixed Amino Acid Cardiac Formulation: No Sodium

Amino acids (4.25%)	42.5 gm
Dextrose (35%)	350 gm
Calcium	4.5 mEq
Magnesium	8 mEq
Potassium	40 mEq
Sodium	45 mEq
Acetate	37.5 mEq
Chloride	4.5 mEq
Phosphorus	12 mM
Sulfate	8 mEq
Heparin sodium	1000 U

Volume: 1050 ml Caloric Value: 1360 kcal
Approx. Osmolarity: 2325 mOsm

Mixed Amino Acid Formulation: Low Potassium and Added Sodium

Amino acids (4.25%)	42.5 gm
Dextrose (25%)	250 gm
Calcium	4.5 mEq
Magnesium	5 mEq
Potassium	23 mEq
Sodium	51 mEq
Acetate	74.5 mEq
Chloride	52.5 mEq
Phosphorus	12 mM
Heparin sodium	1000 U

Volume: 1050 ml Caloric Value: 1020 kcal
Approx. Osmolarity: 1825 mOsm

Mixed Amino Acid Peripheral Formulation

Amino acids (2.5%)	25 gm
Dextrose (10%)	100 gm
Calcium	4.5 mEq
Magnesium	5 mEq
Potassium	23 mEq
Sodium	47 mEq
Acetate	72.5 mEq
Chloride	35 mEq
Phosphorus	9 mM
Heparin sodium	1000 U

Volume: 1050 ml Caloric Value: 440 kcal
Approx. Osmolarity: 880 mOsm
To be infused with fat emulsion

Essential Amino Acid Formulation

Essential amino acids (2%)	15.7 gm
Dextrose (43%)	350 gm
Potassium	1.5 mEq
Acetate	31.5 mEq
Heparin sodium	1000 U

Volume: 800 ml Caloric Value: 1253 kcal
Approx. Osmolarity: 1935 mOsm

From Wesley JR, Khalidi N, Faubion WC, et al: The University of Michigan Hospitals Parenteral and Enteral Nutrition Manual. 4th ed. North Chicago, Ill, Abbott Laboratories, Hospital Products Division, 1986.

a specifically designed electrolyte solution at the appropriate volume, and not by parenteral nutrition solution. Trace elements and vitamins are added to the basic mixture routinely, as indicated in the tables. The TPN solution can be safely increased up to an amount that provides 3.5 gm of protein per kg of body weight per day. Additional calories can be supplied by daily infusion of 10% fat emulsion, up to 60% of the daily caloric budget in adolescents. A maximum of 4 gm of fat per kg per day should be infused to avoid the effect of lipid overdose. A 20% fat emulsion is particularly useful in patients with renal, cardiac, or pulmonary disease requiring fluid restriction.[15] Currently available fat emulsions, containing between 50% and 70% linoleic acid, when administered in amounts to provide 10% or more of the daily caloric budget, easily meet the requirements for essential fatty acids.

Administration of peripheral parenteral nutrition is limited because of the volume necessary to provide the calculated daily energy requirements. Most pediatric trauma victims were healthy before their accidents, and volume administration is not limited by underlying cardiac, pulmonary, or renal disease. Heparin, 1 unit per ml, which is added to the central solution to help prevent clotting at the tip of the catheter, is also added to the peripheral solution to help prevent phlebitis. Unless contraindicated, it is generally advantageous to use an intravenous fat emulsion as a major calorie source in the peripheral feeding regimen for the reasons outlined previously.

Monitoring Nutritional Support

After a specialized enteral or parenteral nutrition regimen has been started, metabolic assessment is performed on an ongoing basis to evaluate the effectiveness of therapy. Essential clinical measurements include daily body weight, weekly body length and head circumference in infants and small children, and accurate intake and output volumes. Urine is monitored for sugar and ketones, initially with each voiding and once each nursing shift after the patient is stable. Table 45–11 lists the recommended blood tests and frequency of monitoring. More frequent monitoring of some parameters may be necessary in patients with specific abnormalities, such as kidney or liver trauma. However, the judicious and sparing use of blood tests is important in infants and smaller pediatric patients because of their small total blood volume and the increased risks of blood transfusion. In addition to monitoring various blood chemistries, the physician must pay careful attention to subjective and objective clinical parameters. For example, improved muscle strength, wound healing, overcoming systemic infections, improved respiratory function, and subsequent weaning from the respirator all indicate improved nutritional status.

Weight changes during parenteral nutrition vary with the patient's overall clinical condition. If an infant or child is severely depleted at the start of treatment, adequate weight gain may not be observed for several days. Patients who are not severely malnourished or septic can be expected to exhibit weight gains more comparable to those of normal infants and children. Increased metabolic demands, such as

Text continued on page 685

THE UNIVERSITY OF MICHIGAN HOSPITALS

DEPARTMENT OF PHARMACY SERVICES
DAILY PARENTERAL NUTRITION (PN)
ORDER AND ADMINISTRATION FORM
FOR **STANDARD** FORMULATIONS

FOR ADOLESCENT AND ADULT PATIENTS

NAME

ADDRESS
(If Outpatient)

LOCATION

REG. NO

If No Plate, Print Name and Reg. #

* Consult your Parenteral and Enteral Nutrition Manual or the back of this form for the concentration of Amino Acids, Dextrose and other additives in each of the available PN solutions. If none of the standard formulations meet the needs of your patient, order the PN solution on the blank PN order form #H-2060401.

* These standard formulations may not provide adequate amounts of vitamins needed in disease induced deficiencies (e.g., thiamine in chronic alcoholics). When indicated, additional electrolytes, trace elements, and vitamins may be ordered with the standard formulation.

* Send yellow and pink copies to the Pharmacy <u>by 9:00 PM the day before</u> PN solutions are to be administered. Only a 24 hour supply can be ordered.

Type of Solution	PN Sequence Number			Any ingredients requested in the space below will be in addition to those already in the solution designated on the left.
CENTRAL FORMULATIONS				PN Sequence No.
Mixed Amino Acid Formulation				
Mixed Amino Acid Formulation; Low Potassium and Added Sodium				
				PN Sequence No.
Mixed Amino Acid Cardiac Formulation; No Sodium				
Essential Amino Acid Formulation				
				PN Sequence No.
PERIPHERAL FORMULATION				
Mixed Amino Acid Peripheral Formulation				
Flow Rate (ml/hr)				

Circle Percentage of Fat Emulsion 500 ml to be Administered Concomitantly   10%   20%

Desired Number of 500 ml Bottles _____

Flow Rate _____ ml/hr

Clerk's Signature   Date   and   Time   AM PM

Physician's Signature   and   Pager Number

Date   Time   AM PM

Date PN to be administered: ____

NURSING ADMINISTRATION RECORD

PN Sequence Number	Date Administered	TIME	AM PM	Administered By	Volume Administered ml
PN Sequence Number	Date Administered	TIME	AM PM	Administered By	Volume Administered ml
PN Sequence Number	Date Administered	TIME	AM PM	Administered By	Volume Administered ml

Fat Emulsion 500 ml Administered	Date	Time AM PM	By	Volume Administered ml	Date	Time AM PM	By	Volume Administered ml

H-2060413 REV 3/86   UNIVERSITY MICHIGAN MEDICAL CENTER   DAILY PN FOR ADOLESCENT AND ADULT PATIENTS - STANDARD

FIGURE 45–6

Protocol for ordering standard total parenteral solutions. (From Wesley JR, Khalidi N, Faubion WC, et al: The University of Michigan Hospitals Parenteral and Enteral Nutrition Manual. 4th ed. North Chicago, Ill, Abbott Laboratories, Hospital Products Division, 1986.)

FIGURE 45–7

Protocol for ordering nonstandard total parenteral solutions for adolescents and adults. (From Wesley JR, Khalidi N, Faubion WC, et al: The University of Michigan Hospitals Parenteral and Enteral Nutrition Manual. 4th ed. North Chicago, Ill, Abbott Laboratories, Hospital Products Division, 1986.)

Table 45–8

Protocol for Calculating Additives in Nonstandard Solutions for Adolescents and Adults (≥30 kg)

1. Base Solution:

Type of Patients	Total Volume of Parenteral Nutrition Solution to be Ordered per Bottle	Final Concentration of Crystalline Amino Acid Solution	Final Concentration of Essential Amino Acid Solution	Final Concentration of Dextrose Solution
Normal liver and renal function	1000 ml	4.25%[1]		25% (Central infusion)
Chronic or acute renal failure	800 ml		2%[2]	43% (Central infusion)
or				
	1000 ml	2.5%[2]		35% (Central infusion)
Liver dysfunction	1000 ml	2.5%[2]		25% (Central infusion)
Cardiac patient with fluid restrictions	1000 ml	4.25%[1]		35% (Central infusion)
Peripheral supplementation for patients with normal renal and liver function	1000 ml	2.5%[2]		10% (Peripheral infusion)

These solutions provide electrolytes in the amounts listed below. Any electrolytes requested on this form will be in addition to those already in the solution.

   (1) Provides 45.0 mEq acetate, 17.5 mEq chloride, and 2.7 mEq potassium.
   (2) Provides 31.5 mEq acetate and 1.5 mEq potassium.
   (3) Provides 43.0 mEq acetate and 2.7 mEq potassium.

2. Additives:
   a. **Electrolytes**

	Recommended Daily Requirement		Compatibility per Liter of Solution
Calcium	10–15 mEq/day	(5 mEq/L)	50 mEq
Magnesium	8–24 mEq/day	(8 mEq/L)	12 mEq
Potassium	90–240 mEq/day	(20–50 mEq/L)	80 mEq
Sodium	60–150 mEq/day	(20–50 mEq/L)	Wide range
Acetate	80–120 mEq/day	(30–50 mEq/L)	Wide range
Chloride	60–150 mEq/day	(20–50 mEq/L)	Wide range
Phosphorus*	30–50 mM/day	(10–15 mM/L)	20 mM

   *1 mM Potassium phosphate provides 1.47 mEq potassium.
    1 mM Sodium phosphate provides 1.33 mEq sodium.

   b. Vitamins:

   The following vitamins should be administered as follows:

   (1) Multivitamin with biotin, B$_{12}$, and folic acid, 2 ml In the first bottle of the day, provides the following vitamins:

Ascorbic acid	100	mg	Pyridoxine HCl (B$_6$)	4 mg	Biotin	60 μg
Vitamin A	3300	IU	Niacinamide	40 mg	Vitamin B$_{12}$	5 μg
Vitamin D	200	IU	Dexpanthenol	15 mg	Folic acid	400 μg
Thiamine HCl (B$_1$)	3	mg	Vitamin E	10 IU		
Riboflavin (B$_2$)	3.6	mg				

   (2) Phytonadione-Vitamin K$_1$, 5 mg should be administered in the parenteral nutrition solution weekly (i.e., Monday), except when the patient is on anticoagulation therapy.

   c. Trace Elements:

   1 ml should be administered in one bottle once a day, except in patients with chronic and acute renal failure, and those with liver dysfunction.

   1 ml of trace elements provides:

Zinc	5 mg	Manganese	0.5 mg	Selenium	0.06 mg
Copper	1 mg	Chromium	0.01 mg		

   d. Heparin:
   1000 U should be ordered with each 1000 ml of parenteral nutrition solution.

   e. Regular Human Insulin:

   To be administered only as indicated by persistent elevation of blood glucose.

3. Fat Emulsion:

   Unless contraindicated, up to 60% of daily caloric intake can be supplemented as fat. Recommended daily dosage is 1–3 gm/kg/day.

From Wesley JR, Khalidi N, Faubion WC, et al: The University of Michigan Hospitals Parenteral and Enteral Nutrition Manual. 4th ed. North Chicago, Ill, Abbott Laboratories, Hospital Products Division, 1986.

THE UNIVERSITY OF MICHIGAN HOSPITALS
DEPARTMENT OF PHARMACY SERVICES
DAILY PARENTERAL NUTRITION (PN)
ORDER AND ADMINISTRATION FORM
FOR PEDIATRIC PATIENTS

NAME

ADDRESS
(If Outpatient)

LOCATION

REG. NO.

If No Plate, Print Name and Reg. #

For patients weighing 10-30 kg.
Send yellow and pink copies to Mott Pharmacy by 9:00 P.M. the day before the PN solution is to be administered. Pharmacy will then deliver by 8:00 A.M. Only a 24 hour supply can be ordered.

STANDARD CENTRAL FORMULATION	STANDARD PERIPHERAL FORMULATION	NON-STANDARD FORMULATION		
PN Sequence Number	PN Sequence Number	PN Sequence Number		
Total Volume of PN Solution Ordered ml	Total Volume of PN Solution Ordered ml	Total Volume of PN Solution Ordered ml		
Flow Rate ml/hr	Flow Rate ml/hr	Flow Rate ml/hr		
Patient's Weight kg	Patient's Weight kg	Patient's Weight kg		
CONTENT PER 1000 ml	CONTENT PER 1000 ml	Final Concentration of Crystalline Amino Acid Solution	g	
Amino Acids (3.5%) 35 g	Amino Acids (2.0%) 20 g	Final Concentration of Special Amino Acids. Specify	g	
Dextrose (25%) 250 g	Dextrose (10%) 100 g	Final Concentration of Dextrose in Solution	%	
Calcium 9 mEq	Calcium 9 mEq			
Magnesium 5 mEq	Magnesium 5 mEq	Calcium Gluconate	mEq	
Potassium 40 mEq	Potassium 30 mEq	Magnesium Sulfate	mEq	
Sodium 35 mEq	Sodium 35 mEq	Potassium Acetate	mEq	
Acetate 82 mEq	Acetate 60 mEq	Potassium Chloride	mEq	
Chloride 35 mEq	Chloride 35 mEq	Potassium Phosphate	mM	
Phosphorus 12 mM	Phosphorus 6 mM	Sodium Acetate	mEq	
Heparin 1000 U	Heparin 1000 U	Sodium Chloride	mEq	
Pediatric Multivitamin 3 ml	Pediatric Multivitamin 3 ml	Sodium Phosphate	mM	
Provides 990 Kcal	Provides 420 Kcal	Pediatric Multivitamin	ml	
Any ingredients requested in the space below will be in addition to those already in the solution designated above.		Pediatric Trace Elements	ml	
Pediatric Trace Elements (0.1 ml/kg) ml	Pediatric Trace Elements ml	Parenteral Iron	mg	
		Heparin	U	

Circle Percentage of Fat Emulsion To Be Administered Concomitantly 10% 20%	Physician's Signature and Pager Number
Volume Ordered ml	
Flow Rate ml/hr	Date Time AM PM
Clerk's Signature Date and Time AM PM	Date PN to be Administered ____ ____

NURSING ADMINISTRATION RECORD					
PN Sequence Number	Date Administered	Time	AM PM	Administered By	Volume Administered ml
PN Sequence Number	Date Administered	Time	AM PM	Administered By	Volume Administered ml
Fat Emulsion 500 ml Administered	Date Administered	Time	AM PM	Administered By	Volume Administered ml

H-2060425 REV. 3/86		UNIVERSITY OF MICHIGAN MEDICAL CENTER	DAILY PN FOR PEDIATRIC PATIENTS

FIGURE 45–8

Protocol for ordering total parenteral solutions for pediatric patients (10 to 30 kg). (From Wesley JR, Khalidi N, Faubion WC, et al: The University of Michigan Hospitals Parenteral and Enteral Nutrition Manual. 4th ed. North Chicago, Ill, Abbott Laboratories, Hospital Products Division, 1986.)

Table 45-9

Protocol for Calculating Additives in Total Parenteral Nutrition Solutions for Pediatric Patients (10-30 kg)

The contents of each standard formulation is listed in Figure 45-8. These formulations provide maintenance requirements for patients over 10 kg. Physicians may request additions but not deletions to the standard parenteral nutrition solutions. When deletions of certain electrolytes or vitamins are indicated, an individualized nonstandard order should be written on this form. Vitamins and heparin are automatically added. Trace elements should be requested daily according to the patient's weight.

1. Base Solution:

Weight	Maintenance Fluid Requirement (ml/kg/24 hr)	Final Concentration of Crystalline Amino Acid Solution Peripheral	Central	Final Concentration of Dextrose Solution (Peripheral Infusion)	Final Concentration of Dextrose Solution (Central Infusion)
10-20 kg	1000 ml + 50 ml/kg over 10 kg	2%	3.5%	10%	25%
20-30 kg	1500 ml + 20 ml/kg over 20 kg	2%	3.5%	10%	25%

Parenteral nutrition should be ordered in multiples of 100 ml to last 24 hr.*

2. Additives:

   a. **Electrolytes**

Electrolytes	Recommended Daily Requirement	Compatibility per Liter of Solution
Calcium	5-20 mEq/day (9 mEq/L)	≤ 10 mEq
Magnesium	4-24 mEq/day (5 mEq/L)	≤ 12 mEq
Potassium	20-240 mEq/day (20-50 mEq/L)	≤ 80 mEq
Sodium	20-150 mEq/day (20-50 mEq/L)	Wide range
Acetate	20-120 mEq/day (30-50 mEq/L)	Wide range
Chloride	20-150 mEq/day (20-50 mEq/L)	Wide range
Phosphate	6-50 mM/day (5-15 mM/L)	≤ 20 mM

   *1 mM Potassium phosphate provides 1.47 mEq potassium.
   1 mM Sodium phosphate provides 1.33 mEq sodium.

Calcium-Phosphate Precipitation Factor
$$\frac{(Calcium\ mEq) + (Phosphate\ mM) \times 1000}{Total\ Infusion\ Volume\ per\ Bottle} \le 30$$
Adjust calcium or phosphate to maintain precipitation factor ≥30 per 1000 ml

   b. Vitamins:

   Pediatric multivitamin injection one vial/day diluted to 3 ml.

   One vial of pediatric multivitamin injection contains:

Ascorbic acid	80	mg	Pyridoxine (B_6)	1	mg	Cyanocobalamin (B_{12})	1	μg
Vitamin A	2300	IU	Niacinamide	17	mg	Phytonadione (K_1)	200	μg
Vitamin D	400	IU	Dexpanthenol	5	mg	Biotin	20	μg
Thiamine (B_1)	1.2	mg	Vitamin E	7	IU			
Riboflavin (B_2)	1.4	mg	Folic acid	140	μg			

   c. Pediatric Trace Elements Formulation: 0.1 ml/kg/day.
   0.1 ml of this formulation provides:

Zinc	100	μg	Copper	20	μg	Selenium	1.2 μg
Manganese	10	μg	Chronium	0.2	μg		

   d. Parenteral iron: Contact parenteral and enteral nutrition team for dosing and additional information.

   e. Heparin: 1.0 U/ml.

   f. Regular Human Insulin: To be administered only as indicated by persistent elevation of blood glucose above 250 mg/dl.

3. Fat Emulsion 10% and 20%:
   Unless contraindicated, up to 50% of daily caloric intake can be supplied as fat.
   Recommended dosage: 1-4 g/kg/day
   Fat emulsion 10% provides 1.1 kcal/ml.
   Fat emulsion 20% provides 2.0 kcal/ml.

From Wesley JR, Kalidi N, Faubion WC, et al: The University of Michigan Hospitals Parenteral and Enteral Nutrition Manual. 4th ed. North Chicago, Ill, Abbott Laboratories, Hospital Products Division, 1986.

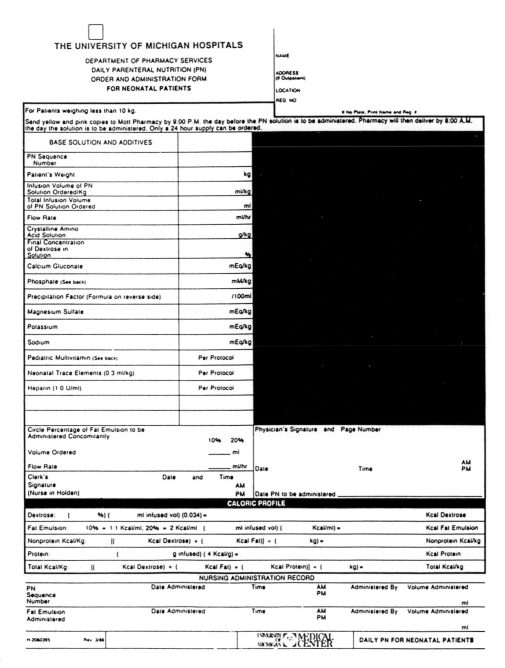

FIGURE 45–9

Protocol for ordering total parenteral solutions infants (up to 10 kg). (From Wesley JR, Khalidi N, Faubion WC, et al: The University of Michigan Hospitals Parenteral and Enteral Nutrition Manual. 4th ed. North Chicago, Ill, Abbott Laboratories, Hospital Products Division, 1986.)

Table 45–10
Protocol for Calculating Additives in Total Parenteral Nutrition Solutions for Infants (<10 kg)

1. Base Solution: Use the table below to estimate volumes to infuse. Overfill will automatically be provided by pharmacy.

   A. Fluids:

Day	Estimated Maintenance (ml/kg/24 hr)			
	Premature		Full Term	Patients under radiant warmers or receiving phototherapy may require an an additional 15–25 ml/kg/24 hr
	< 1250 gm	> 1250 gm		
1	100	75	60–75	
2	100–120	75–100	75–85	
3	Increase as tolerated to meet caloric needs.			

   B. Protein:

   Suggested nonprotein calorie and protein combinations to maximize protein utilization

Protein (gm/kg/24 hr)	Nonprotein Calories (kcal/kg/24 hr)
1	25
2	50
2.5	70+

   C. Dextrose:

   Peripheral concentrations are available in 0.5% increments up to 12.5% (12.5 gm/100 ml).
   Central formulation is available in concentrations up to 35%.
   Use 4–8 mg/kg/min as a baseline glucose infusion rate. Increase as tolerated to provide adequate calories.

2. Fat Emulsion 10% and 20%:

   Unless contraindicated, up to 50% of daily caloric intake can be supplied as fat.
   Recommended dosage: 1–4 gm/kg/day; limit to <3 gm/kg day in infants with respiratory diseases.
   Fat emulsion 10% provides 1.1 kcal/ml.
   Fat emulsion 20% provides 2.0 kcal/ml.

3. Additives:

   A. Electrolytes[c]   Recomended Daily Requirement

Calcium	0.5–3	mEq/kg	[a]Phosphate provided as salt of potassium or sodium. Sodium or potassium used will be subtracted from sodium and/or potassium ordered. Remainder of sodium and/or potassium will be added as chloride salt.
Magnesium	0.5–1	mEq/kg	
Potassium[a, b]	2–4	mEq/kg	
Sodium	2–4	mEq/kg	[b]Sodium and potassium also available as acetate if specifically ordered.
Phosphate[b]	1.0–1.5	mM/kg	[c]Electrolytes should be ordered in whole or half (0.5) units only.

   Calcium Phosphate Precipitation Factor
   $$\frac{(Calcium\ mEq/kg) + (Phosphate\ mM/kg \times Weight\ (kg)) \times 100}{Total\ Infusion\ Volume\ per\ Bottle} \leq 3$$
   Adjust calcium or phosphate to maintain precipitation factor ≤ 3 per 100 ml.

   B. Vitamins provided per protocol: 1 vial if weight of patient > 1750 gm; 0.65 vial if weight of patient < 1750 gm.

   Pediatric multivitamin injection: (1 vial/day) diluted to 3 ml.

   One vial pediatric multivitamin injection contains:

Ascorbic acid	80	mg	Pyridoxine (B_4)	1 mg	Cyanocobalamin (B_{12})	1	μg
Vitamin A	2300	IU	Niacinamide	17 mg	Phytonadione (K_1)	200	μg
Vitamin D	400	IU	Dexpanthenol	5 mg	Biotin	20	μg
Thiamine (B_1)	1.2 mg		Vitamin E	7 IU			
Riboflavin (B_2)	1.4 mg		Folic acid	140 μg			

   C. Neonatal trace elements formulation provided per protocol: 0.3 ml/kg/day.
   0.3 ml of this formulation provides:

Zinc	300 μg	Copper	20 μg	Selenium	1.2 μg
Manganese	10 μg	Chromium	0.2 μg		

   D. Heparin provided per protocol: 1 U/ml.

From Wesley JR, Khalidi N, Faubion WC, et al: The University of Michigan Hospitals Parenteral and Enteral Nutrition Manual, 4th ed. North Chicago, Ill, Abbott Laboratories, Hospital Products Division, 1986.

Table 45-11
Blood Values Routinely Monitored During Total Parenteral Nutrition

At Start of Therapy and Weekly	At Start of Therapy and Every 2 Weeks	As Indicated
Na, K, Cl	SGOT, LDH, alkaline phosphatase	Copper
Urea	Bilirubin, direct and total	Zinc
Glucose	Creatinine	Iron
Magnesium	Triglyceride	Ammonia
Calcium, phosphorus		Osmolarity
Albumin		pH
Hemoglobin, hematocrit, white blood cells, platelets		

Abbreviations: SGOT, Serum glutamic-oxaloacetic transaminase; LDH, lactic dehydrogenase.

that from severe trauma or sepsis, result in a flatter growth curve, which may be counterbalanced to some extent with daily determination of energy needs by indirect calorimetry, if available. Adequate weight gain should average 15 to 25 gm per day in the neonate and infant, or 0.5% of total body weight in kg per day in older children and adolescents. Greater weight gain than this suggests excess fluid administration and retention. Positive nitrogen balance and protein synthesis depend in part on the activity of the patient. Physical exercise is essential for adequate return of muscle strength and cardiovascular function; therefore, physical therapy should not be neglected.

The urine output should be maintained at 1 ml per kg per hour or more, with the urine specific gravity kept between 1.005 and 1.015, and glucosuria should be prevented. If increased gradually, the large amount of intravenous glucose is well-tolerated without the need for exogenous insulin in most pediatric patients. Blood sugar generally remains in the high-normal range, and if hypoglycemia and glucosuria occur, slowing the infusion rate or lowering the concentration of glucose usually temporarily solves the problem unless the patient is septic. Total parenteral nutrition usually results in a greater excretion of solutes in the urine than that observed during enteral feeding, but this increased load does not exceed the concentrating ability of normal kidney. Water balance, even in the face of high rates of TPN administration, is usually maintained.[16, 47]

The transition from parenteral back to oral-enteral nutrition is a very important and often difficult time nutritionally for a recovering patient. If this recovery phase is not managed well, the patient may lose a hard-earned nutritional advantage. During prolonged TPN, the patient may develop hallucinations of taste and smell and become unduly preoccupied with food at meal time. However, TPN frequently suppresses appetite, and the physician should offer reassurance that the patient's appetite will return when the parenteral nutrition is tapered and discontinued. Although it is important that during the transition from parenteral to enteral nutrition, nearly full caloric requirements be supplied before parenteral support is discontinued, it is often necessary to cut back by as much as one half of the daily amount of parenteral nutrition to stimulate a patient's appetite and desire to eat. Traditionally, bland clear liquids are the first foods offered. These are barely acceptable to most patients, and the use of more appetizing food such as popsicles, fudgesicles, hard candy, commercial lactose-free formulas,

cookies and eggnog should be encouraged. A calorie count should be maintained during the transition to measure the patient's progress. Accurate calorie counts are notoriously difficult to obtain in the hospital; if possible, the patient or a member of his or her family should be put in charge of this task and be impressed with its importance. A side benefit is the positive effect this task frequently has on the patient's or parents' psychological well-being.

COMPLICATIONS OF NUTRITIONAL SUPPORT

Technical Complications

Like most effective invasive treatment modalities, TPN, and to a lesser extent specialized enteral nutrition have their share of complications. These are best anticipated and treated by preventive measures centering on the use of detailed protocols, which should be available in any hospital providing this type of nutritional support.[54] The incidence of technical complications due to the placement of central venous lines in infants and children has been greatly reduced by careful attention to technique and by radiologic confirmation of catheter position. The incidence of cardiac arrhythmia due to catheter irritation has been greatly reduced by placing the tip of the catheter at the junction of the superior vena cava and right atrium rather than in the heart. Likewise, radiologic control of catheter placement has removed the risk of hepatic necrosis from direct infusion of hypertonic solutions into the hepatic veins. The replacement of polyvinyl catheters by nonreactive silicone catheters has reduced the incidence of foreign body reactions, vein perforation, and subclavian vein or vena cava thrombosis. Suturing the catheter to the skin at its entry point and checking the security of the catheter at each every-other-day dressing change has greatly reduced the frequency of accidental catheter dislodgement. Even with the proper positioning of a silicone catheter, thrombosis of the vein in which the catheter resides can occur, especially in the critically ill patient with sepsis and reduced circulation. Thrombosis of the superior vena cava can lead to superior vena cava syndrome, but this is uncommon and is usually well-tolerated in children. Although evidence of thromboembolism has been noted at autopsy in children dying with central venous catheters in place, clinical manifestations of this complication are rare. Pulmonary embolism has occasionally been reported in an infant or small child with a central venous catheter for a prolonged period.[8, 52] The use of peripheral parenteral nutrition avoids most of the technical complications inherent in central parenteral nutrition. The most common complications in peripheral intravenous nutrition are phlebitis and superficial skin slough, both of which can be reduced by the simultaneous infusion of a fat emulsion. In addition to reducing the osmolarity and increasing the pH of the solution, infusion of fat appears to provide additional direct mechanical protection of the vein from phlebitis.

Septic Complications

Sepsis is one of the most frequent and serious complications of centrally infused parenteral nutrition in infants and children. Long-term central venous catheters are well-documented sources of bacteremia and septicemia. Microorganisms may enter the blood stream along the catheter tract, via a contaminated intravenous solution, or from a distant septic site with adherence to the catheter, which acts as a foreign-body focus for bacterial growth. The most important factors in reducing the incidence of septic complications are placement of catheters under strict aseptic conditions and meticulous care of the catheter site with every-other-day standardized dressing changes. In addition, use of the catheter for parenteral nutrition alone and strict avoidance of using the catheter for drawing blood, giving blood products, or administering medications minimizes the risk of contamination and mechanical failure. The establishment of a parenteral nutrition team and use of standardized protocols have resulted in a marked decrease in the sepsis rate at the Mott Children's Hospital from 16%, documented before the team started, to 3.2% during the first 2.5 years that the team was in operation.[20] During the 10 years of our team's existence, the TPN central venous catheter sepsis rate has averaged 4.5%.

Catheter sepsis in a patient receiving parenteral nutrition is suggested by fever, leukocytosis, unexplained glucosuria, or any combination of these signs. Infection is confirmed by culturing microorganisms from blood obtained through the central venous line or from another venous site. If the patient is not toxic, the catheter should be left in place during the initial 24 to 48 hours of evaluation, because approximately 50% of febrile patients with central catheters turn out to have another source for their fever. If no other site of sepsis is found, the catheter generally should be removed. Alternatively, intravenous antibiotics may be initiated via the catheter after the appropriate cultures have been made. In many cases, the central venous catheter may be salvaged by 5 to 10 days of intravenous antibiotics.

Febrile patients are frequently those most in need of nutritional support; therefore, it is important to have a protocol for managing central catheters in these high-risk patients. Parenteral nutrition is never an emergency procedure; therefore, a febrile patient should undergo thorough investigation of the source of fever before initiating central parenteral nutrition. Parenteral nutrition should never be initiated during the early stages of uncontrolled infection

and particularly during recurrent septicemia. If parenteral nutrition is begun when a patient is febrile, periodic blood cultures should be drawn every 1 to 3 days until the patient becomes afebrile.

Peripheral parenteral nutrition has the advantage of eliminating most of the septic and technical complications inherent in the use of central venous catheters. At the Mott Children's Hospital, none of the infants and children managed with peripheral intravenous feeding, with or without fat, developed invasive sepsis related to parenteral nutrition.[11–13]

Metabolic Complications

Although almost every conceivable metabolic abnormality has been reported during TPN, Table 45–12 lists the more common ones. Serious consequences may ensue if these complications go undetected for any length of time. However, careful monitoring with appropriate adjustment of the parenteral nutrition solution allows most patients to tolerate TPN quite well.

Hyperglycemia

An elevated blood sugar level may appear during initial parenteral nutrition therapy and should not be treated unless it results in 4+ glucosuria or in a significant osmotic di-

Table 45–12
Potential Metabolic Complications from Total Parenteral Nutrition

Electrolyte Imbalance
  Hyper/hyponatremia
  Hyper/hypokalemia
  Hyper/hypochloremia
  Hyper/hypocalcemia
  Hyper/hypomagnesemia
  Hyper/hypophosphatemia

Carbohydrate Administration
  Hyper/hypoglycemia
  Hyperosmolarity and associated osmotic diuresis with dehydration, leading to nonketotic hyperglycemia coma

Protein Administration
  Cholestatic jaundice
  Azotemia

Lipid Administration
  Hyperlipidemia
  Alteration of pulmonary function
  Displacement of albumin-bound bilirubin by plasma free fatty acid
  Overloading syndrome, characterized by hyperlipidemia, fever, lethargy, liver damage, and coagulation disorders, has been reported in adults but rarely has been recognized in children

Trace Element Deficiencies
  Zinc deficiency
  Copper deficiency
  Chromium deficiency

Essential Fatty Acid Deficiency
  Occurs if lipid emulsions are not used; the major clinical manifestation is a desquamating skin rash

uresis. Endogenous insulin secretion normally adjusts as the parenteral nutrition rate or concentration is increased over a 48- to 72-hour period, and the blood glucose level returns to normal. If hyperglycemia cannot be controlled by this manipulation, regular human insulin may be added to the infusate. Nondiabetic infants and children rarely require added insulin. Patients who are stable on parenteral nutrition and suddenly develop a blood sugar greater than 200 mg/percent or who require increasing doses of insulin should be worked up for other causes of this finding, particularly sepsis.

Hypoglycemia

Although symptoms of hypoglycemia, such as diaphoresis, confusion, or agitation, have been reported when parenteral nutrition is abruptly terminated, we have rarely observed this complication in children despite many accidental interruptions of infusions. Nevertheless, 10% dextrose should always be administered when the TPN solution is interrupted for any reason, and parenteral nutrition should be gradually tapered when nutrition by vein is no longer required.

Patients undergoing major surgical procedures frequently become less glucose tolerant because of endogenous hormone secretion or insulin resistance. Therefore, we recommend that the parenteral nutrition infusion rate be routinely decreased by one half or tapered off altogether when the patient is taken to the operating room. The infusion can usually be brought back to the preoperative rate within 48 hours after surgery, provided that the blood glucose concentration has returned to an acceptable range after the first phase of surgical convalescence.

Hyperkalemia

Patients receiving parenteral nutrition may develop elevated serum potassium levels if they are not adequately anabolic and are unable to fully utilize the administered potassium. Other causes of hyperkalemia include decreased renal function, low cardiac output, tissue necrosis, and systemic sepsis. Potassium should be reduced or withheld from the parenteral nutrition solution until the underlying problem is resolved.

Hypokalemia

As a patient on parenteral nutrition becomes anabolic and begins to synthesize new protein, there is an obligatory requirement for intracellular potassium. Therefore, intravenous potassium is administered at a level of 2 to 4 mEq per kg per day in infants and small children, or 40 mEq per liter in the older child and adolescent. Higher doses may be required, but this will become evident if the patient's serum potassium is monitored on a regular basis.

Hypocalcemia, Hypercalcemia, Hypophosphatemia, and Hyperphosphatemia

Hypocalcemia, hypercalcemia, hypophosphatemia, and hyperphosphatemia have all been reported in patients receiv-

ing TPN. These conditions occur when inappropriate amounts of calcium and phosphorus are added to the TPN solution. These extremes can be avoided by careful monitoring of serum calcium and phosphorus levels. Because of growth requirements, infants and children require relatively more calcium and phosphorus than adolescents or adults.

Hypomagnesemia

Magnesium is required during increased anabolism and protein synthesis, as is the case with potassium and phosphorus. Hallucinations, vertigo, ileus, and hyperreflexia may indicate hypomagenesmia. Addition of appropriate amounts of magnesium to the infusate completely eliminates this complication.

Trace Element Deficiency

Zinc deficiency during long-term parenteral nutrition has been well documented in children and is more likely to occur in patients with diarrhea. It is usually manifested by hair loss, a seborrheic type of dermatitis around the nose and mouth, and occasionally, ileus. Copper deficiency results in hypochromic, normocytic anemia; neutropenia; depigmentation of the skin and hair; hypotonia; psychomotor retardation; and osteoporosis. Chromium deficiency, although very rare, can produce a diabetes-like syndrome. Selenium deficiency, a potential complication of very long-term parenteral nutrition support, is manifested by muscular pain and cardiomyopathy. These deficiencies are rarely observed in patients routinely receiving trace metal additives to the infusate.

Fatty Acid Deficiency or Hyperlipidemia

Chemical signs of essential fatty acid deficiency may occur after as few as 2 to 3 weeks of fat-free parenteral nutrition and consist of a raised serum level of 5,8,11-eicosatrienoic acid, low levels of linoleic and arachidonic acids, and an eicosatrienoic-to-arachidonic (i.e., triene-tetranene) ratio greater than 0.4. Clinical signs usually do not appear until after 2 to 3 months of fat-free therapy.[45] Typically, a flaking, erythematous, papular skin rash develops and is generally limited to the legs, chest, and face. As outlined in a previous section, hyperlipidemia can be corrected by administering at least 4% of the patient's daily caloric requirement in the form of linoleic acid. Because most pediatric patients receiving parenteral nutrition also routinely receive intravenous fat as part of their daily caloric budget, the complication of fatty acid deficiency has largely been eliminated.

Most patients receiving a fat emulsion have normal serum triglyceride and cholesterol levels. A few who receive parenteral nutrition for longer than 1 month have serum triglyceride levels in the range of 300 to 350 mg per percent (normal, 50–150 mg/%) and serum cholesterol values of 150 to 250 mg per percent (normal, 100–150 mg per percent). These elevations appear to be of little consequence, and levels return to normal after the fat infusion is discontinued.[14]

Liver Dysfunction

Although abnormalities in liver functions, such as elevations in serum glumatic-oxaloacetic transaminase (SGOT), lactic dehydrogenase (LDH), serum glutamate pyruvate transaminase (SGPT), and bilirubin levels, have been reported within 2 to 14 days after beginning TPN, histologic examination of the liver does not reveal any consistent pathologic change. These elevations are variable, intermittent, and return to normal in most cases once the parenteral nutrition therapy has been stopped. The abnormalities seen in patients receiving intravenous fat are essentially the same as those seen in patients on fat-free parenteral nutrition regimens. Histologically, fat pigment is usually seen in the Kupffer cells of the liver in most patients receiving intravenous fat for longer than 1 month. The significance of this pigment deposition is not known. Cholestatic jaundice associated with TPN is far more common in premature infants than in older children or adolescents and may be related to the immaturity of the biliary excretory system in the infant. Although this cholestatic jaundice usually clears within 2 to 3 weeks after cessation of intravenous nutrition, in some severe cases, the infant develops hepatic failure and dies.[40]

Allergic Reactions

It is not unusual for patients receiving a fat emulsion as a regular calorie source to develop a peripheral eosinophilia in the range of 5 to 10%, and in a few patients, this level may rise to 35%. This occurrence appears to be of no clinical significance; the eosinophilia is not accompanied by skin rashes or other allergic manifestations and resolves when the intravenous fat is discontinued.[12]

Fluid Overload and Respiratory Failure

Fluid overload in the form of pulmonary edema, peripheral edema, or congestive heart failure is rare in patients treated according to the techniques outlined previously, provided that proper selection and monitoring are carried out. Studies at the Mott Children's Hospital, using the nonradioactive isotope deuterium oxide, have shown that total body water during parenteral nutrition does not increase, but rather decreases, concomitant with an increase in body weight. This strongly supports the hypothesis that weight gain during parenteral nutrition is due to tissue accretion rather than water retention.[16, 47]

In traumatized patients with compromised respiratory function, large dextrose loads associated with parenteral nutrition may contribute to respiratory failure. This is due to the high production of carbon dioxide with the metabolism of carbohydrate (i.e., 1 mol CO_2 produced for every mol of O_2 consumed; RQ = 1), which increases respiratory work. If these patients are already receiving ventilatory assistance, they may be difficult to wean from the ventilator. This complication can be resolved by decreasing the dextrose load and substituting fat calories (RQ = 0.7) for dextrose calories. This complication emphasizes the need for calculating a precise balance between glucose, protein, and fat calories. The necessary formula has been developed for adults and is being worked out for infants and small children.[1, 17, 18]

References

1. Askanazi J, Rosenbaum SH, Hyman AI, et al: Respiratory changes induced by the large glucose loads of total parenteral nutrition. JAMA 243:1444–1447, 1980.
2. Baker JP, Detsky AS, Wesson D, et al: Nutritional assessment: A comparison of clinical judgement and objective measurements. N Engl J Med 306:969–972, 1982.
3. Bartlett RH, Dechert RE, Mault JR, et al: Measurement of metabolism in multiple organ failure. Surgery 92:771–779, 1982.
4. Behkov KJ, Kazlow PG, Waye JE, et al: Percutaneous endoscopic gastrostomies in children. Pediatrics 177:248–250, 1986.
5. Berg RB, Vama RR, Soergel KM: Gastric reflux during perfusion of the small bowel. Gastroenterology 59:890–895, 1970.
6. Benner JW, Coran AG, Weintraub WH, et al: The importance of different calories sources in the intravenous nutrition of infants and children. Surgery 86:429–433, 1979.
7. Brennan MF, Fitzpatrick GF, Cohen KH, et al: Glycerol: Major contributor to the short term protein sparing effect of fat emulsions in normal man. Ann Surg 182:386–394, 1975.
8. Buck JR, Connors RJ, Coon WW, et al: Pulmonary embolism in children. J Pediatr Surg 16:385–391, 1981.
9. Canal DF, Vane DW, Seiichi G: Reduction of lower esophageal sphincter pressure with Stamm gastrostomy. J Pediatr Surg 22:54–57, 1987.
10. Christou NV, McLean APH, Meakins JL: Host defense in blunt trauma: Interrelationships of kinetics of energy and depressed neutrophil function, nutritional status, and sepsis. J Trauma 20:833–841, 1980.
11. Coran AG: The long-term intravenous feeding of infants using peripheral veins. J Pediatr Surg 8:801–807, 1973.
12. Coran AG: Total intravenous feeding of infants and children without the use of central venous catheter. Ann Surg 179:445–449, 1974.
13. Coran AG, Weintraub WH: Peripheral intravenous nutrition without fat in neonatal surgery. J Pediatr Surg 12:195–199, 1977.
14. Coran AG, Edwards B, Zalesk R: The value of heparin in the hyperalimentation of infants and children with a fat emulsion. J Pediatr Surg 9:725–732, 1974.
15. Coran AG, Drongowski RA, Sarahan TM, et al: Studies on the efficacy of a new 20% fat emulsion in pediatric parenteral nutrition. JPEN J Parenter Enteral Nutr 6:222–225, 1982.
16. Coran AG, Drongowski RA, Wesley JR: Changes in total body water and extracellular fluid volume in infants receiving total parenteral nutrition. J Pediatr Surg 19:771–776, 1984.
17. Dechert RE, Wesley JR, Schafer LE, et al: Comparison of oxygen consumption (VO_2), carbon dioxide production (VCO_2), and resting energy expenditure (REE) in premature and full-term infants. J Pediatr Surg 20:765–771, 1985.
18. Dechert RE, Wesley JR, Schafer LE, et al: A water-sealed indirect calorimeter for measurement of oxygen consumption (VO_2), carbon dioxide production (VCO_2), and energy expenditure in infants. JPEN J Parenter Enteral Nutr 12:256–259, 1988.
19. Delany HM, Carnevale N, Garvey JW, et al: Postoperative nutritional support using needle catheter feeding jejunostomy. Ann Surg 186:165–170, 1970.
20. Faubion WC, Wesley JR, Khalidi N, et al: TPN catheter sepsis: Impact of the team approach. JPEN J Parenter Enteral Nutr 10:642–645, 1986.
21. Fonkalsrud EW, Berquist W, Burke M, et al: Long-term hyperalimentation in children through saphenous central venous catheterization. Am J Surg 143:209–211, 1982.
22. Forse RA, Shizgal HM: The assessment of malnutrition. Surgery 88:17–24, 1980.
23. Gallagher MW, Tyson KRT, Ashcraft KW: Gastrostomy in pediatric patients: An analysis of complications and techniques. Surgery 74:536–539, 1973.

24. Gann DS, Robinson HB: Salt, water, and vitamins. In: American College of Surgeons Manual of Surgical Nutrition. Philadelphia, WB Saunders, 1973, pp 73–90.

25. Gauderer ML, Ponsky JL, Izant RJ Jr: Gastrostomy without laparotomy: A percutaneous endoscopic technique. J Pediatr Surg 15:872–875, 1980.

26. Gauderer ML, Picha GJ, Izant RJ: The gastrostomy "button"—a simple skin-level, nonrefluxing device for long-term enteral feedings. J Pediatr Surg 19:803–805, 1984.

27. Gazzaniga AB, Bartlett RH, Shobe JB: Nitrogen balance in patients receiving either fat or carbohydrate for total intravenous nutrition. Ann Surg 182:163–168, 1975.

28. Gustke RF, Vama RR, Soergel KM: Gastric reflux during perfusion of the small bowel. Gastroenterology 59:890–895, 1970.

29. Haws EB, Sieber WK, Kiesewetter WB: Complications of tube gastrostomy in infants and children: 15-year review of 240 cases. Ann Surg 164:284–290, 1966.

30. Heiss K, Hirschl R, Cilley R, et al: Measuring infant metabolism: Design and testing of a miniature gas exchange monitor. J Pediatr Surg 23:543–545, 1988.

31. Heymsfield SB, Bethel RA, Ansley JO, et al: Enteral hyperalimentation—an alternative to central venous hyperalimentation. Ann Intern Med 90:63–71, 1979.

32. Hirschl R, Heiss K, Hultquist K, et al: Right atrial venous saturation: What role can it play in the mechanically ventilated neonate? Paper presented at the Society for Pediatric Research, Toronto, Ontario, September 27, 1987.

33. Jeejeebhoy KN, Marliss EB: Energy supply and total parenteral nutrition. In: Fischer JE (ed): Surgical Nutrition. Boston, Little, Brown & Co., 1983, pp 645–662.

34. Jeejeebhoy KN, Anderson GH, Nakhooda AF, et al: Metabolic studies in total parenteral nutrition with lipid in man: Comparison with glucose. J Clin Invest 57:125, 1976.

35. Kinney JM: Energy requirements for parenteral nutrition. In: Fischer JE (ed): Total Parenteral Nutrition. Boston, Little, Brown & Co., 1976, pp 135–142.

36. Knutrud O: The water and electrolyte metabolism in the newborn child after major surgery. Oslo, Norwegian Monographs on Medical Science, 1965.

37. McLean GK: Radiologic technique of gastrointestinal intubation. In: Rombeau JL, Caldwell MD (eds): Enteral and Tube Feeding. Philadelphia, WB Saunders, 1984, pp 240–252.

38. Meeker IA, Snyder WH: Gastrostomy for the newborn surgical patient: A report of 140 cases. Arch Dis Child 37:159–166, 1962.

39. Mendeloff E, Wesley JR, Deckert RE, et al: Comparison of measured resting energy expenditure (REE) versus estimated energy expenditure (EEE) in infants. JPEN J Parenter Enteral Nutr 10 (Suppl):65, 1986.

40. Merritt RJ: Cholestasis associated with total parenteral nutrition. J Pediatr Gastroenterol Nutr 5:9–21, 1986.

41. Merritt RJ, Suskind RM: Nutritional survey of hospitalized pediatric patients. Am J Clin Nutr 32:1320–1325, 1979.

42. Moore FD: Metabolic Care of the Surgical Patient. Philadelphia, WB Saunders, 1959.

43. Mukherjee D, Emmens RE, Putnam TC: Nonoperative conversion of gastrostomy to feeding jejunostomy in children and adults. Surg Gynecol Obstet 154:881–882, 1982.

44. Nutrition Advisory Group, American Medical Association: Multivitamin preparations for parenteral use. JPEN J Parenter Enteral Nutr 3:258–262, 1979.

45. Paulsrud JR, Pensler L, Whitten CF, et al: Essential fatty acid deficiency in infants, induced by fat-free intravenous feeding. Am J Clin Nutr 25:897–904, 1972.

46. Randall HT, Bauer RH, Hickey MD, et al: Early postoperative feeding (symposium). Contemporary Surgery 30:97–130, 1987.

47. Rhodin AGJ, Coran AG, Weintraub WH, et al: Total body water changes during high-volume peripheral hyperalimentation. Surg Gynecol Obstet 148:196–200, 1979.

48. Rickham PR: The Metabolic Response to Neonatal Surgery. Cambridge, MA, Harvard University Press, 1957.

49. Rombeau JL, Barot LR, Low DW, et al: Feeding by tube enterostomy. In: Rombeau JL, Caldwell MD (eds): Enteral and Tube Feeding. Philadelphia, WB Saunders, 1984, pp 275–291.

50. Shils ME: AMA Department of Foods and Nutrition: Guidelines for essential trace element preparations for parenteral use: A statement by an expert panel. JAMA 241:2051–2054, 1979.

51. Steffee WP, Krey SH: Enteral hyperalimentation of the cancer patient. In: Newell GR, Ellison NM (eds): Nutrition and Cancer: Etiology and Treatment. New York, Raven Press, 1981, pp 7–31.

52. Wesley JR, Keens TG, Miller SW, et al: Pulmonary embolism in the neonate: Occurrence during the course of total parenteral nutrition. J Pediatr 93:113–115, 1978.

53. Wesley JR, Coran AG, Sarahan TM, et al: The need for evaluation of gastroesophageal reflux in brain-damaged children referred for feeding gastrostomy. J Pediatr Surg 16:866–871, 1981.

54. Wesley JR, Khalidi N, Faubion WC, et al: The University of Michigan Hospitals Parenteral and Enteral Nutrition Manual. 4th ed. North Chicago, Abbott Laboratories, Hospital Products Division, 1986.

55. Wesley JR, Tse Y, Dechert RE: Indirect calorimetry on mechanically ventilated rabbits. Paris, European Society of Parenteral and Enteral Nutrition, 1987.

Dennis W. Vane
Jay L. Grosfeld

CHAPTER FORTY-SIX

Ventilatory and Respiratory Support for the Injured Child

Nowhere in the anatomy of the child is the statement "children are not just small adults" more true than in the respiratory system.[11, 17] These striking differences are even more pronounced in the young infant or very small child. The infant's metabolic rate, oxygen consumption, and carbon dioxide production may vary as much as two to three times from that expected in the adult.[19] In addition, anatomic variances in the chest wall and compliance coupled with diminished functional residual capacity contribute to the general problem of reduced respiratory reserve. In instances of traumatic injury, the respiratory system is of primary importance. No matter what the primary injury type or the severity of injury, ensuring an adequate airway and appropriate maintenance of respiratory function is of the highest priority for survival.[6] This chapter provides an overview of recent advances in the maintenance and treatment of pediatric respiratory function in the trauma victim. It is not designed as an in-depth text of critical care, but rather as an overview of current treatment of children who have suffered traumatic injuries. Additional information is provided in the bibliography.

AIRWAY MAINTENANCE

Obstruction of the airway is the most critical medical emergency in any injured patient.[6] It is imperative that physicians dealing with critically injured children have expertise in the management of the pediatric airway and in the use of the numerous techniques available for its maintenance.

Upper Airway

Although maintenance of the airway in an injured child brings to mind endotracheal intubation, other far less complex methods are important to understand and indeed may often suffice. As with all patients who exhibit airway compromise or altered consciousness, the physician must first evaluate the state of the oropharynx. Secretions and foreign bodies must be suspected, looked for, and removed if present.

The posterior oropharyngeal structures of small children are proportionally very large for the oral cavity, and this is often thought to be the reason why small infants cannot breathe as well orally. Occasionally, with edema or perhaps loss of neurologic control of the tongue, the airway may be obstructed when the tongue falls backward. If the child is in the prone position, the tongue can fall forward, relieving any such obstruction. Tilting the head to the side also shifts the tongue forward, allows relief of any intrinsic obstruction, and allows drainage of secretions out of the mouth if the patient must remain in the supine position for additional treatment. If the head cannot be comfortably turned to the side, a backward tilt of the head also elevates the base of the tongue away from the posterior oropharynx. However, these maneuvers are considered by some to be hazardous, as extreme care must be taken to maintain cervical spine integrity if spinal injury has not been ruled out.

Jaw thrust manipulation further increases the diameter of the airway by lifting the mandible and its soft tissue, including the tongue, away from the posterior pharynx, hence relieving simple intrinsic obstructions from minimal edema and loss of tongue control. This is performed by pressing gently behind the angles of the mandible and pushing forward. The chin lift procedure, inserting the thumb behind the lower mandible inside the mouth and gently lifting the jaw, can accomplish the same support of the airway and may be less cumbersome.

In many cases insertion of an oral airway may be desirable. This apparatus acts like a bite block and is inserted to hold the base of the tongue away from the posterior oropharynx and relieve subsequent obstruction. Both size and position are critical for proper function. Care must be taken to avoid pushing the tongue backward and further obstructing the airway.

Insertion is carried out by placing the airway in a curve following the curve of the tongue. This may be accomplished by placing the airway facing superiorly and then rotating the apparatus 180 degrees. Care must be taken to prevent forcing the base of the tongue posteriorly and further obstructing the airway. This method is also useful in providing an airway for infants who have a nasal obstruction but who are of an age (<30 days) that makes them obligate nasal breathers. In these infants, the glossopalatine seal is broken when the airway is properly inserted and the base of the tongue is elevated anteriorly. The mouth is kept open by the bite block.

A nasopharyngeal airway is more useful when the child is awake or semialert, when an oral airway would not be accepted. This apparatus is usually made of a soft plastic material or a rubber compound and is formed into a mild arc. It is inserted in an anatomic arc through the external nares after being adequately lubricated. Resistance may indicate that the tube size is too large and should be replaced with a smaller caliber or that the naris itself is obstructed. In the latter case, the contralateral side may be used. This type of airway provides access to the trachea by maintaining the soft palate away from the posterior airway.

Insertion of the nasopharyngeal airway is not without complications and contraindications. If incorrectly inserted, the epiglottis can be forced against the posterior pharyngeal wall and cause obstructing laryngospasm. Other problems include epistaxis and ulceration of the nasal passage, itself due to traumatic passage of the tube. Specific contraindications to the insertion of this type of airway include patients in whom the integrity of the nasal passage is in question, such as those with basilar skull fractures or cribriform trauma, or any rhinorrhea that may be attributed to a cerebrospinal fluid leak. The presence of a nasal deformity is also a relative contraindication to passage of a nasopharyngeal airway.

Endotracheal Intubation

Indications and Anatomy

Indications for endotracheal intubation are numerous and include maintenance of a compromised or potentially compromised airway or establishment of an avenue for prolonged assisted ventilation.[13] Intubation in children requires some knowledge of the anatomic variants encountered in the infant airway. Familiarity with these variations is essential if potentially serious complications are to be avoided.

In the infant and small child, the larynx lies high in the neck usually at the level of C_3 to C_4. The epiglottis is very soft and mobile and lies at about a 45-degree angle with the anterior oropharynx. The cricoid cartilage is the narrowest part of the airway, and care must be taken to avoid injuring this structure. As the child matures, the larynx falls to the level of C_7 to C_8. The entire structure becomes more cylindric in shape, and the narrowest area becomes the glottis.[13] Because the airway is more anterior in a child, hyperextension of the neck forces the larynx to an even more anterior position, resulting in intubation difficulties. It also predisposes the inexperienced health care provider to perform inadvertent esophageal intubation. For maximal exposure of the airway, the head should be maintained in the neutral position in the young infant. In some cases, gentle flexion of the neck may be useful (beware of cervical spine injury). In addition, it is also useful to have an assistant perform gentle cricoid pressure (Sellick maneuver) that may be necessary to visualize the cords fully. In older children and teenagers, the airway resembles that of the adult, and hyperextension of the neck may be helpful for successful intubation (provided the cervical spine has been cleared).

Preoxygenation

It is preferable to preoxygenate the patient before attempting intubation. This allows the health care provider some reserve should the airway be compromised temporarily or the patient become apneic temporarily during the intubation attempt. Preoxygenation is usually accomplished by allowing the patient to breath 100% oxygen for 4 to 5 minutes. If the patient is not breathing spontaneously, appropriate hand ventilation by mask is needed for a similar period of time.

Sedation and Muscle Relaxants

Under elective and planned conditions, sedation and use of muscle relaxants should be considered. An understanding of the actions of the various available muscular relaxing agents is therefore essential. Depolarizing agents cause persistent depolarization of the neuromuscular junction, whereas nondepolarizing agents compete with acetylcholine for the receptor sites.[3] Acetylcholinesterase inhibits the breakdown of acetylcholine and allows for more of the agent to be available to compete for receptor sites. Although action of the neuromuscular blockers can be reversed, there are no available reversal agents for depolarizing drugs.

Succinylcholine (a depolarizing agent) is commonly employed for elective intubation. It has a relatively short action time, lasting only 3 to 5 minutes, and is generally well tolerated.[7, 15] Infants require significantly higher dosages, most probably because of the water distribution of the drug. The recommended dosages for neonates and small infants is 2 mg per kg intravenously or intramuscularly, whereas older children and infants need only 1 mg per kg for ade-

quate relaxation.[2] The action of the drug varies with metabolic changes in the patient, and a thorough understanding of the medication (as with all drugs) is essential before its utilization.

There are several contraindications to the use of this agent in the injured child. Succinylcholine is commonly associated with bradycardia and other arrhythmias, so atropine may be used concomitantly to provide some protection from the potential resultant arrhythmias. Elevation of serum potassium may occur following the administration of succinylcholine, and its use in patients with hyperkalemia (e.g., burn patients, patients with massive soft tissue injury and bone fractures) should be discouraged. The reason for this reaction of succinylcholine is unclear. It is now recognized, however, that hyperkalemia in trauma victims may persist for up to 3 months and even longer for patients with motor neuron lesions; hence, care must be taken in the use of this agent in this circumstance. In addition, the use of succinylcholine is associated with muscle fasciculations. Fasciculations are more intense after age 4 and can be significant in school-aged children. Aside from causing general pain after anesthesia, these may increase intragastric pressure and predispose a patient to reflux and aspiration.[2] We generally pretreat the patient with diazepam (Valium), 1/10 the normal dose, which theoretically decreases but does not eliminate the problem.

Numerous nondepolarizing agents are available for administration, such as pancuronium, atracurium besylate, D-tubocurarine, and vecuronium. Pancuronium causes paralysis in less than 1 minute and lasts for approximately 1 hour. Dosage is age dependent, ranging from 30 μg per kg intravenously for a neonate up to about 1 week of age, 60 μg per kg for an infant from 1 to 2 weeks of age, and 90 μg per kg for an infant from 2 weeks to 1 month of age. Older children require 0.1–0.15 mg per kg intravenously for adequate paralysis, and duration of action is less than in a neonate because the drug is dependent on glomerular filtration. There is some hepatobiliary degradation of the drug as well, although it is not significant when the child has normal renal function. The drug apparently accumulates with repetitive doses, and smaller and smaller doses are usually required to maintain paralysis over a lengthy period of time. Pancuronium is also associated with a minimal elevation of the heart rate and blood pressure, but these phenomena usually resolve spontaneously.[10]

D-tubocurarine has longer duration of action in the neonate because of its slower rate of renal excretion. It also appears that the neonate requires a lower serum concentration of the medication to achieve adequate paralysis. Usually administered dosages are 0.2–0.4 mg per kg intravenously in the neonate and 0.6 mg per kg in the older infant or child. The side effects of the medication include hypotension and possibly even a direct myocardial depressant effect.

Reversal of action of nondepolarizing agents is dependent on the number of receptors under blockade. Agents utilized for reversal include neostigmine or pyridostigmine. Addition of an anticholinergic is recommended to block the muscarinic effects of these drugs such as bradycardia, bronchospasm, and excessive salivation. Atropine is the most widely used of these drugs, and the normal dosage is 0.02

mg per kg, with a maximum administered amount of 1 mg.[14] Reversal is always more successful if the patient demonstrates some return of neuromuscular function before receiving the reversal agent. Adequate reversal of the agent is determined by sustained tetanus at 50 Hz on the nerve stimulator or the ability to spontaneously generate an inspiratory force of 25 cm of water or more. It should be noted that several exogenous agents can prolong the neuromuscular blockade including hypothermia, magnesium, polymyxin, and the aminoglycosides.

When patients are fully awake and require intubation, sedatives are often helpful to accomplish the procedure successfully. Judicious utilization of sedatives should be employed in the trauma patient only when they do not otherwise compromise the patient's condition. Care must be taken to ensure that evaluation of the mentation of the patient is not compromised, particularly when a head injury is suspected. As a general rule, short-acting drugs are preferable in these situations. Barbiturates with short action, such as thiopental or methohexital, are ideal. The usual dosage of thiopental is 2 to 4 mg per kg intravenously and methohexital 1.5 to 2.0 mg per kg intravenously. Both agents have specific methods of action and side effects. Thiopental lowers cerebral blood flow and has been administered to patients with elevated intracranial pressure. Methohexital apparently may cause epileptiform seizures as well as provoke coughing and hiccupping. Both drugs may be associated with significant tissue necrosis when inadvertent subcutaneous infiltrations from intravenous use occur.[9]

Ketamine has been described as a useful medication for the intubation of patients who are hypovolemic. The drug produces a sympathetic response, with an elevation of both the heart rate and the blood pressure. Ketamine causes a dissociative state that lasts for several minutes. This state is also coupled with a catatonic state that lasts 1 to 2 minutes. The drug has the added benefit of being analgesic in the somatic innervated areas and is useful in cases in which painful procedures are anticipated following intubation. Side effects include hallucinations and dreams; hence, care must be taken not to cloud the neurologic evaluation of a suspected head injury patient. In addition, ketamine increases cerebral blood flow as well as cerebral spinal fluid pressure and must be considered a contraindication in patients with possible elevated intracranial pressure.[18]

Of the hypnotic substances usually employed during intubation, diazepam is the most frequently administered. This drug has been reported to reduce the hallucinogenic effects of ketamine and may be useful as an adjunct in such instances. These medications are often contraindicated in trauma victims with head injury as they may cloud the evaluation of their neurologic findings.[2]

Manipulation of the airway and larynx in preparation for intubation may be associated with several problems. Elevation of intracranial pressure, hypertension, and tachycardia are all well-known complications of laryngoscopy and manipulation of the oropharynx during intubation. Administration of lidocaine (either intratracheally or intravenously) is effective in reducing the risk of these complications. In general, the intravenous route is far more effective than the intratracheal route. Lidocaine (4% concentration) is given at a dose of 1.5 mg per kg intravenously. The drug

is also useful in suppressing the cough reflex and reducing patient intolerance to the endotracheal tube.[1]

Equipment

Appropriate pediatric-sized equipment is necessary for the management of infants and children with airway difficulties. Aside from appropriately sized endotracheal tubes, correct laryngoscopes and blades, suction devices and tubes, and even forceps for nasal intubation are required. Curved or straight laryngoscope blades are the physician's preference. Some investigators have advocated the use of the curved laryngoscope blade, observing that this blade helps keep the tongue out of the physician's field of vision. We have employed the straight blade for most intubations, however, and find it almost mandatory for neonates. For uses other than those in the neonate, the type of laryngoscope is simply the physician's preference.

Selection of the properly sized and type of endotracheal tube is critical in children. Tubes constructed of polyvinylchloride are recommended because they are inert and soft. At normal body temperature they become molded, which theoretically allows for less stress on the airway. In any case, the tube must be of a nontoxic material. This is documented by noting the presence of either "IT" or "Z79" on the tube. These marks indicate assurance that the tube material has been examined and has been found to be neither reactive nor toxic. Other markings on the tube indicate both the internal diameter (i.d.) and the external diameter (o.d.).

Procedures for the selection of a tube of appropriate diameter are somewhat controversial. Numerous formulas have been devised to determine which tube is most appropriate for each patient. As a gross measurement, the tube should be approximately the size of the infant's fifth finger or naris. In addition, the formula 16 + age (in years) = the approximate diameter in mm of the endotracheal tube (Table 46–1). In general, the use of uncuffed endotracheal tubes is recommended in children. Occasionally, a cuffed tube may be required, usually for patients who are difficult to ventilate, but this is the exception rather than the rule. When an uncuffed endotracheal tube is placed, an air leak should be present when ventilatory pressures reach the high teens. This allows for a small area of the airway to remain

Table 46–1

Approximate Endotracheal Tube Size by Patient's Age

Age	Tube Size (mm)
Premature newborn	3.0–3.5
0–12 mo	4.0
12–24 mo	4.5
2–3 yr	5.0
3–5 yr	5.5
5–7 yr	6.0
7–9 yr	6.5
9–11 yr	7.0
11–13 yr	7.5
13–15 yr	8.0

"unfilled" by the endotracheal tube and prevent pressure necrosis of the airway, particularly the subglottic area. The tube should be monitored to ensure that edema of the airway does not occlude the open space and signal the necessity to change it. The rationale for the utilization of the uncuffed tube is that the narrowest portion of the airway in an infant and small child is the cricoid ring. This area may be damaged by the inflated balloon of the cuffed tube, as the cuff normally lies just distal to the cricoid ring. If a cuffed tube is mandated by the child's pulmonary condition, great care must be taken to ensure that the cuff is of the high-volume–low-pressure variety and that it allows for symmetric inflation. Usually the cuff is inflated only until the air leak disappears. It must be noted that inflated pressures higher than 20 mm Hg often cause permanent tracheal damage. In children, repetitive evaluation of the cuff pressure by manometrics is recommended to prevent injury.

Complications

Complications in the use of endotracheal tubes occur mainly when simple safety rules are not followed. Overinflation of the tube may cause herniation of the cuff over the open end of the tube and occlusion of the lumen, with subsequent airway blockage. Also, temperature increases may cause the cuff to dilate in size and pressure and cause tracheal damage. Various methods to determine the changes in size of the airway have been described, including radiologic studies. At present, tables exist that give guidelines for tube diameters. It must be stressed, however, that these are simply guidelines and that nothing substitutes for the physician's clinical acumen. If the tube is inserted and there is no air leak at minimal ventilatory pressures (without the cuff inflated if one is present), it is probably too large and should be replaced expeditiously by one with a smaller diameter. However, if the tube is too small, adequate ventilation may not be possible, particularly if lung compliance is increased. In general, it is important to place the largest endotracheal tube possible to decrease mechanical resistance to ventilation as much as feasible.

Placement of the tip of the tube can also be a problem in children. The airway grows with the child but not always at the same rate. The distance from the cords to the carina in a full-term neonate is generally estimated at 3 cm. It then grows to 5.7 cm in a 3 month old, 7.2 cm at 8 months, and 8.1 cm at about 1 year of age. For children older than 2 years of age, the distance from the alveolar ridge to the carina may be estimated as equal to the age of the child in years divided by 2 plus 12. Flexion and extension of the neck alter these distances, and the tube placement must be checked frequently and confirmed with physical examination (auscultation of the chest) and chest radiograph. Endotracheal tubes are generally marked from the tip with centimeter gradations, and placement can be facilitated by paying attention to these markings.

Technique

The procedure for endotracheal intubation is straightforward as long as certain rules are adhered to. If at all possible, the patient is preoxygenated with 100% oxygen for several minutes. Techniques for preoxygenation with the mask and bag are described earlier in this chapter. Suction is then employed to clear the oral cavity of foreign debris and secretions to provide adequate visualization of the vocal cords. Paralytic agents or sedation are administered if warranted by the child's clinical condition, and the preoxygenation is continued for several minutes with mild hyperventilation utilizing 100% oxygen. The laryngoscope is then introduced.

It is critical to have an array of appropriately sized laryngoscopes available so that if the originally chosen scope is not adequate, a change can be effected quickly. When adequate visualization of the cords is not made with the laryngoscope first selected, it is inadvisable to persist and is clearly recommended to change to a more appropriately sized and shaped apparatus. Stubborn persistence usually only causes trauma to the airway and a low intubation success rate. The child's head is then positioned according to age, the infant in the neutral position, the neonate in slight flexion, and the older child in slight extension, again being aware of the possible threat of a central nervous system injury.[6] Maintaining the oropharyngolaryngeal axis in a straight line improves visualization of the cords. The mouth is opened with gentle pressure on the mandible. The laryngoscope is usually held with the left hand and inserted in the mouth on the right side of the tongue. Care is taken to prevent damage to the teeth or the alveolar ridge in the older infant or young children. The tongue is then moved gently to the left exposing the epiglottis and the vocal cords. If necessary, the blade of the laryngoscope may be advanced carefully over the tongue to improve exposure. Gentle cricoid pressure may be exerted both to assist in preventing aspiration in emergency intubations and to bring the cords more posteriorly to facilitate visualization. In addition, an assistant gently pulling the right side of the lips laterally often aids in visualization of the cords and improvement in the cramped working space in small children, further facilitating placement of the endotracheal tube.

If a straight laryngoscope blade is being used, it is inserted into the mouth and moved under the laryngeal side of the epiglottis. The laryngoscope is then elevated straight up along the axis of the scope (not the blade). It is important not to use the laryngoscope as a crowbar and attempt to pry the back of the throat upward or damage can result that causes bleeding in the posterior oropharynx, thereby reducing exposure. If done correctly, the base of the tongue and epiglottis are carefully raised, exposing the cords. If the larynx remains too anterior for adequate visualization, gentle cricoid pressure as previously described may bring the cords into view.

In some instances, the cords remain too far anterior for easy intubation, and an appropriate stylet may be placed within the endotracheal tube to facilitate its placement. Complications with the use of the stylet are not infrequent and can themselves be life threatening. The stylet is never advanced past the end of the endotracheal tube. It is suggested that the physician performing endotracheal intubation under these circumstances have expertise in the use of stylets to prevent tracheal or laryngeal perforation. Today, new flexible endoscopes exist that may be placed within the endotracheal tube for difficult intubations. These endoscopes are fragile and expensive but provide a great advantage in the management of the difficult pediatric airway.[13]

If the curved laryngoscope blade is employed for visualization of the cords, the blade is inserted until the tip is between the base of the tongue and the valleculae. It then rests behind the epiglottis. With the same upward motion of the laryngoscope as described with the straight blade, the tongue is elevated and the glottis is exposed. The curved blade has the benefit of keeping the tongue out of the field of vision. The curved blade, however, may force the glottis more anteriorly, making intubation more difficult in small infants and children.

Once inserted, the tube is generally fixed to the right side of the mouth. This can be done simply with tape or with one of the many fixation devices presently on the market for this purpose. Personally, we prefer to simply fix the tube to the side of the mouth with an adherent substance such as benzoin or mastisol and adhesive tape. No matter what type of securing device is used, care must be taken to ensure that fixation is firm to prevent unintentional extubation. If further instrumentation of the esophagus or trachea is planned, we prefer to fasten the tube to the left side of the mouth to make access easier.

Tracheostomy

In the past, several clinical situations in trauma patients have required the urgent performance of a tracheostomy. With the introduction of the newer polyvinyl endotracheal tubes, the old maxims that necessitated tracheostomy for patients intubated for a period of 2 weeks are no longer valid. With uncuffed and nonreactive tubes, as well as the large-volume–low-pressure tubes, endotracheal intubation may be maintained for a few weeks. Some studies have questioned whether any time limit for endotracheal intubation is an indication for tracheostomy.[17] The airway usually undergoes fewer traumatic changes after endotracheal intubation than after tracheostomy. Some indications for tracheostomy still exist, however, such as massive airway trauma, and any physician dealing with significant pediatric trauma must be familiar with the indications and the technique.

The purpose of tracheostomy is to relieve an obstructed airway or to allow for long-term ventilatory support. The oropharynx may have been injured and the physician may feel pressure to consider emergency tracheostomy under less than optimal conditions. The temptation to perform an emergency tracheostomy in an unsecured airway must be avoided.[12] Old prejudices against laryngotomy through the cricoid membrane (cricothyroidotomy) have been dispelled, and it is now well accepted that this procedure can be performed in children for temporary airway access.[4] In addition, past data indicate that tracheostomy outside of the operating room should not be considered in children.

Tracheostomy may be performed safely after the airway is controlled with an endotracheal tube or a laryngotomy in the operating room with optimal lighting and the patient under general anesthesia. The child is positioned properly with a folded pad elevating the shoulders and the neck hyperextended to facilitate exposure. The skin is prepared with an antiseptic solution, and sterile towels are applied.

The skin incision can be either transverse or longitudinal. The transverse incision has gained favor recently because it provides equal exposure but gives a better cosmetic result. The incision is placed approximately a fingerbreadth above the sternal notch and rarely needs to be longer than 1.5 cm. The subcutaneous tissue and platysma are divided transversely as well. We generally utilize a fine tip electrocautery for the dissection to minimize blood loss and to keep the tissue planes clear. The dissection is continued in a longitudinal plane. The strap muscles and pretracheal fascia are divided in the midline. This should allow for clear exposure of the trachea. Exposure can be maintained with small Cushing vein retractors or Halsted retractors placed laterally to the trachea. If the isthmus of the thyroid obstructs exposure, it can usually be simply retracted superiorly. In the rare occasion that the isthmus must be divided, it should be suture ligated to prevent subsequent bleeding. The incision is usually carried out through the third, fourth, and fifth tracheal rings and is carried out longitudinally through the rings.

If necessary, the trachea can be stabilized with a skin hook or with lateral sutures. We find that placing 3–0 silk sutures on each side of the trachea and knotting them above the skin level is useful in establishing traction for both placing the tracheostomy tube and also replacing it should inadvertent decannulation occur early in the postoperative course. We remove the sutures at 10 days after the procedure when the tube is first changed by a physician. Excision of a wedge of the trachea should *not* be performed in children as it results in an unacceptable instability of the trachea after decannulation.[12] In addition, we never perform blind emergency replacement of a tracheostomy tube after inadvertent decannulation in a fresh tracheostomy wound. Control of the airway is first obtained with orotracheal intubation if possible. The tracheostomy tube is then reinserted under controlled conditions by the appropriate staff with adequate oxygenation and lighting. This averts the complication of creating a false passage anterior to the trachea in a fresh wound and the possibility of a respiratory arrest secondary to loss of the airway.

Tube size is selected in the same fashion as noted with endotracheal tubes. A comfortable fit is mandatory, and great care should be exercised in ensuring that the tube is not too large for the child. Children present the additional problem of having variable tracheal lengths as well. Standard tubes are usually acceptable for most children, but the physician must be aware that some smaller children may require shorter tubes than those ordinarily available. In an acute situation, the tracheostomy tube can be supported by external means (tracheostomy sponges) to avoid bronchial intubation. The temporary tube can later be changed when a specially ordered tube is obtained from a company that specializes in making these modifications. Cutting tracheostomy tubes to fit is unacceptable, as the cut edge may lacerate the tracheal mucosa and create an ulceration or perforation.

To ensure fixation of the tube in the trachea, cotton tape is attached to the flanges of the tracheostomy tube and tied around the child's neck. The tapes can be passed through an appropriate length of rubber tubing or foam that covers the back of the neck to prevent the tape's cutting the skin of the posterior neck. The tube must be fixed firmly in place to avoid the complication of early decannulation. Appropriate tracheal dressings are commercially available and may be used as necessary to the physician's taste. It is better to use the commercially available tracheostomy dressings than to attempt to cut a standard gauze pad to fit and insert it under the tube. A cut gauze pad will have loose threads present that can be aspirated into the trachea and bronchial tree. The commercial dressing is stitched on its edges to prevent this complication.

Even when performed under optimal conditions, tracheostomy is not without risk. Numerous complications have been reported from the procedure itself, such as infection, airway obstruction, tracheal ulceration, stricture, formation of granulation tissue, hemorrhage, and pneumothorax. Erosion into a major blood vessel can occur but is fortunately rarely seen following pediatric tracheostomy as cuffed tubes are infrequently employed.

Maintenance of Respiratory Function

After the airway is secured, the physician must then ensure adequate ventilation of the child. Before specifics of ventilation techniques are discussed, it is critical that certain definitions and concepts be clear in the physician's mind. A few of the more critical of these are discussed subsequently.

Inadequate Oxygenation

Failure to maintain adequate oxygenation with normal respiration requires investigation as to the cause. In general, these problems result from either alveolar hypoventilation, ventilation-perfusion mismatch, or some other type of impairment of gas diffusion across the alveolar membrane into the pulmonary capillary.

Inadequate Ventilation

An abnormal elevation of arterial carbon dioxide with or without alterations in the arterial oxygen concentration signals failure of alveolar ventilation. This may be related to depression of the respiratory center from a primary effect of the peripheral or central nervous system, musculoskeletal failure, ventilation-perfusion mismatch, or, on very rare occasions, carbon dioxide production in excess of the body's normal minute ventilation capacity to dispose of the gas.

Respiratory Support

The type of respiratory support required in a pediatric patient depends on the gas exchange abnormality and the magnitude of the abnormality that exists. Mild disorders not associated with significant alveolar hypoventilation and accompanied by minimal increases in the alveolar-arterial oxygenation level may often respond to a simple increase in the inspired oxygen content. Loss of lung volume and gas exchange area is the most common cause of hypoxia and is generally easily treated by increasing the distending pressure of the airway.

Ventilation and Ventilators

Ventilation failure occurs when the child develops abnormally elevated arterial carbon dioxide tensions. The causes are varied. In children suffering from trauma, the cause is either an associated central nervous system injury with depression of the respiratory drive, an injury to the musculoskeletal system, or a pulmonary parenchymal injury that causes a mismatch of pulmonary blood flow with alveolar ventilation (given the airway is secured as described earlier). The choice of respiratory support varies with the degree of impairment the child is experiencing. Minimal support can be obtained temporarily with the simple administration of oxygen. However, this solution often does not solve the underlying problems. The limiting factor with this treatment is the level of oxygen that must be administered. Oxygen toxicity may occur with an inspired concentration that is higher than 40%, and this cannot be tolerated for extended periods of time. Other forms of ventilatory assistance may be required. In addition, if metabolic alterations are encountered (e.g., respiratory acidosis), mechanical ventilation and additional respiratory assistance are usually necessary. When all of these conventional methods have been exhausted, the clinician may then have to turn to other less conventional modalities.

The administration of oxygen can be carried out using nasal cannulae, masks, hoods, tents, or any other controlled environment apparatus. Fairly high oxygen concentrations can be obtained using any of these delivery techniques in children (usually higher than adults) because of the child's relatively small tidal volumes (6–10 ml per kg). Humidification is always required with any form of oxygen therapy to prevent desiccation of the mucous membranes and possibly occlusion of the airway. Patients usually prefer cool humidity, because higher levels of water saturation are tolerated with less discomfort. Neonates are an exception to this statement, as administration of cool gas causes problems such as hypothermia and changes in metabolic rate.

When conservative methods fail, the physician is forced to intervene to manage the distending pressure of the patient's alveoli by controlling the delivery of respiratory gases. This may be accomplished with a variety of techniques including those as simple as continuous positive airway pressure (CPAP), intermittent positive pressure breathing (IPPB), or continuous positive pressure ventilation (CPPV).

CPAP requires spontaneous respiratory effort on the part of the patient. This method depends on a high flow of inspired gas, higher than the patient's normal respiratory volume. Connectors and tubing must be of large diameter so that they do not impede the child's respiratory effort. The system employs a valve that closes at a specific predetermined setting during exhalation so that the patient maintains an intrapulmonary pressure that is higher than the ambient atmosphere. The augmented flow diminishes the work of breathing, and increased pressures expand increased numbers of alveoli, thereby increasing respiratory reserve. Unfortunately, CPAP is not without problems. The increase in intrathoracic pressures diminishes venous return and cardiac output. CPAP also requires a relatively closed system, usually with the patient not intubated. This can be modified, however, as nasal prongs or even a mask may be employed occasionally.

Positive end-expiratory pressure, or PEEP, is a modification of CPAP. In this system, a reservoir is utilized to deliver an inspiratory volume. A one-way flow valve prevents exhalation from forcing air back into the reservoir and subsequently preventing rebreathing. The end-expiratory pressure is maintained as with CPAP. The level of PEEP is determined in one of several ways. The most simple and clinically useful method that has been described is the one that determines the pressure that reduces the calculated pulmonary shunt fraction to a minimum without impeding the cardiac output.[8]

When these conservative assist methods fail, the patient must then be placed on controlled ventilation. Controlled ventilation utilizes the sporadic or periodic elevation of the patient's inspiratory pressure and is most useful in the patient with severe neurologic impairment or muscular dysfunction significant enough to prevent adequate respiratory effort. Controlled ventilation is also useful for other patients with severe respiratory insufficiency, which may then require the addition of neuromuscular blocking agents that result in paralysis to be effective (see earlier discussion). In this mode, the ventilator delivers the entire minute ventilation of the patient. The physician regulates the machine to deliver a desired amount of gas during a specific duration of time at a given frequency. The gas concentration can be modified for the specific needs of each patient, particularly if oxygen requirements are deemed necessary. The addition of end-expiratory pressures can also assist in the control of the patient and improve gas exchange even further through the recruitment of additional alveoli. This method is particularly useful in trauma patients who are in the immediate postinjury period. The patient is kept well sedated while respiratory efforts are controlled. In addition, head injury patients can easily have their respiratory rate controlled. The physician can then artificially lower the patient's Pa_{CO_2} to attempt to reduce intracranial pressure. This is a very useful method of ventilation for the severely compromised patient. As the patient's condition improves, or if the patient is not severely compromised, other methods of ventilatory support can be entertained.

When the patient can be relied on to generate a respiratory effort, patient assist modalities can be instituted. Respiratory assist devices have a sensory device installed that can sense changes in pressures or flow that correspond to a breathing effort on the part of the patient. The ventilatory circuit is triggered to deliver a breath or gas pressure and institute a mechanical respiration. The volume (or in some cases the pressure) is accessible to deliver a determined tidal volume for the patient. In this case, the rate is determined by the patient's own ventilatory effort. Although some reports suggest that initial alveolar hyperventilation occurs with this method for a short period of time, it is usually self-limiting and not of major clinical significance.[20] All ventilators in the patient assist mode have the capability of providing a safety device that is preset to a specific minimal ventilatory frequency. In this way, if the patient does not initiate a breath over a prescribed period of time, the machine initiates a breath spontaneously. This is purported to eliminate the danger of apneic spells or respiratory arrest.

When the patient is able to maintain an adequate respiratory rate and can initiate adequate inspiratory volumes, a third type of assisted ventilation may be employed. In these instances, the patient is assisted with supplemental ventilator breaths spaced at a given time sequence. These assists can be delivered at a given rate or timed to the patient's ventilatory efforts. In patients who are awake and alert, timing must coincide with the patient's spontaneous respirations. If this is not done, the assists are extremely uncomfortable for the patient and cause extreme agitation as the patient anticipates the assisted breath.

A new form of this therapy has been developed. In this mode, the machine is set to a preset rate and tidal volume. This gives a specific minute ventilation pattern that is allowed to diminish as the patient makes more and more of a spontaneous respiratory effort. Reports have stated that care must be taken when using this new modality, as a rapid respiratory rate with small volumes may release the machine but still provide inadequate respiratory function. The rapid respiratory rate maintains the prescribed minute volume for the patient while inadequate volumes are delivered. The ventilator then diminishes its support automatically while the child is unable to provide self-maintenance for extended periods of time. This difficulty may be corrected when a maximum rate alarm is installed, which is triggered when the patient is hyperventilating. The automatic correction of the machine to the more rapid rate eliminates the problem.

This summary is simply a brief outline of some of the problems associated with ventilation of the pediatric trauma patient. It is not intended to be a detailed evaluation of ventilator management or availability. For a more in-depth study, the physician should consult one of the many texts devoted to pediatric critical care and respiratory management.

Experimental Approaches

Technologic advances and a more clear understanding of pulmonary and cardiac physiology have led to newer experimental techniques for ventilation. None of these techniques is perfect, and clearly controversy exists over their use in the pediatric trauma patient. It must be noted, however, that their use is limited to situations in which conventional therapy is failing and heroic measures are indicated for preservation of the child's life.

High-Frequency Ventilation. The development of high-frequency ventilation (rate >120 breaths per minute) arose when researchers noted the variance in arterial blood pressure with normal ventilatory volumes. By decreasing the ventilatory volume while increasing the rate, the variations in arterial pressures could be manipulated or eliminated. In addition, it was observed that the normal cardiac function caused some ventilation of the pulmonary parenchyma itself. When volumes are extremely small and the rate is extreme, gas exchange persists in both adults and neonates; in addition, the Venturi effect of the gas insufflation throughout the center of the endotracheal tube also appears to contribute. In essence, the technique depends on high-speed insufflation of a low volume of appropriately oxygenated air under relatively low pressure. Exhalation is not dependent on the elastic recoil of the pulmonary parenchyma or the chest wall but rather is created by the oscillation of gases in the airway. Problems with this technique are numerous, and the retention of carbon dioxide appears to be significant. The process is effective in some cases; however, more data are required to ascertain which children should be candidates for the method.[5]

Extracorporeal Membrane Oxygenation. Extracorporeal membrane oxygenation (ECMO) has gained new favor in the pediatric setting, particularly in the newborn, in whom lung growth and maturation can be relied on to improve respiratory function with time. The technique requires good vascular access; in the newborn the common carotid and internal jugular vein are used for access. Results are impressive in the newborn but not as good in the pediatric patient. Access may be veno-venous or veno-arterial, but the veno-arterial approach appears to be more effective. Sufficient data from trauma patients are not available, but theoretically this system has many advantages and possible uses.[16]

Monitoring. Continuous assessment of the ventilated patient is critical, so adequate monitoring is essential. In critically ill patients, cardiovascular function, respiratory function, and renal function are all interconnected and require instantaneous data flow so that corrective measures for physiologic fluctuations can be made. Cardiovascular evaluation requires assessment of rhythm, rate, filling pressures, systemic blood pressure, and cardiac output. All of these parameters directly influence the ventilatory requirements of the injured child and are critical for adequate management. In addition, any child who is intubated and or ventilated must have arterial blood gas evaluations routinely as well as assessment of continuous arterial oxygen saturations. If these parameters are adhered to, good results from significant pediatric injury become the rule rather than the exception.

References

1. Backofen JE, Rogers MC: Emergency management of the airway. In: Rogers MC (ed): Textbook of Pediatric Intensive Care. Vol. 1. Baltimore, Williams & Wilkins, 1988, pp 57–77.
2. Betts EK, Downes JJ: Anesthesia. In: Welch KJ, Randolph JG, Ravitch MM, et al. (eds): Pediatric Surgery. 4th ed. Chicago, Year Book Medical Publishers, 1986, pp 50–67.
3. Brandom BW, Woelfel SK, Cook DR, et al: Clinical pharmacology of atracurium in infants. Anesthesiology 59:440, 1983.
4. Brantigan CO, Grow JB: Cricothyroidotomy: Elective use in respiratory problems requiring tracheostomy. J Thorac Cardiovasc Surg 71:72–81, 1976.
5. Coghill CH, Haywood JL, Chatburn RL, et al: Neonatal and pediatric high-frequency ventilation: Principles and practice. Respir Care 36:598–608, 1991.
6. Committee on Trauma, American College of Surgeons: Resource Document for Optimal Care of the Injured Patient. Chapter 12, Planning pediatric trauma care. Chicago, American College of Surgeons, 1990, pp 51–54.
7. Cook DR, Fisher CG: Neuromuscular blocking effects of succinylcholine in infants and children. Anesthesiology 42:662–665, 1974.
8. Downs JB, Modell JH: Patterns of respiratory support aimed at pathophysiologic conditions. In: Hershey SG (ed): ASA Refresher Courses in Anesthesiology. Vol. 7. Philadelphia, JB Lippincott, 1977, p 71.
9. Freeman A, Bachman L: Pediatric anesthesia: An evaluation of preoperative medication. Anesth Analg 38:429–437, 1959.
10. Goudsouzian NG, Ryan JF, Savarese JJ: The neuromuscular effects of pancuronium in infants and children. Anesthesiology 41:95–98, 1974.
11. Hazinski MF, van Stralen D: Physiologic and anatomic differences between children and adults. In: Levin DL, Morriss FC (eds): Essentials of Pediatric Intensive Care. St. Louis, Quality Medical Publishing, 1990, pp 5–17.
12. Johnson DG: Lesions of the larynx and trachea—tracheostomy. In: Welch KJ, Randolph JG, Ravitch MM, et al (eds): Pediatric Surgery. 4th ed. Chicago, Year Book Medical Publishers, 1986, pp 622–630.
13. Kingston HGG: Airway problems in pediatric patients. In: Lynn AM (guest ed); Kirby RR, Brown DL (editors-in-chief): Problems in Anesthesia: Pediatric Anesthesia. 2(4):545–565. Philadelphia, JB Lippincott, 1988.
14. Meakin G, Sweet PT, Bevan JC, et al: Neostigmine and edrophonium as antagonists of pancuronium in infants and children. Anesthesiology 59:316–321, 1983.
15. Nightingale DA, Glass AG, Bachman L: Neuromuscular blockade by succinylcholine in children. Anesthesiology 27:736–741, 1966.
16. O'Rourke PP, Stolar CJH, Zwischenberger JB, et al: Extracorporeal membrane oxygenation: Support for overwhelming pulmonary failure in the pediatric population—Collective experience from the extracorporeal life support organization. J Pediatr Surg 28:523–528, 1993.
17. Persky MS: Airway management and post-intubation sequelae. In: Zimmerman SS, Gildea JH (eds): Critical Care Pediatrics. Philadelphia, WB Saunders, 1985, pp 10–15.
18. Ponaman ML, Farrington E, Morris FC: Analgesia and sedation. In: Essentials of Pediatric Intensive Care. St. Louis, Quality Medical Publishing, 1990, pp 911–920.
19. Rowe MI: Fluid and electrolyte management. In: Welch KJ, Randolph JG, Ravitch MM, et al (eds): Pediatric Surgery. 4th ed. Chicago, Year Book Medical Publishers, 1986, pp 22–31.
20. Weng FT: Assisted ventilation. In: Zimmerman SS, Gildea JH (eds): Critical Care Pediatrics. Philadelphia, WB Saunders, 1985, pp 16–31.

Richard J. Andrassy
Robert W. Feldtman
R. Kelly Hill, Jr.

CHAPTER FORTY-SEVEN

Hyperbaric Oxygen Therapy for Childhood Injury

HISTORY

Joseph Priestley discovered oxygen in 1774. Shortly thereafter, in the 1800s, oxygen therapy was thought to be fashionable, and throughout Europe and America, crude hyperbaric oxygen (HBO) tanks were constructed to allow people to breathe this newly discovered gas. Hucksters soon suggested oxygen for every imaginable illness, resulting in HBO rapidly falling into discredit.

In the 1950s, interest in HBO therapy once again flourished.[1] Pediatric cardiovascular operations were performed in a hyperbaric environment. This hyperoxia allowed for longer periods of ischemic in-flow occlusion during congenital cardiac operations. With in-flow times of less than 20 minutes, atrial septal defects and other ''open heart'' operations could be accomplished without neurologic injury.

Oxygen therapy of carbon monoxide poisoning was well established, and several cases of carbon monoxide poisoning were treated successfully in an HBO environment. However, because hyperbaric tanks were not readily available across the country, this therapy was somewhat limited in application.

Recompression of diving-related accidents was understood in the late 1800s when ''caisson disease'' was described. Repressurization of patients suffering from the bends often reduced pain and reversed neurologic deficit. The addition of oxygen to the environment speeded the resolution of symptoms.[3] The U.S. Navy dive tables and treatment tables were in use by the onset of World War II and are used today in both military and civilian diving operations.

High-performance aircraft that arrived on the scene in World War II exposed U.S. Army Air Corps crew members to a rapidly decreasing pressure as high altitudes were reached. Cases of ''the bends'' were seen in air crew members, and this prompted the U.S. Air Force to get involved in decompression research along with the Navy. Air Force flight surgeons were trained in the recognition and treatment of decompression sickness (DCS), and Navy dive tanks were established in several key locations around the world to treat military flyers.

Today's modern applications of HBO therapy were an outgrowth of this military experience, and with this background, physicians at Brooks Air Force Base in San Antonio, Texas, were soon treating a variety of medical and surgical problems. Close cooperation with the Navy and the civilian community resulted in the treatment of a variety of conditions.

As knowledge about HBO disseminated into the medical literature, the method gained further support. Soon it was being used for burns, poisonings, and snake and spider envenomation among other problems. Trauma often causes ischemic, infected wounds, which generally respond well to HBO, so children began to be treated as well.

The pediatric applications of HBO were not new, since one of the earliest uses of HBO was for congenital cardiac disease. Today, modern pumps and oxygenators make this modality unnecessary, and complex congenital cardiac conditions can be corrected with fairly long periods of cardiac standstill without serious neurologic injury. Hyperbaric oxygen is now suited to more specific indications, and these are discussed here.

THEORY AND PHYSIOLOGY OF HYPERBARIC OXYGEN TREATMENT

Physics

Because oxygen is a gas, a brief review of gas laws is in order. *Dalton's law* states that the sum of the partial pressures of a mixture of gases equals the total pressure. As an example, at sea level, the partial pressure of oxygen is 21% of 760 mm Hg, or 159 mm Hg.

Henry's law relates the amount of gas in a solution to its partial pressure and the solubility coefficient of the gas in that solution. It is also inversely related to the temperature of the solution. Because of this law, an amount of oxygen sufficient to maintain life can be obtained by increasing the pressure of the gas to 3 atmospheres absolute (ATA). Breathing 100% oxygen at 3 ATA results in 6.8 vol% of oxygen dissolved in the blood.

Boyle's law states that a volume of gas is inversely proportional to its pressure, assuming the temperature is constant.

Charles' law is related in that if a volume remains constant and pressure increases, temperature rises (adiabatic heating). This is important in the design of hyperbaric chambers to allow for adequate ventilation to prevent hyperpyrexia.

Physiology

Oxygen Binding to Hemoglobin

The hemoglobin molecule is uniquely suited to bind and thus carry oxygen to the tissues. Because 1 gm of hemoglobin can carry 1.34 ml of oxygen, at sea level oxygen is approximately 97% saturated. Increased pressure thus cannot cause hemoglobin to carry more than 100% saturation. Conversely, increased amounts of oxygen can be carried to the tissues by increasing the dissolved oxygen in the blood.

Dissolved Oxygen

As stated in Henry's law, the amount of dissolved oxygen can be increased by increasing the pressure of inspired oxygen. Since average tissue extraction is 6 vol%, oxygen consumption is 300 ml per minute assuming a cardiac output of 5 liters per minute. It is therefore easy to see that at 2000 mm Hg oxygen, tissue oxygen delivery can be increased tremendously.

Closed-Space Problems

As stated in Boyle's law, the volume of a gas expands as the pressure increases. This can be a problem in patients with closed gas spaces. Malfunctioning eustachian tubes can cause tympanic membrane rupture. Pulmonary blebs can burst, causing tension pneumothorax. Other gas spaces above the teeth and in the sinuses can cause pain as pressure (and thus volume) increases.

Hazards Related to Physics and Physiology

Oxygen Toxicity. Up to 15% of normal volunteers suffer grand mal seizures at 30 feet of seawater pressure and on 10% oxygen. Close observation of patients by trained medical personnel can usually forestall seizures by changing the mixture to air.

Nitrogen Narcosis. Just as nitrous oxide can cause sleepiness, gaseous nitrogen at high pressures can cause neurologic abnormality. This is usually seen at pressures of 6 ATA.

Fire Hazards. Because the oxygen environment in the chamber is tremendously enriched, particularly in the monoplace chamber, the risk of combustion and fire is high. Careful choice of clothing, removal of all oil-based cosmetics, and prohibition of all metallic material prevents sparks and fire.[3]

Pharmacology of Oxygen

Although oxygen is necessary for life, it can also be toxic. At high levels, it can be damaging to neurologic tissues as well as bone and pulmonary tissue. Although aerobic bacteria have adequate quantities of the protective enzyme superoxide dismutase, leukocyte phagocytosis is an oxygen-dependent mechanism, requiring a partial pressure of oxygen (P_{O_2}) of 30 to 40 mm Hg. Many bacteria are destroyed by oxygen, and the toxins produced by bacteria are also neutralized by increased levels of oxygen.

By definition, anaerobic bacteria thrive only in an environment devoid of or low in oxygen. Additionally, many bacterial infections are multifactorial, including both aerobic and anaerobic bacteria. Of special interest are the gram-positive anaerobes such as the *Clostridium* species.

Clostridial organisms produce toxins necessary for the spread of bacterial infections. Spreading factor allows for the dissolution of tissue planes as the infection moves along. Partial pressures of oxygen of 250 mm Hg in tissue are sufficient not only to neutralize the toxins but also to destroy the bacteria.

TYPES OF HYPERBARIC CHAMBERS

The distinction between monoplace and multiplace chambers is more than a distinction of size. Many physicians with HBO experience prefer to use one or the other, touting the qualities of their preference and the ''hazards'' of the other. In addition, many referral sources base their choice on the capabilities of a multiplace chamber. Unfortunately, this may affect referral patterns and thus sources of income. The cost of installation of these chambers may also force an administrator to choose a less expensive system in an effort to maximize projected profits.

All of these factors should be considered when planning a new HBO treatment facility. A visit to several facilities will answer many questions about staffing and construction that might not otherwise be considered.

Monoplace Chambers

The monoplace hyperbaric chamber is certainly the most attractive in terms of cost and ease of installation. Several commercially available chambers are in use. One type (Sechrist) is constructed of a clear plastic that has the advantage of decreasing claustrophobia.[4, 11] The metal chamber (Dixie) has only small portholes.[2] Some patients have declined treatment in the metal chamber and have been successfully treated in the plastic chamber.

The small chambers are filled and ventilated with pure oxygen, although most physicians prefer to have a source of compressed breathing air available also so that a hyperbaric air environment can be used as well. Because the volumes are small in the chamber, the chambers can be hooked through appropriate regulators to the hospital's oxygen lines. This oxygen source is usually liquid oxygen. Chamber facilities that rely on bottled oxygen have a major logistic problem with handling compressed oxygen cylinders if many dives, or therapy sessions, are planned.

A disadvantage to the monoplace chamber is the lack of an ''inside tender.'' The inside tender, usually a physician or nurse, can tend to the medical needs of the patient while at depth. This is, however, usually not necessary, and the tender is often there for many hours of boredom, only occasionally for moments of patient anxiety. However, tenders are especially useful with patients who have severe poisoning, gas gangrene, or neurologic impairment. Additionally, critically ill patients may have a variety of tubes and drains that many need attention. Medications may need to be given parenterally during a dive, although preplaced intravenous lines can be used if ''pass-through'' connectors are available. Dressings may become soaked and need to be changed during a dive.

Multiplace chambers afford much more comfort to the patient, solve most of the above problems, and are a convenience to the treating physician, but they are much more expensive. Although most monoplace chambers can be purchased for well under $100,000, the multiplace chambers usually start around $1,000,000, and hospital administrators need to carefully plan for growth and have a reasonably accurate idea as to volume of usage before a large chamber is purchased. Certainly, a large number of patients can justify such an expense. However, one must keep in mind that with a large number of patients, several shifts of nurses and attendants must be paid to provide service to the patients. Also, many patients will need to be treated late at night by necessity because of time and volume constraints. These technicians and nurses need special training by attending an appropriate course to prepare them for safely operating HBO equipment.

REIMBURSEMENT

Generally speaking, patients are charged $200 to $400 per treatment session. Considering that many conditions, such as osteomyelitis, may require daily treatments for a month or more, cost is not small. Most public and private health insurance carriers pay for HBO treatment.

FACILITIES

In addition to the chambers themselves and the oxygen source, several other considerations need to be entertained concerning the construction of an HBO facility. A well-lit reception area with work areas for nurses and physicians, and changing areas for patients, must be provided. The patients should have facilities for removing makeup and changing into clothing of 100% cotton for fire prevention. Fire-fighting equipment should be on hand and include fire extinguishers appropriate to the facility. Large multiplace chambers will probably have a built-in, pressurized-water fire suppression system.

Medical supplies, equipment, and adequate drugs should be on hand to manage the patients treated. All dressings should be removed and the wounds inspected with each treatment. Adequate sterile materials and gloves need to be available for each patient. Topical oxygen may be of use, and some physicians apply a source of oxygen to the wound in patients being treated in an HBO (multiplace chamber) environment.

MEDICATIONS

An emergency cart must be available, with all the appropriate medications for a cardiopulmonary arrest in place. In addition, diazepam and phenytoin (Dilantin) should be available in case of seizures or extreme anxiety. Other medications that the patient may need on a routine basis, such as antibiotics and pain medication, can be sent with the patient to the facility for administration at an appropriate dosing time by a qualified attendant.

Topical antibiotic creams and solutions, such as povidone-iodine, which kills a wide variety of bacteria, fungi, and viruses, should be stocked in the facility for dressing changes. Burn patients may need other types of creams such as silver sulfadiazine and mafenide (Sulfamylon).

PREPARATION OF THE PATIENT FOR HYPERBARIC OXYGEN THERAPY

The most important step in the use of HBO therapy involves thinking about it in the first place. Many physicians have not been trained to think about its use; thus, many patients are denied HBO therapy. There are certain clear-cut indications in which HBO therapy is useful and appropriate. Most often, HBO therapy should be used as an adjunctive therapy to other modalities. Zeal in getting the patient into the tank should not override other medical considerations concerning airway management, shock, blood replacement, and wound care.

CHAMBER LOCATION

As hyperbaric chambers proliferate across the country, the choices increase and the distances patients are required to travel decrease. Many large metropolitan areas have hospital-based chambers available 24 hours a day. Telephone consultation is often available to guide the physician in choosing not only the closest chamber but, more importantly, the most appropriate chamber for the particular patient.

Divers Alert Network

The Divers Alert Network (DAN) is available 24 hours a day by phone at 919/684-8111. DAN provides guidance for physicians, primarily concerning diving accidents. Diving chambers referred to are usually hospital-based, multiplaced chambers that are staffed 24 hours a day.

TRANSPORTATION

Many diving-related or other injuries requiring HBO therapy necessitate transport to a facility for treatment. These accidents often occur hundreds of miles from high-technology medical care, so air evacuation is needed. Diving accidents can be worsened by placing the patient in a cabin environment that is at a pressure below that of sea level. In such situations, the flight crew should be informed of the patient's condition and an attempt made to control cabin pressure to as near that of sea level as possible during transport.

Most conditions that require HBO are benefitted to some degree by face mask oxygen at sea level. The application of oxygen during transport is therefore important whether the patient is traveling by land or air ambulance.

HOSPITALIZATION

On arrival at the HBO facility, prompt evaluation by the physician and possibly other consultants expedites management of the patient. A complete physical examination with special attention to an examination of the tympanic membranes and auscultation of the chest is critical. A history should be taken with special emphasis on pulmonary problems such as chronic obstructive pulmonary disease, previous spontaneous pneumothoraces; ear, nose, and throat problems; or seizure disorders.

An eye examination is important to document any lenticular opacity (cataract) before HBO treatment. Some researchers have suggested that cataracts are worsened by HBO therapy, but this has not been proved.

If the patient is comatose or cannot clear his or her ears, or is very young, a tympanotomy or pressure equalization tube insertion may be needed to prevent space problems in the middle ear. A chest radiograph should be taken to evaluate for unsuspected pulmonary disease or blebs.

If any tubes are in place in the patient, they should be

evaluated for balloon cuffs. Balloon cuffs on endotracheal tubes can rupture if inflated with air, so saline can and should be substituted. Nasogastric decompression tubes should be replaced with simple Cantor, Levin, or Salem sump tubes. Foley catheter balloons can likewise be filled with saline. Intravenous fluids are almost universally supplied in collapsible bags, but caution should be taken to vent glass bottles properly to avoid potential venous air embolism, since gas in a closed space changes volume with the changing pressures.

Familiarizing the patient with the chamber should include a brief conversation aimed at preventing claustrophobia. Some patients have severe claustrophobia, but many can be gently urged to try the chamber. Chambers that are well lighted or constructed with clear plastic allow much easier adaptation to the closed environment. An internal speaker and a visible television may also help ease the patient's nerves during the first few dives. Small children can be joined in the chamber by a nurse or inside attendant who can provide encouragement as they accompany the patient through the treatment.

INDICATIONS

In at least 10 clinical situations, HBO therapy has been shown to be as effective as primary or adjunctive therapy:

1. Decompression sickness
2. Acute gas embolism
3. Gas gangrene
4. Soft tissue infection
5. Compromised skin graft or flap
6. Acute carbon monoxide poisoning (smoke inhalation)
7. Exceptional blood loss when transfusion is delayed or impossible
8. Osteoradionecrosis
9. Soft tissue radionecrosis
10. Crush injury

A second group, in which HBO efficacy is not proved but wherein it may benefit, includes the following:

1. Actinomycosis
2. *Bacteroides* infection
3. Acute peripheral arterial insufficiency or ischemia
4. Head and spinal cord trauma
5. Acute cerebral edema
6. Intestinal obstruction
7. Early or refractory osteomyelitis
8. Renal artery insufficiency
9. Nondiabetic retinopathy
10. Some ulcers
11. Acute thermal burn
12. Limb reanastomosis

Finally, a third group of disorders in which HBO treatment has been suggested but remains extremely controversial includes the following:

1. Bone graft

2. Hydrogen sulfide or acute carbon tetrachloride poisoning
3. Extreme hemodilution in cardiac bypass or valve surgery
4. Diabetic retinopathy
5. Frostbite
6. Migraine headache
7. Nonjoined or nonhealing fracture
8. Intra-abdominal or intracranial abscess
9. Lepromatous leprosy
10. Meningitis
11. Sickle cell hematuria or crisis
12. Brown recluse spider bite

Some of the more common specific indications seen in children are discussed at greater length in the following sections.

Gas Gangrene

Gas gangrene is a clostridial myonecrosis or spreading clostridial cellulitis with systemic toxicity. Clostridia are putrefactive, gram-positive, anaerobic, spore-forming encapsulated bacilli, which can be motile or nonmotile, depending on the species. Most are soil contaminants.

Clostridia have been isolated from the stomach, gallbladder, small bowel, colon, vagina, and skin of healthy individuals. *Clostridium perfringens* has been implicated alone and in combination with other organisms in 50 to 100% of all gas gangrene infections. Clostridia thrive in tissues with low oxygen tension. When tissue is damaged, its vascular supply is compromised, both by direct vascular damage and from an increased diffusion distance due to edema, and tissue oxygen tensions are lowered. Exotoxins are produced by the bacteria with resulting worsening of edema, liquefication of tissues, and systemic responses that further compromise the blood supply.

Most cases are post-traumatic or postoperative, although spontaneous cases have been reported. The classic picture includes an edematous, discolored wound with bronze, gray, or purplish discoloration; brown, watery discharge; hemorrhagic bullae; or any rapidly extending margin of erythema. Palpable crepitation is a late finding and is not a sine qua non for the diagnosis. Early signs of infection include progressive increase in wound or incisional pain disproportionate to the severity of the lesion, tachycardia not in proportion to the fever, mental changes reflected by apathy or indifference, and shiny skin around a wound indicating edema.

The diagnosis of clostridial gas gangrene is made on the basis of clinical suspicion and bacteriologic confirmation. Gram staining of the wound drainage is the most rapid means of confirming the suspected diagnosis. The presence of gram-positive bacilli in conjunction with any of the above-mentioned clinical findings should be considered gas gangrene, and treatment should be instituted immediately.

The management of gas gangrene consists of early institution of antibiotics, surgical débridement, and HBO treatment. Penicillin is the drug of choice for the prophylaxis and treatment of gas gangrene. Broad-spectrum coverage may be indicated in polymicrobial infection. In the presence of penicillin allergy, tetracycline is recommended for older children or adults, but chloramphenicol, erythromycin, and clindamycin have also been advocated. However, surgical débridement of necrotic tissue remains the cornerstone of therapy, and frequent débridement is warranted when indicated.

The addition of HBO therapy to aggressive surgical débridement and appropriate antibiotics is valuable. The mortality rate varies considerably depending on whether the gas gangrene occurred as a posttraumatic, postoperative, or spontaneous event. The degree of injury, extent of involvement, and timing of therapy also affect outcome. Heimbach and colleagues have reported that the mortality rate was 5.1% when HBO therapy was instituted within 24 hours of onset.[6, 7] This reflects the experience of the Air Force at the San Antonio hyperbaric facility. Hart and associates reported on 139 consecutive patients with an *81%* survival rate.[5] Factors favoring survival include patients arriving before shock had developed, an incubation period of less than 12 hours, female gender, youth, and nonspontaneous infection. The HBO treatment used was 2.5 ATA to maximize the oxygen tensions in the infection area so as to immediately halt toxin production and yet not exceed the cerebral oxygen threshold. HBO therapy was continued at 2.5 ATA three times a day for 48 hours, then twice a day at 2 ATA until the infection was controlled (as evidenced by absence of toxicity, cessation of hemolysis, and a clean-appearing wound). This usually required an additional 3 or 4 days of therapy.

A large number of clinical reports have indicated the value of adjunctive HBO therapy in gas gangrene. Other treatment regimens have been used, but the increasing numbers of chambers available make HBO therapy a possibility in most instances. In our experience, children with posttraumatic gas gangrene also benefit from early HBO treatment in conjunction with débridement and antibiotics. They tolerate therapy well and have minimal complications. Unfortunately, although postoperative gas gangrene in children is rare, those afflicted generally are referred for treatment late, so the results are less impressive. Delayed diagnosis and difficulty with transport from the hospital to the chamber in critically ill patients may be another reason for delayed referrals.

Case Example

An 11-year-old white boy was playing in the bayou behind his home and suffered a laceration to the flexor compartment of his right upper extremity. Twelve hours after surgical repair, the skin became tight and the characteristic bronzing of clostridial infection was seen (Fig. 47–1). Gram stain of the exudate was consistent with clostridial infection, and the child experienced tachycardia and severe incisional pain. Although culture results were not available and no gas was present in the tissue on either manual or radiographic examinations, hyperbaric consultation was obtained. The child immediately underwent compression to 3 ATA for 30 minutes, followed by an additional 90 minutes at 2 ATA. There was a prompt decrease in pain and immediate arrest of the spread of the skin changes (Fig. 47–2).

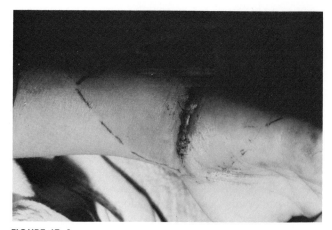

FIGURE 47–1
Pretreatment, demonstrating tight skin from swelling and bronzing.

In view of the response, the surgeon elected not to débride the wound; instead, the patient underwent twice-daily treatments of 90 minutes each in the monoplace chamber for a total of 10 sessions. His wound healed without difficulty or further surgical care.

Carbon Monoxide Poisoning

Carbon monoxide poisoning accounts for almost half of the 3000 fatal poisonings in the United States each year. Carbon monoxide has an affinity for hemoglobin 240 times greater than that of oxygen. After exposure to carbon monoxide, this affinity results in the formation of a significant percentage of hemoglobin existing as carboxyhemoglobin (COHb). Its presence causes a left shift of the oxyhemoglobin dissociation curve and a disruption of intracellular respiratory processes by combining with cytochrome A_3 oxidase. Cellular hypoxia ensues as a result of inadequate extracellular transport and, intracellularly, from disruption of the electron transport system.

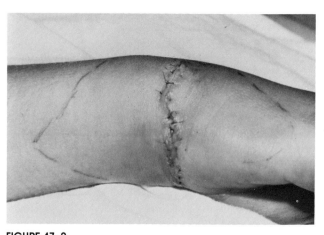

FIGURE 47–2
After treatment, demonstrating decreased swelling and arrest of skin changes.

The rationale for HBO therapy in carbon monoxide poisoning is four-fold:

1. HBO therapy improves tissue oxygenation by increasing the amount of dissolved oxygen in plasma. Although the hemoglobin may be too tightly bound to the carbon monoxide to carry oxygen, enough oxygen can be physically dissolved into the plasma phase to effect improvement and lead to recovery.

2. The HBO treatment increases the rate of dissociation of COHb. When the victim is breathing room air, the half-time (time required to reduce the concentration of COHb to half its starting level) is 320 minutes. When 100% oxygen is breathed at sea-level pressure, this half-time decreases to 80 minutes; when the patient is treated with 100% oxygen at 3 ATA in a hyperbaric chamber, however, the half-time drops to a mere 23 minutes, a reduction of some 93%.

3. Only HBO therapy can reverse the poisoning of the cytochrome A_3 system, thereby normalizing the electron transport system and avoiding or ameliorating long-term neurologic sequelae.

4. HBO treatment has been shown to have a beneficial effect on cerebral edema and intracranial pressure.

The clinical manifestations of carbon monoxide poisoning may vary greatly, depending on a number of factors, including the concentration of carbon monoxide to which the patient was exposed, the duration of exposure, the rate and depth of breathing, the heart rate at the time, and the presence of other cytochrome poisons such as cyanide, carbon tetrachloride. In one study of 115 patients, COHb levels did not correlate with clinical findings, thereby demonstrating the variability between carbon monoxide exposure and impairment of the cellular cytochrome system.[9] Classically, however, there are few symptoms with COHb levels below 10%. Between 10 and 20%, the patient experiences tightness across the forehead and headache. At 20 to 30% saturation, symptoms are more pronounced, with throbbing in the temple regions, and at 30 to 40%, the patient has a severe headache with generalized weakness, dizziness, dimness of vision, nausea and vomiting, and ultimate collapse. With levels approaching 40 to 50%, there may be syncope in addition to the previous symptoms, as well as increases in both pulse and respiratory rate. Concentrations of more than 50% can lead to coma and intermittent convulsions; at 60% saturation, death may accompany the depressed cardiac and respiratory function.

In one study of 28 patients 14 years of age or younger, 27 exposures were secondary to faulty venting or combustion of gas furnaces or stoves.[5] Sixteen of the 28 patients had COHb levels above 15%. Every patient with a COHb level of 24% or higher experienced syncope. All patients with COHb levels higher than 25%, neurologic findings, acidosis, or syncope were considered candidates for HBO treatment and were transferred to an appropriate facility using a 100% oxygen nonrebreathing mask. Smaller children underwent emergency tympanotomy followed by elective placement of pressure equalization tubes, and older children were taught the Valsalva maneuver. No morbidity from HBO therapy was encountered.

In general, the possibility of carbon monoxide poisoning must be considered when there is suspicion of smoke, exhaust fumes, or substances related to carbon monoxide poisoning, and the clinical presentation is one of nausea, vomiting, mental confusion, dizziness, or unconsciousness. The tentative diagnosis should be verified by the measurement of blood COHb saturation in either arterial or venous blood or by analysis of the victim's exhaled air for carbon monoxide. It should be remembered that COHb measurement measures only red blood cell–loaded carbon monoxide; there are no tissue measurements for carbon monoxide. If there has been a long delay from exposure to measurement, the COHb levels may be normal, since the carbon monoxide may have been released from the red blood cells.

Hyperbaric oxygen therapy for carbon monoxide poisoning is recommended in all patients with COHb levels above 40%, even those with no symptoms; in all patients with symptoms; and in those with an abnormal electrocardiogram, altered mental status, shock, focal neurologic findings, or severe acidosis.

Brown Recluse Spider Bite

One interesting application of HBO therapy in children is for brown recluse spider bites. The venom of the brown recluse spider has vasoconstrictive, thrombotic, hemolytic, and necrotizing properties. Early pathologic findings include hemorrhage beneath the epidermis, dermal-epidermal separation, thrombosis of small arterioles, and inflammatory changes with leukocyte infiltration. Later pathologic findings are necrosis, ulceration, and thrombosis of the surrounding dermal and subcutaneous blood vessels. The necrotizing component of the brown recluse venom is probably an enzyme containing sulfhydryl groups that appear to be particularly susceptible to inactivation by HBO.

The suggested indications include (1) a 1-cm diameter or larger blue-black central lesion involving the face, genitalia, hands or feet; (2) a 2½-cm diameter blue-black central lesion involving other areas of the body; (3) lesions progressing despite the usual treatment with antihistamines, corticosteroids, and antibiotics.

Hyperbaric oxygen therapy was initiated first on the theoretic grounds that the necrosis of tissue caused by brown recluse spider bites was at least partially caused by tissue hypoxia secondary to the vasospastic and thrombotic effects of the venom. In one recent series of 15 patients treated with HBO, no patient required surgical excision, there were no skin grafts, most patients were pain-free in 36 to 48 hours, the maximum area of third-degree slough was about 5 mm in diameter, and all lesions healed in 1 month or less.[12] The treatment schedule used was three to four treatments on a twice-a-day schedule at 2 ATA for 90 minutes.

This application should be considered in selected cases, and further clinical evaluation is warranted.

Peripheral Ischemic Injury

Peripheral ischemic injury secondary to injury in older children or as a result of disseminated intravascular clotting or peripheral emboli has been suggested as an indication for HBO therapy for large vessel occlusion, but without ade-

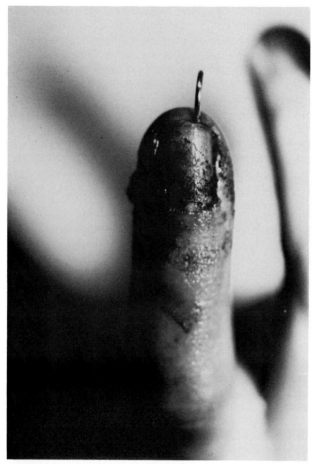

FIGURE 47–3

Postoperative appearance of finger tip, demonstrating cyanosis.

quate collateral circulation these problems will not respond. Occlusion of small peripheral vessels with perhaps marginal collateral circulation may be at least partially benefited by HBO. With oxygen inhalation at 2 ATA or greater, plasma-dissolved oxygen is delivered to marginally perfused tissues in the wound to support tissue viability.

The extensive use of HBO in small infants is restricted by the development of bronchopulmonary dysplasia and convulsions. The development of oxygen toxicity may be delayed by interposing regular, intermittent periods of normal oxygen levels without concurrently reducing the beneficial effects. Another practical limitation in critically ill children is the difficulty of transport to the HBO facility as well as the acute often critical care during the treatment.

In one study of three infants, aged 7, 18, and 24 months, with disseminated intravascular coagulation and gangrene of the fingertips and toes, the researchers concluded that the amount of tissue damage was decreased and resulted in less necrotic tissue with the use of HBO.[10] Before treatment, discoloration extended proximally and in the hands, and the demarcation line had reached the middle and distal phalanges. In the legs, it reached the midtibial area. Hyperbaric oxygen at 2.5 ATA twice daily produced marked improvement, with the demarcation area of discoloration gradually receding after each treatment. (Total treatment was 10 days.)

Case Examples

Case 1. A 12-year-old white boy suffered a near amputation of the distal fifth digit when he fell skateboarding and one of the rear wheels tore off all but a medial bridge of skin. The open, comminuted phalangeal fracture was débrided and reduced with placement of a pin for stabilization. Postoperatively, the tip became cyanotic and the patient was referred for HBO evaluation (Fig. 47–3). He underwent prompt compression to 2 ATA in the monoplace chamber and then completed a course of 21 90-minute treatments on a twice daily basis. Good tissue survival was obtained (Fig. 47–4).

Case 2. A 19-year-old guitarist suffered near amputations of digits two, three, and four of his left hand from an accident with a powersaw. Multiple comminuted fractures were explored, débrided, and stabilized, but vascular compromise of the distal second and fourth digits was noted by the surgeon (Fig. 47–5). The patient underwent 24 90-minute HBO sessions at 2 ATA in the monoplace chamber

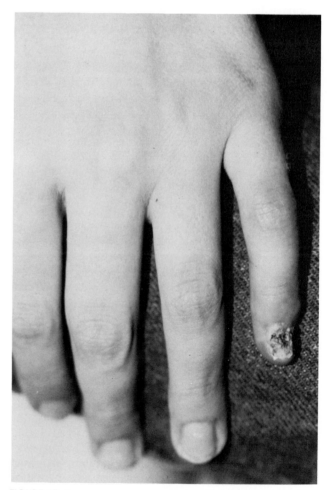

FIGURE 47–4

One month after the injury, demonstrating survival of the finger tip.

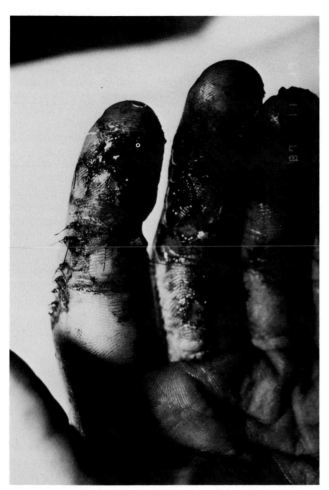

FIGURE 47-5
Pretreatment, demonstrating vascular compromise.

on a twice-daily basis with good salvage of tissue (Fig. 47–6). He returned to his musical career (Fig. 47–7) 2 months after the injury.

Smoke Inhalation

Smoke inhalation is toxic to respiratory function in three ways: (1) as an irritant (e.g., chlorine, phosgene, and ammonia); (2) by decreasing effective oxygen transport by carbon monoxide combining with hemoglobin; and (3) at the cellular level, where cyanide and carbon monoxide combine with cytochrome oxidase, affecting intracellular metabolism. Patients may demonstrate severe metabolic acidoses, have elevated cyanide and carbon monoxide levels, and show pulmonary congestion on radiographs of the chest.

The recommended treatment includes administration of a cyanide antidote kit when patients present from a closed-space fire with findings of metabolic acidosis, elevated COHb levels, and a decrease in arterial oxygen saturation. (Current laboratory methods may require 4 to 6 hours to quantitate cyanide levels.)

When the COHb levels are extremely elevated (i.e.,

above 40%), it may be wise to administer the cyanide antidote kit only *after* the patient is at appropriate pressure in the HBO chamber.

Air Embolism

Air may be introduced into the venous or arterial circulation and result in cerebral air embolism, leading to severe neurologic deficit or death. Indwelling subclavian vein catheters for total parenteral nutrition have been the most common cause in recent years. A sudden change in sensorium is the most common presentation, ranging from disorientation to coma. Focal motor deficits, visual changes, and sensory deficits also occur. With 10 to 15% of the population having at least probe patency of the foramen ovale, right-sided heart gas can readily become arterial emboli.

The rationale for HBO therapy is based on compression of air bubbles to mechanically clear the cerebral circulation and oxygenation of ischemic tissues with large volumes of oxygen dissolved in plasma. According to Boyle's law, the volume of a gas is inversely proportional to the pressure exerted on that gas. Compression to 6 ATA reduces the size of an air bubble obstructing a blood vessel to one sixth of its original volume, effectively relieving the obstruction and restoring perfusion.

In one report of 16 patients who underwent HBO therapy for cerebral air embolism, eight patients had complete relief of symptoms, five had partial relief, and three had no ben-

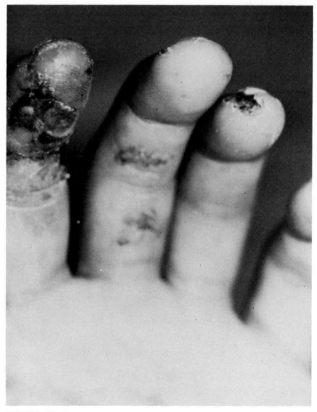

FIGURE 47-6
After 7 days of hyperbaric oxygen treatment.

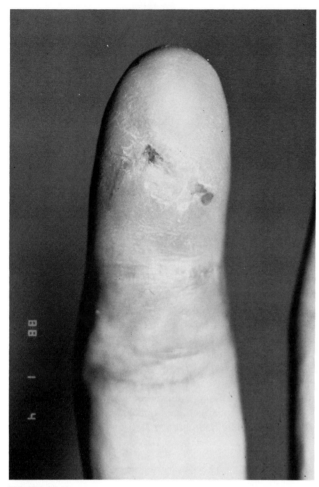

FIGURE 47-7
Two months after the injury.

efit.[8] With an increasing number of HBO chambers in both civilian and military medical facilities, the value and early use of HBO for air embolism should be apparent. Multiple low-pressure (2-ATA) treatments may be required, especially when the initiation of HBO therapy has been delayed.

Refractory Osteomyelitis

Chronic nonhematogenous osteomyelitis, secondary to open fracture or infection at the time of open reduction and internal fixation of closed fractures, continues to be a difficult surgical problem. HBO therapy has been used as an adjunct to débridement, stabilization, and intravenous anti-

biotic therapy. Animal studies have demonstrated hypoxic PO_2s of 0 to 20 mm Hg in infected bone. This can be elevated to normal or above normal bone PO_2 when the animals breathe oxygen in HBO chambers. Periodic elevation of bone PO_2 from hypoxic levels to normal or above promotes fibroblastic division, collagen production, and capillary angiogenesis. For both osteoanagenesis and angiogenesis to occur, a tissue PO_2 of 35 to 40 mm Hg must be available, a level usually readily attainable with HBO. An overall rate of successful arrest of previously refractory cases has been reported to range from 60 to 85%. Because most cases that come to HBO therapy are those in which amputation is the only remaining choice for cure, this is certainly an acceptable arrest rate.

Hyperbaric oxygen must be used as an adjunct to débridement, wound care, and specific bone culture–dictated parenteral antibiotics. Many of the commonly used antibiotics, such as the aminoglycosides and vancomycin, require adequate tissue PO_2 to be effectively taken up by the cells. The growing awareness of the importance of anaerobic bacteria involved in chronic osteomyelitis, as well as the possibility of enhanced osteogenesis, is further reason why HBO therapy may be of value.

References

1. Boerma I, BrummelKamp WH, Meijre NG (eds): Clinical Application of Hyperbaric Oxygen: Proceedings of the First International Congress New York, Elsevier, 1963.
2. ETC Dixie, County Line Industrial Park, Southampton, Pa.
3. Goodman MW: Decompression sickness treated with compression to 2 to 6 atmospheres absolute. Aerospace Med 35:1204, 1964.
4. Hamilton RW, Sheffield PJ: Tissue oxygen measurements in hyperbaric oxygen therapy. In: Davis JC, Hunt TK (eds): Hyperbaric Oxygen Therapy. Bethesda, Undersea Medical Society, 1977, p 53.
5. Hart GB, Strauss MB, Lennon PA, Whitcraft DD: Treatment of smoke inhalation by hyperbaric oxygen. J Emerg Med 3:211–215, 1985.
6. Heimbach RD: Gas gangrene: Review and update. HBO Rev 1:41, 1980.
7. Heimbach RD, Baerema I, BrummelKamp WH, Wolfe WG: Current therapy of gas gangrene. In: Davis JC, Hunt TK (eds): Hyperbaric Oxygen Therapy. Bethesda, Undersea Medical Society, 1977, p 153.
8. Murphy BP, Harford FJ, Cramer FS: Cerebral air embolism resulting from invasive medical procedure. Ann Surg 201:242–245, 1985.
9. Norkool DM, Kirkpatrick JN: Treatment of acute carbon monoxide poisoning with hyperbaric oxygen: A review of 115 cases. Ann Emerg Med 14:1168–1171, 1985.
10. Rosenthal E, Benderly A, Momes-Chass, et al: Hyperbaric oxygenation in peripheral ischemic lesions in infants. Arch Dis Child 60:372–374, 1985.
11. Sechrist Industries, Medical Products Division, Anaheim, Calif.
12. Svendsen FJ: Treatment of clinically diagnosed brown recluse spider bites with hyperbaric oxygen: A clinical observation 83:199–204, 1986.

Kim Massey

CHAPTER FORTY-EIGHT

Nursing Care for the Critically Injured Child

PEDIATRIC TRAUMA NURSING

Pediatric trauma nursing is a unique specialty. Nurses either love it or hate it; there are very few neutral opinions. Caring for vulnerable broken little bodies with hysterical parents in the background conjures up strong images and emotions. It may not be for everyone, but for those who have the knowledge, skill, creativity, compassion, and physical, emotional, and spiritual stamina, it is a wonderful and rewarding profession. Even though pediatric trauma nursing is a most difficult and stressful specialty, an unmatched inner sense of accomplishment and satisfaction is experienced while helping a child and family survive and cope with a traumatic injury.

Infants and children are cared for by nurses in many different settings, such as the scene of the injury, the emergency department, the operating room, the postanesthesia recovery room, the pediatric intensive care unit (ICU), the general trauma care unit, the rehabilitation unit, the outpatient care clinic, and the home. This chapter is devoted to some of the important aspects of hospital-based, pediatric trauma nursing. The focus is the nursing care requirements in the emergency department, the pediatric ICU, and the general trauma care unit.

Throughout hospitalization, nurses have the unusual role of being with the child 24 hours a day. Hence, the expectations and responsibilities placed on the pediatric trauma nurse are extremely high. Children are resilient yet fragile and require special attention and care. The child is part of a family system and must be treated as such, with special attention and planning devoted to involving the family in the management of the child. In this setting, nurses function as patient and family advocates to ensure understanding, support, and compliance with the management regimen.

The pediatric patient's physiologic and psychological responses to injury differ from those of an adult. Understanding the child's responses and needs enables adjustments to be made in nursing care to meet those needs and enhances the overall quality of care.

Nurses have the ability to improve the pediatric trauma patient's outcome considerably by aggressively assessing the child's condition, communicating pertinent findings, and coordinating appropriate interventions. Assessments are based on patient condition and unit policies. The child who is newly injured, hemodynamically unstable, or suffering from respiratory depression may require constant assessment and monitoring. The alert, stable child without respiratory or hemodynamic injury or instability requires regular but less frequent checks. Communication is a vital role of the pediatric trauma nurse because everyone and everything involving the care of the child depends on clear, accurate information being passed on to the appropriate medical personnel, the child, and the family. Coordination of treatment and services for the critically injured child is constant for the nurse. For example, to recover, traumatized children require periods of undisturbed rest, which the nurse arranges by planning and coordinating treatment schedules with different departments such as respiratory therapy and physical therapy.

PEDIATRIC TRAUMA PREVENTION

Historically, the key association with trauma has been "accident" or something beyond the ability to be controlled. Today, the key association is "prevention."[6] A traumatic injury is one that could and should have been prevented.

Traumatic injuries to children present a national health problem. One half of all childhood deaths in the United States among children between 1 and 14 years of age are due to trauma. Even more significant, a very large number of children are permanently disabled each year. The tragedy results in both a present loss and a great loss for the future. The child misses the opportunity to develop, mature, and contribute to society, and society misses out on the child's contribution.

Nurses are becoming more active in pediatric trauma prevention programs. Safety courses for riding bicycles, driving cars, and participating in water sports are becoming increasingly popular. Programs are geared for children and teenagers with the emphasis on preventing injury by teaching safety while still having fun. Nurses are making pediatric trauma prevention a priority within their national, state, and local organizations.

RESUSCITATION OF THE CRITICALLY INJURED CHILD

Nursing Care

The primary cause of cardiac arrest in a child is most often respiratory failure rather than cardiac failure as it is in the adult. Trauma may lead to respiratory failure from upper airway obstruction, pulmonary contusions, pneumothorax, flail chest, or central nervous system depression. Children must be fully immobilized when circumstances are suspicious or mechanisms of injury suggest cervical spine injury. Immobilization devices protect against secondary injuries to the cervical spinal column and cord that may result in paralysis or death.

The respiratory system of a child is more friable and prone to obstruction owing to the large tongue in proportion to the small mouth; the narrow air passages, which can be easily obstructed by mucus or blood; and improper positioning of or pressure on the soft neck and submandibular tissue, which causes obstruction.

The respiratory pattern and heartbeat of a child are normally irregular, and both systems should be monitored for a full minute to obtain an accurate rate. The respiratory rate and heart rate of a child are faster than those of an adult, but the blood pressure is lower. Normal ranges for children vary with age. It is difficult, if not impossible, to memorize all the specific normal rates and ranges for each developmental age; therefore, it is extremely important to have wall charts, flip charts, or cards displaying normal vital signs for infants and children. Tube sizes, medication dosages, and fluid requirements are also difficult to remember when one is stressed by a decompensating child, and these should also be displayed in prominent locations.

Nursing care of the pediatric trauma patient during resuscitation should be centered on assessing, diagnosing, evaluating, and intervening on behalf of the child following a primary survey, a neurologic assessment, and then a secondary survey. The primary survey includes dealing with life-threatening problems with the airway, breathing, or circulation. There is no progression beyond the primary survey until these needs are addressed. The neurologic assessment is brief but essential: to detect abnormalities and to compare changes over time. The secondary survey involves making a full but rapid assessment, including measuring vital signs, determining an initial pediatric trauma score, and making a full head-to-toe evaluation. A focused survey is the next step, in which each injured body part or system is worked up for abnormalities, and treatment is begun. At any point, one can move back to the primary survey to intervene in the most vital of all functions: maintaining an open airway, oxygenating and ventilating, and circulating blood.

Airway

The child's neck (and the adult's) should not be hyperextended if there has been a mechanism of injury that suggests endangerment to the cervical spine. Full immobilization must be maintained until such suspected injury is ruled out. The airway is opened with the jaw thrust or chin lift method, used for all ages. Once cleared of cervical fractures, the infant may require a sniffing position in which the head is extended slightly forward as if sniffing a flower. The shoulders may also need support to align the head and open the airway.

Oral airways are not rotated when inserted in children and are appropriate only for the unconscious or orally intubated child. Nasal airways are better tolerated by the awake or semiconscious child. Endotracheal tubes with cuffs ideally are not used on infants or small children because of their naturally narrowed cricoid ring, which forms a physiologic cuff.

Breathing

Breathing is the act of ventilating or eliminating carbon dioxide from the cells and oxygenating or supplying oxygen to the cells. Respiratory failure results in abnormal respirations, which may be too fast (tachypnea), too slow (bradypnea), or absent (apnea). Trauma to the pulmonary or neuromuscular system can cause respiratory failure by tachypnea. A child who is breathing rapidly and then slowly requires a thorough cardiopulmonary assessment because this pattern may indicate fatigue and impending respiratory arrest rather than improvement. Compensation for respiratory insufficiency is attempted by increased work of breathing with resultant retractions and nasal flaring. Cyanosis is not always present initially when there is respiratory failure, and its absence should not be relied on as an indicator of adequate function.

Circulation

Circulation in a child is assessed by monitoring heart rate; blood pressure; and perfusion of the skin, kidneys, and brain; and by comparing central with peripheral pulses. The traumatically injured child is at great risk of circulatory failure or shock.

Shock

Shock or circulatory failure is the inadequate provision of oxygen to the tissues. The circulating blood volume is less in a child than in an adult, so even small losses can have profound effects. Traumatized children often develop hypovolemic shock from blood loss caused by hepatic or splenic injury, femur fractures, tears of great vessels, lacerations, hemothorax, and occasionally intracranial hemorrhage.

Basically there are two types of hypovolemic shock: compensated and decompensated. In compensated shock, the child maintains a near normal blood pressure as cardiac output drops owing to a compensatory increase in systemic vascular resistance. Children can lose up to 30% of their circulating volume of blood before changes in blood pressure occur. Decompensated shock results in a rapid drop in blood pressure, which is difficult and often impossible to reverse. The usual outcome for decompensated shock is death.

Children compensate and maintain their blood pressure in a normal range longer than adults. When a child's blood pressure falls, it is a late and ominous sign. Delays in resuscitation can have irreversible and devastating results. The child may develop cardiorespiratory arrest or suffer a prolonged death that is due to multiple organ system failure as a direct result of inadequate oxygen delivery.

Assessing the child for shock requires a different approach than the one for an adult. The focus of the assessment must be on peripheral circulation and end-organ perfusion rather than on blood pressure. Changes in pulse quality, level of consciousness, urinary output, and increases in systemic vascular resistance assist in determining the adequacy of perfusion.

The peripheral circulation is evaluated by assessing the volume of peripheral pulses and the adequacy of end-organ perfusion. Peripheral pulses are assessed by comparing the quality of the child's distal pulses to the central pulses. A child with advancing shock shows decreasing or absent pulses in the extremities before the loss of central pulses. Hypothermia associated with trauma causes vasoconstriction and may also cause a difference in volume between peripheral and central pulses. Loss of central pulses may be an irreversible state and must be promptly recognized with immediate and appropriate resuscitation.

Monitoring the brain, kidneys, and skin provides the most reliable assessment of end-organ perfusion. Level of consciousness indicates the adequacy of brain perfusion. Ischemia of the brain causes varying symptoms from pupillary dilation and lethargy or confusion to seizures or complete loss of consciousness. Most children exhibit an alternating pattern of lethargy with combativeness.

A reliable indicator of appropriate alertness and orientation with all ages, even infants, is whether the child recognizes the parents. A parent who says, ''My child doesn't seem to know who I am!'' must be taken seriously; the child should be evaluated immediately for circulatory failure.

Level of consciousness can be assessed with any age infant or child using the modified Glasgow coma scale score or the AVPU (A = alert; V = responds to vocal stimuli; P = responds to painful stimuli; U = unresponsive) method. The Glasgow coma scale provides a numeric score for three criteria: the ability to open the eyes, vocalize, and move. Modified Glasgow coma scale scores adjust each category to fit developmental ability. The AVPU method is useful for observing general alterations of level of consciousness by determining the state of alertness: whether the child is awake, is responsive to voice or pain, or is unresponsive.

The kidneys are excellent windows through which peripheral blood flow can be monitored. Minimal urinary output for a child is 1 ml of urine per kg of body weight per hour, with anything less indicating decreased perfusion.

Changes in skin temperature, capillary refill, or color, such as mottling, pallor, or peripheral cyanosis (often normal in newborns), are early signs of shock. Children are relatively warm to the touch unless they have been exposed to a harsh environment or have experienced a failure of adequate perfusion. A line of demarcation can often be observed on the extremities, with cool skin on one side and warm skin on the other. This line progressively moves up the child's extremities toward the trunk as shock advances. Capillary refill time is normally less than 2 seconds, with any delay indicating perfusion failure.

The nurse is the person who performs regular, repeated cardiopulmonary assessments on the child and must be alert to subtle changes in the child's peripheral circulation and end-organ perfusion. The nurse is usually the first one to recognize symptoms of shock and to begin management.

Children who suffer from or are at risk for hypovolemic shock require immediate intravenous access and volume replacement with 20 ml per kg of crystalloid solutions such as Ringer lactate or normal saline. This fluid is administered as a rapid bolus along with a maintenance drip at 5 ml per hour.[11] The bolus may be repeated until up to 100 to 200 ml per kg is given in the first few hours.[3]

The traumatized child who suffers extensive blood loss often requires blood and colloid infusions, the exact type of fluid being a subject of controversy. The major goal of fluid therapy in hypovolemic shock is the adequate replacement of the volume lost. Each time a bolus is infused, the child must be reassessed for its effect and the present adequacy of circulation.

The quickest method of assessing a critically ill child for shock involves noting the level of consciousness, the heart rate, the urinary output, the volume and quality of peripheral versus central pulses, and the skin temperature and capillary refill. As stated, blood pressure is not a key indicator of shock in children; rather, changes in the peripheral circulation and end-organ perfusion are of paramount importance.

Medications

Resuscitation medications are calculated and dosed on a mg per kg basis. Careful attention must be paid to the admin-

istration of medication, as even small errors may lead to devastating consequences. Wall charts, slide charts, or pocket charts are helpful because even expert pediatric clinicians have difficulty remembering the mg per kg dose of each medication, calculating the child's dosage, and converting the mg dose to ml to withdraw and inject.

The Broselow pediatric resuscitation tapes are extremely valuable during a resuscitation, because of their simplicity of use for obtaining essential information. One places the measuring tape alongside a child and measures from head to toe. The point the child's feet touch has a color-coded area with all tube sizes and resuscitation medication doses outlined on the tape. Corresponding color-coded packs may be made up to save time and reduce the chance of error. Individual resuscitation cards with precalculated medication dosages and tube sizes should be affixed to the child's bed or to the code chart. A pocket calculator should be affixed to each pediatric resuscitation cart.

Heat Loss

Children have a larger body surface area in relation to weight; therefore, they lose heat and develop hypothermia faster than adults. Traumatized children must be kept warm by using overbed warmers, warming pads, or by increasing the ambient room temperature. It is also important to warm intravenous fluids and blood or blood products before administration.

Electrolytes

Abnormalities of glucose, calcium, and potassium often occur in the injured child and must be monitored closely. Extreme imbalances in electrolytes can precipitate an ''arrest'' situation.

Growth and Development

Knowledge of growth and development is important for predicting needs, abilities, and eventual outcome for the traumatically injured child. The child's stage of development affects the methods of communication and comfort that the nurse uses to assist in the child's care.

Support

The nurse provides psychological and emotional assistance to the child and family in crisis. The nurse is the vital link between the child and family and must ensure that their bond is supported. Nurses may also enlist the services of other professionals such as chaplains, psychologists, and social workers to promote the family's coping skills and resources.

Emotions and Feelings of Nurses

Pediatric resuscitations get the adrenalin flowing like nothing else can. There is always a heightened concern for the unstable, critically injured child who may die. Nurses who do not care for children on a routine basis or do not participate regularly in resuscitation attempts on children have the most difficult time. There is always a very emotional element to a pediatric resuscitation. No one wants to see a child die for any reason, and trauma to a child is usually viewed as unfair, unjust, and untimely. In this society, we are supposed to protect our children. When we are unable to do that, we feel cheated and unworthy. Only with experience and personal insight can nurses feel good about a job well done, even if the outcome is unfavorable. If the child dies in a failed resuscitation, there is at least the knowledge that a chance was given, a second chance on life, which every child deserves.

Strong negative feelings and emotions are experienced when a child's injury is presumed or proved to have been inflicted intentionally by another person. The pediatric trauma nurse must often interact with the alleged perpetrator, even if only briefly. This can be very stressful because the instinct to protect the child may be mixed with the desire to bring justice to the perpetrator. Local and state law enforcement and child protection agencies must be contacted to investigate and handle the accusations and facts. Evidence preservation is of utmost importance. Specific policies, procedures, and protocols must be available for nurses to follow in such situations.

FACILITIES

Pediatric trauma nurses require functional facilities, equipment, and supplies to render high-quality, life-saving nursing care. As such, nurses should be included in all phases of the planning, design, and construction of hospital facilities and expansions. Patient and staff traffic flow, bed layout, nursing station placement, equipment location, medication and supply areas, work and storage spaces, and office space must be planned by a multidisciplinary group with nursing having input into all major decisions.

STANDARDS

The Joint Commission on the Accreditation of Healthcare Organizations Standards (1991) guides facility design, equipment, personnel, and functions.[9] The American Academy of Pediatrics has organized specific pediatric standards for design and implementation of pediatric care in "Hospital Care of Children and Youth."[7]

Many states also have specific standards governing designated trauma center facilities, personnel, and equipment. These state standards are usually based on the 1990 document written by the Committee on Trauma of the American College of Surgeons: "Resources for Optimal Care of the Injured Patient."[4] A Trauma Nursing Coalition was formed by a group of specialty nursing organizations including the Emergency Nurses Association, the American Association of Critical Care Nurses, the American Association of Nurse Anesthetists, the Association of Operating Room Nurses, Inc., the American Association of Rehabilitation Nurses, and the National Flight Nurses Association. Together they developed the "Resource Document for Nursing Care of the Trauma Patient," which outlines the optimal conditions for the care of the trauma patient from the nursing perspective.[12]

Other nursing standards address the care of patients in specific areas of practice. The Emergency Nurses Association developed the "Standards of Emergency Nursing Practice" (1991), the American Association of Critical Care Nurses wrote "AACN Standards for Nursing Care of the Critically Ill" (1989), and the American Nurses' Association implemented "Standards of Maternal and Child Health Nursing Practice" (1983).[1, 5, 10]

Most nursing units choose to develop their own individual standards that govern their unique area of practice. These standards are written with the national or state standards, or both, as a reference. The unit-based standards reflect the quality care issues, outcome statements, policies, procedures, and protocols through which the unit or department operates. They guide the nurse in daily practice and ensure quality care for the patient.

EQUIPMENT

Availability of appropriate equipment and supplies is essential to successful care and treatment of the critically injured child. Equipment must be organized and easily accessible with sufficient stock on hand. A resuscitation should never be delayed while a search for equipment is conducted. Disorganization can lead to tragic results with poor patient outcome.

The format for storage of equipment and supplies varies from hospital to hospital; however, everything must be organized so as to allow rapid, easy access to whatever is required. Emergency resuscitation equipment may be stored in a portable pediatric code cart for use within the area. A small portable code box should also be assembled for use during transport to other areas within the hospital such as computed tomography, surgery, or the pediatric ICU.

Other supplies may be stored on exchange carts, wire carts, wall hooks, or shelves or in cabinets, depending on the available space. Each system has advantages and disadvantages; hence, the type of system implemented must meet the needs of the department. It is imperative, however, that nursing time and energy not be utilized to assess and restock supplies. Other nonnursing personnel can be trained to complete this task with great benefits to overall departmental function.

In addition, there must be collaboration and cooperation between nursing and medical personnel to oversee the ordering and stocking of equipment and supplies acceptable to everyone involved in providing care within the area. Each discipline must have input into the selection of appropriate types and amounts of supplies. One person or a defined group of people should take overall responsibility for coordinating the purchasing and stocking of needed items.

PEDIATRIC TRAUMA UNITS

The most successful pediatric trauma units have a clear, well-communicated plan of organization, structure, purpose, and function and encourage close collaboration between physicians and nurses. There must be complete understanding of each others' roles and responsibilities. The medical and nursing directors must communicate openly and work together as a team to ensure a positive impact on quality of care, nurses' sense of professional satisfaction, and patient outcomes.

Nurses maintain continuity of care by coordinating and supervising all unit and patient care activities. Nurses carry out physician orders and provide input and information to assist the physician in management of the patients. The nurse has the unique role of being with the patient more than any other professional and is responsible for overseeing and coordinating that care.

Nonnursing duties should be delegated to ancillary staff to increase personal and professional satisfaction and to make the best use of nursing time. Tasks such as answering the phone, controlling visitation, handling laboratory specimens, obtaining laboratory data, stocking and cleaning equipment and supplies, and clerical duties should be delegated. Nursing time should be concentrated on activities that require nursing skills.

The nursing practice model should incorporate nurse-physician collaboration, decentralized management and operation, shared decision making, and control over scheduling and practice.

Management

The pediatric trauma nurse manager should possess strong administrative skills along with the relevant skills in clinical practice. The very best managers not only have advanced management skills but also are clinical experts. Such individuals are difficult to find, because it is rare for people to excel in more than one area of practice.

Often the clinical experts or the nurses with seniority in years of service are promoted to management positions only to discover that they have no administrative skills or that they miss the nursing aspects of bedside care. This can produce disastrous consequences for a unit if such a manager continues in that role. The nursing staff may lose respect for the manager's decisions and style of authority, and nurses in such a unit often look elsewhere for work.

The terms *nurse manager* and *head nurse* are used interchangeably, depending on the organization, to designate the person responsible for unit management. The nurse manager oversees all aspects of the assigned unit through assessing, planning, organizing, staffing, intervening, directing, controlling, and evaluating.[2] The nurse manager must be knowledgeable, accountable, creative, sensitive, patient, and visionary. He or she must always consider the present and future needs of the unit.

Staff empowerment through participative management, shared governance, and staff autonomy is essential to successful management with today's professional nursing practice. Nurse managers must give staff nurses an active role in making decisions on issues that affect practice and working conditions.

Equally important, nurses need adequate compensation for their work. Traditionally, there has been wage compression with little ability to advance in terms of salary increases. Newly graduated nurses often make almost the same salary as nurses who have been employed for years. Offering a wider range of wages so that experienced nurses can be retained is optimal and necessary. Control over work schedules should be shared with the staff because staff members who can arrange their own work, home, and recreational time have higher job satisfaction.

Nurses want and should have a voice in the major decisions affecting practice and should be responsible for developing and implementing policies, procedures, and protocols; for validating staff competency; and for continuous quality improvement with input from management.

Orientation

Plans must be written, well organized, and specific to include hospital orientation, nursing orientation, and unit orientation for each area in which the nurse may practice. All aspects of nursing care delivery must be included, with some flexibility built in to meet new employees' needs.

The plan should include the orientation program schedule, purpose, duration, overall and weekly objectives, equipment information, clinical competency evaluation tools, and review tools to assess knowledge base and deficits.

Willing, dedicated preceptors are the key to a successful orientation plan. If new nurses do not feel welcome and have difficulty learning the unit-specific procedures, they will not stay. Even the best written orientation plan is useless without staff members who ensure that the plan is understandable, appropriate, and implemented.

Education

The pediatric trauma nurse must apply knowledge and skill to nursing practice. This knowledge and skill can be gained through both education and experience. Currently, there is no basic educational program for pediatric trauma nursing.

Most nursing programs do not specifically teach pediatric trauma nursing but often touch on it with didactic or clinical experiences. There are, however, numerous continuing educational programs concerning pediatric trauma care available throughout the country. Literature regarding childhood injuries and pediatric emergency and critical care is expanding and is available in most hospital or medical libraries.

Continuing Education

Minimal continuing education requirements for nurses caring for critically injured children include completion of courses in basic life support through the American Heart Association, pediatric advanced life support through the American Academy of Pediatrics and the American Heart Association, and the trauma nursing core course developed by the Emergency Nurses' Association.

Additional educational requirements vary depending on basic educational background and clinical experience.

However, all pediatric trauma nurses should obtain a minimum of 6 hours per year in pediatric trauma or critical care continuing education.

SYSTEM OF PEDIATRIC TRAUMA CARE

The system of pediatric trauma care involves a comprehensive, multidisciplinary team approach that utilizes the latest technology, equipment, and personnel expertise to assess, resuscitate, stabilize, treat, and rehabilitate the injured child. From admission until discharge, quality patient care must be provided by a highly trained, caring staff.

Children arrive at a medical center via air ambulance, ground ambulance, or private vehicle. The critically injured child requires the initiation of stabilization and prompt transport to a trauma center if the initial medical center is not equipped and staffed with pediatric trauma specialists. In response, at the referral center the trauma team immediately assembles and prepares for management of the injured child on notification that the child is en route or has arrived. The list of trauma team members, their location at the time of arrival notification, and their response time is described in Table 48–1. It should be noted that level I, level II, and level III trauma centers have varying requirements depending on state standards and these must be appropriately considered.

Responsibilities of Trauma Team Members

Trauma Nurse 1. Checks and stocks the trauma room at the beginning of the shift. Coordinates activities of all allied personnel at the bedside. Inserts and maintains intravenous lines and administers intravenous fluids and blood products. Draws blood specimens for laboratory analysis when inserting lines to minimize the number of sticks. Administers all medications. Performs all duties of the recorder nurse when that position is not filled. Keeps the pediatric trauma surgeon, team director, or both informed of changes in the child's condition and all diagnostic study results. Accompanies the child to other critical areas in the hospital and gives a report to the receiving unit. Cleans and restocks the trauma room (or delegates the job) after patient transfer.

Trauma Nurse 2. Performs the primary and secondary survey and the serial physical assessments. Prepares the trauma room by cleaning and restocking at the beginning of the shift. Removes the child's clothing. Prepares surgical trays and instruments, assists with surgical procedures. Inserts urinary drainage catheters and obtains urine specimen for analysis. Inserts gastric tubes. Assists with cleaning and restocking the trauma room after the patient is transferred.

Recorder Nurse. Documents all patient information on the appropriate forms. Obtains, documents, and secures all patient valuables in the unit safe. Ensures that all laboratory specimens are correctly labeled and transported to the lab-

Table 48–1
Trauma Team

Trauma Team Member	Location	Response
Trauma nurse 1	Inhouse	Immediate
Trauma nurse 2	Inhouse	Immediate
Recorder nurse (when available)	Inhouse	Immediate
Paramedic	Inhouse	Immediate
Pediatric emergency physician	Inhouse	Immediate
Radiology technologist	Inhouse	Immediate
Respiratory therapist	Inhouse	Immediate
Secretary	Inhouse	Immediate
Pediatric trauma surgeon	Inhouse or on call and promptly available	Immediate and/or departs for the trauma center (TC) without delay
Chaplain	Inhouse or on call	Immediate and/or departs for the TC without delay
Pediatric physician	Inhouse or on call	Immediate and/or departs for the TC without delay
Pediatric neurosurgeon	Inhouse or on call	Immediate and/or departs for the TC without delay
Trauma coordinator	Inhouse or on call	Standby
Laboratory technicians	Inhouse or on call	Standby
Blood bank technicians	Inhouse or on call	Standby
Radiologist	Inhouse or on call	Standby/departs for the TC without delay
Child life specialist	Inhouse or on call	Standby
Nursing supervisor	Inhouse	Standby
Administrator	Inhouse or on call	Standby
Computed tomography technologists	Inhouse	Standby
Social services	Inhouse	Standby
Surgery personnel	Inhouse	Standby
Postanesthesia recovery personnel	Inhouse	Standby
Pediatric intensive care personnel	Inhouse	Standby
General trauma unit	Inhouse	Standby

oratory for immediate analysis. Identifies the patient and attaches the armband.

Paramedic. Assists with airway management and cervical spine control. Places the patient on the cardiac monitor. Performs initial and serial vital signs. Assists with patient suctioning. Applies splints and bandages.

Pediatric Emergency Physician. Assists or provides initial resuscitation of the injured child. Assesses, manages, and coordinates patient care until it is assumed by the pediatric trauma surgeon. Provides care for other patients in the emergency department once care is turned over to the pediatric trauma surgeon.

Radiology Technologist. Performs ordered radiologic exams.

Respiratory Therapist. Assists with airway management and ventilation. Assembles and manages ventilators. Performs blood gas analysis.

Secretary. Initiates formation of a patient record using a "trauma alias" until the child's name, age, and other information is known. Prepares labels for blood and urine specimens. Places physician orders in the hospital computer for communication with other departments. Answers the phones and passes information on to the trauma team. Transports specimens to the laboratory (or delegates) and passes results back into the trauma room. Notifies consultants as directed by the pediatric trauma surgeon.

Pediatric Trauma Surgeon. Team leader. Performs trauma resuscitations and surgical interventions necessary to sustain life and preserve vital functions. Directs others in resuscitation and requests and coordinates consultant activities and all diagnostic and therapeutic efforts, including determining patient disposition. Coordinates and provides continued care of the injured child throughout the hospital course.

Chaplain. Assists with patient identification, family location, notification, and continued support.

Pediatric Physician Consultants. Pediatric surgical and medical specialists are available for consultation when requested by the pediatric emergency physician or the pediatric trauma surgeon.

Pediatric Neurosurgeon. Provides diagnostic, therapeutic, and surgical intervention for neural trauma.

Trauma Coordinator. Coordinates and evaluates the response, effectiveness, and outcomes of the multidisciplinary trauma team. Ensures adherence to optimal trauma care standards throughout the trauma system. Participates in quality improvement activities and researches current trauma care issues. Serves as a clinical resource and provides pediatric trauma care education.

Laboratory Technicians. Perform prompt analysis of blood, urine, or other body fluids, giving priority status to trauma patients.

Blood Bank Technicians. Provide immediate type and crossmatching and prepare blood products for the critically injured child.

Radiologist. Available to assist in the evaluation and interpretation of all radiologic studies.

Child Life Specialist. Assists in orienting the stable, conscious child to the hospital experience using a developmental approach.

Nursing Supervisor. Coordinates transfer of patients between units when necessary. Communicates with the media or public relations department when appropriate.

Administrator. Assigned to the trauma service to provide communication between the administration and the trauma team when necessary. Available to make complex administrative and legal decisions.

Computed Tomography Technologists. Perform computed tomography examinations as ordered.

Social Services Personnel. Assist with the management and support of the patient, family, and significant others.

Security Officers. Available for traffic control and security issues.

Surgery Personnel. Prepare the operating suite for the critically ill child's arrival.

Postanesthesia Recovery Personnel. Available to care for the patient immediately after surgery.

Pediatric Intensive Care Unit Personnel. Prepare the pediatric ICU for the critically injured child's arrival.

General Trauma Unit Personnel. A unit designed to care for the stable, noncritically injured child.

General Requirements

Trauma patient care is provided by a multidisciplinary team throughout the hospital course. The care is guided by the policies, procedures, protocols, and standards of care and practice that are specific to or include the pediatric trauma patient.

The number and mix of available personnel must be adequate to meet the needs of the patients and staff. Nurse-to-patient ratios are based on patient acuity and staff qualifications. In each unit, one nurse must have either no assigned patients or a lighter assignment to accept the admission of a critically ill child at a moment's notice and not adversely affect the children already in the unit.

Credentialing

Nurses and paramedics are credentialed for pediatric trauma care by demonstrating specialized skills that are required for care of the critically injured child and by attendance at continuing education programs on trauma care. Skills performance is evaluated by initial, then annual, clinical competency assessments, which are documented and maintained in permanent files. A minimum of 4 contact hours in pediatric trauma topics must be obtained and documented each year.

Documentation

The care provided and the patient's physical findings are documented on a trauma flow sheet in the emergency department. Centers that offer exclusive care to the pediatric population have pediatric-specific forms. Centers that care for adults as well as children often develop a form that meets the needs of both to save time, energy, and cost.

A sample of a combined trauma flow sheet is shown in Figure 48–1. This particular flow sheet begins with the
Text continued on page 721

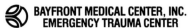

BAYFRONT MEDICAL CENTER, INC.
EMERGENCY TRAUMA CENTER

NAME: _____ AGE: _____ SEX: _____

ED #: _____ BED #: _____ DATE: _____ ED ARRIVAL TIME: _____

CHIEF COMPLAINT: _____

MECHANISM OF INJURY: _____

PREHOSPITAL PROVIDERS: _____ HRS TRAUMA REGISTRY #: _____

PRIMARY SURVEY

ASSESSMENTS AND TREATMENTS	PTA	TIME STARTED	TIME DC'D	PHYSICIAN
AIRWAY		☐ PATENT	☐ OBSTRUCTED	
ORAL/NASAL				
ETT ORAL/NASAL				
CRICO/TRACH				
BREATHING		☐ PRESENT	☐ ABSENT	
OXYGEN				
AMBU BAG				
OXIMETER				
CIRCULATION		☐ PRESENT	☐ ABSENT	
CPR				
CARDIAC MONITOR				
IV				
MAST ☐ INF ☐ DEF				
IMMOBILIZATION				
CERVICAL COLLAR				
BACKBOARD/FERNO				
KED				
SPLINTS ☐ R ☐ L				
H. TRACTION ☐ R ☐ L				
OTHER				
FHT RATE				
ACCUCHECK				
BP	HR	R	T	

GCS/TRAUMA SCORE

ADULT GLASGOW COMA SCALE		PEDIATRIC GLASGOW COMA SCALE ≤ 2 YRS.	
FINDING	**SCORE**	**FINDING**	**SCORE**
EYE OPENING		**EYE OPENING**	
Spontaneous	4	Spontaneous	4
To Voice	3	To Voice	3
To Pain	2	To Pain	3
None	1	None	1
VERBAL RESPONSE		**VERBAL RESPONSE**	
Oriented	5	Coos, Babbles	5
Confused	4	Consolable	4
Inappropriate Words	3	Cries To Pain	3
Incomprehensible Sounds	2	Moans To Pain	2
None	1	None	1
MOTOR RESPONSE		**MOTOR RESPONSE**	
Obeys Commands	6	Normal Spontaneous	6
Localizes (Pain)	5	Withdraws To Touch	5
Withdraw (Pain)	4	Withdraws To Pain	4
Flexion (Pain)	3	Abnormal Flexion	3
Extension (Pain)	2	Abnormal Extension	2
None	1	None	1
TOTAL		**TOTAL**	
TRAUMA SCORE		**PEDIATRIC TRAUMA SCORE**	
GCS CONVERT TO:		**SIZE**	
14-15	5	> 20 KG	2
11-13	4	10-20 KG	1
8-10	3	< 10 KG	-1
5-7	2	**AIRWAY**	
3-4	1	Normal	2
RESPIRATORY RATE:		Oral/Nasal	1
10-24	4	ETT/Trach	-1
25-35	3	**SYSTOLIC BLOOD PRESSURE:**	
≥ 36	2	> 90 (P-Wrist)	2
1-9	1	50-90 (P-Groin)	1
0	0	< 50 (P-O)	-1
RESPIRATORY EFFORT:		**LOC**	
Normal	1	Awake	2
Shallow or Retractive	0	Altered	1
SYSTOLIC BLOOD PRESSURE:		Comatose	-1
≥ 90	4	**OPEN WOUNDS**	
70-89	3	None	2
50-69	2	Minor	1
≤ 49	1	Major or Penetrating	-1
0	0	**FRACTURES**	
CAPILLARY REFILL:		None	2
Normal	2	Single or Closed	1
Delayed	1	Multiple or Open	-1
None	0		
TOTAL		**TOTAL**	

ADDRESSOGRAPH

TRAUMA ALERT

TRAUMA ALERT: ☐ YES ☐ NO

TIME TRAUMA ALERT CALLED: _____

TRAUMA ALERT REASON:

☐ RR <10 OR >29

☐ SBP <90 ☐ GCSS ≤ 12

☐ PENETRATING INJURY

☐ 2nd° OR 3rd° BURNS ≥ 15%

☐ PARALYSIS ☐ AMPUTATION

☐ EJECTION

☐ PEDIATRIC TRAUMA SCORE ≤ 8

TEAM MEMBERS	NAMES	TIME	
		NOTIFIED	ARRIVED
EMERGENCY PHYSICIAN			
TRAUMA SURGEON			
NEURO-SURGEON			
TRAUMA NURSE #1			
TRAUMA NURSE #2			
PARAMEDIC			
X-RAY TECHNOLOGIST			
RESPIRATORY TECHNOLOGIST			
CHAPLAIN			

TRAUMA FLOW SHEET 8/91, 10/91, 1/92 PAGE 1

FIGURE 48–1

Trauma flow sheet. (Courtesy of Bayfront Medical Center, Inc., St. Petersburg, Fla.)

SECONDARY SURVEY

1. = ABRASION
2. = LACERATION
3. = AVULSION
4. = PUNCTURE WOUND
5. = GUNSHOT WOUND
6. = CONTUSION
7. = BURN
8. = SWELLING
9. = DEFORMITY
10. = AMPUTATION
11. = PAIN
12. = (SPECIFY)
_____

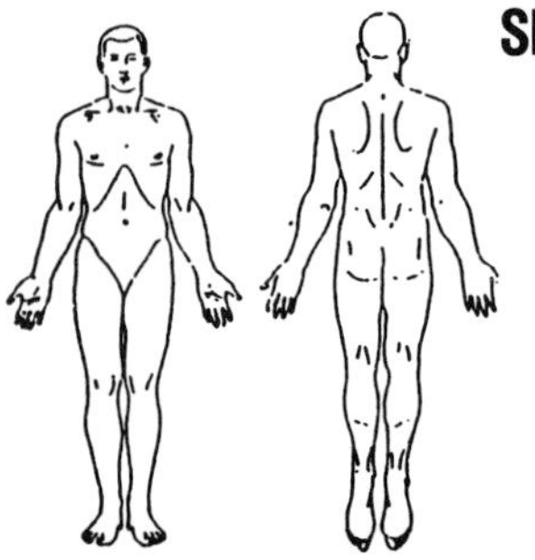

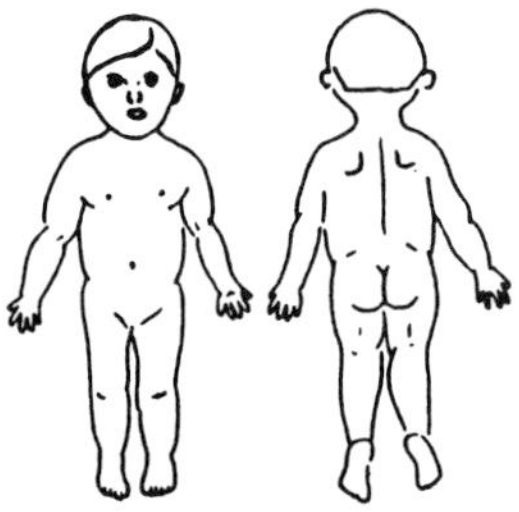

CLOTHING: ☐ CLOTHED ☐ ARRIVED EXPOSED ☐ CUT OFF

PUPILS

REACTION: NONREACTIVE = N
BRISK = B
SLUGGISH = S

• PIN POINT ● 1 ● 2 ● 3 ● 4 ● 5
● 6 ● 7 ● 8

LIMB MOVEMENT: PURPOSEFUL = P
NON-PURPOSEFUL = N
FLEXION = F
EXTENSION = E
NONE = 0

N = NORMAL
A = ABNORMAL
(SEE NARRATIVE)

PAST MEDICAL HISTORY	CURRENT MEDICATIONS
ASTHMA	
CARDIAC	
CVA	
DIABETES	
EMPHYSEMA/COPD	
HEPATITIS	
HIV	
HYPERTENSION	
SEIZURE DISORDER	
SICKLE CELL	

TETANUS STATUS
☐ < 5 YR ☐ > 5 YR
DATE:

ALLERGIES	LAST MENSTRUAL PERIOD
	LAST MEAL
	ESTIMATED WEIGHT

		TIME											
V I T A L S	**S I G N S**	BP											
		HR											
		R											
		SAO2/TEMP											
		CVP/FHT											
N E U R O		EYE											
		VERBAL											
		MOTOR											
		GCS											
		PUPIL: SIZE: R/L											
		RXN: R/L											
		EXT. MOVE: RA/LA											
		RL/LL											
		HEAD AND FACE											
		NECK											
C H E S T		THORAX											
		DYSPNEA											
		RETRACTIONS											
		BREATH SOUNDS: CLEAR											
		EQUAL											
		UNEQUAL											
		CRACKLES											
		WHEEZE											
		HEART SOUNDS: REGULAR											
		IRREGULAR											
		MUFFLED											
ABD		SOFT/NON-DISTENDED											
		RIGID/DISTENDED											
		PELVIS: STABLE											
		UNSTABLE											
		PERIPHERAL PULSES: RADIAL R/L											
		PEDAL R/L											
		POSTERIOR SURFACE											
S K I N		WARM/DRY											
		COOL/MOIST											
		CYANOTIC/PALE											
		CAP REFILL											
		PSYCHO/EMOTIONAL: CALM/COOPERATIVE											
		ANXIOUS/RESTLESS											
		AGITATED/UNCONSCIOUS											

PAGE 2

FIGURE 48-1 Continued

PROCEDURES

PROCEDURES	TIME	SIZE	BY WHOM
ARTERIAL LINE			
AUTOTRANSFUSION			
CENTRAL LINE			
CERVICAL TX			
CHEST TUBES			
CPR			
CRICO/TRACH			
FETAL MONITOR			
INTUBATION			
NEEDLE THORACOSTOMY			
NGT/OGT			
PERITONEAL LAVAGE			
SPLINT			
URINARY CATHETER			

IV FLUIDS

IV SITE	SIZE	BY WHOM	FLUID	WARMER USED	VOLUME HUNG	TIME	TOTAL INFUSED
					TOTAL FLUID		

MEDICATIONS

TIME	DRUG	DOSAGE	ROUTE	DILUTANT	RESPONSE TO MEDICATION	INITIALS

TOTAL DILUTANT/MEDICATION

DIAGNOSTIC STUDIES

LAB SPECIMEN	TIME DRAWN	INITIALS	TIME SENT TO LAB	RESULTS RECEIVED
TRAUMA PACK				
CBC				
T&C SET-UP/HOLD				
ABG				
EMIT				

X-RAYS		TIME DONE
C-SPINE – CROSSTABLE		
LS-SPINE – CROSSTABLE		
CHEST		
PELVIS		
FEMUR	R – L	
TIB/FIB	R – L	
ELBOW	R – L	
WRIST	R – L	
COMPLETE C-SPINE		
COMPLETE L-SPINE		
SKULL		
FACIAL		
KNEE	R – L	
FOOT	R – L	
HAND	R – L	
ANKLE	R – L	

CT SCANS	TIME TO	RETURN
BRAIN		
CHEST		
ABDOMEN		
PELVIS		
CERVICAL		

OTHER TESTS	TIME DONE
EKG	
AORTAGRAM	
CYSTOGRAM	
ULTRASOUND	
ECHOCARDIOGRAM	

ADDRESSOGRAPH

INTAKE / OUTPUT

TOTAL EMERGENCY DEPARTMENT

INTAKE		OUPUT	
IV FLUIDS:		URINE:	
DILUTANT/MEDICATIONS:		GASTRIC:	
PERITONEAL LAVAGE:		CHEST TUBE:	
AUTOTRANSFUSION:		PERITONEAL LAVAGE:	
OTHER:		OTHER:	
TOTAL INTAKE:		TOTAL OUTPUT:	

FIGURE 48–1 *Continued*

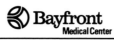
Bayfront
Medical Center

7-3 INITIALS	SIGNATURE/TITLE	3-11 INITIALS	SIGNATURE/TITLE	11-7 INITIALS	SIGNATURE/TITLE

TIME	DISPOSITION
☐ O.R.	☐ PERMIT SIGNED ☐ ID BRACELET ☐ EKG ☐ CBC ☐ UA ☐ T&C ☐ VOIDED ☐ CLOTHING/JEWELRY REMOVED ☐ DENTURES REMOVED ☐ PRE-OP GIVEN
☐ ADMITTED	BED # REPORT CALLED TO: TIME:
☐ LEFT AMA	☐ FORM SIGNED ☐ REFUSED TO SIGN ☐ UNABLE TO LOCATE PATIENT
☐ TRANSFERRED	FACILITY: _____ BED #: _____ ☐ TRANSFER SHEET COMPLETED. REPORT CALLED TO: _____ TIME: _____ SENT WITH PATIENT: ☐ VALUABLES ☐ COPY OF E.D. RECORD ☐ 1ST & 2ND COPIES HRS REGISTRY
☐ DISCHARGED	ACCOMPANIED BY:
☐ EXPIRED	☐ M.E. ☐ ORGAN DONATION
☐ SIGNIFICANT OTHERS	☐ VISITED ☐ CALLED ☐ UNABLE TO LOCATE
☐ CLOTHING	☐ WITH PATIENT ☐ POCKETS CHECKED ☐ TO POLICE ☐ GIVEN TO SIGNIFICANT OTHERS ☐ DISPOSED ☐ CLOTHING LIST COMPLETED
☐ VALUABLES	☐ ENVELOPE # _____ ☐ WITH PATIENT ☐ GIVEN TO SIGNIFICANT OTHERS ☐ SAFE ☐ SEE VALUABLES SHEET
☐ POLICE	☐ NOTIFIED ☐ ACCOMPANIED BY OFFICER:

FIGURE 48-1 *Continued*

720

primary survey, includes an initial neurologic assessment, and then follows with the secondary survey. Serial assessments, procedures, treatments, and the patients' responses are easily and rapidly documented with check boxes; however, space for narrative notes is also provided.

Transport

The critically ill child is resuscitated, stabilized, and transported out of the emergency department as quickly as possible to the computed tomography unit, the operating suite, the pediatric ICU, or the general trauma unit depending on the patient's assessment by the pediatric trauma surgeon. Adequate physician and nursing personnel must accompany the child during transport to continue therapy and respond to emergencies. Oxygen, a cardiac monitor, and a pediatric resuscitation transport box with equipment, supplies, and medications must be present on all transports.

The Pediatric Intensive Care Unit

The pediatric ICU nurse assumes the care of the critically ill child after surgery or stabilization in the emergency department. Necessary equipment is always available and ready for an admission. The nurse performs an initial assessment and then serial assessments to monitor the child's response to the injury and the subsequent management. Actual or pending complications that may result from associated injuries are closely monitored, as the critically injured child may worsen if injuries progress or deterioration occurs.

Traumatic injuries often result in severe pain. The nurse must take care in administering pain medications to the injured child because narcotics may mask neurologic changes or lead to a hypotensive crisis. High doses of narcotics prolong the return of peristalsis and may limit the ability to provide nutrition. Children who are highly sedated cannot clear accumulated secretions from their lungs and may develop atelectasis or pneumonia. Appropriate medication, music therapy, touch, and contact with parents may assist the child who is in pain.

Pulmonary complications may develop from direct pulmonary injuries, fluid overload from overaggressive resuscitation, or multiple blood transfusions. The child requires vigilant pulmonary toilet with ongoing assessments. Unconscious children of any age are provided with chest physiotherapy and suctioning at regular intervals. Conscious, older children can cough and breathe deeply when instructed and often use incentive spirometers without difficulty. The younger child who cannot or will not cough on demand may be willing to take deep breaths by blowing bubbles. This is fun for the child and at the same time improves pulmonary function and toilet.

Wounds from traumatic injuries are often contaminated and require diligent nursing care to prevent infections. Even small lacerations have the potential to become infected and cause local tissue damage, cellulitis, or systemic sepsis.

Nutritional assessments are performed by a registered dietitian. The ordered interventions are carried out by the nurse with consideration to the child's developmental level.

Rehabilitation begins on admission and is a major consideration in the pediatric ICU. Pediatric rehabilitation specialists are often consulted on admission of the child for development of a comprehensive and effective rehabilitation plan. Range of motion exercises, early splinting of extremities, frequent change of position, specialty beds, and pneumatic compression devices are important adjuncts to prevent complications.

The nurse provides constant companionship, comfort, and therapy for the critically injured child, and the family is considered and included in this overall plan of care.

Parental Concerns

Having a child admitted to a trauma center is a very difficult, stressful event for parents, and it presents them with numerous uncertainties. The parents have no time to prepare mentally, physically, or emotionally for the ordeal and are overwhelmed by the suddenness of the child's injury and the possibility that the child may not survive.

The parents must interact with an array of unfamiliar people in a somewhat foreign environment. Their personal lives are placed in turmoil when family, home, work, and financial disruptions occur. The stress of these disruptions results in numerous concerns ranging from everyday worries about other family members to the fear that their child may die. Once the child's condition stabilizes, concern that the child may suffer long-term or permanent disability is common. Parents use different methods to respond to their concerns and display different emotional reactions to the stressful event. Parents are the most important people in a child's world. When there is a serious injury, the child especially needs the emotional and physical support of parents.

Although the child may be well cared for in the trauma center, the parents frequently do not get the attention they need. They must be considered and included in all aspects of the child's care for the outcome to be truly successful, however. When a child is seriously ill, the parents often become very anxious, fearful, confused, and weak. Their energy is rapidly depleted. They need to sleep at night, to eat regular meals, and to relax at intervals throughout the day to maintain their own energy and health to support their child's physical and emotional needs.

Critically injured children need the support of their parents to assist in recovery. However, during the time when the child's condition is most critical, parents literally wear themselves out if they are not given a structured visitation schedule that includes time for resting, eating, and sleeping. Structured visiting times give the parents a way to plan their day during the most uncertain and confusing time of their lives.[8]

The nurse can most assist parents by offering information about all aspects of the child's care. This information must be ongoing and adjusted to the parent's level of understanding and the child's changing condition. The sight of their seriously injured child is often very frightening to parents. Severe bruising, bleeding, edemas, the loss of a limb, fractures, bandages, and monitoring equipment all may drastically alter the child's appearance. If the child is also comatose, the parents may be even more distressed. Preparation of the parents before they are allowed to see the child is extremely important. They need a thorough description of what they are going to see before entering the child's room.

Nurses, then, provide care and support to the parents as well as to the child and serve as parent as well as patient advocates.

SUMMARY

Foresight, planning, knowledge, skills, and teamwork are essential in the provision of nursing care to the critically ill child. Nurses coordinate the efforts of the multidisciplinary team and provide communication regarding all aspects of the patient's treatment and progress. Skilled pediatric nursing care can minimize the physical, psychological, and emotional stress of an injury. Pediatric trauma nurses save lives, preserve ability and function, and improve the expected outcome of the critically injured child.

References

1. American Nurses' Association: Standards of Maternal and Child Health Nursing Practice. Kansas City, American Nurses' Association, 1983.
2. Cardin S, Ward CR (eds): Personnel Management in Critical Care Nursing. Baltimore, Williams & Wilkins, 1989.
3. Chameides L: Textbook of Pediatric Advanced Life Support. Elk Grove Village, Ill, American Heart Association/American Academy of Pediatrics, 1988.
4. Committee on Trauma, American College of Surgeons: Resources for Optimal Care of the Injured Patient. Chicago, American College of Surgeons, 1990.
5. Emergency Nurses Association: Standards of Emergency Nursing Practice. 2nd ed. St. Louis, CV Mosby, 1991.
6. Emergency Nurses Association: Trauma Nursing Core Course. 3rd ed. Chicago, Award Printing, 1991.
7. Evans HE (ed): Hospital Care of Children and Youth. Elk Grove Village, Ill, American Academy of Pediatrics, 1986.
8. Ford DK: An Examination of the Concerns of Parents Who Have Had a Child in a Pediatric Intensive Care Unit. Unpublished master's thesis. Knoxville, University of Tennessee, College of Nursing, 1989.
9. Joint Commission on the Accreditation of Healthcare Organizations: Accreditation Manual for Hospitals. Oakbrook Terrace, Ill, 1991.
10. Sanford SJ, Disch JM (eds): AACN Standards for Nursing Care of the Critically Ill. 2nd ed. East Norwalk, Conn, Appleton & Lange, 1989.
11. Silverman BK: Advanced Pediatric Life Support. Elk Grove Village, Ill, American Academy of Pediatrics/American College of Emergency Physicians, 1989.
12. Trauma Nursing Coalition: Resource Document for Nursing Care of the Trauma Patient. Denver, AORN Inc., Trauma Nursing Coalition, 1992.

The Aftermath of Childhood Injuries

Bruce M. Gans

CHAPTER FORTY-NINE

Rehabilitation Support for the Injured Child

REHABILITATION

Injuries to children are responsible for the largest number of preventable disabilities. It is estimated that 30,000 children experience trauma serious enough to require rehabilitation services on an annual basis. Whereas conventional systems of care for acutely injured children have focused on emergency medical and surgical care, the most advanced systems of trauma care for children also recognize the early need for rehabilitation intervention.[3] In this chapter, the effective use of rehabilitation services for injured children is reviewed, suggestions for proper treatment and preventive care are offered, and strategies to integrate long-term with acute care systems are presented.

Rehabilitation was first developed as a component of the health care system, with Rusk conceiving of it as the "third phase of health care," after diagnosis and definitive treatment.[11] He and others assumed that further cure of the underlying pathophysiology was not possible and that education and adaptation were necessary to allow the patient to resume maximum function in society. Modern rehabilitation practitioners know the value of preventive care, recognizing that early and effective application of rehabilitation interventions may reduce the absolute magnitude of disability and shorten the duration of medical care necessary to achieve optimal function. Thus, early and effective provision of rehabilitation services is deemed essential.

The early involvement of rehabilitation service delivery personnel in the acute care of injured children may be facilitated by standing protocols of care. The practice standards of a level I regional pediatric trauma center should include early (within the first 24 hours) and automatic referral of all seriously injured children for rehabilitation medicine consultation.

Even in this acute stage of care, the physiatrist (a physician specializing in physical medicine and rehabilitation) can evaluate the child for needs related to long-term outcome and function, as well as assist in short-term, immediate management issues. Frequently, the physiatrist pays initial attention to preventive care to avoid secondary disabling complications such as skin breakdown, contractures, compression injuries to peripheral nerves, and secondary neurologic damage due to spinal or cranial injury or edema.

For a child with a serious disabling disorder, such as head and spinal cord injuries, the earlier the physiatrist can establish rapport and contact with the child and family, the better the chances of providing emotional and social support and effecting an efficient program of long-term care through inpatient rehabilitation services and, later, home programs. Also, for those children who ultimately will be transferred to the care of a physiatrist, that care will be facilitated if he or she is fully cognizant of all aspects of the acute care interventions.

PRINCIPLES OF REHABILITATION MANAGEMENT

Providers

The typical structure of any rehabilitation service delivery system includes leadership by a physiatrist or other physician with training and experience in the care of injured children. Because of the severe shortage of pediatric physiatrists, many facilities rely on the services of physiatrists who care primarily for disabled adults (also a shortage specialty) or other physicians who have developed strong practice-based experience in the care of disabled children. Pediatric rehabilitation fellowships and residency training programs leading to dual board certification in both pediatrics and physical medicine and rehabilitation are now available, and it is likely that a greater supply of well-trained pediatric physiatrists will be available over the next 7 to 10 years.[4]

The physiatrist's role is clear. Initially, he or she reviews the medical status of the child and the current management program, offering diagnostic and therapeutic assistance to the attending surgeons. This may include suggestions about the potential value of electrodiagnostic studies (electromyography, nerve conduction velocity studies, and evoked potential studies) for diagnosing peripheral nerve, spinal cord, or brain injuries or to aid in establishing a prognosis in these disorders.

The physiatrist has a special interest in participating in surgical management decisions about either spinal fractures or limb amputation versus salvage procedures. Extensively experienced in the long-term management of paralysis and amputation, the physiatrist can offer helpful insights into issues not usually addressed, such as the possible benefits of amputation or the ideal management of spinal fractures to allow early mobilization and rehabilitation.

In the area of traumatic brain injury, the physiatrist endeavors to establish programs of rehabilitation care as soon as possible and to participate in establishing realistic prognoses for long-term outcome.

Patients with serious burns need rehabilitation services far into the future, and the physiatrist should participate in early decisions about skin care and contracture prevention and management.

In general, the physiatrist is most experienced in facilitating group processes of care. In many settings, the physiatrist acts as the facilitator and coordinator of multiple physicians involved in making acute care decisions (such as ensuring consensus between orthopedists and neurosurgeons about management of spinal column fracture in patients with neurologic deficits).

The physiatrist also leads and facilitates another major group—the allied health professionals who are part of the rehabilitation team. This team typically consists of nurses, physical therapists, occupational therapists, speech and language pathologists, psychologists, social workers, rehabilitation engineers, and assorted other individuals.

The rehabilitation nurse provides more than conventional medical-surgical nursing services. He or she also helps establish and train for bladder and bowel function, care for skin lesions, and in general carry through the training of the other therapists into real-world situations.

In addition to conventional psychological services such as support and cognitive assessment, the rehabilitation psychologist provides services to the patient's family and even the rehabilitation team. This includes cognitive rehabilitation, counseling in adjustment to the disability, and behavior management program development.

The rehabilitation social worker offers family support and also assistance in identifying and using the social and economic resources that exist to aid children with disabilities. He or she may also provide family therapy or counseling.

The physical therapist provides hands-on services involving the applications of exercise and therapy for musculoskeletal injuries. He or she also provides training in gross motor function areas such as transfers and ambulation. When necessary, the physical therapist is also concerned with wheelchair seating and use.

The occupational therapist offers interventions for upper extremity, head and neck, and functional disorders. He or she concentrates on exercises and training for fine motor control. In addition, the occupational therapist pays attention to perceptual motor skills to allow the child to recover age-appropriate self-sufficiency for activities of daily living such as dressing, bathing, and self-feeding.

The speech and language pathologist concentrates on oral motor, swallowing, and language functions. Exercises and training in each of these areas may allow impaired children to make meaningful progress.

The rehabilitation engineer provides expertise for the high-technology resolution of functional limitations in severely disabled children. Technologic advances in rehabilitation include switch controls for power wheelchairs, communication devices, and environmental control systems.

Rehabilitation Process

Each of these professionals offers unique, specialized skills and abilities valuable to the total rehabilitation process. However, they need to be organized and integrated into a unified team that collectively cares for the child in a goal-oriented and efficient manner early on in the care.

This integration is achieved by using a group process dependent on written and verbal communication strategies and directed by the physiatrist. The physiatrist targets initial evaluations by each discipline, focusing on specific major problems that have been identified by the acute care team. These problems also extend beyond the acute health care realm into functional limitations such as ambulation, self-care skills, and cognitive and communicative functions.

After each needed professional has performed an initial assessment of the child, a team meeting is held to share assessments and to establish major goals and objectives for care. These goals may be stated in terms such as "achieve independence in shoe tying" or in quantitative descriptions such as "demonstrate the ability to ambulate 50 feet in less than 30 seconds with only contact guarding." Patients (when old enough) and families participate in this goal-setting process.

Weekly or biweekly team meetings are held to review goals, objectives, progress, needed changes in care, and, of course, discharge planning. This information is documented and shared with families and patients on a regular basis.

Measurement of Function

To quantify progress, measures of physical performance and function are necessary. Although many of these factors appear to be subjective, formal techniques exist or are emerging for this type of quantitative assessment. These are necessary to evaluate the effectiveness of interventions and patient progress once life-threatening illness has passed.

Physiologic Functions

Strength. Strength is measured qualitatively using the Medical Research Council scoring system of 0 to 5. These terms have specific meaning as shown in Table 49–1. Newer methods using quantitative force measurement offer greater sensitivity. With small children who cannot cooperate with manual muscle testing, substantial subjective interpretation is involved in making any strength judgments.

Range of Motion. Range of motion is commonly measured in both casual and formal ways. Casual visual estimates of joint movement angles are only coincidentally accurate. A variety of goniometers are available that measure within ±5 degrees of accuracy for all joints. Electrogoniometers are commercially available but not yet commonly used for clinical measures of this type.

Development

Measures of development on milestone-oriented tools, such as the Denver Developmental Screening Test, are useful in determining the premorbid developmental status of young injury victims. These tests may be only partially helpful in determining developmental deficits that have resulted from injuries. In general, the less severe the deficit, the more likely young children are reasonably assessed using a developmental instrument.

Performance

The quantitative measure of motor and behavioral performance is a more complex task. No widely used, standardized tests of motor performance of seriously disabled children exist. One emerging tool for this purpose is the Tufts Assessment of Motor Performance (TAMP).[8, 9] The TAMP is a standardized test that consists of 32 tasks that disabled children (and adults) commonly perform. Criterion-referenced scores for each aspect of the behavior are assigned by the observing rater, and summary scores of performance along several different domains are computed. The TAMP

Table 49–1
Medical Research Council Strength-Scoring System

Numeric Score*	Descriptive	Gravity	Resistance	Movement
0	Absent	Eliminated	None	None
1	Trace	Eliminated	None	Palpable or visible
2	Poor	Eliminated	None	Full range
3	Fair	Present	None	Full range
4	Good	Present	Moderate	Full range
5	Normal	Present	Full	Full range

*A + or − sign may be added to each score except 0.

is sensitive to changes in motor performance and is useful for the quantitative assessment of motor performance of children over the age of 5 years.

In addition to testing of motor performance, evaluation of cognitive, linguistic, and social skills is necessary. Various quantitative measurement instruments are available for each of these skills.

Functional Assessment

Measures of function are even less available than measures of performance in the pediatric age group. In the measure of functional assessment of adults, more than 40 different tools have been published, but few are in current use, and even fewer have been formally validated and shown to be reliable. The most widely accepted available measurement tool is the Functional Independence Measure (FIM), developed by a consortium led by Granger and others.[7] The currently available version is not useful for children under age 6. A pediatric version of the FIM (the WeeFIM) is also available.[6] Another functional assessment tool specifically designed for children is the PEDI.[2]

Patterns of Recovery

The time pattern of recovery from any impairment that causes disability and handicap is shown in Figures 49–1 and 49–2. The curve shows that an early plain of low-level function is followed by a rapid recovery phase, which gradually slows and ultimately reaches a plateau of function. Superimposed on the recovery process is the growth and development of the child. These two processes frequently are not readily distinguishable. Judgments about the effectiveness of a rehabilitation program are based on both the level of need or severity of the problem as well as the rate of progress being achieved toward the measurable rehabilitation objectives. Thus, the trajectory or slope of the curve

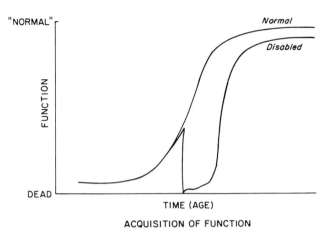

FIGURE 49-2

The time pattern for the acquisition of function of a child with a later acquired traumatic disability shows a rapid recovery phase with a higher slope than that of Figure 49–1 but not quite as high as normal. A distinction among recovery, the effects of rehabilitation treatment, and growth and development may be difficult.

showing rate of change is an important tool in utilization review and program evaluation.

SYSTEMS OF CARE

Rehabilitation services are provided at a number of locations within the health care delivery system. The judgment as to which setting is appropriate is based on an assessment of the needs of the child, the availability of family and insurance resources, and the accessibility of the service delivery method. Usually, the overriding goal is to discharge a child to home as soon as possible. However, this should not be done at the expense of the child's best interests in achieving improved function or before the family is able to effectively provide care for the child in the home setting.

Inpatient Comprehensive Rehabilitation

The most labor-intensive rehabilitation programs are possible only when the child is an inpatient in an organized pediatric rehabilitation hospital or unit.[10] The coordinated services of physicians, nurses, therapists, social workers, psychologists, and other providers are most readily available and effectively integrated in this setting.

Inpatient rehabilitation programs are considered appropriate when the patient needs multiple and differing therapies on a daily basis, an integrated program of goal-directed care, and significant medical and nursing input. Families may need to board at the facility or at least be available to learn rehabilitation techniques as part of the rehabilitation program.

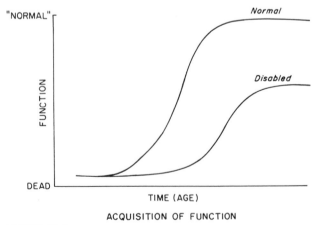

FIGURE 49-1

The time pattern for the acquisition of function of a child with a congenital or early acquired traumatic disability reveals an early plane of delayed onset of improvement. This is followed by improvement, and then the final stage of stable level of function is the plateau. The trajectory or slope of the curve showing rate of change is an important tool in evaluation.

Outpatient Rehabilitation Programs

When slower rates of progress are expected, less labor-intensive therapeutic programs (i.e., two or three times weekly) may be provided on an outpatient basis when the child can be cared for at home and can be transported to the outpatient facility by the family. The availability of medical services is less than when the child is an inpatient, and medical stability must be achieved for this type of care to be effective.

Home Care Programs

When possible, therapists may travel to the home of the child to provide care and services. This is generally more expensive than facility-based outpatient services but may be the most effective method of assessing the home setting and providing interventions that specifically match the environmental needs of the child and family. When frequent multidisciplinary therapeutic services are needed, home care is usually inadequate to meet the needs.

School-Based Programs

Many times children with serious, disabling disorders are eligible for special-needs services through the local public school system. These services may include all the rehabilitation therapies in addition to special education. The balance to be achieved in this setting is the distinction between medical and educational needs. Frequently, school systems are reluctant to provide any services that are more medically than educationally necessary, and an integration of the two types of providers is necessary. Advocacy by the physicians and other acute and rehabilitation providers may be necessary to facilitate adequate service delivery by the school system.

INDICATIONS FOR REFERRAL TO REHABILITATION MEDICINE

The rehabilitation team and physiatrist can make important contributions to the care and management of any child with central or peripheral neurologic damage.[1]

Neurologic Injuries

Diagnostic information may be obtained from the rehabilitation team in a number of areas, including electrodiagnostic studies, formal assessments of function, level of consciousness, and prognosis.

Electrodiagnostic studies performed by the physiatrist are helpful in both peripheral and central injuries. For peripheral nerve injuries, the nature, extent, and prognosis may be determined with nerve conduction velocity and electromyographic studies. Traumatic brain injuries may be assessed by evoked potential studies. Spinal cord injuries may be assessed for both level and degree of severity using electromyography, evoked potentials, and cortical stimulation techniques.

Routine assessment of the mental status of the child by therapists according to behavioral scales (such as the Rancho Los Amigos Coma Scale) offers useful information to the acute care team.

For children with major neurologic deficits, rehabilitation programs are of great importance. The earlier started, the better their likely effectiveness. In the case of traumatic brain injuries, early intervention with bracing or casting may prevent lower extremity contractures from developing. Early aggressive management of spasticity with drugs or nerve blocks may also optimize long-term care.[5]

Children with major neurologic injuries are at risk for decubitus ulcers, so the rehabilitation team provides preventive care measures, including attention to bed positioning and skin care.

Bowel and bladder dysfunction also should receive attention. Promotion of safe and developmentally appropriate bladder and bowel function is an important rehabilitation focus.

Limb Injuries and Amputation

Early appropriate use of braces and prostheses as necessary is accomplished by the rehabilitation team. The use of braces to stabilize paralyzed limbs and restore function is an early objective of the rehabilitation program for a child with a brachial plexus injury for example. Immediate postoperative prosthetic fitting reduces postoperative complications in stump management and allows early mobilization and recovery of function.

MAJOR FUNCTIONAL PROBLEMS

Each child is unique, and vast differences exist between specific injuries. Nevertheless, many aspects of rehabilitation programs cross diagnostic boundaries. This is especially true for functional problem management. The rehabilitation team deals with many functional problem areas in the care of injured children.

Positioning

Proper positioning of the acutely injured child is an important aspect of overall care. Benefits include prevention of contracture and skin breakdown, control of spasticity, improved arousal (by upright positioning), and oral motor function, and enhanced feeding.

Seating

For children with impaired or developmentally deficient postural control, adapted seating systems provide improved upright posture and stability. This makes care easier, allows mobility devices to be used, and facilitates developmental and therapeutic progress. Simple, commercially available systems may suffice. If not, more complex commercial or custom-made system prescriptions may be developed by the rehabilitation team.

Mobility

Assisting the child to recover independent mobility is a major goal. When ambulation is feasible, intensive work is focused on this objective. Gait training may need to be supplemented by the prescription of braces, ambulation aids, or prostheses.

When ambulation is impractical, wheelchair prescription and training are necessary. Whenever possible, manual wheelchairs should be chosen. In extreme cases, however, powered wheelchairs may be prescribed and used, even by children as young as 18 to 24 months.

Transfers

Training a child to get on and off seats, beds, and other objects sometimes requires significant attention by the rehabilitation team. Education of the family also is necessary. At times, it is necessary to teach families what not to do for a child to facilitate greater ultimate independence; transfer skill building is a common area where this management strategy may be necessary.

Self-Care Activities

A number of self-care skills are lumped under the descriptive term *activities of daily living,* including self-dressing, self-feeding, bathing, grooming, personal hygiene, and related tasks. The occupational therapist may develop complex treatment programs to retrain, educate, and adapt the child or the task. Adaptations may include new methods (such as changing choice of clothing closures) or the use of specialized tools (e.g., a universal cuff to hold eating utensils). Family education may again be of major importance.

Communication

Augmentative communication aids or techniques may be necessary for severely communicatively handicapped children. These range from simple communication boards to complex computerized speech output communication devices. The choice of these interventions requires a sophisticated and experienced treatment team.

Psychosocial Features

The emotional adaptation of a child to a permanent disability may be difficult or surprisingly easy. Treatment of the child's adaptation usually goes hand in hand with treatment of the parents' adaptation. Younger children in particular tend to be adaptive and tolerant of changes in function.

During adolescent or preadolescent years, however, greater emotional turmoil is common. The rehabilitation program attempts to provide specific psychological and social interventions as necessary and, in general, to anticipate these difficulties in adaptation. Providing a child with new abilities and functions through the rehabilitation process is one of the most effective preventive methods of managing the difficulties of adaptation.

TOOLS AND METHODS OF REHABILITATION

The types of treatment needs and opportunities described above use a number of methods and devices, many of which are newly available because of technologic advances.

Orthotics and Prosthetics

Sophisticated new materials and fabrication methods are routinely used for the fabrication of braces and artificial limbs. Heat-moldable materials, advanced computer-aided fitting techniques, and sophisticated electronics have allowed the use of dynamic braces and myoelectric prostheses. These more-sophisticated devices (especially powered prostheses) should be fit by experienced treatment teams in regional centers.

Exercise

The traditional adult methods of exercise usually do not engage the attention or cooperation of smaller children. Much of the exercise programming for children is camouflaged as play. Games, races, and group activities may achieve more practical success for strengthening and endurance training than do standard repetitive activities.

Active strength building through functional electrical stimulation is also gaining acceptance in the adult rehabilitation program. The physiologic feasibility of external stimulation to achieve muscle hypertrophy is clear. The practical application of this method in children is still in question, however. Children may be less tolerant of the sensory experience of external stimulation than adults are. Further experience is needed before the routine application of functional electrical stimulation to children can be recommended.

Newer exercise devices that allow isokinetic muscle contractions (isokinetic dynamometers such as those manufactured by Cybex or Lido) have limited applications to children. These devices need adaptation for size and programming before being useful for children.

High-Technology Aids and Devices

Sophisticated, electric-powered wheelchairs with joystick controls are readily available for disabled children. In addition to providing mobility, some of the newest designs also allow vertical adjustment of the seat height and assistance with coming to the standing position from a seated one.

Environmental control systems allow a severely disabled child to regain control over electrical appliances. Single switches may be hooked into systems that allow everything from turning on lights to changing channels on a television or controlling battery-operated toys.

Access to computers is possible for even the most severely physically disabled child through simple switches, voice recognition, or even eye-gaze detection. With these adaptations, the use of computers for education, communication, work, and play is feasible.

LONG-TERM OUTCOME

The survival of severely injured children will lead to a continuing increase in the prevalence of severely disabled children in homes, residential facilities, and acute care institutions. Many children, even though severely disabled, are medically stable and look forward to essentially normal life expectancies. The challenge to the trauma care and rehabilitation systems is to provide meaningful quality-of-life options for these children and their families.

By focusing on function and quality of life of the survivors of serious injuries, it is possible to provide the scope of rehabilitation and acute care services described earlier in an effort to provide for the physical, psychological, social, and functional needs of these children and their families. Through close collaboration and even integration of the acute and rehabilitative systems of care, technically sophis-

ticated yet humane care may be delivered in a cost-effective manner to all children in need following serious disabling injuries.

References

1. DiScala C, Osberg JS, Gans BM, et al: Children with traumatic head injury: Morbidity and postacute treatment. Arch Phys Med Rehabil 72:662–666, 1991.
2. Feldman AB, Haley SM, Coryell J: Concurrent and construct validity of the Pediatric Evaluation of Disability Inventory. Physical Ther 70:602–610, 1990.
3. Gans BM, DiScala C: Rehabilitation of severely injured children. West J Med 154:566–568, 1991.
4. Gans BM, Nagy JM: Survey and commentary on fellowship training for pediatric rehabilitation. Am J Phys Med Rehabil 67:273–274, 1988.
5. Glenn MB, Whyte J: The Practical Management of Spasticity in Children and Adults. Philadelphia, Lea & Febiger, 1990.
6. Granger CV, Hamilton BB, Kayton R: Guide for the Use of the Functional Independence Measure (WeeFIM) of the Uniform Data Set for Medical Rehabilitation. Buffalo, Research Foundation, State University of New York, 1988.
7. Granger CV, Hamilton BB, Sherwin FS: Guide for the Use of the Uniform Data Set for Medical Rehabilitation. Buffalo, Research Foundation, State University of New York, 1986.
8. Haley SM, Ludlow LH, Gans BM, et al: Tufts assessment of motor performance: An empirical approach to identifying motor performance categories. Arch Phys Med Rehabil 72:359–366, 1991.
9. Ludlow LH, Haley SM, Gans BM: A hierarchical model of functional performance in rehabilitation medicine: The Tufts assessment of motor performance. Eval Health Prof 15:59–74, 1992.
10. Osberg JS, DiScala C, Gans BM: Utilization of inpatient rehabilitation services among traumatically injured children discharged from pediatric trauma centers. Am J Phys Med Rehabil 69:67–72, 1990.
11. Rusk HA: Rehabilitation Medicine. 4th ed. St Louis, CV Mosby, 1977.

Steven Stylianos
Burton H. Harris

CHAPTER FIFTY

Long-Term Disability and Morbidity after Childhood Injuries

"If only the ambulance had arrived 5 minutes earlier . . . or 5 minutes later . . ."

Advances in prehospital, emergency surgical, and intensive care have resulted in improved survival of patients with serious multisystem injuries. As the delivery of pediatric trauma care has improved, an enlarging group of survivors with significant long-term care issues is being recognized. We are beginning to learn about the morbidity of pediatric trauma beyond the initial hospitalization and the consequences for the injured children and their families.

THE PATIENTS

Fewer than 3% of pediatric trauma patients die of their injuries, but there is a paucity of information about what happens to those who survive.[6, 8] We do know that for the more than 100,000 children who are admitted to hospitals each year with head injuries, morbidity after the initial convalescence remains the most significant problem of long-term care and quality of life.

In 1983, Mahoney and colleagues reported a long-term outcome study of 46 children with significant head injuries who had remained comatose more than 24 hours.[7] The average length of coma among the 34 survivors was 15 days, and the follow-up period was 1 to 4 years (mean = 21 months). Almost one third of the survivors eventually returned to normal. An additional 53% had cognitive or behavioral problems, some of whom had evidence of similar problems before injury. Nine percent of survivors had residual motor deficits with normal intellect. Mahoney and colleagues concluded that, despite violent injury and prolonged coma, most children survive and retain the potential for excellent recovery.

Although children fare much better than comparably brain-injured adults, cognitive, psychomotor, emotional, and behavioral sequelae can pose significant long-term problems.[7, 10] Adults and children with head injuries often need to relearn skills, and although children are said to "outgrow" residual impairments, the evidence suggests contrary findings, revealing that children may actually "grow into" additional deficits as the developmental demands of language and reasoning become more complex and abstract. There is a particularly vulnerable period when a child with posttraumatic deficits reaches adolescence and confronts issues of personal identity, peer acceptance, and sexuality.

Wesson and co-workers studied 250 consecutive children hospitalized with severe injuries to determine their functional outcomes at discharge and 6 months after injury.[10] Sixty-two percent of the cases were caused by motor vehicle accidents. Severe injury was defined as involvement of at least one organ system with an Abbreviated Injury Score (AIS) greater than 4 or two or more systems with AIS scores greater than 2. The mean age was 9 years, and the mean Injury Severity Score (ISS) was 24. The investigators used the RAND Health Insurance Study categories for physical activity, role-appropriate activity, and self-care activities and the Glasgow Outcome Scale to define early and late morbidity. For the 217 surviving patients, the mean hospital stay was 22 days, and 190 (88%) patients had one or more functional limitations at discharge. Only one third of the children were found to be without a neurologic deficit. A substantial portion (54%) of the whole group had ongoing physical disabilities that limited participation in normal activities 6 months after discharge. This study emphasizes the late consequences for injured children. A subsequent prospective study by this group found functional impairment in 71% of severely injured children (ISS >15) at 6 months after injury and 55% at 1 year.[7]

The psychological effects of nonneurologic trauma on children are poorly defined. Basson and colleagues surveyed the parents of 80 children who had experienced relatively minor injuries (mean ISS = 4.5; mean hospital stay = 3.5 days).[1] In 30% of this group, substantial behavioral disability was identified by a modification of Achenbach's Child Behavioral Checklist. Diagnoses included phobias, major scholastic difficulties, rage attacks, and episodic depression. Most children with these disabilities eventually returned to "normal," but the duration of symptoms averaged 19 months (range, 3–72 months).

If these studies are representative, millions of children in the United States may suffer from posttraumatic behavior dysfunction. In many instances, the behavioral and emotional complications of pediatric injuries appear more debilitating than the injury itself. Early assessment and intervention may ameliorate the psychological stress of the patients and families.

PARENTS AND SIBLINGS

A study from the Kiwanis Pediatric Trauma Institute disclosed unpleasant surprises concerning the late effects of trauma on injured children and their families.[3] In an attempt to characterize the physical, emotional, and behavioral consequences of severe multisystem injury for pediatric trauma patients and members of their immediate families, 54 trauma patients and their families were studied 1 year or more after discharge. The mean age of the patients was 8 years, the mean length of hospital stay was 31 days, and 68% of the patients had been involved in motor vehicle accidents. More than half had speech or emotional impairment and deficits in attention, memory, or learning. Eighty percent needed special education or a school setting that appropriately adjusted social interaction.

The effects of trauma on families was profound. At the end of 1 year, the composition of the family unit had changed in 40% of 50 families. The changes included separations, divorce, and occasional return of a previously estranged parent. Those reporting marital discord were usually mothers who felt that their husbands had emotionally withdrawn from the situation and left them to bear the burden.

Family finances were strikingly affected by trauma. After recovery, 58% of families reported that one family member stopped working to care for the injured child, and 25% of families had used all their savings. The mean hospital bill for the study group patients was $44,800.

An unexpected finding was the effect of trauma on uninjured siblings. Almost half had developed emotional reactions, school problems, or aggressive personality changes. Unlike adults, siblings often lack the emotional maturity or verbal abilities to express their feelings. Isolated from the patient during hospitalization and receiving vague explanations of their sibling's condition, the brother or sister can experience intense resentment about the added responsibilities, reduced parental attention, and limits on their own socialization and recreation.

Patients are not the only victims of pediatric trauma. The family members also suffered from the behavioral and intellectual deficits of the injured child, and they experienced drastic shifts in the usual roles and responsibilities among family members. The constellation of emotional and behavioral problems presented by these injured children can tax any parent's ability to cope with adversity. The community and academic resources available to help families in these situations are very limited.

After injury to a child, parents experience periods of shock, denial, anger, guilt, depression, and anxiety about the future. Intense feelings of guilt and blame may jeopardize their ability to assist their child and each other through the event and the difficulties that lie ahead. Meeting the needs of family members must be part of the comprehensive treatment plan for all pediatric trauma victims.

FAMILY SUPPORT

Family members need a clear and compassionate explanation of their child's condition and treatment, an understanding of realistic expectations, and the knowledge that they will not be alone in dealing with the sequelae of the trauma. The treatment of injured children should include educating parents about the cognitive sequelae, expectations for recovery, and socioeconomic implications of their child's injuries.

During the child's hospitalization, parents should be encouraged to participate actively in therapies and the development of behavior-intervention strategies. Early communication with home intervention specialists can alleviate a major source of parental anxiety. In New England, the Kiwanis Family Care Network also addresses nonmedical issues raised by injury and prolonged hospitalization.[4]

Many parents recall the pain and guilt of silently wishing their child had died from his or her injuries rather than becoming severely disabled.[9] Most would not discuss this with anyone, only to learn months or years later that their spouse or other parents had had the same thoughts. Support groups can be valuable for those trying to cope with ambivalence and are a meaningful experience for many parents. Meeting on a regular basis, parents can share information on programs and resources, provide emotional support for each other, and exchange thoughts and ideas. There is much to be learned from the experience of others.

School can be a major rehabilitation and socialization environment for injured children. Successful educational reentry is a predictor of the difficulty of the postinjury period. Federal legislation passed in 1975 and amended in 1986 mandated that each state thoroughly assess the educational needs of disabled children, involve parents in the development of each child's education program, and pro-

vide education in the least restrictive setting. Public Law 94-142 has had an enormous impact on the funding and provision of educational programs and services for children with disabilities.

Most young children have a difficult time grasping the concept of death, particularly the death of someone their own age. Children look to adults for help with questions and feelings. Children involved in or witnessing an accident in which others are seriously injured or killed have predictable problems, but most teachers, coaches, and counselors have little training in providing this kind of help.

The Good Grief Program at Boston's Judge Baker Children's Center (see Appendix) was designed as a mental health effort to help schools and community groups support children and adolescents facing the terminal illness or death of a friend. Techniques involve in-service training, consultation, educational programs, and crisis intervention.[2] In 7 years, this program has served over 30,000 children in 25 states and 13 countries. The goal of Good Grief is to keep bereaved children and adolescents psychologically healthy and prevent the development of later emotional problems. The program helps parents, teachers, and children accomplish four important tasks: understand death through sensible definitions; grieve while expressing sadness, anger, and guilt; commemorate in ways emphasizing the value of a tragically shortened life; and move on with the everyday activities of living and caring.

Every year, almost 300,000 children sustain injuries requiring hospital admission, at a cost of about $1 billion.[5] These costs are paid by private sources (63%) or Medicaid programs (28%), with only 9% remaining uninsured. Approximately 1500 children die yearly of injuries, representing a loss to society of 88,000 life-years and an estimated $350 million in lost productivity. These costs highlight the importance of pediatric trauma as a major public health concern. Greater resources are needed to develop and implement effective prevention strategies, and if that fails to ensure optimal acute care, resources are needed to provide physical, emotional, and educational rehabilitation.

CONCLUSION

There is a hidden morbidity in pediatric trauma. It manifests itself as physical disability, as changes in cognition, personality, behavior, and family stress. Because success in pediatric trauma care is the restoration of the child and his or her family to the premorbid state, these findings suggest that more attention and resources should be directed to the late consequences of multisystem injury children. The clinician must also be an advocate, educator, therapist, friend, and community networker. Those with hospital trauma program responsibilities should add skilled counselors to help provide long-term continuity of care to the injured patients and recruit appropriate support services for these children and their families.

References

1. Basson MD, Guinn JE, McElligott J, et al: Behavioral disturbances in children after trauma. J Trauma 31:1363–1368, 1991.

2. Fox SS: Good Grief: Helping groups of children when a friend dies. Boston, The New England Association for the Education of Young Children, 1988.

3. Harris BH, Schwaitzberg SC, Seman TM, et al: The hidden morbidity of pediatric trauma. J Pediatr Surg 24:103–106, 1989.

4. Lockwood DT, Harris BH: Family care in pediatric trauma. Emerg Care Q 3:61–64, 1987.

5. MacKenzie EJ, Morris JA, de Lissovoy GV, et al: Acute hospital costs of pediatric trauma in the United States: How much and who pays. J Pediatr Surg 25:970–976, 1990.

6. Mahoney WJ, D'Souza BJ, Haller JA, et al: Long-term outcome of children with severe head trauma and prolonged coma. Pediatrics 71:756–762, 1983.

7. Scorpio RJ, Wesson DE, Spence LJ, et al: The physical, psychological, and socio-economic cost of pediatric trauma. J Trauma 33:252–255, 1992.

8. Tepas JJ, DiScala D, Ramenofsky ML, et al: Mortality and head injury: The pediatric perspective. J Pediatr Surg 25:92–96, 1990.

9. Waaland PK, Kreutzer JS: Family response to childhood traumatic brain injury. J Head Trauma Rehabil 3:51–63, 1988.

10. Wesson DE, Williams JI, Spence LJ, et al: Functional outcome in pediatric trauma. J Trauma 29:589–592, 1989.

Appendix
Support Groups

National Head Injury Foundation: Provides a variety of support and educational programs for families through local and state chapters; 1-800-444-NHIF.

Research and Training Center in Rehabilitation and Childhood Trauma: Multiple research and educational programs available to meet the physical and emotional needs of the injured child and family. An extensive bibliography is available. Research and Training Center in Rehabilitation and Childhood Trauma, Kiwanis Pediatric Trauma Institute, Box 75K-R, 750 Washington Street, Boston MA 02111; (617) 956-5032.

The Good Grief Program: A preventive mental health program designed to help schools and community groups become a locus of support for children and adolescents facing terminal illness or death. Techniques include in-service training, consultation, educational programs, and crisis intervention. An extensive bibliography and video library is available. Judge Baker Children's Center, 295 Longwood Avenue, Boston MA 02115; (617) 232-8390.

New Medico Head Injury System: Treatment of closed or penetrating head injuries, spinal cord injuries, and nontraumatic central nervous system catastrophes in hospital units, nursing facilities, community reentry programs, or supervised apartments. 14 Central Avenue, Lynn MA 01901; 1-800-CARE TBI, ext. 3053.

Mothers Against Drunk Driving (MADD): Focuses national attention and provides support to victims and their families. MADD, 669 Airport Freeway, Suite 310, Hurst TX 76053.

CHAPTER FIFTY-ONE

Sandra Loucks

Psychological Consequences of Trauma

The psychological impact of physical trauma on the child can be profound and long lasting. As with adults, children are vulnerable to negative long-term psychological sequelae due to the experience and meaning of the trauma itself, including severity of injury and organ system involvement; the subsequent pain and suffering; the negative aspects of emergency and ongoing medical interventions and hospitalization; the rehabilitative demands of injuries; and any resulting disabilities. Unfortunately, the available research literature has seldom discriminated among these variables when reporting follow-up data on psychological or behavioral functioning in children who have been hospitalized. It has long been clearly established, however, that a significant number of children do experience psychological symptoms after leaving the hospital (Table 51–1), such as eating problems, sleep disturbances, enuresis, encopresis, regressive behavior in general, tics, depression, hyperactivity, anxiety, death fears and fantasies, withdrawal, somatic preoccupations, hysterical reactions, fear of all medical personnel, separation anxiety, increased aggression toward authority figures, speech defects, and nervousness.[2, 9, 23, 39, 47] These symptoms often last for months and occasionally for years. A follow-up study during the adolescence of children who had been hospitalized at a young age demonstrated continued deficits in academic skills, behavior problems, and juvenile delinquency. Frequency and duration of hospitalization before the age of 5 years was the most potent predictive variable of problems in adolescence.[9]

Both the child's and the family's mental health are affected by childhood trauma (Table 51–2). When a child's illness has been unexpected and life threatening, parents report feelings at follow up of loss of control, helplessness, lack of self-confidence with regard to decisions about their children, incomplete mourning reactions to the threatened loss of their child, and death fantasies.[2] If debility is chronic, family interaction patterns can be altered permanently, producing the "vulnerable child syndrome" in which the family centers its life around the previously ill child and is consistently overprotective of this child at the expense of other members of the family.[16]

In light of these data on psychological morbidity, it is surprising that only modest efforts at psychological intervention and research have followed. Improvements in the psychological management of physical trauma and the

Table 51–1
Posthospital Psychological Sequelae in Children

Eating problems
Sleep disorders
Enuresis and encopresis
General regressive behavior
Tics and mannerisms
Depression
Hyperactivity
General anxiety
Separation anxiety
Death fears and fantasies
Fear of medical personnel
Inncreased aggression toward authority figures
Speech defects
Nervousness

Table 51–2
Posthospital Psychological Sequelae in Families

Loss of control
Pervasive feelings of helplessness
Lack of self-confidence regarding decisions about their children
Incomplete mourning reactions to the threatened loss of their child
Death fantasies

trauma treatment process should inevitably lead to improved outcome both mentally and physically, after discharge.

The psychology of childhood physical trauma is more complex than it is in the adult. The psychological adjustment to physical trauma must be understood in terms of the psychological processes elicited by the necessity of adjusting to injury and treatment. In addition, the child's emotional and cognitive development level and the child's family context, especially the nature of the child's relationship with the parents, are central factors. This chapter presents a synopsis of theory and empirical data pertaining to those factors most relevant in reducing the negative consequences of trauma and its treatment.

WHY CHILDREN ARE PARTICULARLY VULNERABLE

Healthy psychological development requires a milieu of relative safety, allowing the child to acquire a basic trust in the adequacy of the physical and social environment to meet his or her needs for survival. This acquisition of basic trust is the foundation of the child's ability to relax and concentrate efforts on the development of higher order skills and psychological functions. Children are more vulnerable psychologically than their adult counterparts because they are more instrumentally and emotionally dependent for their survival on an adult world over which they exercise relatively little control and about the workings of which they comprehend very little. This relative lack of competence in comparison with that of adults requires continual protection and nurturing by committed caregivers for optimal physical and psychological development, without which the child would be crippled by overwhelming fear and anxiety.

The occurrence of trauma constitutes a major breakdown in the protective and nurturing environment so necessary for ongoing psychological development and maturation; trauma constitutes an injury to the child's psychological and physical sense of self. Whether the negative psychological impact of this injury is profound and chronically debilitating depends on many factors, a number of which are under the control of the medical professions. The primary thrust of intervention must be toward returning the child to a psychological state in which he or she feels nurtured, protected, and safe and as free from injury-related anxiety as possible.

UNIVERSAL STRESSORS ASSOCIATED WITH TRAUMA

The occurrence of injury is psychologically stressful owing to the magnification of life-preserving instincts and associated pain, triggering shock, denial, fear, and anger. Injury always constitutes a narcissistic insult to the self, bringing home with full force one's vulnerability and lack of omnipotence. Because it is associated with debility, whether due to pain or to restriction and impairment of function of the affected organ or organs, the narcissistic insult is ongoing past the point of initial injury. In accidental injury, the need to live in a relatively predictable environment is unmet. In nonaccidental injury, as in child abuse or a suicide attempt, the stress of the injury is compounded by issues of rage, disrupted family relationships, distrust, anxiety, extreme depression, and poor self-concept.

Change is stressful. In the classic Holmes and Rahe study of sources of stress leading to later illness, major personal injury or illness ranked number six out of a possible 43 major life events as requiring major social readjustment.[18] The disruption in daily functioning and family routine compounded by the necessity of engaging in special activities, such as hospital visitation and medical intervention, and spending time and money to repair the damage done creates potentially traumatizing stress. Fear of the unknown; of loss of control; of dependence on potentially incompetent, uncaring, or unreliable caregivers; and of permanent disfigurement, disability, or death are all experienced to some degree by the victim of injury and the injured party's family and friends.

The all too universal human need to attribute blame aggravates an already bad situation in that both parents and children tend to blame themselves, each other, health care professionals, outside parties involved in the accident, God, society, or any other available target for anger. Although this blame may be temporarily therapeutic, it can interfere with appropriate health promoting behaviors and adequate resolution of the traumatic incident.

PHYSICAL TRAUMA AND PSYCHOLOGICAL TRAUMA

There is no one-to-one correspondence between physical trauma and psychological trauma. The psychological impact of any injury depends on the individual's ability to cope with, work through, and eventually recover from the painful and negative aspects of the traumatic event. Therefore, there is an important interaction between the patient's abilities and skills and the nature and meaning of the injury to that patient, including the meaning of the ensuing medical and social interventions. Even the experience of pain itself appears to be dependent on the individual's coping mechanisms and cognitions regarding that pain rather than simply on the extent of injury.[30]

When any stressful event occurs, there are two possible outcomes, one positive and one negative. When an individual—child or adult—is able to master or cope with a stressful, challenging event successfully, psychological growth results and benefit accrues. However, when an individual's emotional and cognitive abilities are such that the stressful event cannot be mastered adequately, whether emotionally, cognitively, physically, or socially, psychological trauma ensues and the individual becomes relatively debilitated by the "traumatic" experience. Whether a child or adolescent is traumatized psychologically by a physical injury depends on an interaction among the coping abilities and competencies that the individual brings to the injuring event; the severity and quality of the injury itself; and the assistance and support the individual receives from the caregiving environment, primarily family and health care professionals, in managing the stresses of the injury and treatment. All intentional injuries, whether child abuse, suicide, or peer assault, are psychologically damaging.

PRINCIPLES OF PSYCHOLOGICAL MANAGEMENT DURING PHASES OF TRAUMA

To prevent or reduce the negative psychological impact of trauma, it is important to integrate an assessment of all of these areas with an eye toward intervening to build up areas of deficit and increase areas of strength, whether in the child's coping skills and competencies, in the family's support abilities, or in reducing the stress of the injury itself. The following principles are important:

1. Interventions, just as in physical and medical management, should begin early and continue throughout the process of recovery rather than late during the child's hospital stay, after the child evidences the aftereffects of psychological trauma.

2. The family is also the patient; the child's ability to cope will indirectly reflect the family's ability. When parents are anxious, distressed, and poorly functioning, the child's experience is much more traumatic.

3. Parents should be counseled after emergency care about expected needs and changes in their child's behavior; parents and nurses should encourage the appropriate expression of negative feelings by the patient.

4. A team approach in which psychological supportive interventions are based on a rational assessment of the child's and the family's needs and coordinated among the various staff is usually the most effective approach and requires a designated team leader to ensure this coordination.

5. To achieve this, the groundwork must be laid well before the assessment and intervention is needed by a particular child through staff education and procedural planning. The usual emergency nature of trauma makes prior training and planning essential so that these ameliorative interventions are a matter of routine and are integrated into the ongoing plan of medical management.

Psychological Developmental Overview

Phases in the trauma treatment process hold their own unique psychological stresses and, therefore, require their own interventions. In parallel fashion, developmental phases throughout childhood and adolescence likewise are associated with their own unique psychological tasks, qualities of cognitive functioning, emotional needs, and predominant fears and vulnerabilities. It is the interplay of the child's developmental level and the phase of trauma and its treatment that makes psychological management so complex. Thus, to understand the basis for psychological management during the phases of trauma management, it is important to first review the general principles of emotional and cognitive functioning at various age levels, important developmental tasks at these ages, and health-related issues. The psychological meaning of an injury changes with age, as does the child's ability to understand and work through the psychological issues involved. Table 51–3 presents a developmental schema based upon Jean Piaget's hallmark research findings on the development of cognitive functions in children and Eric Erickson's developmental schema of emotional and general psychological development, combined with a synopsis of health-related concerns.[11, 37, 38]

Infancy

The period from birth to 1 year is characterized by the basic developmental psychological task of establishing what Er-

ickson terms "basic trust."[11] This important psychological task forms the basis for all later development and is related to drive and to hope in life. Basic trust is formed out of interactions with the world that are positive, nurturing, and comforting and are related to "good enough" mothering. Negative, depriving, frustrating, and painful states or encounters lay the basis for basic mistrust. The greatest fear associated with this period is a profound and primitive one: the fear of loss of self and annihilation. Because the infant gradually gains the ability to attach to its mother, distinguish self from mother, and discriminate mother from strangers, this period is also characterized by an intense need for and closeness (symbiosis) to the mother and a concomitant distress when separated from her. Stranger anxiety also appears during this period.

Trauma Issues. Trauma experienced during infancy is especially problematic owing to the negative impact of pain on the establishment of basic trust in a safe, positive world; the separation from mother that may be necessitated by treatment; the necessary interaction with strangers in the caregiving role (e.g., physicians and nurses); and the disruption of cognitive and emotional development due to the debilitating effects of injury and treatment. If the infant is physically immobilized or restricted or if the infant becomes highly anxious owing to separation, stranger anxiety,

Table 51–3
Developmental Approach to Children's Health Care*

Age Level	Chronologic Age	Piagetian Cognitive Level	Ericksonian Psychological Tasks	Greatest Psychological Fears	Health-Related Issues
Infancy	Birth–1.5 year	Sensorimotor Magical thinking	Basic trust Basic mistrust Establishment of drive and hope	Loss of self Separation anxiety Stranger anxiety	Motor restriction Developmental delays Painful world view Separation anxiety Stranger anxiety Perceptual instability and confusion
Toddler	1.5 yr–2.5 yr	Sensorimotor Magical thinking Prelogical and egocentric	Autonomy and shame and doubt Establishment of self-control and willpower	Loss of love and approval Fear of punishment, abandonment Loss of control	Motor restriction Loss of control of bodily function Regression Abandonment Punishment Painful world view
Preschool	2.5 yr–6.5 yr	Preoperational Magical thinking Prelogical and egocentric	Initiative and guilt Establishment of direction and purpose	Humiliation Debilitation and mutilation Regression	Purpose of procedures distorted Hospitalizations and injury as punishment Loneliness Fear of regression
Schoolage	6.5 yr–12 yr	Concrete Operational	Industry and inferiority	Failure and rejection	Academic achievement Social acceptance Need for peers Need for social play Worry about failure and rejection Death anxiety Surrogate parents more satisfying
Adolescence	12 yr–18 + yr	Formal Operational	Identity and role confusion	Reiteration of all	Disfigurement Death anxiety Importance of peer group Need for privacy Self-consciousness

or disruption in the maternal-infant bond associated with the trauma, exploration of objects in the environment, repetitive psychomotor activities, and the subsequent elaboration of mental representations through mental processes of assimilation and accommodation may become extremely limited. Intellectual, motor, and emotional development suffer. Research investigations have demonstrated that disruptions in infant-mother attachment often lead to infant withdrawal, apathy, and "anaclitic depression."[4, 5, 44, 45] Failure to thrive or less extreme developmental delays may result in maternal separation or deprivation if extended.

Management. If separation has occurred, the older infant is likely to protest by crying and screaming for its mother, to refuse consolation from others, and to continue this behavior for hours or days to the point of exhaustion if the mother is not returned. Separation occurs most frequently in automobile accidents in which the mother and other family members are also injured. After the first stage of protest, the infant enters a state of despair in which withdrawal ensues, characterized by a disinterest in play, food, and others and a depressive-like apathy. The final stage is detachment and denial, in which the infant becomes livelier and evidences greater interest in its surroundings, a period often mistaken as a return to "normalcy."[49] Over the short run, there is no substitution for the infant's mother, although primary nursing helps. Co-rooming with mother in the hospital greatly assists the infant's return to good behavior and reduces the harmful psychological sequelae. If impossible, having another family member room in is recommended. Transitional objects should accompany the infant, such as blankets, pillows, stuffed animals. Tone of voice and physical contact comfort are important in soothing and comforting the infant.

Infants need stimulation and are especially responsive to visual cues. Mobiles on cribs for the younger infant and brightly colored, age-appropriate toys for the older infant to view and manipulate are important. Because bodily exploration is also important during this period in establishing an internalized body schema, the infant makes attempts to view hands and feet. Injuries requiring immobilization interfere with this development of internalized body schema. Physical rehabilitation, that is, infant stimulations, should make use of those body parts available for the infant to explore and encourage this activity; when possible, orthopedic interventions should be made with these infant needs taken into consideration. Little self-control has been established in this age group so that the mother's or a family member's assistance in restraining the infant during procedures is important and makes procedures less frightening and, therefore, less painful and psychologically traumatic.

The Toddler Period

The transition from infancy to toddlerhood occurs from approximately 1.5 to 2.5 years. During this period cognitive functioning is characterized by prelogical, magical thinking and is still based on sensorimotor functions. Language is gradually becoming part of the thought process, with comprehension of receptive language outdistancing language expression. The toddler lives in an egocentric world bearing little resemblance to that of the adult. It is during this period

that the need to establish one's self as separate from others is at its height. This period embraces most of the "terrible twos" where "no" becomes the child's favorite response. Toddlers feel omnipotent, and their ability to move about leads to an increasingly independent exploration of newly emerging abilities and of the environment. This period, therefore, is especially high risk for accidents: falls, ingestions, electric shocks, and the like.

Just as the toddler is enjoying newfound independence, the mother begins in earnest to make necessary demands on her child for obedience and inhibition of impulses. Toilet training usually begins during this period. What follows is a struggle for autonomy on the part of the child and a struggle for safety and socialization on the part of the parent. This inevitable struggle results in the fear of loss of parental love and approval if obedience and inhibition of impulses are not forthcoming. It is through the mother's prohibitions and the child's compliance and noncompliance with them that self-control and willpower are established. Loss of control and disobedience lead to experiences of shame and doubt. Potent fears of punishment, abandonment, and loss of control are also established during this period.

Trauma Issues. Trauma during the toddler years may be experienced as loss of love and punishment for disobedience. Health-related issues also revolve around pain, separation, and physical limitations, but the impact of these issues is different from those in infancy. Although separation anxiety is not as intense, it is still an issue, experienced as fear of abandonment. Because the child can now understand that what disappears can return and can verbalize needs, the toddler will communicate goal-directed wishes for the return of a parent and for greater mobility. The child's continued prelogical, limited understanding of events and vivid imagination may result in significant distortions surrounding the injury, its cause, and the treatment process. The child's willful noncompliance and experimentation may have led to the accident so that the child may be inhibited in future necessary exploration and exercise of abilities, regressing to a clinging, insecure attachment to the mother. It is also possible in this age group that the injury and subsequent pain may become associated nonrationally with a host of irrelevant, incidental cues that later induce anxiety and regressive behavior in the toddler. The child's invariable loss of control and autonomy during the trauma management process also frequently results not only in regressive behaviors, as in loss of previously acquired bladder control or demands to be fed, but also in demanding behavior toward parents and health care personnel as a way of substituting autonomous mobility with social control of others.

Management. Toddlers need the continued presence of their parent or parents, physical comforting, and firm but modulated limit setting (i.e. disciplining), because oppositional behavior and negativism are common reactions. Children at this age are little ready to be reasoned with and should not be expected to control behaviors based on rational explanation, although simple reasons for limit setting and commands should be given when possible. Parents hesitant to discipline their injured child should be encouraged to do so as long as limits are not too strictly set.

Toddlers should be given as much mobility as their injuries allow and as many choices within circumscribed limits as can be permitted ("Would you rather hold your blanket or your bear while the doctor listens to your heart?"). Caution must be exercised even when parents are present that the child's tendency to explore does not lead to compromise of treatment or further accidental injury. Two year olds have been known to climb out of bed and roam the ward while parents are asleep in the child's room. Even the most alert nursing staff may be otherwise occupied at these times. If immobility is important, as in head or orthopedic trauma, restraints are often necessary but should be avoided when possible. Transitional objects such as favorite blankets and toys can be comforting, especially when parents must be absent.

Toddlers and preschoolers thrive on routine; if hospital staff and parents can provide it, the child benefits. Part of established routine in the toddler may be certain rituals, often established around meals, baths, and bedtimes. These should be followed as much as possible. Parents should be encouraged to remain involved with their child and provide as much of the caregiving as is possible after initial phases of treatment. Parents should also be counseled about the normality of angry, oppositional, and clinging, repressive behaviors. Primary nursing in which consistency of nursing personnel is provided is optimal so that the nurse becomes a source of security and can be familiarized with the child's special qualities, rituals, and the like. Children at this age are especially sensitive to the anxiety and distress communicated by family and caregivers and may also distort and personalize the reasons for the distress. Efforts should be made to communicate support and concern and to minimize demonstrations of negative affect.

Because intrusive procedures, whether painful or not, are especially anxiety provoking at this age, it is important to approach the child gradually and gently when not in emergency situations. Allowing the child to sit on the mother's lap, having the mother assist with the examination or distract the toddler during procedures, and playing with the child when feasible around the examination or procedure often helps quell some of the child's fears and tendency to physically resist. If parents cannot tolerate active involvement at the time of painful procedures, they should be close at hand to console the child after the intervention. Many of the preparatory procedures used in older age groups are relatively ineffective in the toddler.

The Preschool Child

The preschool period from ages of approximately 2.5 to 6.5 years is characterized by a lively exuberance, growing socialization, cooperation, and peer interaction, vivid imagination, and preoperational thinking sometimes termed "magical thinking."[12, 37] Thinking, which is housed firmly in language, continues to be prelogical and egocentric and yet more realistic than previously. Emotionally, the child is now concerned with both parents and is identifying increasingly with the same-sexed parent in role appropriate behaviors. Modeling behavior, begun in the prior period, is supplemented at an increasing rate by language-mediated learning. Social skills are acquired at a rapid rate. Behavior

appears more goal directed as the child plans more and is more "attacking" in undertaking tasks, a quality that Erickson calls "initiative."[11] The child takes pleasure in attack and conquest and in acts of aggressive manipulation. Children during this period often appear boastful and exaggerate their aggressive abilities.

The preschool child is increasingly guided by internalized parental values, prohibitions, and reality limitations that are conceptualized as the child's conscience or superego. He or she is increasingly able to delay, channel, and guide impulses into complex behavior; instantaneous gratification is no longer the order of the day. The greatest fear associated with this developmental period is the fear of social humiliation and, secondarily, the fears of debilitation, mutilation, and regression to former states of dependency. It is at this age that the child first becomes aware of death although without understanding its permanence, irreversibility, or universality.

Trauma Issues. The preschool child, although a bit more realistic and able to communicate, still lacks the reasoning capacity of the school-aged child. Thinking is magical and personalized, making the reasoning about health and illness prelogical. For example, this age group has been reported to believe in the occurrence of illness as punishment.[3, 34] Thinking about the accident may be distorted by incidental associations to which the child attributes cause and effect. For example, a child who was angry at a sibling may feel punished by an accident that occurs shortly thereafter. Responsibility for the accident may be exaggerated and associated in illogical ways with the pain of trauma and ensuing treatment. The child may consider the pain of treatment as deliberately imposed because of minor misbehavior the day of the accident. The child's ability to reason may seem deceptively adequate due to the modeling of adult language usage; the adult may not ascertain without careful exploration that the child does not use or understand conceptual words such as "because" in the same ways that older children and adults do.[38] Therefore, children may appear to understand explanations of medical procedures or directions given when they do not.

Even at this stage, behavior is still often insufficiently under the control of cognition. Even when children do understand the reasons for certain prohibitions or for medical procedures, they are often unable and unwilling to cooperate owing to the overwhelming nature of their fears and anxieties. The intense fear of debilitation and mutilation that appears at this age makes the occurrence of trauma and its treatment much more painful. Another characteristic of the preschool-aged child's thinking is animism, that is, the child geocentrically attributes human feelings, thoughts, and motivations to inanimate objects. This tendency may increase fear of medical equipment especially when the child projects anger, generated by the pain and scariness of the treatment situation, onto the world at large. Radiographic equipment may be seen as diabolical and mutilating.

Management. Because these children do have an increased capacity to reason and plan, explanations for interventions and information about injuries are important to counteract the child's tendency to imagine the worst. Explanations must be simple, short, and concrete. The child should be asked to repeat or explain what she or he understands. The child's fears about permanent debilitation and mutilation should be dealt with by providing direct reassurance of recovery when valid and, when possible, an estimate of time needed for such. Children may need time to adjust to the sight of an injury and can be encouraged to refer to "it" or "that leg" as though foreign, allowing time for psychological adjustment once bandages are removed.

Children have difficulty estimating time at this age so that time estimates should be presented concretely whenever possible through use of a calendar on which the days are marked off; for shorter time intervals, major events of the day may be given as markers, for example, "You'll be able to go in the wheelchair to the playroom after lunch." Children during this period often misunderstand the meaning of words and take things literally. Attempts at minor surgery may be seen as potentially castrating events in which the injured foot or hand is being amputated. Open-ended questions about the child's fears by parents and care providers can often lead to the discovery of important misunderstandings and distortions that can be addressed through the provision of better information, reassurance, empathy with the child's concerns, and directed educational play.

Children during this period usually have more control of their behavior in the face of pain than toddlers but still tend to become aggressive or withdrawn. When children cannot control their behavior because of pain or anxiety, direct suggestion that they will soon be able to relax and control themselves can be effective if the atmosphere surrounding them remains relatively calm and the intervention is made soon enough. Limit setting is often helpful if done in a nonhostile, nonpunitive manner. Anger by staff or family only serves to increase the fear and resistance. Children also fear regression, which is a reality at this age. In response to the stress, children lose their newly captured maturity and exhibit clinging and whining behaviors and loss of control. They should not be humiliated by pointing out the "babyish" nature of this regression but rather should be supported in regaining control through lowering stress and increasing their understanding of the situation and the time involved for intervention, when the pain will get better, and ultimate outcome (e.g., "Your pain will start easing up in about ten minutes; we're going to make your arm fine again.").

The School-Aged Child

The school-aged period, from approximately 6.5 years to 12 years, encompasses a broad span often termed *latency* because the child becomes primarily involved in issues of "industry" and the "entrance into life," which first takes place at school.[11] The child is now more capable of logical reasoning and has a better grasp of concepts that express relationships, such as "because," which allows greater and more accurate incorporation of information about injury, illness, and its causes. Cognition during this period is still, however, tied to perception and termed by Piaget *concrete operational*.[37] This is the period in which the child learns to win admiration and recognition from parent surrogates in the form of teachers and from peers, especially same-sexed peers, by producing things, such as good academic work, entertaining behaviors, or good athletic performance. It is during this period that sustained attention and diligence lead to internalization of the work ethic, and the child becomes ready to handle the tools, weapons, and technology of the adult world. Socially, the child learns to work alongside others cooperatively so that teamwork begins. If the child is hindered in the ability to rudimentarily master these tools and become a productive member of a "team," whether in the classroom, neighborhood group, or athletic team, the child is in danger of developing an inordinate sense of inferiority and inadequacy. The school-aged child greatly fears failure in productivity and rejection by the social group and parent surrogates.

Trauma Issues. It is during this period that children are able to gradually conceptualize the meaning and permanence of death and that children develop anxieties about their own deaths. Yet, they do not usually ask direct questions or express these concerns, probably owing to the greater, overriding fear of debilitation and further pain. The school-aged child appears to be most affected by anything that hinders the ability to produce and take a place alongside same-sexed peers in work and social ventures. Thus, the necessity of removal from the classroom and social unit brings about realistic and fantasied loss of place, belonging, and the feeling of and fear of growing inferiority and inadequacy. Children worry about the permanence of injury and loss of ability that may result. Peer group rejection is an ongoing fear when scarring, disfigurement, or decreased skills result. Separation from parents is still an issue at this age, but there is a greater ability to rely on surrogate parents, such as teachers, nurses, or child life workers. The peer group is much more important, and there is a high need for continued social play during treatment and recovery phases.

Management. Children are much better able to utilize information for behavioral self-control and management of anxiety and pain during this period, especially at the upper end of this period from ages 10 to 12 years. Explanations can be more extensive, although they should be kept in simple language. Unfortunately for medical staff, children have relatively little prior information about their bodies, illness, or health care personnel. A study of 100 school children, aged 6 to 12, conducted through the University of Tennessee Medical Center at Knoxville revealed that children's understanding of their bodies does parallel cognitive development. Questions about internal organ function revealed that only 50% were correct in what the heart and lungs did, and only 5% of the group knew what heart, lungs, kidneys, and brain did. It would appear that the educational system is not laying even rudimentary groundwork for medical explanations to children in these age groups.[26] Pain control techniques are generally more effective in this age group because the child is able to cooperate in them.

For extended hospital stay, it is essential that school-aged children continue their school studies for two reasons: (1) to continue the acquisition of academic skills, and, just as important, (2) to "renormalize" life as much as possible and allow the child the sense of continued belonging to the productive peer group. Likewise, social play is important and should be promoted, through interhospital unit contacts or flexible visitation from school and neighborhood friends. As with younger children, family support and comforting is important, as is sensitive disciplinary limit setting. Preparatory play therapy techniques can be quite effective in reducing fear of painful or threatening medical procedures, whether a computed tomography scan, a lumbar puncture, or surgery.

Although some regression in the face of stress and loss of control inherent in medical treatment is inevitable, the school-aged child has a somewhat greater reserve of coping skills in place and can acquire even more with intervention. Familiar objects brought from home can be helpful. Frequent telephone contacts with peers also increase support and reduce stress. Food preferences should be honored whenever possible, especially since the loss of appetite is a common reaction to illness and to stress. A frequent complaint of most school-aged children about hospital stay is the food. Children especially need company during meals, so parents should be encouraged to stay at mealtime and also to bring favorite foods for sharing from home; consultation with the nutritionist for this home-hospital food planning is recommended.

The Adolescent

It is finally with the onset of puberty that the transition from child to adult thinking takes place. Logical, symbolic, formal operational thought is acquired from ages 12 to 15 years and represents the culmination of human reasoning. This rather rapid acquisition of the ability to reason abstractly and in adult fashion and the enormous physical and sexual changes of puberty are responsible for what has been commonly thought of as the turmoil of the adolescent years. It is fortunate that most teenagers handle these profound changes quite well. Adolescence is also the period in which individual, adultlike identity is stabilized as the child becomes further psychologically and socially differentiated from the family in preparation for the adoption of a career and independent living. In some ways, all previous psychological issues are reiterated during this period and integrated into the adolescent identity. The adolescent must struggle to master his newly reawakened impulses and drives, especially sexual, and begin forming heterosexual love relationships. Adolescents become less concerned with what they feel they are themselves and more preoccupied with how they appear to be in the eyes of others. Thus, this is a time in which the peer group is all important, and there is much mutual sharing of perceptions. As Erickson stated:

In their search for a new sense of continuity and sameness, adolescents have to re-fight many of the battles of earlier years, even though to do so they must artificially appoint perfectly well-meaning people to play the roles of adversaries. . . .[11]

Trauma Issues. The "perfectly well-meaning people to play the roles of adversaries" are often the members of the trauma management team and associated hospital staff. Adolescents are exquisitely sensitive to issues of autonomy, privacy, and body image. The occurrence of trauma and its treatment insults these areas of sensitivity in that the adolescent is required to forego his or her newfound increase in independence and allow adults to make decisions, intrude physically into body boundaries, and invade physical and psychological privacy. Young adolescents, who are particularly prone to deny physical vulnerability to the point of engaging in high-risk behaviors, may deny the impact of trauma and actively resist medical intervention. The concern with how others see one and the newly acquired sexual maturity naturally leads to self-consciousness and makes physical exposure to strangers, especially of the opposite sex, excruciating. The fear of disfigurement because of the need to be like everyone else, that is, normal, is great, as is the fear of death when it is not deniable. The adolescent tends to vocalize concerns about the immediate future with regard to both.

Management. Because adolescents are humiliated when treated like children, every effort should be made to address the adolescent's adult reasoning capacity while also recognizing his or her childlike emotional needs for reassurance, comforting, and the physical presence of friends or family members. Adolescents, like adults, need information in appropriate digestible doses concerning extent of injury, interventions to be made, and probable outcomes. Even though consent for intervention must be obtained from parents in nonemergency situations, the adolescent needs to be included in the consent process for intervention. Every attempt should be made to respect the adolescent's need for privacy and physical integrity. Draping whenever possible is important and doors to public areas should not be left open. Well-meant joking for tension release among the staff may easily be misconstrued by the adolescent patient and should be avoided.

When hospitalization is necessary, every attempt should be made to place the adolescent patient within easy proximity of other adolescents. The older adolescent may feel more comfortable on an adult unit. Rebelliousness should be understood by staff and families as related to the need for independence. Interventions with adolescent patients should emphasize vocalizing the adolescent's concerns and needs while setting firm limits with reasons attached. Asking the adolescent patient to help and enlisting the adolescent's cooperation as a patient-colleague is usually a very effective approach because the adolescent's tendency to idealize and act altruistically can be brought to bear on his or her ability to help the staff do their jobs. In so doing, an unnecessary power struggle can be averted. Unfortunately for the busy medical staff, there is no substitute for time spent physically present with the adolescent in building up an alliance. When circumstances have made this impossible because of the emergency nature of the situation or demands on staff time, then enlisting the assistance of someone who already has an alliance with the teenager may be essential, for example, a friend or family member. Families need information so that they may prepare the adolescent for interventions and enlist cooperation, but the adolescent should be included and consulted about information dispersal owing to privacy and autonomy needs.

PHASES OF TRAUMA INTERVENTION

Psychological Processes in Response to Injury

The psychological response to physical trauma has been likened by a number of researchers to "shell shock," more recently reconceptualized as "posttraumatic stress syndrome" in which the subject experiences emotional dissociation or numbing, feelings of derealization and depersonalization, ideational avoidance, or denial with episodic breakthroughs of vivid, emotional memories, intrusive and unwelcome thoughts, and disturbing dreams.[8, 19, 24] The stage of denial is associated with poor cognitive functioning, selective inattention, amnesia, decrease in reality testing, and either frantic overactivity or withdrawal. Intrusion states are characterized by ruminations, repetitions, cognitive confusion and disorganization, inability to concentrate owing to preoccupations, and hypervigilance and arousal.[19] These processes are elicited in both the victim of injury and in the injured's family when the injury is serious; victim and family alternate between these two states and, it is hoped, can be assisted in working through the psychological trauma by medical staff. Failure to recognize these states leads to much misunderstanding by the medical management team members when dealing with children and their families until normal functioning is reacquired. The length of time needed for this process is highly individual. Nevertheless, the early phases of physical trauma are most certainly characterized by them.

Phase One: The Injuring Event and Transport

Depending on the degree of central nervous system involvement, the most typical initial responses to the injuring event are fear and shock, an adaptive mechanism based on the primitive need to fight or flee the scene of danger. This serves as a pain-delaying or pain-reducing mechanism, allowing time for taking defensive action. Even individuals who are not injured, as in a family automobile accident, are usually in emotional shock. Accompanying symptomatology is often coldness, feelings of derealization as though in a dream, confusion, disorientation, poor memory, and an ensuing inability to exercise normal skills and judgment. Although the child's initial response to injury is likely to be alarm and help-seeking behavior, shock often follows. Multisystem injuries are, of course, more likely to result in these stress-related responses. Both physical and psychological insults create this cognitively debilitating condition in most cases of serious trauma.

Psychological intervention at the scene and during transport should consist of minimizing the ensuing alarm and confusion on the part of the child and, when present, the family. The child's reaction to injury is greatly influenced by the family's reaction. Thus, psychological management includes attempts to reassure and calm the distressed family, secondary to those interventions necessary for medical management, so that the family can help intervene to calm the child. Communication to the child must be simple, direct, and redundant. If a parent or other family member is on the scene and is able, then the family member should be kept in close proximity to the child or adolescent. The family member should be encouraged to reassure and to help distract the child from the injury during transport, setting limits gently but firmly. As medical interventions are made at the scene that are necessary for life saving and transport, a running commentary in the simplest language

possible of what is being done and how it will help is reassuring to all. It is at the initial stages of trauma that children and family need information the most; this information is usually not retained but has a calming effect and allows the child and parent to regain greater cognitive control of emotions and behavior. Parents need information so that they can intervene with their child.

It is important for transport personnel to remember that neither children nor families are "themselves" at these times of catastrophic stress. They are likely to be dazed or hysterical and cannot be expected to react in rational ways owing to the alarm experienced. Especially in the presence of a clouded sensorium, the child or adolescent may become aggressive as a result of pain and fear. High emotion, especially hostility and panic, can be contagious and should be guarded against; emergency staff who can quickly acknowledge the child and family's distress in a calm and controlled manner and then go on to tell the child and family what is being done and will be done are the most effective interveners. When physical restraint is necessary, it should be administered with accompanying direct messages about needed compliance and why it is being done. Good intentions and rationales for interventions that staff members think are obvious and that, indeed, might be obvious to children or parents during normal circumstances will not be obvious during times of high stress. Therefore, stating the obvious is often helpful.

If family members are interfering with medical treatment or are further stressing the child, direct messages about what the family member should do differently and why are most helpful. Criticism should be avoided. Asking the parent, for example, to hold the child's hand and stroke the child's forehead while in transport may be comforting to both parent and child.

The older infant, toddler, and preschool-aged child most desperately require the presence of a parent at the scene and during transport. Pain is heightened by anxiety and fear so that unnecessary separations compound the stress on the physiologic systems. Children at these young ages have little information about the world at large and reason illogically. They are easily overwhelmed by the emergency situation, which may evoke fantasies of annihilation and bodily mutilation related to the medical personnel and medical interventions (see Table 51–3). Telling children of this age, or having a parent tell a child, that the procedures are being done to make them well helps, but they cannot help but be skeptical when the pain is increased. The instinctive flight from pain, especially in the presence of neurologic insult, overwhelms the child; children of this age should not be expected to exercise the cognitive control over their own behavior that older children have. Parental or staff punishment and anger rarely assist the child in gaining control and may make the fearful fantasies and ensuing resistance even worse. It is better to physically and verbally reassure the child, using physical restraint only when absolutely necessary.

Phase Two: The Emergency Department—Emergency Surgery

A unique exploratory study of pediatric trauma center interactions among children, their parents, and management staff found that the predominant behaviors exhibited by children in the emergency department are protest and withdrawal.[15] Protest behaviors consist of kicking, crying, and resisting the procedures in general. Younger children exhibited this type of response significantly more frequently than did older children. Withdrawing behaviors consisted of reticence and lack of eye contact and were exhibited equally by all age groups.

Age was also an important variable in the area of delaying tactics by children. School-aged children tended to attempt to stall treatment by asking for irrelevant materials, such as toys or water. Gender differences were not found; boys and girls protest and withdraw in response to emergency treatment at equal rates. Verbalization of fears was found significantly more frequently in preschool and school-aged children, whereas preteens tended not to give evidence of these fears. Preteens expressed significantly more concern about the immediate future. This study provides empirical confirmation of increased cognitive control over behavior in emergency situations with increasing age.

The behavior of parents was also interesting. Again, age of child was a principal determinant of parental response to the emergency department situation. Parents were more caretaking and responsible toward the younger child, feeling guilty and verbalizing self-blame for the child's injury. The older child seemed to elicit verbalizations pertaining to the child's own responsibility for the injury. More than half (54%) of all parents gave a guilt-inducing or punishing-type message to their child; 67% of the school-aged child's parents and 69% of the preteen's parents did so. Of concern is the finding that although 93% of parents displayed concern and affection for their preschool child and 56% of parents did the same toward their school-aged child, only 13% of the preteens' parents evidenced this concern or affection. Surprisingly, there were no differences in this affectionate, comforting behavior. Thus, it appears that parents respond to the need for greater comfort and support in the preschool child, blaming themselves for the injuries incurred. However, parents tend to punish or blame the school-aged child, both in terms of the responsibility for the injury itself and for any uncooperative behavior in the emergency department.

The lack of comforting or affection evidenced toward the preteen is of concern. Although one explanation might lie in the greater independence and potential embarrassment of the preteen if the parent were comforting, the occurrence of trauma and its management should be a time when this behavior is sanctioned because it is definitely needed by the older child. Parents should be encouraged to provide this when they do not; trauma center staff should be on the alert for this lack of support and provide as much of it as possible when the parents do not, modeling for parents by doing so.

Even more alarming findings resulted from a study by Roskies and colleagues in which they compared the stress of emergency pediatric admissions to that of elective admissions.[42] Given that children undergoing emergency admissions were sicker than those undergoing elective admissions, they underwent significantly more painful and more frequent medical procedures. The child in emergency encountered almost twice as many "white-robed strangers"

and underwent many more changes of physical location than the child in the nonemergency situation. This study found that children in emergency received much less support from those in the environment than the children in nonemergency admissions. Separation from parents tended to occur much earlier in the child's hospital experience, for many children less than 3 hours after hospital arrival. Even when the mother was present, the child derived less comfort from her presence. Although mother-child interactions in the elective group were evenly distributed among positive, neutral, and negative interchanges, only 15% of the mother-child interactions in the emergency group were positive; 85% were neutral or negative.

These findings point out that emergency situations are more stressful to the child and that even resources that could support the child's coping abilities are negatively altered, that is, the family's supportive function. In a fascinating analysis of the role of parents in hospital, these investigators observed that there appears to be an abrogation of the parental role, neither a caregiver nor a protector but rather a passive information-giver to the child and an instrument for making the child more compliant with hospital routine and more acceptable to nurses. They state, "The parent seemed to share the child's view of the hospital as a terrifying monster and his sense of helplessness in relation to it."

Children were little prepared for the painful procedures they underwent or for the emergency surgeries. The parents were little able to serve as models of coping ability for their children, feeling out of control and inadequate in the situation. Thus, although there is some necessity for parents to move aside and allow the emergency medical staff to take control, research observations confirm that too many parents give up too much of their caregiving function, which leads to negative psychological developments in the child and in the family. Just as the family should be encouraged to stay within close proximity to the child in the emergency department whenever feasible, family members should be given a caregiving role as soon as possible in the management process and as soon as the parent can handle it psychologically.

Even though there is pressure to perform emergency care in the most efficient manner possible, this care should also include psychological care. Both child and family should be given information about what is going to be done, how it will be done, and why it is being done and information about the duration of pain. If the mother is the designated person to support the child in the emergency department, this information should be given to her, and she should be encouraged to convey it to her child in a way that is comprehensible to the child.

If emergency surgery is necessary, prior psychological preparation is not really possible. However, it is important to inform the child of the pending move to the surgery area and to give the child some information regarding what to expect there, what is to be done, and why. The child should be reassured about the procedures and, when appropriate, informed of what the procedures feel like and how long they take. Older children should be told that they will wake up in the recovery room and whether the parent will be present.

Management of Painful Procedures

Pain is a psychological phenomenon. There is no one-to-one correspondence between tissue damage and the experience of pain.[7] The degree to which a given child experiences pain is determined not only by the nature and extent of the injury, but also by that child's emotional state, the meaning of the injury to the child, the fantasies activated by the injury, and the social context in which the injury has occurred. The word *pain* itself is derived from the Greek word meaning "punishment," and there is a primitive psychological link between the two in the mind of humans.

Unfortunately, significant evidence exists that pain is undertreated in hospital settings and that medical staff members have unrealistic fears regarding addiction.[10, 22, 28, 35, 48] A study by Schechter and Allen of physicians' attitudes toward pain in children found that pediatricians are more likely than surgeons or family practitioners to recognize that younger children have adultlike pain and to prescribe narcotics in their younger patients.[43] All physicians were more generous in endorsing analgesia usage outside of their own areas of clinical practice, for example, pediatricians for postsurgery and surgeons for lumbar punctures. The researchers concluded that it is both confusing and disturbing that concerned physicians continue to perform procedures in children without prescribing anesthesia or analgesia for which adults are automatically medicated.

Pain avoidance is a most basic behavioral principle. Whenever an injury occurs, the natural instinct is to avoid further manipulation of or injury to the area; it is a protective instinct. Treatment of injuries usually violates this most primitive instinct. Thus, it comes as no great surprise that young children protest and fight against medical personnel attempting to treat their wounds and react to them as though they were evil torturers and potential mutilators when the pain is increased.

Unfortunately, the necessity of speedy intervention and the fear generated by the injuring event tend to increase pain and might render psychological techniques that could easily reduce it ineffective. The reason for this statement is that effective psychological interventions to reduce pain consist of methods of distraction and suggestion, suggestion that is best accomplished when the patient is in a state of deep relaxation and concentration. Because the basic meaning of pain is danger-injury, its presence serves as a powerful signal to protective action, the antithesis of relaxation. Nevertheless, many opportunities are missed in emergency treatment for lessening the pain of children and adolescents and, thereby, lessening the long-term negative impact of trauma.

The principles of psychological pain management are straightforward and, of course, are somewhat dependent on the age of the child. Brown and associates studied the types of cognitions 8- to 16-year-old children reported in response to personal stressors including pain, both constructive "coping" cognitions and destructive "catastrophizing" cognitions.[6] As predicted, they found that coping strategies increased with age, older children using coping strategies more often and a more varied array. Strategies were positive self-talk (e.g., "I can take this; it's not so bad"), attention diversion (i.e., thinking about something else), relaxation, and thought stopping (i.e., blocking negative thoughts). Unfortunately, an alarming number of children of all ages were "catastrophizers," children who responded to pain by focusing attention on it and engaging in thoughts of avoidance, escape, and exaggerated negative fantasies of destructive outcome or intent from the caregiver (e.g., "Is this guy trying to kill me?"). Children who catastrophize, like adults, are more likely to feel greater pain and stress than children who can utilize cognitive coping strategies.

Cognitive coping strategies are attention diversion or distraction techniques, as is storytelling or focusing on something else in the room; positive self-talk, which consists of making positive and minimizing statements about the situation; negative thought blocking; and systematic relaxation. These coping techniques are best acquired before they are needed in a real-life situation.

Perhaps the most effective pain management technique is the most misunderstood: hypnosis. Hypnosis consists simply of an altered state of consciousness that combines focused attention and concentration with suggestion and mental imagery. It is often accomplished with the patient in a state of deep relaxation. It is probably so effective because it combines many coping strategies into one—positive thoughts, distractions, relaxation—and accomplishes negative thought blocking automatically. For many children and adolescents, suggestion under hypnosis can achieve pain blocking in which the subject is aware of the pain but no longer concerned by it. Hypnosis has been used effectively in a wide array of pediatric pain problems.[14, 17, 21, 50]

I have used hypnosis effectively to manage pain in burn patients before and after débridment to minimize discomfort during painful procedures such as the placement of a subclavian line, and to decrease fears prior to radiologic procedures such as magnetic resonance imaging. Studies have consistently demonstrated the efficacy of hypnosis for the management of pain in children, including reduction in the amount of pain medication required.

These pain management techniques, summarized in Table 51–4, can be applied in many emergency situations in which the child's life is not in imminent danger, in the intensive care unit, and in the general hospital unit. Distraction techniques, positive self-talk, and the like can be accomplished while medical procedures are being conducted if the person assisting the child can be given a few minutes alone with the child to explain what will happen and how to use these techniques before the child views the threatening equipment and before the painful procedures are initiated. Even hypnotic induction can be accomplished in as little as 15 minutes if the child is reasonably calm and can be continued during anesthesia administration or during a procedure. Unfortunately, it is difficult to predict which children will respond to hypnotic induction and which will not, but any effective means of alleviating pain decreases the long-term psychological sequelae of injury.

Phase Three: Pediatric Intensive Care Unit

If the child's injuries require hospitalization and placement in the pediatric intensive care unit, several additional stress-

Table 51–4
Pain Management Techniques

Toddler	Preschooler	School-Aged	Adolescent
Bubble blowing Pre- and postprocedural play Modeling	Pop-up books, story books Favorite stories Talking through	Distraction techniques Relaxation techniques Cognitive techniques: A. Thought-stopping B. Positive self-statements C. Emotive and pleasant scene imagery	Distraction techniques Relaxation techniques Cognitive techniques
Music distraction	Active play Hypnosis (4–5 year old) Behavioral Rehearsal	Biofeedback Hypnosis	Biofeedback Hypnosis

ors come into play. The child tends to be stressed by the continual level of noise in the unit, by the exotic nature and abundance of monitoring equipment, by the lack of privacy, by the limited visitation by family, and by the lack of cues available for orientation to day and time. Even the diurnal rhythm is disrupted; sleep deprivation is not uncommon. It is indeed difficult to separate the more severe pain and suffering associated with greater illness, a greater number of more painful procedures, and the unit-related issues.

Another complication occurs when children hear the suffering of others and conversations of medical staff about others or themselves. Children in subalert states may incorporate overheard remarks into nightmares, unbeknownst to staff. The first week after the injury, children often have nightmares related to working through the stress of the injury and emergency treatment. The psychological reaction to the pain of others is complicated by the ''misery loves company'' and ''glad it's not me'' reactions, which may be followed by guilt. Empathy with others in older children may increase anxiety and depression.

Here, as much attendance by the mother as possible, plus primary nursing, is helpful. Children should be given as many opportunities as possible to ventilate feelings as injuries and medical equipment allow. Parents need support in overcoming fear of ventilators, tubes, and the like in interacting with their child. Explanations of the equipment, the psychological preparation for procedures, and the use of pain-reducing techniques should begin at admission. Calendars, clocks, familiar toys, and family pictures are helpful to older children. Another phenomenon, which in adults is associated with ''intensive care unit psychosis'' is ''stimulus habituation,'' often termed *stimulus deprivation* in the medical literature. The sameness of a bland environment may lead to understimulation and possibly to compensatory hallucinatory phenomena. Some change in bed position or strategic placement of a mirror to take advantage of a new view may be helpful in avoiding this in addition to the other interventions mentioned.

When transfer must occur from the unit, children must also be prepared for this because of the dependency on and the trust of the medical staff that develops. Transfer, although representing increased recovery, also constitutes a loss of valuable relationships for the child. A visit from one of the general unit nurses may bridge the gap from the pediatric intensive care unit to the general unit. Children

who further recover away from the pediatric intensive care unit should be allowed and encouraged to return for a visit before leaving the hospital.

Phase Four: Prolonged Hospitalization—The General Unit

A survey of all long-term care pediatric hospitals in the United States demonstrated that 70% of hospitals offer a prehospital preparation program to reduce psychological trauma.[36] Unfortunately, emergency hospitalization offers little opportunity for such intervention. In addition, studies indicate that brief hospitalization, especially elective admissions, are not particularly psychologically traumatic to the child over the long run. However, prolonged hospitalization of more than a few days does result in the trauma described at the beginning of this chapter. Sources of these stressors have also been described for each developmental age level. It is at this stage that children and adolescents attempt to reverse the regression that has invariably occurred at earlier stages, and they may be perceived as troublemakers by staff. However, these attempts to exert control and independence are usually psychologically healthful developments if they are not too extreme.

The gradual realization of the impact of injury, perhaps begun in the pediatric intensive care unit, may lead not only to further anger but also to sadness and depression. Children should be encouraged to voice their feelings and should be provided as many opportunities as possible to make choices. The opportunities for formal intervention programs are probably greatest at this stage and can alleviate medical staff by providing creative outlets for emotional catharsis and self-assertion. For children having significant difficulties in working through their negative emotions toward acceptance of the injury and its sequelae, a pediatric psychologist or child psychiatrist may be of assistance in providing therapeutic services and consultation to staff.[40]

Recreational and ''occupational'' therapies also relieve boredom and anxiety in all children. A staff person designated for these activities is essential and is usually termed the *child life coordinator*. In addition, therapeutic play has been used effectively to prepare children for surgery and other therapeutic and diagnostic procedures. Realistic play equipment, dolls, puppets, films, coloring books, and play or discussion groups have been found effective in reducing anxiety and the resulting trauma of interventions.[31, 46] Modeling techniques, cognitive control, and more traditionally verbal therapeutic programs are also effective.[36, 41] The hospital pediatric psychologist, pediatric social worker, child life worker, and nursing staff can form an effective psychological intervention team in implementing these programs.

It is important to establish an area on the hospital unit where children are safe from interventions and can engage in play activities—the hospital playroom. Optimal designs for these are available in the psychological literature.[25, 33] Even for children who are bedridden, every attempt should be made to provide some stimulus change from week to week, even if it consists simply of moving the bed to a new position.

Of great concern during hospitalization to patients and families is the amount of contact and information received from the admitting physician and consultants. In a study by Freiberg, mothers gave as the reasons for their anxiety when their children were hospitalized that they were not given sufficient information about diagnosis and procedures and treatments.[13] Fears about procedures and treatments were given as the top reason for anxiety. It is difficult to quell one's fears, much less those of one's child, if ignorance reigns. The mind tends to fill an information vacuum with imagined facts, often negative. There is also evidence that lack of communication is one of the chief reasons for a majority of lawsuits. Patient education materials can supplement physician contact as a means of imparting helpful information but cannot substitute for personal contact and involvement.

Phase Five: Discharge and Beyond

By the time of discharge, strong relationships have often developed among medical staff, patients, and families. The loss represented by discharge should not be underestimated nor the new stress involved in the demands on child and family for a return to ''normal'' functioning. Although the relationship between the hospital and the patient and family may be an ambivalent one, loss of support and security is always experienced no matter how joyful the return to home. Therefore, follow-up during the next week or two is psychologically reassuring and also allows the physician an opportunity to check on problematic emotional reactions and life adjustment difficulties. The rehabilitation phase may be quite prolonged for multiple trauma patients, and the child's and family's hopes of a speedy return to their previous lifestyle and circumstances may be dashed on the rock of reality all too quickly. Anticipatory guidance at the time of discharge strengthens the family's ability to cope with the inevitable disappointment and depression that follow recognition of the long road to recovery. As much as rehabilitation and debility allow, it is essential that the family resume as much of its prior ''normal'' functioning as possible. Family therapy can be a potent tool in returning a traumatized family to healthier functioning and can begin well before discharge and continue after.

STAFF CONFLICTS

Treatment situations, especially when life is threatened, are often high pressure, high risk, and exciting and therefore are tension, anxiety, and fatigue inducing unless group cohesiveness, group skill, and group morale are high. Sources of staff conflict, especially between surgeon and nurse, are usually due to problems in interstaff administrative procedures, especially those affecting communication; poor communication skills among staff; professional role conflict; or inappropriate and unconscious displacement of personal emotional stress, frustrations, or expectations onto staff members. These problems are inherent in all workplaces but are especially debilitating in medical care facilities owing to the need for complex, coordinated, and timely service delivery in an overall atmosphere of perfect competence.

Nurses often feel like low-status, undervalued, and ignored members of the health care team, which makes the low pay level and the long hours particularly apt to induce resentment. Role conflict occurs most frequently when nurses are caught between the goal of quickly carrying out physician orders versus the goal of comforting and minimizing stress in child and family. Children, families, and nurses often form strong affectionate bonds so that families confide concerns and problems. Because nurses are more available, the family often makes demands on them for explanations of interventions, treatment plan, and prognosis that are not made on the busy surgeon and that the nurse may feel uncomfortable about or unable to answer. The nurse then often assumes the role of advocate for the family and patient to the surgeon and may seem to, or may in reality, challenge the surgeon's expertise.

The best management techniques for ensuring smooth interstaff functioning are based on a large body of group process and management research. Again, reality is the best foe of negative fantasy. There must be structured, formal, and effective methods for information dispersal not only through charting but also through face-to-face meetings. The surgeon must provide sanction for the voicing of problems, anxieties, and concerns in private.

A team approach requires two-way consultation when appropriate. Finding an opportunity for group problem solving, for asking the nurse's opinion on an appropriate issue, for verbally recognizing a job well done, or for giving timely negative feedback is a way to lay aside negative fantasies and passive-aggressive, sabotaging behaviors. Group meetings held standing can promote efficient communication.

The surgeon should welcome nursing input but also feel free to set limits on role function. When a nurse has lost objectivity in caring for a child, whether in a negative or positive direction, the nurse should be made aware of this fact in private and be asked to seek help from co-workers or a consultant. Change in patient assignment may be helpful but should be used as a last resort.

Joint meetings with family, surgeon, and primary nurse promote accurate communication, ensure mutual understanding, and build team alliance.[1] These joint meetings can also be used to make difficult patients and families aware of the destructiveness of their behavior and what new behaviors would be helpful. If all else fails, a communications facilitator, such as a psychologist or a psychiatrist with group process expertise, may provide valuable assistance.

ACCIDENT PREVENTION

How can accidents be prevented, and which children are at highest risk? Because accidents are the number one cause of death in children from 1 to 21 years old, major efforts at prevention are warranted. Preschool children are most endangered by poisonings and school-aged children by guns and drownings. The teenager is endangered by automobile accidents and by nonaccidental trauma by suicide.

Boys are at greater risk than girls. Matheny has shown that among toddlers, maleness is predictive of accidental injury, along with less tractable and manageable behavioral traits, a lower socioeconomic level home, and a mother who feels emotionally overwhelmed and with less energy.[29] A Boston study showed that accidents tend to occur when increased stress is present that is associated with hunger or fatigue; behavioral hyperactivity; illness, pregnancy, or menstruation of the mother; recent change in child caretaker; illness or death in the family; marital tension; changes of environment; and maternal preoccupation.[32] Although an accident-prone personality has yet to be identified, there are identifiable accident repeaters. These children are generally male, highly active, risk takers, hard to discipline, and live in homes characterized by disorganization, stress, and lack of parental understanding of child development.[20, 27] Thus, there is an interaction among temperament, personality trait, stress level, and parental supervision.

In addition to public campaigns for safety devices and precautions from professional and civic organizations (e.g., lower speed limits, limit of alcohol consumption, car seat usage, childproof bottles), anticipatory guidance should include not only information about child age-related limitations, need for supervision, and safety interventions but also an assessment of general stress and the family's ability to consistently supervise and protect the child. Supportive counseling to enable families to establish and promote safety is more effective than fact-based educational efforts.

References

1. Atkinson JH Jr, Stewart N, Gardner D: The family meeting in critical care settings. J Trauma 20(1):43–46, 1980.
2. Benjamin PY: Psychological problems following recovery from acute life-threatening illness. Am J Orthopsychiatry 48:284–290, 1978.
3. Bibace R, Walsh ME: Development of children's concepts of illness. Pediatrics 66:912–917, 1980.
4. Bowlby J: Attachment and Loss. New York, Basic Books, 1969.
5. Bowlby J: Separation, Anxiety, and Anger. New York, Basic Books, 1973.
6. Brown JM, O'Keeffe J, Sanders SH, Baker B: Developmental changes in children's cognition to stressful and painful situations. J Pediatr Psychol 11:343–357, 1986.
7. Burstein AG: Reactions to physical illness and life stress. In: Bowden CL, Burstein AG: Psychosocial Basis of Health Care. Baltimore, Williams & Wilkins, 1983, pp 55–76.
8. Cohen F: Personality, stress, and the development of physical illness. In: Stone G, Cohen F, Adler N (eds): Health Psychology: A Handbook. San Francisco, Jossey-Bass, 1979.
9. Douglas JW: Early hospital admissions and later disturbances of behaviour and learning. Dev Med Child Neurol 17:456–480, 1975.
10. Eckhardt LO, Prugh DG: Preparing children psychologically for painful medical and surgical procedures. In: Gellert E (ed): Psychosocial Aspects of Pediatric Care. New York, Grune & Stratton, 1978.
11. Erickson E: Childhood and Society. 2nd ed. New York, WW Norton & Co, 1978.
12. Fraiberg SH: The Magic Years. New York, Charles Scribners Sons, 1959.
13. Freiberg KH: How parents react when their child is hospitalized. Am J Nurs 72:1270–1272, 1972.
14. Gardner GG, Olness K: Hypnosis and Hypnotherapy with Children. New York, Grune & Stratton, 1981.
15. Gratz RR: Children's responses to emergency department care. Ann Emerg Med 13:322–333, 1984.
16. Green M, Solnit AJ: Reactions to the threatened loss of a child: A vulnerable child syndrome. Pediatrics 34:58–66, 1964.
17. Hilgard JR, LeBaron S: Relief of anxiety and pain in children and adolescents with cancer: Quantitative measures and clinical observations. Int J Clin Exp Hypn 30:417–442, 1982.
18. Holmes TH, Rahe RH: The social readjustment rating scale. J Psychosom Res 11:213–218, 1967.
19. Horowitz MJ: Psychological processes induced by illness, injury, and loss. In: Millon T, Greer C, Mesgher R (eds): Handbook of Clinical Health Psychology. New York, Plenum Press, 1982.
20. Husband P, Hinton PE: Families of children with repeated accidents. Arch Dis Child 47:396–400, 1972.
21. Katz ER, Kellerman J, Ellenberg L: Hypnosis in the reduction of acute pain and distress in children with cancer. J Pediatr Psychol 12:379–394, 1987.
22. Keeri-Szanto M, Heaman S: Postoperative demand analgesia. Surg Gynecol Obstet 134:647–651, 1972.
23. Kenny TJ: The hospitalized child. Pediatr Clin North Am 22:583–593, 1975.
24. Lazarus RS: Psychological Stress and the Coping Process. New York, McGraw-Hill, 1966.
25. Lindheim R, Glaser HH, Coffin C: Changing Hospital Environments for Children. Cambridge, Harvard University Press, 1972.
26. Loucks S, House J: Developmental Changes in Children's Health Beliefs and Knowledge. In progress.
27. Manheimer DI, Mellinger GD: Personality characteristics of the child accident repeater. Child Dev 38:491–513, 1967.
28. Marks RM, Sachar EJ: Undertreatment of medical inpatients with narcotic analgesics. Ann Intern Med 78:173–181, 1973.
29. Matheny AP Jr: Injuries among toddlers: Contributions from child, mother, and family. J Pediatr Psychol 11:163–176, 1986.
30. Meinhart NT, McCaffery M: Preexisting psychological factors. In: Pain: A Nursing Approach to Assessment and Analysis. East Norwalk, Conn, Apple-Century-Crofts, 1983, pp 146–168.
31. Melamed BG, Siegel LJ: Reduction of anxiety in children facing hospitalization and surgery by use of filmed modeling. J Consult Clin Psychol 43:511–521, 1975.
32. Mofensen HC, Greensher J: Childhood accidents. In: Friedman SB, Hoekelman RA (eds): Behavioral Pediatrics: Psychosocial Aspects of Child Care. New York, McGraw-Hill, 1980, pp 407–410.
33. Olds AR: Psychological considerations in humanizing the physical environment of pediatric outpatient and hospital settings. In: Gellert E (ed): Psychosocial Aspects of Pediatric Care. New York, Grune & Stratton, 1978, pp 111–131.
34. Perrin EC, Gerrity PS: There's a demon in your belly: Children's understanding of illness. Pediatrics 67:841–849, 1981.
35. Perry SW: Undermedication for pain on a burn unit. Gen Hosp Psychiatry 6:308–316, 1984.
36. Peterson L, Ridley-Johnson R, Tracy K, Mullins LL: Developing cost-effective presurgical preparation: A comparative analysis. J Pediatr Psychol 9:439–455, 1984.
37. Piaget J: Judgement and Reasoning in the Child. Totawa, NJ, Littlefield, Adams, and Company, 1976.
38. Piaget J: The Psychology of Intelligence. Totawa, NJ, Littlefield, Adams, and Company, 1976.
39. Prugh DE: Investigations dealing with the reactions of children and families to hospitalization and illness: Problems and potentialities. In: Caplan G (ed): Emotional Problems of Early Childhood. New York, Basic Books, 1955.
40. Ravenscroft K: Psychiatric consultation to the child with acute physical trauma. Am J Orthopsychiatry, 52:298–307, 1982.

41. Roberts MC, Wurtele SK, Boone RR, et al: Reduction of medical fears by use of modeling: A preventive application in a general population of children. J Pediatr Psychol 6:298–300, 1981.

42. Roskies E, Bedard P, Gauverau-Guilbault H, LaFortune D: Emergency hospitalization of young children: Some neglected psychological considerations. Med Care 13:570–581, 1975.

43. Schechter NL, Allen D: Physicians' attitudes toward pain in children. J Dev Behav Pediatr 7:350–354, 1986.

44. Spitz RA: The First Year of Life. New York, International Universities Press, 1965.

45. Suhr MA: Trauma in pediatric populations. Adv Psychosom Med 16:31–47, 1986.

46. Tisza VB, Hurwitz I, Angoff K: The use of a play program by hospitalized children. J Am Acad Child Psychiatry 9:515–531, 1970.

47. Vernon DT, Schulman JL, Foley JM: Changes in children's behavior after hospitalization. Am J Dis Child 111:581–593, 1966.

48. Weis OF, Sriwatanakul K, Alloza JL, et al: Attitudes of patients, housestaff, and nurses toward postoperative analgesic care. Anesth Analg 62:70–74, 1983.

49. Wong DL: Childhood trauma: Its developmental aspects and nursing interventions. Crit Care Quarterly 5:47–60, 1982.

50. Zeltzer LK, LaBarron S: The hypnotic treatment of children in pediatrics. In: Routh D, Wolraich M (eds): Advances in Developmental Behavioral Pediatrics. Vol. 7. Greenwich, Conn, JAI Press, 1986, pp 197–234.

Mitchell H. Goldman

CHAPTER FIFTY-TWO

Organ Procurement in the Fatally Injured Child

Pediatric organ transplantation presents many unique problems that transcend humanitarian, ethical, legal, biomedical, and technical endeavors.[20, 31] Often, humanistic imperatives find themselves in conflict; for example, physicians feeling the compelling need for pediatric livers for transplantation in a population predominantly made up of pediatric recipients often are confronted with the difficulty of determining brain function in young victims of anoxic cerebral injury. In the trauma environment of tragedy, many factors—the presence of an anguished family, the sense of failure among medical personnel, the potential use of extensive hospital and intensive care resources, and the lack of familiarity of staff and community with the organ donation process—can mask the ultimate beneficial effect of organ donation on the donor family, the hospital, and the recipients.[21, 22] It is precisely in the arena of the pediatric trauma victim that organ donation is so important.[8]

Transplantation technology has extended the potential for successful liver, kidney, heart, heart-lung, and pancreas transplantations with increasing long-term success, to the extent that there exists a significant shortfall of these organs (Table 52–1).[5, 9, 12, 26, 27] That only 20% of patients meeting cadaveric donor criteria ever donate represents a failure of the medical community to recognize the benefits of organ donation and to organize efficient organ procurement efforts on a local level.[2] Public requests by anguished parents of children needing transplants illustrates this failure and has culminated in state and federal legislation designed, ostensibly, to promote organ donation. In addition to whole organs, eye, bone marrow, skin, musculoskeletal tissue, heart valves, and blood vessels are being used as well.[4, 10, 14, 25]

The National Organ Transplant Act of 1984 mandates professional and community education through its Organ Procurement and Transplantation Network (OPTN) contract with the United Network for Organ Sharing (UNOS).[15] Federal legislation, the Omnibus Budget Reconciliation Act of 1986, ties Medicare reimbursement to the hospitals having policies and procedures for requesting consent for organ and tissue donation from all persons dying in the hospital environment.[18] Most states have followed suit with similar "required requests" laws.[17, 24] The effect will be mandatory penalties for noncompliance. Hospitals, specifically hospitals engaged in large volumes of trauma, should respond to these imperatives by doing the following:

1. Educating physicians in the recognition of potential organ and tissue donors
2. Educating nursing staff in the recognition and care of organ and tissue donors
3. Educating all staff in the sympathetic approach to obtaining consent for organ and tissue donation
4. Establishing close contact with organ and tissue procurement agencies and using the educational and support services available through these agencies
5. Enlisting chaplains, social services, and transplant support groups for the publicizing of organ and tissue donation issues
6. Participating in community educational ventures

In short, organ and tissue donation should be part of the trauma curriculum, enabling the trauma team to present accurate, supportive, sensitive, informative messages to the family of a trauma victim to maximize the beneficial effects of donation. Organ and tissue donation depends both on the altruism of the donor family and the commitment of the trauma team to promote donation as an integral part of the care of the donor and his or her family.[1, 3]

DONORS

Criteria for Brain Death in Children

Organ and tissue donors are either living or dead. Living donors are relatives or in some instances emotionally related individuals who are willing to donate an organ such as kidney or segmental pancreas, or a tissue such as bone, skin, or bone marrow. Cadaveric donors are either dead by brain death criteria or by prolonged absence of heartbeat or respirations. If either criterion is met, the patient is dead.

Table 52–1
Organ and Tissues for Transplantation

Organ	Transplants per Year	Age (yr)	Preservation Time	Time After Cessation of Heartbeat	Specific Criteria
Kidney	10,000	0–60	72 hr	<20 min	Creatinine 2.0–2.5
Heart	1000	0–40	4 hr	0	Electrocardiogram, echocardiogram, angiogram
Liver	1000	0–50	12 hr	0	Liver function tests
Pancreas	200	5*–50	12 hr	0	Amylase, blood sugar
Heart/lung and lung	<50	≤40	0–4 hr	0	PO_2 of 250 mm Hg on FI_{O_2} 100%; bronchoscopy and Gram stain
Intestine	<10	0–?	0–4 hr	0	
Musculoskeletal	30,000	14†–65	Indefinite	12–24 hr	
Bone marrow	Unknown	Unknown	Unknown	0	
Eye	30,000	<5 mo	3–7 days	12 hr	
Skin	2–5000	0–65	Indefinite	12–24 hr	

*Pancreatic islets from younger donors, including aborted fetuses, may be used.
†Epiphyseal areas in children who are still growing are not used where viable bone is to be transplanted; however, younger donors may be used as ground or nonviable bone donors.

The liberal use of words such as *brain death* and *coma*, which do not emphasize the concept of death by brain death criteria as death, generally confuses families, especially in the setting of life-support apparatus. In general, when talking about a cadaveric donor, it is simply best to say that he or she is dead. The somewhat controversial brain death criteria recommended by the Task Force for the Determination of Brain Death in Children[28] are as follows:

1. Physical examination criteria
   a. Coexistence of coma and apnea with complete loss of consciousness, vocalization, and volitional activity
   b. Absence of brain stem function by demonstration of a midposition or fully dilated pupils unresponsive to light
2. Absence of spontaneous eye movements, including those induced normally by oculocephalic and oculovestibular testing
3. Absence of bulbar muscular movement, including facial and oropharyngeal movement, and absence of corneal, gag, cough, sucking, and rooting reflexes
4. Absence of respiratory movement
5. Flaccid tone and absence of spontaneous or induced movement; reflex withdraw and spinal myoclonus are not included
6. Hypotension, hypothermia, central nervous system abnormality, depressant drugs, hypoxemia, hypovolemia must be excluded

The observation period should be at least 48 hours for patients aged 7 days to 2 months, 24 hours for patients aged 2 months to 1 year, and 12 hours for patients over 1 year old. If the patient is initially examined soon after an acute event, especially in situations in which it is difficult to assess the extent and reversibility of brain damage (specifically hypoxic-ischemic encephalopathy), a longer observation period may be necessary. Electroencephalography performed at the beginning and end of the two observations confirms brain death. Cerebral radionuclide angiography and contrast angiography that indicate absent cerebral flow may confirm brain death. The basic essentials of knowing how to determine brain death include knowledge of the cause of cessation of brain function (i.e., trauma) and the exclusion of the possibility of return of any function.[11]

Donor Screening

Organ and tissue donors should be screened for infections such as human immunodeficiency virus (HIV), hepatitis B, cytomegalovirus, urinary tract infection, pulmonary infection, septicemia, or central nervous system infection. Specifically, in trauma victims, a pretransfusion HIV antibody test is safest to prevent missing an HIV infection because of a dilutional effect of transfusion or large volume replacement. *It should be the policy of the hospital to save a serum sample until a trauma victim is no longer a potential donor.* With the present technology, ELISA and Western blot for HIV antibody are the available tests. Until a reliable antigen test is available, there may be a window of 3 to 6 months between the time the patient is infected and the time antibody appears. Thus, careful patient and family histories are

necessary to rule out possibly infected patients as donors (Table 52–2). History of hemophilia, recent transfusion, drug abuse, sexual contacts, or parenterally equivalent risk factors should be considered.

Testing for hepatitis B core antigen and serum alanine aminotransferase testing should be performed to rule out hepatitis B. Other infections—such as Reye syndrome and rabies, collagen vascular diseases, and other systemic diseases such as malignancy—mitigate against donation. Creutzfeldt-Jacob disease precludes donation of tissue or organs. Diseases of and trauma to specific organs such as heart, liver, pancreas, kidney, bones, eyes, lungs, may eliminate these organs from consideration. Although some organs may not be suitable for organ transplantation because of trauma, other organs or tissues in the same potential donor may be procured and used.

The minimum age requirements for donated tissues are specific to the tissues (see Table 52–1). Common baseline tests for donation should include urinalysis, creatinine, blood urea nitrogen, chest radiography, electrocardiography, and serum amylase; hepatitis screening including core antibody, Venereal Disease Research Laboratory, serum alanone aminotransferase, HIV, and arterial blood gases; and cultures of urine, lung, and blood. Echocardiography and angiography may be necessary to rule out congenital or traumatic cardiac disease. Bronchoscopy may be necessary for lung and heart-lung evaluation. In the end, no donor should be eliminated from consideration until consultation with an organ and tissue procurement or recipient center has been made. Some factors that might ordinarily eliminate a potential donor from consideration may be waived in circumstances in which a specific organ is urgently needed.

Consent for organ and tissue donation can be obtained from donor cards, driver's licenses, wills, and next of kin. The last is most often the source. Spouses, parents, and siblings may give consent, in that order. In the absence of an adult able to give consent, a court-appointed guardian may be sought. Consent of the medical examiner should be obtained in appropriate situations.

Donor Maintenance

Maintenance of Hemodynamic Stability

Once a donor has been identified and consent obtained, it is important to maintain hemodynamic stability for the preservation of solid organ function while the procurement team assembles. Volume replacement usually is necessary. A urine output of 30 to 100 ml per hour or 1 ml per kg per hour is appropriate. Central venous or pulmonary artery

Table 52–2
General Unacceptable Donor Criteria

1. Current malignancy, other than cerebral or skin
2. Untreated infection, viral infections
3. Systemic disease—diabetes mellitus, autoimmune disease
4. Specific trauma
5. Prolonged ischemia

pressures should be monitored. Diabetes insipidus may result from cerebral ischemia and pressure on the pituitary. Vasopressin with chlorobutanol (Pitressin), up to 20 mg intravenously, may be used to correct diabetes insipidus and to prevent excessive urinary output and concomitant need for replacement.[19] Dextrose-containing solutions may be contraindicated when urinary output is excessive. The osmotic load serves to increase diuresis. Some centers give steroids before surgery to help stabilize cellular membranes during preservation and perhaps to have an effect on presentation of donor antigen by dendritic or antigen-presenting cells. Often, a tight line must be followed between hydration in an effort to preserve renal function and pulmonary edema or overdistention of the heart and liver and subsequent functional impairment of those tissues. Here, pulmonary artery pressures may enable optimal management. Vasoconstrictors in the form of pressors, especially alpha-acting agents, should be avoided in favor of low-dose dopamine or dobutamine.[30] Transfusion may be necessary to maintain adequate oxygen-carrying capacity. Often, the transplant coordinator from an organ procurement agency can take some of the nursing care responsibilities from an intensive care unit staff, lightening their load and forming good rapport.[7]

Tissue Typing

Occasionally, predonation tissue typing is necessary to match organs with specific individuals. This is especially so when the potential recipient has a significant amount of preformed antibodies to potential donors as a result of previous transplants, transfusions, or pregnancy. This is determined by screening the serum of recipients against a panel of known cell types of a variety of HLA antigens. In heart and liver donation, predonation crossmatching may be required before a recipient center will accept the organ.

Inguinal Node Retrieval

Because of the short time permitted for ex vivo preservation of hearts and livers, inguinal nodes may be retrieved in the intensive care unit. The groin area is prepared and draped with sterile drapes, and an incision is made in the thigh at the fossa ovalis. The femoral artery is identified, and the chain of nodes medial to the artery is dissected. The nodes are placed in sterile tissue culture medium. Saline may be acceptable in the absence of tissue culture medium. The nodes should be kept on ice. The incision is then closed and dressed neatly (Fig. 52–1).

Donor Operation

Organization and Technique

With multiple organ donors, there is often some confusion in the operating room, especially if the procedure is new to the operating room staff. Care must be taken to understand the feelings and emotional responses of the operating room staff to make the procurement effort as minimally traumatic as possible to the staff. It may be important to emphasize

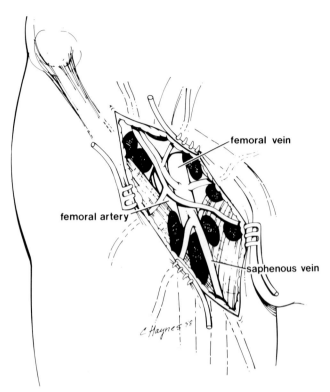

FIGURE 52–1

Dissection of the inguinal area to obtain nodes for tissue typing.

that the patient is already dead and will *not* be "pronounced" at the end of the procedure.

Organization is key. The procedures usually can be performed using a major abdominal kit with the addition of a sternal retractor, a sternal saw, and some vascular instruments. Procurement teams usually bring whatever specialty instruments or equipment they require. It is helpful for the donor hospital to provide such things as sterile ice or slush and cold lactated Ringer solution or saline solution. When more than one organ is being procured, separate back tables are necessary with large basins for back table bench surgery and further ex vivo perfusion. These nuances can be discussed with the organ procurement coordinators from the individual teams so that the surgery proceeds with coordination and ease. All tissues and specimens should be accurately labeled with the donor's name and a hospital identification number. Sterile technique is mandatory in all instances.

With the procuring team present, the donor is prepared from the neck to the thighs and draped appropriately. The median sternotomy and midline abdominal incision offer the best exposure for all organs (Fig. 52–2). These incisions will not hamper the subsequent procurement of eye, bone, and skin. To gain access to the liver, the diaphragm may be taken down to expose the caval hiatus and the back of the liver. A transverse paraumbilical incision may be added from colic gutter to colic gutter to facilitate exposure of the kidneys.

There are separate preservation techniques for each organ. All involve in situ perfusion. EuroCollins intracellular

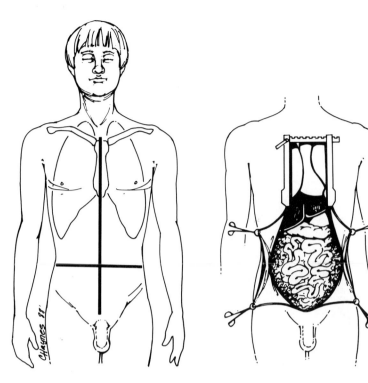

FIGURE 52-2

Incision for combined cardiac and abdominal organ procurement. Usually a median sternotomy extending down the midline of the abdomen coupled with a transverse abdominal incision provides more than adequate exposure for organ donation.

solution and lactated Ringer solution are commonly used for kidneys, liver, and pancreas. They are given through an aortic cannula or the portal vein. Cardioplegia solution is given through the ascending aorta and coronary arteries with aortic cross-clamping in cardiac and cardiopulmonary donation. Anticoagulation with 100 to 300 mg per kg of heparin is performed before cross-clamping and insertion of perfusion cannulae. An alpha-blocker such as phentolamine (Regitine), 5 to 25 mg, or chlorpromazine (Thorazine), 25 to 50 mg, may be administered to prevent renal vasospasm. However, with profound hypotension during the procedure, these may be withheld. Furosemide (Lasix) and mannitol are given before clamping for renal procurement. Large volumes of crystalloid solution and blood may need to be given to maintain pressure. Again, care must be taken to avoid overdistending the heart and liver given the large volumes of fluid that must be administered to maintain adequate perfusion of the organs. At the end of the organ retrieval, the spleen and mesenteric lymph nodes are obtained for tissue typing. The incisions are neatly closed in a single layer.

En Bloc Nephrectomy

The kidneys are mobilized by entering the retroperitoneal area along the line of Toldt on each side (Fig. 52–3). The ureters are dissected to the bladder, preserving the periureteric fat and blood vessels. The gonadal veins are ligated and divided. On the left, the colon is swept medially, exposing the renal vein. After the adrenal, gonadal, and lumbar veins are divided and the adrenal gland is dissected off the kidney, the aorta above the renal vein is cleared of lymphatics and neural tissue, exposing the superior mesenteric artery (SMA). It is sometimes necessary to divide fibers of the crux of the diaphragm. If pancreatic procurement is contemplated, the SMA is preserved. Also, the SMA is preserved in the situation in which an accessory right hepatic artery originates from the SMA or its branches. This may occur in 17% of the potential donors. If neither of these situations occurs, the SMA may be divided, as is the crux of the diaphragm, to ensure aortic control above all potential renal arteries. The ureter is mobilized to the bladder by sweeping all periureteric fat toward the ureter to preserve the ureteral vascular supply originating from the kidney. Injuring the ureteral artery may result in necrosis on reimplantation. The ureters are divided distally and cultured, and urine output is assessed.

The right kidney is mobilized in a similar fashion, bringing the right colon and duodenum all the way to the left, exposing the aorta from the right side. The cava is exposed, the renal vein identified, and the gonadal vein divided. With concomitant liver dissection, a spot that does not compromise the right renal vein and still gives adequate length to the hepatic cava is chosen at this time for subsequent division. After dividing the inferior mesenteric artery and vein, the whole mesentery can be mobilized upward so that the kidneys can be removed en bloc either from the right or left. Care is taken not to divide aortic side branches that may be inferior polar renal arteries. A large renal infarct may result in ureteric necrosis and a complicated posttransplantation course.

The patient is given heparin. The aorta and cava are cannulated at the bifurcations. If cardiac donation is occurring in conjunction with renal donation, the cava may be vented into the pericardium at the time the heart is removed, obviating the need for caval drainage inferiorly. Mannitol, 12.5 gm, and furosemide, 80 mg, are administered. After the aorta is cross-clamped, preservation solution is infused. If kidneys alone are procured, a minimum of 1 liter of Collin solution should be infused to ensure

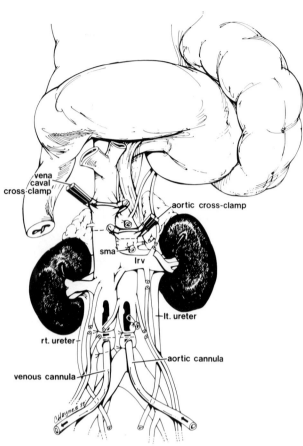

FIGURE 52–3

Nephrectomy. The en bloc nephrectomy is performed by cannulating both the aorta and the inferior vena cava below the level of the renal vessels. Preservation solution is infused while cross-clamping the aorta above the level of the superior mesenteric artery (sma). After in situ perfusion, the kidneys may be removed en bloc on an aortic and vena caval pedicle.

adequate cooling. The kidneys are removed still on the aortic and caval pedicles and placed in ice solution. The aorta and cava are divided such that a patch of each including all vessels to that side is left with each kidney.

Hepatectomy

Median sternotomy and midline abdominal incisions are used (Fig. 52–4). The diaphragm may be taken down. The round ligament is divided. The porta hepatis is inspected and palpated to identify aberrant left and right hepatic arteries. The hepatic artery is dissected retrograde to the celiac artery, and the origin of the celiac artery is identified on the aorta. Each step in dividing the tissues in the porta hepatis and around the celiac artery must be accompanied by meticulous hemostasis. The portal vein is exposed distally beyond the confluence of the splenic and superior mesenteric veins. The coronary veins are ligated. The pancreas is divided and ligated en masse unless segmental pancreatectomy is planned.[16] The splenic vein is cannulated for portal perfusion solutions. The gallbladder is incised and the bile irrigated completely from the area to prevent subsequent

necrosis of the gallbladder. The common bile duct is divided as close to the duodenum as possible. The ligaments of the liver are taken down, and the phrenic veins at the hiatus of the diaphragm are ligated. If cannulae have not been placed in the aorta and cava by the renal procedure, they are placed at the iliac bifurcations. Cold perfusion solutions are begun after heparin is administered and cross-clamping is achieved above the celiac artery. At least 3 liters is given in the aorta and the portal vein. The liver is palpated to ensure that it is cooling. It is then removed en bloc with care (1) to reserve adequate suprahepatic cava by including the diaphragm and (2) to provide a cuff of aorta with the celiac artery.

Pancreatectomy

Total pancreatectomy is performed basing the arterial pedicle on both the celiac and mesenteric arteries and the venous pedicle on the portal vein[16] (Figs. 52–5, 52–6). However, when hepatectomy is being performed concomitantly, a segmental pancreatectomy may be done, with reconstruction of the splenic artery and vein provided by using donor iliac artery and vein. Alternatively, the iliac artery and vein may be used to lengthen the portal vein and hepatic arteries when there is some imperative to preferentially use a whole pancreatic graft. The greater omentum is freed from the colon and the whole pancreas mobilized, preserving the middle colic vessels. The right colon is mobilized toward the left, and the duodenum is mobilized by an extensive Kocher maneuver. The duodenal and pancreatic areas are dissected, and the body and tail dissected inferiorly and posteriorly to the spleen. The SMA is identified at the base of the mesentery and exposed distally to the colic branches, preserving the inferior pancreaticoduodenal artery and other arteries on the right side of the SMA leading to the duodenum. The fourth part of the duodenum is fully mobilized. The upper borders of the duodenum and pancreas are dissected, exposing the bile duct, hepatic artery, and portal vein, and ligating the right gastric artery. The celiac artery is exposed at its origin on the aorta by dividing the left gastric artery and opening the arcuate ligament of the diaphragm. The spleen is freed medially, using it as a handle to mobilize the pancreas to the right (Fig. 52–7). The short gastric arteries and the inferior mesenteric vein are divided. The aorta and vena cava are cannulated, and the pancreas is perfused with Collin or EuroCollins solution after clamping the aorta cephalad to the celiac artery. The portal structures and the mesenteric artery distal to the duodenal branches are divided. The mesenteric and celiac arteries are removed on a Carrel patch of aorta. The duodenum is stapled and divided proximal and distal to the pancreas. A duodenotomy is performed to facilitate irrigating the lumen with solution containing 0.5% neomycin to prevent autolysis by bile and pancreatic contents.

Cardiectomy

After median sternotomy, the superior vena cava is mobilized proximally, and a tape is placed around it (Fig. 52–8). Sufficient length of the superior vena cava is important to protect the sinoatrial node on closing the superior vena cava

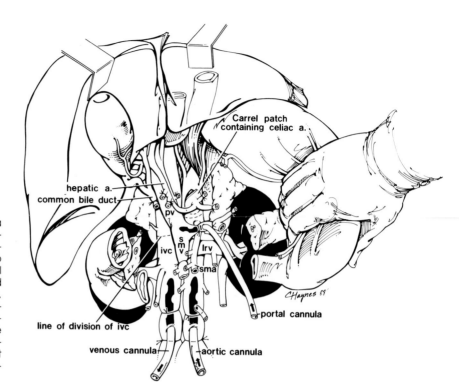

FIGURE 52-4

Hepatectomy. The aorta and vena cava are cannulated in a similar fashion as for the nephrectomy. An additional cannula is placed in the stump of the splenic vein to perfuse the portal vein (pv). The celiac axis is removed from the aorta on a Carrel patch. Cross-clamping above the celiac artery at the time of in situ perfusion permits perfusion of both the liver and the kidneys. smv, Superior mesenteric artery; ivc, inferior vena cava; lrv, left renal vein; sma, superior mesenteric artery.

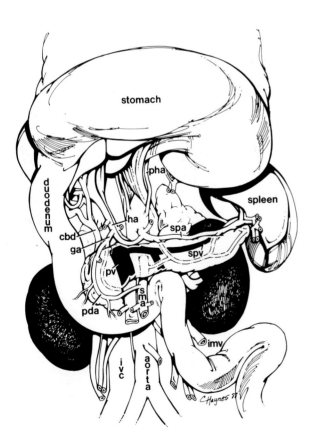

FIGURE 52-5

Dissection of the pancreas involves mobilizing the superior mesenteric artery (sma) including the pancreaticoduodenal artery (pda). The celiac axis is dissected as well and includes the right gastric artery (ga) and the superior pancreaticoduodenal artery. The splenic artery (spa) and the splenic vein (spv) are included in the dissection. The common bile duct (cbd) is ligated. ha, Hepatic artery; ivc, inferior vena cava; imv, inferior mesenteric artery; pha, phrenic artery; cbd, common bile duct; pv, portal vein.

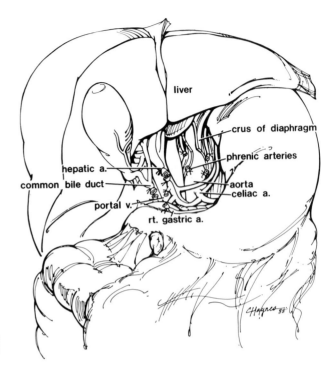

FIGURE 52–6

Pancreatectomy. The exposure of the celiac artery is done through the lesser omentum. The celiac artery is dissected and the hepatic artery ligated.

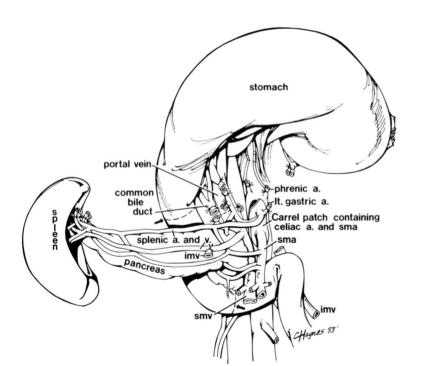

FIGURE 52–7

The spleen is freed medially, using it as a handle to mobilize the pancreas to the right. sma, Superior mesenteric artery; imv, inferior mesenteric vein; smv, superior mesenteric vein.

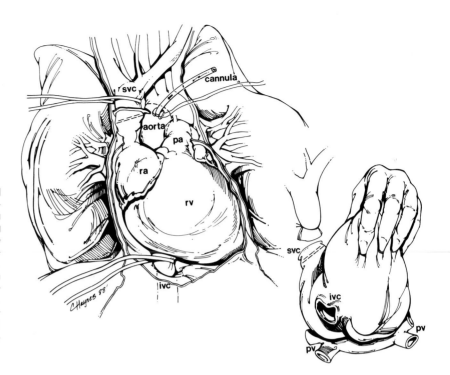

FIGURE 52-8

Cardiectomy. The pericardium is opened through a median sternotomy. The superior vena cava (svc) and inferior vena cava (ivc) are encircled after dissecting some of the pericardium off the svc. The cannula is placed in the aorta for administration of the cardioplegia solution. After the cardioplegia solution has been administered and the aorta cross-clamped, the svc and ivc are divided. The heart is lifted anteriorly, and the pulmonary veins (pv) are divided *(right)*. pa, Pulmonary artery; ra, right atrium; rv, right ventricle.

during reimplantation. Central venous lines should be withdrawn before dividing the superior vena cava. The inferior vena cava is encircled. The ascending aorta is freed distally so that cardioplegic solution may be given (not all centers use cardioplegia during cardiac procurement). The heart is now ready to be removed. When all teams are ready, heparin is administered. The superior vena cava is ligated or stapled caudally and clamped cephalad and divided. The inferior vena cava is clamped at the right atrium, leaving the inferior vena cava for the liver team. The inferior vena cava is divided caudal to the clamp. Once the heart is emptied, cardioplegia is begun and the aorta cross-clamped. During this time, in situ preservation of the abdominal organs is proceeding. Ice slush may be placed in the pericardium to facilitate cooling. After 1 liter of cardioplegia, the heart is removed by dividing the vena cava, the pulmonary veins, the right and left pulmonary arteries, and finally the aorta, leaving a minimum of a 5-cm aortic remnant. The heart is placed in iced lactated Ringer solution and triple-bagged for transportation.

Tissue Procurement

Enucleation of the eye is performed under sterile conditions by circumferentially separating the conjunctiva from the corneal limbus. The conjunctiva is undermined, and scissors are passed beneath the Tenon capsule to form a plane in each quadrant identifying the rectus muscles. The muscles are divided 2 to 3 mm from the sclera. The oblique muscles are divided. Using the medial rectus as a retractor, the globe is lifted, the adhesions are divided, and the optic nerve divided. The eye is rinsed with saline and placed in a holding basket. Alternatively, a corneoscleral rim may be excised when the globe must be left in place.

Skin is procured from the back, chest, abdomen, and thighs. A standard dermatome may be used. Thorough cleansing of the skin is necessary before it is harvested.

Bones are removed after extensive preparation of the skin. The lower extremity incision begins at the anterior superior iliac spine and extends over the greater trochanter, lateral femoral shaft, and lateral femoral condyle, and then extends anteriorly to the tibial tubercle and the ankle. If the articular surfaces are to be preserved, the joints are disarticulated, leaving capsules and ligaments intact. The hemipelvis is removed by proximal extension of the incision posteriorly over the posterior iliac spine along the crest. Disarticulation of the hemipelvis is performed at the sacroiliac joint and symphysis pubis. Care must be taken to avoid bladder and bowel perforation. The upper extremity bones are removed through a lateral upper arm incision extended posteriorly in the lower arm to just short of the wrist. Usually, either the ulna or radius is left behind to aid in reconstruction of the limb for funeral purposes. Ribs and carpal and tarsal bones are also removed. The mandible may be removed through an anterior neck skin flap or intraorally. Dowels are inserted to replace the long bones, and a plastic mandible is used to replace the jaw. The incisions are meticulously sutured closed.

RESULTS

The advent of cyclosporine has had dramatic impact on cadaveric renal and liver transplantation in the pediatric age group.[32] Although cardiac transplantations in children have been sporadic, the results have been good, leading to use in younger patients with congenital cardiac disease.[13] Pancreatic transplantation has not yet been adapted to the pediatric population. However, if it can be shown to mollify the ravages of juvenile-onset diabetes mellitus—eliminating the renal, ocular, neurologic, and vascular complications—it may have a significant effect on the pediatric population. Lung and heart–lung transplantations have not been used extensively in children. Bowel transplantations have been sporadic and have had limited success.[29] Should they become more successful, they will be a useful solution to the problem of short-gut syndrome.

Numerous bone and skin transplantations have been performed in children, and as tissue banks continue in their proliferation, more allograft skin and bone will be used. Thousands of corneal transplantations have been performed. Kidney, liver, heart, pancreas, and other tissues from children may also be used in adults.[6, 23] Thus, the success of transplantation and its impact on a wide spectrum of diseases and populations support even more the imperative for pediatric trauma teams to promote organ and tissue donation and transplantation.

References

1. Bart KJ, Macon EJ, Humphries AL, et al: Increasing the supply of cadaveric kidneys for transplantation. Transplantation 32(5):383–387, 1981.
2. Bart KJ, Macon EJ, Whittier FC, et al: Cadaveric kidneys for transplantation. Transplantation 31(5):379–382, 1981.
3. Bartucci MR, Seller MC: Donor family responses to kidney recipient letters of thanks. Transplant Proc 18(3):401–405, 1986.
4. Baxter C, Aggarwal S, Diller KR: Cryopreservation of skin: A review. Transplant Proc 17(6)(suppl 4):112–120, 1985.
5. Clark AGB, Rigden SPA, Haycock GB, et al: Renal transplantation in children. Transplant Rev 1:101–131, 1987.
6. Dafoe DC, Campbell DA Jr, Merion RM, et al: Pancreatic transplantation. Transplant Proc 19(4)(suppl 4):55–62, 1987.
7. Denney DW: The nonphysician coordinator's contribution to the development of an organ procurement program. Transplant Proc 17(6)(suppl 4):83–87, 1985.
8. Dickerman RM, Dunn EL, White MG: The impact of an air evacuation system on cadaver kidney retrieval. Transplant Proc 18(3):413–415, 1986.
9. Dunn JM, Cavarocchi NC, Balsara RK, et al: Pediatric heart transplantation at St. Christopher's Hospital for Children. J Heart Transplant 6(6):334–342, 1987.
10. Graham CR: Eye banking: A growth story. Transplant Proc 1985, 17(6)(suppl 4):105–111.
11. Guidelines for the determination of death. JAMA 246:2184–2186, 1981.
12. Jamieson SW, Starkey T, Sakakibara N, et al: Procurement of organs for combined heart-lung transplantation. Transplant Proc 18(3):616–617, 1986.
13. Lawrence KS, Fricker FJ: Pediatric heart transplantation: Quality of life. J Heart Transplant 6(6):329–333, 1987.
14. Mugishima H, Terasaki P, Sueyoshi A: Bone marrow from cadaver donors for transplantation. Blood 65(2):392–396, 1985.
15. National Organ Transplant Act. P.L. 98-507, Oct 19, 1984.
16. Nghiem DD, Schulak JA, Corry RJ: Duodenopancreatectomy for transplantation. Arch Surg 122:1201–1206, 1987.
17. Oh HK, Uniewski MH: Enhancing organ recovery by initiation of required request within a major medical center. Transplant Proc 18(3):426–428, 1986.
18. Omnibus Budget Reconciliation Act of 1986. P.L. 99-509, Oct 21, 1986.
19. Outwater KM, Rockoff MA: Diabetes insipidus accompanying brain death in children. Neurology 34:1243–1845, 1984.
20. Rapaport FT, Miller CM, Starzl TE: Medical, ethical and legal implications of current trends in clinical transplantation: An assessment of the respective roles of government and the private sector in the regulation of transplantation. Transplant Proc 19(4):3525–3537, 1987.
21. Robinette MA, Stiller CR, Marshall WJS: Barriers to organ donation within hospitals and involving health care professionals: Findings of the Ontario government task force on kidney donation. Transplant Proc 18(3):397–398, 1986.
22. Sales CM, Burrows L: Cadaveric organ procurement: An investigation of a source of kidney shortage. Transplant Proc 18(3):416–418, 1986.
23. Savatierra O, Belzer F: Pediatric cadaver kidneys. Arch Surg 110:181–183, 1975.
24. Senate Bill No. 1140: An Act Relative to Anatomical Gifts, and to Amend Tennessee Code Annotated, Title 68, Chapter 30, Part 1, and Section G8-3-502 passed April 29, 1986.
25. Snyder SO, Wheeler JR, Gregory RT, et al: Freshly harvested cadaveric venous homografts as arterial conduits in infected fields. Surgery 101(3):283–291, 1987.
26. Starzl TE, Esquivel C, Gordon R, et al: Pediatric liver transplantation. Transplant Proc 19(4):3230–3235, 1987.
27. Sutherland DER, Moudry KC: Pancreas transplant registry report. Transplant Proc 19(4)(suppl 4):5–7, 1987.
28. Task Force for the Determination of Brain Death in Children: Guidelines for the determination of brain death in children. Arch Neurology 44:587–588, 1987.
29. Wassef R, Makowka M, Burnstein M, et al: Harvesting the human small bowel for transplantation purposes. Transplant Proc 18:491–493, 1986.
30. Welchel JD, Diethelm AG, Phillips MG, et al: The effect of high-dose dopamine in cadaver donor management in delayed graft function and graft survival following renal transplantation. Transplant Proc 18(3):523–527, 1986.
31. Younger SJ, Allen M, Bartlett ET, et al: Psychosocial and ethical implications of organ retrieval. N Engl J Med 313(5):321–324, 1985.
32. Zitelli BJ, Gartner JC, Malatack JJ, et al: Pediatric liver transplantation: Patient evaluation and selection, infectious complications, and life style after transplantation. Transplant Proc 19(4):3309–3316, 1987.

William L. Buntain
John M. Templeton, Jr.

Expectations for the Future

Trauma is a multisystem disease and, as such, benefits from almost any advance in medical science. As more is learned about the physiology and biochemistry of various organ systems, better management will ensue. However, advancing scientific knowledge is only part of our responsibilities for the future.

Trauma is expensive, and it involves all of society, not just the injured and their families. Recognition of trauma as the unsolved epidemic of modern society must be appreciated and accepted by the public, the government, and the medical profession as an important social issue. The public and its governing bodies, nevertheless, still resist helmet and seatbelt laws, gun control, fire safety, and serious consideration of the extreme morbidity, mortality, and social impact of injuries. Many of the following suggested (and hoped for) improvements would help prevent needless pain and suffering, as well as death.

CURRENT PERCEPTIONS

The report "Injury in America" resulted in the development of a center for injury control, which is housed in the Centers for Disease Control and is administered through its offices.[2] Financing for this center has been increased by congressional appropriation, and the center seems to be well on its way to providing support for research of all types of injury control. However, the focus at present for national health care reform primarily conveys the perception that methods to control or reduce costs while improving access to care are of primary importance, a philosophic approach very difficult for most physicians to accept because too often the impression is that the patient's well-being is not the primary concern.

In the future physicians also must recognize the extreme importance and impact on society of the critically injured and not just give the issue lip service and incorporate it into their busy schedules as simply another area of concern. Physicians must accept that not everyone can successfully manage a critically ill or injured patient, particularly a small child. It requires a considerable degree of expertise on the part of the physician and resolute support from the proper backup facilities with committed personnel. Physicians usually do not and should not undertake the care of a disease that they believe is outside their area of expertise. Such specialization must also apply to management of the injured.

At the same time physicians who focus primarily on critical care must accept that busy and eminently competent and successful generalists cannot meet the stringent requirements sometimes forced on them by well-meaning but perhaps overly enthusiastic and idealistic committees. For too long those of us who focus on the injured have believed that anything done for the trauma patient is better than nothing, but this is not necessarily true.[3] It is time for the critical care–oriented physicians, particularly those who specialize in the care of the injured, to move to the next level of maturity and sophistication, where multidisciplinary critical care is truly understood, appreciated, respected, and desired by all health care professionals.[5]

CURRENT ISSUES AND POSSIBLE SOLUTIONS

In the Spring 1987 issue of *Concern,* the newsmagazine of the Society of Critical Care Medicine (SCCM), Norma Shoemaker wrote on nursing considerations relating to critical care in the next 20 years, addressing issues very general to care of the critically ill or injured.[9] The article had actually been written in 1976, and at publication in 1987, the editor remarked, "what a short distance we have traveled in 11 years." Now, in 1994, 18 years from the concepts and suggestions that follow, remarkably little has changed.

Addressing the problems then, which are similar to those today, Shoemaker pointed out that "to predict the course of Critical Care over the next two decades it is essential to identify the most pressing problems inherent in the discipline today and then attempt to describe reasonable and rational solutions." From a nursing perspective, in 1976 as now, there was a severe shortage of nursing personnel.

1. The American Nurses Association (ANA) claimed that only 980,000 of the 1.4 million licensed nurses in the United States were in the work force, 70% of the total.
2. From 1965 to 1975 the number of critical care beds increased from 15,000 to 40,000, or by 266%.
3. Forty thousand critically ill patients cared for ideally with an optimal ratio of 1 nurse to 2 patients over three shifts a day would require a pool of 160,000 nurses, or 16.3% of the work force.

Present increases have perhaps compounded these problems, particularly since cost containment is certainly upon us. Current figures are based on 1992 data, the most recent available, from the American Nurses Association and the American Hospital Association.

1. There are now 2,239,816 licensed nurses in the United States, and of these 82.7%, or 1,853,025, are in the work force, 12.7% more than were working in 1976, meaning an overall increase in available working nurses of 873,025, or nearly twice as many.
2. At the same time, the number of critical care beds now available has risen to 96,707, more than doubling the availability of such beds in 1976 despite only a 12.7% increase in nurses to care for these patients.
3. Using the same calculations, 96,707 critically ill patients cared for ideally with an optimal ratio of 1 nurse to 2 patients over three shifts a day, including time off and holidays, would require a pool of 386,828 nurses, nearly 2.5 times the number required 16 years ago and 21% of the available nurses working today.

Hence, although the number of critical care beds has more than doubled in the 16 years from 1976 to 1992, the number of available nurses has only increased by 12.7%, and now 1 in 5, or 20%, of the available working nurses is working in critical care, up from the 16% in 1976.

In addition, in 1976, critical care units, new, old, or remodeled, were not designed for patient comfort, nursing or medical personnel efficiency, supply, or backup facility priority. This has improved today with critical care unit guidelines requiring, among other things, that every patient have access to a window to the natural outside environment. This has been accomplished with nursing administrators, architects, and physicians working in concert to improve the environment with the interests of efficiency and the welfare of the patient and staff in mind.

Also, the team approach, although popular as a slogan, was not being utilized appropriately in 1976 or in 1987 and is not even today in surgical situations. Ideally, charge nurses and patient care individuals would do medical rounds with the medical team daily, but as surgeons, our time is hard to schedule on a regular basis, and we cannot and should not expect nurse managers to drop everything and do rounds when we suddenly appear from the operating room.

Another problem noted in 1976 that is still unsolved in 1994 is the waste occurring in terms of resources and supplies. With the increased awareness of infection, prepackaging has replaced multiple-use equipment, but many of these packs are poorly designed—too much or too little—which adds cost to each procedure.

Shoemaker also predicted that cost, space, and personnel will dictate that "patients with a very poor prognosis, low social value (alcoholics, drug abusers and the elderly) and those who do not want extreme measures will not be treated in critical care facilities." Will we as physicians be asked to accept this? Are we being asked to do that now by being required to do more with less in this age of severe cost containment? Will the public—the consumer—accept this when at present the public considers it its "right" to have access to everything that can be done.

Acute or tertiary care facilities will have a much higher percentage of their total bed capacity devoted to critically ill or injured patients, and it is conceivable that 30 to 40% of all beds in teaching hospitals will be critical care beds, utilized for step-down patients and for those whose illness or injuries lend themselves easily to research-oriented workup. The public must be educated regarding the meaning of tertiary care so they will go to the right place for the proper care and so that acute care hospitals are not inundated with patients who have chronic illnesses. The ability of the consumer to do this is very limited, some would say purposely, as present day medical politics seemingly demand that each hospital present and advertise itself as a "full service" facility.

As predicted in 1976, and gradually becoming a reality now, the future should see an increase in the trend toward centers, such as the trauma, burn, neuro, cancer, and women's centers of today. As the consumer becomes better informed concerning survival statistics in a designated center versus the local hospital, positive pressure in the media and on lawmakers and insurance carriers should increase, and regionalized centers of excellence for care will and should flourish. This process may be slow, however, because of the individual community's sense of pride and prestige at having local facilities and by the political perceptions of the administrators of these institutions who may perceive that they are being left behind.

PEDIATRIC SURGEONS' PERCEPTIONS

A 1989 survey of pediatric trauma specialists from 17 cities and 14 states (including Ontario in Canada) was conducted to elicit perceived recent and predicted future improvements in pediatric trauma management.[11] There was an 89% response rate, 24 of the 27 surveyed. Two questions were asked: "What two things are *significant* improvements in the *present* management of pediatric trauma victims which were not routinely being done two years ago," and "What two things will we be doing for pediatric trauma patients 3 to 5 years from now which we do not routinely do *at present*."

There were 19 different perceived improvements in existing management at the time, broadly separated into two categories: improvements in systems approaches to pediatric injuries and improvements in the normal continuum of care from prehospital triage and transport through resuscitation, stabilization, definitive management, and rehabilitation. The establishment of designated pediatric trauma centers, particularly the recognition of the need for a trauma program in every children's hospital, and training and continuing medical education review of prehospital care providers regarding pediatric trauma care standards were considered important systems improvements, reflecting 10 of the 34 (29%) opinions cast in this category. Improvements in the systems approach and the truly comprehensive continuum of care approach, from injury scene through rehabilitation and recovery, were reflected in improvements in field triage utilizing trauma scores, recognition that cardiopulmonary resuscitation and stabilization were the keys to improved outcome (especially in the child with a head injury), and utilization of a team approach based on common standards of certification (such as the Advanced Trauma Life Support course and the Pediatric Advanced Life Support course). The advantages of incorporating pediatric surgeons, emergency physicians and intensive care specialists as a comprehensive team were recognized by eight of the 34 (24%) opinions. Increased awareness of utilization of intraosseous access to the circulation, of lap belt injuries to the viscera and spine, of associated injuries contributing to the morbidity and mortality of head injuries, and of aggressive early definitive care of burns with cultured skin and early excision and grafting were recognized as major contributions to improvements in management by another six of the 34 (18%).

Important other perceived improvements from the previous 2 years included the preferential use of abdominal computed tomography with double contrast as opposed to diagnostic peritoneal lavage, the use of percutaneous computed tomography–guided drainage of intra-abdominal abscesses and pseudocysts, the use of magnetic resonance imaging for the evaluation of possible spine injuries, and the immediate or early fixation of long bone fractures. In addition, the increased utilization of nonoperative management of liver injuries, the toleration of lower hematocrit values before transfusion, and the improved comprehensive use of the pediatric critical care unit were also appropriately considered important improvements.

With regard to future advancements or changes in the care of injuries to children, 18 such improvements were predicted, 75% of which were positive and dealt with improvements in systems of trauma care and clinical management and 25% of which predicted negative trends in these areas. Predicted improvements in systems of trauma care largely dealt with prehospital management, in particular resuscitation of the airway and circulation and triage, preferably to designated pediatric trauma centers.

Predicted improvements in clinical management centered around diagnosis and monitoring in the emergency department, operating room, and critical care units. A variety of breakthroughs were suggested, including the discovery and use of mediator antagonists, for example, in patients with axonal shearing injuries or in patients with severe multisystem injuries; the clinical use of new methods to combat sepsis, such as glutamine enteral feeding; new extracorporeal membrane oxygenation technology that would permit such treatment for life-threatening adult respiratory distress syndrome in patients with survivable injuries; the use of synthetic oxygen-carrying blood substitutes to enable acceptance of lower hematocrit levels to avoid transfusion of blood or blood products; the enhancement of the nonoperative approach to management because of improved and selective blood component replacement; the use of growth factors in the management of burns and wound problems; and the development of improved techniques and drugs to control intracranial pressure. Some additional trauma systems improvements predicted included quantitative outcome measurements for assessing quality assurance, for example, the use of the Delta score to measure medium- and long-term disability and improved rehabilitation with routine neuropsychological assessment for all head injuries; early intervention programs designed to identify and prevent posttraumatic stress; and the development of remedial educational services designed to meet the needs of clearly defined levels of mental and physical dysfunction.

Negative predictions were offered by 25% of the respondents and appeared to reflect future trends that may or may not be considered ideal. First, the spread of the trauma center movement to smaller regional hospitals was viewed as a threat to quality of care because it would require significant change in the makeup of what is viewed by some as the ideal trauma team for the care of seriously injured children. Specifically, nonsurgeons, such as pediatricians, and specialists in adult surgery would play an increased role in the initial assessment and resuscitation of the injured child.

There are two sides to this concern, both important and both valid. Some argue that the failure to admit seriously injured children to a designated pediatric trauma center raises important considerations regarding quality assurance. In general, the number of seriously injured children is a small proportion of the total population of trauma patients, and real progress in pediatric trauma care has come from cohorting seriously injured children in specialized pediatric centers. An example of this is the successful nonoperative management of spleen or liver injuries, which resulted largely from work in centers in which this cohorting approach took place. This somewhat idealistic approach predicts that future progress in pediatric trauma will require cohorting of the two most challenging and expensive problems we are faced with in childhood injuries: survival and recovery of children with severe head injuries and comprehensive short-term and long-term rehabilitation.

However, it can be argued that of the approximately 450 pediatric surgeons in North America, few have dedicated themselves exclusively to the care of injured children. Many others believe they cannot ethically guarantee first priority care to these children with all of their other responsibilities and are unwilling to dedicate all of their free time to do this. These equally idealistic individuals believe that general surgeons should be well schooled in the issues of injury in children because the bulk of delivery of care is provided by them. At the same time, many, if not most, trauma surgeons, equally idealistic and sincerely interested in providing superior quality care to the injured, believe that the concept of the injured child being cared for only in pediatric trauma centers is hopelessly impractical, there being at most perhaps a dozen such centers in the country that in the aggregate care for perhaps 1% of the trauma patients.

Most pediatric surgeons live at least 30 minutes from the hospital, and few, if any, are willing to move to accommodate the stringent requirements some standards require. Hence, even if some pediatric surgeons are willing to devote their time exclusively to the injured child, very few are in house. In this regard, is it preferable to have a pediatric trauma surgeon 20 to 30 minutes away or an adult trauma surgeon in house? Also, is a fourth-year general surgery resident preferable to an adult trauma surgeon or an in-house pediatric emergency physician? Requirements that impose such standards on a system that is generally giving good pediatric trauma care may detract from the systems that really need improvement, the community hospitals.

The regionalization of critical care services may be a solution to these concerns. Federal legislation and regulation could create a regionalized system to provide high-quality patient care in an efficient and cost-effective manner with the regionalization of critical care sources and the establishment of critical care centers of excellence.

Second, some believe that initial resuscitation decisions should be based on predicted outcome, which would be derived from analysis of current outcome data. In critique of "do not resuscitate" policies based on current outcome data, it is important to understand and accept that children are more resilient to the initial impact of trauma than are adults. Seemingly fixed and dilated pupils in the emergency department may not be permanent in children and are therefore not a valid criterion of brain death. In addition, progress is hampered when yesterday's or today's results become the norm. For example, success in the ventilation of small premature infants and the use of extracorporeal membrane oxygenation for neonatal lung failure grew from 20% to 80% because initial outcome results were not accepted as normal.

There was also concern that mandatory policies and institutional interests, rather than the welfare of patients, will play a major role in decisions to limit therapy and allow patients to die. In response to this, practitioners will have to change their practices because of legal ambiguities and societal attitudes surrounding ethical issues, and physicians, perhaps fearful of the legal consequences, may allow these to influence commonsense decisions.[10]

An example of this concern is the Nancy Beth Cruzan case. Injured in an automobile accident in 1983 at age 25 and living in a Missouri State Hospital exhibiting motor reflexes but showing no indication of possessing significant cognitive function, she breathes spontaneously through a natural airway and receives nutrition and hydration via a gastrostomy. The State of Missouri bears the cost of her care. Her father and mother, parents and co-guardians, acted on her behalf and sought a court order directing the withdrawal of her artificial nutrition and hydration. The Circuit Court of Missouri authorized this, but the attorney general of that state, her guardian ad litem, appealed this decision to the Missouri Supreme Court and the Circuit Court's decision was reversed. On June 25, 1990, the United States Supreme Court, in a five to four decision, upheld the Missouri Supreme Court's decision denying Ms. Cruzan's parents the right to disconnect their daughter from artificial nutritional support.

How does this decision influence our practice of caring for the critically injured? This decision may cause some family and health care professionals to decide to withhold treatment that might prove effective if instituted, yet others may refrain from withdrawing such therapy unless a written directive from the patient specifically indicates a wish to forego any therapy in such a situation, the so-called living will. However, not all patients will have chosen to execute advance directives like this, and even those who do will fail to deal adequately with all therapeutic options. Neonates and older children do not have the option of preparing such a directive in advance. Those who care for them will by necessity have to turn to their parents, for within the family unit a strong presumption exists in favor of parents as primary decision makers for their minor children. In states that follow the Missouri position, requiring clear and convincing evidence and rejecting substituted judgment, *practitioners and parents* may have no choice about continuing therapy that they believe does not serve the best interests of the child.[8]

A major goal of critical care research has been to develop a method of predicting which patients will benefit from the intensive care environment.[7] Some patients develop an acute illness that can clearly be treated effectively by applying the technology available in an intensive care unit. Others have an illness or injury so life threatening that it cannot be reversed by any known treatment available. Most, however, fall between these two extremes, and as candidates for admission to an intensive care unit there is considerable ambiguity as to whether this technology can, in fact, reverse their acute problems. Moreover, the monitoring and therapeutic interventions available in an intensive care unit have certain inherent risks. Hence, some believe that in the future, increased emphasis must be placed on developing methods to define prospectively who will benefit from intensive care with a reduced morbidity and mortality and who will not.

Other potential trends for the future, because of cost, might see diagnostic peritoneal lavage reemerge as a first choice in the assessment of blunt abdominal trauma in children and a swing to earlier operative intervention in children with intra-abdominal bleeding to minimize the use of blood or blood products. In our thinking, both would be serious setbacks to quality care for injured children, and it behooves all pediatric surgeons, not only those with a special interest in childhood injuries, to resist such changes.

One area of future improvement in the field of pediatric trauma received broad support from the respondents: 50% cited the development of *effective trauma prevention programs* as the most important future contribution to the care of injured children. This conviction is supported by the 1989 Report to Congress entitled "Cost of Injury in the United States." Figures from 1985 in this report document 10,200 pediatric deaths due to trauma and 317,000 pediatric hospitalizations in the age range of 0 to 14 years. The estimated lifetime cost of this death and disability is $13.8 billion. Half of the deaths and half of the costs are believed to be preventable.

NURSES

An important tenant in our overall concept of care is the critical care nurse, so important that this book has been dedicated to them. The very nature of critical care nursing demands that these nurses spend a great deal of time at the bedside.[10] Any wish for the future should include mechanisms to allow these dedicated people to spend even more time at the bedside. Inherent in this request is the realization that the ability and the technology to do this already exist, but cost restraints contain it. In the cardiac surgery intensive care unit at the University of Alabama in Birmingham, most charting is done by computer, a plan that was developed and put into effect by Dr. John Kirklin, the now-retired Chairman of the Department of Surgery and Chief of the Cardiac Surgery section, leaving the nurses free to provide what is more important: nursing care and time with the patient. They can become even closer to the patient and family and can hear their concerns, their questions and fears, and their need to be involved in the decision-making process—one of the most important roles of the critical care nurse—and can make sure their wishes are known. Such a computerized system would free nurses' time for nursing care and at the same time be cost-effective.

WHAT WE MUST DO

The old Chinese curse "may you live in interesting times" could be taken then in one of two ways: on the one hand, these times could be considered uncharted and potentially dangerous territory for health care policy; on the other hand, they may provide great opportunity to modify the existing system and create and influence legislation and regulation leading to a more efficient and cost-effective health care system.[1]

We *must* see increased training for those managing the prehospital phase of patient care and the development of an integrated transport system, including ground and air vehicles. Simultaneously, we *must* categorize hospitals according to their ability to manage the patient, including staffing and support services capable of managing the most severely injured. Inherent in this is the belief that no one individual has the background and knowledge to practice critical care alone. As in all patient care situations, however, there should be one physician of record, in the case of pediatric trauma care preferably a pediatric surgeon with a strong interest in trauma or a general trauma surgeon, to establish and monitor priorities in care and to communicate with the family. This is a multidisciplinary effort, then, that requires the involvement of all health care professionals, including other physicians, nurses, and paramedical personnel.[4]

An example of how such a cooperative approach works is illustrated by the actions of the SCCM at the time of the Persian Gulf War.[6] As the largest multidisciplinary critical care organization, the SCCM is committed to providing critical care assistance in times of crisis. Establishing a national resource was not the intent, but with the Persian Gulf War, the SCCM began organizing multidisciplinary critical care teams to be available to care for military casualties. Responding to this wartime need, critical care professionals across the nation stepped forward to volunteer their time and talents to provide services for those in need, and 35 multidisciplinary teams were organized and available, a significant and impressive turnout. It does not require much to see the usefulness and importance of such a response in times of national crisis such as the recent natural disasters we have all witnessed.

Critical care of the injured child *must* be incorporated into the national health care plan, and appropriate reimbursement *must* be ensured for those looking after these critically injured children. Scientific and outcomes research in this regard *must* receive the attention and federal funding it deserves, and the policymakers and staff who create legislation and regulation *must* develop a greater understanding of this care as a complete health care delivery system and see its life-saving benefits to all of society.

References

1. Cerra FB: Winds of change equal new opportunity for critical care. In Session; The Legislative and Public Policy Newsletter of the Society of Critical Care Medicine. December 1992.
2. Committee on Trauma Research, National Research Council, and the Institute of Medicine: Injury in America. Washington, DC, National Academy Press, 1985.
3. Davis JH: History of trauma. In: Moore EE, Mattox KL, Feliciano DV (eds): Trauma. East Norwalk, Conn, Appleton & Lange, 1991, p 12.
4. Gallagher TJ: Education, outreach, communication are vital. Concern, Summer 1990, p 12.
5. Gallagher TJ: Society of Critical Care Medicine's vision for the future of critical care. Concern, Spring 1991, p 6.
6. Gallagher TJ: Building a national critical care resource. Concern, Winter 1991, p 6.
7. Parrillo J: Multidisciplinary aspect of critical care stressed in research testimony. Concern, Summer 1990, p 16.
8. Raphaely RC: What will the Supreme Court's decision mean to critical care? Concern, Summer 1990, pp 14, 15.
9. Shoemaker NJ: Critical care in the next twenty years. Concern, Spring 1987, pp 14, 15.
10. Sprung CL, Jameton A, White S: Ethics in critical care: What will the future hold? Panel discussion. Concern, Fall 1989, pp 14, 15.
11. Templeton JM: The present and future of pediatric trauma. Survey conducted of pediatric trauma specialists, 1989. Personal communication.

Index

Note: Page numbers in *italics* refer to illustrations; page numbers followed by t refer to tables.